The Medical Management *of*

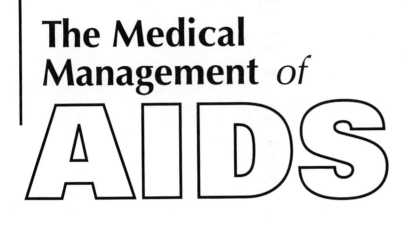

The Medical Management *of*

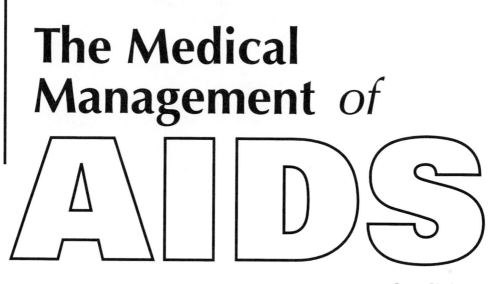

AIDS

6th Edition

Merle A. Sande, MD
Professor and Chairman
Department of Internal Medicine
University of Utah
Salt Lake City, Utah

Paul A. Volberding, MD
Professor, Department of Medicine
University of California, San Francisco
Director, AIDS Program
San Francisco General Hospital
San Francisco, California

W.B. SAUNDERS COMPANY
A Division of Harcourt Brace & Company
Philadelphia • London • Toronto • Montreal • Sydney • Tokyo

W.B. SAUNDERS COMPANY
A Division of Harcourt Brace & Company

The Curtis Center
Independence Square West
Philadelphia, Pennsylvania 19106

Library of Congress Cataloging-in-Publication Data

The medical management of AIDS / [edited by] Merle A. Sande, Paul A.
  Volberding. — 6th ed.
     p. cm.
   Includes bibliographical references and index.
   ISBN 0-7216-8102-6
   1. AIDS (Disease)—Treatment.   I. Sande, Merle A.
  II. Volberding, Paul.
    [DNLM: 1. Acquired Immunodeficiency Syndrome.   2. HIV Infections.
  WC 503 M489   1999]
  RC607.A26M43   1999
  616.97′92—dc21
  DNLM/DLC   98-43930

NOTICE

Medicine is an ever-changing field. Standard safety precautions must be followed, but as new research and clinical experience broaden our knowledge, changes in treatment and drug therapy become necessary or appropriate. Readers are advised to check the product information currently provided by the manufacturer of each drug to be administered to verify the recommended dose, the method and duration of administration, and contraindications. It is the responsibility of the treating physician relying on experience and knowledge of the patient to determine dosages and the best treatment for the patient. Neither the Publisher nor the editor assumes any responsibility for any injury and/or damage to persons or property.

THE PUBLISHER

Contributors

Donald I. Abrams, MD
Professor of Clinical Medicine, University of California, San Francisco; Assistant Director, AIDS Program, San Francisco General Hospital, San Francisco, California
Alternative Therapies

John G. Bartlett, MD
Professor of Medicine, The Johns Hopkins University School of Medicine; Chief, Division of Infectious Diseases; Director, HIV Care Program, The Johns Hopkins University School of Medicine, Baltimore, Maryland
Other HIV-Related Pneumonias

Karen P. Beckerman, MD
Assistant Professor, Department of Obstetrics, Gynecology, and Reproductive Sciences, University of California, San Francisco; Director, University of California, San Francisco Bay Area Perinatal AIDS Center, San Francisco, California
Conception, Pregnancy, and Parenthood: Maternal Health Care and the HIV Epidemic

Bradley S. Bender, MD
Professor of Medicine, University of Florida; Staff Physician, Geriatric Research, Education and Clinical Center, VA Medical Center, Gainesville, Florida
AIDS in Older Persons

David W. Bentley, MD
Professor, Department of Internal Medicine and Director of Training Programs, St. Louis University; Director, Nursing Home Care Unit, St. Louis VA Medical Center, St. Louis, Missouri
AIDS in Older Persons

Marina Berenguer, MD
Assistant Professor in Hepatology, Hospital Universitario LA FE, Valencia, Spain
Hepatitis C Infection

Timothy G. Berger, MD
Clinical Professor, University of California, San Francisco; Clinic Chief, Dermatology Service, San Francisco General Hospital, San Francisco, California
Dermatologic Care of the AIDS Patient

v

Gail Bolan, MD
Assistant Clinical Professor of Medicine, University of California, San Francisco; Staff Physician, San Francisco General Hospital; Director, STD Prevention and Control, San Francisco Department of Public Health, San Francisco, California
Management of Syphilis in HIV-Infected Persons

Lisa Capaldini, MD
Associate Clinical Professor of Medicine, University of California, San Francisco, San Francisco, California
Psychosocial Issues and Psychiatric Complications of HIV Disease

Andrew Carr, MD
Senior Lecturer in Medicine, University of New South Wales; Staff Specialist in HIV Medicine/Immunology, St. Vincent's Hospital, Sydney, Australia
Primary HIV Infection

Willard Cates, Jr., MD
President, Family Health International, Research Triangle Park, North Carolina
The Global Prevention of HIV

Henry F. Chambers, MD
Professor, Department of Medicine; Chief, Division of Infectious Diseases, San Francisco General Hospital, University of California, San Francisco, San Francisco, California
Tuberculosis in the HIV-Infected Patient

Melvin D. Cheitlin, MD
Emeritus Professor of Medicine, University of California, San Francisco; Former Chief, Cardiology Division, San Francisco General Hospital, San Francisco, California
Cardiovascular Complications of HIV Infection

Margaret A. Chesney, PhD
Professor of Medicine, Center for AIDS Prevention Studies, University of California, San Francisco, San Francisco, California
Adherence to HIV Therapy

John C. Christenson, MD
Professor of Pediatrics, University of Utah; Chief, Division of Pediatric Infectious Diseases and Geographic Medicine, University of Utah, Salt Lake City, Utah
Pediatric AIDS

Myron S. Cohen, MD
Chief, Division of Infectious Disease and Professor of Medicine, Microbiology, and Immunology, University of North Carolina at Chapel Hill, Division of Infectious Diseases, Chapel Hill, North Carolina
The Global Prevention of HIV

David A. Cooper, DSc, MD, FRACP, FRCPA
Professor of Medicine, National Centre in HIV Epidemiology and Clinical Research, University of New South Wales; Director, HIV Medicine Unit, St. Vincent's Hospital, Sydney, Australia
Primary HIV Infection

Emmett T. Cunningham, Jr., MD, PhD, MPH
Assistant Professor, Department of Ophthalmology; Co-Director, The Uveitis
Service; Director, The Pearl and Samuel J. Kimura Ocular Immunology
Laboratory, University of California, San Francisco School of Medicine and the
Francis I. Proctor Foundation, San Francisco, California
Ocular Complications of HIV Infection

Gina Dallabetta, MD
Director, Technical Support, HIV/AIDS Prevention and Care Department, Family
Health International, Arlington, Virginia
The Global Prevention of HIV

Kevin M. DeCock, MD, FRCP, DTM&H
Visiting Professor (Medicine and International Health), London School of Hygiene
and Tropical Medicine, London, England; Director, Division of HIV/AIDS
Prevention, Centers for Disease Control and Prevention, Atlanta, Georgia
Current Trends in the Epidemiology of HIV/AIDS

Steven G. Deeks, MD
Assistant Clinical Professor of Medicine, University of California, San Francisco;
University of California, San Francisco AIDS Program; San Francisco General
Hospital, San Francisco, California
Antiretroviral Therapy

Douglas T. Dieterich, MD
Associate Professor of Medicine, New York University School of Medicine,
New York, New York
Gastrointestinal and Hepatic Manifestations of HIV Infection

W. Lawrence Drew, MD, PhD
Professor of Laboratory Medicine and Medicine, University of California,
San Francisco; Director, Clinical Microbiology and Infectious Diseases,
Mt. Zion Medical Center of the University of California, San Francisco,
San Francisco, California
Management of Herpesvirus Infections (CMV, HSV, VZV)

Kim S. Erlich, MD
Assistant Clinical Professor of Medicine, University of California, San Francisco,
California; Consultant in Infectious Diseases, Northern Peninsula Infectious
Diseases, Seton Medical Center, Daly City, California
Management of Herpesvirus Infections (CMV, HSV, VZV)

Gerald Friedland, MD
Professor of Medicine and Epidemiology and Public Health, Yale University
School of Medicine; Director, AIDS Program, Yale New Haven Hospital,
New Haven, Connecticut
HIV Disease in Substance Abusers: Treatment Issues

Romas Geleziunas, PhD
Staff Research Investigator, Gladstone Institute of Virology and Immunology,
San Francisco, California
Molecular Insights into HIV-1 Infection and Pathogenesis

Julie Louise Gerberding, MD, MPH
Associate Professor of Medicine (Infectious Diseases) and Epidemiology and
Biostatistics, University of California, San Francisco
  HIV Exposure Risk Assessment and Prophylactic Treatment

Philip C. Goodman, MD
Professor of Radiology, Chief, Division of Thoracic Imaging, Department of
Radiology, Duke University Medical Center, Durham, North Carolina
  The Chest Film in AIDS

Robert M. Grant, MD, MPH
Assistant Adjunct Professor of Medicine, University of California, San Francisco;
Director, Gladstone Institute of Virology and Immunology, Laboratory of Clinical
Virology, San Francisco, California
  Laboratory Testing for HIV-1

Warner C. Greene, MD, PhD
Professor of Medicine, Microbiology, and Immunology, University of California,
San Francisco; Director, Gladstone Institute of Virology and Immunology,
San Francisco, California
  Molecular Insights into HIV-1 Infection and Pathogenesis

Deborah Greenspan, BDS, DSc, FDS, ScD(hon)
Professor of Clinical Oral Medicine, Department of Stomatology, and Clinical
Director, Oral AIDS Center, School of Dentistry, University of California,
San Francisco, San Francisco, California
  Oral Complications of HIV Infection

John S. Greenspan, BSc, BDS, PhD, FRCPath, ScD(hon)
Professor and Chair, Department of Stomatology, and Director, Oral AIDS Center,
School of Dentistry; Professor of Pathology and Director, AIDS Clinical Research
Center, School of Medicine, University of California, San Francisco, San
Francisco, California
  Oral Complications of HIV Infection

Carl Grunfeld, MD, PhD
Professor of Medicine, University of California, San Francisco; Co-Director,
Special Diagnostic and Treatment Unit, Department of Veteran's Affairs Medical
Center, San Francisco, California
  Endocrinologic Manifestations of HIV Infection

Julie Hambleton, MD
Assistant Clinical Professor of Medicine, Director, Hemostasis and Thrombosis
Center, University of California, San Francisco, San Francisco, California
  Hematologic Complications of HIV Infection

Frederick M. Hecht, MD
Assistant Professor of Medicine, AIDS Program at San Francisco General Hospital,
University of California, San Francisco, San Francisco, California
  Adherence to HIV Therapy

Harry Hollander, MD
Professor of Clinical Medicine, University of California, San Francisco; Director,
Categorical Medicine Residency Program, University of California, San Francisco,
San Francisco, California
  Primary and Preventive Care for the HIV-Infected Adult

King K. Holmes, MD, PhD
Professor of Medicine, Adjunct Professor of Microbiology and Epidemiology;
Director, University of Washington, Center for AIDS & STD; Head, Infectious
Diseases, Harborview Medical Center, Seattle, Washington
  The Global Prevention of HIV

Laurence Huang, MD
Assistant Professor of Medicine, University of California, San Francisco; Medical
Director, San Francisco General Hospital, Inpatient AIDS Unit; Chief, San
Francisco General Hospital AIDS Chest Clinic, San Francisco, California
  Pneumocystis carinii Pneumonia

Michael H. Humphreys, MD
Professor of Medicine, School of Medicine, University of California, San
Francisco; Chief, Division of Nephrology, San Francisco General Hospital,
San Francisco, California
  Renal Complications of HIV Infection

Mark A. Jacobson, MD
Associate Professor of Medicine in Residence, University of California, San
Francisco; Attending Physician, San Francisco General Hospital, San Francisco,
California
  *Disseminated Mycobacterium avium Complex and Other Atypical Mycobacterial
  Infections*

Harold W. Jaffe, MD
Clinical Instructor, Department of Medicine, Emory University School of
Medicine; Associate Director for HIV/AIDS, National Center for Infectious
Disease; Director, Division of AIDS, STD, TB Laboratory Research, Centers for
Disease Control and Prevention, Atlanta, Georgia
  Current Trends in the Epidemiology of HIV/AIDS

Christine M. Jamjian, DPharm
Assistant Professor (Clinical) of Pharmacy Practice, University of Utah College of
Pharmacy; HIV Clinical Pharmacist, University of Utah Hospital and Clinics,
Salt Lake City, Utah
  *Antiretroviral Adverse Effects and Interactions: Clinical Recognition
  and Management*

Jeffrey L. Jones, MD, MPH
Chief, Special Projects Section, Surveillance Branch, Division of HIV/AIDS
Prevention, Centers for Disease Control and Prevention, Atlanta, Georgia
  Current Trends in the Epidemiology of HIV/AIDS

Lawrence D. Kaplan, MD
Associate Professor of Medicine, University of California, San Francisco; Director,
AIDS-Malignancies Program, San Francisco General Hospital, San Francisco,
California
  Malignancies Associated with AIDS

Malika Kheraj, MD
Infectious Diseases Fellow, University of California San Francisco Mt Zion
Medical Center, San Francisco, California
  Management of Herpesvirus Infections (CMV, HSV, VZV)

Kathryn Kocurek, MD
Assistant Clinical Professor of Medicine, University of California, San Francisco;
Director, University of California San Francisco HIV Case Management Program;
Co-Chair, HIV Advisory Panel for Brown and Toland Medical Group; Associate
Director, Primary Care Internal Medicine Residency, University of California
San Francisco-Stanford Health Care, San Francisco, California
  Primary and Preventive Care for the HIV-Infected Adult

Jane E. Koehler, MD
Associate Professor of Medicine, Division of Infectious Diseases, University of
California, San Francisco, San Francisco, California
  *Bacillary Angiomatosis and Other Unusual Infections in HIV-Infected
  Individuals*

Shantel M. Mullin, DPharm
Assistant Professor (Clinical) of Pharmacy Practice, University of Utah College of
Pharmacy; Clinical Pharmacist and Drug Information Specialist, University of
Utah Hospitals and Clinics, Salt Lake City, Utah
  *Antiretroviral Adverse Effects and Interactions: Clinical Recognition
  and Management*

Meg D. Newman, MD
Assistant Professor of Medicine, University of California, San Francisco; Director,
San Francisco General Hospital, AIDS Education Unit, (SFGH), San Francisco,
California
  Women and HIV Disease

Donald W. Northfelt, MD
AIDS Oncologist, Pacific Oaks Medical Group, Palm Springs, California
  Malignancies Associated with AIDS

Andrew T. Pavia, MD
Associate Professor of Pediatrics and Medicine, University of Utah; Director for
Clinical Research, University AIDS Center, Salt Lake City, Utah
  Pediatric AIDS

Richard W. Price, MD
Professor and Vice Chair, Department of Neurology, University of California,
San Francisco; Chief, Neurology Service, San Francisco General Hospital,
San Francisco, California
  Management of the Neurologic Complications of HIV-1 Infection and AIDS

Jack S. Remington, MD
Professor of Medicine, Division of Infectious Diseases and Geographic Medicine,
Stanford University School of Medicine; Marcus A. Krupp Research Chair and
Chairman, Department of Immunology and Infectious Disease, Research Institute,
Palo Alto Medical Foundation, Palo Alto, California
  AIDS-Associated Toxoplasmosis

Rudolph A. Rodriguez, MD
Assistant Clinical Professor, University of California San Francisco; Medical
Director, San Francisco General Hospital, San Francisco, California
  Renal Complications of HIV Infection

Michael S. Saag, MD
Professor of Medicine, and Director, AIDS Outpatient Clinic, University of
Alabama at Birmingham, Birmingham, Alabama
  *Laboratory Testing for HIV-1; Cryptococcosis and Other Fungal Infections
  (Histoplasmosis, Coccidioidomycosis)*

Morris Schambelan, MD
Professor of Medicine, University of California, San Francisco; Chief, Division
of Endocrinology and Metabolism, and Program Director, General Clinical
Research Center, San Francisco General Hospital, San Francisco, California
Endocrinologic Manifestations of HIV Infection

Deborah E. Sellmeyer, MD
Assistant Adjunct Professor of Medicine, University of California, San Francisco,
San Francisco, California
Endocrinologic Manifestations of HIV Infection

Spotswood L. Spruance, MD
Professor of Medicine, Department of Internal Medicine, Division of Infectious
Disease, University of Utah School of Medicine; Medical Staff, University of Utah
Hospital, Salt Lake City, Utah
*Antiretroviral Adverse Effects and Interactions: Clinical Recognition
and Management*

John D. Stansell, MD
Assistant Professor of Medicine, University of California, San Francisco; Medical
Director, AIDS Program, San Francisco General Hospital, San Francisco,
California
Pneumocystis carinii Pneumonia

Mary Jean Stempien, MD
Director, Medical Research, Roche Global Development, Palo Alto, California
Management of Herpesvirus Infections (CMV, HSV, VZV)

Carlos S. Subauste, MD
Assistant Professor of Medicine, Division of Infectious Diseases, University of
Cincinnati College of Medicine, Cincinnati, Ohio
AIDS-Associated Toxoplasmosis

Andrew H. Talal, MD, MPH
Research Associate and Clinical Scholar, The Rockefeller University, New York,
New York
Gastrointestinal and Hepatic Manifestations of HIV Infection

Paul A. Volberding, MD
Professor of Medicine, University of California, San Francisco; Director, AIDS
Program, San Francisco General Hospital, San Francisco, California
Antiretroviral Therapy

Constance B. Wofsy, MD*
Professor of Medicine, University of California, San Francisco; Co-Director, AIDS
Program, and Associate Director, Infectious Disease, San Francisco General
Hospital, San Francisco, California
Women and HIV Disease

Teresa L. Wright, MD
Associate Professor of Medicine, University of San Francisco; Chief,
Gastrointestinal Unit, Veterans Affairs Medical Center, San Francisco, California
Hepatitis C Infection

---

*Deceased.

Preface

This is the sixth edition of *The Medical Management of AIDS*, whose sole purpose over the past 12 years of this terrible epidemic has been to bring up-to-date clinical information to the many dedicated health care workers around the world to help them to provide the very latest, cutting edge care to their HIV-infected patients. In order to accomplish this objective, this textbook has been published every 2 years, which is again the case with this edition.

Publication in 1999 is particularly timely because the changes that have taken place in the last several years since the introduction of highly active antiretroviral therapy (HAART) and the use of HIV viral RNA (vRNA) plasma levels have totally changed our approach to the care of HIV-infected patients. The availability of HAART and the ability to directly measure its effect in vivo are unique in the entire field of clinical infectious diseases. This has allowed investigators to develop new therapeutic approaches without waiting for results of large, cumbersome trials that used only clinical endpoints and required large numbers of patients and years to complete. However, it has been necessary to take some of the assumptions central to current therapeutic strategies on the basis of faith, without complete clinical validation, although each day more information becomes available that tends to support currently recommended guidelines.

As of the writing of this edition, the current wisdom suggests that antiretroviral therapy should be initiated when the CD4 count is less than 500 cells/mm^3 and the viral load is greater than 5000 copies of vRNA/ml of plasma; the exact numbers are debated, but these values fit with most recommendations. Most experts initially recommend three drugs, two nucleoside reverse transcriptase inhibitors and a protease inhibitor (or a non-nucleoside reverse transcriptase inhibitor), and accept as an adequate response a reduction of vRNA to less than detectable levels at 6 to 10 weeks. Reaching fewer than 500 copies of vRNA/ml of plasma appears to drive the total body viral load to levels near or below which the virus is less likely to develop resistant mutations to the drugs and escape from the antiretroviral effect of the triple therapy. Recent analysis of ongoing studies with the new supersensitive assays suggests that levels of less than 20 to 50 copies of vRNA/ml of plasma are associated with more prolonged suppression than 500 copies, but these results must be confirmed with future clinical studies. The analogy to therapeutic strategies for tuberculosis is striking.

HAART has proven to be successful in reducing viral load to undetectable levels in up to 80% of patients who have not previously received antiretroviral therapy and who adhere to their therapy, according to a trial involving zidovudine, lamivudine, and indinavir, for which we now have up to 2 years of follow-up data. Mortality rates have dropped dramatically, and formerly bedridden AIDS patients have been able to go back to work. Inpatient admissions have decreased markedly and many of the opportunistic infections have essentially disappeared. But in 1998, we have begun to ask questions: Are things really as amazing as they seem? How long will this euphoria be sustained? The first indication that all was not as it seemed was reported in 1997 from the clinic population at San Francisco General Hospital. When data on nearly 200 patients who had been started on triple therapy 1 year previously were analyzed, viral loads were still effectively suppressed (vRNA less than detectable) in only 50% of patients. Most failures were attributed to poor compliance with HAART. In addition, some patients had had previous antiretroviral therapy, and several had been started on a single drug to augment a previously failing multidrug regimen, practices that risked rapid emergence of resistant viral subpopulations.

When we consider the complexities of these regimens—twice- and thrice-daily dosing schedules, some drugs to be taken with food and others without, many drugs interacting adversely with other drugs, and now the emergence of significant side effects such as lipodystrophies, diabetes mellitus, and hyperlipidemias—is it realistic to expect our patients to faithfully comply with these treatments for life? There are also data to indicate that, if the drugs are not taken as recommended, resistance will develop and the therapeutic effect will not be sustained. In addition, new isolates from antiretroviral-naive patients are showing increased resistance to all three classes of drugs (zidovudine resistance ranges from 10% to 20%), indicating that these resistant populations of HIV are being transmitted from person to person. New effective drugs that can be given once a day without bothersome side effects are desperately needed if the advances we are currently celebrating are to continue, and before the drugs we have lose their efficacy.

However, even as we temper some of the optimism brought about by our recent successful therapeutic attack on HIV with these latest data on resistance and side effects, it is critically important to remember that, for the vast majority of infected individuals in the world who would benefit from these drugs, cost is prohibitive and access to currently available drugs will not be possible with the current economic structure. The sobering reality is that the HIV epidemic worldwide continues its relentless progression: 50 million cases by the end of the millennium, countries in sub-Saharan Africa experiencing a negative population growth, millions of orphans resulting from AIDS-associated death of young parents, and dramatic reversals in hard-won advances in infant mortality and duration of life expectancy. It is now obvious that, without a cheap and effective vaccine, this epidemic will continue its relentless course. What can we expect in the year 2010? 100 million, 500 million, or 1 billion infected persons dead from HIV? The vaccine effort has been weak, and to date there are few candidates on the horizon for which the outlook is optimistic. The virus appears to be much smarter and more facile in evading immunization strategies than is the collective scientific brain power of the western world in developing them. The grim prospect is that it seems unlikely that we will have an effective preventive vaccine in the field within the next 10 years.

Worrisome trends continue in the United States, which has been far more heavily affected by HIV/AIDS than any other industrialized nation. Heterosexual sex is still the fastest growing method of transmission, increasingly so in younger women. The greatest increases in AIDS incidence in 1995 were among women who were 14 to 18 years old back in 1988, when they were likely to have been infected. These young populations of women require *urgent* outreach and intervention methods.

We will continue to publish our textbook and try to keep our dedicated AIDS providers up to date with clinically relevant information on recent advances in the care of HIV-infected individuals. New to this edition are chapters on maximizing adherence to antiviral therapy, ocular complications of HIV, HIV-related pneumonias other than *Pneumocystis carinii* pneumonia, hepatitis C infection, global prevention of HIV, pregnant women with HIV, HIV in substance abusers, and in geriatric patients. We will also continue our efforts to keep our public informed that the epidemic is neither over nor controlled, and that it can rightfully take its place as one of the most devastating natural disasters in the history of mankind.

We thank the Hoffman–La Roche and Glaxo Wellcome Companies for continued educational support for the "Clinical Care of the AIDS Patient" conference, which is held in San Francisco in early December every year, and from which this publication results. We also wish to thank the staffs in the Division of Medicine at San Francisco General Hospital; in Continuing Medical Education and the Department of Medicine at the University of California, San Francisco; and in the Department of Medicine at the University of Utah. Finally, we wish to thank our editor, Pamela Derish.

MERLE A. SANDE, MD
PAUL A. VOLBERDING, MD

COLOR PLATE IA. Maculopapular rash on trunk of an individual with acute HIV infection. (See page 68.)

COLOR PLATE IB. Hairy leukoplakia on tongue. (See page 162.)

COLOR PLATE IC. Giemsa stain of induced sputum demonstrating cysts and trophozoites of *Pneumocystis carinii*. There is no uptake of stain by cyst wall; therefore, walls appear as clear-to-white circles. Trophozoites appear as dark dots. (×960.) (See page 306.)

COLOR PLATE ID. Acid-fast stain of lymph node tissue demonstrating large numbers of red-staining *Mycobacterium avium-intracellulare*. (See page 344.)

COLOR PLATE IE. Severe edema complicating advanced lower extremity cutaneous Kaposi's sarcoma. (See page 470.)

COLOR PLATE IF. Cytomegalovirus-associated retinitis. Note characteristic hemorrhages and exudates. (See page 429.)

COLOR PLATE IG. Widespread cutaneous Kaposi's sarcoma in a Caucasian individual; typical violaceous appearance of skin lesions. (See page 470.)

COLOR PLATE IH. Typical appearance of early Kaposi's sarcoma involving the palate. (See page 470.)

COLOR PLATE IIA. Bacillary angiomatosis of the upper thigh in an AIDS patient who was seen initially 6 months earlier with subacute cellulitis. (See page 187.)

COLOR PLATE IIB. Widespread maculopapular eruption typical of rashes seen with trimethoprimsulfamethoxazole and other antibiotics. (See page 190).

COLOR PLATE IIC. Ampullary biopsy—AIDS papillary stenosis. Note large cells with intranuclear inclusions characteristic of cytomegalovirus (*arrows*). (See page 207.)

COLOR PLATE IID. Wright-Giemsa stain of circulating phagocyte with intracellular *Histoplasma capsulatum*. (See page 371.)

COLOR PLATE IIE. Papanicolau stain of sputum demonstrating spherules (one intact, one partially collapsed) of *Coccidioides immitis*. (See page 374.)

COLOR PLATE IIF. Atypical chronic HSV infection at the gluteal cleft in a patient with AIDS. Note the clinical resemblance to a pressure decubitus. (See page 440.)

COLOR PLATE IIG. Small noncleaved-cell Burkitt's lymphoma involving lymph node. (Original mangnification, ×100.) (See page 479.)

COLOR PLATE IIH. Hematoxylin and eosin staining of a biopsied cutaneous BA lesion demonstrating a dermal vessel. The vessel is lined with protuberant endothelial cells surrounded by myxoid connective tissue containing neutrophils and amphophilic granular material in close proximity to the vascular lumen. (See page 416.) (From Koehler JE, LeBolt PE, Eghert BM, et al: Cutaneous vascular lesions and disseminated catscratch-disease in patients with the acquired immunodeficiency syndrome (AIDS) and AIDS-related complex. Ann Intern Med 109:449–455, 1988.)

COLOR PLATE IIIA. Fundus photograph showing HIV microvasculopathy, also called HIV retinopathy or AIDS retinopathy. Note the characteristic nerve fiber layer infarcts, or "cotton-wool spots," and the single, small intraretinal hemorrhage temporal to the optic nerve head. (See page 176.)

COLOR PLATE IIIB. Fundus photograph showing active CMV retinitis. Note the characteristic "satellite" lesions at the advancing edges of the lesion. Vitreous inflammation is typically mild, but may be more severe in patients on combination antiretroviral therapy. (See page 176.)

COLOR PLATE IIIC. Fundus photograph showing progressive outer retinal necrosis (PORN). Note the simultaneous involvement of large areas of retina, as well as the absence of a blood-column in some of the large retinal vessels near the optic nerve head due to vascular occlusion, both characteristic PORN. Vitreous inflammation is typically mild. Most cases are due to VZV infection, although HSV retinitis has been described as well. (See page 177.)

COLOR PLATE IIID. Fundus photograph showing active toxoplasmic retinitis. Note the moderate vitreous inflammation, as well as the adjacent, pigmented retinal scar immediately temporal to the area of retinitis, both characteristic for toxopolasmosis. (See page 177.)

PLATE I

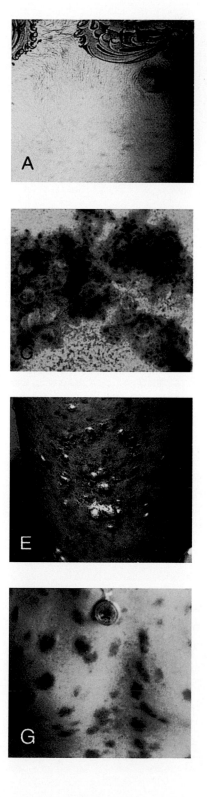

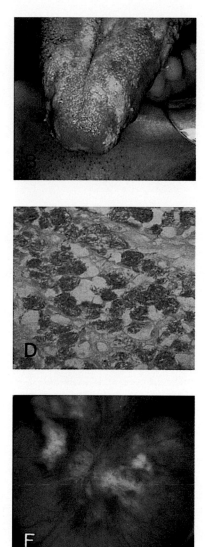

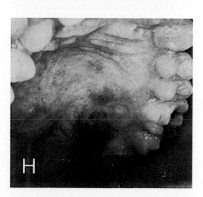

PLATE II

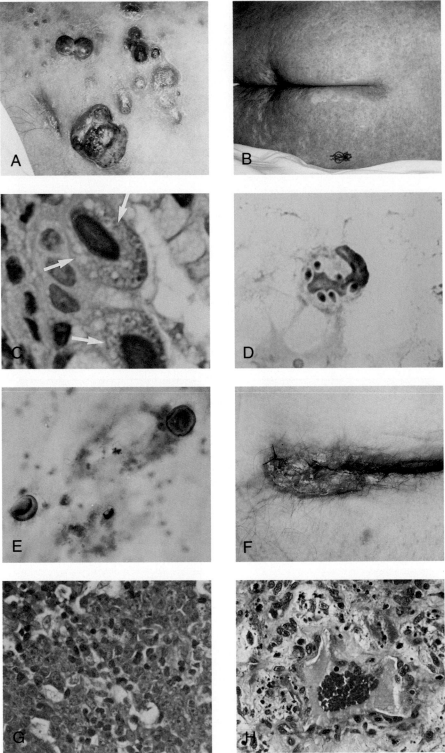

PLATE III

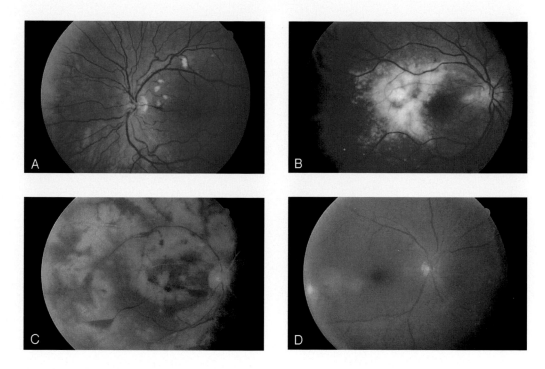

Contents

S E C T I O N   I
HIV: Transmission and Biology 1

CHAPTER 1   Current Trends in the Epidemiology of HIV/AIDS   3
JEFFREY L. JONES • KEVIN M. DeCOCK • HAROLD W. JAFFE

CHAPTER 2   Molecular Insights into HIV-1 Infection
and Pathogenesis   23
ROMAS GELEZIUNAS • WARNER C. GREENE

S E C T I O N   I I
Treatment of HIV Infection 41

CHAPTER 3   Laboratory Testing for HIV-1   43
ROBERT M. GRANT • MICHAEL S. SAAG

CHAPTER 4   Primary HIV Infection   67
ANDREW CARR • DAVID A. COOPER

CHAPTER 5   Antiretroviral Adverse Effects and Interactions: Clinical
Recognition and Management   79
SHANTEL M. MULLIN • CHRISTINE M. JAMJIAN
SPOTSWOOD L. SPRUANCE

CHAPTER 6   Antiretroviral Therapy   97
STEVEN G. DEEKS • PAUL A. VOLBERDING

CHAPTER 7   Adherence to HIV Therapy   117
FREDERICK M. HECHT • MARGARET A. CHESNEY

SECTION III
Management of Patients with HIV Infection and Its Complications 123

CHAPTER 8   Primary and Preventive Care for the HIV-Infected Adult   125
KATHRYN KOCUREK • HARRY HOLLANDER

CHAPTER 9   The Chest Film in AIDS   139
PHILIP C. GOODMAN

CHAPTER 10   Oral Complications of HIV Infection   157
JOHN S. GREENSPAN • DEBORAH GREENSPAN

CHAPTER 11   Ocular Complications of HIV Infection   171
EMMETT T. CUNNINGHAM, JR.

CHAPTER 12   Dermatologic Care of the AIDS Patient   185
TIMOTHY G. BERGER

CHAPTER 13   Gastrointestinal and Hepatic Manifestations of HIV Infection   195
ANDREW H. TALAL • DOUGLAS T. DIETERICH

CHAPTER 14   Management of the Neurologic Complications of HIV-1 Infection and AIDS   217
RICHARD W. PRICE

CHAPTER 15   Psychosocial Issues and Psychiatric Complications of HIV Disease   241
LISA CAPALDINI

CHAPTER 16   Hematologic Complications of HIV Infection   265
JULIE HAMBLETON

CHAPTER 17   Cardiovascular Complications of HIV Infection   275
MELVIN D. CHEITLIN

CHAPTER 18   Endocrinologic Manifestations of HIV Infection   285
MORRIS SCHAMBELAN • DEBORAH E. SELLMEYER • CARL GRUNFELD

CHAPTER 19   Renal Complications of HIV Infection   297
RUDOLPH A. RODRIGUEZ • MICHAEL H. HUMPHREYS

SECTION IV
Specific Infections and Malignancies in HIV Disease 303

CHAPTER 20   *Pneumocystis carinii* Pneumonia   305
LAURENCE HUANG • JOHN D. STANSELL

C H A P T E R **21**   Other HIV-Related Pneumonias   331
JOHN G. BARTLETT

C H A P T E R **22**   Disseminated *Mycobacterium avium* Complex and Other
Atypical Mycobacterial Infections   343
MARK A. JACOBSON

C H A P T E R **23**   Tuberculosis in the HIV-Infected Patient   353
HENRY F. CHAMBERS

C H A P T E R **24**   Cryptococcosis and Other Fungal Infections
(Histoplasmosis, Coccidioidomycosis)   361
MICHAEL S. SAAG

C H A P T E R **25**   AIDS-Associated Toxoplasmosis   379
CARLOS S. SUBAUSTE • JACK S. REMINGTON

C H A P T E R **26**   Hepatitis C Infection   399
MARINA BERENGUER • TERESA L. WRIGHT

C H A P T E R **27**   Bacillary Angiomatosis and Other Unusual Infections in
HIV-Infected Individuals   411
JANE E. KOEHLER

C H A P T E R **28**   Management of Herpesvirus Infections (Cytomegalovirus,
Herpes Simplex Virus, and Varicella-Zoster Virus)   429
W. LAWRENCE DREW • MARY JEAN STEMPIEN
MALIKA KHERAJ • KIM S. ERLICH

C H A P T E R **29**   Management of Syphilis in HIV-Infected Persons   453
GAIL BOLAN

C H A P T E R **30**   Malignancies Associated with AIDS   467
LAWRENCE D. KAPLAN • DONALD W. NORTHFELT

S E C T I O N **V**
Special Aspects of HIV and Population-Specific Management 497

C H A P T E R **31**   The Global Prevention of HIV   499
MYRON S. COHEN • GINA DALLABETTA • WILLARD CATES, JR.
KING K. HOLMES

C H A P T E R **32**   HIV Exposure Risk Assessment and Prophylactic
Treatment   513
JULIE LOUISE GERBERDING

C H A P T E R **33**   Pediatric AIDS   525
ANDREW T. PAVIA • JOHN C. CHRISTENSON

CHAPTER 34   Women and HIV Disease 537
MEG D. NEWMAN • CONSTANCE B. WOFSY

CHAPTER 35   Conception, Pregnancy, and Parenthood: Maternal Health
Care and the HIV Epidemic 555
KAREN P. BECKERMAN

CHAPTER 36   HIV Disease in Substance Abusers:
Treatment Issues 575
GERALD FRIEDLAND

CHAPTER 37   AIDS in Older Persons 593
BRADLEY S. BENDER • DAVID W. BENTLEY

CHAPTER 38   Alternative Therapies 601
DONALD I. ABRAMS

Index 613

SECTION

1

HIV:
Transmission
and Biology

1

Current Trends in the Epidemiology of HIV/AIDS

JEFFREY L. JONES • KEVIN M. DeCOCK • HAROLD W. JAFFE

INTERNATIONAL ASPECTS

Global Impact of HIV/AIDS

Through the end of 1997, the Joint United Nations Programme on HIV/AIDS (UNAIDS) estimated that, worldwide, 30.6 million persons were living with HIV infection.[1] Of these persons, most reside in sub-Saharan Africa (68%) or South and Southeast Asia (20%), with less than 3% living in North America and less than 2% in western Europe (Fig. 1–1). Of the estimated 16,000 persons becoming newly infected with HIV each day, more than 40% are women, more than 50% are 15- to 24-year-olds, and 10% are children age 14 years or younger. The HIV epidemic has left an estimated 8.2 million children orphaned and 1.1 million children living with HIV. In 1997 alone, UNAIDS estimated that 5.8 million persons became infected with HIV and 2.8 million persons died with AIDS, with more than 90% of new infections and 89% of deaths occurring in sub-Saharan Africa and South and Southeast Asia.

Since the beginning of the epidemic, an estimated 11.7 million persons throughout the world have died with AIDS.[1] Life expectancy at birth has been markedly reduced in many sub-Saharan African countries; in Botswana, for example, it is projected to be reduced to 50 years in the year 2000, down from 62 years in 1990.[1] Clearly, the HIV epidemic has had a vast global impact, especially in developing countries in sub-Saharan Africa, and is rapidly emerging in countries in South and Southeast Asia.

Overall patterns of HIV transmission vary throughout the world. In Europe, for example, the majority of reported AIDS cases in Scandinavia and the United Kingdom have occurred among homosexual men, whereas in Spain and Italy most persons with AIDS have been injection drug users (IDUs).[7] In sub-Saharan Africa, the spread of HIV has occurred primarily through heterosexual contact, although transfusion-related infections still occur in areas that transfuse unscreened or inadequately screened blood.[3] Although the predominant mode of transmission in South and Southeast Asia is heterosexual contact, especially between female sex workers and their customers, injection drug use accounts for a large proportion of cases in northeastern India,[4] Burma,[5,6] and Thailand.[7,8] Central and eastern Europe are also experiencing an emerging HIV epidemic, with injection drug use the predominant mode of transmission.[9–11] In this region of Europe, the increasing syphilis incidence is also raising concern about sexual spread of HIV.[11]

HIV seroprevalence rates have been among the highest in regions of sub-Saharan Africa. For example, serologic surveys conducted among pregnant women in Botswana, Uganda, Zambia, Malawi, and South Africa have commonly found infection rates of 20% to 35% in urban areas.[12,13] Even in rural areas, rates in pregnant women often exceed 10%.[13] Among commercial sex workers in southern, eastern, and western Africa, seroprevalence rates often exceed 40%.[12] The high rates of HIV infection in Africa have been associated with multiple sexual partners, prostitution and contact with prostitutes,[14–16] and sexually transmitted diseases (STDs), especially genital ulcer disease.[17,18]

HIV Genetic Types and Subtypes

HIV-2

HIV-2, a second AIDS-related retrovirus, has contributed to the AIDS epidemic in limited

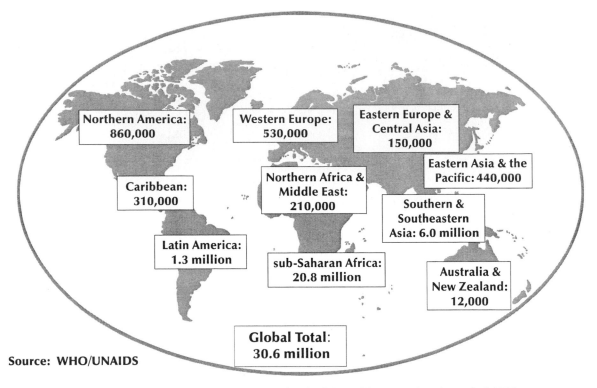

FIGURE 1–1. Adults and children estimated to be living with HIV/AIDS at the end of 1997.

parts of the world. This virus was first isolated from two West African AIDS patients.[19] Subsequent studies established that HIV-2 was present throughout West Africa and was more common than HIV-1 in Guinea-Bissau, The Gambia, and Senegal.[20] Outside of West Africa, HIV-2 has been diagnosed most often among persons in France and Portugal,[20,21] Angola and Mozambique (two former Portuguese colonies),[13,19] and, most recently, India.[22,23] In the United States, infections with HIV-2 are rare, with only 77 cases reported through December 1997.[24] Most of these U.S. cases occurred in persons who were born in, had traveled to, or had a sex partner from West Africa.

While HIV-2 is clearly pathogenic and produces a spectrum of illness that is similar to that seen with HIV-1 infection, the two viruses have important biologic differences. For example, in studies of prostitutes in Senegal, Marlink et al. have shown that CD4+ T-lymphocyte counts decline significantly faster in persons with HIV-1 infection compared to those with HIV-2 infection.[25]

HIV-2 also appears to be less easily transmitted than HIV-1. Studies of young women in Abidjan, Ivory Coast, showed that, from 1988 to 1992, HIV-1 seroprevalence increased from 5.0% to 9.2%, while HIV-2 seroprevalence decreased from 2.6% to 1.5%.[26] Additionally, rates of perinatal transmission are much lower for HIV-2 than for HIV-1.[27,28] In another study from Ivory Coast, the perinatal transmission rate was 1.2% for HIV-2 infection, compared with 24.7% for HIV-1 infection.[29] DeCock et al. have suggested that these differences in transmission rates are a consequence of lower concentrations of HIV-2 than HIV-1 in the blood of persons in the early stages of infection.[26] Researchers have also reported a slower rate of heterosexual spread of HIV-2 compared to HIV-1.[30]

HIV-1 Genetic Subtypes

Based on phylogenetic analysis of the HIV envelope gene sequences, HIV-1 has been categorized into two major groups, group M and group O. Group M has been further categorized into at least 10 subtypes (denoted A through J) based on isolates from many areas of the world[31,32] (Fig. 1–2). Subtype B predominates in the United States and western Europe.[31] The greatest number of different group M subtypes have been identified in Africa.[32] Recombination has been found to occur between specific subtypes, for example, E and G.[33]

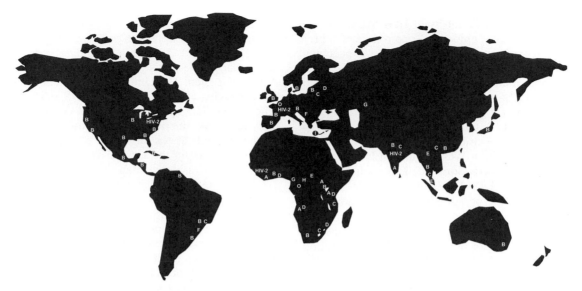

FIGURE 1–2. Geographic regions where various HIV isolates have been reported. HIV-1 group M subtypes A through I are represented on the map by letters A through I; HIV-1 group O is represented by the letter O. The points on the map represent approximate locations where persons infected with certain HIV strains have been reported and do not imply the actual distribution of HIV strains, which is not well known. This map is not an exhaustive list of all reported subtypes and does not include isolated reports of single cases or recently imported cases. (Adapted from Hu DJ, Dondero TJ, Rayfield MA, et al: The emerging genetic diversity of HIV: The importance of global surveillance for diagnostics, research, and prevention. JAMA 275:210, 1996, with permission.) Subtype J (not shown) has been found in several persons from Western Africa and in immigrants from Central Africa.

Currently, no conclusive evidence has been found for differential rates of transmission or progression associated with various group M HIV-1 genetic subtypes. A study demonstrating that subtype E and C viruses replicate in Langerhans' cells significantly more efficiently than do subtype B strains,[34] and the increasing prevalence of subtype E versus B in Bangkok IDUs[35] have been cited as possible evidence for differential transmission of group M HIV subtypes. However, other researchers have disputed whether replication in vitro varies by specific viral subtypes,[36] and evidence against differential transmission includes (1) the presence of non-B subtypes in Europe without rapid spread; (2) similar rates of perinatal transmission without intervention in different parts of the world; and (3) similar estimates of per-sex-act transmission among couples in Europe, North America, and northern Thailand.[37]

Group O HIV-1 viruses are highly divergent and mainly found in Africa, especially in Cameroon, where the frequency of group O relative to group M ranged from 1% to 6.3% in 1994–1995,[38] in countries neighboring Cameroon, and in western and southeast Africa.[39] Group O viruses have also been identified in other areas of the world, but most group O HIV infections have occurred in Africa or in persons from Africa. Of the two group O infections identified in the United States,[40,41] both occurred in persons originally from Africa. No group O HIV was detected in stored serum samples obtained from persons in both high- and low-prevalence HIV risk groups in the United States and Puerto Rico that were analyzed by peptide-specific enzyme immunoassay (EIA).[42] Therefore, group O HIV is thought to be rare in the United States.[40] The natural history of group O HIV infection appears to be similar to that of group M infections.[43] The public health importance of group O HIV infections stems from the lack of sensitivity of some HIV diagnostic tests, including EIA screening tests, to detect infection.[40,44–46]

Summary

Through the end of 1997, UNAIDS estimated that 30.6 million persons were living with HIV infection worldwide. Most HIV-infected persons live in sub-Saharan Africa or in South and Southeast Asia. The HIV epidemic has left an estimated 8.2 million children orphaned and 1.1

million children living with HIV. Since the beginning of the epidemic, approximately 11.7 million persons have died and life expectancy in some sub-Saharan African countries has dropped markedly. HIV infection has spread rapidly in South and Southeast Asia by heterosexual contact and injection drug use and is spreading to central and eastern Europe primarily by injection drug use. HIV-2 is contributing to the epidemic in West Africa but has a limited worldwide distribution and is less easily transmitted than HIV-1. Finally, specific genetic types and subtypes of HIV-1 may predominate in specific regions of the world, but currently there is no direct evidence for differential rates of transmission or progression of disease among them.

THE EPIDEMIC IN THE UNITED STATES

AIDS Case Surveillance

Through December 1997, 641,086 persons with AIDS had been reported to the Centers for Disease Control and Prevention (CDC) by state and local health departments.[47] Of these, 83.4% (534,532) were men, 15.4% (98,468) were women, and 1.2% (8086) were children less than 13 years old. As of this same date, 385,968 adults and adolescents and 4724 children with AIDS have died. The United States has been far more heavily affected by HIV/AIDS than any other industrialized nation; using a comparable case definition, the rate per 1 million population in the United States in 1996 was 8.0 times higher than that in the United Kingdom or Germany, 3.0 times higher than that in France, and 1.2 times higher than in Spain, Europe's most heavily affected country.[2,48]

Of the 60,634 U.S. persons with AIDS reported to the CDC in 1997, the largest proportion (45%) were blacks, with whites comprising 33%, Hispanics 21%, and American Indian/Alaskan Native or Asian/Pacific Islanders 1%. In 1997, 22% of adult/adolescent AIDS cases occurred in women, an increase from 20% in 1996.[49] In 1997, rates of reported AIDS cases per 100,000 population were 83.7 among blacks, 37.7 among Hispanics, 10.4 among whites, and 10.4 among American Indians/Alaskan Natives, with the lowest rate (4.5) occurring in Asian/Pacific Islanders. AIDS rates in the United States by states and territories for 1997 are shown in Figure 1-3.

By HIV exposure category, among adults and adolescents in 1997, men who have sex with

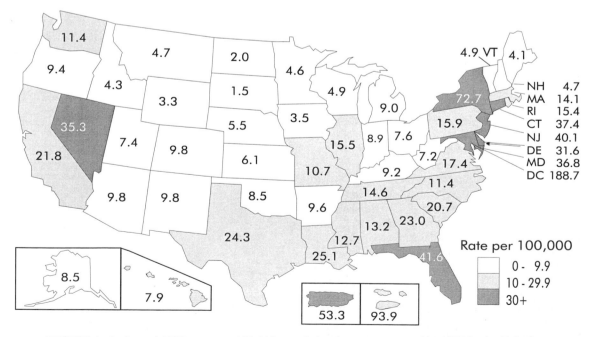

FIGURE 1-3. Annual AIDS rates per 100,000 population for cases reported in 1997 in the United States.

men (MSM) continued to be the largest single group of persons reported with AIDS (35%).[47] IDUs were the second largest group (24%), followed by persons exposed through heterosexual contact (13%), MSM who also injected drugs (4%), and recipients of blood and blood products, including persons with hemophilia (1%). However, the proportional distribution of cases in each exposure category will increase over time as the 22% of persons initially reported with unspecified exposure category are later reclassified into known risk categories after additional reviews of medical records.

Significant differences exist between racial and ethnic groups in the distribution of AIDS cases by exposure category. Among MSM reported in 1997, more than twice as many were white as were black; however, among male IDUs or men exposed by heterosexual contact, nearly three times as many were black as were white. A greater proportion of AIDS cases among blacks and Hispanics than among whites is directly or indirectly associated with injection drug use, which emphasizes the importance of drug use prevention in combating the HIV epidemic among U.S. minority populations. Although national AIDS surveillance collects information about race and ethnicity, it does not collect information about socioeconomic status. However, studies by Hu et al. in New Jersey[50] and Simon et al. in Los Angeles[51] have shown that, for all racial groups, poverty is independently associated with higher AIDS rates. It is well documented that a disproportionate proportion of U.S. minority populations live below the poverty level.[52]

A geographic analysis in 1995 found that the largest numbers of U.S. AIDS cases were reported from the South and the largest proportionate increase in cases were reported from the South and Midwest.[53] Increases were also occurring in rural areas, with a higher proportion of AIDS cases occurring among adolescents and young adults in small cities and rural areas in the South and Midwest than in similar areas in the West or Northeast.[53]

Of the 678 children (<13 years old) reported with AIDS in 1997, 91% had a mother with or at risk for HIV infection, 8% were infected through blood or blood products, and 2% had other or no reported risks.[47] Of the children who had a mother with or at risk for HIV infection, 67% had mothers who either were IDUs or had sex with an IDU. When the children reported in 1997 were stratified by race/ethnicity, 62% were black, 23% Hispanic, 13% white, and less than 2% other racial/ethnic groups.

Trends in AIDS Morbidity and Mortality

The CDC's AIDS surveillance case definition was revised in 1985, 1987, and 1993 to incorporate additional severe illnesses found to be associated with HIV infection and to reflect changes in medical management of persons with AIDS.[54–56] The criteria in the 1993 revision also included HIV-infected adults and adolescents with a CD4+ T-lymphocyte count less than 200 cells/μl or a percentage of total lymphocytes less than 14. These immunologic criteria were rapidly implemented by local AIDS reporting sources and were the basis for a large increase in reported cases, representing almost half of the AIDS cases reported in 1993 and 1994[57,58] and 57% of AIDS cases reported in 1996.[49] Following the expansion of the case definition, some of the increase in AIDS cases included HIV-infected persons reported using the immunologic criteria who would have been reported as having AIDS-related opportunistic illnesses (AIDS-OIs) when these subsequently developed. To take the expanded surveillance criteria into account for analysis of temporal trends, a statistical adjustment is required to estimate when persons who were reported using the immunologic criteria will develop an AIDS-OI.[59] Estimated AIDS-OIs are then used to describe the trends in the AIDS epidemic among different populations.

Throughout the early 1990s, the annual incidence of AIDS-OIs increased about 2%. However, during 1996, AIDS-OIs were diagnosed in an estimated 56,730 persons, a decline of 6% compared with 1995[60] (Fig. 1–4). This was the first year that the AIDS-OI incidence did not increase in the United States. From 1995 to 1996, AIDS-OI incidence declined in all four geographic areas of the United States (West [12%], Midwest [10%], Northeast [8%], and South [1%]), as well as in men, non-Hispanic whites, Hispanics, all 5-year age groups, IDUs, and MSM who also inject drugs. However, continuing increases in AIDS-OI incidence occurred among heterosexually exposed persons in the following groups: non-Hispanic black men (19%), Hispanic men (13%), non-Hispanic black women (12%), and Hispanic women (5%).[60]

Trends in the estimated AIDS-OI incidence rate per 100,000 population during 1990–1996 for men showed a leveling, then a decline, for MSM and for IDUs but no decline for men exposed by heterosexual contact (Fig. 1–5). Over-

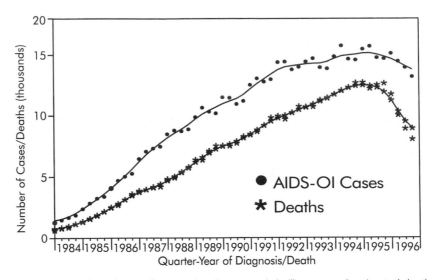

FIGURE 1–4. Estimated incidence of AIDS-related opportunistic illnesses and estimated deaths among persons with AIDS, adjusted for delays in reporting, by quarter-year of diagnosis/death, United States, 1984–1996. Points represent quarterly incidence; lines represent "smoothed" incidence. Estimates are not adjusted for incomplete reporting of AIDS cases.

all declines for 1990–1995 have also been observed in the number of AIDS cases among young MSM 13 to 25 years of age,[61] but these declines occurred mainly among whites. Among women, since 1995, rates in those exposed by heterosexual contact have exceeded rates in those directly exposed through injection drug use and continue to rise (Fig. 1–6). However, nearly half of women exposed by heterosexual contact report sex with an IDU.[47] For 1991–1995, the greatest increases in AIDS-OI incidence rates have occurred in women in the South exposed by heterosexual contact and the highest incidence rates have occurred in black women and women in the Northeast.[62,63]

Examining 1990–1996 data by race for both men and women combined for the United States reveals that, in the past several years, estimated AIDS-OI incidence rates have leveled among black persons, leveled then decreased in Hispanic and white persons, and leveled among Asian/Pacific Islanders and American Indians/ Alaskan Natives (Fig. 1–7).

Deaths among persons with AIDS have also recently decreased, declining 23% in 1996 compared with deaths in 1995[60] (Fig. 1–4). Deaths declined in all four geographic regions (West [33%], Midwest [25%], Northeast [22%], and South [19%]), among men and women, among all racial and ethnic groups, and in all risk/

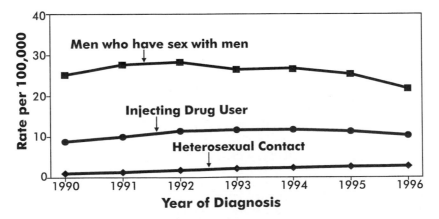

FIGURE 1–5. Estimated AIDS-related opportunistic illnesses incidence rate by HIV exposure risk among men per 100,000 population, United States, 1990–1996.

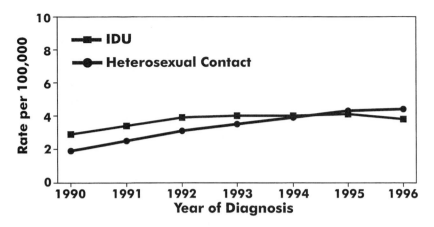

FIGURE 1–6. Estimated AIDS-related opportunistic illnesses incidence rate by HIV exposure risk among women per 100,000 population, United States, 1990–1996. IDU indicates injection drug user.

exposure categories; however, deaths in women, blacks, and persons exposed by heterosexual contact decreased the least. From 1993 to 1995, HIV infection was the leading cause of death among Americans 25 to 44 years of age. However, in 1996, HIV dropped to the number two position, below unintentional injuries, as a cause of death in this age group (Fig. 1–8) (CDC, unpublished data). Decreases in deaths from HIV infection have also been reported from New York City,[64] in a multisite clinic population,[65] and by others nationally.[66]

Temporal trends in AIDS cases and deaths result from changes in the rate of new HIV infections, AIDS diagnoses resulting from the progression of HIV to AIDS, and deaths among HIV-infected persons. Therefore, the declines in AIDS-OI incidence and deaths reflect the impact of antiretroviral therapies, AIDS-OI prophy-

laxis, and HIV prevention efforts. These declines are consistent with reports that recent improvements in HIV care are preventing or delaying the onset of AIDS-OIs and deaths among many populations of HIV-infected persons.[67,68] Recent declines in AIDS incidence have also been reported in several western European countries and have been attributed to widespread use of combination antiretroviral therapies.[69] Data from the CDC's Adult/Adolescent Spectrum of HIV Disease (ASD) project,[70] a longitudinal HIV surveillance project conducted in 11 U.S. cities, indicated that the proportion of HIV-infected persons in clinical care receiving combination therapy increased from 24% in the second half of 1995 to 65% in the second half of 1996 (CDC, unpublished data). Use of combination antiretroviral therapy is expected to increase because revised HIV treat-

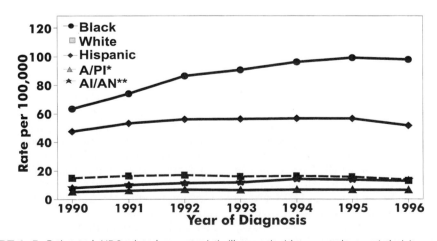

FIGURE 1–7. Estimated AIDS-related opportunistic illnesses incidence rate by race/ethnicity per 100,000 population, United States, 1990–1996. *A/PI indicates Asian/Pacific Islander; **AI/AN indicates American Indian/Alaskan Native.

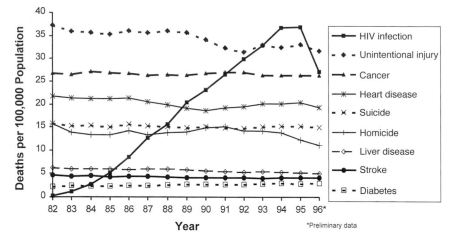

FIGURE 1–8. Trends in rates of death from leading causes of death among persons 25 to 44 years old, United States, 1982–1996.

ment guidelines recommend earlier initiation of this therapy in HIV-infected persons.[71,72]

The prolonged time from HIV infection to AIDS and AIDS to death resulting from new therapies is limiting the usefulness of AIDS case reporting as an indicator of trends in the HIV epidemic.[60,73] As of February 1998, 31 states monitor trends more directly in adults/adolescents or children with HIV case reporting in addition to AIDS case and mortality reporting. National HIV infection reporting by name has been recommended by the Council of State and Territorial Epidemiologists to more completely monitor HIV incidence and trends.[74] Although many states are now pursuing HIV infection reporting, some states are using or considering unique identifiers rather than names for reporting because of concerns about confidentiality.[75] However, evaluations in Maryland and Texas indicated that unique identifiers limit completeness of reporting, completeness of data on HIV exposure, and ability to eliminate duplicate reports.[75]

Approximately 235,470 persons in whom AIDS has been diagnosed were estimated to be living in 1996,[60] and from 1995 to 1996 the prevalence of AIDS increased 11%. This increase in AIDS prevalence reflects declines in AIDS deaths that are greater than declines in AIDS incidence. The increase in AIDS prevalence (Fig. 1–9) indicates the need for medical and other services for persons with HIV infection and for prevention programs to reduce the number of persons becoming infected with HIV.[73]

Perinatally Transmitted AIDS

Perinatal transmission accounts for virtually all new HIV infections in children.[49] Starting in 1993, the estimated number of children with perinatally acquired AIDS declined, decreasing 43% from 1992 through 1996[76] (Fig. 1–10). The declines occurred in all racial/ethnic groups and in all regions of the United States, including urban and rural areas, but were somewhat greater among whites (50%) than among blacks (42%) or Hispanics (43%). The decline was also much greater among children who were younger than 5 years of age at AIDS diagnosis (51%) than in older children (7%). In 1994, clinical trials demonstrated a two-thirds reduction in the risk for perinatal HIV transmission among HIV-infected pregnant women and their infants receiving a regimen of zidovudine (ZDV).[77] The Public Health Service issued guidelines for the use of ZDV to reduce perinatal transmission in 1994[78] and for universal HIV counseling and voluntary testing of pregnant women in 1995.[79] In an analysis of data from the 29 states that report both HIV infection and AIDS, the proportion of mothers who were known to be prescribed prenatal ZDV increased from 24% in 1994 to 64% in 1996.[76] These percentages should be considered a minimal estimate because the ZDV prescription status was not reported for all women; for example, nearly 20% of the women reported with HIV/AIDS in 1996 did not have their ZDV status reported. The widespread decline in perinatally acquired AIDS is temporally associated with the HIV counseling and voluntary testing

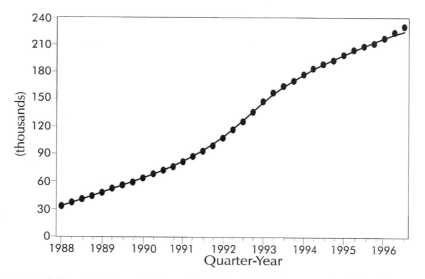

FIGURE 1–9. Adults and adolescents living with AIDS, adjusted for reporting delays, by quarter-year, United States, 1988–September 1996. Points represent quarterly prevalence; the line represents "smoothed" prevalence. Estimates are not adjusted for incomplete reporting of diagnosed AIDS cases or AIDS-related deaths.

recommendations and the increasing use of ZDV therapy by health care providers. The ZDV regimen recommended in the United States may be too complex and expensive for use in some areas of the world. However, in an evaluation among Thai women, a short course of ZDV consisting of 3 weeks of oral prenatal therapy and intrapartum therapy was found to be effective in reducing the risk of perinatal HIV transmission by 51%.[80]

TRENDS IN SPECIFIC AIDS-OIs

Researchers recently examined data from more than 20,000 patients from the ASD project to determine incidence trends for the 13 AIDS-OIs most frequently reported among MSM and IDUs in 1991–1996.[81] Among MSM, decreasing trends occurred for 11 of the most frequent AIDS-OIs: *Mycobacterium avium* complex disease (MAC), *Pneumocystis carinii* pneumonia (PCP), cytomegalovirus retinitis, Kaposi's sarcoma (KS), esophageal candidiasis, cytomegalovirus disease, extrapulmonary cryptococcosis, toxoplasmic encephalitis, tuberculosis, chronic herpes simplex, and disseminated histoplasmosis. Among IDUs, decreasing trends occurred for 5 AIDS-OIs (PCP, esophageal candidiasis, tuberculosis, chronic herpes simplex, and chronic cryptosporidiosis), but an increase occurred in recurrent pneumonia. In this same analysis, combination antiretroviral therapy and

MAC prophylaxis increased more for MSM than for IDUs, and PCP prophylaxis was prescribed at a fairly high level in both these groups. During the study period, MSM made more outpatient visits per year than IDUs (nine versus six, respectively). The overall decreases in AIDS-OI incidence are likely to be due to antiretroviral therapy and opportunistic infection prophylaxis, whereas the differences in trends between MSM and IDUs are likely to be due to differences in exposure (e.g., tuberculosis), medical care, and adherence to preventive medications. Recommendations for prevention of opportunistic infections in HIV-infected persons were published in 1995[82] and updated in 1997.[83]

In a separate analysis using data from the ASD project, prolonged survival was observed among persons with AIDS who were prescribed antiretroviral therapy (including triple combination therapy), PCP prophylaxis, and MAC prophylaxis.[68] Other researchers have reported survival benefits associated with these medications[84–92] and have found a decrease in preventable opportunistic infections such as PCP and MAC.[65,93–98]

For KS, the most common AIDS-related cancer, investigators have found a general downward trend from U.S. surveillance data,[99] in San Francisco cohorts,[100,101] in New York,[102] in a European multicenter retrospective cohort study,[103] and in Germany,[104] although several studies have not shown this trend.[105–107] In the Multicenter AIDS Cohort Study, antiretroviral

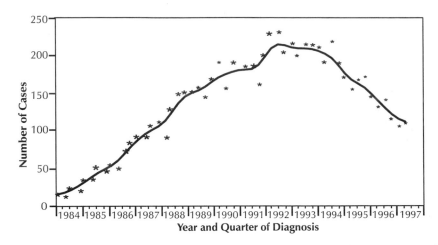

FIGURE 1–10. Number of perinatally acquired AIDS cases by quarter-year of diagnosis, United States, 1984–March 1997. Estimates were based on cases reported through September 1997, adjusted for reporting delay and unreported risk but not for incomplete reporting of diagnosed AIDS cases. Points represent quarterly incidence, and the line represents "smoothed" incidence.

therapy was found to have a possible protective effect on KS[108] and a downward trend in KS was observed from 1985 to 1991.[93] Most of the above studies evaluated trends in KS before the era of combination antiretroviral therapy.

An evaluation of the incidence from January 1994 through June 1997 of seven HIV-associated cancers (KS, immunoblastic lymphoma, primary brain lymphoma, Burkitt's lymphoma, other non-Hodgkin's lymphoma, Hodgkin's lymphoma, and invasive cervical cancer) from the ASD observational cohort found decreasing trends for KS and primary brain lymphoma, particularly during follow-up time, when patients were prescribed antiretroviral therapy.[109] Although recent data from the Multicenter AIDS Cohort Study showed a marked decline in KS in 1996 and 1997 compared to earlier years, an overall increase was found in non-Hodgkin's lymphoma.[110] Another possible factor in the decline of KS is the effect of antiherpesvirus medications.[111] Large observational cohort studies are now collecting data on the effect of new antiherpesvirus medications such as cidofovir on KS. Because of the expanding use of combination antiretroviral therapy in the United States, the incidence of KS and of some other cancers will likely decline in HIV-infected persons in the future.

Prevalence and Incidence of HIV

The overall prevalence and incidence of HIV infection in the United States have been estimated using data from three sources:[112] (1) a statistical procedure based on back-calculation[113,114] using national AIDS surveillance data, (2) a national survey of childbearing women,[115,116] and (3) a household survey of current health status.[117] Researchers estimated that, in 1992, approximately 0.3% of U.S. residents (650,000 to 900,000 persons) were HIV infected (with or without AIDS), including 0.6% of men, 2% of non-Hispanic black men, 1% of Hispanic men, 0.1% of women, and 0.6% of non-Hispanic black women. Approximately half of all infected persons were estimated to be MSM, and 25% IDUs. In addition, investigators estimated that, in 1992, approximately 40,000 new HIV infections were occurring annually.[118]

Since 1988, the CDC has been monitoring HIV seroprevalence in populations at risk for HIV infection.[119,120] These include persons attending STD clinics[121–123] and drug treatment centers[124–126] and adolescents and adults in other clinical settings.[127–130] In addition, HIV testing of filter paper specimens collected for newborn metabolic screening has been used to estimate seroprevalence among childbearing women[115,131–136] and children.[116] All of these serosurveys use unlinked (blinded) HIV testing in which personally identifying information is removed from blood specimens. Overall, these seroprevalence data suggest that, by the late 1980s and early 1990s, HIV prevalence among U.S. men had stabilized and may have started to decrease in some groups, and among women had stabilized overall.

STD clinic surveys provide most of the national data about HIV infection prevalence among MSM. Among MSM attending STD

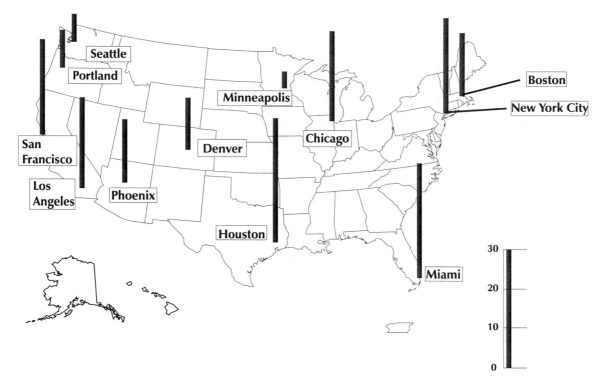

FIGURE 1–11. HIV seroprevalence among MSM attending STD clinics by metropolitan statistical area, 1996. Includes only metropolitan areas with clinics reporting at least 50 eligible specimens from MSM.

clinics in 16 U.S. cities in 1996, median seroprevalence was the highest of any group in the CDC's National Serosurveillance Program (19.5%) and ranged from a low of 3.7% in Minneapolis to a high of 31.4% in Houston (Fig. 1–11) (CDC, unpublished data). However, median seroprevalence decreased overall from 1990 through 1996 among MSM (Fig. 1–12) to well below the 1988 median of 36%.[137] A report analyzing data from 1988 through 1992 found that white MSM had a lower HIV seroprevalence rate (22%) than black (40%) or Hispanic (28%) MSM and that the decrease in seroprevalence during these years was greater for

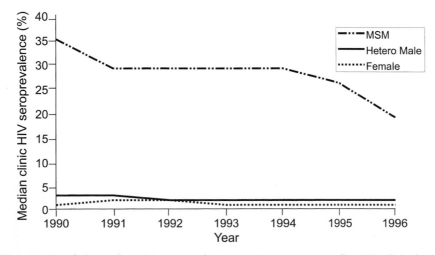

FIGURE 1–12. Trends in median HIV seroprevalence among persons attending STD clinics by selected HIV exposure mode and sex, 1990–1996. MSM indicates men who have sex with men, hetero male indicates heterosexual male, female indicates heterosexual female.

white MSM compared to black and Hispanic MSM.[137]

Although HIV seroprevalence appears to have stabilized or decreased in many populations of MSM, HIV infections are continuing to occur and the prevalence is still high in this group. The CDC-sponsored Young Mens Survey conducted among young men in street locations, dance clubs, and bars in six urban counties (Dade, Florida; Dallas, Texas; and Alameda, Los Angeles, San Francisco, and Santa Clara, California) from 1994 through January 1996 found a median HIV seroprevalence rate of 7% among 17 to 22-year-old MSM, with higher rates among blacks (11%) and Hispanics (7%) than among whites (4%).[138] Researchers from New York City and Pittsburgh have also found high levels of HIV infection in young adult gay and bisexual men, with prevalences ranging from 7% to 9%.[139,140] Studies in San Francisco in 1992–1993 found an HIV prevalence of 9.4% among men ages 17 to 22 years recruited from public parks, bars, and other congregating areas[141] and an HIV prevalence of 18% and annual incidence rate of 2.7% in a household survey of unmarried men ages 18 to 29 years who reported having sex with other men.[142] Rosenberg et al. estimated that, between 1987 and 1991, one in four new HIV infections occurred among men younger than age 22 who had sex with men.[143]

STD clinics also provide data on high-risk heterosexuals. In this group, seroprevalence has remained lower than in other groups (median 1.7% for men, 1.2% for women) and has been stable from 1990 through 1996 (Fig. 1–12). These figures probably overestimate the seroprevalence among heterosexuals attending STD clinics because some gay and bisexual men and some IDUs probably did not acknowledge their behaviors and were misclassified as having heterosexual activity as their only risk factor. Seroprevalence rates among heterosexuals have been highest in black and Hispanic persons[137,144] and in persons in the Northeast and South.[144,145]

The primary source of national seroprevalence data for IDUs is ascertainment at entry into drug treatment centers. In 1996, the median seroprevalence rate in 13 U.S. cities was 9.5% (CDC, unpublished data). Infection is concentrated along the East Coast and in the South, with the highest HIV seroprevalence occurring in Baltimore (32.2%), New York City (28.5%), and Atlanta (25%) and relatively low rates occurring in the West (e.g., San Francisco, 1.6%; Los Angeles, 1.5%) (Fig. 1–13). The reasons

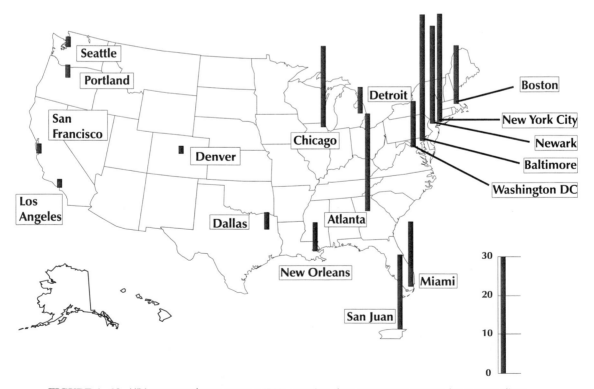

FIGURE 1–13. HIV seroprevalence among IDUs entering drug treatment centers by metropolitan area, 1996. Includes only centers reporting at least 50 eligible specimens from IDUs.

for the geographic differences in seroprevalence are not completely understood but are related to factors such as the frequency of sharing injection equipment, the number of needle-sharing partners, the use of "shooting galleries," and the mobility of IDUs.[126,146–152] Among IDUs entering treatment, seroprevalence declined from 1990 through 1996 in the Northeast and increased somewhat from 1994 through 1996 in the South to a level that exceeded the Northeast prevalence in 1996 (Fig. 1–14). HIV seroprevalence has remained stable in other geographic areas. Overall, rates have been higher in black and Hispanic IDUs than in white IDUs.

The CDC-sponsored survey of childbearing women was conducted in the United States through 1994. In that year, seroprevalence was 0.15% among childbearing women, with a distribution similar to that of IDUs, being highest along the Atlantic coast and in the South (Fig. 1–15). The overall seroprevalence rate remained stable from 1989 through 1994.[153] The highest seroprevalence rates among childbearing women were in Washington, DC (6.9/1000), New York (5.2/1000), and Florida (4.6/1000), with large differences by race/ethnicity; for example, compared to rates among white women, rates among black women were 22 times higher in New York and 16 times higher in Florida. From 1989 through 1994, seroprevalence decreased among childbearing women from 4.1/1000 to 3.2/1000 in the Northeast; in the South the rate increased from 1.6/1000 in 1989 to 1.9/1000 in 1991, then remained stable through 1994. During this time, seroprevalence rates

were relatively low (<1/1000) and stable in the West and Midwest.

Populations that are routinely tested provide another opportunity to monitor seroprevalence. Such populations include applicants to the Job Corps Residential Training Program, civilian applicants for military service, and blood donors. Although these sources are valuable, they are biased to the degree that persons at high risk for HIV infection are excluded from these populations. For example, persons who have used intravenous drugs and homosexual and bisexual men are actively discouraged from donating blood and enlisting in the armed forces. Consequently, the seroprevalence rate in high-prevalence areas in the United States was very low among voluntary blood donors (0.008%) in 1992–1993[154] and in 1995[155] and low (0.3%) among those applying for military service in 1996.[156] Among persons applying for military service, the highest rates in 1996 were among black men and women, but overall rates in this population have been fairly stable since 1991.

Persons who enter the Job Corps training programs tend to be economically disadvantaged, racial and ethnic minority youths from both rural and urban areas.[157] Among persons ages 16 to 21 years who entered the program from January 1990 through December 1996, the HIV prevalence rate was 2.3/1000.[158] The prevalence rate was higher among women (2.8/1000) than among men (2.0/1000) and highest among blacks (3.8/1000), especially black women in the South (6.4/1000). From 1990 through 1996, the prevalence in persons in this population de-

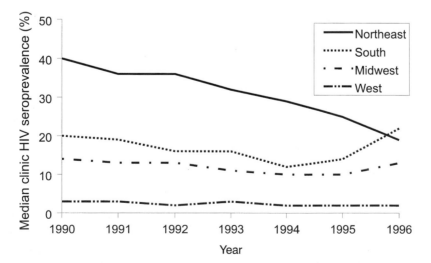

FIGURE 1–14. Trends in median HIV seroprevalence among IDUs in drug treatment centers by region of the United States, 1990–1996.

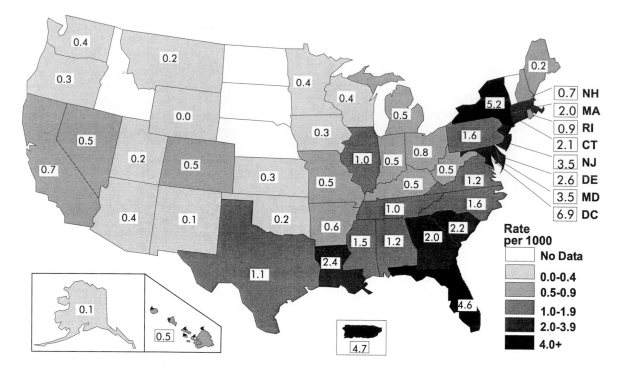

FIGURE 1–15. Prevalence of HIV infection among childbearing women in the United States, 1994.

clined for both women (4.1/1000 to 2.1/1000) and men (2.8/1000 to 1.4/1000).

A number of studies also provide useful information about incidence rates in specific populations. Weinstock and colleagues[159] evaluated more than 16,000 repeat STD clinic attendees in six cities from 1988 through 1995 and found incidence rates among MSM that ranged from 2.1 to 9.8 HIV infections per 100 person-years, with the highest rates among those in the younger age groups. Incidence rates in heterosexual men and women ranged from 0.08 to 1.1 per 100 person-years. Overall, HIV incidence was higher in men than in women (except heterosexual women had a higher rate than heterosexual men) and in blacks and Hispanics than in whites. Having other STDs was a risk factor for seroconversion in MSM and heterosexuals, while the use of illicit drugs and the exchange of drugs or money for sex were also associated with acquisition of HIV infection among heterosexuals. There was a fairly high rate of new STDs among HIV-infected persons, indicating that a substantial proportion of HIV-infected persons in this population continued to engage in high-risk behavior after HIV diagnosis.[160] This finding has been documented in other settings as well.[161–163]

Seroincidence surveys are also being conducted among repeat attendees at drug treatment centers. Among more than 2500 IDUs admitted to drug treatment centers and undergoing HIV counseling and testing, the annual incidence was 1.1% in New York (1990–1996) and 1.2% in New Jersey (1994–1996), compared with 0.5% in Seattle (1994–1996) and 0% in Los Angeles (1994–1996) (CDC, unpublished data). Because persons attending drug treatment centers most likely do not represent IDUs at highest risk for HIV infection,[164,165] the true HIV incidence in IDUs may be higher than those found in these studies.

The HIV incidence data described above come from persons tested more than once. However, researchers are developing a new tool for incidence ascertainment known as the "detuned assay" or "less sensitive assay."[166] By modifying the performance characteristics of a highly sensitive EIA to make it less sensitive, the "window period" for seroconverting specimens is extended. Discordantly positive specimens (i.e., those positive on the sensitive assay and negative on the less sensitive assay) represent seroconverting specimens in which the antibody response has not yet fully developed. This allows identification of recently infected persons and enables incidence to be calculated from cross-sectional studies that otherwise would yield only prevalence data.

SUMMARY

In the United States, AIDS-OIs and AIDS-related deaths decreased for the first time in 1996. By HIV-exposure category, the decreases were largest among MSM. However, AIDS-OIs continued to increase in heterosexually exposed minority men and women, particularly in the South. The declines in AIDS-OI incidence and AIDS-related deaths reflect the impact of anti-retroviral therapies and AIDS-OI prophylaxis. These declines have caused an increase in the number of persons living with HIV/AIDS who will need medical and other services. The prolonged time from HIV infection to AIDS is limiting the usefulness of AIDS case reporting and necessitates a shift in emphasis to HIV infection reporting. Among women, AIDS-OI rates have been declining overall. Since 1995, AIDS-OI rates in women exposed by heterosexual contact have exceeded rates in those exposed directly by injection drug use, although many women infected heterosexually are infected by IDUs. Among children, the number with perinatally acquired AIDS has declined since 1993. In adults and adolescents, the major AIDS-OIs are declining, but not equally in all groups, raising issues of differential access to medical care and adherence to preventive medications. Seroprevalence trends are similar to those occurring in AIDS case surveillance. HIV prevalence is declining overall in MSM (but not necessarily in young MSM). However, HIV prevalence is not declining in heterosexuals or in the South. Seroprevalence trends in IDUs show a decline in the Northeast but an increase in the South, with rates relatively stable in the West and Midwest. Finally, HIV seroprevalence rates remain consistently higher in racial and ethnic minority populations.

Acknowledgments

We would like to thank Robin Moseley for review of the chapter and helpful suggestions.

References

1. Joint United Nations Programme on HIV/AIDS and World Health Organization: Report on the Global HIV/AIDS Epidemic. Geneva, World Health Organization, 1997

2. European Centre for the Epidemiological Monitoring of AIDS: HIV/AIDS Surveillance in Europe: Quarterly Report No. 55. Saint-Maurice, France, European Centre for the Epidemiological Monitoring of AIDS, 1997, p 1

3. McFarland W, Mvere D, Shandera W, Reingold A: Epidemiology and prevention of transfusion-associated human immunodeficiency virus transmission in sub-Saharan Africa. Vox Sang 72:85, 1997

4. Lalvani A, Jayanthi S: HIV epidemic in India: Opportunity to learn from the past. Lancet 347:1349, 1996

5. Monitoring the AIDS Pandemic: The Status and Trends of the HIV/AIDS/STD Epidemics in Asia and the Pacific. Report from the 4th International Conference on AIDS in Asia and the Pacific, Official Satellite Symposium, Manila, October 1997

6. Hooton MT, Lwin HH, San KO, et al: HIV/AIDS in Myanmar. AIDS 8(Suppl 2):S105, 1994

7. Brown T, Sittitrai W, Vanichseni S, Thisyakorn U: The recent epidemiology of HIV and AIDS in Thailand. AIDS 8(Suppl 2):S131, 1994

8. Vanichseni S, Kitayaporn D, Mastro TB, et al: HIV-incidence, subtypes, and follow up in a prospective cohort of injecting drug users (IDUs) in Bangkok, Thailand. In Abstracts of the 4th International Congress on AIDS in Asia and the Pacific, Manila, 1997, Abstract A[P]043

9. Pimenov A: Some epidemiological aspects of HIV infection revealed in the Republic of Belarus. In Abstracts of the XIth International Conference on AIDS, Vancouver, 1996, Abstract Tu.C.202

10. Kobyshcha Y, Sccherbinskaya A, Khodekevitch L, et al: HIV infection among drug users in Ukraine: The beginning of the epidemic. In Abstracts of the XIth International Conference on AIDS, Vancouver, 1996, Abstract Tu.C.204

11. Gromyko A: Epidemiological trends of AIDS and other sexually transmitted diseases in the Eastern part of Europe. In Abstracts of the XIth International Conference on AIDS, Vancouver, 1996, Abstract Tu.C.205

12. U.S. Bureau of the Census: Recent HIV Seroprevalence Levels by Country: Research Note No. 24. Washington, DC, U.S. Bureau of the Census, 1998

13. U.S. Bureau of the Census: HIV/AIDS in Africa: Research Note No. 20. Prepared for the 9th International Conference on AIDS and STDs in Africa, Kampala, Uganda. Washington, DC, U.S. Bureau of the Census, 1995

14. Kreiss JK, Koech D, Plummer FA, et al: AIDS virus infeciton in Nairobi prostitutes: Spread of the epidemic to East Africa. N Engl J Med 314:414, 1986

15. Piot P, Plummer FA, Rey MA, et al: Retrospective seroepidemiology of AIDS virus infection in Nairobi prostitutes. J Infect Dis 155:1108, 1987

16. Ryder RW, Ndilu M, Hassig SE, et al: Heterosexual transmission of HIV-1 among employees and their spouses at two large businesses in Zaire. AIDS 4:725, 1990.

17. Greenblatt RM, Lukehart SA, Plummer FA, et al: Genital ulceration as a risk factor for human immunodeficiency virus infection. AIDS 2:47, 1988

18. Laga M, Nzila N, Goeman J: The interrelationship of sexually transmitted diseases and HIV infection: Implications for the control of both epidemics in Africa. AIDS 5(Suppl 1):S55, 1991

19. Clavel F, Guetard D, Brun-Vezinet F, et al: Isolation of a new human retrovirus from West African patients with AIDS. Science 233:343, 1986

20. Kanki PJ, DeCock KM: Epidemiology and natural history of HIV-2. AIDS 8(Suppl 1):S85, 1994

21. DeCock KM, Brun-Vezinet F: Epidemiology of HIV-2 infection. AIDS 3(Suppl 1):S89, 1989

22. Pfutzner A, Dietrich U, von Eichel U, et al: HIV-1 and HIV-2 infections in a high risk population in Bombay, India: Evidence for the spread of HIV-2 and presence of divergent HIV-1 subtype. J Acquir Immune Defic Syndr 5:972, 1992

23. Dietrich U, Maniar JK, Rubsamen-Waigmann H: The epidemiology of HIV in India. Trends Microbiol 3: 17, 1995

24. Centers for Disease Control and Prevention: Facts about Human Immunodeficiency Virus Type 2. Atlanta, Centers for Disease Control and Prevention, 1988

25. Marlink R, Kanki P, Thior I, et al: Reduced rate of disease development after HIV-2 infection as compared to HIV-1. Science 265:1587, 1994

26. DeCock KM, Adjorlolo G, Ekpini E, et al: Epidemiology and transmission of HIV-2: Why there is no HIV-2 pandemic. JAMA 270:2083, 1993

27. Andreasson PA, Dias F, Naucler A, et al: Prospective study of vertical transmission of HIV-2 in Bissau, Guinea Bissau. AIDS 7:989, 1993

28. The HIV Infection in Newborns French Collaborative Study Group: Comparison of vertical human immunodeficiency virus type 2 and human immunodeficiency virus type 1 transmission in the French prospective cohort. Pediatr Infect Dis J 13:502, 1994

29. Adjorlolo-Johnson G, DeCock KM, Ekpini E, et al: Prospective comparison of mother-to-child transmission of HIV-1 and HIV-2 in Abidjan, Ivory Coast. JAMA 272:462, 1994

30. Kanki PJ, Travers KU, Mboup S, et al: Slower heterosexual spread of HIV-2 than HIV-1. Lancet 343: 943, 1994

31. Hu DJ, Dondero TJ, Rayfield MA, et al: The emerging genetic diversity of HIV: The importance of global surveillance for diagnostics, research, and prevention. JAMA 275:210, 1996

32. Expert Group of the Joint United Nations Programme on HIV/AIDS: Implications for HIV variability for transmission: Scientific and policy issues. AIDS 11: UNAIDS1, 1997

33. McCutchan FE, Salminen MO, Carr JK, Burke DS: HIV-1 genetic diversity. AIDS 10(Suppl 3):S13, 1996

34. Soto-Ramirez LE, Renjifo B, McLane MF, et al: HIV Langerhans' cell tropism associated with heterosexual transmission of HIV. Science 271:1291, 1996

35. Wasi C, Herring B, Raktham S, et al: Determination of HIV-1 subtypes in injecting drug users in Bangkok, Thailand, using peptide-binding immunoassay and heteroduplex mobility assay: Evidence of increasing infection with HIV-1 subtype E. AIDS 9:843, 1995

36. Pope M, Ho DD, Moore JP, et al: Different subtypes of HIV-1 and cutaneous dendritic cells [letter]. Science 278:786, 1997

37. Mastro TD, de Vincenzi I: Probabilities of sexual HIV-1 transmission. AIDS 10(Suppl A):S75, 1996

38. Mauclere P, Loussert-Ajaka I, Damond F, et al: Serological and virological characterization of HIV-1 Group O infection in Cameroon. AIDS 11:445, 1997

39. Peeters M, Gueye A, Mboup S, et al: Geographical distribution of HIV-1 group O viruses in Africa. AIDS 11:493, 1997

40. Centers for Disease Control and Prevention: Identification of HIV-1 group O infection—Los Angeles County, California, 1996. MMWR Morb Mortal Wkly Rep 45:561, 1996

41. Sullivan PS, Do AN, Robbins K, et al: Surveillance for variant strains of HIV: Subtype G and group O HIV-1 [letter]. JAMA 278:292, 1997

42. Pau CP, Hu DJ, Spruill C, et al: Surveillance for human immunodeficiency virus type 1 and group O infections in the United States. Transfusion 36:398, 1996

43. Simon OF, Mauclere P, Fagot P, et al: Virological and serological characterization of HIV-1 group O. In Abstracts of the 4th Conference on Retroviruses and Opportunistic Infections, Washington, DC, 1997, Abstract 30

44. Loussert-Ajaka I, Ly TD, Chaix ML, et al: HIV-1/HIV-2 seronegativity in HIV-1 subtype O infected patients. Lancet 343:1393, 1994

45. Schable C, Leopold Z, Pau C-P, et al: Sensitivity of United States antibody tets for detection of HIV-1 group O infections. Lancet 344:1333, 1994

46. Simon F, Ly TD, Baillou-Beaufils A, et al: Sensitivity of screening kits for anti-HIV-1 subtype O antibodies. AIDS 8:1628, 1994

47. Centers for Disease Control and Prevention: U.S. HIV and AIDS cases reported through December 1997. HIV/AIDS Surveill Rep 9(No. 2):1, 1997

48. Centers for Disease Control and Prevention: U.S. HIV and AIDS cases reported through June, 1997. HIV/AIDS Surveill Rep 9(No. 1):1, 1997

49. Centers for Disease Control and Prevention: U.S. HIV and AIDS cases reported through December 1996. HIV/AIDS Surveill Rep 8(No. 2):1, 1996

50. Hu DJ, Frey RF, Costa SJ, et al: Geographical AIDS rates and sociodemographic variables in the Newark, New Jersey, metropolitan area. AIDS Public Policy J 9:20, 1994

51. Simon PA, Hu DJ, Diaz T, Kerndt PR: Income and AIDS rates in Los Angeles County. AIDS 9:281, 1995

52. U.S. Bureau of the Census: Poverty 1996—Poverty Estimates by Selected Characteristics: 1995 and 1996. Tables on U.S. Bureau of the Census Web page *http://www.census.gov/hhes/www/povty96.html* Poverty Highlights, Poverty Estimates by Selected Characteristics: 1995 and 1996. (accessed 25 March 1998)

53. Centers for Disease Control and Prevention: First 500,000 AIDS cases—United States, 1995. MMWR Morb Mortal Wkly Rep 44:849, 1995

54. Centers for Disease Control: Revision of the case definition of acquired immunodeficiency syndrome for national reporting—United States. MMWR Morb Mortal Wkly Rep 34:373, 1985

55. Centers for Disease Control: Revision of the CDC surveillance case definition for acquired immunodeficiency syndrome. MMWR Morb Mortal Wkly Rep 36(Suppl 1):1S, 1987

56. Centers for Disease Control and Prevention: 1993 revised classification system for HIV infection and expanded surveillance case definition for AIDS among adolescents and adults. MMWR Morb Mortal Wkly Rep 41(RR-17):1, 1992

57. Centers for Disease Control and Prevention: Update: Impact of the expanded AIDS surveillance case definition for adolescents and adults on case reporting—United States. MMWR Morb Mortal Wkly Rep 43: 161, 1994

58. Centers for Disease Control and Prevention: Update: Acquired immunodeficiency syndrome—United

States, 1994. MMWR Morb Mortal Wkly Rep 44:64, 1995

59. Karon JM, Green TA, Hanson DL, Ward JW: Estimating the number of AIDS-defining opportunistic illness diagnoses from data collected under the 1993 AIDS surveillance definition. J Acquir Immune Defic Syndr Hum Retrovirol 16:116, 1997

60. Centers for Disease Control and Prevention: Update: Trends in AIDS incidence—United States, 1996. MMWR Morb Mortal Wkly Rep 46:861, 1997

61. Denning PH, Jones JL, Ward JW: Recent trends in the HIV epidemic in adolescent and young adult gay and bisexual men. J Acquir Immune Defic Syndr Hum Retrovirol 16:374, 1997

62. Wortley PM, Fleming PL: AIDS in women in the United States. JAMA 278:911, 1997

63. Centers for Disease Control and Prevention: Update: AIDS among women—United States, 1995. MMWR Morb Mortal Wkly Rep 44:81, 1995

64. Chiasson M, Gerenson L, Li W, et al: Declining AIDS mortality in New York City. In Abstracts of the 4th Conference on Retroviruses and Opportunistic Infections, Washington, DC, 1997, Abstract 376

65. Palella FJ, Delaney KM, Moorman AC, et al: Declining morbidity and mortality among patients with advanced human immunodeficiency virus infection. N Engl J Med 338:853, 1998

66. National Center for Health Statistics: Births, marriages, divorces, and deaths for July 1996. Monthly Vital Stat Rep 45:1, 1997

67. Hammer SM, Squires KE, Hughes MD, et al: A controlled trial of two nucleoside analogues plus indinavir in persons with human immunodeficiency virus infection and CD4 cell counts of 200 per cubic millimeter or less. N Engl J Med 337:725, 1997

68. McNaghten AD, Hanson DL, Jones JL, et al: The effects of antiretroviral therapy and opportunistic illness primary chemoprophylaxis on survival after AIDS. In Abstracts of the 5th Conference on Retroviruses and Opportunistic Infections, Chicago, 1998, Abstract 10

69. Hamers F, Downs A, Alix J, Brunet JB: AIDS trends in Europe: Decrease in the west, increase in the east. Eurosurveillance 2:36, 1997

70. Farizo KM, Buehler JW, Chamberland ME, et al: Spectrum of disease in persons with human immunodeficiency virus infection in the United States. JAMA 267:1798, 1992

71. Carpenter CC, Fischl MA, Hammer SM, et al: Antiretroviral therapy for HIV infection in 1997: Updated recommendations of the International AIDS Society–USA Panel. JAMA 277:1962, 1997

72. Centers for Disease Control and Prevention: Report on the NIH panel to define principles of therapy of HIV infection and guidelines for the use of antiretroviral agents in HIV-infected adults and adolescents. MMWR Morb Mortal Wkly Rep 47(RR-5):1, 1998

73. Centers for Disease Control and Prevention: Update: Trends in AIDS incidence, deaths, and prevalence, United States, 1996. MMWR Morb Mortal Wkly Rep 46:165, 1997

74. Council of State and Territorial Epidemiologists: CSTE: Position statement ID-4. National HIV surveillance: Addition to the National Public Health Surveillance System. Atlanta, Council of State and Territorial Epidemiologists, 1997

75. Centers for Disease Control and Prevention: Evaluation of HIV case surveillance through the use of non-name unique identifiers—Maryland and Texas, 1994–1996. MMWR Morb Mortal Wkly Rep 46:1254, 1998

76. Centers for Disease Control and Prevention: Update: Perinatally acquired HIV/AIDS—United States, 1997. MMWR Morb Mortal Wkly Rep 46:1086, 1997

77. Connor EM, Sperling RS, Gelber R, et al: Reduction of maternal-infant transmission of human immunodeficiency virus type 1 with zidovudine treatment. N Engl J Med 331:1173, 1994

78. Centers for Disease Control and Prevention: Recommendations of the U.S. Public Health Service Task Force on the use of zidovudine to reduce perinatal transmission of human immunodeficiency virus. MMWR Morb Mortal Wkly Rep 43(RR-11):1, 1994

79. Centers for Disease Control and Prevention: U.S. Public Health Service recommendations for human immunodeficiency virus counseling and voluntary testing for pregnant women. MMWR Morb Mortal Wkly Rep 44(RR-7):1, 1995

80. Centers for Disease Control and Prevention: Administration of zidovudine during late pregnancy and delivery to prevent perinatal HIV transmission—Thailand, 1996–1998. MMWR Morb Mortal Wkly Rep 47:151, 1998

81. Jones JL, Hanson DL, Dworkin MS, et al: Trends in AIDS-related opportunistic infections among men who have sex with men and among injecting drug users, 1991–1996. J Infect Dis 178:114, 1998

82. Centers for Disease Control and Prevention: U.S. Public Health Service/Infectious Diseases Society of America guidelines for the prevention of opportunistic infections in persons infected with human immunodeficiency virus: A summary. MMWR Morb Mortal Wkly Rep 44(RR-8):1, 1995

83. Centers for Disease Control and Prevention: 1997 U.S. Public Health Services/Infectious Diseases Society of America guidelines for the prevention of opportunistic infections in persons infected with human immunodeficiency virus. MMWR Morb Mortal Wkly Rep 46(RR-12):1, 1997

84. Graham NMH, Zeger SL, Part LP, et al: The effects on survival of early treatment of human immunodeficiency virus infection. N Engl J Med 326:1037, 1992

85. Saah AJ, Hoover DR, He Y, et al, for the Multicenter AIDS Cohort Study: Factors influencing survival after AIDS: Report from the Multicenter AIDS Cohort Study (MACS). J Acquir Immune Defic Syndr 7:287, 1994

86. Chaisson RE, Kerruly JC, Moore RD: Race, sex, drug use, and progression of human immunodeficiency virus disease. N Engl J Med 333:751, 1995

87. Osmond D, Charlebois E, Lang W, et al: Changes in AIDS survival time in two San Francisco cohorts of homosexual men, 1983 to 1993. JAMA 271:1083, 1994

88. Horsburgh CR Jr, Metchock B, Gordon SM, et al: Predictors of survival in patients with AIDS and disseminated *Mycobacterium avium* complex disease. J Infect Dis 170:573, 1994

89. Ives DI, Davis RB, Currier JS: Impact of clarithromycin and azithromycin on patterns of treatment and survival among AIDS patients with disseminated *Mycobacterium avium* complex. AIDS 9:261, 1995

90. Chin DP, Reingold AL, Stone EN, et al: The impact of *Mycobacterium avium* complex bacteremia and its treatment on survival of AIDS patients—a prospective study. J Infect Dis 170:578, 1994

91. Campo RE, Campo CE: *Mycobacterium kansasii* disease in patients infected with human immunodeficiency virus. Clin Infect Dis 24:1233, 1997

92. Hoover DR, Saah AJ, Bacellar H, et al: Clinical manifestations of AIDS in the era of *Pneumocystis* prophylaxis. N Engl J Med 329:1922, 1993
93. Munoz A, Schrager LK, Bacellar H, et al: Trends in the incidence of outcomes defining acquired immunodeficiency syndrome (AIDS) in the Multicenter AIDS Cohort Study: 1985–1991. Am J Epidemiol 137:423, 1993
94. Delmas MC, Schwoebel V, Heisterkamp SH, et al: Recent trends in *Pneumocystis carinii* pneumonia as an AIDS-defining disease in nine European countries: Coordinators for AIDS Surveillance. J Acquir Immune Defic Syndr Hum Retrovirol 9:74, 1995
95. Moore RD, Chaisson RE: Natural history of opportunistic disease in an HIV-infected urban clinical cohort. Ann Intern Med 124:633, 1996
96. Weiss PJ, Wallace MR, Olson PE, Rossetti R: Changes in the mix of AIDS-defining conditions [letter]. N Engl J Med 329:1962, 1993
97. Smith E, Orholm M: Danish AIDS patients 1988–1993: A recent decline in *Pneumocystis carinii* as an AIDS-defining disease related to the period of known HIV positivity. Scand J Infect Dis 26:517, 1994
98. Wall PG, Porter K, Noone A, Goldberg DJ: Changing incidence of *Pneumocystis carinii* pneumonia as initial AIDS defining disease in the United Kingdom. AIDS 7:1523, 1993
99. Biggar RJ, Rabkin CS: The epidemiology of AIDS-related neoplasms. Hematol Oncol Clin North Am 10: 997, 1996
100. Katz MH, Hessol NA, Buchbinder SP, et al: Temporal trends of opportunistic infections and malignancies in homosexual men with AIDS. J Infect Dis 170:198, 1994
101. Rutherford GW, Schwarcz SK, Lemp GF, et al: The epidemiology of AIDS-related Kaposi's sarcoma in San Francisco. J Infect Dis 159:569, 1989
102. Des Jarlais DC, Stoneburner R, Thomas P, et al: Declines in the proportion of Kaposi's sarcoma among cases of AIDS in multiple risk groups in New York City. Lancet 2:1024, 1987
103. Hermans P, Lundgren J, Sommereigns B, et al: Epidemiology of AIDS-related Kaposi's sarcoma in Europe over 10 years. AIDS 10:911, 1996
104. Schwartlander B, Horsburgh CR, Hamouda O, et al: Changes in the spectrum of AIDS-defining conditions and decrease in CD4+ lymphocyte counts at AIDS manifestation in Germany from 1986 to 1991. AIDS 6:413, 1992
105. Jacobson LP, Munoz A, Fox R, et al: Incidence of Kaposi's sarcoma in a cohort of homosexual men infected with the human immunodeficiency virus type 1. J Acquir Immune Defic Syndr 3(Suppl 1):S24, 1990
106. Lundgren JD, Melbye M, Pedersen C, et al: Changing patterns of Kaposi's sarcoma in Danish acquired immunodeficiency syndrome patients with complete follow-up: The Danish Study Group for HIV Infection (DASHI). Am J Epidemiol 141:652, 1995
107. Selik RM, Chu SY, Ward JW: Trends in infectious diseases and cancers among persons dying of HIV infection in the United States from 1987 to 1992. Ann Intern Med 123:933, 1995
108. Bacellar H, Munoz A, Hoover DR, et al: Incidence of clinical AIDS conditions in a cohort of homosexual men with CD4+ cell counts <100/mm³. J Infect Dis 170:1284, 1994
109. Jones JL, Hanson DL, Ward JW: Effect of antiretroviral therapy on recent trends in cancers among HIV-infected persons. In Abstracts of the 2nd Annual National AIDS Malignancy Conference, Bethesda, MD, 1998, Abstract S1
110. Jacobson LP: Impact of highly effective anti-retroviral therapy on the incidence of malignancies among HIV-infected individuals. In Abstracts of the 2nd Annual National AIDS Malignancy Conference, Bethesda, MD, 1998, Abstract S5
111. Jones JL, Hanson DL, Chu SY, et al: AIDS-associated Kaposi's sarcoma [letter]. Science 267:1078, 1995
112. Karon JM, Rosenberg PH, McQuillan G, et al: Prevalence of HIV infection in the United States, 1984 to 1992. JAMA 276:126, 1996
113. Brookmeyer R: Reconstruction and future trends of the AIDS epidemic in the United States. Science 253: 37, 1991
114. Rosenberg PS: Backcalculation models of age-specific HIV incidence rates. Stat Med 13:1975, 1994
115. Gwinn M, Pappaioanou M, George JR, et al: Prevalence of HIV infection in childbearing women in the United States. JAMA 265:1704, 1991
116. Davis SF, Byers RHJ, Lindegren ML, et al: Prevalence and incidence of vertically acquired HIV infection in the United States. JAMA 274:952, 1995
117. McQuillan GM, Khare M, Ezzati-Rice TM, et al: The seroepidemiology of human immunodeficiency virus in the United States household population: NHANES III, 1988–1991. J Acquir Immune Defic Syndr 7: 1195, 1994
118. Rosenberg PS: Scope of the AIDS epidemic in the United States. Science 270:1372, 1995
119. Dondero TJ, Pappaioanou M, Curran JW: Monitoring the levels and trends of HIV infection: The Public Health Service's HIV surveillance program. Public Health Rep 103:213, 1988
120. Pappaioanou M, Dondero TJ, Petersen LR, et al: The family of HIV seroprevalence surveys: Objectives, methods, and use of sentinel surveillance for HIV in the United States. Public Health Rep 105:113, 1990
121. McCray E, Onorato IM, for the Field Services Branch: Sentinal surveillance of human immunodeficiency virus infection in sexually transmitted disease clinics in the United States. Sex Transm Dis 19:235, 1992
122. Onorato IM, McCray E, Pappaioanou M, et al: HIV seroprevalence surveys in sexually transmitted disease clinics. Public Health Rep 105:119, 1990
123. Cannon RO, Schmid GP, Moore PS, Pappaioanou M: Human immunodeficiency virus (HIV) seroprevalence in persons attending STD clinics in the United States, 1985–1987. Sex Transm Dis 16:184, 1989
124. Allen DM, Onorato IM, Green TA, Forrester WR: Human immunodeficiency virus infection in intravenous drug users entering drug treatment, United States, 1988–89. Am J Public Health 82:541, 1992
125. Jones TS, Allen DM, Onorato IM, et al: HIV seroprevalence surveys in drug treatment centers. Public Health Rep 105:125, 1990
126. Prevots DR, Allen DM, Lehman JS, et al: Trends in HIV seroprevalence among injection drug users entering drug treatment centers, United States 1988–1993. Am J Epidemiol 143:733, 1996
127. Onorato IM, McCray E: Prevalence of human immunodeficiency virus infection among patients attending tuberculosis clinics in the United States. J Infect Dis 165:87, 1992
128. Wendell D, Onorato IM, McCray E, et al: Youth at risk: Sex, drugs, and human immunodeficiency virus. Am J Dis Child 146:76, 1992
129. Janssen RS, St. Louis ME, Satten G, et al: HIV infection among patients in U.S. acute-care hospitals:

Strategies for the counseling and testing of hospital patients. N Engl J Med 327:445, 1992

130. St. Louis ME, Rauch KJ, Petersen LR, et al: Seroprevalence rates of human immunodeficiency virus infection at sentinel hospitals in the United States. N Engl J Med 323:213, 1990

131. Gwinn M, Redus MA, Granade TC, et al: HIV-1 serologic test results for one million newborn dried blood specimens: Assay performance and implications for screening. J Acquir Immune Defic Syndr 5:505, 1992

132. Morse DL, Medvesky MG, Glebatis DM, Novick LF: Geographic distribution of newborn HIV seroprevalence in relation to four sociodemographic variables. Am J Public Health 81(Suppl):25, 1991

133. Novick LF, Berns D, Stricof R, et al: HIV seroprevalence in newborns in New York State. JAMA 261:1745, 1989

134. Novick LF, Glebatis DM, Stricof RL, et al: Newborn seroprevalence study: Methods and results. Am J Public Health 81(Suppl):15, 1991

135. Pappaioanou M, George JR, Hannon WH, et al: HIV seroprevalence surveys of childbearing women—objectives, methods, and uses of the data. Public Health Rep 105:147, 1990

136. Wasser SC, Gwinn M, Fleming P: Urban-nonurban distribution of HIV in childbearing women in the United States. J Acquir Immune Defic Syndr 6:1035, 1993

137. Weinstock HS, Sidhu J, Gwinn M, et al: Trends in HIV seroprevalence among persons attending sexually transmitted disease clinics in the United States, 1988–1992. J Acquir Immune Defic Syndr Hum Retrovirol 9:514, 1995

138. Valleroy LA, MacKeller D, Janssen R, Jacobs T: HIV and risk behavior prevalence among young men who have sex with men sampled in six urban counties in the U.S.A. In Abstracts of the 11th International AIDS Conference, Vancouver, 1997, Abstract Tu.C.2407

139. Dean L, Meyer I: HIV prevalence and sexual behavior in a cohort of New York City gay men (aged 18–24). J Acquir Immune Defic Syndr Hum Retrovirol 8:208, 1995

140. Silvestre AJ, Kingsley LA, Wehman P, et al: Changes in HIV rates and sexual behavior among homosexual men, 1984 to 1988/92. Am J Public Health 83:578, 1993

141. Lemp G, Hirozawa AM, Givertz D, et al: Seroprevalence of HIV and risk behaviors among young homosexual and bisexual men: The San Francisco/Berkeley Young Men's Survey. JAMA 272:449, 1994

142. Osmond DH, Page K, Wiley J, et al: HIV infection in homosexual and bisexual men 18 to 29 years of age: The San Francisco young men's study. Am J Public Health 84:1933, 1994

143. Rosenberg PS, Biggar RJ, Goedert JJ: Declining age at HIV infeciton in the United States. N Engl J Med 330:789, 1994

144. Centers for Disease Control and Prevention: National HIV Serosurveillance Summary: Results Through 1992, Vol 3. Atlanta, GA: Centers for Disease Control and Prevention, 1993

145. Centers for Disease Control and Prevention: National HIV Serosurveillance Summary: Update–1993, Vol 3. Atlanta, GA: Centers for Disease Control and Prevention, 1995

146. Nelson KE, Vlahov D, Cohn S, et al: Sexually transmitted diseases in a population of intravenous drug users: Association with seropositivity to the human

immunodeficiency virus (HIV). J Infect Dis 164:457, 1991

147. De Jarlais DC, Friedman SR, Novick DM, et al: HIV-1 infection among intravenous drug users in Manhattan, New York City, from 1977 through 1987. JAMA 261:1008, 1989

148. Diaz T, Chu SY, Byers RH, et al: The types of drugs used by HIV-infected injection drug users in a multistate surveillance project: Implications for intervention. Am J Public Health 84:1971, 1994

149. Koblin BA, McKlusker J, Lewis BF, et al: Racial/ethnic differences in HIV-1 seroprevalence and risky behaviors among intravenou drug users in a multisite study. Am J Epidemiol 132:837, 1990

150. Chaisson RE, Bacchetti P, Osmond D, et al: Cocaine use and HIV infection in intravenous drug users in San Francisco. JAMA 261:561, 1989

151. Kerndt PR, Weber M, Ford W, et al: HIV incidence among injection drug users enrolled in a Los Angeles methadone program [letter]. JAMA 273:1831, 1995

152. Des Jarlais DC, Hagan H, Friedman SR, et al: Maintaining low HIV seroprevalence in populations of injecting drug users. JAMA 274:1226, 1995

153. Davis SF, Steinberg S, Jean-Simon M, et al: HIV prevalence among U.S. childbearing women, 1989–1994. In Abstracts of the 11th International AIDS Conference, Vancouver, 1996, Abstract Mo.C.331

154. Lackritz EM, Satten GA, Aberle-Grasse J, et al: Estimated risk of transmission of the human immunodeficiency virus by screened blood in the United States. N Engl J Med 333:1721, 1995

155. Jacobs T, Kennedy M, Sullivan M, et al: Trends in HIV prevalence and risk behaviors among U.S. blood donors: A multicenter study. In Abstracts of the 125th American Public Health Association Conference, Indianapolis, 1997, Abstract 2223

156. Centers for Disease Control and Prevention: Prevalence of HIV-1 infection in civilian applicants for military service, October 1995–September 1997, Department of Defense: Selected tables prepared by the Division of HIV/AIDS Prevention. Atlanta, Centers for Disease Control and Prevention, 1997

157. St. Louis ME, Conway GA, Haymann CR, et al: Human immunodeficiency virus infection in disadvantaged adolescents. JAMA 266:2387, 1991

158. Valleroy LA, Mackellar DA, Karon JM, et al: HIV infection in disadvantaged out-of-school youth: prevalence for U.S. Job Corps entrants, 1990 through 1996. J Acquir Immune Defic Syndr Hum Retrovirol 19:67, 1998

159. Weinstock HS, Sweeney S, Steinberg S, Gwinn M: HIV seroincidence among persons attending sexually transmitted disease (STD) clinics in the United States. In Abstracts of the 11th International Conference on AIDS, Vancouver, 1996, Abstract Tu.C.2409

160. Warner DL, Weinstock HS, Sweeney SJ, Gwinn M: Continued risk behavior among patients receiving HIV testing in sexually transmitted disease (STD) clinics, 1988–1996. In Abstracts of the 125th Annual Meeting and Exposition of the American Public Health Association, Indianapolis, 1997, Abstract 1016

161. Simon P, Thometz E, Bunch G, et al: Risk factors for unprotected sex among men reported with AIDS in Los Angeles County: Implications for HIV prevention. In Abstracts of the 5th Conference on Retroviruses and Opportunistic Infections, Chicago, 1998, Abstract 14

162. De Vincenzi I, for the European Study Group on Heterosexual Transmission of HIV: A longitudinal study

of human immunodeficiency virus transmission by heterosexual partners. N Engl J Med 331:341, 1994

163. Diaz T, Chu SY: Crack cocaine use and sexual behavior among people with AIDS [letter]. JAMA 269:2845, 1993

164. Waters JK, Cheng YT: Toward comprehensive studies of HIV in intravenous drug users: Issues in treatment-based and street-based samples. In: Longitudinal Studies of HIV Infection in Intravenous Drug Users.

National Institute on Drug Abuse Research Monograph 109. Rockville, MD: U.S. Department of Health and Human Services, 1991

165. Des Jarlais DC, Marmor M, Paone D, et al: HIV incidence among injecting drug users in New York City syringe-exchange programs. Lancet 348:987, 1996

166. Janson RS, Satten GA, Stramer SL, et al: New testing strategy to detect early HIV-1 infection for use in incidence estimates and for clinical and prevention purposes. JAMA 280:42, 1998

2 | Molecular Insights into HIV-1 Infection and Pathogenesis

ROMAS GELEZIUNAS • WARNER C. GREENE

HIV-1 is now established as the primary cause of AIDS. The magnitude of the expanding global epidemic continues to be sobering. Worldwide, 16,000 new infections occur daily, including 1600 in children. More than 90% of these new HIV infections occur in developing countries, most commonly in young adults 15 to 25 years of age. Only 10% of these infected persons know that they harbor HIV. As a consequence of this epidemic, more than 9 million children have already been orphaned by HIV infection of their parents. This virus has now spread to all of the continents of the world. The epidemic is now focused principally in sub-Saharan Africa, the Indian subcontinent, and southeast Asia.[1]

HIV-1 is spread by sexual contact, by exposure to infected blood or blood products, and by perinatal transmission from mother to child.[2] Although the incidence of AIDS in the homosexual population has received great public attention, worldwide more than two thirds of the estimated 30 million cases of HIV-1 infection have been heterosexually acquired.

Infection with HIV-1 induces a progressive loss of CD4+ T cells. The decline of these critical lymphocytes squarely underlies the profound immunodeficiency that characterizes advanced AIDS.[3] CD4+ T cells serve as both essential regulators and effectors of the normal immune response. HIV-1 infects monocytes and macrophages as well, but its cytopathic effects in these cells are much less pronounced.[4,5] Infected monocytes may, in fact, serve as a cellular reservoir for HIV-1, allowing further dissemination of the pathogen to the brain and other organs of the body. The recent finding of high-level dynamic viral replication and a concomitant high level of cell replacement suggests that HIV-1 has a direct cytopathic effect on its host cells.[6–9] These findings also suggest that

earlier treatment of HIV-infected individuals may prevent irreversible damage to the immune system.

One in vitro mechanism of HIV-1 induced cytopathicity involves cell fusion and the formation of syncytia mediated by the gp41 Env protein.[10–12] This fusion process requires only the presence of the HIV-1 Env proteins on the surface of infected cells and thus may involve uninfected CD4+ cells that inadvertently come in contact with cells expressing these proteins.[13] Subsequent fusion of these cells leads to the formation of multinucleated giant cells that ultimately die.[14,15] Cells expressing low levels of CD4 receptors appear less susceptible to this form of cell death, a finding that may underlie the relative paucity of cytopathic effects produced by HIV-1 in monocytes and macrophages. Additionally, HIV may induce programmed cell death in its cellular targets as well as in bystander CD8+ T-lymphocytes through the concomitant action of viral envelope proteins able to bind the CXCR4 chemokine receptor and the type II INFα receptor.[16–21,21a] Nevertheless, despite considerable effort, the precise mechanism by which HIV induces CD4+ T cell death remains unresolved. It seems increasingly likely that this process is multifactorial. Recent findings suggest that HIV infection may also result in reduced production of T cells.[21b,21c,21d]

The rational design and development of drug therapies to control the virus in infected individuals and the preparation of an effective vaccine to prevent infection represent public health goals of the highest priority. Additionally, these therapies and interventions must be cost effective so that they can be readily introduced into developing countries where the virus is flourishing. Substantial progress in these areas will likely hinge on achieving a more complete understanding, in molecular and biochemical terms, of HIV-1 and the nature of its frequently cytopathic interplay with its cellular host. Only through such studies will new drug targets be identified and the correlates of protective immunity against HIV delineated. In the following sections, we review our current understanding of the molecular biology of HIV-1 infection and viral pathogenesis.

HIV-1 GENOMIC STRUCTURE

HIV-1 is a member of the Lentivirinae subfamily of retroviruses. Lentiviruses characteristically cause indolent infections notable for nervous system involvement, long periods of clinical latency, and weak humoral immune responses complicated by persistent viremia.[22] Other lentiviruses include the simian immunodeficiency virus (SIV), which causes an AIDS-like disease in Asian monkeys; the visna and maedi viruses, which cause severe demyelinating encephalomyelitis and interstitial pneumonia in sheep; the caprine arthritis-encephalitis virus; the equine infectious anemia virus; and the feline immunodeficiency virus.

One feature that distinguishes the lentiviruses from other retroviruses is the remarkable complexity of their viral genomes. Most replication-competent retroviruses contain only three genes, *gag*, *pol*, and *env*. The *gag* and *env* genes encode the inner core polypeptides and envelope proteins of the virus, respectively, whereas the *pol* gene gives rise to the viral reverse transcriptase, integrase, and protease activities (Fig. 2–1). HIV-1, however, contains within its 9-kilobase pair (kb) RNA genome not only these three essential genes but at least six additional genes (*vif, vpu, vpr, tat, rev,* and *nef*) (Fig. 2–1). The proviral DNA is flanked by long terminal repeats (LTRs), which are important for both transcriptional regulation and polyadenylation. It is the distinct but concerted actions of these additional genes that probably underlie the profound pathogenicity of HIV-1. From a therapeutic standpoint, this same genomic complexity may also be the Achilles heel of the virus should effective antagonists specific for these HIV-1 gene products be successfully isolated.

THE HIV-1 VIRION

High-resolution electron microscopy has shown that the HIV-1 virion contains an inner conical structure and 72 external spikes formed by the

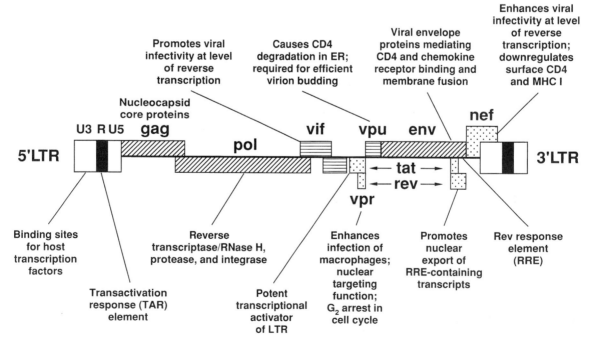

FIGURE 2–1. Genomic structure of HIV-1. The nine known genes of HIV-1 are shown, and their recognized primary functions are summarized. The 5′ and 3′ long terminal repeats (LTRs) containing regulatory sequences recognized by various host transcription factors are also depicted, and the positions of the Tat and Rev RNA response elements—transactivation response (TAR) element and Rev response element (RRE)—are indicated. ER, endoplasmic reticulum; MHC I, major histocompatibility complex class I.

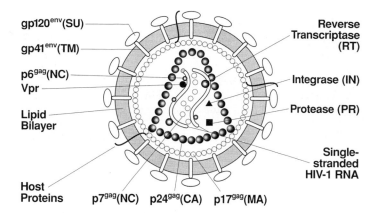

FIGURE 2–2. Schematic of the HIV-1 virion. Each of the virion proteins making up the envelope (gp120^{env} and gp41^{env}) and inner core (p24^{gag}, p17^{gag}, p7^{gag}, and p6^{gag}) is identified. In addition, the diploid RNA genome is shown associated with reverse transcriptase (RT), an RNA- and DNA-dependent DNA polymerase. Integrase (IN) and protease (PR) are also found in the mature HIV-1 virion. The auxiliary protein Vpr is incorporated into the HIV-1 virion through an interaction with the p6^{gag} protein, which comprises the carboxyl terminus of the p55^{gag} precursor protein. CA, capsid protein; MA, matrix protein; NC, nucleocapsid protein; SU, surface protein; TM, transmembrane protein.

two major viral envelope proteins, gp120 and gp41.[23] The HIV-1 lipid bilayer is also studded with a number of host proteins, including class I and class II major histocompatibility complex (MHC) antigens, acquired during virion budding. The viral core contains four proteins: the p24 capsid protein, the p17 matrix protein, and the p7 and p6 nucleocapsid proteins, each of which is proteolytically cleaved from a 55-kDa Gag precursor by the HIV-1 protease. The capsid protein forms the chief component of the inner shell of the virion (Fig. 2–2), whereas the myristylated matrix protein is associated with the inner surface of the lipid bilayer and probably stabilizes the exterior and interior components of the virion. The p7 nucleocapsid protein binds directly to the genomic RNA through a zinc-finger structural motif and, together with the p6 nucleocapsid, forms the retroviral core. Importantly, this retroviral core also contains two copies of the single-stranded HIV-1 genomic RNA that are associated with the various preformed viral enzymes, including reverse transcriptase, integrase, and protease (Fig. 2–2).

THE LIFE CYCLE OF HIV-1

Attachment of the HIV-1 Virion: Receptor Utilization

Infection with HIV-1 begins with the binding of virions to a specific combination of receptors displayed on host cells. CD4+ T lymphocytes and monocyte-derived macrophages are the major cellular targets for HIV-1 infection in vivo.[3]

HIV-1 specifically infects these cells because the CD4 membrane antigen present on each is a high-affinity cellular receptor[24,25] (Fig. 2–3). In fact, the HIV-1 surface envelope protein gp120 binds directly to CD4 with an affinity of approximately 4×10^{-9} M. However, soon after the discovery that CD4 was essential for HIV-1 entry, it became evident that this transmembrane receptor alone was not sufficient.[26] The recent identification of certain seven transmembrane G-protein–coupled chemokine receptors as cofactors for viral entry and fusion has led to a better understanding of the process of HIV entry and cellular tropism.[27–32]

Certain strains of HIV-1 preferentially infect macrophages, whereas others preferentially infect transformed CD4+ T-cell lines. Both types of viruses infect and replicate in activated primary CD4+ T cells. Viral tropism for particular cell types reflects the chemokine receptor utilized for viral entry.[27–32] HIV-1 strains that display tropism for transformed T-cell lines generally use the CXCR4 chemokine receptor.[32] Infection of such cells by these viruses can be blocked by the natural ligand of this receptor, stromal-derived factor 1.[33] Macrophage-tropic strains of HIV-1 generally use the CCR5 chemokine receptor.[27,29,31] Infection of macrophages by these viruses can be blocked by the β or CC chemokines RANTES, MIP-1α, and MIP-1β,[27,29,31,34] which form the physiologic ligands for CCR5. According to current nomenclature, HIV-1 strains that utilize CCR5 are termed R5 viruses and those that utilize CXCR4 are termed X4 viruses.[35,36] The failure of R5 viruses to infect transformed T-cell lines reflects the absence

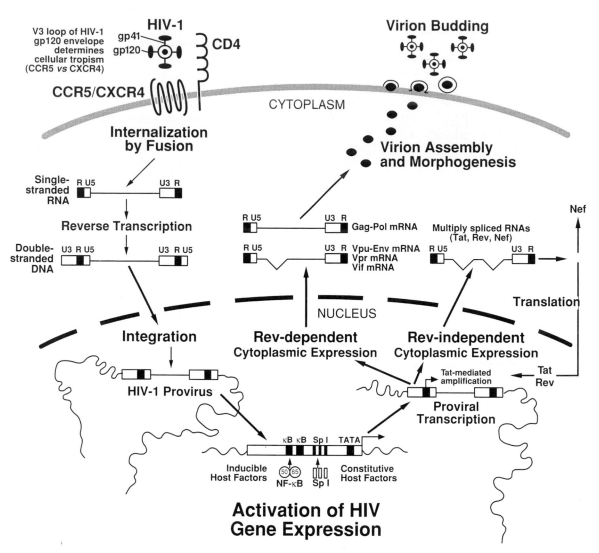

FIGURE 2–3. Life cycle of HIV-1. After the interaction of gp120 with CD4 and a chemokine receptor (CCR5 or CXCR4), gp41-mediated membrane fusion occurs, leading to the entry of HIV-1 into the cell. After uncoating, reverse transcription of viral RNA begins, resulting in the production of the double-stranded viral DNA. In turn, HIV-1 integrase promotes the insertion of this viral DNA duplex into the host genome, thereby giving rise to the HIV-1 provirus. The expression of HIV-1 genes is stimulated initially by the action of select inducible (NF-κB) and constitutive (Sp1) host transcription factors with cognate binding sites in the long terminal repeat. The action of these enhancer-binding proteins leads to the sequential production of various viral mRNAs. The first mRNAs produced correspond to the multiply spliced species of approximately 2 kb encoding the Tat, Rev, and Nef regulatory proteins. Tat shuttles back to the nucleus and strongly up-regulates the activity of the long terminal repeat. Subsequently, in the presence of Rev, the viral structural proteins are produced, allowing the assembly and morphogenesis of virions. The HIV-1 virions that are produced bud from the host cell and can then reinitiate the retroviral life cycle by infecting other CD4+ cells.

of CCR5 on the surfaces of these cells. However, it is less clear why X4 viruses cannot infect macrophages since these cells express small amounts of CXCR4 at their surface.[35,36] Perhaps complete infection in the macrophage requires an additional action of CCR5 beyond entry.

A particular subregion of the HIV-1 gp120 surface envelope protein, termed the V3 loop, appears to play a dominant role in determining viral tropism.[37–39] In fact, single amino acid changes within the V3 loop may completely alter the tropism of HIV-1 from CCR5 to CXCR4 and vice versa.[40] It remains unclear whether the V3 loop directly binds to a chemokine receptor.

Evidence indicates that R5 viruses are preferentially transmitted and are present in the early stages of infection. In contrast, isolates obtained later in the course of the disease, often at the time of significant CD4 decline and emergence of clinical symptoms, are of the X4 type.[41-44] Strikingly, cells from subjects who are homozygous for a 32-base pair deletion mutation in CCR5 are highly resistant to infection by R5 viruses.[45-47] Despite exposure to HIV-1, these subjects generally remain free of HIV-associated disease. These findings suggest that entry of HIV via CCR5 is essential for the establishment of early infection. The essential role of CCR5 in primary HIV transmission and its apparent dispensability for proper immunologic function further suggest that strategies aimed at blocking CCR5 function may help control HIV transmission.

Internalization of the HIV-1 Virion

After the HIV-1 virion attaches to the host cell, the viral envelope must fuse with the target cell to gain entry. Receptor-bound HIV-1 virions are internalized by pH-independent membrane fusion mediated by the gp41 Env protein (Fig. 2-3). This gp41 polypeptide contains a membrane-spanning region that anchors both envelope proteins (gp41 and gp120) in the lipid bilayer of the virion envelope and an amino-terminal fusogenic domain resembling the F proteins of the paramyxoviruses (e.g., mumps virus and parainfluenza virus). Conformational changes induced by the interaction of gp120 with CD4 and a chemokine receptor lead to the activation of the gp41 fusogenic domain, which enables the viral and host cell membranes to fuse.[48] Clinical trials of a potential fusion inhibitor (T-20 peptide) corresponding to a portion of gp41 are now underway.[148a]

Reverse Transcription and Integration

After internalization, the HIV-1 virion is partially uncoated in preparation for the replicative phase of its life cycle. Viral replication in a cytoplasmic particle retaining nucleocapsid proteins begins with the generation of a first-strand DNA copy of the viral RNA mediated by the HIV-1 encoded reverse transcriptase (Fig. 2-3). Second-strand DNA synthesis is also controlled by reverse transcriptase but proceeds only after its ribonuclease H activity partially degrades the original RNA template. After completion of a strand switch whereby reverse transcriptase jumps from one strand of the diploid RNA genome to the other, a double-stranded DNA replica of the original RNA genome is created that contains LTRs at each end of the DNA. This viral DNA duplex is then imported into the nucleus as part of the preintegration complex (PIC) (see below) and inserted into the host genome by the viral integrase, another enzymatic product of the *pol* gene (Fig. 2-3).

Considerable therapeutic attention has focused on the clinical use of dideoxynucleosides, agents that specifically inhibit the action of reverse transcriptase.[49,50] These compounds include 3'-azido-2',3'-dideoxythymidine (zidovudine), 2',3'-dideoxycytidine (zalcitabine), 2',3'-dideoxyinosine (didanosine), stavudine, and lamivudine.[51-59] Each of these agents must be phosphorylated to an active triphosphate form after entry into the cell, and each acts either as a chain terminator of the nascent DNA strand produced by reverse transcriptase or as a simple competitor blocking the incorporation of the respective normal deoxynucleoside 5'-triphosphate.[49] Reverse transcriptase appears to incorporate these dideoxynucleoside analogs preferentially, which probably explains their therapeutic effectiveness. Unfortunately, the error-prone nature of the HIV reverse transcriptase (at least one mutation per replication cycle) and the high level production of virus (up to 10 billion virions/day in untreated persons) lead to the generation of a swarm of HIV mutants. Certain mutants exhibit resistance to these nucleoside antagonists and rapidly become the preponderant strain in the viral population when a single drug is employed.[49,60-64] Because resistance to the antiviral agents is encoded at different amino acid sites in the reverse transcriptase, combinations of reverse transcriptase inhibitors are significantly more effective.[53] When specific inhibitors of the HIV-1 protease are used in conjunction with reverse transcriptase inhibitors, truly remarkable reductions in viral load have been observed.[65] These potent antiviral therapies have led to a lengthening of life and a significant improvement in the quality of life.[66] However, the mutability of HIV and problems with patient adherence with the complex antiretroviral regimens will almost certainly lead to the emergence of resistant viruses. Accordingly, the search for new antiviral therapies must continue, even though currently used drugs are still rather effective.

Nef and Vif in Proviral DNA Synthesis

Two of the auxiliary proteins encoded by HIV-1, Nef and Vif, enhance the reverse transcription process.[67-69] In SIV-infected adult rhesus macaques and in HIV-infected humans, defects in the *nef* gene lead to a markedly delayed time course for development of disease.[70-72] In tissue culture models, HIV production in the presence of Nef yields virions that have greater infectious potential.[73,74] Importantly, expression of Nef in target cells does not enhance the infectivity of incoming Nef-defective viruses.[75] However, Nef-defective proviruses are complemented by expression of Nef in the virus-producer cell to generate particles of comparable infectivity to those produced from proviruses carrying an intact Nef gene.[76,77] These findings strongly suggest that, although Nef is required during the efferent portion of the viral life cycle (the viral production and assembly phase), its effect is manifested during the afferent portion of the life cycle (binding to the target cell and establishment of a provirus). An intact proline-rich region, reminiscent of an SH3 ligand domain, located in the central conserved core of Nef is essential for Nef enhancement of HIV infectivity.[78-80] Viruses produced in the absence of Nef display a normal complement of virion proteins, including reverse transcriptase. Further, these Nef-deficient viruses bind to and enter target cells like Nef-positive viruses.[77] However, Nef-deficient HIV is defective in synthesizing proviral DNA.[67,76,81] Nef-associated serine phosphorylation of matrix protein in producer cells has also been observed.[82] Moreover, Nef associates with a serine kinase that shares certain properties with members of the p21-activated kinase family.[83-85] Binding of this kinase to Nef involves the proline-rich region in Nef; therefore, kinase binding appears to correlate with the production of viral particles displaying enhanced infectious potential.[80] This posttranslational modification of matrix may somehow lead to enhanced proviral DNA synthesis, permitting completion of the viral life cycle. However, the importance of Nef's proline-rich region for pathogenesis in SIV-infected macaques is still unclear.[86,87] A tyrosine kinase of the Src family, named Hck, also interacts with the proline-rich region of Nef via its SH3 domain.[79,88,89] This interaction appears to augment the enzymatic activity of Hck,[90,91] but the biologic relevance of this interaction to HIV replication or infectivity has not yet been es-

tablished. Other reports suggest that mitogen-activated protein kinase (MAPK) is incorporated into virions and phosphorylates matrix.[92,93] Modulation of the activity of MAPK has also been shown to affect HIV-1 infectivity.[93]

Vif-deficient HIV also replicates poorly in primary T-cells in vitro. This impairment appears attributable to diminished viral infectivity.[94,95] In contrast to Nef, which is generated from completely spliced genomic transcripts in a Rev-independent manner, Vif is synthesized from partially spliced mRNAs and accordingly requires Rev for expression (see below). Thus, Vif appears later in the infected cells than Nef, at a time when the various viral structural and enzymatic proteins are also expressed (see below). Like Nef, the presence of Vif is required during the efferent portion of the viral life cycle, but its effects are only observed during the afferent portion of the cycle. Again, like Nef-defective HIVs, Vif-deficient virions appear to bind and enter cells in the same fashion as wild-type virions, but may be impaired in their ability to complete proviral DNA synthesis.[68,69,96] Recent evidence suggests that Vif acts to counteract an intracellular antiviral activity that inhibits virus replication.[96a]

Karyophilic Properties of the HIV-1 PIC

Among retroviruses, lentiviruses are unique because they can infect terminally differentiated and nondividing cells, such as macrophages. Such cells can be infected successfully because the PICs of lentiviruses, unlike those of simple oncoretroviruses such as murine leukemia virus, are actively transported across the nuclear pore complex.[97,98] It is believed that at least three proteins of HIV that are found in the PIC exhibit karyophilic properties: Vpr, matrix, and integrase.[99-102] Vpr is a small auxiliary protein of HIV that is stoichiometrically packaged into virions with Gag through its interaction with the carboxyl-terminal p6 nucleocapsid protein component of Gag.[103] However, Vpr does not contain a classic nuclear localization sequence (NLS); instead, it appears to contain noncanonical NLSs that may utilize novel pathways of nuclear import.[103a] These signals may directly engage one or more of the nucleoporin proteins present in the nuclear pore complex.[104-107] Vpr enhances the replication rate of HIV in macrophages.[101] However, because Vpr-deficient viruses can replicate to a certain degree in non-dividing cells, it is believed that other constituents of the PIC possess NLSs that act in concert with Vpr. At its amino terminus, matrix was shown to contain an NLS that resembles the prototypical NLS of the simian virus 40 large T antigen.[99,108,109] Furthermore, phosphorylation of a tyrosine residue in the carboxyl terminus of matrix was required for it to associate with integrase, enabling matrix to associate with the PIC.[110,111] However, each of these observations has recently been challenged.[112–114] Finally, integrase was also shown to possess karyophilic properties and to be required for HIV replication in nondividing cells.[100] The contribution of each of these NLSs is likely central to successful nuclear uptake and integration of the viral PIC.

Viral Latency

Studies of plasma levels of HIV-1 in infected persons have suggested a dynamic pattern of HIV replication and CD4+ T-cell turnover during the period of clinical latency that follows primary infection and precedes the development of disease.[6–9] The initial immune response to primary infection reduces the level of circulating virus to a variable extent. Recent studies suggest that the magnitude of the viral load after the immune response (viral set point) predicts the time course of disease progression.[115] Sensitive measurements of viral RNA load after treatment with antiviral agents revealed that the plasma half-life of HIV was less than 6 hours.[8] In contrast, the half-life of productively infected T cells was calculated to be approximately 1 to 2 days.[8] Up to 10 billion new virions are produced daily, but the vast majority of these viral particles are noninfectious, presumably because of errors in reverse transcription or because of their inactivation by the host immune system. It is believed that most of this plasma virus emanates from recently infected CD4+ lymphocytes present in the peripheral lymphoid tissues, such as lymph nodes and spleen.[116,117]

After entry into the CD4+ cell, HIV-1 may establish a productive or latent form of infection.[118,119] With sensitive techniques of DNA and RNA amplification based on the polymerase chain reaction, it has been found that less than 1 in 1000 peripheral blood CD4+ T cells from patients with AIDS harbor stably integrated, replication-competent virus.[120] In contrast, approximately 1 in every 100 resting CD4+ T cells contains unintegrated HIV-1 DNA.[118,120] However, the fraction of HIV-1–infected lymphocytes was significantly higher in lymph nodes.[117]

Productive HIV replication generally results from infection of activated CD4+ lymphocytes. However, HIV infection can also lead to viral latency in vivo.[121–123] For instance, HIV cannot complete its life cycle in resting CD4+ lymphocytes because reverse transcription or nuclear import of the PIC is blocked.[119,124] If such cells are activated before decay of the PIC, a productive infection ensues. Another form of latency may result from the reversion of infected memory CD4+ lymphocytes to a resting state.[120,125] Because of their long life span, memory T-cells appear to form a long-lived latent reservoir in vivo. This cellular reservoir of latent virus has thwarted eradication of HIV with powerful combination therapies. Attempts are now underway to induce the virus in the 1 to 10 million cells that form this latent reservoir.

Activation of latently infected T cells by antigens, mitogens, select cytokines (tumor necrosis factor-α or interleukin-1), or various gene products of different viruses (human T-cell leukemia virus type I, herpes simplex virus, cytomegalovirus, and human herpesvirus type 6) creates a permissive cellular environment that promotes a high level of HIV-1 replication[126] (Fig. 2–4). Many of these activating agents induce the expression of select host transcription factors, notably members of the NF-κB/Rel family of enhancer-binding proteins.[127,128] These NF-κB/Rel factors, which normally regulate the expression of various T-cell genes involved in growth, including interleukin-2 and the alpha subunit of the interleukin-2 receptor, bind to and activate the two κB enhancer elements present in the U3 region of the proviral LTR.[129] It seems likely that the induced expression of NF-κB/Rel, which accompanies T-cell activation, may play an important part in the initial stimulation of latent or persistent proviral forms of HIV-1. Various constitutively expressed host transcription factors such as Sp1 also are required for HIV-1 transcription.

Early Expression of HIV-1 Regulatory Genes: Role of Tat as a Potent Transcriptional Activator of the HIV-1 LTR

The binding of inducible and constitutive host transcription factors to sites in the HIV-1 LTR stimulates a low but important level of expression of the HIV-1 genes (Fig. 2–4). Analyses of

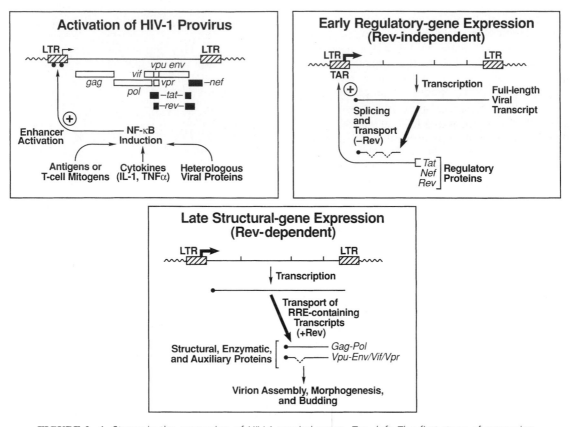

FIGURE 2–4. Stages in the expression of HIV-1 proviral genes. *Top, left,* The first stage of expression of the HIV-1 genes involves activation of the provirus by various T-cell mitogens, antigens, cytokines (tumor necrosis factor α [TNFα] or interleukin-1 [IL-1]), or other viral gene products. Among the many other transcriptional events, the NF-κB family of DNA-binding proteins is induced, binds to the HIV-1 enhancer in the long terminal repeat (LTR), and augments the expression of the HIV-1 genes. *Top, right,* The resultant low-level transcription of HIV-1 allows early synthesis of the products of the HIV-1 regulatory genes, including the Tat protein. Acting through the transactivation response (TAR) element, Tat potently amplifies viral gene expression, leading to a high level of expression of all sequences linked to the HIV-1 LTR. *Bottom,* The HIV-1 Rev protein then activates the expression of the HIV-1 structural, enzymatic, and certain auxiliary genes while simultaneously inhibiting the production of early regulatory proteins, which allows the assembly, morphogenesis, and budding of infectious virions. Rev is thus important in governing the transition from the expression of early regulatory genes to the expression of late genes. RRE, Rev response element.

one-step HIV-1 growth curves reveal that the initial population of genomic-length viral mRNA molecules reaches the cytoplasm exclusively as fully spliced, approximately 2-kb viral transcripts.[130] These viral mRNAs uniquely encode three regulatory proteins of HIV-1: Tat, Rev, and Nef (Fig. 2–4).

Tat is an 86-amino-acid nuclear protein that is essential for the replication of HIV-1.[131–133] By acting on the HIV LTR, Tat potently transactivates the expression of all viral genes.[131–133] Specifically, this viral regulatory protein functions by binding to an RNA stem-loop structure termed the transactivation response (TAR) element, located at the beginning of all HIV-1

mRNAs. The Tat protein appears to contain two important functional domains: a proline-rich, amino-terminal activation domain and a positively charged (arginine-rich) segment responsible for TAR RNA binding and nuclear localization. The preponderance of evidence suggests that Tat acts primarily at the level of transcriptional elongation by augmenting the processivity of the already bound RNA polymerase II complex,[134] giving rise to full-length HIV-1 transcripts. In the absence of Tat, short, truncated transcripts are formed as a result of a lack of polymerase processivity. Tat binds directly to a bulge region in the stem of the TAR element and recruits a cellular cofactor termed cyclin T, which in turn interacts with the loop of TAR and binds to the amino-terminal activation domain of Tat.[135] Importantly, cyclin T also binds to a kinase termed CDK9/PITALRE, which effectively phosphorylates the carboxyl terminus of RNA polymerase II.[135–139] This modification enables the polymerase to switch from a nonprocessive to a processive form. Thus, it appears that Tat recruits to nascent viral mRNAs a cellular factor that modifies the RNA pol II complex, making it more competent to complete the synthesis of the 9-kb genomic-length viral RNA (Fig. 2–5). HIV-1 Tat does not function well in rodent cells. However, this defect can be repaired by the introduction of human chromosome 12 into these cells.[140] Interestingly, the human cyclin T gene is encoded on chromosome 12, and its expression in rodent cells restores Tat function.[135]

Vpr also appears capable of mildly enhancing transcription from the HIV-1 LTR as well as from many other promoter elements.[141] Recent studies have demonstrated that Vpr expression leads to an arrest of cells in the G2 phase of the cell cycle.[142–146] It has been suggested that the transcriptional environment provided during G2 leads to augmented LTR activity, which is significant for virus production during the brief life span of the productively infected T lymphocyte.[147]

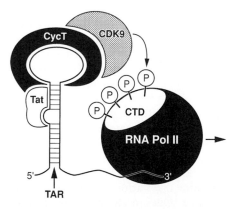

FIGURE 2–5. Mechanism of action of HIV-1 Tat. Tat directly interacts with a bulge in the stem of the transactivation response (TAR) element and recruits to the loop of TAR a cellular protein called cyclin T (CycT). CycT, in turn, associates with a cellular kinase termed CDK9, which phosphorylates the carboxyl-terminal domain (CTD) of RNA polymerase II. This post-translational modification to RNA polymerase II (RNA Pol II) renders it more processive. This strategy appears to ensure that the long (9-kb) genomic-length viral mRNAs are synthesized to completion.

Late Expression of HIV-1 Structural and Enzymatic Genes: Role of Rev as a Viral RNA Export Factor

The early phase of expression of HIV-1 genes is characterized by the cytoplasmic expression of the multiply spliced 2-kb class of viral mRNAs uniquely encoding the three HIV-1 regulatory proteins (Tat, Rev, and Nef) (Fig. 2–4). For the assembly of infectious HIV-1 virions, however, structural and enzymatic proteins must also be produced. The Gag and Pol proteins are translated from the full-length unspliced genomic mRNA, whereas Vpu and the envelope proteins as well as Vif and Vpr are generated from singly spliced subgenomic mRNAs. The transition from early to late gene product synthesis appears critically dependent on the HIV-1 Rev protein (Fig. 2–4). Rev is a 19-kDa nuclear phosphoprotein, that, like Tat, is essential for the replication of HIV-1.[131–133] The Rev protein appears to exert its regulatory activity at a post-transcriptional level by inhibiting viral RNA splicing and by activating cytoplasmic transport of the unspliced and singly spliced forms of HIV-1 RNA.[148,149,149a] In the absence of Rev, these incompletely spliced viral mRNAs remain sequestered in the nucleus, where they are either degraded or completely spliced.

Like Tat, Rev functions by binding to a highly structured RNA stem-loop structure, termed the Rev response element (RRE). This RNA motif is located in the *env* gene and, because of the pattern of HIV-1 splicing, is present only in mRNA species whose expression is regulated by Rev.[149–153] Mutational analyses have revealed that a positively charged, arginine-rich domain in the amino terminus of Rev mediates its direct binding to the RRE.[154] This arginine-rich segment also serves as a nuclear targeting signal. Rev contains a second leucine-rich domain that is uniquely required for its functional activity.[154] Mutations in this activation domain result in dominant-negative mutant proteins that not only lack Rev's intrinsic biologic activity but also block the action of wild-type Rev.[154] The potential use of such transdominant Rev mutants as a genetic therapy to attenuate HIV infection is now being evaluated in clinical trials.[154a] The leucine-rich domain forms a nuclear export signal that interacts with a cellular protein called Exportin 1/Crm1.[155–159] Exportin 1/Crm1 mediates nuclear export by directly associating with nucleoporins. This association of Rev with Exportin 1/Crm1 is dependent on the small GTPase Ran in its GTP-bound state. Thus

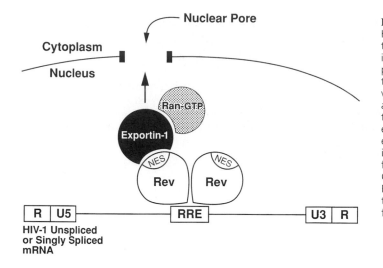

FIGURE 2–6. Mechanism of action of HIV-1 Rev. Multimers of Rev interact with the Rev-response element (RRE) situated in the *env* open reading frame. The RRE is present in unspliced genomic-length viral transcripts as well as in the singly spliced viral mRNAs that encode Vpu-Env, Vpr, and Vif. Splicing leads to the exclusion of the RRE from doubly spliced viral mRNAs encoding Tat, Rev, and Nef. The nuclear export signal (NES) in Rev mediates an interaction with the cellular nuclear export factor Exportin-1. In the presence of the GTP-bound form of the small G protein Ran, this RNA protein complex enables the export of RRE-containing viral mRNAs from the nucleus to the cytoplasm.

it appears that Rev recruits the cellular protein Exportin 1/Crm1 together with Ran GTP to the HIV RRE-containing RNAs that encode the late viral products (Fig. 2–6). This interaction promotes the export of these RNAs to the cytoplasm, allowing their translation and the assembly of infectious virions.

Morphogenesis of the HIV-1 Virion

The products of the HIV-1 *gag* and *pol* genes form the core of the mature HIV-1 virion, whereas the products of the *env* gene form the principal exterior coat proteins (Fig. 2–2). These coat proteins are synthesized as a gp160 precursor that is subsequently cleaved by a cellular protease (possibly furin) in the Golgi apparatus to yield gp120 and gp41. Although gp160 is extensively modified by glycosylation, these added sugars are not essential for subsequent CD4 ligation. Similarly, the HIV-1 Gag proteins are derived from a 55-kDa precursor protein that is specifically cleaved by the HIV-1–derived protease, yielding the p24 capsid, p17 matrix, and the p7 and p6 nucleocapsid Gag proteins (Fig. 2–2). Inhibiting the myristylation of the matrix protein appears to block the assembly of the HIV-1 virion and renders the virus noninfectious. As with the *rev* gene, dominant-negative mutants of the HIV-1 *gag* gene have been identified and shown to inhibit the replication of HIV-1 in tissue culture systems.[160]

The HIV-1 Pol polyprotein is translated from the same transcript as the Gag precursor by a ribosomal frameshifting mechanism with a −1 nucleotide change of frame.[161] In general, approximately 20-fold more Gag precursor protein than Pol precursor protein is produced, reflect-ing the relative inefficiency of this frameshifting process. Inhibition of this ribosomal frameshifting reaction would be an attractive approach to therapy, but agents with activity against mRNA pseudoknots have not been identified. Once translated, the Pol precursor is cleaved to produce several critical viral enzymes, including reverse transcriptase, integrase, and an aspartyl protease (Fig. 2–2). Both the reverse transcriptase and protease proteins have been crystallized, and data regarding their intrinsic three-dimensional structures have been collected and deciphered.[162–166] In the case of the HIV-1 protease, this structural information has permitted exciting progress in the rational development of specific active site inhibitors.[167,168] The combination of protease inhibitors with reverse transcriptase inhibitors has made HIV therapy radically more effective.[65] Logical next targets for drug development include the HIV integrase enzyme, the interaction between viral envelope and CCR5, and the viral regulatory proteins.

Assembly of infectious HIV virions proceeds in a stepwise manner, initially involving aggregation of the ribonucleoprotein cores beneath the plasma membrane. These retroviral cores are composed of the HIV-1 genomic RNA, Gag proteins, and the various enzymes encoded by the *pol* gene. Once assembled, these cores bud through the plasma membrane, where they acquire their lipid membranes, complete with the two protein products of the HIV-1 *env* gene, gp120 and gp41 (Fig. 2–3). Only after this final budding do the cleavage events mediated by HIV-1 protease occur, leading to maturation of the infectious viral particle. It is at this step that the protease inhibitors exert their antiviral effects.

Roles of Vpu and Nef in Enhancing the Formation of Infectious Particles

The Vpu protein of HIV-1 appears to exert an important function during the late stages of virion morphogenesis. Specifically, the Vpu protein promotes the efficient release of the budding virions from the surface of the cell.[169]

Along with two other gene products of HIV (gp160 and Nef), Vpu can down-regulate CD4.[170] Vpu binds to the cytoplasmic tail of CD4, which is sequestered in the endoplasmic reticulum by the viral envelope precursor gp160, targeting it for proteolysis via the ubiquitin-proteasome pathway.[171-173] Vpu produces CD4 degradation by connecting CD4 to a protein termed β-TrCP, which in turn interacts with Skp1p, a targeting factor for ubiquitin-mediated proteolysis.[174]

The HIV-1 Nef protein also down-regulates CD4, but it does so through a different mechanism. Nef appears to form a bridge between CD4 and the cellular adaptor protein complex AP-2, promoting accelerated endocytosis of CD4 through clathrin-coated pits[175-177] (Fig. 2–7). Nef via a dileucine motif present in its carboxyl terminus likely engages the μ2 chain of the AP-2 complex.[177,177a] A dileucine motif in the cytoplasmic tail of CD4 is also required for Nef-mediated internalization of CD4.[178] By acting together to down-regulate CD4 expression, Nef and Vpu may enhance viral particle infectivity

by reducing the trapping or shedding of virion-associated gp120 by CD4 during egress of viral particles from the infected cell. Nef also prevents the expression of cell-surface MHC class I antigens.[176,179,180] This function relies on an intact proline stretch within Nef that is also required for the generation of optimally infectious HIV particles.[179] This function of Nef may be mediated through an interaction with the Golgi-associated adaptor protein complex AP-1[176,177,179,180a] (Fig. 2–7). It is unclear if, or how, MHC class I down-regulation contributes to the morphogenesis of virions displaying greater infectious potential. Alternatively, Nef-associated MHC class I down-regulation may permit infected cells to partially evade lysis mediated by cytotoxic CD8+ T lymphocytes.[181]

SUMMARY

Although AIDS remains incurable, remarkable progress has been made in our overall understanding of this fatal immunodeficiency syndrome and its retroviral cause. The application of modern techniques of molecular and cellular biology has yielded new information about the structural, enzymatic, and regulatory genes of HIV-1 and its frequently lethal interplay with its cellular host. These studies have identified several promising points of attack to interdict the

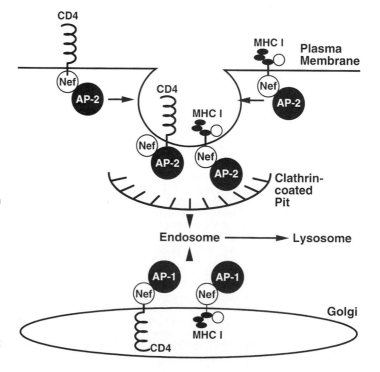

FIGURE 2–7. Mechanism of action of HIV-1 Nef. Nef appears to engage the cytoplasmic tail of CD4 and the clathrin adaptor protein 2 (AP-2). This interplay leads to the rapid endocytosis of cell-surface CD4 through the formation of clathrin-coated pits and the ensuing lysosomal degradation of CD4. Elimination of CD4 seems to represent an important objective in the life cycle of HIV-1. However, the purpose of CD4 down-regulation remains unclear, although diminished superinfection is one possibility. It is believed that the interaction between Nef and the adaptor protein 1 (AP-1) complex may also play a role in diminishing the expression of major histocompatibility complex class I (MHC I) antigens on the cell surface, thus blunting lysis mediated by CD8+ cytotoxic lymphocytes.

HIV-1 life cycle, including the attachment and internalization of the virion, reverse transcription, integration, viral transcription, viral RNA splicing and transport, and virion morphogenesis and budding. These insights have already led to successful combination therapies that allow people with AIDS to live longer, return to work, gain weight, and avoid opportunistic infections. However, this therapeutic advantage may be short lived unless new antiviral agents are developed that can halt the emergence of drug-resistant mutants of HIV. In addition, we must develop therapies that can be practically used in developing areas of the world, where the virus is spreading most rapidly. Finally, work continues on the development of an HIV vaccine to protect uninfected persons. Unfortunately, this work is proceeding slowly, in part because of the unique abilities of HIV to alter its genetic composition. In the final analysis, our greatest weapon against this virus will continue to be the prevention of its transmission.

Acknowledgments

We thank John Carroll and Neile Shea for preparation of the figures, Stephen Ordway and Gary Howard for editorial assistance, and Robin Givens for preparation of the manuscript.

References

1. World Health Organization/Joint United Nations Programme on HIV/AIDS: Global HIV/AIDS and STD Surveillance: Report on the Global HIV/AIDS Epidemic. Geneva, World Health Organization, 1998
2. Curran JW, Jaffe HW, Hardy AM, et al: Epidemiology of HIV infection and AIDS in the United States. Science 239:610, 1988
3. Fauci AS: Multifactorial nature of human immunodeficiency virus disease: Implications for therapy. Science 262:1011, 1993
4. Gartner S, Markovits P, Markovitz DM, et al: The role of mononuclear phagocytes in HTLV-III/LAV infection. Science 233:215, 1986
5. Ho DD, Rota TR, Hirsch MS: Infection of monocyte/macrophages by human T lympotropic virus type III. J Clin Invest 77:1712, 1986
6. Ho DD, Neumann AU, Perelson AS, et al: Rapid turnover of plasma virions and CD4 lymphocytes in HIV-1 infection. Nature 373:123, 1995
7. Perelson AS, Essunger P, Cao Y, et al: Decay characteristics of HIV-1-infected compartments during combination therapy. Nature 387:188, 1997
8. Perelson AS, Neumann AU, Markowitz M, et al: HIV-1 dynamics in vivo: Virion clearance rate, infected cell life-span, and viral generation time. Science 271:1582, 1996
9. Wei X, Ghosh SK, Taylor ME, et al: Viral dynamics in human immunodeficiency virus type 1 infection. Nature 373:117, 1995
10. Frankel SS, Wenig BM, Burke AP, et al: Replication of HIV-1 in dendritic cell-derived syncytia at the mucosal surface of the adenoid. Science 272:115, 1996
11. Lifson JD, Reyes GR, McGrath MS, et al: AIDS retrovirus induced cytopathology: Giant cell formation and involvement of CD4 antigen. Science 232:1123, 1986
12. Sodroski J, Goh WC, Rosen C, et al: Role of the HTLV-III/LAV envelope in syncytium formation and cytopathicity. Nature 322:470, 1986
13. Yoffe B, Lewis DE, Petrie BL, et al: Fusion as a mediator of cytolysis in mixtures of uninfected CD4+ lymphocytes and cells infected by human immunodeficiency virus. Proc Natl Acad Sci USA 84:1429, 1987
14. Maldarelli F, Sato H, Berthold E, et al: Rapid induction of apoptosis by cell-to-cell transmission of human immunodeficiency virus type 1. J Virol 69:6457, 1995
15. Sylwester A, Murphy S, Shutt D, Soll DR: HIV-induced T cell syncytia are self-perpetuating and the primary cause of T cell death in culture. J Immunol 158:3996, 1997
16. Ameisen JC, Capron A: Cell dysfunction and depletion in AIDS: The programmed cell death hypothesis. Immunol Today 12:102, 1991
17. Groux H, Torpier G, Monte D, et al: Activation-induced death by apoptosis in CD4+ T cells from human immunodeficiency virus-infected asymptomatic individuals. J Exp Med 175:331, 1992
18. Herbein G, Van LC, Lovett JL, Verdin E: Distinct mechanisms trigger apoptosis in human immunodeficiency virus type 1-infected and in uninfected bystander T lymphocytes. J Virol 72:660, 1998
19. Katsikis PD, Wunderlich ES, Smith CA, et al: Fas antigen stimulation induces marked apoptosis of T lymphocytes in human immunodeficiency virus-infected individuals. J Exp Med 181:2029, 1995
20. Meyaard L, Otto SA, Jonker RR, et al: Programmed death of T cells in HIV-1 infection. Science 257:217, 1992
21. Terai C, Kornbluth RS, Pauza CD, et al: Apoptosis as a mechanism of cell death in cultured T lymphoblasts acutely infected with HIV-1. J Clin Invest 87:1710, 1991
21a. Herbein G, Mahlknecht V, Batliwalla F, et al: Apoptosis of CD8+ T cells is mediated by macrophages through interaction of HIV gp120 with chemokine receptor CXCR4. Nature 395:189, 1998
21b. Hellerstein M, Hanley MB, Cesar D, Siler S, et al: Directly measured kinetics of circulating T lymphocytes in normal and HIV-1-infected humans. Nature Med 5:83, 1999
21c. Sachsenberg N, Perelson AS, Yerby S, Schockmel GA, et al: Turnover of CD4+ and CD8+ T lymphocytes in HIV-1 infection as measured by Ki67 antigen. J Exp Med 187:1295, 1998
21d. Fleury S, deBoer RJ, Rizzard GP, Wolthers KC, et al: Limited CD4+ T cell renewal in early HIV-1 infection: Effect of highly active antiviral therapy. Nature Med 4:794, 1998
22. Letvin NL: Animal models for AIDS. Immunol Today 11:322, 1990
23. Gelderblom HR, Hausmann EH, Ozel M, et al: Fine structure of human immunodeficiency virus (HIV) and immunolocalization of structural proteins. Virology 156:171, 1987

24. Dalgleish AG, Beverley PC, Clapham PR, et al: The CD4 (T4) antigen is an essential component of the receptor for the AIDS retrovirus. Nature 312:763, 1984

25. Klatzmann D, Champagne E, Chamaret S, et al: T-lymphocyte T4 molecule behaves as the receptor for human retrovirus LAV. Nature 312:767, 1984

26. Maddon PJ, Dalgleish AG, McDougal JS, et al: The T4 gene encodes the AIDS virus receptor and is expressed in the immune system and the brain. Cell 47:333, 1986

27. Alkhatib G, Combadiere C, Broder CC, et al: CC CKR5: A RANTES, MIP-1α, MIP-1β receptor as a fusion cofactor for macrophage-tropic HIV-1. Science 272:1955, 1996

28. Choe H, Farzan M, Sun Y, et al: The β-chemokine receptors CCR3 and CCR5 facilitate infection by primary HIV-1 isolates. Cell 85:1135, 1996

29. Deng H, Liu R, Ellmeier W, et al: Identification of a major co-receptor for primary isolates of HIV-1. Nature 381:661, 1996

30. Doranz BJ, Rucker J, Yi Y, et al: A dual-tropic primary HIV-1 isolate that uses fusin and the β-chemokine receptors CKR-5, CKR-3, and CKR-2b as fusion cofactors. Cell 85:1149, 1996

31. Dragic T, Litwin V, Allaway GP, et al: HIV-1 entry into CD4+ cells is mediated by the chemokine receptor CC-CKR-5. Nature 381:667, 1996

32. Feng Y, Broder CC, Kennedy PE, Berger EA: HIV-1 entry cofactor: Functional cDNA cloning of a seven-transmembrane, G protein-coupled receptor. Science 272:872, 1996

33. Bleul CC, Farzan M, Choe H, et al: The lymphocyte chemoattractant SDF-1 is a ligand for LESTR/fusin and blocks HIV-1 entry. Nature 382:829, 1996

34. Cocchi F, DeVico AL, Garzino-Demo A, et al: Identification of RANTES, MIP-1α, and MIP-1β as the major HIV-suppressive factors produced by CD8+ T cells. Science 270:1811, 1995

35. Cairns JS, D'Souza MP: Chemokines and HIV-1 second receptors: The therapeutic connection. Nature Med 4:563, 1998

36. Littman DR: Chemokine receptors: Keys to AIDS pathogenesis? Cell 93:677, 1998

37. Hwang SS, Boyle TJ, Lyerly HK, Cullen BR: Identification of the envelope V3 loop as the primary determinant of cell tropism in HIV-1. Science 253:71, 1991

38. O'Brien WA, Koyanagi Y, Namazie A, et al: HIV-1 tropism for mononuclear phagocytes can be determined by regions of gp120 outside the CD4-binding domain. Nature 348:69, 1990

39. Shioda T, Levy JA, Cheng MC: Macrophage and T cell-line tropisms of HIV-1 are determined by specific regions of the envelope gp120 gene. Nature 349:167, 1991

40. Speck RF, Wehrly K, Platt EJ, et al: Selective employment of chemokine receptors as human immunodeficiency virus type 1 coreceptors determined by individual amino acids within the envelope V3 loop. J Virol 71:713, 1997

41. Connor RI, Mohri H, Cao Y, Ho DD: Increased viral burden and cytopathicity correlate temporally with CD4+ T-lymphocyte decline and clinical progression in human immunodeficiency virus type 1-infected individuals. J Virol 67:1772, 1993

42. Schuitemaker H, Koot M, Kootstra NA, et al: Biological phenotype of human immunodeficiency virus type 1 clones at different stages of infection: progression of disease is associated with a shift from monocytotropic to T-cell-tropic virus population. J Virol 66:1354, 1992

43. Tersmette M, de GR, Al BJ, Winkel IN, et al: Differential syncytium-inducing capacity of human immunodeficiency virus isolates: frequent detection of syncytium-inducing isolates in patients with acquired immunodeficiency syndrome (AIDS) and AIDS-related complex. J Virol 62:2026, 1988

44. Zhu T, Mo H, Wang N, et al: Genotypic and phenotypic characterization of HIV-1 patients with primary infection. Science 261:1179, 1993

45. Dean M, Carrington M, Winkler C, et al: Genetic restriction of HIV-1 infection and progression to AIDS by a deletion allele of the CKR5 structural gene: Hemophilia Growth and Development Study, Multicenter AIDS Cohort Study, Multicenter Hemophilia Cohort Study, San Francisco City Cohort, ALIVE Study. Science 273:1856, 1996

46. Liu R, Paxton WA, Choe S, et al: Homozygous defect in HIV-1 coreceptor accounts for resistance of some multiply-exposed individuals to HIV-1 infection. Cell 86:367, 1996

47. Samson M, Libert F, Doranz BJ, et al: Resistance to HIV-1 infection in Caucasian individuals bearing mutant alleles of the CCR-5 chemokine receptor gene. Nature 382:722, 1996

48. Chan DC, Kim PS: HIV entry and its inhibition. Cell 93:681, 1998

48a. Kilby JM, Hopkins S, Venetta TM, et al: Potent suppression of HIV-1 replication in humans by T-20, a peptide inhibitor of gp41-mediated virus entry. Nature Med 4:1302, 1998

49. Arts EJ, Wainberg MA: Mechanisms of nucleoside analog antiviral activity and resistance during human immunodeficiency virus reverse transcription. Antimicrob Agents Chemother 40:527, 1996

50. Yarchoan R, Mitsuya H, Broder S: Immunologic issues in anti-retroviral therapy. Immunol Today 11:327, 1990

51. Coates JA, Cammack N, Jenkinson HJ, et al: The separated enantiomers of 2'-deoxy-3'-thiacytidine (BCH 189) both inhibit human immunodeficiency virus replication in vitro. Antimicrob Agents Chemother 36:202, 1992

52. Dahlberg JE, Mitsuya H, Blam SB, et al: Broad spectrum antiretroviral activity of 2',3'-dideoxynucleosides. Proc Natl Acad Sci USA 84:2469, 1987

53. Fischl MA, Stanley K, Collier AC, et al: Combination and monotherapy with zidovudine and zalcitabine in patients with advanced HIV disease: The NIAID AIDS Clinical Trials Group. Ann Intern Med 122:24, 1995

54. Hamamoto Y, Nakashima H, Matsui T, et al: Inhibitory effect of 2',3'-didehydro-2',3'-dideoxynucleosides on infectivity, cytopathic effects, and replication of human immunodeficiency virus. Antimicrob Agents Chemother 31:907, 1987

55. Kahn JO, Lagakos SW, Richman DD, et al: A controlled trial comparing continued zidovudine with didanosine in human immunodeficiency virus infection: The NIAID AIDS Clinical Trials Group. N Engl J Med 327:581, 1992

56. Kinloch-De Loes S, Hirschel BJ, Hoen B, et al: A controlled trial of zidovudine in primary human immunodeficiency virus infection. N Engl J Med 333:408, 1995

57. Mitsuya H, Weinhold KJ, Furman PA, et al: 3'-Azido-3'-deoxythymidine (BW A509U): An antiviral

agent that inhibits the infectivity and cytopathic effect of human T-lymphotropic virus type III/lymphadenopathy-associated virus in vitro. Proc Natl Acad Sci USA 82:7096, 1985

58. Soudeyns H, Yao XI, Gao Q, et al: Anti-human immunodeficiency virus type 1 activity and in vitro toxicity of 2'-deoxy-3'-thiacytidine (BCH-189), a novel heterocyclic nucleoside analog. Antimicrob Agents Chemother 35:1386, 1991

59. Volberding PA, Lagakos SW, Grimes JM, et al: A comparison of immediate with deferred zidovudine therapy for asymptomatic HIV-infected adults with CD4 cell counts of 500 or more per cubic millimeter: AIDS Clinical Trials Group. N Engl J Med 333:401, 1995

60. Emini EA, Graham DJ, Gotlib L, et al: HIV and multidrug resistance. Nature 364:679, 1993

61. Frost SD, McLean AR: Quasispecies dynamics and the emergence of drug resistance during zidovudine therapy of HIV infection. AIDS 8:323, 1994

62. Mitsuya H, Yarchoan R, Kageyama S, Broder S: Targeted therapy of human immunodeficiency virus-related disease. FASEB J 5:2369, 1991

63. Najera I, Holguin A, Quinones-Mateu ME, et al: Pol gene quasispecies of human immunodeficiency virus: Mutations associated with drug resistance in virus from patients undergoing no drug therapy. J Virol 69:23, 1995

64. St. Clair M, Martin JL, Tudor WG, et al: Resistance to ddI and sensitivity to AZT induced by a mutation in HIV-1 reverse transcriptase. Science 253:1557, 1991

65. Collier AC, Coombs RW, Schoenfeld DA, et al: Treatment of human immunodeficiency virus infection with saquinavir, zidovudine, and zalcitabine: AIDS Clinical Trials Group. N Engl J Med 334:1011, 1996

66. Palella FJ, Delaney KM, Moorman AC, et al: Declining morbidity and mortality among patients with advanced human immunodeficiency virus infection: HIV Outpatient Study Investigators. N Engl J Med 338:853, 1998

67. Chowers MY, Pandori MW, Spina CA, et al: The growth advantage conferred by HIV-1 *nef* is determined at the level of viral DNA formation and is independent of CD4 downregulation. Virology 212:451, 1995

68. Goncalves J, Korin Y, Zack J, Gabuzda D: Role of VIF in human immunodeficiency virus type 1 reverse transcription. J Virol 70:8701, 1996

69. Simon JH, Malim MH: The human immunodeficiency virus type 1 VIF protein modulates the postpenetration stability of viral nucleoprotein complexes. J Virol 70:5297, 1996

70. Deacon NJ, Tsykin A, Solomon A, et al: Genomic structure of an attenuated quasi species of HIV-1 from a blood transfusion donor and recipients. Science 270:988, 1995

71. Kestler HWD, Ringler DJ, Mori K, et al: Importance of the nef gene for maintenance of high virus loads and for development of AIDS. Cell 65:651, 1991

72. Kirchhoff F, Greenough TC, Brettler DB, et al: Absence of intact nef sequences in a long-term survivor with nonprogressive HIV-1 infection. N Engl J Med 332:228, 1995

73. Chowers MY, Spina CA, Kwoh TJ, et al: Optimal infectivity in vitro of HIV-1 requires an intact nef gene. J Virol 68:2906, 1994

74. Miller MD, Warmerdam MT, Gaston I, et al: The HIV-1 nef gene product: A positive factor for viral infection and replication in primary lymphocytes and macrophages. J Exp Med 179:101, 1994

75. Pandori MW, Fitch NJS, Craig HM, et al: Producer-cell modification of human immunodeficiency virus type 1: Nef is a virion protein. J Virol 70:4283, 1996

76. Aiken C, Trono D: Nef stimulates human immunodeficiency virus type 1 proviral DNA synthesis. J Virol 69:5048, 1995

77. Miller MD, Warmerdam MT, Page KA, et al: Expression of the human immunodeficiency virus type 1 (HIV-1) nef gene during HIV-1 production increases progeny particle infectivity independently of gp160 or viral entry. J Virol 69:570, 1995

78. Goldsmith MA, Warmerdam MT, Atchison RE, et al: Dissociation of the CD4 downregulation and viral infectivity enhancement functions of human immunodeficiency virus type 1 Nef. J Virol 69:4112, 1995

79. Saksela K, Cheng G, Baltimore D: Proline-rich (PxxP) motifs in HIV-1 Nef bind to SH3 domains of a subset of Src kinases and are required for the enhanced growth of Nef+ viruses but not for downregulation of CD4. EMBO J 14:484, 1995

80. Wiskerchen M, Cheng MC: HIV-1 Nef association with cellular serine kinase correlates with enhanced virion infectivity and efficient proviral DNA synthesis. Virology 224:292, 1996

81. Schwartz O, Marechal V, Danos O, Heard JM: Human immunodeficiency virus type 1 Nef increases the efficiency of reverse transcription in the infected cell. J Virol 69:93, 1995

82. Swingler S, Gallay P, Camaur D, et al: The Nef protein of human immunodeficiency virus type 1 enhances serine phosphorylation of the viral matrix. J Virol 71:4372, 1997

83. Lu X, Wu X, Plemenitas A, et al: CDC42 and Rac1 are implicated in the activation of the Nef-associated kinase and replication of HIV-1. Curr Biol 6:1677, 1996

84. Nunn MF, Marsh JW: Human immunodeficiency virus type 1 Nef associates with a member of the p21-activated kinase family. J Virol 70:6157, 1996

85. Sawai ET, Khan IH, Montbriand PM, et al: Activation of PAK by HIV and SIV Nef: Importance for AIDS in rhesus macaques. Curr Biol 6:1519, 1996

86. Khan IH, Sawai ET, Antonio E, et al: Role of the SH3-ligand domain of simian immunodeficiency virus Nef in interaction with Nef-associated kinase and simian AIDS in rhesus macaques. J Virol 72:5820, 1998

87. Lang SM, Iafrate AJ, Stahl HC, et al: Association of simian immunodeficiency virus Nef with cellular serine/threonine kinases is dispensable for the development of AIDS in rhesus macaques. Nature Med 3:860, 1997

88. Lee CH, Leung B, Lemmon MA, et al: A single amino acid in the SH3 domain of Hck determines its high affinity and specificity in binding to HIV-1 Nef protein. EMBO J 14:5006, 1995

89. Lee CH, Saksela K, Mirza UA, et al: Crystal structure of the conserved core of HIV-1 Nef complexed with a Src family SH3 domain. Cell 85:931, 1996

90. Briggs SD, Sharkey M, Stevenson M, Smithgall TE: SH3-mediated Hck tyrosine kinase activation and fibroblast transformation by the Nef protein of HIV-1. J Biol Chem 272:17899, 1997

91. Moarefi I, LaFevre BM, Sicheri F, et al: Activation of the Src-family tyrosine kinase Hck by SH3 domain displacement. Nature 385:650, 1997

92. Cartier C, Deckert M, Grangeasse C, et al: Association of ERK2 mitogen-activated protein kinase with

human immunodeficiency virus particles. J Virol 71: 4832, 1997

93. Jacque JM, Mann A, Enslen H, et al: Modulation of HIV-1 infectivity by MAPK, a virion-associated kinase. EMBO J 17:2607, 1998

94. Gabuzda DH, Lawrence K, Langhoff E, et al: Role of vif in replication of human immunodeficiency virus type 1 in CD4+ T lymphocytes. J Virol 66:6489, 1992

95. Gabuzda DH, Li H, Lawrence K, et al: Essential role of vif in establishing productive HIV-1 infection in peripheral blood T lymphocytes and monocyte/macrophages. J Acquir Immune Defic Syndr 7:908, 1994

96. von Schwedler U, Song J, Aiken C, Trono D: Vif is crucial for human immunodeficiency virus type 1 proviral DNA synthesis in infected cells. J Virol 67: 4945, 1993

96a. Simon JHM, Gaddis NC, Fouchier RAM, Moliar MH: Evidence for a newly discovered cellular anti-HIV-1 phenotype. Nature Med 4:1397, 1999

97. Bukrinsky MI, Sharova N, Dempsey MP, et al: Active nuclear import of human immunodeficiency virus type 1 preintegration complexes. Proc Natl Acad Sci USA 89:6580, 1992

98. Lewis P, Hensel M, Emerman M: Human immunodeficiency virus infection of cells arrested in the cell cycle. EMBO J 11:3053, 1992

99. Bukrinsky MI, Haggerty S, Dempsey MP, et al: A nuclear localization signal within HIV-1 matrix protein that governs infection of non-dividing cells. Nature 365:666, 1993

100. Gallay P, Hope T, Chin D, Trono D: HIV-1 infection of nondividing cells through the recognition of integrase by the importin/karyopherin pathway. Proc Natl Acad Sci USA 94:9825, 1997

101. Heinzinger NK, Bukinsky MI, Haggerty SA, et al: The Vpr protein of human immunodeficiency virus type 1 influences nuclear localization of viral nucleic acids in nondividing host cells. Proc Natl Acad Sci USA 91:7311, 1994

102. von Schwedler U, Kornbluth RS, Trono D: The nuclear localization signal of the matrix protein of human immunodeficiency virus type 1 allows the establishment of infection in macrophages and quiescent T lymphocytes. Proc Natl Acad Sci USA 91:6992, 1994

103. Paxton W, Connor RI, Landau NR: Incorporation of Vpr into HIV-1 virions: Requirements for the p6 region of Gag and mutational analysis. J Virol 67: 7229, 1993

103a. Jenkins Y, McEntee M, Weis K, Greene WC: Characterization of HIV-1 Vpr nuclear import. Analysis of signals and pathways. J Cell Biol 143:875, 1998

104. Fouchier RA, Meyer BE, Simon JH, et al: Interaction of the human immunodeficiency virus type 1 Vpr protein with the nuclear pore complex. J Virol 72: 6004, 1998

105. Popov S, Rexach M, Ratner L, et al: Viral protein R regulates docking of the HIV-1 preintegration complex to the nuclear pore complex. J Biol Chem 273: 13347, 1998

106. Popov S, Rexach M, Zybarth G, et al: Viral protein R regulates nuclear import of the HIV-1 pre-integration complex. EMBO J 17:909, 1998

107. Vodicka MA, Koepp DM, Silver PA, Emerman M: HIV-1 Vpr interacts with the nuclear transport pathway to promote macrophage infection. Genes Dev 12:175, 1998

108. Gallay P, Stitt V, Mundy C, et al: Role of the karyopherin pathway in human immunodeficiency virus type 1 nuclear import. J Virol 70:1027, 1996

109. Gulizia J, Dempsey MP, Sharova N, et al: Reduced nuclear import of human immunodeficiency virus type 1 preintegration complexes in the presence of a prototypic nuclear targeting signal. J Virol 68:2021, 1994

110. Gallay P, Swingler S, Aiken C, Trono D: HIV-1 infection of nondividing cells: C-terminal tyrosine phosphorylation of the viral matrix protein is a key regulator. Cell 80:379, 1995

111. Gallay P, Swingler S, Song J, et al: HIV nuclear import is governed by the phosphotyrosine-mediated binding of matrix to the core domain of integrase. Cell 83:569, 1995

112. Fouchier RA, Meyer BE, Simon JH, et al: HIV-1 infection of non-dividing cells: Evidence that the amino-terminal basic region of the viral matrix protein is important for Gag processing but not for post-entry nuclear import. EMBO J 16:4531, 1997

113. Freed EO, Englund G, Maldarelli F, Martin MA: Phosphorylation of residue 131 of HIV-1 matrix is not required for macrophage infection. Cell 88:171, 1997

114. Reil H, Bukovsky AA, Gelderblom HR, Gottlinger HG: Efficient HIV-1 replication can occur in the absence of the viral matrix protein. EMBO J 17:2699, 1998

115. Mellors JW, Kingsley LA, Rinaldo CRJ, et al: Quantitation of HIV-1 RNA in plasma predicts outcome after seroconversion. Ann Intern Med 122:573, 1995

116. Embretson J, Zupancic M, Ribas JL, et al: Massive covert infection of helper T lymphocytes and macrophages by HIV during the incubation period of AIDS. Nature 362:359, 1993

117. Pantaleo G, Graziosi C, Demarest JF, et al: HIV infection is active and progressive in lymphoid tissue during the clinically latent stage of disease. Nature 362:355, 1993

118. Bukrinsky MI, Stanwick TL, Dempsey MP, Stevenson M: Quiescent T lymphocytes as an inducible virus reservoir in HIV-1 infection. Science 254:423, 1991

119. Zack JA, Arrigo SJ, Weitsman SR, et al: HIV-1 entry into quiescent primary lymphocytes: Molecular analysis reveals a labile, latent viral structure. Cell 61: 213, 1990

120. Chun TW, Carruth L, Finzi D, et al: Quantification of latent tissue reservoirs and total body viral load in HIV-1 infection. Nature 387:183, 1997

121. Finzi D, Siliciano RF: Viral dynamics in HIV-1 infection. Cell 93:665, 1998

122. Garcia-Blanco MA, Cullen BR: Molecular basis of latency in pathogenic human viruses. Science 254: 815, 1991

123. McCune JM: Viral latency in HIV disease. Cell 82: 183, 1995

124. Stevenson M, Stanwick TL, Dempsey MP, Lamonica CA: HIV-1 replication is controlled at the level of T cell activation and proviral integration. EMBO J 9: 1551, 1990

125. Finzi D, Hermankova M, Pierson T, et al: Identification of a reservoir for HIV-1 in patients on highly active antiretroviral therapy. Science 278:1295, 1997

126. Greene WC: Regulation of HIV-1 gene expression. Annu Rev Immunol 8:453, 1990

127. Greene WC, Bohnlein E, Ballarc DW: HIV-1, HTLV-1 and normal T-cell growth: Transcriptional strategies and surprises. Immunol Today 10:272, 1989

128. Thanos D, Maniatis T: NF-kappa B: A lesson in family values. Cell 80:529, 1995

129. Nabel G, Baltimore D: An inducible transcription factor activates expression of human immunodeficiency virus in T cells. Nature 326:711, 1987

130. Kim SY, Byrn R, Groopman J, Baltimore D: Temporal aspects of DNA and RNA synthesis during human immunodeficiency virus infection: Evidence for differential gene expression. J Virol 63:3708, 1989

131. Cullen BR: Regulation of HIV-1 gene expression. FASEB J 5:2361, 1991

132. Cullen BR: Regulation of HIV gene expression. AIDS 9(Suppl A):S19, 1995

133. Cullen BR, Greene WC: Functions of the auxiliary gene products of the human immunodeficiency virus type 1. Virology 178:1, 1990

134. Kao SY, Calman AF, Luciw PA, Peterlin BM: Antitermination of transcription within the long terminal repeat of HIV-1 by tat gene product. Nature 330:489, 1987

135. Wei P, Garber ME, Fang SM, et al: A novel CDK9-associated C-type cyclin interacts directly with HIV-1 Tat and mediates its high-affinity, loop-specific binding to TAR RNA. Cell 92:451, 1998

136. Herrmann CH, Rice AP: Lentivirus Tat proteins specifically associate with a cellular protein kinase, TAK, that hyperphosphorylates the carboxyl-terminal domain of the large subunit of RNA polymerase II: Candidate for a Tat cofactor. J Virol 69:1612, 1995

137. Mancebo HS, Lee G, Flygare J, et al: P-TEFb kinase is required for HIV Tat transcriptional activation in vivo and in vitro. Genes Dev 11:2633, 1997

138. Yang X, Gold MO, Tang DN, et al: TAK, an HIV Tat-associated kinase, is a member of the cyclin-dependent family of protein kinases and is induced by activation of peripheral blood lymphocytes and differentiation of promonocytic cell lines. Proc Natl Acad Sci USA 94:12331, 1997

139. Zhu Y, Pe'ery T, Peng J, et al: Transcription elongation factor P-TEFb is required for HIV-1 tat transactivation in vitro. Genes Dev 11:2622, 1997

140. Alonso A, Derse D, Peterlin BM: Human chromosome 12 is required for optimal interactions between Tat and TAR of human immunodeficiency virus type 1 in rodent cells. J Virol 66:4617, 1992

141. Cohen EA, Terwilliger EF, Jalinoos Y, et al: Identification of HIV-1 vpr product and function. J Acquir Immune Defic Syndr 3:11, 1990

142. Bartz SR, Rogel ME, Emerman M: Human immunodeficiency virus type 1 cell cycle control: Vpr is cytostatic and mediates G2 accumulation by a mechanism which differs from DNA damage checkpoint control. J Virol 70:2324, 1996

143. He J, Choe S, Walker R, et al: Human immunodeficiency virus type 1 viral protein R (Vpr) arrests cells in the G2 phase of the cell cycle by inhibiting p34cdc2 activity. J Virol 69:6705, 1995

144. Jowett JB, Planelles V, Poon B, et al: The human immunodeficiency virus type 1 vpr gene arrests infected T cells in the G2 + M phase of the cell cycle. J Virol 69:6304, 1995

145. Re F, Braaten D, Franke EK, Luban J: Human immunodeficiency virus type 1 Vpr arrests the cell cycle in G2 by inhibiting the activation of p34cdc2-cyclin B. J Virol 69:6859, 1995

146. Rogel ME, Wu LI, Emerman M: The human immunodeficiency virus type 1 vpr gene prevents cell proliferation during chronic infection. J Virol 69:882, 1995

147. Goh WC, Rogel ME, Kinsey CM, et al: HIV-1 Vpr increases viral expression by manipulation of the cell cycle: A mechanism for selection of Vpr in vivo. Nature Med 4:65, 1998

148. Malim MH, Hauber J, Fenrick R, Cullen BR: Immunodeficiency virus rev trans-activator modulates the expression of the viral regulatory genes. Nature 335:181, 1988

149. Malim MH, Hauber J, Le SY, et al: The HIV-1 rev trans-activator acts through a structured target sequence to activate nuclear export of unspliced viral mRNA. Nature 338:254, 1989

149a. Powell DM, Amaral MC, Wu HY, et al: HIV-Rev-dependent binding of SF4 ASF to the Rev response element: Possible role in Rev-mediated inhibition of HIV RNA splicing. Proc Natl Acad Sci USA 94:973, 1997

150. Daly TJ, Cook KS, Gray GS, et al: Specific binding of HIV-1 recombinant Rev protein to the Rev-responsive element in vitro. Nature 342:816, 1989

151. Dayton ET, Powell DM, Dayton AI: Functional analysis of CAR, the target sequence for the Rev protein of HIV-1. Science 246:1625, 1989

152. Heaphy S, Dingwall C, Ernberg I, et al: HIV-1 regulator of virion expression (Rev) protein binds to an RNA stem-loop structure located within the Rev response element region. Cell 60:685, 1990

153. Zapp ML, Green MR: Sequence-specific RNA binding by the HIV-1 Rev protein. Nature 342:714, 1989

154. Malim MH, Bohnlein S, Hauber J, Cullen BR: Functional dissection of the HIV-1 Rev trans-activator—derivation of a trans-dominant repressor of Rev function. Cell 58:205, 1989

154a. Woffendin C, Rango V, Yang Z, et al: Expression of a protective gene—prolongs survival of T cells in human immunodeficiency virus-infected patients. Proc Natl Acad Sci USA 93:2889, 1996

155. Fischer U, Huber J, Boelens WC, et al: The HIV-1 Rev activation domain is a nuclear export signal that accesses an export pathway used by specific cellular RNAs. Cell 82:475, 1995

156. Fornerod M, Ohno M, Yoshida M, Mattaj IW: CRM1 is an export receptor for leucine-rich nuclear export signals. Cell 90:1051, 1997

157. Fukuda M, Asano S, Nakamura T, et al: CRM1 is responsible for intracellular transport mediated by the nuclear export signal. Nature 390:308, 1997

158. Neville M, Stutz F, Lee L, et al: The importin-beta family member Crm1p bridges the interaction between Rev and the nuclear pore complex during nuclear export. Curr Biol 7:767, 1997

159. Stade K, Ford CS, Guthrie C, Weis K: Exportin 1 (Crm1p) is an essential nuclear export factor. Cell 90:1041, 1997

160. Trono D, Feinberg MB, Baltimore D: HIV-1 Gag mutants can dominantly interfere with the replication of the wild-type virus. Cell 59:113, 1989

161. Jacks T, Power MD, Masiarz FR, et al: Characterization of ribosomal frameshifting in HIV-1 gag-pol expression. Nature 331:280, 1988

162. Jacobo MA, Ding J, Nanni RG, et al: Crystal structure of human immunodeficiency virus type 1 reverse transcriptase complexed with double-stranded DNA at 3.0 A resolution shows bent DNA. Proc Natl Acad Sci USA 90:6320, 1993

163. Kohlstaedt LA, Wang J, Friedman JM, et al: Crystal structure at 3.5 A resolution of HIV-1 reverse transcriptase complexed with an inhibitor. Science 256:1783, 1992

164. Lapatto R, Blundell T, Hemmings A, et al: X-ray analysis of HIV-1 proteinase at 2.7 A resolution confirms structural homology among retroviral enzymes. Nature 342:299, 1989

165. Smerdon SJ, Jager J, Wang J, et al: Structure of the binding site for nonnucleoside inhibitors of the reverse transcriptase of human immunodeficiency virus type 1. Proc Natl Acad Sci USA 91:3911, 1994

166. Wlodawer A, Miller M, Jaskolski M, et al: Conserved folding in retroviral proteases: Crystal structure of a synthetic HIV-1 protease. Science 245:616, 1989

167. McQuade TJ, Tomasselli AG, Liu L, et al: A synthetic HIV-1 protease inhibitor with antiviral activity arrests HIV-like particle maturation. Science 247:454, 1990

168. Meek TD, Lambert DM, Dreyer GB, et al: Inhibition of HIV-1 protease in infected T-lymphocytes by synthetic peptide analogues. Nature 343:90, 1990

169. Klimkait T, Strebel K, Hoggan MD, et al: The human immunodeficiency virus type 1-specific protein vpu is required for efficient virus maturation and release. J Virol 64:621, 1990

170. Chen BK, Gandhi RT, Baltimore D: CD4 down-modulation during infection of human T cells with human immunodeficiency virus type 1 involves independent activities of vpu, env, and nef. J Virol 70:6044, 1996

171. Bour S, Schubert U, Strebel K: The human immunodeficiency virus type 1 Vpu protein specifically binds to the cytoplasmic domain of CD4: Implications for the mechanism of degradation. J Virol 69:1510, 1995

172. Fujita K, Omura S, Silver J: Rapid degradation of CD4 in cells expressing human immunodeficiency virus type 1 Env and Vpu is blocked by proteasome inhibitors. J Gen Virol 78:619, 1997

173. Willey RL, Maldarelli F, Martin MA, Strebel K: Human immunodeficiency virus type 1 Vpu protein induces rapid degradation of CD4. J Virol 66:7193, 1992

174. Margottin F, Bour SP, Durand H, et al: A novel human WD protein, h-βTrCP, that interacts with HIV-1 Vpu connects CD4 to the ER degradation pathway through an F-box motif. Molec Cell 1:565, 1998

175. Greenberg ME, Bronson S, Lock M, et al: Co-localization of HIV-1 Nef with the AP-2 adaptor protein complex correlates with Nef-induced CD4 downregulation. EMBO J 16:6964, 1997

176. Le Gall S, Erdtmann L, Benichou S, et al: Nef interacts with the μ subunit of clathrin adaptor complexes and reveals a cryptic sorting signal in MHC I molecules. Immunity 8:483, 1998

177. Piguet V, Chen YL, Mangasarian A, et al: Mechanism of Nef-induced CD4 endocytosis: Nef connects CD4 with the μ chain of adaptor complexes. EMBO J 17:2472, 1998

177a. Greenberg M, DeTulleo L, Rapoport I, et al: A dileucine motif in HIV-1 Nef is essential for sorting into clathrin-coated pits and for downregulation of CD4. Curr Biol 8:1239, 1998

178. Aiken C, Konner J, Landau NR, et al: Nef induces CD4 endocytosis: Requirement for a critical dileucine motif in the membrane-proximal CD4 cytoplasmic domain. Cell 76:853, 1994

179. Greenberg ME, Iafrate AJ, Skowronski J: The SH3 domain-binding surface and an acidic motif in HIV-1 Nef regulate trafficking of class I MHC complexes. EMBO J 17:2777, 1998

180. Schwartz O, Marechal V, Le Gall S, et al: Endocytosis of major histocompatibility complex class I molecules is induced by the HIV-1 Nef protein. Nature Med 2:338, 1996

180a. Bresnahan PA, Yomemoto W, Ferrell S, et al: A dileucine motif in HIV-1 Nef acts as an internalization signal for CD4 downregulation and binds the AP-1 clathrin adaptor. Curr Biol 8:1235, 1998

181. Collins KL, Chen BK, Kalams SA, et al: HIV-1 Nef protein protects infected primary cells against killing by cytotoxic T lymphocytes. Nature 391:397, 1998

SECTION
II

Treatment of HIV Infection

3 Laboratory Testing for HIV-1

ROBERT M. GRANT • MICHAEL S. SAAG

When considering what is the optimum "AIDS test," AIDS testing must be placed into appropriate historical context. AIDS was first described as a syndrome, a collection of clinical features that were the result of a weakened immune system. It was not until the causative agent of AIDS, human immunodeficiency virus type 1 (HIV-1), was discovered in 1984 that "tests for AIDS" became available. However, because AIDS is a clinical syndrome, there is no such thing as a laboratory test for AIDS per se. Rather, all "AIDS tests" are designed to detect, either directly or indirectly, the presence of underlying HIV-1 infection.

The first test developed to detect HIV-1 infection was isolation of the virus through tissue culture. This was the technique used originally to establish HIV-1 as the causative agent of AIDS. Unfortunately, although sensitive for viral isolation, the tissue culture procedure is expensive, time consuming, and labor intensive. As a result, soon after the initial discovery of HIV-1, several tests were developed using protein products of the newly discovered virus to detect antibodies produced by the infected host. Through these newer techniques, the immunologic "footprints" (i.e., antibodies) to the viral infection are detected rather than the virus itself.

The two antibody tests used most commonly are the enzyme-linked immunosorbent assay (ELISA) and the Western blot. In addition to being less expensive, faster, and easier to perform than viral culture, the ELISA and the Western blot test do not require working with live virus and are therefore safer. Nonetheless, no test is perfect, and the HIV-1 antibody tests are limited by their reliance on the production of

antibody by the host and the absence of cross-reacting antibodies.

Over the last 5 to 6 years, several novel techniques have been developed that directly detect viral protein products or amplify minute fragments of viral RNA and DNA to avoid the pitfalls of antibody testing and the dangers and expense of live virus culture.[1,2] Yet these tests have their own limitations, not the least of which is the interpretation of the results by the clinician ordering the test.

The best way to minimize errors in interpretation of laboratory findings is to understand the methodology of the test, the advantages and limitations of the testing technology, and the application of the test in the context of what is known about the epidemiology and pathogenesis of the underlying disease. This chapter reviews the methodologies of currently available tests for HIV-1, examines their appropriate use and limitations, and discusses the role of each test in the context of diagnosis and as measurements of response to antiretroviral therapy.

METHODOLOGIES

HIV-1 tests can be divided into several groups: virus culture techniques, antibody detection tests, antigen detection tests, viral genome amplification tests, drug resistance assays, and immune function tests.

Virus Culture Techniques

Peripheral Blood Mononuclear Cell Co-culture for HIV-1 Isolation

This technique was used initially to establish HIV-1 as the causative agent of AIDS.[3,4] Viable peripheral blood mononuclear cells (PBMCs) from HIV-1−infected patients are obtained via

This work was supported in part by the University of Alabama at Birmingham General Clinical Research Center (RR00032), the University of Alabama at Birmingham AIDS Center (AI27767), the University of California, San Francisco Center for AIDS Research (MH59037), and the J. David Gladstone Institutes.

centrifugation of anticoagulated whole blood (collected in either acid citrate dextran [ACD] tubes or syringes containing preservative-free heparin) over Ficoll-Hypaque lymphocyte separation medium. Infected PBMCs then are co-cultured with PBMCs derived from an uninfected human donor that have been stimulated previously for 24 to 48 hours with phytohemagglutinin (PHA). Growth of the cells in tissue culture is supported by a special medium (RPMI-1640) that has been supplemented with L-glutamine, fetal bovine serum, gentamicin, and interleukin-2 (to stimulate expression of CD4 receptors for enhanced viral replication and proliferation of lymphocytes). The cultures are observed for evidence of syncytium formation (i.e., multinucleated giant cell formation) as a sign of viral infection in vitro, and for the presence of either HIV-1 reverse transcriptase (RT) activity or HIV-1 p24 antigen production in the culture supernatant. Cultures are declared "positive" when at least two consecutive assays detect the presence of RT or p24 antigen in increasing magnitude above a predetermined cutoff value. When performed properly, HIV-1 isolation by PBMC co-culture is positive in 95% to 99% of HIV-1–infected patients.[1,2]

Quantitative Cell Culture

Quantitative cell culture is a technique that measures the relative amount of viral load within cells. The cell culture technique is the same as described previously. However, in addition to co-cultivating 10^6 patient cells with 10^6 donor cells, serial dilutions of patient cells are also set in culture in decreasing amounts (e.g., 10^6, 10^5, 10^4, 10^3) with 10^6 donor cells[5] (Fig. 3–1A). In this way fewer patient cells are introduced into the co-culture system, thereby allowing measurement of relative viral burden. The last positive culture with the fewest number of patient cells represents the endpoint. The reciprocal of the endpoint dilution indicates the relative number of infected cells in the patient. For example, if the last positive titer is 1×10^4 (10,000), the relative burden signifies 1 of every 10,000 patient cells is infected. If the endpoint titer is 1×10^3 (1000), approximately 1 of 1000 cells is infected. This procedure can be improved further by using serial dilutions on a 1:3 basis rather than a 1:10 basis.

Quantitative Plasma Culture

Another means of measuring viral load is through the measurement of free infectious virus in the plasma.[5–8] This is accomplished through quantitative plasma culture techniques (Fig. 3–1B). Serial dilutions of plasma are prepared by mixing 0.6 ml of plasma with 2.4 ml of culture medium consisting of RPMI-1640, supplemented with L-glutamine, gentamicin, fetal bovine serum, and interleukin-2. One milliliter of each of the dilutions is added to 2×10^6 PHA-stimulated PBMCs from an uninfected donor in a microtiter, 96-well tissue culture plate. Culture supernatants are monitored for viral replication at days 7 and 14 after cultivation by an HIV-1 p24 antigen test. The endpoint dilution is defined as the smallest volume of plasma that yields a positive culture result. The reciprocal of the smallest volume of plasma indicates the titer expressed as the tissue culture infectious dose per milliliter of plasma. As shown in Fig. 3–1B, a positive dilution of 1:3125 implies that there are more than 3000 free infectious virions per milliliter of plasma in that patient. To ensure accuracy, these tests usually are performed in duplicate and, under special circumstances, in quadruplicate.

Ultrasensitive Cell Culture

The advent of antiretroviral therapy that suppresses plasma viral RNA below detectable limits prompted a search for tissue reservoirs that could provide sanctuary for HIV-1. One such reservoir was found in resting memory CD4+ T lymphocytes that were found to be persistently infected with HIV-1 that could be induced to replicate under optimal circumstances in the laboratory.[9–11] These optimal culture conditions increased the sensitivity of the standard methods, thereby allowing HIV-1 to be cultured from nearly 100% of subjects with suppressed plasma HIV-1 RNA, even those with fewer than 20 HIV-1 RNA copies/ml of plasma and those who had been treated for as long as 30 months. Several variations of the ultrasensitive culture methods were used, but all involved depletion of CD8+ T lymphocytes from the subject's blood cells and from the uninfected donor cells used in the culture. These CD8+ cells could suppress HIV-1 growth in the culture by killing CD4+ cells that HIV-1 uses for replication or by secreting chemokines that may compete with HIV-1 for entry through chemokine receptors. In addition, ultrasensitive cultures used potent and relatively natural techniques for stimulating lymphocytes from the subject, including anti-CD3 and anti-CD28 antibodies or irradiated cells from allogeneic donors. These ultrasensitive cultures can be performed qualitatively us-

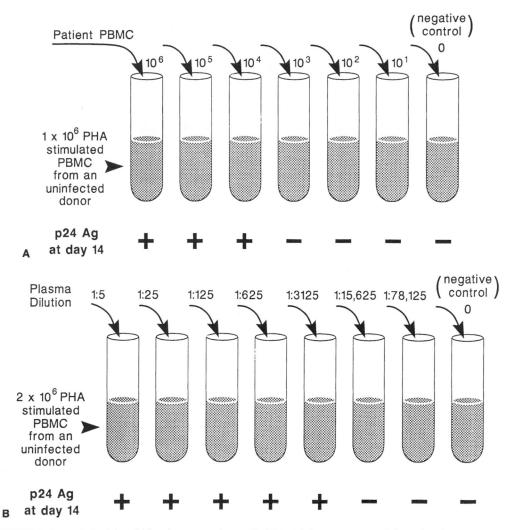

FIGURE 3–1. *A*, Peripheral blood mononuclear cells (PBMCs) from an HIV-1–infected patient are added in 10-fold serial dilutions to a standard amount (e.g., 1×10^6) of phytohemagglutin (PHA)-stimulated PBMCs from an uninfected donor. The lowest dilution yielding a positive result, as determined by p24 antigen (p24 Ag) positivity in the culture supernatant, represents the endpoint. In this example, the endpoint dilution is 1×10^4 cells/mm³. *B*, Serial fivefold dilutions of plasma from an HIV-1–infected patient are co-cultivated with a standard amount (e.g., 2×10^6) of PBMCs from an uninfected donor. As in the quantitative cell dilution assay, the least amount of plasma required to yield a positive culture result represents the endpoint. In this example, the endpoint titer is 1:3125.

ing at least 2 million cells enriched for CD4+ cells, or quantitatively using a dilution series of cells.

The clinical utility of these ultrasensitive cultures remains uncertain. The assay modifications required to achieve nearly 100% positive results in subjects with suppressed plasma viremia involve expensive supplies and technical sophistication, thereby restricting the availability of these assays to research laboratories. Furthermore, these methods have not performed reproducibly in a wide range of laboratories that do have the necessary resources. From a basic

biologic perspective, it remains unclear whether the persistance of replication-competent HIV-1 after suppression of plasma viral RNA represents ongoing low-level viral replication or the long-term survival of cells that were infected prior to starting therapy and remain latently infected. Finally, although it is reasonable to expect that persisting reservoirs of replication-competent HIV-1 could re-ignite viral replication even after long periods of suppression, available information is inadequate to assess the clinical importance of the results of ultrasensitive viral cultures.

HIV Antibody Tests

Standard ELISA

The technology to perform the ELISA was available before the discovery of HIV in 1983 and 1984. This technology was applied rapidly for use as an HIV-1 diagnostic test and was in widespread use by the summer of 1985.[12] As shown in Figure 3–2, this test uses HIV antigens (proteins) produced in a tissue culture system or through recombinant molecular technology. After the virus has been grown to high titers, the cell culture is lysed. The soluble antigens are then coated onto the wells of a microtiter plate. The test is initiated by adding patient serum to the antigen-coated wells. Anti–HIV–1-specific antibody present in the patient's serum will bind very tightly and specifically with the HIV-1 antigens in the plate. After a washing procedure to remove unbound materials, the specific anti–HIV-1 antibodies that have bound to the coated antigen are detected through the addition of a goat anti-human antibody that binds very tightly and specifically to any anti–HIV-1 human antibody bound to HIV-1 antigens on the plate. The goat anti-human antibody has been conjugated to an enzyme that specifically cleaves a colorless substrate into a product with color (usually yellow). After a washing proce-

dure, the substrate for the enzyme is added. The amount of color present in the well is proportional to the amount of conjugated enzyme bound to the human antibody present. By spectrophotometrically measuring the optical density in the sample well versus that in the negative control well, the amount of HIV-1 antibody can be determined quantitatively.

Through examination of large panels of known HIV-positive sera and comparison of their optical densities with those of known seronegative controls, a cutoff optical density measurement can be determined that distinguishes between a positive and negative result. To make the test more sensitive, the optical density cutoff is established at a lower value. Conversely, to improve specificity, the cutoff can be established at a higher value.

Western Blot Test

The Western blot test is also designed to detect the presence of anti–HIV-1 antibodies. However, in addition to identifying the presence of such antibodies, the Western blot test allows determination of the specific antigen against which the antibody is directed. As shown in Figure 3–3A, HIV-1 antigens are prepared from a lysate of HIV-1–infected cells and are separated

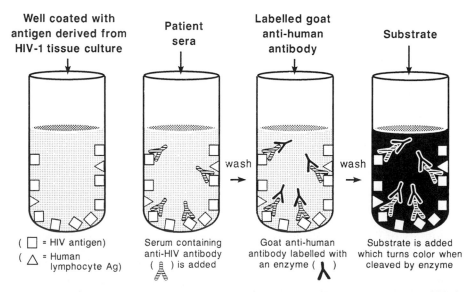

FIGURE 3–2. In the HIV-1 enzyme-linked immunosorbent assay (ELISA), patient serum is added to a microwell plate that has been coated with antigens derived from an HIV-1 tissue culture lysate. Bound anti-HIV antibody from the infected patient is detected via a goat anti-human antibody that has been labeled with an enzyme designed to react with a specific substrate. The cleaved substrate product yields a color that can be measured photometrically. Because the HIV-1 antigens are derived from tissue culture, some human lymphocyte antigens (Ag) may also be present in the well, potentially yielding a false-positive test result (see text for details).

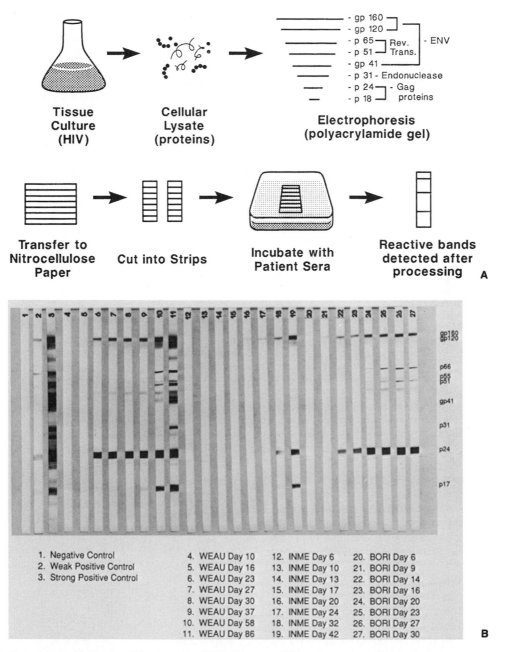

FIGURE 3–3. *A*, Western blot test is performed by separating tissue culture–derived HIV-1 proteins (p) and glycoproteins (gp) via polyacrylamide gel electrophoresis, transferring (blotting) the separated proteins onto nitrocellulose paper, incubating the cut strips of nitrocellulose paper with patient serum, and detecting anti-HIV antibodies that have bound to the HIV-1–associated proteins at the precise point at which they migrated in the gel. Through this procedure, the antibody reactivity against specific antigens can be determined (e.g., anti-Gag, anti-Env, or anti-endonuclease antibodies). *B*, Examples of Western blot tests from three patients (WEAU, BORI, and INME) identified at the time of acute HIV-1 infection (seroconversion). Each lane represents a time point (in days) from the time of presentation with symptomatic acute HIV-1 disease or a positive or negative control (lanes 1 to 3).

electrophoretically in a polyacrylamide gel. The electrophoretic procedure separates the antigens according to their size: the larger fragments remain toward the top of the gel and the smaller fragments migrate further down the gel, thereby creating a gradient of antigen by size within the gel. The proteins within the gel are then transferred (blotted) onto nitrocellulose filter paper, which holds the antigens in place for further testing. The nitrocellulose filter is cut into strips that can be incubated with the patient's serum. Anti–HIV-1 antibodies present in this serum bind tightly and specifically to the antigens on the nitrocellulose paper at the point where the antigens migrated. The anti–HIV-1 antibodies can then be detected by goat anti-human antibody, which is conjugated to either an enzyme or a radioactive probe. Once processed, bands appear at the location where the antibody has bound to antigen. Through the use of reference bands produced as a positive control, the reactivity of the antibodies against specific antigens can be determined (Fig. 3–3B).

The precise criteria for what constitutes a positive Western blot test remain controversial.[13-16] In general, positive bands from two of the three major antigen groups, the Gag, Pol, and Env regions of the virus, are required for a positive test. The Gag proteins consist of p55, p24, and p18 proteins (p stands for protein), the Pol region codes for RT (p66 and p51) and an endonuclease (p31), and the Env region codes for the envelope glycoprotein gp160 (the precursor product) and its two major subunits, gp120 and gp41 (gp stands for glycoprotein). Most laboratories use the criteria developed by the Centers for Disease Control and Prevention and the Association of State, Territorial, and Public Health Laboratory Directors (CDC/ASTPHLD) as the most appropriate for judging results of the Western blot tests.[12,14] The CDC/ASTPHLD criteria require the presence of at least two of the following bands—p24, gp41, or gp160/120—for a positive result, the presence of no bands for a negative result, and the presence of any HIV-1–related (or non–HIV-1–related) band(s) not meeting the criteria for a positive result as an indeterminate result.[16]

Radioimmunoprecipitation Assay

The radioimmunoprecipitation assay (RIPA) is a more time-consuming and labor-intensive test than the Western blot, yet it provides much finer resolution of the high-molecular-weight envelope proteins than the Western blot test.[17] The RIPA requires ongoing cell culture of HIV-1 to provide the appropriate substrate for the assay. HIV-1 replication in lymphocytic cell lines occurs in the presence of radiolabeled amino acids (e.g., ^{35}S-methionine or ^{35}S-cysteine). The radiolabeled amino acids are incorporated into viral proteins during viral replication. A cell lysate is prepared via homogenization of infected cells, and the lysate is then incubated in the presence of patient serum. Anti–HIV-1 antibodies present in the serum react with the radiolabeled antigens and form immune complexes. These complexes are removed by incubating the reaction mixture with protein A–coated Sepharose beads, which bind the Fc portion of immunoglobulin molecules. The beads are separated from the reaction mixture through centrifugation, and the antibody–antigen complexes are eluted from the separated beads by adding a detergent and heating. The immunoprecipitants are then run through an electrophoretic gel, which separates them according to their molecular weight (as in the Western blot procedure). An audioradiograph of the gel yields a banding pattern very similar to that of the Western blot test.

The RIPA is considered more sensitive and specific than the Western blot test.[17-20] However, the time, expense, and need for active cell lines and radioactive materials make the RIPA a poor choice for routine testing in commercial laboratories. Rather, its use is best reserved for difficult-to-diagnose cases.

Indirect Immunofluorescence Assay

Like the RIPA, the indirect immunofluorescence assay (IFA) requires preparation of HIV-1 antigens that are expressed on infected cells and are stained subsequently.[1] Infected cells are placed on glass slides in a fixed monolayer and are incubated with patient serum. Anti–HIV-1 antibodies present within the serum bind to antigens expressed on the surface of cells, and these bound antibodies are then detected with anti-human antibody that has been labeled with fluorescein isothiocyanate (FITC), an ultraviolet-activated dye compound. After appropriate processing, the slide is viewed under a fluorescent microscope, and the number of cells, the intensity of staining, and the staining pattern are assessed. IFA can detect the earliest serologic response against the virus (immunoglobulin M [IgM] antibodies) during acute infection.[21] However, the time, expense, and expertise required for the IFA procedure make its routine use in a commercial laboratory impractical.

Other Anti–HIV-1 Antibody Tests

Important modifications of the standard anti-HIV ELISA have increased the sensitivity, specificity, and convenience of HIV-1 antibody testing. Increased sensitivity has been achieved in the third-generation, double antigen-capture ELISA tests, which are based on using labeled HIV-1 antigen to detect binding of patient antibodies to beads also covered by HIV-1 antigens. In this way, these assays detect antibodies of all classes, including IgM antibodies that arise early after infection. These assays are more sensitive, thereby allowing detection of HIV-1 seroconversion earlier after HIV-1 infection.

Assay modifications that intentionally make the ELISA anti-HIV antibody assay less sensitive were evaluated to allow detection of subjects who recently seroconverted.[22] The less sensitive ELISA assay, or "detuned ELISA," involves specific modification of the sample dilution and sample incubation time. Empiric analysis of specimens from subjects with known dates of infection determined that the less sensitive ELISA assay remains negative for an average of 129 days (range 109 to 149 days) after seroconversion can be detected using the more sensitive assay. This assay allows identification of recent HIV-1 seroconversion from a single serum sample, which has important applications for studies of HIV-1 incidence surveillance and biologic studies of recently infected subjects. The clinical utility of identifying subjects who are within 129 days of seroconversion remains to be determined, although some have proposed that early treatment may help preserve immune function.

Increased specificity of antibody testing has been achieved by using recombinant purified HIV-1 antigens rather than lysates of viruses. Virus lysates contain substantial amounts of antigens derived from the host cells that may cross-react with the patient's serum and produce a false-positive test. Recombinant virus proteins are more pure, thereby eliminating serum reactions with the host cells from which the virus lysates are derived. This increased specificity was important in the re-evaluation of serum collected in Africa in the 1960s, which initially indicated evidence for prevalent HIV-1 antibodies that was later shown to be due to false-positive antibody testing. Use of recombinant HIV-1 antigens also allows inclusion of antigens from a wide range of HIV variants, including type 2, which is common in West Africa, and subtypes of HIV-1 found throughout Africa, Asia, Brazil, and Europe.

The convenience of HIV-1 antibody testing has improved with the development of rapid antibody tests and tests that use specimens other than blood, such as oral secretions and urine. Rapid tests often involve embedding HIV-1 antigens on filter paper, then passing the serum to be tested through the paper. After a wash step removes any antibodies that did not bind to the filter paper, the secondary antibodies are passed over the filter, allowing binding to anti-HIV antibodies that were retained. A final step allows detection of the presence of secondary antibodies. These rapid tests can be performed outside of sophisticated laboratory settings in less than an hour.[23] Furthermore, the tests are designed to be performed one at a time, which eliminates the need to accumulate sufficient samples for batch testing. Like all HIV-1 antibody tests, rapid tests that indicate the presence of anti-HIV antibodies have to be confirmed using confirmatory tests (see below). Nevertheless, the preliminary results of rapid tests can be discussed with the subject during the initial visit, which may improve the effectiveness of counseling.[24] To further increase the convenience of antibody testing, tests based on oral secretions and urine have been developed.[23,25] These assays may further increase the convenience of antibody testing by eliminating the expense and discomfort of venipuncture.

p24 Antigen Assays

HIV p24 Antigen Test

This assay measures the amount of free viral protein (p24) present in the plasma or tissue culture supernatant.[26] Although this protein may be present in the plasma of patients at all stages of HIV infection, p24 antigenemia is most prevalent during the time of initial seroconversion and again later in the course of more advanced HIV disease.[6,8,27–29] The test uses an ELISA sandwich technique in which antibodies to p24 are bound to the bottom of a microtiter well or onto polystyrene beads (Fig. 3–4). The bound antibodies are incubated with patient serum or plasma. If free p24 antigen is present in the serum, the antigen is bound tightly and specifically to the capture anti-p24 antibody. After a washing procedure, a second detector anti-p24 antibody is added, followed by addition of an enzyme-linked immunoglobulin, which is directed against the second p24 antibody. With the addition of substrate, the conjugated enzyme cleaves the substrate into a color-generating

| Well with anti-HIV capture antibody | → Add sera containing HIV antigen (p 24) | → Add rabbit anti-HIV detection antibody | → Add goat anti-rabbit antibody (labeled) | → Add substrate; measure color photometrically |

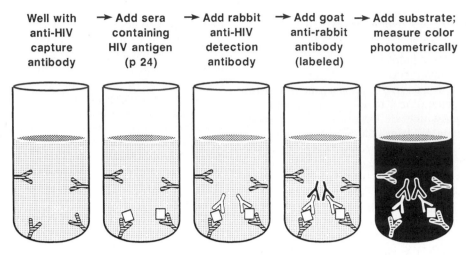

FIGURE 3–4. HIV-1 antigen capture assay is an ELISA-based test that detects the presence of free HIV-1 p24 antigen in patient serum. Free antigen is bound (captured) by specific anti-p24 capture antibodies that have been coated onto a microwell. Bound antigen is detected by specially designed rabbit anti-HIV p24 (detection antibodies), which, in turn, are detected by goat anti-rabbit antibodies. The goat antibodies have been conjugated with an enzyme that cleaves a specific substrate, yielding a colored product. By photometrically measuring the degree of color in the well, the amount of HIV-1 p24 antigen can be determined quantitatively.

product that can be measured spectrophotometrically (as in the ELISA anti-HIV antibody procedure). This test was originally developed with the second anti-p24 antibody having a polyclonal nature. More recently, the use of monoclonal anti-p24 antibodies has increased the sensitivity of the assay substantially. With the more advanced test, p24 antigen levels as low as 7 to 10 pg/ml can be detected reliably.

Acidified p24 Antigen Procedure

A modification of the p24 antigen test was introduced that further increases the test's sensitivity. This modification is based on the concept that p24 antigen, when produced in the presence of significant amounts of anti-p24 antibody, forms antigen–antibody complexes that bind free antigen and prevent detection. Through acidification of plasma, the antigen–antibody complexes can be disrupted, releasing free antigen for detection by the antigen assay.[30–32]

The procedure is performed by pretreating patient plasma (or serum) with glycine and incubating it for 1 hour at 37°C. After stabilization of the plasma, the plasma is analyzed for the presence of p24 antigen as described previously. Studies are underway to assess the degree of increased sensitivity achieved by using this technique. Preliminary results indicate that it may be especially helpful in detecting p24 antigen in HIV-1–infected infants in the perinatal

period. The acidified p24 antigen assay also may be useful in following patient responses to antiretroviral therapy in clinical trials, although more recent data indicate that regular p24 antigen testing may yield more information.

Quantitative Viral RNA and DNA Assays

Currently available data indicate that viral load measurements should be used routinely in clinical practice.[33] Quantitative polymerase chain reaction (PCR) and branched-chain DNA (bDNA) have demonstrated *independent* predictive value in determining the relative risk of clinical progression and/or survival when compared to other markers, including CD4 lymphocyte counts.[33–37] In these studies, viral load measures were better predictors of clinical outcome than other markers, whether using either baseline values or change in the marker in response to antiviral therapy. As all of the viral load assays become more standardized and more readily available, clinicians will be able to make decisions regarding the effectiveness of antiretroviral therapy based on measurements of viral load rather than indirect assessments of antiretroviral therapy effects, such as CD4 counts. Viral load assays have been based on the PCR, bDNA, and nucleic acid sequence–based amplification (NASBA) techniques. Although these techniques differ fundamentally, all serve to quantify the concentration of virus in blood and other tissues by measuring viral RNA.

Polymerase Chain Reaction Technique

The PCR technique, introduced in the late 1980s, represents a major advance in the diagnosis of many disorders, including HIV infection.[29,38] This powerful technique can amplify target DNA existing in very small quantities (as few as one copy of HIV per 100,000 cells) through a series of binary replicative cycles (Fig. 3–5).[29,38] Oligonucleotide primers, approximately 25 to 30 bp in length, are carefully designed to bind to a known sequence of the target DNA. These complementary primers bind to highly conserved regions of the genome, usually spaced 150 to 600 bp apart.

Each PCR cycle consists of a period of denaturation (during which the temperatures reach 95°C), followed by an annealing period during which the primers bind to the target DNA (typically with temperatures of 55°C to 60°C) and finally by an extension period during which complementary sequences are generated (temperature 72°C). The key to the entire reaction is the Taq polymerase, a unique DNA polymerase derived from the bacterium *Thermus aquaticus*, which maintains its activity at high temperatures (72°C). In addition to the Taq polymerase enzyme and primers, the reaction mixture contains the necessary phosphorylated nucleotide products (dATP, dGTP, dCTP, and dTTP), appropriate concentrations of divalent cations (e.g., magnesium), buffers, and the target DNA to allow optimum amplification to occur.

The duration of each portion of the cycle is generally 1 to 3 minutes. At the end of each completed cycle, the amount of DNA in the region of interest is doubled. After a total of a specified number (N) of cycles, the amplified region of DNA exists at 2^N power (usually 20 to 30 cycles are used). Therefore, even if the target DNA initially exists in only a small copy number, the PCR reaction magnifies it several hundred millionfold (e.g., 2^{30} after 30 cycles). The amount of amplified product is easily detected on agarose gel electrophoresis.

The PCR procedure can also be applied to RNA.[39–41] In such an instance, RNA is reversed transcribed into cDNA with an animal retrovirus RT (e.g., murine leukemia virus RT), and the cDNA product is then amplified as described previously. In the case of HIV, proviral HIV-1 DNA, genomic RNA, and mRNA have all been amplified successfully.

The major problem with PCR amplification, ironically, is also its greatest strength—its incredible sensitivity. When performed properly, there is probably no more powerful molecular biologic technique. Unfortunately, inadvertent contamination of reagents or target DNA or both can lead to false-positive results even in labo-

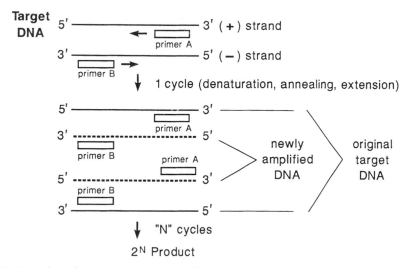

FIGURE 3–5. In the polymerase chain reaction (PCR) technique, target DNA is amplified through a series of cycles, each consisting of (1) denaturation of the double-stranded target DNA, (2) annealing of specially designed complementary primers (A and B) to the target DNA, and (3) extension of the primers into complementary new strands of DNA through the use of a unique heat-stable DNA polymerase (Taq polymerase). By repeating the cycles N times, the amount of original target DNA is amplified exponentially, 2^N (see text for details).

ratories with the most experienced personnel.[42] The problem with contamination is the limiting obstacle to the widespread use of the PCR technique in clinical practice. Nonetheless, when used properly in laboratories with experienced personnel, this technique allows early detection of infection before the development of a serologic response.[43,44]

QUANTITATIVE PCR. Several laboratories have developed techniques to quantitate the amount of HIV proviral DNA and genomic RNA as relative measures of viral load.[41,43,45–50] Previously, serial dilutions of target DNA (or cDNA) were PCR amplified and the relative intensities of the PCR products were compared to a standard curve. Even with co-amplification of highly conserved cellular products (such as the β-globin gene) as positive controls, a high degree of variability was observed. Inefficient RNA extraction, RNAse or DNAse contamination, and variability in PCR efficiency all have contributed to the unreliability of early quantitative PCR techniques.

More recently, several new approaches have been developed that circumvent many of the previously identified obstacles. Competitive PCR techniques, which use an internal standard consisting of known RNA or DNA template matched to the target sequence of interest, have shown more promise in initial studies. One such technique, quantitative competitive PCR (QC-PCR), was first applied to a cohort of 66 patients that covered the spectrum of HIV infection.[50] The dynamic range of this assay was from 100 copies/ml of plasma to over 21,000,000 copies/ml, varying with stage of disease. The mean plasma HIV-1 RNA value for patients with early asymptomatic disease was 78,200 copies/ml, for those with symptomatic disease (AIDS-related complex) 352,100 copies/ml, and for those with advanced disease (AIDS) 2,448,000 copies/ml; the highest value, 5,178,000 copies/ml, was observed in patients with acute seroconversion syndrome (formerly CDC stage I). Of special interest, the QC-PCR assay was applied to a small number of patients who had been treated with antiretroviral therapy (Table 3–1). Treatment with zidovudine resulted in an 80% to 95% reduction in viral burden as measured by QC-PCR, which was readily reversible within 1 week after cessation of therapy. These data demonstrated both the potential use of more sophisticated viral markers in future clinical studies and the dynamic nature of HIV replication in vivo.

The Amplicor HIV-1 RNA Monitor assay (Roche Molecular Systems) is a commercially available assay that is based on PCR, quantified by serially diluting the test plasma and comparing the amplified products with a standard that is spiked into the test plasma and amplified in parallel. The assay can be readily modified to increase sensitivity for low viral loads by addition of a centrifugation step that concentrates the virus prior to loading into the assay.

Branched-Chain DNA

A novel non–PCR-based technique has been developed by investigators at Chiron. The so-called bDNA technique is an ELISA-like assay that amplifies signal from target HIV RNA or DNA using a series of branched probes. The signal amplification approach is fundamentally different from PCR, which amplifies the target, and is theoretically less prone to contamination because the amplified signal in bDNA assays cannot contaminate new assays. The bDNA assay for HIV-1 is now in its third version, which has a lower limit of detection of 50 HIV-1 RNA copies/ml of plasma, with good specificity at that level. The advantages of the bDNA approach over other methods include relative ease of use and capacity to analyze non–clade B subtypes of HIV-1, as are commonly found outside of North America. Despite obvious differences in technique, a remarkable correlation exists between values obtained via quantitative PCR versus bDNA ($r = .89$, $p < .001$)[51] (see Fig. 3–6).

Nucleic Acid Sequence–Based Amplification

Assays based on NASBA are similar to PCR-based assays in that the target is amplified rather than the signal. The NASBA assays involve amplification of RNA targets at a single temperature using RNA transcriptases, which differs from PCR-based assays, wherein RNA is transcribed once into DNA followed by DNA amplification using DNA polymerases. An important characteristic of the NASBA assays being developed by Organon Teknica is the inclusion of an RNA extraction step that uses activated silica. This method yields highly purified viral RNA from samples of human tissues. Although this may not be important for analysis of blood plasma, the silica-based extraction of RNA is important for analysis of viral RNA in semen and possibly other tissues where assay inhibitors may be present.

TABLE 3–1. Virologic Effect of Zidovudine Therapy over 6 Weeks as Measured by QC-PCR and p24 Antigen Techniques

PATIENT NO.	HIV RNA (copies/ml)	HIV p24 Ag		ZIDOVUDINE (AZT)*	TIME ON TREATMENT
		ICD (pg/ml)	Reg (pg/ml)		
1	84,900	0	0	−	Week 0*
	18,000	0	0	+	Week 1
	33,500	0	0	+	Week 2
	28,100	0	0	+	Week 6
	72,700	0	0	−	Week 7
2	49,100	0	0	−	Week 0
	7,300	0	0	+	Week 1
	6,500	0	0	+	Week 2
	11,200	0	0	+	Week 6
	58,400	0	0	−	Week 7
3	173,600	79	0	−	Week 0
	21,900	28	0	+	Week 1
	10,900	24	0	+	Week 2
	9,200	31	0	+	Week 6
	136,300	47	0	−	Week 7

*For kinetic analysis of viral load over a 6-week period of treatment with zidovudine, patients were studied before initiation of treatment (week 0), after 1, 2, and 6 weeks of treatment, and 1 week after temporary discontinuation of treatment (week 7).

Adapted from Pistak M Jr, Saag MS, Yang LC, et al: High levels of HIV-1 in plasma during all stages of infection determined by competitive PCR. Science 259:1749, 1993. Copyright 1993 American Association for the Advancement of Science, with permission.

Viral RNA Assay Sensitivity and Specificity

The sensitivity of viral RNA assays is continually improving to allow evaluation of plasma viral load in subjects being treated with antiretroviral therapy. Assay sensitivity can be defined as either the "limit of detection," or the "limit of quantitation." The limit of detection refers to the lowest viral load that can be reliably distinguished from uninfected specimens, whereas the limit of quantitation refers to the lowest viral load that can be precisely (i.e., reproducibly) measured. In either case, the criteria used to establish the limits of detection and quantitation will depend on the clinical and research setting. Hence, the same assay may be noted to have a limit of quantitation of 20 HIV RNA copies/ml

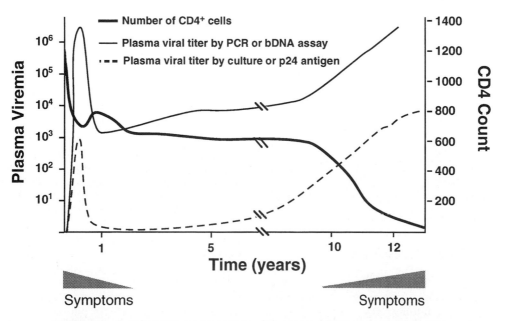

FIGURE 3–6. Schematic representation of the natural history of HIV-1 infection.

in a research paper but be approved for clinical use with a much higher limit. In general, the precision of all viral load assays decreases as the viral load decreases, making viral load fluctuations in the low range more likely to be due to random assay variation.

The sensitivity of the assays is usually improved by adding a centrifugation step that concentrates the viral particles prior to extraction of viral RNA. By analysis of a larger volume of plasma, the sensitivity of the assays can be increased proportionately. Preliminary data indicate that differences in viral loads that occur in the very low range may predict the duration of virologic suppression on therapy. For example, subjects with plasma viremia less than 20 HIV-1 RNA copies/ml of plasma had a decreased risk of virologic failure and less evidence of viral sequence evolution than subjects with plasma viral loads between 20 and 400 HIV-1 RNA copies/ml.[52] Correlation between differences in viremia in the low range and clinical outcomes remains to be documented. Furthermore, the feasibility and clinical benefit of driving plasma viremia below detection by intensifying antiretroviral therapy in subjects with low but detectable viremia have not yet been determined.

The specificity of viral RNA-based assays is of concern when these assays are used to identify subjects in research studies who have been recently infected with HIV-1. All of the viral load assays that are currently available have false positive rates up to 5%, although the mechanism underlying false-positive test results differs between assays. Contamination is likely to contribute to false-positive test results in PCR-based assays, especially if the assay detection involves opening the reaction tubes after amplification. Nonspecific signal amplification is likely to contribute to false-positive bDNA results. In practice, the specificity of viral load assays for diagnosing HIV-1 infection is typically between 95% and 99%, which is considerably worse than the specificity of p24 antigen assays and antibody assays. Hence, HIV-1 antibody assays remain the gold standard for diagnosing HIV-1 infection.

Drug Resistance Assessment

HIV-1 variants with decreased susceptibility to antiretroviral therapy frequently emerge at the time of virologic failure. HIV susceptibility to drugs can be assessed phenotypically, by culturing the virus in the presence of the drugs, or genotypically, by detecting viral genetic mutations that have been associated with decreased resistance. In general, genotyping assays are less expensive and less demanding technically than phenotyping assays. For these reasons, drug resistance genotyping assays are becoming widely available in research laboratories and clinical reference laboratories, whereas phenotyping assays are less readily available. The phenotyping assays, however, are more direct measures of the susceptibility of HIV-1 to the drugs that are tested. The results are reported as the concentration of drug that inhibits the virus by 50% (IC_{50}), which is more intuitive to physicians accustomed to antibacterial resistance testing.

Genotypic Drug Resistance Assays

Genotypic assessment of drug resistance is possible because there are well-defined viral mutations associated with decreased drug susceptibility to some drugs (Fig. 3–7).[53] For some drugs, such as lamivudine and the non-nucleoside RT inhibitors, there are single mutations that increase viral resistance to high levels. For other drugs, such as zidovudine and the protease inhibitors, there are several mutations that are associated with drug resistance. Accumulation of mutations in these settings is associated with decreasing susceptibility to the drug. For yet other drugs, such as stavudine, the viral genetic mutations associated with resistance remain to be determined. Taken together, the viral mutation information derived from drug resistance genotypic assays has good predictive failure for susceptibility to some drugs but not others.

Genotypic drug resistance assays involve PCR amplification of the protease and RT genes of HIV-1 followed by determination of the nucleotide sequence. The sequence of the PCR products can be determined using cycle sequencing methods. These methods identify the nucleotide at each position of the gene by copying the gene, with an enzyme such as Taq polymerase, in the presence of low concentrations of nucleotides that have been chemically modified so that the DNA copying is terminated whenever one of the modified nucleotides is incorporated. Separate reactions using each of the four modified nucleotides (dCTP, dTTP, dATP, dGTP) are performed, or the nucleotides are labeled with different fluorescent markers to allow identification of the nucleotide at which the DNA copy was prematurely terminated. During polyacrylamide gel electrophoresis, the lengths of the prematurely terminated copies reflect the

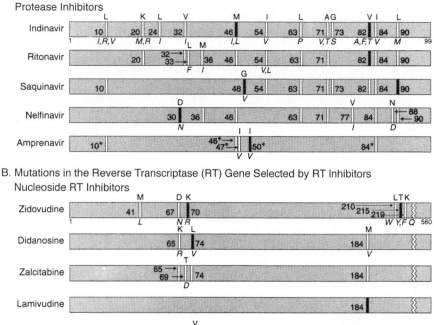

FIGURE 3–7. The most common human immunodeficiency virus 1 mutations selected by protease inhibitors (*A*), and nucleoside and non-nucleoside reverse transcriptase inhibitors (*B*). For each amino acid residue listed, the *letter* above the listing indicates the amino acid associated with the wild-type virus. The *italicized letter* below the residue indicates the substitution that confers drug resistance. The drug-selected mutations are categorized as "primary" (*black bars*) or "secondary" (*white bars*). (The *black-and-white bar* indicates a mutation selected in vitro, but rarely seen in specimens from patients in whom therapy fails.) Primary mutations generally decrease inhibitor binding and are the first mutations selected. For indinavir, the mutations listed as primary may not be the first mutations selected, but they are selected in most patients' isolates in combination with other mutations. For zalcitabine, all mutations are listed as secondary because of inadequate clinical data to determine a common initial mutation. For nevirapine and delavirdine, each mutation can occur as either an initial or subsequent mutation and affect inhibitor binding. The asterisk indicates that the mutation has been reported in vitro, but relevance for clinical drug failure is uncertain. Amino acid abbreviations are as follows: A, alanine; C, cysteine; D, aspartate; E, glutamate; F, phenylalanine; G, glycine; H, histidine; I, isoleucine; K, lysine; L, leucine; M, methionine; N, asparagine; P, proline; Q, glutamine; R, arginine; S, serine; T, threonine; V, valine; W, tryptophan; Y, tyrosine. Multinucleoside resistance viruses have phenotypic resistance to most nucleoside reverse transcriptase inhibitors. Current listings are also available at http://hiv-web.lanl.gov/ or at http://www.viral-resistance.com. (From Hirsch MS, Conway B, D'Aquila RT, et al: Antiretroviral drug resistance testing in adults with HIV infection: Implications for clinical management. International AIDS Society–USA Panel. JAMA 279:1984, 1998. Copyright 1998, American Medical Association, with permission.)

positions of each of the bases in the original sequence.

The sequence of the PCR products containing the gene for protease and RT can also be determined using hybridization methods rather than cycle sequencing.[54–56] Hybridization methods are based on the principle that two strands of DNA, or RNA, will hybridize more tightly if the strands are exact complements of each other, whereas hybridization is weaker if the two strands are mismatched at one or more nucleotide positions. Hybridization is usually measured using fluorescently labeled DNA or through chemical enzyme activity. In hybridization-based assays, DNA of unknown sequence from the patient is mixed with probes that have mutant and wild-type (e.g., naturally occurring) sequences. The presence of a mutation is inferred when the DNA derived from the patient's virus binds better to the mutant probe than to the wild-type probe. Assays based on the principle of differential hybridization may be less technically demanding than assays based on cycle sequencing, thereby allowing greater acceptance in clinical laboratories where molecular biologic assays are not already widely applied. Furthermore, hybridization-based assays may have increased capacity to identify mutant variants that exist infrequently (<20%) in the virus population. Nevertheless, the utility of hybridization assays is limited by the extremely high diversity of HIV-1, which often results in more than one mutation being present in the sequence that is probed. Even high-density arrays of several thousand probes require some similarity of the HIV-1 to the class B subtype consensus sequence upon which the probes are based.

Phenotypic Assays

Direct measurement of HIV susceptibility to drugs requires use of a drug resistance phenotyping assay. These assays involve culture of HIV-1 in a series of wells containing a dilution series of the drug. The IC_{50} is calculated by interpolation of a graph in which drug concentration is plotted against percent viral inhibition.

The standard AIDS Clinical Trials Group drug resistance phenotyping assay involves three separate HIV culture steps. First, HIV-1 is isolated from the blood of the subject using qualititative culture methods described earlier in this chapter. Second, the virus isolate is titered by serial dilution on uninfected blood mononuclear cells to determine the concentration of infectious virus present in the stock, measured as the tissue culture infectious dose 50% ($TCID_{50}$). Third, a constant titer of the virus stock is incubated in a dilution series of the drug. Each step requires between 2 and 4 weeks; consequently, the entire assay can require between 6 and 8 weeks. Furthermore, each culture step produces opportunities for virus selection in the laboratory such that mixtures of wild-type and drug-resistant HIV-1 could be overgrown by wild-type virus. Finally, only one drug is tested at a time. Synergistic and antagonistic effects require additional testing. Hence, these assays do not directly measure the virus that is present in the patient.

Novel approaches to drug resistance phenotyping based on molecular biology have been developed to address limitations of the standard assay.[57–59] One such approach involves PCR amplification of protease and RT genes directly from the patient's blood, thereby avoiding the time, cost, and selection associated with virus isolation. These PCR-amplified subgenomic segments are then combined with the remaining HIV genes taken from laboratory-adapted HIV-1 to construct chimeric viruses that are infectious. The constructed viruses can carry markers that facilitate detection of viral infection. These viruses are then evaluated using a serial concentration of drug as in the standard assay. These assays can be performed in shorter periods of time because virus culture steps are eliminated. Nevertheless, these techniques are much more specialized than standard phenotyping assays, which restricts their availability to only a few laboratories worldwide.

Clinical Use of Drug Resistance Assessment

The appropriate clinical use of drug resistance testing is still being evaluated. Both genotypic and phenotypic drug resistance assays have excellent explanatory value in that the majority of subjects with recurrent viremia who are on therapy will have at least some markers of drug resistance,[60] although exceptions have been described.[61] The predictive value of these assays is less well documented. Preliminary information indicates that drug resistance patterns after virologic failure predict short-term virologic responses after changes in therapy,[62] although in many situations a good medication history might be equally predictive. In one study of 54 subjects who changed antiretroviral therapy after virologic failure, drug resistance genotyping results in combination with antiretroviral history were more predictive of short-term virologic response than was antiretroviral history alone.[63]

Prospective randomized trials are underway to compare virologic responses to therapy guided by drug resistance assessment with therapy guided only by medication history. Ultimately, evaluation of the effect of these tests on clinical outcomes would be ideal, but most laboratory assays are widely used in clinical practice without demonstration that their use improves clinical outcomes.

Evaluation of Immunologic Status

CD4 Cell Count

Human lymphocytes possess specific glycoproteins on their surface that play an important role in cell activity and function. Although many surface glycoproteins have been identified, the CD3, CD4, and CD8 cell surface markers are used most often in the context of HIV infection.[64] The CD3 (T3) cell marker is present on all adult human lymphocytes. The CD8 (T8) cell marker is present on the subset of suppressor or cytotoxic lymphocytes that control or suppress specific ongoing immunologic activity. In contrast, the lymphocytes bearing the CD4 (T4) cell surface marker help or induce immunologic reactions.

CD4 cells respond to the class II major histocompatibility complex (MHC) antigens and release cytokines that activate and augment the immunologic response. CD4+ lymphocytes are the primary targets of HIV infection, and the CD4 receptor is the primary binding site of HIV-1. Throughout the course of chronic HIV-1 infection, the number of CD4 lymphocytes is depleted, and the loss of these cells is associated with development of the characteristic opportunistic infections and malignancies of AIDS.[1,65-71] Thus the measurement of CD4+ lymphocytes is one of the most important determinants for clinically staging the disease status of HIV-1–infected patients.

The numbers of CD4 and CD8 cells are measured through the use of specific monoclonal antibodies directed against the surface glycoprotein. These monoclonals are labeled with fluorescent markers, which can be detected when light is passed through the sample. Specialized fluorescent antibody cell sorting (FACS) machines have been developed that automatically count the number of cells labeled with the monoclonal antibody. Using this flow cytometric technique, the percentage of cells bearing the CD4 or CD8 cell surface markers can be determined.

The FACS analysis yields the percentage of cells carrying a certain surface marker. The absolute CD4 count cannot be measured directly but is calculated by the following formula:

$$\text{Absolute CD4 count} = \text{Total white blood count} \times \% \text{ Lymphocytes} \times \% \text{ CD4 cells}$$

Clinical staging can be based on either the CD4 percent or the absolute CD4 count. However, most clinical studies have used the absolute CD4 count, even though the percentage value is less subject to fluctuations.[72,73]

Variability in the CD4 percent and the absolute CD4 cell count can be a significant problem both over time and with repeated determinations. CD4 counts normally undergo diurnal variation, with fluctuations of as much as a 150- to 300-cell/mm^3 difference between morning and evening values in normal hosts.[72] Additionally, the longer samples set before processing, the more likely CD4 count values will be artificially elevated. Refrigeration also dramatically increases CD4 cell count values. Such variation has posed difficulties both in clinically staging patients and in following response to therapy in clinical trials.

Another means of clinically following patients is to use the CD4/CD8 ratio.[73] It is determined by dividing the number of CD4 cells by the number of CD8 cells. In uninfected controls, normal values for the CD4/CD8 ratio are 0.5 to 2.0. Normal values for CD4 percent are 40% to 70%, and CD4 counts are generally 500 to 1600 cells/mm^3 in adults.

$β_2$-Microglobulin

$β_2$-Microglobulin is a protein present on the surface of all nucleated cells and serves as the light chain of the class T MHC complex.[1] Measurable levels of $β_2$-microglobulin are increased whenever mononuclear cell activation or cell destruction occurs, as is the case with HIV-1 infection. Serum levels of $β_2$-microglobulin are determined through radioimmunoassay determination or through an enzyme immunoassay. Several clinical studies have shown that levels greater than 3 mg/L are associated with increased risk of progression to AIDS among HIV-infected patients.[74-77] When levels are greater than 5 mg/L, the likelihood of occurrence of new opportunistic diseases or death increases further.[78,79] Unfortunately, $β_2$-microglobulin levels are too nonspecific and not sufficiently predictive of clinical outcome to be of value in clinical practice.

Serum Neopterin

Neopterin is produced during guanosine triphosphate metabolism and is increased during periods of cellular activation. The primary source of neopterin apparently is cells of the monocyte-macrophage lineage that release increased amounts of neopterin after stimulation with interferon-γ. Neopterin levels can be determined through high-pressure liquid chromatography or by competitive radioimmunoassay and can be detected in both serum and urine. Like β_2-microglobulin, elevated levels of neopterin have been correlated to advancing clinical HIV disease.[80-82] Levels greater than 15 ng/ml are noted in patients with AIDS as compared to levels in the 3- to 5-ng/ml range for asymptomatic seropositive patients.[83] Like β_2-microglobulin, neopterin levels are not sufficiently predictive of clinical events to be of use in clinical practice.

TEST INTERPRETATION

To interpret results of any HIV-related test appropriately, the natural history of HIV infection and the host immune response must be understood. After initial primary infection with HIV, there is an immunologically silent window period before the development of detectable antibody (Fig. 3–6). The median time from initial infection to the development of detectable antibody is 2.1 months, with 95% of individuals developing antibody within 5.8 months of initial infection.[84] Although the majority of individuals notice very few, if any, symptoms associated with seroconversion, an estimated 40% to 60% of individuals will develop symptoms of an acute mononucleosis-like syndrome, consisting of sore throat, headache, fever, myalgias, lymphadenopathy, and skin rash.[6,85-88] When such symptomatic patients have been studied carefully, virus replication is typically quite high, as demonstrated by high levels of plasma HIV RNA, infectious free virus in plasma, and plasma p24 antigen levels.[6,43,50,89] (Fig. 3–8). Within 14 to 21 days after the onset of symptoms, anti−HIV-1 antibodies become detectable, and titers rise very rapidly against both the envelope glycoproteins and p24. Once a patient develops a mature antibody response, it usually remains detectable for life. The rise in detectable antibody response is associated with a rapid decline in both the p24 antigenemia and plasma viremia (culturable virus), usually to undetectable levels within weeks. The p24 antigenemia and plasma viremia generally return to detecta-

ble levels as the patient approaches more advanced disease.[5,7,8] However, viral burden as measured by quantitative PCR remains detectable throughout the course of the disease.[50] Indeed, studies demonstrate continued, ongoing, viral replication throughout *all* stages of HIV infection with extraordinarily high rates of viral replication (~1 billion virions provided daily with a half-life of 1.2 days).

The CD4 count generally decreases during the acute viral-like illness of acute seroconversion (as CD4 counts do with most acute viral syndromes) but usually returns toward normal levels as a healthy immune response is established. Over a period of many years, the CD4 count declines.[71] As the cell count drops below 500/mm³, antiretroviral therapy usually is initiated.[90] The risk of serious opportunistic infections and death increases substantially as CD4 counts drop below 200/mm³.[65-67,69,70] Prophylactic therapy against the development of *Pneumocystis carinii* pneumonia is indicated when the CD4 cell count approaches 200/mm³.[90] Much controversy still exists about routine prophylaxis of other opportunistic diseases when CD4 counts drop below 50/mm³, although current data suggest initiation of routine preventative therapy against *Mycobacterium avium* complex disease (see Chapter 22).

SENSITIVITY, SPECIFICITY, AND MISLEADING TEST RESULTS

Any discussion of HIV testing must address the questions of sensitivity, specificity, positive predictive value, and negative predictive value (Table 3–2). By definition, *sensitivity* refers to the ability to detect accurately an individual with a particular disorder among those individuals who truly have the disorder. In contrast, *specificity* is the ability to identify accurately all those individuals who truly do not have the disorder out of all of those individuals within a population who are unaffected. The sensitivity and specificity of a given test are test specific and are not dependent on the population being tested. Positive and negative predictive values, in contrast, refer to the test's ability to predict accurately who does or does not have a particular disorder and are critically related to the prevalence of the disorder within the population being tested.

False-negative antibody test results can occur any time an individual is within that 1- to 3-month seronegative window period between the

FIGURE 3–8. Detailed analysis of plasma viremia titers (*open squares*), HIV-1 p24 antigen levels (*closed circles*), and anti-p24 antibody levels (*open circles*) in three patients with acute primary HIV-1 infection. The *arrows* indicate the time of first detection of both gp160 and p24 antibodies by Western blot technique (see Fig. 3–3*B*). (From Clark SJ, Saag MS, Decker WD, et al: High titers of cytopathic virus in plasma of patients with symptomatic primary HIV-1 infection. N Engl J Med 324:956, 1991, with permission.)

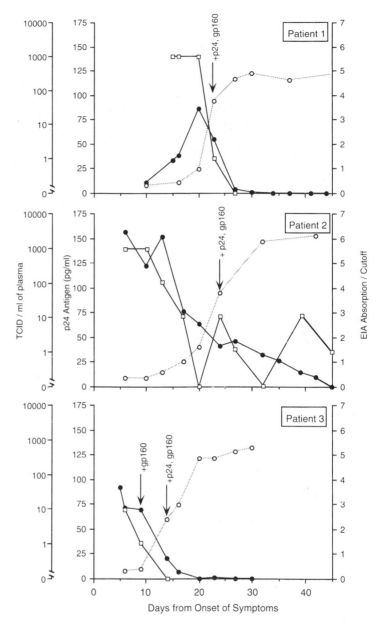

time of initial infection and the development of a detectable immune response. Fortunately, this time period is short, and, based on blood bank transfusion data, the number of false-negative results among low-risk populations is approximately 1 in 40,000 to 1 in 150,000.[91] Other causes of false-negative ELISA reactions to HIV-1 include replacement transfusions, bone marrow transplantation, and commercially available test kits that detect antibody to p24 only (e.g., the ELISA test using recombinant p24 antigen).

False-positive ELISA reactions generally result from cross-reacting antibodies, such as those against class II human leukocyte antigens (HLA-DR-4 and DQw-3).[92–94] Such antibodies are most often observed in multiparous women and in individuals who have received multiple transfused units of blood. Other autoantibodies (e.g., those against smooth muscle or parietal cells, antimitochondrial antibodies, antinuclear antibodies, and anti–T-cell antibodies) can lead to false-positive results.[96–98]

A common misconception is that a false-positive ELISA will always be corrected by the confirmatory Western blot test. In fact, false-positive Western blot results do occur, although the frequency of false-positive Western blot re-

TABLE 3–2. HIV Testing Results

	HIV INFECTION	
TEST RESULT	Present	Absent
Positive	True-positive (A)	False-positive (B)
Negative	False-negative (C)	True-negative (D)

Sensitivity (%) = $A/(A + C)(\times 100)$
Positive predictive value (%) = $A/(A + B)(\times 100)$
Specificity (%) = $D/(D + B)(\times 100)$
Negative predictive value (%) = $D/(D + C)(\times 100)$

sults is generally less common than with ELISA results.[97] Antibodies against HLA class I antigens may lead to false-positive gp41 bands, whereas antibodies to class II HLA antigens cause false-positive bands at p31. Other auto-antibodies (e.g., antimitochondrial, antinuclear, anti–T-cell, and antileukocyte antibodies) that react with proteins present in the T-lymphocyte cell line that propagated the virus used in the Western blot test also may lead to false-positive test results.[96,97]

The most important parameter when interpreting HIV tests is the positive predictive value. The probability of a positive test result occurring in a truly infected individual is critically dependent on the prevalence of HIV infection of the population tested.[99] As an example, assuming tests (ELISA and Western blot) of 100% sensitivity and a joint false-positive rate of 0.01%, the rates of truly infected patients among those with positive ELISA and Western blot results vary dramatically, depending on who is tested. In testing intravenous drug users from a major U.S. metropolitan center in which the seroprevalence is 50%, the positive predictive value would approach 100%. Conversely, in screening female schoolteachers from a rural area in the United States where the prevalence of HIV infection is 0.01%, 50% of the women testing positive would have false-positive test results. If the joint false-positive rate increases to 0.1%, 90% of the women with positive ELISA and Western blot results would be falsely labeled as HIV infected[99] (Fig. 3–9).

Although test specificity has improved over the last 3 to 5 years, the specificities do not equal 100% and in some instances, depending on the experience of the laboratory personnel, may be 99.9% (false-positive rate, 0.1%). For most other tests, this is an acceptable false-positive rate; however, when considering the difficulties in counseling an individual who has a low risk of HIV infection who has just been

diagnosed as HIV positive, it becomes quite difficult to know what precisely to tell the patient. In such instances in which the test result does not match the clinical presentation, it is best initially to repeat both the ELISA and the Western blot test at a different laboratory. If the results do not change or are indeterminate, testing at specialized laboratories using either RIPA, IFA, HIV-1 isolation by cell culture, or, preferably, PCR techniques may be of benefit.

Another difficult problem in antibody test interpretation is how to deal with an indeterminate Western blot result. As described earlier, this situation is created when bands are present on the Western blot that do not meet criteria of a definitively positive test. Several algorithms have been proposed in the literature for dealing with indeterminate Western blots. However, the applied concepts of assessing the risk to the patient combined with repeat testing in another laboratory are a common theme with all these algorithms.[100,101] When retesting a patient who has had an indeterminate result at more than one laboratory, it is recommended that the individual be retested at 3 and 6 months to determine whether he or she was in the process of seroconverting at the original time of testing.

Use of Markers in Clinical Trials and Clinical Practice

Since the discovery of zidovudine as an effective antiretroviral agent (Table 3–1), it is no longer ethically appropriate to have untreated placebo groups in patients with advanced HIV infection. Neither is it appropriate to rely on gross measurements of antiviral efficacy, such as advancing morbidity or mortality, as a means of assessing relative antiviral activity of one compound versus another. As a result, markers of viral replication, such as p24 antigenemia, plasma viremia, quantitative cell culture, and quantitative PCR, along with indirect markers such as CD4 cell count are being used in various combinations to assess the relative antiretroviral activity of one compound or regimen versus another (Table 3–1). Although the definitions of how to use each test most appropriately are still being clarified, viral load measurements, via quantitative PCR or bDNA, are the best measures of antiretroviral activity and can demonstrate the relative antiviral effect of a given regimen within 2 weeks. The long-term clinical benefit of a short-term virologic assessment is still under investigation; however, viral load

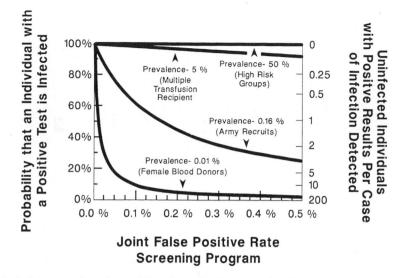

Joint False Positive Rate
Screening Program

FIGURE 3–9. Interpretation of a positive HIV antibody test result. The joint false-positive rate from the ELISA and Western blot tests is shown on the *horizontal axis*. The *left vertical axis* demonstrates the probability that a person with a positive test result is truly infected with HIV. The *right vertical scale* shows the number of uninfected individuals falsely identified as infected for every infected person correctly identified. The four *bold lines* represent four populations that might be screened (high-risk groups, transfusion recipients, army recruits, and female blood donors), each of which has a different prevalence of HIV infection (listed accordingly). (From Meyer KB, Pauker SG: Sounding board: Screening for HIV: Can we afford the false positive rate? N Engl J Med 317:240, 1987, with permission.)

changes at 8 weeks of therapy have been associated with clinical benefit over time.[34,35]

From a clinical standpoint, however, it is important to separate the goals of experimental therapeutics and the goals of optimum patient care. The goal of antiretroviral therapy is to keep the viral load as low as possible for as long as possible. Based on the predictive nature of viral load and its rapid response to changes in antiretroviral regimens, measurement of viral load in clinical practice should be performed on a routine basis.[33] Table 3–3 summarizes how the

measures might be used to initiate antiretroviral therapy, monitor the response to therapy, and determine when a given regimen may be failing. Plasma HIV RNA levels should be obtained every 3 to 4 months, preferably in conjunction with CD4 cell counts or at shorter intervals as critical decision points are neared. Proper specimen handling is essential for ensuring accurate RNA values, including use of plasma (as opposed to serum), use of EDTA or ACD (rather than heparin) as an anticoagulant, prompt specimen processing (within 2 to 4 hours of phle-

TABLE 3–3. Summary of Current Recommendations

CHARACTERISTIC	RECOMMENDATION
Plasma HIV RNA level that suggests initiation of treatment	More than 5000–10,000 copies/ml and a CD4+ count/clinical status suggestive of progression; >20,000–50,000 copies/ml regardless of laboratory/clinical status
Target level of HIV RNA after initiation of treatment	Undetectable; <50 copies/ml is an ideal target
Minimal decrease in HIV RNA indicative of antiviral activity	>0.5 log decrease
Change in HIV RNA that suggests drug treatment failure	A confirmed return to detectable levels or a return toward baseline
Suggested frequency of HIV RNA measurement	At baseline: 2 measurements, 2–4 weeks apart every 3–4 months or in conjunction with CD4+ counts. Shorter intervals as critical decision points are neared 3–4 weeks after initiating/changing therapy

Data from Carpenter CC, Fischl MA, Hammer SM, et al: Antiretroviral therapy of HIV infection in 1998: Updated recommendations of the International AIDS Society–USA Panel, JAMA 280:78, 1998.

botomy), and, ideally, consistent use of the same type of assay (bDNA or quantitative PCR). Plasma HIV RNA assays substantially improve the ability to determine when an antiretroviral regimen is no longer active and, therefore, are likely to reduce the overall cost of care by minimizing continued use of ineffective and expensive treatment regimens.

Acknowledgment

Thanks to Ms. Jane Garrison for her assistance in the preparation of this manuscript, to Katharine Coleman for preparation of the figures, and to Dr. Victoria Johnson for her critical review.

References

1. Davey RT Jr, Lane HC: Laboratory methods in the diagnosis and prognostic staging of infection with human immunodeficiency virus type 1. Rev Infect Dis 12:912, 1990
2. Sloand EM, Pitt E, Chiarello RJ: HIV testing—state of the art. JAMA 266:2861, 1991
3. Barre-Sinoussi F, Chermann JC, Rey F, et al: Isolation of a T-lymphotropic retrovirus from a patient at risk for acquired immune deficiency syndrome (AIDS). Science 220:868, 1983
4. Popovic M, Sarngadharan MG, Read E, et al: Detection, isolation, and continuous production of cytopathic retroviruses (HTLV-III) from patients with AIDS and pre-AIDS. Science 224:497, 1984
5. Ho DH, Moudgil T, Alam M: Quantitation of human immunodeficiency virus type 1 in the blood of infected persons. N Engl J Med 321:1621, 1989
6. Clark SJ, Saag MS, Decker WD, et al: High titers of cytopathic virus in plasma of patients with symptomatic primary HIV-1 infection. N Engl J Med 324:954, 1991
7. Coombs RW, Collier AC, Allain J-P, et al: Plasma viremia in human immunodeficiency virus infection. N Engl J Med 321:1626, 1989
8. Saag MS, Crain MJ, Decker WD, et al: High-level viremia in adults and children infected with human immunodeficiency virus: Relation to disease stage and CD4+ lymphocyte levels. J Infect Dis 164:72, 1991
9. Finzi D, Hermankova M, Pierson T: Identification of a reservoir for HIV-1 in patients on highly active antiretroviral therapy. Science 278:1295, 1997
10. Wong J, Hezareh M, Gunthard H: Recovery of replication-competent HIV despite prolonged suppression of plasma viremia. Science 278:1291, 1997
11. Chun T, Stuyver L, Mizell S: Presence of an inducible HIV-1 latent reservoir during highly active antiretroviral therapy. Proceedings of the National Academy of Science 94:13193, 1997
12. Centers for Disease Control: Update: Serologic testing for antibody to human immunodeficiency virus. MMWR Morbid Mortal Wkly Rep 36:833, 1988
13. Barnes DM: New questions about AIDS test accuracy. Science 238:884, 1987
14. Centers for Disease Control: Interpretation and use of the Western blot assay for serodiagnosis of human

15. immunodeficiency virus type 1 infections. MMWR Morbid Mortal Wkly Rep 38:1, 1989
15. Consortium for Retrovirus Serology Standardization: Serological diagnosis of human immunodeficiency virus infection by Western blot testing. JAMA 260:674, 1988
16. O'Gorman MRG, Weber D, Landis SE, et al: Interpretive criteria of the Western blot assay for serodiagnosis of human immunodeficiency virus type 1 infection. Arch Pathol Lab Med 115:26, 1991
17. Carlson JR, Yee J, Hinrichs SH, et al: Comparison of indirect immunofluorescence and Western blot for detection of antihuman immunodeficiency virus antibodies. J Clin Microbiol 25:494, 1987
18. Chiodi F, Bredberg-Raden U, Biberfeld G, et al: Radioimmunoprecipitation and Western blotting with sera of human immunodeficiency virus infected patients: A comparative study. AIDS Res Hum Retroviruses 3:165, 1987
19. Gallo D, Diggs JL, Shell GR, et al: Comparison of detection of antibody to the acquired immune deficiency syndrome virus by enzyme immunoassay, immunofluorescence, and Western blot methods. J Clin Microbiol 23:1049, 1986
20. Hedenskog M, Dewhurst S, Ludvigsen C, et al: Testing for antibodies to AIDS-associated retrovirus (HLTV-III/LAV) by indirect fixed cell immunofluorescence: Specificity, sensitivity, and applications. J Med Virol 19:325, 1986
21. Cooper DA, Imrie AA, Penny R: Antibody response to human immunodeficiency virus after primary infection. J Infect Dis 155:1113, 1987
22. Janssen RS, Satten GA, Stramer SL, et al: New testing strategy to detect early HIV-1 infection for use in incidence estimates and for clinical and prevention purposes. JAMA 280:42, 1998
23. Grant RM, Piwowar EM, Katongole-Mbidde E, et al: Comparison of saliva and serum for human immunodeficiency virus type 1 antibody testing in Uganda using a rapid recombinant assay. Clin Diagn Lab Immunol 3:640, 1996
24. Centers for Disease Control and Prevention: Update: HIV counseling and testing using rapid tests—United States, 1995. MMWR Morbid Mortal Wkly Rep 47:211, 1998
25. Hashida S, Hashinaka K, Ishikawa S, Ishikawa E: More reliable diagnosis of infection with human immunodeficiency virus type 1 (HIV-1) by detection of antibody IgGs to Pol and Gag proteins of HIV-1 and p24 antigen of HIV-1 in urine, saliva, and/or serum with highly sensitive and specific enzyme immunoassay (immune complex transfer enzyme immunoassay): A review. J Clin Lab Anal 11:267, 1997
26. Allain J-P, Laurian Y, Paul DA, et al: Long-term evaluation of HIV antigen and antibodies to p24 and gp41 in patients with hemophilia. N Engl J Med 317:1114, 1987
27. Allain J-P, Laurian Y, Paul DA, et al: Serological markers in early stages of human immunodeficiency virus infection in hemophiliacs. Lancet 2:1233, 1986
28. Goudsmit J, DeWolf F, Paul DA, et al: Expression of human immunodeficiency virus antigen (HIV-Ag) in serum and cerebrospinal fluid during acute and chronic infection. Lancet 2:177, 1986
29. Paul DA, Falk LA, Kessler HA, et al: Correlation of serum HIV antigen and antibody with clinical status in HIV-infected patients. J Med Virol 22:257, 1987
30. Kestens L, Goofd G, Gigase PL, et al: HIV antigen detection in circulating immune complexes. J Virol Methods 31:67, 1991

31. Nishanian P, Huskins KR, Stehn S, et al: A simple method for improved assay demonstrates that HIV p24 antigen is present as immune complexes in most sera from HIV-infected individuals. J Infect Dis 162: 21, 1990

32. Portera M, Vitale F, La Licata R, et al: Free and antibody-complexed antigen and antibody profile in apparently healthy HIV-seropositive individuals and in AIDS patients. J Med Virol 30:30, 1990

33. Saag MS, Holodniy M, Kuritzkes DR, et al: HIV viral load markers in clinical practice. Nat Med 2:625, 1996

34. Coombs RW, Welles SL, Hooper C, et al: Association of plasma human immunodeficiency virus type 1 RNA level with risk of clinical progression in patients with advanced infection. J Infect Dis 174:704, 1996

35. Hammer SM, Katzenstein DA, Hughes MD, et al: Virologic markers and outcome in ACTG 175 [Abstract 524]. In: Abstracts of the 3rd Conference on Retroviruses and Opportunistic Infections, Washington, DC, 1996, p 175

36. Mellors JW, Rinaldo CR Jr, Gupta P, et al: Prognosis in HIV-1 infection predicted by the quantity of virus in plasma. Science 272:1167, 1996

37. O'Brien WA, Hartigan PM, Martin D, et al: Changes in plasma HIV-1 RNA and CD4 lymphocyte counts and the risk of progression to AIDS. N Engl J Med 334:426, 1996

38. Saiki RK, Gelfand DH, Stoffel S, et al: Primer-directed enzymatic amplification of DNA with a thermostable DNA polymerase. Science 239:487, 1988

39. Hart C, Schochetman G, Spira T, et al: Direct detection of HIV RNA expression in seropositive subjects. Lancet 2:596, 1988

40. Hewlett IK, Gregg RA, Ou CY, et al: Detection in plasma of HIV-1-specific DNA and RNA by polymerase chain reaction before and after seroconversion. J Clin Immunoassay 11:161, 1988

41. Holodniy M, Katzenstein DA, Sengupta S, et al: Detection and quantification of human immunodeficiency virus RNA in patient serum by use of the polymerase chain reaction. J Infect Dis 163:862, 1991

42. Lifson AR, Stanley M, Pane J, et al: Detection of human immunodeficiency virus DNA using the polymerase chain reaction in a well-characterized group of homosexual and bisexual men. J Infect Dis 161: 436, 1990

43. Daar ES, Moudgil T, Meyer RD, et al: Transient high levels of viremia in patients with primary immunodeficiency type 1 infection. N Engl J Med 324:961, 1991

44. Wolinsky SM, Rinaldo CR, Kwok S, et al: Human immunodeficiency virus type 1 (HIV-1) infection a median of 18 months before a diagnostic Western blot. Ann Intern Med 111:961, 1989

45. Abbott MA, Poiesz BJ, Byrne BC, et al: Enzymatic gene amplification: Qualitative and quantitative methods for detecting proviral DNA amplified in vitro. J Infect Dis 158:1158, 1988

46. Becker-Andre M, Hahlbrock K: Absolute mRNA quantification using the polymerase chain reaction (PCR): A novel approach by a PCR aided transcript titration assay (PATTY). Nucleic Acids Res 17:9437, 1989

47. Dickover RE, Donovan RM, Goldstein E, et al: Quantitation of human immunodeficiency virus DNA by using the polymerase chain reaction. J Clin Microbiol 28:2130, 1990

48. Holodniy M, Katzenstein D, Winters M, et al: Measurement of HIV virus load and genotypic resistance by gene amplification in asymptomatic subjects treated with combination therapy. J Acquir Immune Defic Syndr 6:366, 1993

49. Oka S, Urayama K, Hirabayashi Y, et al: Quantitative analysis of human immunodeficiency virus type 1 in asymptomatic carriers using the polymerase chain reaction. Biochem Biophys Res Commun 167:1, 1990

50. Piatak M Jr, Saag MS, Yang LC, et al: High levels of HIV-1 in plasma during all stages of infection determined by competitive PCR. Science 259:1749, 1993

51. Cao Y, Ho DD, Todd J, et al: Clinical evaluation of branched DNA signal amplification for quantifying HIV type-1 in human plasma. AIDS Res Hum Retroviruses 11:353, 1995

52. Raboud JM, Montaner JS, Conway B, et al: Suppression of plasma viral load below 20 copies/ml is required to achieve a long-term response to therapy. AIDS 12:1619, 1998

53. Hirsch MS, Conway B, D'Aquila RT, et al: Antiretroviral drug resistance testing in adults with HIV infection: Implications for clinical management. International AIDS Society–USA Panel [see comments]. JAMA 279:1984, 1998

54. Eastman P, Boyer E, Mole L, et al: Nonisotopic hybridization assay for determination of relative amounts of genotypic human immunodeficiency virus type 1 zidovudine resistance. J Clin Microbiol 33: 2777, 1995

55. Lipshutz R, Morris D, Chee M, et al: Using oligonucleotide probe arrays to access genetic diversity. Biotechniques 19:442, 1995

56. Schmit JC, Ruiz L, Stuyver L, et al: Comparison of the LiPA HIV-1 RT test, selective PCR and direct solid phase sequencing for the detection of HIV-1 drug resistance mutations. J Virol Meth 73:77, 1998

57. Mammano F, Petit C, Clavel F: Resistance-associated loss of viral fitness in human immunodeficiency virus type 1: Phenotypic analysis of protease and gag coevolution in protease inhibitor-treated patients. J Virol 72:7632, 1998

58. Hertogs K, de Béthune MP, Miller V, et al: A rapid method for simultaneous detection of phenotypic resistance to inhibitors of protease and reverse transcriptase in recombinant human immunodeficiency virus type 1 isolates from patients treated with antiretroviral drugs. Antimicrob Agents Chemother 42:269, 1998

59. Whitcomb J, Limoli K, Wrin T, et al: Phenotypic and genotypic analysis of stavudine-resistant isolates of HIV-1. In 2nd International Workshop on HIV Drug Resistance and Treatment Strategies. Lago Maggiore, Italy, International Medical Press, 1998, p 14

60. Deeks SG, Grant RM, Beatty GW, et al: Activity of a ritonavir plus saquinavir-containing regimen in patients with virologic evidence of indinavir or ritonavir failure. AIDS 12:F97, 1998

61. Havlir DV, Marschner IC, Hirsch MS, et al: Maintenance antiretroviral therapies in HIV infected patients with undetectable plasma HIV RNA after triple-drug therapy: AIDS Clinical Trials Group Study 343 Team [see comments]. N Engl J Med 339:1261, 1998

62. Deeks S, Parkin N, Petropoulos C, et al: Correlation of baseline phenotypic drug susceptibility with 16 week virologic response in a pilot combination therapy study in HIV-infected patients who failed indinavir therapy. In 2nd International Workshop on HIV Drug Resistance and Treatment Strategies. Lago Maggiore, Italy, International Medical Press, 1998, p 36

63. Zolopa A, Shafer R, Warford A, et al: Predictors of antiviral response to saquinavir/ritonavir therapy in a

clinic cohort who have failed prior protease inhibitors: A comparison of clinical characteristics, antiretroviral drug history, and HIV genotype. In 2nd International Workshop on HIV Drug Resistance and Treatment Strategies. Lago Maggiore, Italy, International Medical Press, 1998, p 37

64. Lane HC, Fauci AS: Immunologic abnormalities in the acquired immunodeficiency syndrome. Annu Rev Immunol 3:477, 1985
65. El-Sadr W, Marmor M, Zolla-Pazner S, et al: Four year prospective study on homosexual men: Correlation of immunologic abnormalities, clinical status and serology to human immunodeficiency virus. J Infect Dis 155:789, 1987
66. Eyster ME, Gail MH, Ballard JO, et al: Natural history of human immunodeficiency virus infection in hemophiliacs: Effects of T-cell subsets, platelet counts, and age. Ann Intern Med 107:1, 1987
67. Goedert JJ, Biggar RJ, Melbye M, et al: Effect of T4 count and cofactors on the incidence of AIDS in homosexual men infected with human immunodeficiency virus. JAMA 257:331, 1987
68. Moss AR, Bacchetti P, Osmond D, et al: Seropositivity for HIV and the development of AIDS or AIDS-related condition: Three year follow-up of the San Francisco General Hospital cohort. BMJ 296:745, 1988
69. Polk BF, Fox R, Brookmeyer R, et al: Predictors of the acquired immunodeficiency syndrome developing in a cohort of seropositive homosexual men. N Engl J Med 316:61, 1988
70. Redfield RR, Wright DC, Tramont EC: The Walter Reed staging classification for HTLV-III/LAV infection. N Engl J Med 314:131, 1986
71. Stein DS, Korvick JA, Vermund SH: CD4+ lymphocyte cell enumeration for prediction of clinical course of human immunodeficiency virus disease: A review. J Infect Dis 165:352, 1992
72. Malone JL, Simms TE, Gray GC, et al: Sources of variability in repeated T-helper lymphocyte counts from human immunodeficiency virus type 1-infected patients: Total lymphocyte count fluctuations and diurnal cycle are important. J Acquir Immune Defic Syndr 3:144, 1990
73. Taylor JMG, Fahey JL, Detels R, et al: CD4 percentage, CD4 number, and CD4:CD8 ratio in HIV infection: Which to choose and how to use. J Acquir Immune Defic Syndr 2:114, 1989
74. Calabrese LH, Proffitt MR, Gupta MK, et al: Serum β_2-microglobulin and interferon in homosexual males: Relationship to clinical findings and serologic status to the human T lymphotropic virus (HTLV-III). AIDS Res 1:423, 1984
75. Klein E, Gindi EJ, Brown DK, et al: Cross-sectional study of immunologic abnormalities in intravenous drug abusers on methadone maintenance in New York City. AIDS 3:235, 1989
76. Lazzarin A: Raised serum β_2-microglobulin levels in different stages of human immunodeficiency virus infection. J Clin Lab Immunol 27:133, 1988
77. Taylor CR, Krailo MD, Levine AM: Serum beta-2 microglobulin levels in homosexual men with AIDS and with persistent, generalized lymphadenopathy. Cancer 57:2190, 1986
78. Anderson RE, Lang W, Shiboski S, et al: Use of β_2-microglobulin level and CD4 lymphocyte count to predict development of acquired immunodeficiency syndrome in persons with human immunodeficiency virus infection. Arch Intern Med 150:73, 1990
79. Moss AR, Bacchetti P: Natural history of HIV infection. AIDS 3:550, 1989
80. Fahey JL, Taylor JMG, Detels R, et al: The prognostic value of cellular and serologic markers in infection with human immunodeficiency virus type 1. N Engl J Med 322:166, 1990
81. Fuchs D, Hausen A, Reibnegger G, et al: Neopterin as a marker for activated cell-mediated immunity: Application in HIV infection. Immunol Today 9:150, 1988
82. Fuchs D, Spira TJ, Hausen A, et al: Neopterin as a predictive marker for disease progression in human immunodeficiency virus type 1 infection. Clin Chem 35:1746, 1989
83. Reddy MM, Grieco MH: Neopterin and alpha and beta interleukin 1 levels in sera of patients with human immunodeficiency virus infection. J Clin Microbiol 27:1919, 1989
84. Horsburgh CR Jr, Ou CY, Jason J, et al: Duration of human immunodeficiency virus infection before detection of antibody. Lancet 2:637, 1989
85. Cooper DA, Gold J, Maclean P, et al: Acute AIDS retrovirus infection. Lancet 1:537, 1985
86. Isaksson B, Albert J, Chiodi F, et al: AIDS two months after primary human immunodeficiency virus infection. J Infect Dis 158:866, 1988
87. Tindall B, Barker S, Donovan E, et al: Characterization of the acute clinical illness associated with human immunodeficiency virus infection. Arch Intern Med 148:945, 1988
88. Ward JW, Bush TJ, Perkins HA, et al: The natural history of transfusion-associated infection with human immunodeficiency virus: Factors influencing the rate of progression to disease. N Engl J Med 321:947, 1989
89. Mulder J, McKinney N, Christopherson C, et al: Rapid and simple PCR assay for quantitation of human immunodeficiency virus type 1 RNA in plasma: Application to acute retroviral infection. J Clin Microbiol 32:292, 1994
90. NIH State-of-the-Art Conference: State-of-the-Art Conference on azidothymidine therapy for early HIV infection. Am J Med 89:335, 1990
91. Ward JW, Holmberg SD, Allen JR, et al: Transmission of human immunodeficiency virus (HIV) by blood transfusions screened as negative for HIV antibody. N Engl J Med 318:473, 1988
92. Ameglio F, Dolei A, Benedetto A, et al: Antibodies reactive with nonpolymorphic epitopes on HLA molecules interfere in screening tests for the human immunodeficiency virus. J Infect Dis 156:1034, 1987
93. Blanton M, Balakrishnan K, Dumaswala U, et al: HLA antibodies in blood donors with reactive screening tests for antibody to the immunodeficiency virus. Transfusion 27:118, 1987
94. Kuhnl P, Seidl S, Holzberger G: HLA DR4 antibodies cause positive HTLV-III antibody ELISA results. Lancet 1:1222, 1985
95. Biberfeld G, Bredberg-Raden U, Bottinger B, et al: Blood donor sera with false-positive Western blot reactions to human immunodeficiency virus. Lancet 2:289, 1986
96. Saag MS, Britz J: Asymptomatic blood donor with a false positive HTLV-III Western blot. N Engl J Med 314:118, 1986
97. Schleupner CJ: Diagnostic tests for HIV-1 infection. In Mandell GL, Douglas RG, Bennet JE (eds): Principles and Practice of Infectious Diseases, Update 1. New York, Churchill Livingstone, 1989, p 3

98. Smith DM, Dewhurst S, Shepherd S, et al: False-positive enzyme-linked immunosorbent assay reactions for antibody to human immunodeficiency virus in a population of Midwestern patients with congenital bleeding disorders. Transfusion 127:112, 1987

99. Meyer KB, Pauker SG: Sounding board: Screening for HIV: Can we afford the false positive rate? N Engl J Med 317:238, 1987

100. Celum CL, Coombs RW, Lafferty W, et al: Indeterminate human immunodeficiency virus type 1 Western blots: Seroconversion risk, specificity of supplemental tests, and an algorithm for evaluation. J Infect Dis 164:656, 1991

101. Dock NL, Kleinman SH, Rayfield MA, et al: Human immunodeficiency virus infection and indeterminate Western blot patterns. Arch Intern Med 151:525, 1991

4 | Primary HIV Infection

ANDREW CARR • DAVID A. COOPER

Primary HIV infection defines a brief period soon after inoculation with HIV that is characterized by intense viremia, a subsequent immune response, and, in the majority of patients, a brief, febrile illness.[1] Understanding primary HIV infection has improved our understanding of the two-way interaction between HIV and the immune system. Evolution in molecular diagnostics has transformed the speed and accuracy of diagnosing primary HIV infection, although the most appropriate diagnostic algorithm has not been defined. Zidovudine monotherapy initiated during primary HIV infection confers modest clinical benefit.[2] Preliminary reports now suggest that combination antiretroviral therapy of primary HIV infection is safe, tolerated, and far more effective in suppressing viral replication[3–5] and results in greater preservation of immune function.[6] The clinical impact of early combination therapy, however, is unknown. Whether such therapy can eradicate HIV or is more effective than delayed therapy is currently under investigation. Because there are minimal data on primary HIV-2 infection, only primary HIV-1 infection is considered in this review; nevertheless, the same biologic, diagnostic, and therapeutic principles are likely to apply.

CLINICAL FINDINGS

General Features

An acute clinical illness associated with primary HIV infection occurs in 53% to 93% of individuals.[7–12] In a prospectively studied group of homosexual men, primary HIV-1 infection was the second most common cause (after influenza) of an acute febrile illness lasting more than 3 days.[11] Although asymptomatic primary HIV infection does occur, a high index of clinical suspicion and prior experience with primary

HIV infection greatly increase the recognition rate. Indeed, in our experience many patients present because they believe that they may have primary HIV infection, reflecting high awareness in both primary care physicians and high-risk groups.

The vast majority of individuals are infected sexually, by sharing infected needles, or peripartum. Nevertheless, infection in a health care setting,[13] including by patient-to-patient transmission,[14] and from breast milk[15] can occur; there is also potential for infection across undamaged oral mucosa.[16] The time from exposure to HIV-1 until the onset of the acute clinical illness is typically 2 to 4 weeks,[7–12,17–19] although incubation periods of 6 days to 6 weeks are not rare. There are isolated reports of primary HIV illness and seroconversion 12 months after presumed inoculation.[20] The clinical illness is acute in onset and lasts from 1 to 2 weeks.[7–12,17–19,21–25] In the largest analysis to date, Vanhems et al. reported a median illness duration of 20 days that was not influenced by age, gender, or risk factor.[9]

Clinical Manifestations

The main clinical features of primary HIV infection reflect the broad cellular tropism of HIV-1 during this period. A review of 139 cases of primary HIV-1 infection[17] found that the most common physical signs and symptoms were fever (97%), adenopathy (77%), pharyngitis (73%), rash (70%), and myalgia or arthralgia (58%). In another series of 46 patients,[25] the most common features were fever (94%), fatigue (90%), pharyngitis (72%), weight loss (70%), myalgias (60%), and headaches (55%). Nevertheless, most patients in these reports were diagnosed not at the time of their illness but at subsequent routine testing, stressing the need for awareness on the part of the diagnosing doctor, particularly the primary care physician.

In a larger, unselected cohort of patients with primary HIV infection,[9] the most common features were different: fever (77%), fatigue (66%), rash (56%), myalgia (55%), and headache (51%) (Table 4–1). These findings emphasize that many patients with primary HIV infection do not have the classic "mononucleosis-like" illness. In fact, only 16% of patients with primary HIV infection had what might be described as classic features, namely fever, pharyngitis, and cervical lymphadenopathy. The most common features in febrile patients without pharyngitis or lymphadenopathy were headaches (52%), mouth ulcers (25%), abdominal pain (25%), and diarrhea (17%). Furthermore, 10% of patients had none of these three features. These data suggest that increasing awareness by experienced diagnosing physicians increases the likelihood of diagnosis in those individuals with few or atypical symptoms.

Other important clinical features of primary HIV infection[1] are listed below:

- Most clinical manifestations are self-limited, although some symptoms, such as fatigue, may persist for months.
- The illness is generally of rapid onset.
- Fever may or may not be associated with night sweats.
- Lymphadenopathy develops most commonly in the second week of the illness and may be generalized, but the axillary, occipital, and cervical nodes are most commonly involved. Splenomegaly has also been reported.
- The classic erythematous, nonpruritic, maculopapular rash (Fig. 4–1 and Color Plate 1A) is generally symmetrical, has lesions 5 to 10 mm in diameter and affects the face or trunk,

TABLE 4–1. Clinical Manifestations of Primary HIV-1 Infection in 218 Patients*

	FREQUENCY (%)	DURATION (mean days)
>50%		
Fever >38°C	77	17
Fatigue	66	24
Erythematous maculopapular rash	56	15
Myalgia	55	18
Headache	51	26
25%–50%		
Pharyngitis	44	12
Cervical lymphadenopathy	39	15
Arthralgia	31	23
Oral ulcer	29	13
Odynophagia	28	16
5%–25%		
Axillary lymphadenopathy	24	164
Weight loss	24	29
Nausea	24	18
Diarrhea	23	13
Night sweats	22	15
Cough	22	18
Anorexia	21	15
Inguinal lymphadenopathy	20	9
Abdominal pain	19	15
Oral candidiasis	17	10
Vomiting	12	10
Photophobia	12	11
Sore eyes	12	13
Genital ulcer	7	14
Tonsillitis	7	13
Depression	6	23
Dizziness	6	11

*Only 16% of patients had the "classic" triad of fever, pharyngitis and cervical lymphadenopathy and 10% of patients had none of these features.

Modified from Vanhems P, Allard R, Cooper DA, et al: Acute HIV-1 disease as a mononucleosis-like illness: Is the diagnosis too restrictive? Clin Infect Dis 24:965, 1997, with permission.

FIGURE 4–1. Rash of primary HIV infection.

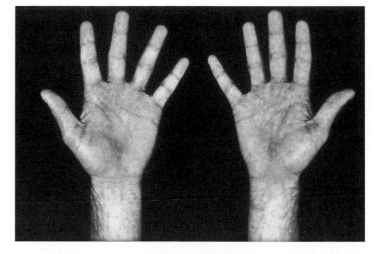

but can affect the extremities or be generalized.

- Other skin lesions noted include a roseola-like rash; diffuse urticaria; a vesicular, pustular exanthem; desquamation of the palms and soles; alopecia; and erythema multiforme (desquamation and alopecia typically occur in the second month).
- Ulceration of the oropharynx is common (and may less commonly involve the esophagus, anus, or penis) and is generally oval and well demarcated.
- Although headache is very common in many acute viral illnesses, retro-orbital pain exacerbated by eye movements appears fairly specific for primary HIV infection.
- Photophobia may reflect an underlying aseptic meningitis.
- Oral or esophageal candidiasis, often self-limiting, may occur and probably reflects an appreciable decline in CD4+ lymphocyte count.
- The presence of candidiasis or neurologic involvement during primary HIV infection has been found to have adverse prognostic significance (Table 4–5).
- An illness lasting longer than 14 days is also associated with a worse prognosis.[8]

Predisposing Factors

Several factors have been associated with an increased relative risk for symptomatic primary HIV infection, including a low pre-existing CD4+ cell count or CD4+:CD8+ ratio, anergy to the neoantigen dinitrochlorobenzene (but not to "recall" antigens), and infection from an index case with advanced HIV-1 disease.[26–28] Because acute infection with other viruses such as cytomegalovirus (CMV) often causes similar symptoms, acute co-infection should increase the likelihood of symptomatic illness as well as accelerate the expression of HIV.[29,30]

Diagnosis

The most important step in the diagnosis of primary HIV infection is to suspect the possibility (Table 4–2). In turn, the most important clinical data are the knowledge that an individual has had an HIV exposure, usually in the preceding 2 to 8 weeks, and the presence of one or more suggestive symptoms or signs. Once the possibility is considered, the diagnosis can be confirmed in the laboratory usually within days of presentation.

There are several advantages of early diagnosis of HIV infection. First, it enables the patient to access therapies at a time when the immune system has suffered the least amount of damage. Second, some clinical and laboratory variables at or soon after primary HIV infection have prognostic value and help define patients who might merit early or more aggressive antiretroviral therapy. Third, a positive diagnosis (combined with counseling and perhaps antiviral therapy) should help minimize further transmission of HIV.

Although originally described as "mononucleosis-like"[7] and described as such in the Centers for Disease Control and Prevention classification system of HIV disease,[31] symptomatic primary HIV infection is a distinct and recognizable clinical syndrome. The major symptoms

TABLE 4–2. Diagnosis of Primary HIV Infection

Setting(s)
At least 1 clinical feature of primary HIV infection
  and/or
Exposure to HIV within preceding 12 weeks
  and/or
Indeterminate HIV ELISA antibody
Algorithm
HIV-specific antibodies (at least one ELISA)*
  and
HIV Western blot*
  and
HIV-1 p24 antigen[†]
  and
T-cell subset enumeration[‡]
  and
HIV DNA PCR (especially if serology indeterminate)
  ? and
HIV RNA quantitation (especially if antiviral therapy
  contemplated)
  and
Exclude other causes of viral illness (eg. CMV, EBV)
For inconclusive samples, retest every 2 to 4 weeks
  until diagnosis confirmed or excluded (most sensitive
  and cost effective interval unknown)
Assays of uncertain utility
Genotypic/phenotypic assays for antiretroviral drug
  resistance
Virus isolation
SI/NSI phenotyping

*An overnight incubation method should be used to maximize assay sensitivity; either the ELISA(s) or Western blot should be able to detect HIV-2.

[†]If antibody assays are inconclusive, sample should be neutralized to ensure p24 assay specificity.

[‡]A small number (percentage unknown) p24 negative/antibody negative patients may have CD4+ lymphocyte counts <500 or inverted CD4+ : CD8+ ratios (<1.0).

From Carr A, Cunningham P, Kelleher A, Cooper DA: Diagnosis and treatment of primary HIV infection. J HIV Comb Ther 2:49, 1997.

TABLE 4–3. Major Differential Diagnoses

Primary HIV-1 infection
Epstein-Barr virus mononucleosis
Cytomegalovirus mononucleosis
Toxoplasmosis
Rubella
Viral hepatitis
Secondary syphilis
Disseminated gonococcal infection
Primary herpes simplex virus infection
Other viral infection
Drug reaction

and signs that strengthen the diagnosis include mucocutaneous ulceration, maculopapular rash, lymphadenopathy, and nonsuppurative pharyngitis.

The differential diagnoses of primary HIV infection are listed in Table 4–3. Skin eruptions are rare in patients with Epstein-Barr virus (EBV) or CMV infections (unless antibiotics such as amoxicillin have been given) or toxoplasmosis, do not affect the palms and soles in patients with rubella, and are typically scaly and pruritic in pityriasis rosea. Mucocutaneous ulceration is unusual in most of the other differential diagnoses. Clinical evidence of immune compromise, such as candidiasis or *Pneumocystis carinii* pneumonia, is highly suggestive of HIV infection rather than of other viral infections.

The major differences between primary HIV infection and EBV mononucleosis have been detailed by Gaines et al.[24] and are summarized

in Table 4–4. Although serologic testing for HIV and EBV usually provides the definitive diagnosis, clinicians should be aware that false-positive tests for heterophil antibodies may occur during primary HIV infection. Of course, patients can have primary HIV infection and infection with another virus such as CMV or EBV.[29,30]

Because HIV remains predominantly a sexually transmitted disease (STD) and because the incubation period of primary HIV infection is comparable to that of most common STDs, primary care physicians managing other STDs should be particularly alert to the clinical manifestations of primary HIV infection and include this in their differential diagnosis. Patients suspected of sexually acquired HIV infection should also be screened for other STDs; for example, rash, mouth ulcers, and lymphadenopathy can also occur with syphilis, and pharyngitis with orally acquired gonorrhea.

In patients with meningoencephalitis, other causes of aseptic meningoencephalitis should be excluded rapidly.

LABORATORY FEATURES

A number of laboratory variables should be measured during primary HIV infection to assist in diagnosis. Some of these should be measured in the ensuing months to assist in determining prognosis and so identify those individuals most likely to gain from intervention with antiretroviral therapy.

Serology

Antibody Testing

Primary HIV infection must be confirmed serologically by the detection of serum antibodies directed against specific internal and surface proteins of HIV.[32] Such antibodies are usually

TABLE 4–4. Clinical Differences Between Primary HIV-1 Infection and Epstein-Barr Virus (EBV) Mononucleosis

PRIMARY HIV-1 INFECTION	EBV MONONUCLEOSIS
Acute onset	Insidious onset
Little or no tonsillar hypertrophy	Marked tonsillar hypertrophy
Enanthema on hard palate	Enanthema on border of hard and soft palates
Exudative pharyngitis uncommon	Exudative pharyngitis common
Mucocutaneous ulcers common	No mucocutaneous ulcers
Rash common	Rash rare (in absence of ampicillin)
Jaundice rare	Jaundice (8%)
Diarrhea possible	No diarrhea
Opportunistic infections occasionally	No opportunistic infections

Modified from Gaines H, von Sydow M, Pehrson PO, Lundbergh P: Clinical picture of primary HIV infection presenting as a glandular-fever-like illness. BMJ 297:1363, 1988, with permission.

detectable within 4 weeks of inoculation and the first few weeks of onset of the acute illness by enzyme-linked immunosorbent assay (ELISA).[32–35] Immunoglobulin M (IgM) antibodies to HIV Gag or Env proteins appear within 2 weeks of infection, precede the immunoglobulin G (IgG) response, reach peak titers at 2 to 5 weeks, and then decline to undetectable levels within approximately 3 months. IgG antibody is then detected, usually 2 to 6 weeks after the onset of illness. Separate detection for HIV-specific IgM is not required because most antibody ELISAs detect both HIV-specific IgG and IgM. Differences in the length of the "window period" according to the type

TABLE 4–5. Useful Prognostic Variables at or Soon After Primary HIV Infection (PHI)

Clinical (during PHI)
  Presence of symptoms
  Duration of symptoms (>14 days)
  Number of symptoms (3 symptoms)
  Acquisition of HIV from an index with advanced
    HIV disease
  Candidiasis
  Neurologic involvement
  Immunodeficiency at time of infection
Laboratory (at or after 3 months' onset of PHI)
  CD4+ lymphocyte count
  HIV RNA
  β_2 microglobulin
  Infection with SI viral strain
  Persistent p24 antigenemia
  Higher HIV RNA viremia postseroconversion
Reported but not usually evaluated
  Low p24 antibody titers
  High gp120 antibody titers
  Plasma IgM level before the appearance of specific
    antibodies
  Presence of specific anti–HIV-1 IgM and IgA after
    infection
  High CD38 expression on CD8+ lymphocytes
Infection with zidovudine-resistant HIV does affect
  medium-term prognosis.

of the ELISA screening tests mandates the consistent use of sensitive screening tests.

The 3- to 6-month window period of seroconversion commonly cited is by necessity conservative, particularly if other tests are used in conjunction. Rare reports of up to 12 months of HIV infection without seroconversion[20] have important implications for public health and our understanding of HIV immunopathogenesis. HIV ELISAs are designed for maximum sensitivity. Nevertheless, negative results in early primary HIV infection are not uncommon. Clinical information on a request form that suggests possible primary HIV infection (e.g., "febrile illness" or "flu-like illness") should result in automatic testing as per Table 4–2, maximizing diagnostic sensitivity and allowing for rapid turnaround time. IgG detection in saliva samples may have comparable sensitivity for HIV seroconversion as compared with licensed serum ELISAs.[36] Antibodies to regulatory proteins (including those produced from the *rev, tat, nef, vpu,* and *vpr* genes) develop early in infection but are not measured routinely.[1]

Immunoblotting

Figure 4–2 shows the typical evolution of antibody development demonstrated by serial immunoblotting in a patient with primary HIV infection. Immunoblotting usually first shows antibody to p24 or gp41, with virtually all sera obtained 2 weeks or more after onset of the acute illness being positive.[32–34] Patients can rarely have positive immunoblots prior to ELISA reactivity, perhaps because most immunoblots involve an overnight incubation of patient serum rather than a few hours in most ELISAs.

Immunoblotting is essential to confirm the diagnosis of HIV infection because biologic false-positive or inconclusive ELISA results are not

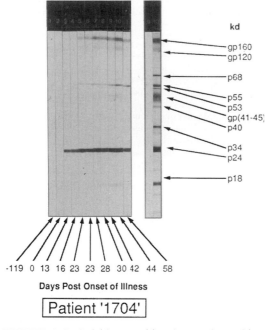

kd

gp160
gp120

p68

p55
p53
gp(41-45)
p40

p34
p24

p18

-119 0 13 16 23 23 28 30 42 44 58

Days Post Onset of Illness

Patient '1704'

FIGURE 4–2. Serial immunoblots in a patient with primary HIV infection.

the level of serum HIV antibodies increase[1,22,35] and immune complexes develop.[23] Persistent antigenemia or the reappearance of antigenemia at a later time is associated with an increased risk for the development of severe HIV disease.[11,39]

Assay for serum HIV-1 p24 antigen is essential if the differential diagnosis includes primary HIV infection. The assay is easy, cheap, widely available, sensitive, and specific and can be performed in a few hours. False-positive p24 antigen tests rarely occur, however, and the specificity should be confirmed by neutralization.

To minimize the risk of transfusion-associated HIV infection (estimated at 1 in 493,000 in the United States), blood banks in the United States now screen for HIV antibodies and p24 antigen in a single assay.[40] In developing countries such as Thailand, where the risk of transfusion-associated HIV infection has been estimated to be much greater (1 in 2644),[41] such combined assays may be of greater value. One alternative strategy practiced in some countries is to not pay blood donors, eliminating any financial incentive to high-risk individuals to donate blood.

rare. Immunoblots, however, can also yield indeterminate results (e.g., the presence of one or more nonglycoprotein bands), especially during primary HIV infection or advanced HIV disease or in those patients with biologic false-positive ELISA results, but the pattern of reactivity and the clinical history can usually distinguish between these possibilities. One possible cause for an indeterminate result may be abortive HIV infection, suggested from molecular and virologic analyses of recipients of HIV-infected blood products,[37] although abortive perinatal infection appears to be a very rare phenomenon.[38]

For patients with a history suggestive of primary HIV infection, an equivocal ELISA and immunoblot should also suggest the possibility of primary HIV-2 infection, although some commercially available HIV immunoblot strips can detect both HIV-2 and HIV-1 infection.

Virology

HIV-1 p24 Antigen

HIV-1 p24 antigen can be detected in serum and cerebrospinal fluid (CSF) in the period before *gag* and *env* seroconversion, in most patients during the first few weeks of symptoms, as early as 24 hours after the onset of acute illness, and a mean of 7 days prior to HIV antibodies.[1,22] Serum p24 antigen levels typically decrease as

HIV RNA and Proviral DNA Detection

During primary HIV infection, there are very high HIV RNA levels (about 10^6 copies/ml of plasma). These levels decreased spontaneously and precipitously concurrently with resolution of symptoms and the appearance of anti–HIV-1 antibodies. Nadir ("set point") levels are not reached for an average of 3 to 4 months, however, and levels measured prior to the nadir have been shown not to have prognostic value.[25,42,43] The viral clearance during primary HIV-1 infection is likely to be due to the emergence of an effective host immune response, but may also reflect reduced numbers of infectable target cells.[44]

Assays to detect HIV-specific RNA or DNA have revolutionized HIV diagnosis and therapy (see also Chapter 4). With respect to diagnosis, HIV DNA or RNA may be detected 2 to 3 days prior to p24 antigen.[45] HIV DNA polymerase chain reaction detection is cheaper than HIV RNA detection and rapidly assists in resolving sera with indeterminate immunoblot reactivity and diagnosis of perinatal transmission. Therefore, although the sensitivity and specificity of such an approach is currently unclear, we routinely perform HIV DNA detection in those with indeterminate or negative serology as part of our diagnostic algorithm of primary HIV infection. This has the potential to shorten the period of diagnostic uncertainty from several weeks to a few days.

HIV RNA should probably be measured only in those patients who are contemplating antiretroviral therapy at this time, with the aim of determining the most appropriate combination of antivirals to use; the higher the viral load, the more potent a therapy would probably be appropriate.[2]

Strain Selection During Transmission

A single strain of HIV is transmitted in general,[46] although co-infection has been described in individual cases of sexual and transfusional transmission.[45,47] Transmitted strains tend to have a nonsyncytium-inducing (NSI) phenotype[46,48,49] but may not be the most common strain in the blood or semen of the source subject,[50] suggesting that one or more structural, viral, or immunologic features may influence strain transmission. One such factor is the presence of the CXCR4 chemokine receptor on the surface of macrophages and dendritic and Langerhans' cells that allows for preferential transmission of NSI virus.[51]

Viral Phenotype

The ability of HIV to be syncytium inducing (SI) in MT-2 cell culture correlates with a worse prognosis.[52] However, the vast majority of HIV isolates at seroconversion are NSI, and determining whether a virus is SI or NSI is slow and unlikely to alter therapy.[48]

Transmission of zidovudine-,[48,53] nevirapine-,[54] and protease inhibitor[55]−resistant HIV has been documented. In Sydney, Australia, 10% of seroconverters infected since 1990 had phenotypic and genotypic evidence of infection with high-level zidovudine-resistant HIV.[48] A rapid, simple genotypic assay can detect mutations associated with resistance to most reverse transcriptase inhibitors.[56] If antiretroviral therapy is to be used during primary HIV infection, it would be advantageous to determine the drug susceptibility prior to therapy. Similar assays assessing protease inhibitor resistance are in development.

Immunology

T-Cell Subsets

Primary HIV infection is characterized by rapid changes in peripheral T-cell subsets.[57−60] During the first 1 to 2 weeks there is characteristically lymphopenia affecting both CD4+ and CD8+ subsets. The nadirs of total, CD4+, and CD8+ lymphocytes occur a median of 9 days following onset of illness and may approach those seen with advanced HIV disease.[1] This transient lymphopenia is followed at 3 to 4 weeks by lymphocytosis; in less than 50% of patients atypical lymphocytes are seen in the peripheral blood film.[24,61] The decrease in CD4+ lymphocyte numbers mostly represents a decline in those expressing CD45RA (i.e., "naive" T lymphocytes).[58] Although both CD4+ and CD8+ cells contribute to the lymphocytosis, the increase in CD8+ cells is relatively greater, leading to a sustained inversion of the CD4:CD8 ratio. Many CD8+ lymphocytes also express the activation markers HLA-DR, CD38, and CD11a/CD18, markers that correlate with a cytotoxic phenotype.

The inverted CD4:CD8 ratio may have some diagnostic value for primary HIV infection, because an inverted ratio is not seen in most other acute viral illnesses (except acute EBV infection) and may develop prior to detectable HIV-specific antibodies or p24 antigenemia.[58] Nevertheless, the changes in CD8+ lymphocyte counts are similar to those seen in primary CMV and EBV infections.[62,63]

β₂ Microglobulin

Elevated serum β_2 microglobulin levels a mean of 4 months after primary HIV infection correlate with a worse prognosis.[64] Nevertheless, the values during primary infection, like CD4+ counts and RNA levels at this time, have no known prognostic value.

Other Laboratory Findings

Lymph node biopsies typically show a reduction of extrafollicular B cells, CD8+ cell follicular infiltration, and only little activation and proliferation of the germinal center cells.[65] The Env proteins gp120 and gp160 have been found in interfollicular and follicular lymphocytes, endothelial cells, and interdigitating and dendritic reticulum cells. The relative normality of the structure of the germinal centers during primary HIV-1 infection contrasts with the follicular hyperplasia associated with established HIV-1 infection.

Elevated serum levels of hepatic transaminases, which are infrequently associated with clinical hepatitis, have been noted.[1,30] These generally return to normal within 3 months of presentation.

IMMUNE RESPONSE TO HIV

CD8 Cell Responses

The increase in the number of CD8+ cells during primary HIV-1 infection occurs concomitant with resolution of clinical symptoms and a decrease in the detectable levels of serum p24 antigen,[61] suggesting that the CD8+ cell response to primary HIV-1 infection has a role in controlling viral replication in vivo, as it has been shown to have in vitro.[66]

Roos et al. reported that activated CD8+ cells were found in all patients with primary HIV-1 infection but were only transiently elevated in those patients infected with SI variants of HIV.[60] They hypothesized that SI variants may be selectively cleared by the host immune response and that the persistent isolation of SI variants may reflect failure of the CD8+ response.

HIV-specific, CD8+ lymphocyte–mediated, HLA-restricted cytotoxic activity appears early in HIV seroconversion at a time when HIV-specific neutralizing antibody activity cannot be detected.[67–72] These cytotoxic cells appear to present with relatively high precursor frequency (0.1 to 1%), thereby predicting prognosis.[73,74] Nevertheless, some cytotoxic T-cell clones may not be clinically useful because they may rapidly disappear despite high antigenic load (immune tolerance) or accumulate within lymphoid tissue away from the site of HIV replication.[72,75–77]

Analysis of V-β T-cell receptor gene usage in these CD8+ lymphocytes has demonstrated different responses between individuals. The V-β response may be monoclonal, oligoclonal, or polyclonal, with patients generating a polyclonal response appearing to have the best CD4+ count outcome over the medium term.[75]

CD8+ lymphocytes may also suppress HIV replication by secretion of one or more soluble noncytolytic chemokines such as RANTES, macrophage inflammatory proteins 1α and 1β, and interleukin-16, which inhibit HIV replication.[78,79] This soluble suppressor activity has been observed in a small number of HIV seroconverters.[80] This activity was also observed in some individuals months prior to seroconversion, suggesting that this activity is not sufficient to prevent infection.

Proliferative Responses

Severe lymphocytic proliferative hyporesponsiveness to both mitogens and antigens occurs during primary HIV-1 infection[59,81,82] and persists after resolution of the acute illness in the absence of therapy. Pokeweed mitogen responses were depressed in most patients at some point in the acute illness, and reached the lowest levels at 6 to 8 weeks after onset of illness. Responses subsequently improved but remained subnormal at 1 year of follow-up. Phytohemagglutinin responses showed a similar pattern but were less affected. Persistent impairment of B-cell function also rapidly follows primary HIV-1 infection.[83]

Neutralizing Antibodies

Neutralizing antibodies may contribute to viral clearance,[77,84–86] although a direct correlation between decline in viral load and development of neutralizing antibody has not been demonstrated. Limited data suggest that serum neutralizing antibodies are not present when viral load falls.[68,86,87] Antibodies that inhibit syncytium formation and antibodies that mediate antibody-dependent cellular cytotoxicity against virally infected cells also develop soon after infection.[88] HIV-1 immune complexes appear in the blood during the period of declining concentrations of p24 antigen and increasing concentration of IgM and IgG antibodies[89] and may be detected before overt seroconversion.

Cytokines

Increased levels of interferon-α (IFN-α), tumor necrosis factor-α, neopterin, and β$_2$ microglobulin have been detected in blood and CSF during primary HIV-1 infection, reflecting activation of the cellular immune system.[90–93] High circulating levels of these cytokines are also presumably responsible for the pathogenesis of some of the major clinical manifestations of primary HIV-1 infection (e.g., the symptoms of primary HIV-1 infection, such as fevers, chills, myalgia, headache, fatigue, leukopenia, and weight loss, are very similar to those found in people receiving exogenous IFN-α).

Levels of p24 antigen rapidly declined following the IFN-α peak response that in turn occurred before the development of HIV-specific antibodies and before the CD8+ cell lymphocytosis, suggesting that it is a first line of defense against HIV-1 infection, a finding that has some support in a murine model.[94]

PROGNOSIS

After resolution of the acute clinical illness, most patients enter a stage of asymptomatic infection that lasts from many months to years. The development of severe HIV-1–related disease within the first 2 years after infection is unusual. Several studies have highlighted clinical, virologic and immunologic parameters at or soon after primary HIV infection that have prognostic significance (Table 4–5). In contrast, infection with zidovudine-resistant HIV-1 (i.e., HIV with a 90% inhibitory concentration of greater than 1 μM did not affect the clinical or CD4+ lymphocyte outcome at 1 year after documented seroconversion.

MANAGEMENT

Antiretroviral Therapy

Antiretroviral therapy of primary HIV infection has progressed greatly in recent years. Although not yet proven, it is possible that antiretroviral intervention during primary HIV-1 infection might prevent persistent HIV-1 infection or lessen the initial viral load and subsequently improve long-term prognosis. Several observations suggest that HIV could be eradicated at this time: the reduction in perinatal transmission of HIV by 70% by the use of zidovudine monotherapy,[95] the reduction in occupational transmission of HIV after needlestick injury by 80% by zidovudine monotherapy,[96] and, in some animals, antiretroviral therapy, given at or prior to inoculation, having prevented persistent infection.[97,98] By the time symptomatic primary HIV-1 infection develops, widespread viral dissemination has already occurred, so treatment at this stage is unlikely to eradicate infection. Nevertheless, studies evaluating the possibility of eradicating HIV at this time are in progress.

A double-blind, placebo-controlled trial of zidovudine 250 mg bid for 6 months found that zidovudine was safe, although it did not shorten the duration of seroconversion illness.[2] After 6 months of therapy, patients receiving zidovudine had higher CD4+ lymphocyte counts (by about 140 cells/mm³), lower HIV RNA load (by about 0.5 log), and a significant reduction in the number of HIV-related minor opportunistic infections during 18 months of follow-up.

More recent reports have showed that combination therapy yields more potent antiviral effects.[3–5,99,100] Patients who received and toler-

ated zidovudine, lamivudine, and one of the protease inhibitors (ritonavir, indinavir, or nelfinavir) all had RNA levels fall to undetectable within 6 months, similar to responses seen in those with established HIV infection. Enthusiasm for such therapy has been dampened by anecdotal reports of viral replication becoming detectable within weeks in those who interrupted therapy. Current antiretroviral therapy consensus guidelines recommend combination therapy including a protease inhibitor treatment for patients with primary HIV infection, but there are no clinical endpoint data to justify this approach. It may be that delaying therapy until the patient has recovered from the illness and has addressed the numerous psychosocial and economic issues that arise at this time (or even until the CD4 count falls to below 350 to 500 cells/mm³) may have similar clinical outcome (see also Chapter 6).

The immunologic consequences of such therapy are not known. It is noteworthy, however, that the combination of zidovudine and didanosine appeared to result in less intense bands on immunoblots, suggesting substantial reduction in HIV antigen presentation. Although the antiretroviral effects of combination therapy appear similar to those seen later in disease, such therapy during acute HIV infection results in greater preservation of HIV-specific immune function than in those patients with established infection who receive the same therapy.[6] The clinical significance of this finding is unknown but suggests that patients treated during primary HIV infection may have a greater chance of withdrawing therapy with the hope of an intact immune response suppressing any rebound in viral replication.

Other unresolved treatment issues include whether initiation of therapy can be withheld for any length of time (e.g., until symptoms resolve) without compromising the immunologic outcome, whether therapy can be safely reduced to maintenance doses, what combination is most potent in those with drug-resistant HIV at primary HIV infection, and what potent combination is best tolerated.

References

1. Carr A, Cooper DA. Primary HIV infection. In Sande M, Volberding P (eds): The Medical Management of AIDS, 5th ed. Philadelphia, WB Saunders Company, 1997, p 89
2. Kinloch-Löes S, Hirschel BJ, Hoen B, et al: A controlled trial of zidovudine in primary HIV infection. N Engl J Med 333:408, 1995

3. Perrin L, Markowitz M, Calandra G, Chung M, and the MRL Acute HIV Infection Study Group: An open treatment study of acute HIV infection with zidovudine, lamivudine and indinavir sulfate. In: Abstracts of the 4th Conference on Retroviruses and Opportunistic Infections, Washington, DC, 1997, Abstract 238

4. Hoen B, Harzic M, Fleury S, et al: ANRS053 trial of zidovudine, lamivudine and ritonavir combination in patients with symptomatic primary HIV-1 infection: Preliminary results. In: Abstracts of the 4th Conference on Retroviruses and Opportunistic Infections, Washington, DC, 1997, Abstract 232

5. Markowitz M, Cao Y, Vesanen M, et al: Recent HIV infection treated with AZT, 3TC, and a protease inhibitor. In: Abstracts of the 4th Conference on Retroviruses and Opportunistic Infections, Washington, DC, 1997, Abstract LB8

6. Rosenberg ES, Billingsley JM, Caliendo AM, et al: Vigorous HIV-1-specific CD4+ T cell responses associated with control of viremia. Science 324:1447, 1997

7. Cooper DA, Gold J, Maclean P, et al: Acute AIDS retrovirus infection: Definition of a clinical illness associated with seroconversion. Lancet 1:537, 1985

8. Pedersen C, Lindhardt BO, Jensen BL, et al: Clinical course of primary HIV infection: Consequences for subsequent course of infection. BMJ 299:154, 1989

9. Vanhems P, Allard R, Cooper DA, et al: Acute HIV-1 disease as a mononucleosis-like illness: Is the diagnosis too restrictive? Clin Infect Dis 24: 965, 1997

10. Ho DD, Sarngadharan MG, Resnick L, et al: Primary human T-lymphoptropic virus type III infection. Ann Intern Med 103:880, 1985

11. de Wolf F, Lange JMA, Bakker M, et al: Influenza-like syndrome in homosexual men: A prospective diagnostic study. J R Coll Gen Pract 38: 443, 1988

12. Tindall B, Barker S, Donovan B, et al: Characterization of the acute clinical illness associated with human immunodeficiency virus infection. Arch Intern Med 148:945, 1988

13. Anonymous: Needlestick transmission of HTLV-III from a patient infected in Africa. Lancet 2:1376, 1984

14. Chant K, Lowe D, Rubin G, et al: Patient-to-patient transmission of HIV in private surgical consulting rooms. Lancet 1:8886, 1993

15. Ziegler JB, Cooper DA, Johnson RO, Gold J: Postnatal transmission of AIDS-associated retrovirus from mother to infant. Lancet 1:896. 1985

16. Baba TW, Trichel AM, An L, et al: Infection and AIDS in adult macaques after nontraumatic oral exposure to cell-free SIV. Science 272:1486, 1996

17. Clark SJ, Saag MS, Decker WD, et al: High titers of cytopathic virus in plasma of patients with symptomatic primary HIV-I infection. N Engl J Med 324: 954, 1991

18. Daar ES, Moudgil T, Meyer RD, Ho DD: Transient high levels of viremia in patients with primary human immunodeficiency virus type I infection. N Engl J Med 324:961, 1991

19. Valle S-L: Febrile pharyngitis as the primary sign of HIV infection in a cluster of cases linked by sexual contact. Scand J Infect Dis 19:13, 1987

20. Ridzon R, Gallagher K, Ciesielski C, et al: Simultaneous transmission of human immunodeficiency virus and hepatitis C virus from a needle stick injury. N Engl J Med 336:919, 1997

21. Brehmer-Andersson E, Torssander J: The exanthema of acute (primary) HIV infection: Identification of a characteristic histopathological picture? Acta Derm Venereol (Stockh) 70:85, 1990

22. Kessler HA, Blaauw B, Spear J, et al: Diagnosis of human immunodeficiency virus infection in seronegative homosexuals presenting with an acute viral syndrome. JAMA 258:1196, 1987

23. Sinicco A, Palestro G, Caramello P, et al: Acute HIV-1 infection: Clinical and biological study of 12 patients. J Acquir Immune Defic Syndr 3:260, 1990

24. Gaines H, von Sydow M, Pehrson PO, Lundbergh P: Clinical picture of primary HIV infection presenting as a glandular-fever-like illness. BMJ 297:1363, 1988

25. Schacker TW, Coolier AC, Hughes J, et al: Clinical and epidemiologic features of primary HIV infection. Ann Intern Med 125:257, 1997

26. Ludlam CA, Tucker J, Steel CM, et al: Human T-lymphotropic virus type III (HTLV-III) infection in seronegative haemophiliacs after transfusion of factor VIII. Lancet 2:233, 1985

27. Marion SA, Schechter MT, Weaver MS, et al: Evidence that prior immune dysfunction predisposes to human immunodeficiency virus infection in homosexual men. J Acquir Immune Defic Syndr 2:178, 1989

28. Ward JW, Bush TJ, Perkins HA, et al: The natural history of transfusion-associated HIV infection: Factors influencing progression to disease. N Engl J Med 321:947, 1989

29. Bonnetti A, Weber R, Vogt MW, et al: Co-infection with human immunodeficiency virus-type 1 (HIV-1) and cytomegalovirus in two intravenous drug users. Ann Intern Med 111:293, 1989

30. Raffi F, Boudart D, Billaudel S: Acute co-infection with human immunodeficiency virus (HIV) and cytomegalovirus. Ann Intern Med 112:234, 1990

31. Centers for Disease Control: CDC classification system for human T-lymphotropic virus type III/lymphadenopathy-associated virus infections. MMWR Morb Mortal Wkly Rep 35:334, 1986

32. Cooper DA, Imrie AA, Penny R: Antibody response to human immunodeficiency virus following primary infection. J Infect Dis 155:1113, 1987

33. Gaines H, von Sydow M, Sonnetborg A, et al: Antibody response in primary human immunodeficiency virus infection. Lancet 1:1249, 1987

34. Gaines H, von Sydow M, Parry JV, et al: Detection of immunoglobulin M antibody in primary human immunodeficiency virus infection. AIDS 2:11, 1988

35. Lange JMA, Parry JV, de Wolf F, et al: Diagnostic value of specific IgM antibodies in primary HIV infection. Br Med J 293:1459, 1986

36. Burgess-Cassler A, Barriga-Angulo G, Wade SE, et al: A field test for the detection of antibodies to human immunodeficiency virus types 1 and 2 in saliva or plasma. Clin Diagn Lab Immunol 3:480, 1996

37. Georgoulias VA, Malliaraki NA, Theodoropoulou M, et al: Indeterminate human immunodeficiency virus type 1 Western blot may indicate abortive infection in some low risk blood donors. Transfusion 37:65, 1997

38. Frenkel LM, Mullins JI, Learn GH, et al: Genetic evaluation of suspected cases of transient HIV-1 infection of infants. Science 280:1073, 1998

39. Pedersen C, Nielsen CM, Vestergaard BF, et al: Temporal relation of antigenaemia and loss of antibodies to core antigens to development of clinical disease in HIV infection. Br Med J 295:567, 1987

40. Schreiber GB, Busch MP, Kleinman SH, Korelitz JJ: The risk of transfusion-transmitted viral infections: The retrovirus epidemiology donor study. N Engl J Med 334:1685, 1996

41. Kitayporn D, Kaewkungwal J, Bejrachandra S, et al: Estimated rate of HIV-1 infectious but seronegative

blood donations in Bangkok, Thailand. AIDS 10: 1157, 1996

42. Mellors JW, Kingsley LA, Rinaldo CR Jr, et al: Quantitation of HIV-1 RNA in plasma predicts outcome after seroconversion. Ann Intern Med 122:573, 1995

43. Craib KJP, Strathdee SA, Hogg RS, et al: Serum levels of human immunodeficiency virus type 1 (HIV-1) RNA after seroconversion: A predictor of long-term mortality in HIV infection. J Infect Dis 176:798, 1997

44. Phillips AN: Reduction of HIV concentration during acute infection: Independence from a specific immune response. Science 271:497, 1996

45. Busch MP, Lee LL, Satten GA, et al: Time course of detection of viral and serologic markers preceding human immunodeficiency virus type 1 seroconversion: Implications for screening of blood and tissue donors. Transfusion 35:92, 1995

46. Zhu T, Mo H, Wang N, et al: Genotypic and phenotypic characterization of HIV-1 in patients with primary infection. Science 261:1179, 1993

47. Zhu T, Wang N, Carr A, et al: Evidence for coinfection by multiple strains of human immunodeficiency virus type 1 infection subtype B in an acute seroconvertor. J Virol 69:1324, 1995

48. Imrie A, Carr A, Duncombe C, et al: Primary infection with zidovudine-resistant HIV-1 does not adversely affect outcome at one year. J Infect Dis 174:195, 1996

49. Schacker TW, Hughes JP, Shea T, et al: Biological and virologic characteristics of primary HIV infection. Ann Intern Med 128:613, 1998

50. Zhu T, Wang N, Carr A, et al: Genetic characterization of human immunodeficiency virus type 1 in blood and genital secretions: Evidence for viral compartmentalization and selection during sexual transmission. J Virol 70:3098, 1996

51. Zaitseva M, Blauvelt A, Lee S, et al: Expression and function of CCR5 and CXCR4 on human Langerhans' cells and macrophages: Implications for primary HIV infection. Nature Med 3:412, 1996

52. Richman DD, Bozzette SA: The impact of the syncytium-inducing phenotype of human immunodeficiency virus on disease progression. J Infect Dis 169:968, 1994

53. Erice A, Mayers DL, Strike DG, et al: Primary infection with zidovudine-resistant human immunodeficiency virus type 1. N Engl J Med 328:1163, 1993

54. Imrie A, Beveridge A, Genn W, et al and the Sydney Primary HIV Infection Study Group: Transmission of human immunodeficiency virus type 1 resistant to nevirapine and zidovudine. J Infect Dis 175:1502, 1997

55. Hecht F, Grant RM, Petropoulos CJ, et al: Sexual transmission of an HIV-1 variant resistant to multiple reverse transcriptase inhibitors and protease inhibitors. N Engl J Med 339:307, 1998

56. Stuyver L, Wyseur A, Rombout A, et al: Line probe assay for rapid detection of drug-selected mutations in the human immunodeficiency virus type 1 reverse transcriptase gene. Antimicrob Agents Chemother 41: 284, 1997

57. Cooper DA, Tindall B, Wilson EJ, et al: Characterization of T lymphocyte responses during primary HIV infection. J Infect Dis 157:889, 1988

58. Zaunders J, Carr A, McNally L, et al: Effects of primary HIV-1 infection on subsets of CD4+ and CD8+ T lymphocytes. AIDS 9:561, 1995

59. Pedersen C, Dickmeiss E, Gaub J, et al: T-cell subset alterations and lymphocyte responsiveness to mitogens and antigen during severe primary infection with HIV: A case series of seven consecutive HIV seroconverters. AIDS 4:523, 1990

60. Roos MTL, Lange JMA, Goede REY, et al: Virus phenotype and immune response in primary human immunodeficiency virus type 1 (HIV-1) infection. J Infect Dis 165:427, 1992

61. Steeper TA, Horwitz CA, Hanson M, et al: Heterophil-negative mononucleosis-like illnesses with atypical lymphocytosis in patients undergoing seroconversion to the human immunodeficiency virus. Am J Clin Pathol 89:169, 1988

62. Carney WP, Rubin RH, Hoffman RA, et al: Analysis of T lymphocyte subsets in cytomegalovirus mononucleosis. J Immunol 126:2114, 1981

63. de Waele M, Thielmans C, Van Camp BKG: Characterization of immunoregulatory T cells in EBV-induced infectious mononucleosis by monoclonal antibodies. N Engl J Med 304:460, 1981

64. Phillips AN, Sabin CA, Elford J, et al: Serum beta-2 microglobulin at HIV-1 seroconversion as a predictor of severe immunodeficiency during 10 years of followup. J Acquir Immune Defic Syndr Hum Retrovir 13:262, 1996

65. Sinicco A, Palestro G, Caramello P, et al: Acute HIV-1 infection: Clinical and biological study of 12 patients. J Acquir Immune Defic Syndr 3:260, 1990

66. Walker CM, Moody DJ, Stites DP, Levy JA: CD8+ lymphocytes can control HIV infection *in vitro* by suppressing virus replication. Science 234:1563, 1986

67. Ariyoshi K, Harwood E, Chiengsong-Popov R, Weber J: Is clearance of HIV-1 at seroconversion mediated by neutralising antibodies? Lancet 340:1257, 1992

68. Koup RA, Safrit JT, Cao Y, et al: Temporal association of cellular immune responses with the initial control of viremia in primary human immunodeficiency virus type 1 infection. J Virol 68:4650, 1994

69. Borrow P, Lewicki H, Hahn BH, et al: Virus-specific CD8+ cytotoxic T-lymphocyte activity associated with control of viraemia in primary human immunodeficiency virus type 1 infection. J Virol 68:6103, 1994

70. Yang OO, Kalams SA, Rosenzweig M, et al: Efficient lysis of human immunodeficiency virus type 1-infected cells by cytotoxic T lymphocytes. J Virol 67: 1707, 1993

71. Yasutomi Y, Reimann KA, Lord CI, et al: Simian immunodeficiency virus-specific CD8+ lymphocyte response in acutely infected rhesus monkeys. J Virol 67: 1707, 1993

72. Borrow P, Lewicki H, Wei X, et al: Antiviral pressure exerted by HIV-1-specific cytotoxic T lymphocytes (CTLs) during primary HIV infection demonstrated by rapid selection of CTL escape virus. Nature Med 3:205, 1997

73. Musey L, Hughes J, Schacker T, et al: Cytotoxic-T-cell responses, viral load and disease progression in early human immunodeficiency virus type 1 infection. N Engl J Med 337:1267, 1997

74. Ogg GS, Jin X, Bonhoeffer S, et al: Quantitation of HIV-1-specific cytotoxic T lymphocytes and plasma load of viral RNA. Science 279:2103, 1998

75. Pantaleo G, Demarest JF, Schacker T, et al: The qualitative nature of the primary immune response to HIV infection is a prognosticator of disease progression independent of the initial level of plasma viremia. Proc Natl Acad Sci USA 94:254, 1997

76. Pantaleo G, Soudeyns H, Demarest JF, et al: Evidence for rapid disappearance of initially expanded HIV-specific CD8+ T cell clones during primary

HIV infection. Proc Natl Acad Sci USA 94:9848, 1997

77. Pantaleo G, Soudeyns H, Demarest JF, et al: Accumulation of human immunodeficiency virus-specific cytotoxic T lymphocytes away from the predominant site of virus replication during primary infection. Eur J Immunol 27:3166, 1997

78. Baier M, Werner A, Bannert N, et al: HIV suppression by interleukin-16. Nature 378:563, 1995

79. Cocchi F, de Vico AL, Garzino-Demo A, et al: Identification of RANTES, MIP-1a and MIP-1b as the major HIV-suppressive factors produced by CD8+ T cells. Science 270:1811, 1995

80. Mackewicz CE, Yang LC, Lifson JD, Levy JA: Noncytolytic CD8 T-cell anti-HIV responses in primary HIV-1 infection. Lancet 344:1671, 1994

81. Daar ES, Moudgil T, Meyer RD, Ho DD: Transient high levels of viremia in patients with primary human immunodeficiency virus type I infection. N Engl J Med 324:961, 1991

82. Teeuwsen VJP, Siebelink KHJ, de Wolf F, et al: Impairment of in vitro immune responses occurs within 3 months after HIV-1 seroconversion. AIDS 4:77, 1990

83. Terpstra FG, AI BMJ, Roos MTL, et al: Longitudinal study of leukocyte function in homosexual men seroconverted for HIV: Rapid and persistent loss of B cell function after HIV infection. Eur J Immunol 19:667, 1989

84. Albert J, Abrahamsson B, Nagy K, et al: Rapid development of isolate-specific neutralizing antibodies after primary HIV-1 infection and consequent emergence of virus variants which resist neutralization by autologous sera. AIDS 4:107, 1990

85. Boucher CAB, de Wolf F, Houweling JTM, et al: Antibody response to a synthetic peptide covering a LAV-I/HTLV-IIIB neutralization epitope and disease progression. AIDS 3:71, 1989

86. Tsang MI, Evans LA, McQueen P, et al: Neutralizing antibodies against sequential autologous human immunodeficiency virus type 1 isolates after seroconversion. J Infect Dis 170:1141, 1994

87. Pilgrim AK, Pantaleo G, Cohen OJ, et al: Neutralizing antibody responses to human immunodeficiency virus type 1 in primary infection and long-term-nonprogressive infection. J Infect Dis 176:924, 1997

88. Bolognesi DP: Prospects for prevention of and early intervention against HIV. JAMA 261:3007, 1989

89. von Sydow M, Gaines H, Sonnerborg A, et al: Antigen detection in primary HIV infection. Br Med J 296:238, 1988

90. Gaines H, von Sydow MAE, von Stedingk LV, et al: Immunological changes in primary HIV infection. AIDS 4:995, 1990

91. Sonnerborg AB, von Stedingk L-V, Hansson L-O, Strannegard OO: Elevated neopterin and beta2-microglobulin levels in blood and cerebrospinal fluid occur early in HIV-1 infection. AIDS 3:277, 1989

92. von Sydow M, Sonnerborg A, Gaines H, Strannegard O: Interferon-alpha and tumor necrosis factor in serum of patients in varying stages of HIV-1 infection. AIDS Res Hum Retroviruses 7:375, 1991

93. Graziosi C, Gantt KR, Vaccarezza M, et al: Kinetics of cytokine expression during primary human immunodeficiency virus type 1 infection. Proc Natl Acad Sci USA 93:4386, 1996

94. Ruprecht RM, Chou T-C, Chipty F, et al: Interferon-alpha and 3′-azido-3′-deoxythymidine are highly synergistic in mice and prevent viremia after acute retrovirus exposure. J Acquir Immune Defic Syndr 3:591, 1990

95. Connor EM, Sperling RS, Gelber R, et al: Reduction of maternal-infant transmission of human immunodeficiency virus type 1 by zidovudine treatment. N Engl J Med 331:173, 1994

96. Cardo DM, Culver DH, Ciesielski CA, et al: A case-control study of HIV seroconversion in health care workers after percutaneous exposure. N Engl J Med 337:1485, 1997

97. McCune JM, Namikawa R, Shih C-C, et al: Suppression of HIV infection in AZT-treated SCIDhu mice. Science 247:564, 1990

98. Tsai CC, Follis KE, Sabo A, et al: Prevention of SIV infection in macaques by (R)-9-(2-phosphonylmethoxypropyl)adenine. Science 270:1197, 1995

99. Perrin L, Rakik A, Yerly S, et al: Combined therapy with zidovudine and L-697,661 in primary HIV infection. AIDS 10:1233, 1996

100. Lafeuillade A, Poggi C, Tamelet C, et al: Effects of a combination of zidovudine, didanosine and lamivudine on primary human immunodeficiency virus type 1 infection. J Infect Dis 175:1051. 1997

5 | Antiretroviral Adverse Effects and Interactions: Clinical Recognition and Management

SHANTEL M. MULLIN • CHRISTINE M. JAMJIAN • SPOTSWOOD L. SPRUANCE

Three classes of antiretrovirals are currently available for patient use: nucleoside reverse transcriptase inhibitors (NRTIs), non-nucleoside reverse transcriptase inhibitors (NNRTIs), and protease inhibitors (PIs). The combined use of these agents shows great promise in reducing viral load and increasing longevity; however, significant toxicities and drug–drug interactions complicate therapeutic decisions. Patients tend to be on multiple drug regimens (polypharmacy) for a variety of HIV-related conditions, and individuals with an AIDS diagnosis have a higher incidence of drug reactions than the general population. This chapter endeavors to list the most common and/or serious adverse effects and interactions of drugs used to treat HIV infection. The clinical management of these adverse effects and interactions is also described.

ADVERSE REACTIONS OF ANTIRETROVIRALS (Table 5–1)

Nucleoside Reverse Transcriptase Inhibitors

Zidovudine

The major toxicities associated with zidovudine are anemia and neutropenia.[1] They are inversely related to the CD4 lymphocyte count, hemoglobin concentration, and granulocyte count and directly related to dosage and duration of therapy.[2] Significant anemia most commonly occurs after 4 to 6 weeks of treatment. Granulocytopenia usually develops after 6 to 8 weeks of therapy. Therefore, frequent monitoring of complete blood counts with differentials, hemoglobin, and hematocrit is recommended during the first 8 weeks of treatment.[3]

Although lithium and hematopoietic factors (e.g., filgrastim, sargramostim) have been used in the management of neutropenia, the current data are insufficient to support the efficacy and safety of these agents. The treatment of severe anemia requires multiple blood transfusions. Erythropoietin is indicated for the treatment of anemia associated with zidovudine. The recommended dose is 100 U/kg intravenously or subcutaneously three times a week for 8 weeks. If the response is not adequate after 8 weeks, the dose can be increased by 50 to 100 U/kg three times a week. Doses higher than 300 U/kg three times a week are unlikely to be effective. Patients with low baseline endogenous erythropoietin concentrations (≤ 500 IU/L) tend to respond better to erythropoietin.[4,5]

Severe headache, myalgia, nausea, malaise, and insomnia also may occur in zidovudine-treated patients. These side effects tend to wane despite continued therapy.[6] Seizures, macular edema, and the Stevens-Johnson syndrome were reported with zidovudine, although the causal relationship is uncertain.[7] Zidovudine was also associated with rare but potentially fatal cases of lactic acidosis in the absence of hypoxemia, in addition to severe hepatomegaly with steatosis. If a patient receiving zidovudine develops tachypnea, dyspnea, or a fall in serum bicarbonate concentrations, lactic acidosis should be suspected and the drug should be discontinued. Caution should also be exercised when zidovudine is prescribed to patients with hepatomegaly, hepatitis, or other risk factors for liver disease.[8]

TABLE 5–1. Adverse Effects of Antiretroviral Agents

DRUG	MAJOR ADVERSE REACTIONS
Zidovudine (AZT, ZDV)	Anemia, neutropenia, myopathy, anorexia, nausea, fatigue, headache, malaise, myalgia, insomnia
Didanosine (ddI)	Pancreatitis, peripheral neuropathy, hyperamylasemia, diarrhea (caused by antacid), hyperuricemia, transaminase elevation
Zalcitabine (ddC)	Peripheral neuropathy, pancreatitis, vomiting, rash, stomatitis
Stavudine (d4T)	Peripheral neuropathy, pancreatitis, arthralgia, hypersensitivity, myalgia, asthenia, gastrointestinal disturbances, headache, and insomnia
Lamivudine (3TC)	Rash, cough, dizziness, fatigue, gastrointestinal distress, headache, insomnia, and hair loss. (The pancreatitis and peripheral neuropathy are more common in pediatric patients)
Nevirapine	Severe rash, headache, nausea, fever, and elevated γ-glutamyltranspeptidases
Delavirdine	Moderate to severe rash, headache, fatigue, nausea, vomiting, and increased liver function test values
Saquinavir	Diarrhea, abdominal discomfort, nausea, asthenia, rash, paresthesia, elevated transaminases, hypertriglyceridemia
Indinavir	Nephrolithiasis, dyslipidemias (Crixbelly), asymptomatic hyperbilirubinemia, abdominal pain, asthenia/fatigue, flank pain, malaise, nausea, diarrhea, vomiting, anorexia, dry mouth, headache, insomnia, dizziness, somnolence, and taste perversion
Ritonavir	Nausea, vomiting, diarrhea, asthenia, taste perversion, circumoral paresthesia, headache, dyslipidemias, hyperglycemia
Nelfinavir	Diarrhea, abdominal pain, nausea, flatulence, rash

Didanosine (2′,3′-Dideoxyinosine)

The major clinical toxicities associated with didanosine therapy include peripheral neuropathy and pancreatitis. In a Phase I study,[9] reversible neuropathy was related to both daily dosage and total dose of drug administered. The incidence of neuropathy was 34% of all Phase I patients treated with doses at or below the currently recommended dose but was 14.2% in controlled trials. Didanosine-associated neuropathy includes a tingling, burning, or aching sensation in the hands and lower extremities, especially the soles of the feet. An intermittent, shooting "electrical" pain in the legs that lasts for longer than 1 hour is also described. The drug should be withheld in individuals developing severe neuropathic pain. Two to 12 weeks may be required before the peripheral neuropathy subsides. After the drug is discontinued, the pain tends to progress or worsen before it improves.[10] The drug can be restarted at a lower dose in those patients whose pain abates.

In one study, acute pancreatitis occurred in 5 of 37 patients (13.5%)[9] and was not clearly related to the dose of didanosine. In the U.S. Expanded Access Program, 13.8% of 166 persons developed pancreatitis, of whom 2 died.[11] However, in randomized controlled trials, frequency of pancreatitis has been lower, approximately 2.3%. Predisposing factors to the development of pancreatitis with administration of didanosine include alcohol ingestion, a prior history of pancreatitis, advanced HIV disease, and low CD4 count (<50 cells/mm³).[12] Pancreatitis normally occurs during the first 1 to 6 months of didanosine therapy and resolves within 1 to 3 weeks after discontinuing the drug. Patients present with symptoms of vague abdominal pain, nausea, and vomiting. Certain patients also experience an increase in serum triglyceride or glucose concentrations prior to the onset of pancreatitis. Amylase and lipase concentrations should be checked at baseline and then periodically or as needed if pancreatitis is suspected.

Retinal changes, optic neuritis,[13] and fulminant hepatitis[14] have been associated with didanosine therapy. Patients should undergo periodic retinal examinations. Other dose-limiting toxicities include elevation in liver function test (LFT) values, diarrhea, and asymptomatic hyperuricemia.

Zalcitabine

The most common adverse effect reported with zalcitabine is a dose-dependent sensorimotor peripheral neuropathy, with a "stocking–glove" distribution primarily in the feet, occurring in 17% to 31% of treated patients.[15,16] The neuropathy experienced with zalcitabine is characterized by numbness and burning dysesthesia.[17] These symptoms usually become apparent during the first 7 to 24 weeks of therapy. If the drug is continued despite complaints, sharp shooting pains or severe continuous burning pain may develop, requiring opiate analgesics for relief. In addition, patients may experience gait disturbances. When the drug is stopped, pain may progress or worsen for an additional 3 to 4 weeks. Recovery might require up to 3 to 18 weeks following interruption of therapy.[17,18] Damage can become irreversible if the drug is not discontinued or the dose reduced (0.375 mg three times per day) as soon as the initial manifestations are noted. Other potential adverse effects include esophageal ulceration,[19] congestive cardiomyopathy,[20] arthralgias,[15] and dermatologic eruptions.[21] Rash occurs fairly commonly and develops during the first 4 to 6 weeks of therapy, but usually resolves despite continued therapy.[21] There are isolated case reports of acute pancreatitis caused by zalcitabine, but the incidence is less than 1%. However, caution must be observed in patients with a prior history of pancreatitis and in those with other risk factors for pancreatitis, such as alcohol abuse. Baseline serum amylase and lipase concentrations should be checked in these situations.[16]

Stavudine

The most frequently reported adverse effect with stavudine is peripheral neuropathy. Peripheral neuropathy occurs in 15% to 21% of patients treated with stavudine. As with zalcitabine, the neuropathy is characterized by numbness, tingling, or pain in the feet or hands. The drug should be withdrawn promptly at the onset of neuropathy. Patients should be counseled that symptoms may get worse when the drug is discontinued. Once the neuropathy resolves, the drug can be resumed at half the recommended dose (15 to 20 mg twice daily).[22,23]

Fewer than 1% of patients enrolled in clinical trials developed pancreatitis. Other adverse effects that occur less frequently with stavudine include arthralgia, hypersensitivity, myalgia, anemia, asthenia, gastrointestinal (GI) disturbances, headache, and insomnia.[23] One case report of fatty liver has been published.[24]

Lamivudine

In one study, 14 of 97 pediatric patients (14%) being treated with lamivudine monotherapy developed pancreatitis. Pancreatitis was seen in only 3 of 656 adult patients (<0.5%) who received lamivudine. Paresthesias and peripheral neuropathy are also reported, and occur more frequently in children. Other adverse effects that have been reported include rash, cough, dizziness, fatigue, GI distress, headache, insomnia, and hair loss.[25]

Non-nucleoside Reverse Transcriptase Inhibitors

Nevirapine

The major adverse effect associated with nevirapine is rash, which occurs in 33% of patients. Stevens-Johnson syndrome, which may be a severe and even life-threatening reaction, may develop in up to 0.5% of patients.[26-28] Most rashes reported in clinical trials were mild to moderate, maculopapular, erythematous cutaneous eruptions, with or without pruritus, located on the trunk, face, and extremities.[29] Although 7% of patients stopped taking nevirapine because of rash development, only 1% with mild to moderate rashes stopped the drug.[26,27]

A lead-in period for dosing appears to decrease the frequency of rash. Patients should initially receive 200 mg/day for 14 days. If the drug is tolerated with no rash developing, the dose can be increased to 200 mg twice daily. If mild to moderate rash (e.g., erythema, pruritus, diffuse erythematous macular or maculopapular cutaneous eruption) develops, nevirapine can still be continued but the dose should not be increased until the rash abates. This type of rash requires about 2 to 4 weeks before complete resolution.[26] In the case where nevirapine is withheld for longer than 7 days, the agent should be reintroduced at the lower dose of 200 mg/day for 14 days. If a patient develops urticaria, the same guidelines for mild to moderate rash management should be followed; however, if therapy is interrupted, nevirapine cannot be reintroduced. If severe rash (e.g., extensive erythematous or maculopapular rash or moist desquamation, angioedema, serum sickness—like reactions, Stevens-Johnson syndrome, toxic epidermal necrolysis) or rash accompanied by constitutional symptoms (e.g., fever >39°C, edema, myalgia/arthralgia, lymphadenopathy, general malaise, LFT value elevations) develops, the drug should be stopped immediately and should not be reinitiated. The rash usually develops within the first 6 weeks of therapy; patients should be monitored carefully during that period.

Liver toxicity was also noted with nevirapine. Any moderate or severe LFT value elevation necessitates discontinuing the drug. When the LFT values return to normal, the medication can be reintroduced at a lower dose. If the LFT values increase again, the drug should be stopped permanently. Other common side effects noted with nevirapine include headache, nausea, fever, and elevated γ-glutamyltranspeptidase (GGT).[29,30]

Delavirdine

As with nevirapine, rash is the most common adverse effect noted with delavirdine and generally occurs within the first 3 weeks of therapy.[31,32] Rash rarely develops after 1 month of therapy, and, unlike nevirapine, dose escalation is not useful in reducing the incidence of rash. In Phase II/III trials, 18% of subjects presented with rash, with fewer than 5% developing a severe rash (e.g., grade 3 or 4), including Stevens-Johnson syndrome. Rash is associated with a lower CD4 count. Skin reactions generally present as diffuse, maculopapular, erythematous, pruritic lesions located on the upper body and proximal arms, with decreasing intensity on the neck, face, trunk, and limbs. Symptoms associated with the rash respond to oral antihistamines (e.g., diphenhydramine, hydroxyzine) and/or topical corticosteroids, and rashes tend to resolve within 10 to 14 days of onset. Patients should be advised to stop delavirdine therapy and call their physician at the first sign of severe rash with fever, oral lesions, blistering, arthralgia, myalgia, or swelling.[32]

Other reactions occurring in more than 2% of patients include headache, fatigue, nausea, vomiting, and increased LFT values. These reactions may be moderate to severe, and prescribers and pharmacists should educate patients on how to recognize these toxicities when they occur. In addition, patients receiving a combination of delavirdine with PIs should be monitored frequently for the development of hepatotoxicity (e.g., elevated LFT values).[32]

Protease Inhibitors

Saquinavir

Saquinavir was initially studied as an adjunct to NRTI therapy in a hard capsule formulation. Recently a soft-gel capsule (SGC) replaced the original formulation, improving saquinavir absorption and increasing the potential for dose-related adverse effects.[33] Saquinavir produced diarrhea, nausea, abdominal discomfort, flatulence, and rash in several studies.[33,34] In an open-label safety study of 442 patients, significantly elevated LFT values (i.e., aspartate transaminase, alanine transaminase, and GGT values

more than 5 times the upper limit of normal) occurred in approximately 4% to 6% of patients; however, fewer than 1% of patients discontinued the SGC for these abnormalities. Other laboratory abnormalities included hyper- and hypoglycemia, hypertriglyceridemia, and elevated calcium, potassium, and creatine kinase levels. Rarely, patients developed anemia, thrombocytopenia, jaundice, or severe skin rashes.[33]

When prescribing saquinavir, providers should evaluate baseline and follow-up chemistry and hematology panels, particularly LFT values, triglyceride levels, and blood sugar levels. Saquinavir should be discontinued for significant aberrations in blood chemistries if no other explanation of the alteration can be found. Rechallenge is recommended when the initial event was not life threatening.

Indinavir

In the initial safety and efficacy studies of indinavir, more than 2% of patients developed abdominal pain, asthenia, fatigue, nausea, diarrhea, insomnia, and taste perversion.[35] These reactions tend to be tolerable and may diminish with time. Indinavir may also produce mild elevations in bilirubin concentration that are not associated with liver damage or hepatitis.[35,36]

The most common, preventable adverse effect of indinavir is nephrolithiasis, which presents with flank pain with or without hematuria in approximately 4% of patients within the first year of treatment.[35] The formation of stones is generally painful but does not produce any permanent renal damage. The renal calculus is largely composed of a urinary precipitate of pure indinavir.[37] Patients should be advised to drink 1.5 liters (48 oz) of fluid daily to prevent the development of stones. Patients should also stop indinavir therapy and call their physician immediately when severe back pain or bloody urine develops.[35,38]

In postmarketing reports, indinavir was associated with a redistribution of subcutaneous fat, resulting in increased abdominal girth and reduced fat in the arms and legs that is commonly referred to as "Crix-belly."[39,40] All patients on indinavir may develop a collection of fat on the back commonly called a buffalo hump, and women may also experience breast swelling.[41,42] The reaction is similar to the lipid redistribution noted with Cushing's syndrome, however, the mechanism of altered fat distribution is not understood.

Ritonavir

Ritonavir is the least tolerated protease inhibitor: 4% to 17% of patients discontinue the drug within the first few weeks of therapy because of adverse reactions.[43,44] The most frequently reported adverse effects of ritonavir include nausea, diarrhea, vomiting, anorexia, abdominal pain, taste perversion, and circumoral and peripheral paresthesias.[45] Patients should be informed that these effects tend to be mild to moderate and diminish with time in most cases. Additionally, clinicians should monitor patients for significant elevations in triglycerides, blood glucose, and LFT values.[45]

Ritonavir's dose-related adverse effects are diminished by two methods. First, ritonavir is initiated and slowly titrated to full dose within 2 weeks, starting at no less than 300 mg twice daily and increasing by 100-mg twice daily increments to 600 mg twice daily. Additionally, when ritonavir and one or more reverse transcriptase inhibitors are to be taken simultaneously, fewer GI effects are noted when ritonavir is started first, followed by the other agents within 1 to 2 weeks. Second, ritonavir must be taken with food, both for improved bioavailability and for decreased nausea and vomiting.[36,45]

Nelfinavir

Nelfinavir is the best tolerated protease inhibitor. The most notable side effect of nelfinavir is diarrhea, which occurs in up to 40% of patients and is generally controlled with oral antidiarrheal agents (e.g., loperamide).[46,47] In addition to diarrhea, more than 2% of patients may develop abdominal pain, nausea, flatulence, or rash.[47]

Adverse Reactions Potentially Associated with PIs

As of May 1997, over 80 cases of hyperglycemia were reported to the Food and Drug Administration (FDA) involving each of the four PIs, 27 of which required hospitalization. As a result, the FDA issued a public health advisory warning to health care providers to use PIs cautiously.[48] The patients involved were diagnosed not only with exacerbation of existing diabetes but with new-onset diabetes mellitus, which was recently confirmed for all four PIs.[49] As a result, all patients starting PI therapy should be taught to watch for the symptoms of hyperglycemia (e.g., fatigue, polyuria, and polydipsia). Patients who take insulin should increase their monitoring of glucose levels for a few weeks after a PI is initiated.

In addition to hyperglycemia, patients taking PIs tend to develop hypercholesterolemia and hypertriglyceridemia within a few weeks of initiation.[33,45,47,50] Several case reports have been published describing vascular complications in patients receiving PIs including angina pectoris, myocardial infarction, and ischemia.[50a,50b,50c]

The mechanism by which PIs cause peripheral lipodystrophy and hyperlipidemia is not fully elucidated. One hypothesis is that these agents contain a catalytic region that is about 60% homologous to regions within two proteins that regulate the lipid metabolism. PIs may alter these proteins and lead to hyperlipidemia.[50d]

Recently, clinicians noted increased bleeding in patients with hemophilia types A and B treated with PIs. By January 1997, 55 cases had been reported worldwide, including hemarthrosis, hematomas, and intracranial bleeds.[51,52] Some patients required additional Factor VIII to stop bleeding, and clinicians should warn hemophiliac patients to note any increase in bleeding or bruising when initiating PI therapy.[53]

DRUG–DRUG INTERACTIONS

Patients with HIV infection commonly use multiple-drug regimens. As the number of drugs increases, the risk for drug–drug interactions also increases. Drug–drug interactions are classified as either pharmacodynamic or pharmacokinetic based on the nature of the interaction.

Pharmacodynamic Interactions

Pharmacodynamic interactions occur when the therapeutic effect or adverse effect of one agent is amplified (synergy) or diminished (antagonism) by another agent without alterations in drug concentration or distribution in the body. For example, the concomitant use of two agents that may cause nephrotoxicity (e.g., aminoglycosides and amphotericin) will increase the potential for renal toxicity.[54,55]

Pharmacokinetic Interactions

Pharmacokinetic interactions (Table 5–2) include altered absorption, protein binding, metabolism, or excretion of one drug by another,

TABLE 5–2. Pharmacokinetic Drug Interaction Mechanisms

MECHANISMS OF DRUG INTERACTIONS	EXAMPLES
Absorption	Excipients in the didanosine tablet formulation bind to fluoroquinolones to form nonabsorbable chelates.
Gastric motility	Metoclopramide reduces digoxin absorption from the GI tract by decreasing GI motility.
Gastric pH	Ketoconazole requires an acidic pH for appropriate dissolution. Histamine$_2$ antagonists and didanosine decrease the absorption of ketoconazole.
Gastric bacterial flora	Certain antibiotics can reduce the enterohepatic circulation of oral contraceptives, leading to a decreased efficacy.
Protein binding	The addition of chloral hydrate to warfarin therapy can lead to a transient increase in warfarin hypothrombinemic effect by displacing warfarin from protein binding sites.
Excretion	The renal tubular secretion of cidofovir can be reduced by the addition of probenecid.

and are the primary source of most interactions noted with HIV drug treatments.

Absorption

Several mechanisms affect how GI absorption of one drug may influence another. Certain drugs act as adsorbents and prevent the passage of other drugs through the intestinal wall. Other medications form insoluble, nonabsorbable complexes or chelates with drugs. For example, cholestyramine and colestipol, bile-acid resins used to treat hypercholesterolemia, bind to other drugs and reduce their absorption. Drugs that affect GI motility can also modify the absorption of another agent. For instance, drugs that decrease gastric emptying will increase the bioavailability of agents that do not dissolve well in GI fluids. Gastrointestinal pH influences the absorption of several drugs that require a specific pH to be adequately absorbed. Bacterial flora present in the GI tract also play a role in the absorption of certain agents. Bacteria are involved in the deactivation and hydrolysis of certain drugs. The intestinal wall plays a role in the metabolism of certain drugs and therefore affects absorption.[55,56]

Distribution

The distribution of drugs to active sites in the body is largely affected by the degree to which these agents bind to plasma proteins. Drugs highly bound to plasma proteins have limited access to the extravascular space and site of drug action. When two highly protein-bound drugs (>90%) are administered concomitantly, an increase in the free plasma concentration of one of the two drugs can occur. Drug interactions involving highly protein-bound agents usually cause a transient increase in plasma concentrations of free drug. Only those drugs with restrictive clearance and narrow therapeutic indices may cause a significant and toxic elevation in free drug. Restrictive clearance implies that only free drug is cleared or metabolized by the liver. Drugs that influence metabolism as well as protein binding tend to have the most significant interactions.[55,57]

Excretion

Interactions related to modified drug excretion occur primarily in the kidney. Several acidic and basic drugs are subject to renal tubular secretion. Secretion is achieved by the anion or cation binding to a specific protein before it is excreted. Interactions occur at this level when two agents compete for the same transport protein, resulting in accumulation of one or both interacting drugs. An example of a beneficial interaction is probenecid binding to the transport protein necessary for cidofovir (Vistide) elimination. As a result, higher cidofovir blood concentrations are achieved for treating cytomegalovirus infection. Passive renal tubular reabsorption can also affect drug excretion. For instance, alkalinization of the urine can increase the excretion of a weak acid (e.g., aspirin).[55]

Hepatic Biotransformation

Interference with drug metabolism is the most common cause of serious drug interactions with the NNRTIs and PIs. In order to clear most lipophilic drugs, hepatic enzymes transform them into substances that are more easily removed from the body. This is accomplished by two general classes of enzyme reactions, designated Phase I and Phase II. Phase I reactions oxidize, reduce, or hydrolyze the drug or other foreign substance. Phase II reactions then link these metabolites with highly water-soluble molecules (e.g., glucuronides) that have low protein binding and are rapidly removed by the kidney.[58] Most significant drug–drug interactions with NNRTIs and PIs involve phase I reactions mediated by a group of heme-containing micro-oxygenases called the cytochrome P-450 (CYP) isoenzymes. Over 90% of drug oxidation in humans is attributed to six CYP isoforms designated 1A2, 2C9/10, 2C19, 2D6, 2E1, and 3A4.[54,59,60]

Substrates of these micro-oxygenase enzymes (e.g., NNRTIs or PIs) may induce or inhibit CYP enzyme function. Chemicals that induce either CYP or phase II reaction enzymes, such as phenobarbital and rifampin, do so by increasing the de novo production of the isoenzyme. This tends to take place over an extended period of time (i.e., days to weeks) of exposure to the drug or environmental pollutant.[54,61] As the number of enzymes increases, other substrates of the enzyme are more efficiently biotransformed and eliminated from the body, resulting in therapeutic failure.

Unlike enzyme induction, inhibition of enzymes by drugs such as ketoconazole occurs immediately and may result in toxic concentrations of co-administered medications. Patients avoid severe health consequences by using alternative medications not affected by enzyme induction or by adjusting doses based on expected increases or decreases in drug concentration.

Enzyme inhibition accounts for the majority of interactions with the newest classes of HIV medications. The PIs and delavirdine utilize the CYP3A enzyme family for metabolism to active and inactive metabolites, and the high affinity of these agents for CYP3A may result in competitive inhibition of the metabolism of other medications oxidized by this pathway. For example, the use of PIs with cisapride (Propulsid) may result in the prevention of cisapride metabolism, increased blood concentrations, and possibly arrhythmias and death.

In addition to CYP3A4 inhibition, ritonavir also inhibits other enzymes in the CYP2C9, 2C19, 2D6, and 3A3 subgroups to varying degrees. This accounts for the larger number of potential interactions with this medication as compared with the other PIs.

Both ritonavir and nevirapine induce the subsets of enzymes in the CYP3A family, and ritonavir alone induces CYP1A2 activity. Induction of enzyme activity by nevirapine or ritonavir may decrease the blood concentrations of other agents that are metabolized by one of these isoenzymes. For example, nevirapine may induce enzymes responsible for the metabolism of oral contraceptives, resulting in reduced efficacy and an increased risk of pregnancy.

The following sections provide information on common drug–drug interactions with each agent used to treat HIV infection. The clinical management of each interaction is also described.

Nucleoside Reverse Transcriptase Inhibitors (Table 5–3)

Zidovudine

Zidovudine is rapidly absorbed from the GI tract, with a bioavailability of 65%. Thirty-four percent to 38% of the drug is bound to plasma proteins. Zidovudine is predominantly metabolized to the inactive metabolite 5′-glucuronyl zidovudine by the uridine diphosphoglucuronosyltransferase system. A small quantity of zidovudine is converted to 3′-amino-3′-deoxythymidine (AMT), which may play a role in the cytotoxicity reported with the parent drug.[62] Zidovudine and its metabolites are eliminated renally by glomerular filtration and tubular secretion. Drug interactions with zidovudine are mainly due to interference with glucuronidation and renal excretion of the parent compound, as well as additive or synergistic side effects.[63,64]

Several drugs can inhibit the glucuronidation of zidovudine, which can result in an elevation in serum zidovudine and AMT concentrations and therefore increase the risk for adverse effects. Drugs that have been shown to decrease the glucuronidation of zidovudine include aspirin, atovaquone,[65] fluconazole,[66] indomethacin,[67] interferon-β and -β1A,[68] methadone,[69] phenytoin,[70] probenecid,[58,71,72] and valproic acid.[73] The use of zidovudine with any of the above-listed agents is not contraindicated. Appropriate monitoring should be established to circumvent any problems arising from highly elevated serum concentrations.

Rifampin enhances zidovudine glucuronidation, which can result in a drop in serum concentrations and therapeutic failure.[74] Zidovudine should not be administered with this agent. The manufacturer of rifabutin states that the antiretroviral effect of zidovudine may diminish when the two drugs are given together, but a recent study showed no clinically significant interaction.[74a]

The renal excretion of zidovudine can be diminished by several agents, including probenecid,[71,72] sulfamethoxazole, and trimethoprim.[75] Because only 14% to 18% of zidovudine is excreted unchanged by the kidney, this interaction becomes clinically significant only in the pres-

TABLE 5–3. NRTI Interactions*

NRTI	INTERACTING AGENTS
Didanosine (ddI, Videx)	Antacids, alcohol, chloramphenicol, cisplatin, dapsone, delavirdine, disulfiram, ethionamide, ganciclovir, glutethimide, gold, hydrazine, indinavir, iodoquinol, isoniazid, itraconazole, ketoconazole, metronidazole, nitrofurantoin, pentamidine (intravenous), phenytoin, quinolones, tetracycline, valproic acid, vincristine, zalcitabine
Lamivudine (3TC, Epivir)	Trimethoprim-sulfamethoxazole
Stavudine (d4t, Zerit)	**Ribavirin**, chloramphenicol, cisplatin, dapsone, didanosine, disulfiram, ethionamide, glutethimide, gold, hydrazine, iodoquinol, isoniazid, metronidazole, nitrofurantoin, phenytoin, vincristine
Zalcitabine (ddC, Hivid)	**Ribavirin**, alcohol, cimetidine, probenecid, chloramphenicol, cisplatin, dapsone, disulfiram, ethionamide, glutethimide, gold, hydrazine, iodoquinol, isoniazid, metronidazole, nitrofurantoin, pentamidine (intravenous), phenytoin, valproic acid, vincristine, zalcitabine
Zidovudine (AZT, ZDV, Retrovir)	**Ribavirin**, **rifampin**, **stavudine**, amphotericin B, aspirin, atovaquone, dapsone, doxorubicin, fluconazole, flucytosine, foscarnet, ganciclovir, indomethacin, interferon-α, interferon-β and -β1A, methadone, pentamidine, phenytoin, probenecid, pyrimethamine, sulfadiazine, trimethoprim-sulfamethoxazole, trimetrexate, rifabutin, valproic acid, vinblastine, vincristine

*Drugs in bold type should not be used in combination with the specified NRTI.

ence of agents that affect glucuronidation or in the presence of liver disease. The result is a rise in serum zidovudine concentrations that necessitates careful clinical and laboratory monitoring for increased incidence of toxicologic consequences.

Anemia and granulocytopenia are the most common adverse events associated with zidovudine. Agents with adverse hematologic effects similar to zidovudine can cause an additive or synergistic effect when combined with zidovudine. Anemia and neutropenia occur more frequently when zidovudine is used simultaneously with amphotericin B, dapsone, doxorubicin, flucytosine, foscarnet, ganciclovir,[76,77] interferon-α, interferon-β, interferon-β1A, pentamidine, pyrimethamine, sulfadiazine, trimethoprim-sulfamethoxazole, trimetrexate, vinblastine, or vincristine. The use of such drugs should be avoided, but, when no alternatives exist, frequent monitoring of hematocrit, hemoglobin, and white blood cell count with differential is recommended.

Two other drugs alter the pharmacodynamic activity of zidovudine. Ribavirin inhibits the phosphorylation of zidovudine to the active moiety that is responsible for its antiretroviral effect.[78] Therefore, these two agents should not be administered together. In addition, stavudine antagonizes the antiretroviral activity of zidovudine in peripheral blood mononuclear cells.[79] The concurrent use of these two drugs is not recommended.

Didanosine

Didanosine is acid labile, therefore, the commercially available preparations either are combined with buffering agents (magnesium hydroxide and dihydroaluminum sodium carbonate) or should be mixed with antacids prior to administration. Didanosine is rapidly absorbed after oral administration and has a bioavailability of 33% to 43%. The drug is less than 5% bound to plasma proteins. Although animal studies showed didanosine to be extensively metabolized, data in humans are lacking. Approximately 40% to 60% of didanosine is excreted unchanged in the urine after intravenous administration. The most common drug interactions noted with didanosine are due to altered absorption. Addictive or synergistic side effects are encountered when the drug is used with agents possessing a similar toxicologic profile.

The administration of didanosine with antacids was shown to increase bioavailability and potentially serum concentrations. Antacids reduce degradation of didanosine in the stomach by maintaining an elevated gastric pH.[80] Patients using antacids along with didanosine should be counseled about an increased risk for side effects. The use of didanosine with dapsone,[81] indinavir,[35] quinolones,[82,83] or tetracycline can lead to a reduced absorption of these agents. The buffer in the didanosine formulation can bind to these drugs and prevent dissolution and absorption. If these medications are prescribed with didanosine, they should be taken at least 2 hours apart. Quinolones should be taken 2 hours before or 6 hours after didanosine. The concomitant administration of didanosine and delavirdine reduces the area under the concentration–time curve (AUC) of both drugs by approximately 20%.[84] The current recommendation is to separate these two drugs by at least 1 hour.[32]

Itraconazole and ketoconazole require an acidic environment for adequate absorption. Therefore, when given simultaneously with didanosine, their serum concentrations can drop significantly, leading to therapeutic failure.[85] These agents should be taken 2 hours prior to ingesting didanosine.[86]

In a study evaluating the effect of ganciclovir on didanosine, the AUC of didanosine increased by 70% while its peak plasma concentration rose by 60%.[55] Therefore, the concomitant administration of these two agents requires careful monitoring for increased side effects of didanosine.

Certain drugs, when administered with didanosine, can increase the risk for peripheral neuropathies (e.g., chloramphenicol, cisplatin, dapsone, disulfiram, ethionamide, glutethimide, gold, hydrazine, iodoquinol, isoniazid, metronidazole, nitrofurantoin, phenytoin, vincristine, and zalcitabine). A higher potential for pancreatitis may occur when didanosine is co-administered with intravenous pentamidine, alcohol, zalcitabine, or valproic acid.[87] The use of any of these agents with didanosine is discouraged, but, when obligatory, patients should be monitored carefully for signs of toxicity.

Zalcitabine

Zalcitabine is greater than 80% bioavailable. The drug is not significantly metabolized by the liver. About 60% of an oral dose is excreted unchanged in the urine. Drug interactions with zalcitabine are mainly due to reduced renal clearance or to synergistic or additive adverse effects.[88]

Cimetidine and probenecid can decrease the renal tubular elimination of zalcitabine, which may result in an elevation in serum concentrations.[89] When placed on this combination, patients should be counseled about the increased risk for toxicity (e.g., peripheral neuropathies, pancreatitis). Dose reduction of zalcitabine may be necessary.

As with didanosine, the administration of zalcitabine with agents that cause peripheral neuropathies is discouraged. Similarly, the combination of zalcitabine with drugs that have the potential to cause pancreatitis should be avoided.[87,90]

Stavudine

Stavudine is rapidly absorbed from the GI tract, with a bioavailability of $86.4 \pm 18.2\%$. Protein binding is negligible. The metabolism of stavudine in humans has not been elucidated. The urinary excretion of unchanged drug accounts for about $39 \pm 23\%$. As a result, the only type of interactions expected with stavudine are pharmacodynamic in nature. Because peripheral neuropathy is the major clinical toxicity associated with stavudine, administration with neurotoxins, such as cisplatin, didanosine, and vincristine, may increase the overall frequency of neuropathies.[87]

Lamivudine

After oral administration, lamivudine shows rapid absorption. Lamivudine binding to plasma protein is low (<36%). The drug is not metabolized to a significant extent. Approximately 70% of the drug is excreted unchanged in the urine. The only reported interaction with lamivudine is with trimethropim-sulfamethoxazole. The AUC of lamivudine increased by 43% when the two agents were administered concomitantly for 5 days.[91] The mechanism of interaction was postulated to be a competitive inhibition of renal tubular secretion by trimethoprim. Lamivudine has no significant toxicity; therefore, this interaction is minor. The effect of higher doses of trimethoprim-sulfamethoxazole, such as those used to treat *Pneumocystis carinii* pneumonia, were not evaluated.[87,91]

Non-nucleoside Reverse Transcriptase Inhibitors (Table 5–4)

Nevirapine

More than 90% of a nevirapine dose is rapidly absorbed from the GI tract. Once absorbed, approximately 50% of a dose binds to plasma proteins. Autoinduction of CYP enzymes during the first 2 to 4 weeks of nevirapine therapy results in increased biotransformation and elimination from the body. Nevirapine is the only antiretroviral agent that acts exclusively as an inducer of CYP3A enzymes; as a result, this agent may reduce the concentrations of any CYP3A4-metabolized drug. Of particular concern is the possibility of reduced concentrations of oral

TABLE 5–4. NNRTI Interactions*

NNRTI	DRUG INTERACTIONS
Delavirdine (Rescriptor): CYP3A inhibitor, CYP2C9 inhibitor	INCREASED CONCENTRATION OF **alprazolam, amphetamines, astemizole, cisapride, dihydropyridines, calcium channel blockers (e.g., nifedipine), ergot derivatives, midazolam, quinidine, rifampin, terfenadine, triazolam**; clarithromycin, dapsone, fluoxetine, indinavir, ketoconazole, nelfinavir, rifabutin, saquinavir, warfarin DECREASED DELAVIRDINE CONCENTRATIONS WITH **carbamazepine, phenobarbital, phenytoin, rifabutin, rifampin**; antacids, didanosine, histamine₂ antagonists, nelfinavir
Nevirapine (Viramune): CYP3A inducer	INCREASED NEVIRAPINE CONCENTRATIONS WITH erythromycin, cimetidine REDUCED CONCENTRATIONS OF **ketoconazole, oral contraceptives**; indinavir, nelfinavir, rifampin, rifabutin, saquinavir

*Drugs in bold type should not be used in combination with the specificed NNRTI.

contraceptive, ketoconazole, and PIs. For patients taking hormonal contraceptives, alternative methods of contraception should be used while the patient is on concurrent nevirapine therapy. In a study of the effect of nevirapine on ketoconazole pharmacokinetics at steady state, median plasma AUC decreased 63% and maximum plasma concentration (C_{max}) decreased 40% as compared to baseline (Roxane Laboratories, Inc. Data on file. 1998). Combined use of nevirapine with ketoconazole is therefore contraindicated.

The original labeling for nevirapine indicated it should only be used with nucleoside analogs; however, recent studies demonstrate that interactions with the PIs may be managed by increased monitoring for efficacy or dosage adjustment. Minor reductions in AUC and C_{max} were noted with nelfinavir and ritonavir, whereas significant decreases in saquinavir AUC (27%) and indinavir AUC (28%) may necessitate an increase in the doses of these PIs to prevent therapeutic failure. When used with nevirapine, indinavir may be increased to 1000 mg three times daily to compensate for the interaction as long as the patient is able to accept the potential increase in adverse effects and drug cost. No recommendations are available for increasing the dose of the saquinavir SGC when used in combination with nevirapine.[27]

Potent inhibitors and inducers of CYP3A also affect nevirapine metabolism. Enzyme inhibitors, such as cimetidine and erythromycin, produce small increases in nevirapine concentrations. If alternative agents cannot be used, prescribers should monitor for increased nausea, headache, and LFT values associated with nevirapine toxicity. Both rifampin and rifabutin induce the metabolism of nevirapine, resulting in decreased steady-state through nevirapine

plasma concentrations of 37% when co-administered with rifampin and 16% when co-administered with rifabutin (Roxane Laboratories, Inc. Data on file. 1998). In a situation that requires the use of a rifamycin, rifabutin is the drug of choice for the patients also receiving nevirapine. Additional clinical and laboratory monitoring of therapeutic efficacy is recommended when either rifabutin or rifampin is added to nevirapine therapy.[27]

Delavirdine

Delavirdine is rapidly absorbed after oral administration. The drug is extensively bound to plasma proteins (98%). Delavirdine is primarily metabolized by cytochrome CYP3A. In vitro data suggest that CYP2D6 may also be involved in the metabolism of the drug. Less than 5% of delavirdine is recovered in the urine as unchanged drug. Studies showed that delavirdine can inhibit CYP3A, CYP2C9 and CYP2C19 activity.[32] Drug interactions reported with delavirdine are due to absorption and protein binding, as well as metabolism disturbances.[32]

In a single-dose study,[32] the AUC of delavirdine was reduced by $41\pm19\%$ in the presence of antacids. Therefore, antacids and delavirdine should be taken at least 1 hour apart. The use of long-term histamine₂ antagonists is also discouraged because of the potential for reduced delavirdine absorption.[32]

Because delavirdine is an inhibitor of CYP3A, co-administration with certain agents that are metabolized by this enzyme system is contraindicated as a result of toxic increases in plasma concentrations. Terfenadine, astemizole, sedative-hypnotics (i.e., alprazolam, midazolam, triazolam), dihydropyridine, calcium channel blockers (e.g., nifedipine), ergot alkaloid derivatives, amphetamines, cisapride, quinidine, and warfarin are contraindicated with delavirdine.[32]

The administration of delavirdine with PIs can increase both agents' serum concentrations as a result of CYP3A inhibition. When given with delavirdine, indinavir serum concentrations increased by twofold. Therefore a dose reduction of indinavir to 600 mg three times daily is warranted. The AUC of saquinavir increased by fivefold when it was combined with delavirdine. Currently, no recommendations for dosing adjustment are available when these two agents are used concomitantly. Ritonavir and delavirdine co-administration does not appear to alter the pharmacokinetics of either drug. Data from a prospective drug–drug interaction study in normal volunteers and a community practice setting showed that delavirdine increases nelfinavir steady-state plasma concentrations by up to 110%. Delavirdine plasma concentrations dropped by about 50%. Neutropenia was reported in two of the normal volunteers. Dosing adjustment when delavirdine is combined with nelfinavir is not recommended. Absolute neutrophil count should be monitored carefully when the combination of the two drugs is used.[32]

The concomitant use of delavirdine with CYP3A4 enzyme inducers (e.g., rifampin, rifabutin, phenytoin, phenobarbital, carbamazepine) is not recommended because of a substantial decrease in the delavirdine AUC. Delavirdine also increases the serum concentrations of rifampin.[32]

When combined with clarithromycin, delavirdine AUC increases by approximately 44%. When used with either fluoxetine or ketoconazole, delavirdine trough concentrations increase by about 50%. The clinical significance of these interactions is currently unknown. Patients should be counseled about an increased risk for adverse effects if these drugs are added to a regimen that includes delavirdine.[32]

PI Interactions

Pharmacokinetic Parameters (Table 5–5)

With the exception of saquinavir, the PIs are rapidly absorbed from the GI tract. Four percent of initial saquinavir formulations were absorbed on an empty stomach.[33] The SGC formulation had a 331% greater absorption,[33] and, as a result, is the preferred agent. Once absorbed, the lipophilic PI molecules bind to plasma proteins and undergo extensive metabolism in the liver to primarily inactive metabolites. These metabolites are removed by both bile and urine, with only 1% to 10% eliminated unchanged in the urine.

Common PI Interactions (Table 5–6)

The majority of significant drug–drug interactions with PIs occur as a result of enzyme inhibition. In recent studies, the relative potency of the PIs as inhibitors of CYP3A4 function ranked ritonavir first, followed by indinavir, saquinavir, and nelfinavir (in descending order of potency).[92,93] Medications metabolized by CYP3A4 potentially become elevated in plasma and target tissues when co-administered with a PI. Medications that become toxic when CYP3A enzymatic metabolism is blocked include astemizole, cisapride, ergot derivatives, midazolam, pimozide, and triazolam.[33,35,45,47,94] These medications should not be administered with PIs, and alternative agents should be selected. In a rep-

TABLE 5–5. Pharmacokinetic Parameters of PIs

PARAMETER	SAQUINAVIR (Invirase, Fortovase)	INDINAVIR (Crixivan)	RITONAVIR (Norvir)	NELFINAVIR (Viracept)
Absorption	4% (hard-shell cap)*[†]	Rapidly absorbed	80%[†]	Rapidly abosrbed[†]
Protein binding	97%	60%	99%	99%
Metabolism	Extensive (CYP3A); 2 inactive oxidative metabolites	Extensive (CYP3A4); 6 oxidative metabolites, 1 glucuronide metabolite	Extensive (CYP3A4 > 2D6); active oxidative metabolite isopropylthiazole (M-2)	Extensive (CYP3A); 1 active oxidative metabolite, several inactive metabolites
Elimination	1–3% urine UC 88% feces total	9.4% urine UC 19.1% feces UC 83% feces total	3.5% urine UC 11.4% urine total 86% feces total	1–2% urine UC 22% feces UC 99% feces total

UC = unchanged drug.
*The SGC is 331% more bioavailable than the hard-gel formulation.[33]
[†]Absorption is improved if taken with food.

TABLE 5–6. Contraindicated PI–Drug Combinations

CATEGORY	CONTRAINDICATED MEDICATIONS	RESULT OF CO-ADMINISTRATION
Antihistamines	Astemizole (Hismanal), terfenadine (Seldane)	Cardiotoxicity, torsades de pointes
Antipsychotics	Pimozide (Orap)	Cardiotoxicity, torsades de pointes
Ergot derivatives	Dihydroergotamine mesylate (D.H.E. 45)	Arrhythmia, vasospasm
Prokinetic agents	Cisapride (Propulsid)	Cardiotoxicity, torsades de pointes
Sedatives	Midazolam (Versed), triazolam (Halcion)	Oversedation, confusion

resentative case, a follow-up bone marrow biopsy requiring pretreatment with midazolam resulted in profound, prolonged sedation in a patient taking saquinavir. The reaction did not occur after the initial marrow biopsy with midazolam sedation 8 weeks prior; the only difference was the addition of saquinavir after the first biopsy.[95] This reaction could be prevented by selecting an alternative agent such as lorazepam or a short-acting barbiturate.

Induction of the CYP3A4 system by other medications also accounts for common interactions within the PI class (Table 5–7). Rifampin and rifabutin both induce the metabolism of PIs by CYP3A4 resulting in lower antiretroviral concentrations, development of viral resistance, and therapeutic failure.[33,35,45,47,96] Other enzyme inducers that patients should avoid while taking PIs include carbamazepine, phenobarbital, phenytoin, and dexamethasone.[97] When no alternative agents exist, however, increasing the doses of PIs may compensate for the interaction. At this time, no standard recommendations are available for dosage adjustments with these combinations.

Potent inhibitors of the CYP3A subfamily of enzymes include ketoconazole and erythromycin. These agents may increase PI concentrations and toxicity. While on ketoconazole or clarithromycin during PI therapy, patients should be cautioned to report any additional PI-related adverse effects to prescribers or pharmacists.[97]

Saquinavir

In addition to the drugs listed above, each PI has unique interactions. Most drugs that interact

TABLE 5–7. CYP3A4 Inducers

CATEGORY	DRUGS THAT MAY REDUCE PI EFFICACY
Antiepileptics	Carbamazepine, phenytoin, phenobarbital
Antimycobacterials	Rifampin, rifabutin
Corticosteroids	Dexamethasone

with saquinavir involve CYP3A4 enzyme inhibition. Saquinavir may elevate the blood concentration of calcium channel antagonists (e.g., amlodipine, diltiazem), clarithromycin, clindamycin, dapsone, and quinidine. Although these combinations may result in increased drug effect and adverse reactions, the interactions tend not to be significant and may be managed by monitoring patients for signs of increased adverse effects, and reducing the dose of combined medication accordingly.[33]

Drugs that induce or inhibit the activity of the CYP3A subfamily of enzymes may alter the concentration of saquinavir. Rifabutin and rifampin decrease saquinavir AUCs 43% and 84%, respectively, and are not recommended.[33] Ritonavir, conversely, inhibits saquinavir metabolism, resulting in a 121% increase in AUC after 14 days and a 17-fold greater AUC value for saquinavir after 4 weeks of combined therapy. In order to avoid toxicity and to benefit from therapeutic synergy, the dose of ritonavir is 400 mg twice daily with saquinavir SGC 400 mg twice daily. Nelfinavir increases saquinavir SGC exposure fivefold; however, the significance of this interaction is not known and no specific guidelines are available for dosing adjustment.[33,98] Ketoconazole, clarithromycin, and delavirdine increase saquinavir's AUC by 131%, 177%, and fivefold, respectively, with short-term co-administration. These increases are not generally associated with toxicity, however, patients taking the combinations should be monitored for saquinavir-induced adverse effects (e.g., elevated LFT values).[33]

Indinavir

Altered metabolism and absorption are the pharmacokinetic pathways responsible for indinavir's drug interactions. Indinavir, like saquinavir, inhibits CYP3A drug metabolism; however, it has stronger affinity for this enzyme. As a result, combined use of indinavir with saquinavir may result in a five- to eightfold increase in saquinavir concentrations. In vitro studies also suggest that indinavir and saquinavir have synergy at low concentrations; however, higher concentrations may be antagonistic, particularly in zidovudine-resistant viral isolates.[99] In addition to saquinavir, indinavir significantly reduces the metabolism of rifabutin, resulting in a 204% increase in rifabutin AUC and a 32% decrease in indinavir AUC due to enzyme induction.[35] This interaction is managed by reducing the rifabutin daily dose by half and by increasing indinavir's dose to 1000–1200 mg every 8 hours.

Agents that significantly alter indinavir concentrations in the blood require indinavir dosage adjustments. When used concomitantly with nevirapine, an enzyme inducer, indinavir may be dosed at 1000 mg three times daily. Conversely, delavirdine and ketoconazole inhibit indinavir metabolism, producing elevated indinavir concentrations and toxicity. When used with either medication, the indinavir dose is reduced to 600 mg three times daily.[35]

A commonly overlooked interaction with indinavir involves medications that alter indinavir absorption from the GI tract. Indinavir requires an acid medium to be well absorbed. When taken simultaneously with antacids or buffered agents (e.g., didanosine), indinavir absorption may be significantly reduced. Patients should be counseled to take these agents at least 1 hour apart.[35]

Ritonavir

Interactions with ritonavir fall into four general mechanistic categories: CYP enzyme inhibition/induction by ritonavir (phase I reactions), induction of ritonavir metabolism by other chemicals (phase I), glucuronosyltransferase induction by ritonavir (phase II), and disulfiram-type reactions.[45] A study by Kumar et al demonstrated ritonavir's high affinity for several CYP isoforms, resulting in inhibition of CYP3A, 2D6, and 2C, in descending order of inhibitory activity.[100] In a few cases, the inhibition of drug metabolism may result in dangerously elevated concentrations of medications, and alternative agents should be prescribed (Table 5–8). With ritonavir-inhibited drug metabolism, practitioners may avoid interactions by educating patients to note drug-related adverse reactions and reducing doses when these reactions occur. For example, ritonavir may inhibit amitriptyline (Elavil) metabolism, resulting in elevated blood concentrations that manifest as increased anticholinergic activity, sedation, and confusion. If these reactions are noted, the practitioner should

reduce the tricyclic dose based on amitriptyline levels and/or side effects.

In addition to CYP manipulation, ritonavir also increases the elimination of some agents that are directly glucuronidated following absorption. Induction of the glucuronosyltransferase enzymes by ritonavir may play a role in the reduced efficacy of drugs such as morphine and naproxen, and may necessitate higher dosing of these medications.[45]

Agents that induce ritonavir metabolism and potentially reduce efficacy include carbamazepine, dexamethasone, nevirapine, phenobarbital, phenytoin, rifampin, and tobacco. These medications may be used concomitantly only when alternatives do not exist. Monitoring antiretroviral efficacy (e.g., viral load) after initiating the combination is essential in determining whether to increase the dose of ritonavir or reduce the dose of the inducer.[45] Physicians and pharmacists should advise all patients who use tobacco to discontinue its use while taking ritonavir.

Finally, ritonavir's SGC and liquid formulations contain alcohol and may produce flushing, nausea, and palpitations when used with disulfiram (Antabuse).[45] Metronidazole (Flagyl) and chlorpropamide (Diabinese) produce disulfiram-like reactions and may induce these symptoms when used with ritonavir.

Nelfinavir

In addition to the general list of contraindicated medications, nelfinavir may not be used with oral contraceptives. When used concurrently with nelfinavir, norethindrone and ethinyl estradiol plasma concentrations decrease 18% and 47%, respectively. Patients should be advised to use an additional or alternative method of birth control while on nelfinavir. When used in combination with nelfinavir, half-dose rifabutin is warranted as well as an increase in nelfinir's dose to 1000 mg three times daily.[47]

Antiretroviral–Nutrient Interactions

The most clinically significant interactions that are reported between food and drugs include the absorption process. The presence of food in the GI tract can increase, delay, or decrease the absorption of antiretroviral medications. The mechanism of these interactions varies. Nutrients can directly bind to drugs, change luminal pH, affect gastric emptying, influence intestinal transit time, modify mucosal absorption, or alter splanchnic–hepatic blood flow.[101] For some

TABLE 5–8. Potential Drug–Drug Interactions Associated with Ritonavir

INTERACTION MECHANISM	INTERACTING DRUG OR DRUG CATEGORY		

Contraindicated Medication Combinations

CYP2C, 2D6, and/or 3A4 inhibition	Amiodarone	Estazolam	Propoxyphene
	Astemizole	Flecainide	Quinidine
	Bupropion	Flurazepam	Rifabutin
	Cisapride	Meperidine	Terfenadine
	Clorazepate	Midazolam	Triazolam
	Clozapine	Pimozide	Zolpidem
	Diazepam	Piroxicam	
	Encainide	Propafenone	

Drugs Requiring Additional Monitoring for Toxicity and/or Dosage Reductions

CYP2C, 2D6, and/or 3A4 inhibition	*Anti-infectives*	*Neuropsychiatric Agents*	*Sedative-Analgesics*
	Albendazole	Alprazolam	Alfentanil
	Chloroquine	Amitriptyline	Fentanyl
	Clarithromycin	Carbamazepine	Hydrocodone
	Erythromycin	Chlorpromazine	Methadone
	Itraconazole	Clomipramine	Nabumetone
	Ketoconazole	Clonazepam	Oxycodone
	Metronidazole	Desipramine	Sulindac
	Miconazole	Doxepin	Tramadol
	Nelfinavir	Ethosuximide	
	Primaquine	Fluvoxamine	*Miscellaneous*
	Pyrimethamine	Haloperidol	Cimetidine
	Quinine	Imipramine	Dexamethasone
	Rifampin	Maprotiline	Dronabinol
	Saquinavir	Nefazodone	Loratadine
		Nortriptyline	Methamphetamine
	Cardiovascular Agents	Paroxetine	Pentoxifylline
	Atrovastatin	Perphenazine	Prednisone
	β-Adrenergic blockers:	Prochlorperazine	
	acebutolol, metoprolol,	Promethazine	
	propranolol	Risperidone	
	Calcium channel antagonists:	Sertraline	
	amlodipine, diltiazem,	Thioridazine	
	nifedipine, verapamil	Trazodone	
	Digoxin	Venlafaxine	
	Disopyramide		
	Doxazosin	*Oncology/Hematology*	
	Fluvastatin	Cyclosporine	
	Gemfibrozil	Doxorubicin	
	Lidocaine	Etoposide	
	Lovastatin	Ondansetron	
	Mexiletine	Tacrolimus	
	Prazosin	Tamoxifen	
	Simvastatin	Vinblastine	
	Terazosin	Vincristine	
	Tocainide	Warfarin	

Drugs Requiring Additional Monitoring for Efficacy and/or Dosage Increases

Increased drug glucuronidation and elimination	Atovaquone	Hydromorphone	Metoclopramide
	Clofibrate	Ketoprofen	Morphine
	Codeine	Ketorolac	Naproxen
	Diphenoxylate	Lamotrigine	
Enhanced elimination	Oral contraceptives	Theophylline	Valproic acid

Drugs That May Significantly Reduce Ritonavir Concentrations

Induction of CYP enzymes	Carbamazepine	Phenobarbital	Rifampin
	Dexamethasone	Phenytoin	Tobacco
	Nevirapine		

TABLE 5–9. Recommended Dosing with Regard to Meals

TAKE ON AN EMPTY STOMACH	TAKE WITH FOOD	TAKE WITH OR WITHOUT FOOD	
Didanosine	Nelfinavir	Delavirdine*	Stavudine
Indinavir	Ritonavir	Lamivudine	Zalcitabine
	Saquinavir	Nevirapine	Zidovudine

*Delavirdine absorption may be enhanced when taken with acidic juices (e.g., orange or cranberry).

drugs, rapid absorption leads to saturation of CYP enzymes responsible for their metabolism and leading to significant blood concentrations of the agent; whereas nutritional circumstances that prolong absorption allow the enzymes to effect nearly complete degradation of the agent immediately after entering the bloodstream.

Zidovudine, zalcitabine, stavudine, lamivudine, nevirapine, and delavirdine can be administered with or without food (Table 5–9). Pharmacokinetic studies showed that the presence or absence of nutrients in the GI tract does not affect the AUC.[10,16,102,103] Although delavirdine pharmacokinetics are not affected by the presence of food, absorption is enhanced by the presence of acidic beverages (e.g., orange juice or cranberry juice).[32]

Didanosine and indinavir are the two agents that require administration on an empty stomach. Significant reductions in didanosine's AUC and C_{max} were reported when the drug was given with a meal or within 2 hours of a meal.[104,105] When indinavir was administered with a meal high in calories, fat, and protein, the AUC and C_{max} dropped by $77\pm8\%$ and $84\pm7\%$, respectively. Lighter meals (e.g., a meal of dry toast with jelly, apple juice, and coffee with skim milk and sugar, or a meal of corn flakes, skim milk, and sugar) did not produce any significant changes in AUC and C_{max}. Therefore, indinavir should be taken on an empty stomach. If the patient is unable to tolerate the drug on an empty stomach, lighter meals are acceptable.

Saquinavir, ritonavir, and nelfinavir are generally better absorbed when taken with a meal. In a study of saquinavir absorption with a "light" meal versus a "heavy" meal, the larger meal delayed absorption but resulted in a doubling of saquinavir oral absorption as measured by AUC and C_{max}.[106] When administered with a meal, ritonavir capsules produce a 15% increase in absorption. The absorption of the liquid ritonavir formulation may decrease 7% when taken with food; therefore, the liquid should be diluted in chocolate milk, Ensure, or Advera immediately prior to administration to avoid altered absorption while masking the ritonavir flavor.[45] In a study of absorption pharmacokinetics, nelfinavir absorption was 27% to 50% lower in fasting versus fed volunteers.[107] Patients should be counseled to schedule doses of saquinavir, ritonavir capsules, and nelfinavir with meals or snacks in order to maximize treatment benefit.

Grapefruit Juice

Recently, studies of grapefruit juice demonstrated inhibition of the CYP3A isoenzymes. Of particular concern is its use with saquinavir and indinavir. When grapefruit juice was taken within 1 hour following saquinavir, increases of 50% to 150% were noted. When grapefruit was taken within 1 hour following saquinavir, increases of 50% to 150% were noted in AUC.[108,108a] Indinavir's AUC, however, is noted to be decreased by 26% when taken with grapefruit juice.[108]

SUMMARY

Therapeutic agents used in the treatment of HIV infection produce a wide variety of adverse effects. In addition to antiretroviral therapy, most patients require a host of medications to treat both related and unrelated illnesses. Polypharmacy in this population requires practitioners to vigilantly manage drug toxicities and interactions that may compromise patient safety or therapeutic efficacy.

Three general rules apply in prescribing new drugs to HIV patients. First, prescribers must familiarize themselves with agents that are contraindicated with antiretroviral therapy and avoid their combined use. In almost all cases, alternative agents that do not interact with current therapies are available and should be utilized. Second, many drug–drug interactions may be managed by increasing or decreasing doses to compensate for altered drug concentrations. Finally, patients should be educated about the adverse effects of agents and when to contact their physician when these reactions occur. Patient feedback is essential for deciding when to stop medications, switch to alternative agents, or alter doses.

References

1. Fischl MA, Parker CB, Pettinelli C, et al: A randomized controlled trial of a reduced daily dose of zidovudine in patients with the acquired immunodeficiency syndrome. N Engl J Med 323:1009, 1990
2. Collier AC, Bozzette S, Coombs RW, et al: A pilot study of low-dose zidovudine in human immunodeficiency virus infection. N Engl J Med 323:1015, 1990
3. Retrovir® (zidovudine) package insert. Research Park Triangle, NC, Glaxo Wellcome; 1996
4. Kuehl AK, Noormohamed SE: Recombinant erythropoietin for zidovudine-induced anemia in AIDS. Ann Pharmacother 29:778, 1995
5. Perrella O, Finelli E, Perrella A, et al: Combined therapy with zidovudine, recombinant granulocyte colony stimulating factors and erythropoietin in asymptomatic HIV patients. J Chemother 8:63, 1996
6. Gelmon K, Montaner JSG, Fanning M, et al: Nature, time course and dose dependence of zidovudine-related side effects: Results from the Multicenter Canadian Azidothymidine Trial. AIDS 3:555, 1989
7. McLeod GX, Hammer SM: Zidovudine: Five years later. Ann Intern Med 117:487, 1992
8. Sundar K, Suarez M, Banogon PE, et al: Zidovudine-induced fatal lactic acidosis and hepatic failure in patients with acquired immunodeficiency syndrome: Report of two patients and review of the literature. Crit Care Med 25:1425, 1997
9. Lambert JS, Seidlin M, Reichman RC, et al: 2′,3′-Dideoxyinosine (ddI) in patients with the acquired immunodeficiency syndrome or AIDS-related complex. N Engl J Med 322:1333, 1990
10. Shelton MJ, Portmore A, Blum MR, et al: Prolonged but not diminished, zidovudine absorption induced by a high-fat breakfast. Pharmacotherapy 14:671, 1994
11. Steinberg JP, Gunthel CJ, White RL, et al: Outcomes and toxicities on 2′,3′-dideoxyinosine (ddI) in the expanded access program. In: Abstracts of the 31st Interscience Conference on Antimicrobial Agents and Chemotherapy, Chicago, 1991, Abstract 707
12. Whitefield RM, Bechtel LM, Starich GH: The impact of ethanol and Marinol/marijuana usage on HIV+/-AIDS patients undergoing azidothymidine, azidothymidine/dideoxycytidine, or dideoxyinosine therapy. Alcohol Clin Exp Res 21:122, 1997
13. Lafeuillade A, Aubert L, Chaffanjon P, et al: Optic neuritis associated with dideoxyinosine. Lancet 337:615, 1991
14. Lai KK, Gang DL, Zawacki JK, Cooley TP: Fulminant hepatic failure associated with 2′,3′-dideoxyinosine (ddI). Ann Intern Med 115:283, 1991
15. Merigan TC, Skowron G, for the ddC Study Group of the AIDS Clinical Trials Group of the National Institute for Allergy and Infectious Diseases: Safety and tolerance of dideoxycytidine as a single agent. Am J Med 88(Suppl 5B):11S, 1990
16. Hivid® (zalcitabine) package insert. Nutley, NJ, Roche Laboratories, 1996
17. Whittington R, Brogden RN: Zalcitabine: A review of its pharmacology and clinical potential in acquired immunodeficiency syndrome (AIDS). Drugs 44:656, 1992
18. Blum AS, Dal Pan GJ, Feinberg J, et al: Low-dose zalcitabine-related toxic neuropathy: Frequency, natural history, and risk factors. Neurology 46:999, 1996
19. Indorf AS, Pegram PS: Esophageal ulceration related to zalcitabine (ddC). Ann Intern Med 117:133, 1992
20. Herskowitz A, Willoughby SB, Baughman KL, et al: Cardiomyopathy associated with antiretroviral therapy in patients with human immunodeficiency virus infection: A report of 6 cases. Ann Intern Med 116:311, 1992
21. Broder S, Yarchoan R: Dideoxycytidine: Current clinical experience and future prospects. Am J Med 88(Suppl 5B):31S, 1990
22. Skowron G: Biologic effects and safety of stavudine: Overview of phase I and II clinical trials. J Infect Dis 171(Suppl 2):S113, 1995
23. Zerit® (stavudine) package insert. Princeton, NJ, Bristol-Meyers Squibb Immunology, 1996
24. Lenzo NP, Garas BA, French MA: Hepatic steatosis and lactic acidosis associated with stavudine treatment in an HIV patient: A case report [letter]. AIDS 11:1294, 1997
25. Epivir® (lamivudine) package insert. Research Triangle Park, NC, Glaxo Wellcome, 1997
26. Mascolini M: Nevirapine: New drug, new class, new questions. J Int Assoc Phys AIDS Care 2:8, 1996
27. Viramune® (nevirapine) package insert. Columbus, OH, Roxane Laboratories, 1996
28. D'Aquila RT, Hughes MD, Johnson VA, et al: Nevirapine, zidovudine, and didanosine compared with zidovudine and didanosine in patients with HIV-1 infections. Ann Intern Med 124:1019, 1996
29. Havlir D, Cheesman SH, McLaughlin M, et al: High-dose nevirapine: Safety, pharmacokinetics, and antiviral effects in patients with human immunodeficiency virus infection. J Infect Dis 171:537, 1995
30. Carr A, Vella S, de Jong MD, et al: A controlled trial of nevirapine plus zidovudine versus zidovudine alone in p24 antigenamic HIV-infected patients. AIDS 10:635, 1996
31. Freimuth WW: Delavirdine mesylate, a potent non-nucleoside HIV-1 reverse transcriptase inhibitor. In: Mills J, Volberding PA, Corey L (eds): Antiviral Chemotherapy 4. New York, Plenum Press, 1996, p 279
32. Rescriptor® (delavirdine mesylate) package insert. Kalamazoo, MI, Pharmacia & Upjohn, 1997
33. Fortovase® (saquinavir) package insert. Nutley, NJ, Roche Laboratories, 1997
34. Collier AC, Coombs RW, Schoenfeld DA, et al, for the AIDS Clinical Trials Group: Treatment of human immunodeficiency virus infection with saquinavir, zidovudine, and zalcitabine. N Engl J Med 334:1011, 1996
35. Crixivan® (indinavir) package insert. West Point, PA, Merck & Co, 1996
36. Deeks SG, Smith M, Holodniy M, et al: HIV-1 protease inhibitors: A review for clinicians. JAMA 277:145, 1997
37. Kopp JB, Miller KD, Mican JA, et al: Crystalluria and urinary tract abnormalities associated with indinavir. Ann Intern Med 127:119, 1997
38. Rich JD, Ramratnam B, Chiang M, et al: Management of indinavir associated nephrolithiasis. J Urol 158:2228, 1997
39. Hengel RL, Watts NB, Lennox JL: Benign symmetric lipomatosis associated with protease inhibitors [letter]. Lancet 350:1596, 1997

40. Miller K, Jones E, Yanovski J, et al: Increased intra-abdominal fat deposits in patients on indinavir. In: Abstracts of the 5th Conference on Retroviruses and Opportunistic Infections, Chicago, 1998, Abstract 413

41. Henry I, Bernard L, de Truchis P, et al: Hypertrophy of the breasts in a patient treated with indinavir. Clin Infect Dis 25:937, 1997

42. Mulligan K, Tai VW, Algren H, et al: Buffalo hump in HIV-infected patients on antiretroviral therapy. In: Abstracts of the 5th Conference on Retroviruses and Opportunistic Infections, Chicago, 1998, Abstract 409

43. Cameron W, Heath-Chiozzi M, Kravcik S, et al: Prolongation of life and prevention of AIDS in advanced HIV immunodeficiency with ritonavir. In Program and abstracts of the 3rd Conference on Retroviruses and Opportunistic Infections, Washington, DC, 1996, Abstract LB6a

44. Danner SA, Carr A, Leonard JM, et al, for the European-Australian Collaborative Ritonavir Study Group: A short-term study of the safety, pharmacokinetics, and efficacy of ritonavir, an inhibitor of HIV-1 protease. N Engl J Med 333:1528, 1995

45. Norvir® (ritonavir) package insert. North Chicago, IL, Abbott Laboratories, 1997

46. Gathe J, Burkhardt B, Hawley P, et al: A randomized phase II study of viracept, a novel HIV protease inhibitor, used in combination with stavudine versus stavudine alone. In Program and abstracts of the XIth International Conference on AIDS, Vancouver, 1996, Abstract MoB413

47. Viracept® (nelfinavir) package insert. La Jolla, CA, Agouron Pharmaceuticals, 1997

48. Nightingale SL: Public health advisory on protease inhibitors for HIV treatment. JAMA 278:377, 1997

49. Eastone JA, Decker CF: New-onset diabetes mellitus associated with use of protease inhibitor. Ann Intern Med 127:948, 1997

50. Sullivan AK, Nelson MR: Marked hyperlipidemia on ritonavir therapy [letter]. AIDS 11:938, 1997

50a. Behrens G, Schmidt H, Meyer D, et al: Vascular complications associated with use of HIV protease inhibitors. Lancet 351:1958, 1998

50b. Gallet B, Pulik M, Genet P, et al: Vascular complications associated with use of HIV protease inhibitors. Lancet 351:1958, 1998

50c. Vittecoq D, Escaut L, Monsuez JJ. Vascular complications associated with use of HIV protease inhibitors. Lancet 351:1959, 1998

50d. Carr A, Samaras K, Chisholm DJ. Pathogenesis of HIV-1 protease inhibitor-associated peripheral lipodystrophy, hyperlipidaemia, and insulin resistance. Lancet 351:1881, 1998

51. HIV protease inhibitors and increased bleeding in hemophilia [news]. CMAJ 156:90, 1997

52. Ginsburg C, Salmon-Ceron D, Vassilief D, et al: Unusual occurrence of spontaneous hematomas in three asymptomatic HIV-infected haemophilia patients a few days after the onset of ritonavir treatment. AIDS 11:388, 1997

53. FDA protease inhibitor letter urges monitoring of hemophiliacs [news]. FDC Rep 57:T&G 3, 1996

54. Benet LZ, Kroetz DL, Sheiner LB: Pharmacokinetics: The dynamics of drug absorption, distribution, and eliminiation. In Hardman JG, Limbird LE (eds): Goodman & Gilman's The Pharmacological Basis of Therapeutics, 9th ed. New York, McGraw-Hill, 1996, p 3

55. Hansten PD, Horn JR: Drug Interactions Analysis and Management. Vancouver, WA, Applied Therapeutics Inc, 1997

56. Welling PG: Interactions affecting drug absorption. Clin Pharmacokinet 9:404, 1984

57. Sansom LN, Evan AM: What is the true clinical significance of plasma protein binding displacement interactions? Drug Saf 12:227, 1995

58. Kroemer HK, Klotz U: Glucuronidation of drugs: A re-evaluation of the pharmacological significance of the conjugates and modulating factors. Clin Pharmacokinet 23:292, 1992

59. Guengerich FP: Role of cytochrome P450 enzymes in drug-drug interactions. Adv Pharmacol 43:7, 1997

60. Wrighton SA, Steven JC: The human hepatic cytochromes P450 involved in drug metabolism. Crit Rev Toxicol 22:1, 1992

61. Park BK, Breckenride AM: Clinical implications of enzyme induction and enzyme inhibition. Clin Pharmacokinet 6:1, 1981

62. Veal GJ, Back DJ: Metabolism of zidovudine. Gen Pharmacol 26:1469, 1995

63. Heylen R, Miller R: Adverse effects and drug interactions of medications commonly used in the treatment of adult HIV positive patients. Genitourin Med 72:237, 1996

64. Robertson-Dallas S, Read SE, Bendayan R: New drug interactions with zidovudine. Pharmacotherapy 17:1198, 1997

65. Lee BL, Tauber MG, Sadler B, et al: Atovaquone inhibits the glucuronidation and increases the plasma concentrations of zidovudine. Clin Pharmacol Ther 59:14, 1996

66. Sahai J, Gallicano K, Pakuts A, et al: Effect of fluconazole on zidovudine pharmacokinetics in patients infected with human immunodeficiency virus. J Infect Dis 169:1103, 1994

67. Barry M, Howe J, Back D, et al: The effects of indomethacin and naproxen on zidovudine pharmacokinetics. Br J Clin Pharmacol 36:82, 1993

68. Nokta M, Loh JP, Douidar SM, et al: Metabolic interaction of recombinant interferon-beta and zidovudine in AIDS patients. J Interferon Res 11:159, 1991

69. Schwartz EL, Brechbuhl AB, Kahl P, et al: Pharmacokinetic interactions of zidovudine and methadone in intravenous drug-using patients with HIV infection. J Acquir Immune Defic Syndr 5:619, 1992

70. Burger DM, Meenhorst PL, Napel CH, et al: Pharmacokinetic variability of zidovudine in HIV-infected individuals: Subgroup analysis and drug interactions. AIDS 8:1683, 1994

71. DeMiranda P, Good SS, Yarchoan R, et al: Alteration of zidovudine pharmacokinetics by probenecid in patients with AIDS or AIDS-related complex. Clin Pharmacol Ther 46:494, 1989

72. Kornhauser DM, Petty BG, Hendrix CW, et al: Probenecid and zidovudine metabolism. Lancet 2:473, 1989

73. Lertora JJ, Rege AB, Greenspan DL, et al: Pharmacokinetic interaction between zidovudine and valproic acid in patients infected with human immunodeficiency virus. Clin Pharmacol Ther 56:272, 1994

74. Burger DM, Meenhorst PL, Koks CH, et al: Pharmacokinetic interaction between rifampin and zidovudine. Antimicrob Agents Chemother 37:1426, 1993

74a. Li RC, Nightingale S, Lewis RC, et al: Lack of effect of concomitant zidovudine on rifabutin kinetics in patients with AIDS-related complex. Antimicrob Agents Chemother 40:1397, 1996

75. Chatton JY, Munafo A, Chave JP, et al: Trimethoprim, alone or in combination with sulphamethoxazole, decreases the renal excretion of zodivudine and its glucuronide. Br J Clin Pharmacol 34:551, 1992

76. Hochster H, Dieterich D, Bozzettee S, et al: Toxicity of combined ganciclovir and zidovudine for cytomegalovirus associated with AIDS. Ann Intern Med 113:111, 1990

77. Millar AB, Miller RF, Patou G, et al: Treatment of cytomegalovirus retinitis with zidovudine and ganciclovir in patients with AIDS: Outcome and toxicity. Genitourin Med 66:156, 1990

78. Vogt MW, Hartshorn KL, Furman PA, et al: Ribavirin antagonizes the effect of azidothymidine on HIV replication. Science 235:1376, 1987

79. Merrill DP, Moonis M, Chou TC, et al: Lamivudine or stavudine in two- and three-drug combinations against human immunodeficiency virus type I replication in vitro. J Infect Dis 173:355, 1996

80. Hartman NR, Yarchoan R, Pluda JM, et al: Pharmacokinetics of 2',3'-dideoxyinosine in patients with severe human immunodeficiency infection. II. The effects of different oral formulations and the presence of other medications. Clin Pharmacol Ther 50:278, 1991

81. Metroka CE, McMechan MF, Andrada R, et al: Failure of prophylaxis with dapsone in patients taking dideoxyinosine. N Engl J Med 325:737, 1991

82. Knupp CA, Barbhaiya RH: A multiple-dose pharmacokinetic interaction study between didanosine (Videx) and ciprofloxacin (Cipro) in male subjects seropositive for HIV but asymptomatic. Biopharm Drug Dispos 18:65, 1997

83. Sahai J, Gallicano K, Oliveras L, et al: Cations in the didanosine tablet reduce ciprofloxacin bioavailability. Clin Pharmacol Ther 53:292, 1993

84. Morse GD, Fischl MA, Shelton MJ, et al: Single-dose pharmacokinetics of delavirdine mesylate and didanosine in patients with human immunodeficiency virus infection. Antimicrob Agents Chemother 41:169, 1997

85. May DB, Drew RH, Yedinak KC, et al: Effect of simultaneous didanosine administration on itraconazole absorption in healthy volunteers. Pharmacotherapy 14:509, 1994

86. Knupp CA, Brater DC, Relue J, et al: Pharmacokinetics of didanosine and ketoconazole after coadministration to patients seropositive for the human immunodeficiency virus. J Clin Pharmacol 33:912, 1993

87. Tseng Al, Foisy MM: Management of drug interactions in patients with HIV. Ann Pharmacother 31:1040, 1997

88. Adkins JC, Peters DH, Faulds D: Zalcitabine: An update of its pharmacodynamic pharmacokinetic properties and clinical efficacy in the management of HIV infection. Drugs 53:1054, 1997

89. Massarella JW, Nazareno LA, Passe S, et al: The effect of probenecid on the pharmacokinetics of zalcitabine in HIV-positive patients. Pharm Res 13:449, 1996

90. LeLacheur SF, Simon GL: Exacerbation of dideoxycytidine-induced neuropathy with dideoxyinosine. J Acquir Immune Defic Syndr 4:538, 1991

91. Moore KH, Yuen GJ, Raasch RH, et al: Pharmacokinetics of lamivudine administered alone and with treimethoprim-sulfamethoxazole. Clin Pharmacol Ther 59:550, 1996

92. Eagling VA, Back DJ, Barry MG: Differential inhibition of cytochrome P450 isoforms by the protease inhibitors, ritonavir, saquinavir and indinavir. Br J Clin Pharmacol 44:190, 1997

93. Lee CA, Liang BH, Grettenberger HM, et al: Prediction of nelfinavir mesylate (Viracept) clinical drug interactions based on in vitro human P450 metabolism studies. In Abstracts of the 4th Conference on Retroviruses and Opportunistic Infections, Washington, DC, 1997, Abstract 373

94. Caballero-Granado FJ, Viciana P, Cordero E, et al: Ergotism related to concurrent administration of ergotamine tartrate and ritonavir in an AIDS patient. Antimicrob Agents Chemother 41:1207, 1997

95. Merry C, Mulcahy F, Barry M, et al: Saquinavir interaction with midazolam: Pharmacokinetic considerations when prescribing protease inhibitors for patients with HIV disease. AIDS 11:268, 1997

96. Centers for Disease Control and Prevention: Clinical update: Impact of HIV protease inhibitors on the treatment of HIV-infected tuberculosis patients with rifampin. MMWR 45:921, 1996

97. Wilkinson GR: Cytochrom P4503A (CYP3A) metabolism: Prediction of in vitro activity in humans. J Pharmacokinet Biopharm 24:475, 1996

98. Merry C, Barry MG, Mulcahy F, et al: Saquinavir pharmacokinetics alone and in combination with nelfinavir in HIV-infected patients. AIDS 11:F117, 1997

99. Merrill DP, Manion DJ, Chou TC, Hirsch MS: Antagonism between human immunodeficiency virus type 1 protease inhibitors indinavir and saquinavir in vitro. J Infect Dis 176:265, 1997

100. Kuman GN, Rodrigues AD, Buko AM, et al: Cytochrome P450-mediated metabolism of the HIV-1 protease inhibitor ritonavir (ABT-538) in human liver microsomes. J Pharmacol Exp Ther 277:423, 1996

101. Tschanz C, Stargel W, Thomas JA: Interactions between drugs and nutrients. Adv Pharmacol 35:1, 1996

102. Nazareno LA, Holazo AA, Limjuco R, et al: The effect of food on pharmacokinetics of zalcitabine in HIV-positive patients. Pharm Res 12:1462, 1995

103. Sahai J, Gallicano K, Garber G, et al: The effect of a protein meal on zidovudine pharmacokinetics in HIV-infected patients. Br J Clin Pharmacol 33:657, 1992

104. Knupp CA, Milbrath R, Barbhaiya RH: Effect of time of food administration on the bioavailability of didanosine from a chewable tablet formulation. J Clin Pharmacol 33:568, 1993

105. Shyu WC, Knupp CA, Pittman KA, et al: Food-induced reduction in bioavailability of didanosine. Clin Pharmacol Ther 50:503, 1991

106. Muirhead GJ, Shaw T, Williams PEO, et al: Pharmacokinetics of the HIV-proteinase inhibitor, Ro 318959, after single and multiple oral doses in healthy volunteers. Br J Clin Pharmacol 34:170P, 1992

107. Shetty BV, Kosa MB, Khalil DA, et al: Preclinical pharmacokinetics and distribution to tissue of AG1343, an inhibitor of human immunodeficiency virus type 1 protease. Antimicrob Agents Chemother 40:110, 1996

108. Rodvold KA, Meyer J: Drug-food interactions with grapefruit juice. Infect Med 13:868, 1996

108a. Kupferschmidt HH, Fattinger KE, Ha HR, et al: Grapefruit juice enhances the bioavailability of the HIV protease inhibitor saquinavir in man. Br J Clin Pharmacol 45:355, 1998

6 | Antiretroviral Therapy

STEVEN G. DEEKS • PAUL A. VOLBERDING

Antiretroviral therapy is a key element of the overall management of HIV disease. When properly used, antiretroviral therapy delays the onset of AIDS and improves quality of life. Despite these advantages, antiretroviral therapy has clear limitations. The drugs are expensive, are often inconvenient to take, and usually result in significant side effects and drug interactions. Perhaps most importantly, current therapies fail to achieve durable viral suppression in a large number of patients. To avoid drug failure, it is critical to manage therapy carefully and to base therapeutic decisions on the most current information. Therefore, this chapter reviews HIV pathogenesis and viral load testing, establishing the platform upon which antiretroviral strategies are based. Each drug is then summarized, focusing on practical issues such as dosing strategies, side effect management, drug interactions, and resistance profiles. The chapter concludes with a discussion on several unanswered questions in this rapidly evolving area of HIV medicine.

HIV PATHOGENESIS

The treatment of HIV infection is increasingly based on an understanding of HIV pathogenesis.[1-4] By understanding the relationship between viral replication and disease pathogenesis, clinicians should be able to translate scientific advances directly into clinical practice.[4]

HIV infection is a dynamic process, characterized by a high rate of viral replication (as many as 10 billion viral particles are produced daily).[57] Because of the error-prone nature of HIV reverse transcriptase, each cycle of viral replication results in the production of at least one mutation per genome (on average), resulting in as many as 10^4 to 10^5 mutations at each site in the HIV genome each day.[8]

Unless HIV replication is fully suppressed, viral evolution is continuous. In the face of incomplete viral suppression, each antiretroviral agent selects for drug-specific genotypic resistance. Treatment strategies are designed to prevent the emergence of drug resistance by suppressing viral replication as much as possible.[4-9]

HIV disease progression is characterized by progressive loss of CD4 T cells. Despite years of research, the mechanism of HIV-induced T-cell depletion remains controversial. One model assumes that disease progression occurs as a result of virally mediated CD4 T-cell death, either through a direct cytopathic effect or via increased apoptosis. A second model assumes that CD4 T-cell depletion occurs as a result of decreased T-cell production, either through the effects of HIV on hematopoietic cells (stem cells) or through the effect of HIV on the infrastructure required for T-cell maturation (lymphoid tissue; thymus)[10] Regardless of the mechanism, it remains clear that inhibiting viral replication prevents disease progression, and that sustained viral suppression restores CD4 T-cell number and function.[11,12]

Based on these observations, several therapeutic principles have been proposed.[4] First, antiretroviral therapy should be initiated early in the natural history of HIV infection, before the development of divergent and potentially more virulent viral strains. Second, at least three drugs to which the patient is naïve should be initiated simultaneously. Theoretically, mutations that cause resistance to each of the available antiretroviral drugs exist at baseline. Individual virions with resistance to multiple agents are probably rare. Therefore, three or more drugs initiated simultaneously may suppress all viral replication. Finally, therapy should be initiated early, with the goal of maintaining immune function before irreversible defects arise.

TABLE 6–1. Clinical Glossary of Antiretroviral Drugs

	DRUG	OTHER NAMES	DOSE	TOXICITY	COMMENTS
Nucleoside Analogs	Zidovudine	ZDV, AZT, Retrovir	200 mg tid or 300 mg bid	Anemia, neutropenia, nausea, vomiting, fatigue, malaise	May prevent AIDS dementia complex. Prevents perinatal transmission; may reduce transmission after occupational exposure.
	Didanosine	ddI, Videx	200 mg bid (fasting); 400 mg once daily under evaluation	Gastrointestinal (GI) disturbances, pancreatitis, peripheral neuropathy	Less neurotoxic than zalcitabine. Requires gastric neutralization with antacids, which can interfere with absorption of other drugs. Avoid use in patients with high potential for pancreatitis (drugs, alcohol, prior history).
	Zalcitabine	ddC, HIVID	0.75 mg tid	Oral ulcers, peripheral neuropathy, pancreatitis	Most effective in previously untreated patients, particularly in combination with zidovudine.
	Stavudine	d4T, Zerit	40 mg bid	Peripheral neuropathy	Less neurotoxic than didanosine or zalcitabine; generally well tolerated.
	Lamivudine	3TC, Epivir	150 mg bid	None	Resistance develops rapidly but may restore zidovudine sensitivity. No clear side effects.
	Abacavir	ABC, Ziagen	300 mg bid	Nausea, hypersensitivity reaction	More potent than other nucleoside analogs. Patients who experience a hypersensitivity reaction to abacavir should never be rechallenged.
Protease Inhibitors	Saquinavir	Fortovase	1200 mg tid with food	Nausea, abdominal cramping, diarrhea	Often used in combination with ritonavir or nelfinavir.
	Indinavir	Crixivan	800 mg every 8 h fasting	Nephrolithiasis, hyperbilirubinemia	Elevated bilirubin common and typically benign. Aggressive hydration recommended to prevent renal stones. May be given with low-fat, low-protein snacks.
	Ritonavir	Norvir	600 mg bid with food	Circumoral paresthesias, nausea, headache, fatigue, taste disturbance	Dose escalation recommended (see package insert). Liquid formulation associated with significant taste disturbances; it may be mixed with chocolate milk or nutritional supplements to improve tolerability.
	Nelfinavir	Viracept	750 mg tid (with meals)	Diarrhea	Nelfinavir is commonly dosed twice daily (1250 mg twice daily)
	Amprenavir	Agenerase	1200 mg bid	Rash, GI side effects	
Non-nucleoside Reverse Transcriptase Inhibitors	Nevirapine	Viramune	200 mg bid	Rash	Rapid resistance. Dose escalation commonly recommended to prevent rash (200 mg qd × 14 days, then 200 mg bid).
	Delavirdine	Rescriptor	400 mg tid	Rash	Rapid resistance. Dose escalation to prevent rash is not recommended.
	Efavirenz	Sustiva	600 mg qd	Central nervous system (CNS) symptoms, rash	Rapid resistance. CNS symptoms generally resolve after first few weeks of dosing.

HIV QUANTITATION

The number of HIV RNA molecules per milliliter of plasma (viral load) is an important predictor of disease progression.[13,14] In one large cohort, plasma viral load was a more accurate and stable predictor of disease progression than the baseline CD4 T-cell count.[13] Changes in viral load occur rapidly after the initiation of effective antiretroviral drugs, with reductions ranging from approximately 0.5 log with monotherapy zidovudine to 3 or more logs with combination therapy. There is a close correlation between therapy-induced reduction in viral load and the delay in disease progression.[14,15] Based on these observations, clinical guidelines recommend that antiretroviral therapy should be managed based largely on viral load determinations.[1-4] The level of immune function, reflected by the CD4 T-cell count, remains an important factor in deciding when to initiate therapy.

NUCLEOSIDE ANALOGS

As outlined in Table 6–1, there are six widely available nucleoside analogs (zidovudine, didanosine, zalcitabine, stavudine, lamivudine, and abacavir). Each drug must first undergo intracellular phosphorylation to an active triphosphate metabolite. In their active forms, these drugs compete with endogenous nucleotides at the active site of HIV reverse transcriptase. In general, the nucleoside analogs are less potent inhibitors of HIV-1 replication in vivo than are the protease inhibitors and non-nucleoside reverse transcriptase inhibitors (NNRTIs). Plasma viral load reductions of 0.5 to 1.0 log RNA copies/ml are typically seen with nucleoside analog monotherapy. When nucleoside analogs are used in combination with each other, durable (>1 year) viral suppression of approximately 1 log is commonly achieved. Despite their modest individual anti-HIV effects, nucleoside analogs remain a critical component of combination therapy.[1-3]

The pharmacokinetics, safety, and activity of each nucleoside analog are outlined below and in Table 6–1. Commonly associated resistance mutations are outlined in Table 6–2. Clinical trials illustrating the clinical efficacy of these drugs are presented in Table 6–3. In contrast to the protease inhibitors and the NNRTIs, drug interactions involving the nucleoside analogs are rare, and are not covered in this review.

Zidovudine (Retrovir, AZT)

Zidovudine was approved for use in patients with advanced disease in 1987. It has an oral bioavailability of approximately 60% and is the only antiretroviral agent readily available for parental administration. Zidovudine is commonly given twice daily (300 mg bid, either fasting or with food). Zidovudine crosses the blood–brain barrier and prevents AIDS dementia complex (for reviews see Price[16]).

TABLE 6–2. Common Mutations Associated with Antiretroviral Therapies

DRUG	CRITICAL MUTATIONS	OTHER MUTATIONS*,†
Zidovudine	M41L, D67N, K70R, T215Y/F	L210W, K219E/Q
Didanosine	L74V	K65R, V75T, M184V
Zalcitabine	K65R	T69D, L74V, V75GT, M184V
Stavudine	I50T, V75T	
Lamivudine	M184V	
Abacavir	M184V, L65R, L74V, Y115F	
Nevirapine	K103N, Y181C/I	A98G, V106A, V108I, Y188C, G190A
Delavirdine	K103N/T, Y181C	P236L, others
Efavirenz	K103N	V108I, L100N, Y181C, G190S, others
Saquinavir	G48V, L90M	L10I, I54V, A71V, L63P, V82A, I84V, others
Ritonavir	V82A/F	L10I, K20R, M36I, M46I, I54V/L, L63P/H/Q, A71V/L, I84V, L90M, others
Indinavir	V82A/F, M46I/L	L10I, K20M, I54V/T, L63P/H/Q, A71T/V, I84V, L90M, others
Nelfinavir	D30N	M36I, L63P, A71V, V77I, N88D, L90M, others
Amprenavir	I50V, others	L10I, M46I, I54, I84V, others

*Partial list; see Schinazi RF, Larder BA, Mellors JW: Mutations in retroviral genes associated with drug resistance. Int Antiviral News 5:129, 1997, for complete list of reported resistance mutations.

†The 151M mutation and 69 S-S insertion complex (both within reverse transcriptase gene) are associated with broad cross-resistance among all nucleoside analogs.

TABLE 6–3. Key Trials of Selected Drugs or Drug Combinations

TRIAL	SELECTED DRUG OR DRUG COMBINATION	POPULATION (APPROXIMATE)	COMMENTS
ACTG 019 (baseline CD4 <500)	ZDV monotherapy	1500 asymptomatic subjects (CD4 <500)	ZDV delayed disease progression over first year
Concorde	ZDV monotherapy	1700 asymptomatic subjects with any CD4 cell count at entry	Early use of ZDV not associated with a clinical benefit when compared to delayed ZDV monotherapy; reanalysis suggested measurable benefit if baseline CD4 below 500/mm^3
ACTG 116B/117	ZDV vs. ddI	1000 ZDV-experienced patients	After prolonged exposure to ZDV, switching to ddI was associated with a clinical benefit when compared to continued ZDV
ACTG 175	ZDV vs. ZDV/ddI vs. ZDV/ddC vs. ddI	Most asymptomatic; CD4 <500; 40% of overall group ZDV naïve	Progression to AIDS, death, or CD4 loss decreased significantly with ZDV/ddI, ZDV/ddC, and ddI monotherapy when compared to ZDV monotherapy, ZDV/ddC effective only in treatment-naïve patients; ZDV/ddI most effective arm
Delta	ZDV vs. ZDV/ddI vs. ZDV/ddC	More advanced disease than ACTG 175	Combination therapy was superior to ZDV monotherapy in delaying disease progression
NUCA 3001	ZDV vs. 3TC vs. ZDV/3TC	366 ZDV-naïve patients, CD4 200–500	ZDV/3TC resulted in 1 log reduction in viral load through week 52
CEASAR	ZDV/3TC	1400 patients with moderate disease	In ZDV-experienced patients, addition of 3TC to ZDV-based regimen delayed disease progression
ACTG 306	d4T; ddI; d4T/3TC; ddI/3TC; ZDV/3TC	300 treatment-naïve patients	ZDV/3TC and d4T/3TC had similar efficacy (approximate 1 log decrease in viral load at week 48); ddI monotherapy similar to ZDV/3TC (at week 24)
ACTG 290	d4T vs. ZDV/d4T vs. ddI vs. ZDV/ddI	150 ZDV-experienced patients	The combination of ZDV and d4T should not be used concurrently
BMS	d4T/ddI	89 treatment-naïve patients (CD4 200–500)	Combination of d4T/ddI resulted in approximate 1 log decrease in viral load over 1 year; peripheral neuropathy rare
Swiss Cohort Study	d4T/ddI vs. d4T/ddI/hydroxyurea	150 treatment naïve subjects, CD4 200–500	Combination of d4T/ddI and hydroxyurea resulted in potent HIV suppression; hydroxyurea blunted CD4 T-cell response to therapy; follow-up limited

Study	Regimen	Patient population	Results
CNAA3003	ZDV/3TC vs. ZDV/3TC/ABC	175 treatment-naïve subjects	Combination of ZDV, 3TC, and ABC resulted in potent anti-HIV effect; limited follow-up
ACTG 229	ZDV, ddC, SQV	Moderate-advanced disease	Modest benefit when SQV hard-gel capsule added to ZDV/ddC
ACTG 241	ZDV, ddI, nevirapine	400 treatment-experienced (ZDV) patients with moderate disease	ZDV/ddI/nevirapine had similar efficacy as ZDV/ddI in treatment-experienced patients
INCAS	ZDV/ddI with nevirapine	150 treatment-naïve patients	ZDV, ddI, and nevirapine resulted in sustained viral suppression in the majority of patients; medication adherence critical in achieving durable suppression
Pharmacia and Upjohn 021	ZDV/3TC with delavirdine	375 treatment-naïve patients; mean baseline CD4 350	Combination of ZDV, 3TC, and delavirdine resulted in significant and durable viral suppression (68% of patients remained at CD4 <400 through week 52)
Dupont 006	ZDV/3TC/indinavir vs. ZDV/3TC/efavirenz vs. indinavir/efavirenz	450 asymptomatic treatment-naïve patients	ZDV/3TC/efavirenz as effective as an indinavir-based regimen in suppressing viral replication; first study to compare NNRTI- and PI-based regimens
Merck 035	ZDV+3TC vs. indinavir vs. ZDV/3TC/indinavir	90 ZDV-experienced patients (mean CD4 142)	85% patients had viral RNA <500 at 2 years (intent to treat); first study to demonstrate that simultaneous use of combination therapy is superior to sequential use
ACTG 320	ZDV/3TC vs. ZDV/3TC/indinavir	1100 ZDV-experienced patients with advanced disease (CD4 <200)	ZDV/3TC + indinavir delayed disease progression and prolonged life in patients with advanced disease when compared to ZDV/3TC; virologic failure common in patients with CD4 <50 at baseline
Abbott 247	RTV added to stable nucleoside analog regimen	1100 patients CD4 <100	RTV, when added to a failing NRTI regimen, delayed disease progression in patients with advanced disease and improved quality of life
Agouron 511	ZDV/3TC with NFV	300 treatment-naïve patients	ZDV, 3TC, and NFV (750 mg tid) resulted in durable viral suppression through week 48; NFV was well tolerated
Abbott 462	RTV/SQV	140 PI-naïve patients	RTV + SQV, with d4T/3TC added early for virologic failure, was highly effective in suppressing viral replication
SPICE	NFV/SQV	150 PI-naïve patients	The 4-drug combination of NFV, SQV, and 2 nucleoside analogs more effective than either 3-drug combination

ABC, abacavir; ddC, zalcitabine; ddI, didanosine; d4T, stavudine; NFV, nelfinavir; NNRTI, non-nucleoside reverse transcriptase inhibitor; NRTI, nucleoside reverse transcriptase inhibitor; PI, protease inhibitor; RTV, ritonavir; SQV, saquinavir; 3TC, lamivudine; ZDV, zidovudine.

Zidovudine is generally well tolerated, particularly in patients with early-stage disease. Nausea, anorexia, fatigue, malaise, headaches, and other nonspecific constitutional symptoms may occur. Neutropenia and anemia are common in patients with advanced disease. Proximal myopathy is an uncommon but potentially serious complication of zidovudine therapy.

As monotherapy, zidovudine results in a moderate anti-HIV effect (0.5 log decline in viral load), reduces perinatal transmission, and prevents AIDS-associated dementia complex.[16-18] In asymptomatic patients with CD4 T-cell counts less than 500 cells/mm^3, zidovudine monotherapy delays disease progression over the first year of therapy.[19] This modest effect may not be durable.[20] Resistance to zidovudine occurs after prolonged exposure, and is associated with mutations at positions 41, 67, 70, and 215, among others (see Table 6–2). High-level zidovudine resistance probably confers cross-resistance to other nucleoside analogs, including didanosine, stavudine, and abacavir.

Didanosine (Videx, ddI)

The U.S. Food and Drug Administration approved didanosine in 1991. Because of the prolonged half-life of its active metabolite, didanosine is given twice daily. The standard dose is 200 mg bid fasting for patients who weigh 60 kg or more and 125 mg twice daily for patients who weigh less than 60 kg. Preliminary data indicate that didanosine may be given once daily (400 mg qd fasting; two 150-mg tablets plus one 100-mg tablet). Because didanosine is inactivated by acid, it is formulated with a buffer. Didanosine should be taken on an empty stomach (1 hour before or 1 hour after a meal). A soft gel formulation (which can be administered once daily with meals) has been developed.

Diarrhea (typically mild) is common with didanosine. Peripheral neuropathy occurs, particularly in patients with advanced disease or in patients receiving other neurotoxic medications. Patients commonly present with tingling, burning, pain, and/or numbness in the distal extremities. Unless therapy is discontinued, symptoms may progress and become irreversible. Pancreatitis is a rare but potentially fatal toxicity associated with didanosine use. It occurs more commonly in patients with a prior history of pancreatitis or with active alcohol abuse.

Didanosine may be more active in vivo than other nucleoside analogs. Didanosine prevents disease progression in patients previously treated with zidovudine.[21] In the ACTG 306 trial, didanosine monotherapy was as effective as zidovudine and lamivudine in decreasing viral load over 24 weeks. There was no clear additional benefit when lamivudine was added to didanosine.[22] In ACTG 175, didanosine monotherapy was as effective as the combination of zidovudine plus didanosine or zidovudine plus zalcitabine in delaying disease progression.[23] Resistance to didanosine occurs and is commonly associated with a mutation at position 74, among others (see Table 6–2). It is unclear to what degree didanosine resistance compromises future responses to other nucleoside analogs.

Zalcitabine (Hivid, ddC)

Zalcitabine was approved by the U.S. Food and Drug Administration in 1992. Because of its short plasma half-life, it should be given three times daily (the standard dose is 0.75 mg every 8 hours). As with didanosine, the major toxicities associated with zalcitabine treatment are pancreatitis and peripheral neuropathy. Pancreatitis has been reported but appears to very uncommon. Stomatitis (oral ulcerations) may also occur.

Zalcitabine has no proven efficacy as monotherapy. Most studies have used zalcitabine in combination with zidovudine. Because of concerns of toxicity (neuropathy, pancreatitis), zalcitabine should not be given concurrently with didanosine or stavudine. Resistance to zalcitabine in vivo has been poorly characterized.

Stavudine (Zerit, d4T)

Stavudine was approved by the U.S. Food and Drug Administration in 1994. It is typically dosed at 40 mg twice daily (fasting or with food). Lower doses (20 to 30 mg twice daily) have been used clinically, particularly for patients who have a history of peripheral neuropathy or who weigh less than 60 kg. As with didanosine and zalcitabine, the major clinical toxicity associated with stavudine use is peripheral neuropathy. The drug is otherwise very well tolerated.

Stavudine is commonly given in combination with lamivudine or didanosine. Zidovudine and stavudine should not be used together. As thymidine analogs, both drugs undergo intracellular phosphorylation by thymidine kinase. Zidovudine monophosphate inhibits the activity of this enzyme. Because the thymidine kinase step is rate limiting for stavudine (but not zidovudine), zidovudine appears to prevent stavudine activation.[24] This effect was studied in ACTG 290, where patients received both nucleoside analogs concurrently.[24,25] As predicted, the triphosphate form of stavudine was lower than normal. Patients on this combination experienced a rapid decline in CD4 T-cell levels, presumably as a consequence of this negative interaction. The combination of stavudine and zalcitabine has not been studied, and is not recommended because of concerns over increased risk of peripheral neuropathy.

Resistance to stavudine in vivo is poorly characterized. Although stavudine selects for a mutation at position 75 in vitro, this rarely occurs in vivo.

Lamivudine (Epivir, 3TC)

Lamivudine was approved by the U.S. Food and Drug Administration in November 1995. The intracellular half-life is approximately 10 to 15 hours, allowing for twice-daily dosing. The standard dose is 150 mg twice daily (either fasting or with food). There are no clear side effects associated with lamivudine use.

As monotherapy, lamivudine results in a dramatic decrease in viral load over the first few weeks of therapy. However, high-level resistance to lamivudine occurs rapidly and is associated with a mutation at position 184. For unclear reasons, this mutation delays the development of zidovudine resistance.[26] In fact, HIV carrying the 184V mutation shows enhanced susceptibility to both zidovudine and the nucleotide analogs (adefovir, phosphonylmethoxypropyladenine). Zidovudine and lamivudine are commonly used together (a single tablet containing lamivudine 150 mg and zidovudine 300 mg is available). The combination of zidovudine and lamivudine results in sustained viral suppression (approximately 1 log over 52 weeks)[27] and delays disease progression.[28] In addition to its anti-HIV activity, lamivudine is effective in suppressing hepatitis B replication.[29]

Abacavir (ABC, Ziagen)

Abacavir, a guanosine analog, has several unique characteristics. It is dosed 300 mg twice daily (either fasting or with food). Nausea, anorexia, and other constitutional symptoms have been reported; however, they appear to be mild and uncommon. The major toxicity associated with abacavir therapy is a hypersensitivity reaction. This potentially fatal reaction typically presents during the first few weeks of dosing with nonspecific flu-like symptoms (nausea, abdominal pain, diarrhea, fevers, and fatigue). A rash may or may not be present. Symptoms generally progress until the patient is very ill. Once abacavir is discontinued because of an expected hypersensitivity reaction, it should never be restarted. Severe, potentially life-threatening reactions have been reported after re-exposure to the drug.

Abacavir appears to be more potent than other nucleoside analogs. As monotherapy, it decreases viral load by as much as 2 log over 12 weeks. In combination with zidovudine and lamivudine, abacavir therapy results in a sustained decrease in viral load. High-level resistance to abacavir can occur but requires the development of multiple mutations (see Table 6–2). High-level zidovudine resistance, or resistance to multiple nucleoside analogs, confers cross-resistance to abacavir in vitro and possibly in vivo.

PROTEASE INHIBITORS

HIV-1 protease inhibitors are potent inhibitors of viral replication. When used in combination with nucleoside analogs, durable viral suppression is commonly achieved. As shown in Table 6–1, there are now five protease inhibitors available (saquinavir, ritonavir, indinavir, nelfinavir, amprenavir). Although the protease inhibitors have similar chemical structures, each has a unique side effect and resistance profile.[30] Drug interactions are common with protease inhibitors and are discussed in a separate section below.

Saquinavir (Invirase, Fortovase)

Saquinavir was the first HIV-1 protease inhibitor licensed for use in the United States (approval date December 1996). Because the initial hard-gel formulation (Invirase) had limited oral bioavailability (approximately 4%), it was difficult to achieve optimal serum concentrations. As a result, a soft-gel formulation (Fortovase) was developed and approved by the U.S. Food and Drug Administration in November 1997. Although both remain available, only the soft-gel formulation has been recommended for use as a single protease inhibitor in combination with nucleoside analogs.

The saquinavir soft-gel capsule (sgc) is dosed at 1200 mg three times daily with food. Preliminary data indicate that 1600 mg twice daily may be as effective; however, this dose is still considered experimental. Reported side effects with saquinavir-sgc include diarrhea, nausea, gastrointestinal discomfort, and rash, all typically mild.

One large study indicated that the combination of saquinavir hard-gel capsule and zalcitabine prevented disease progression and prolonged life when compared to either drug alone.[31] Viral load suppression, however, was limited with the saquinavir hard-gel capsule.[31] Saquinavir sgc (in combination with two nucleoside analogs) may be as effective in suppressing viral replication as other protease inhibitor–based regimens.[32] Because of its susceptibility to cytochrome P-450 isoform 3A (CYP3A) metabolism, saquinavir is commonly used in combination with other protease inhibitors (see below).

In vitro and in vivo, saquinavir selects for several mutations, particularly at positions 48 and 90. Although this is controversial,[33] saquinavir resistance appears to confer cross-resistance to other protease inhibitors.[34]

Ritonavir (Norvir)

Ritonavir, developed by Abbott Laboratories, was the second HIV protease inhibitor licensed in the United States (approval date March 1996). Ritonavir is given as 600 mg twice daily (with a full meal). The drug is available both in capsule form (100-mg capsules) and as a liquid (80 mg/ml). A new soft gel formulation has been developed.

Because ritonavir has potent and often unpredictable effects on cytochrome P-450 activity, drug interactions are common. Notably, ritonavir induces its own metabolism over time. To prevent side effects, the manufacturer recommends initiating ritonavir therapy at 300 mg twice daily, then increasing the dose by 100 mg/day as tolerated until a level of 600 mg twice daily is achieved. Like saquinavir, ritonavir is commonly used in combination with other protease inhibitors.

Side effects are common with ritonavir, particular during the first few weeks of dosing. Diarrhea, nausea, vomiting, anorexia, headaches, asthenia (loss of strength and energy), fatigue, and circumoral paresthesia are common. Taste disturbance is particularly common with the oral

suspension. Elevations in triglycerides, creatinine kinase, and liver transaminases occur. Finally, some metabolic abnormalities, including abnormal fat distribution (lipodystrophy), may be associated with ritonavir therapy.

As monotherapy, ritonavir results in a significant but transient decrease in plasma viral load. In combination with two nucleoside analogs, this potent anti-HIV effect is sustained. When added to a stable nucleoside analog regimen in patients with advanced disease, ritonavir delays disease progression[35] and improves quality of life.[36] Despite this, the clinical development of ritonavir has increasingly focused on its use in dual protease inhibitor combinations (see below).

Although multiple mutations have been associated with ritonavir resistance, an initial mutation at position 82 appears to be necessary for the subsequent development of other mutations.[37] Resistance patterns for ritonavir are similar to those for indinavir,[38] suggesting that failure of one drug may predict failure of the second drug. Resistance to ritonavir probably confers broad cross-resistance to other protease inhibitors.

Indinavir (Crixivan)

Indinavir, the third HIV protease inhibitor to be licensed in the United States, received U.S. Food and Drug Administration approval in March 1996. Because of its short half-life, indinavir should be given every 8 hours. The recommended dose is 800 mg every 8 hours with the patient in a fasting condition (2 hours after or 1 hour before meals). To increase compliance, indinavir may be given with a low-protein, low-fat snack. Twice-daily dosing of indinavir is not as effective as the three-times-a-day dose and is not recommended.

Approximately 5% of patients develop renal stones while receiving indinavir. To prevent nephrolithiasis, patients should drink large quantities of water throughout the day (approximately 48 oz/day, or six 8-oz glasses). Indinavir therapy has also been associated with abdominal pain, nausea, vomiting, and gastroesophageal reflux. Mild to moderate elevation of bilirubin is common, although not associated with hepatic damage.

In a Phase II study, 78 subjects naïve to lamivudine and protease inhibitor therapy were randomized to one of three arms: zidovudine plus lamivudine; indinavir alone; or zidovudine, lamivudine, and indinavir. The majority of patients who received all three drugs concurrently had sustained viral suppression (for over 2 years). In contrast, most patients in whom zidovudine plus lamivudine was initiated first, followed by indinavir, experienced virologic failure.[39] In patients with advanced disease (CD4 T-cell count <200 cells/mm^3), zidovudine, lamivudine, and indinavir delayed disease progression when compared to zidovudine and lamivudine.[40] Based largely on these studies, combination therapy with two nucleoside analogs and a potent protease inhibitor became standard of care in 1997.[41]

Resistance to indinavir requires the development of multiple mutations (see Table 6–2).[42] Mutations at positions 46 and/or 82 may be critical. Indinavir resistance has been associated with high-level phenotypic cross-resistance to all other protease inhibitors.[43]

Nelfinavir (Viracept)

Nelfinavir, approved by the U.S. Food and Drug Administration in March 1997, was the fourth HIV-1 protease inhibitor to be developed clinically. Nelfinavir is dosed at 750 mg three times daily with food (dosing exactly every 8 hours is not required). Preliminary data indicate that nelfinavir 1250 mg twice daily may be as effective as the standard three-times-a-day dose. In general, nelfinavir is well tolerated. In Phase III studies, the most common side effect was mild to moderate diarrhea.

When used in combination with two nucleoside analogs (zidovudine and lamivudine), nelfinavir results in a sustained decrease in viral load.[44] In vivo and in vitro, nelfinavir resistance is associated with a mutation at position 30. Other mutations (including L90M) have been observed.[38] Preliminary data from uncontrolled studies suggest that salvage therapy with ritonavir/saquinavir-based regimens may be possible after nelfinavir-based regimens fail.

Amprenavir (Agenerase)

Safety and efficacy data regarding amprenavir are limited. Because of its long half-life (approximately 7 hours), amprenavir may be dosed twice daily (1200 mg bid either with or without food). Like the other protease inhibitors, amprenavir is metabolized by CYP3A, resulting in important drug interactions. In small studies, rash, nausea, diarrhea, and headache were all reported with amprenavir therapy. Most cases of

rash have been mild. However, more severe rashes (including Stevens-Johnson syndrome) have been reported.

Amprenavir monotherapy results in a significant but transient decrease in viral load. In combination with two nucleoside analogs, amprenavir results in durable viral suppression in the majority of treatment-naïve patients studied.[45]

In vitro and occasionally in vivo, amprenavir selects for a unique resistance mutation at position 50; this mutation may not confer cross-resistance to other protease inhibitors. Mutations at other positions have also been reported (including 10, 46, 47, 54, and 84). Whether amprenavir will be effective for patients who have developed resistance to current therapies remains to be determined.

Dual Protease Inhibitor Therapy

Because of complex drug interactions, protease inhibitors are often used together.[30] For example, ritonavir dramatically increases serum concentrations of saquinavir, allowing the two drugs to be used together at lower doses. In theory, the use of two protease inhibitors with non-overlapping resistance patterns may result in increased efficacy. Of the possible combinations (see Table 6–4), ritonavir plus saquinavir[46] and nelfinavir plus saquinavir sgc[47] have been validated in large clinical studies.

Protease Inhibitors and Drug Interactions

Drug interactions are common with protease inhibitors.[30] To varying degrees, each protease inhibitor is both a substrate and an inhibitor of CYP3A. Drugs that induce CYP3A4 activity will enhance the metabolism of all protease inhibitors, thus leading to reduced blood levels. Rifampin, a known inducer of CYP3A4, decreases steady-state serum concentrations of each protease inhibitor. Rifabutin (300 mg/day) may have a similar effect. In general, co-administration of any of these drugs with a protease inhibitor should be avoided. In contrast, agents that inhibit cytochrome P-450 activity will increase serum concentrations of each protease inhibitor. Notably, the protease inhibitors themselves are among the most potent inhibitors of cytochrome P-450 activity, leading to potential beneficial drug interactions when used together.

TABLE 6–4. Antiretroviral Drugs: Alternative Dosing Regimens Under Evaluation

DRUG REGIMEN	UNDER EVALUATION*
Didanosine (once daily)	400 mg qd (fasting)
	Two 150-mg tablets + one 100-mg tablet (dose adjust for weight)
Nevirapine (NVP) (once daily)	400 mg qd
Nelfinavir (NFV) (twice daily)	1250 mg bid
Indinavir (IDV) (twice daily)	Not recommended[†]
Saquinavir (SQV) sgc (twice daily)	1600 mg bid (with food)
Ritonavir (RTV)/saquinavir[‡]	400 mg bid (RTV) and 400 mg bid (SQV)
Ritonavir/indinavir	400 mg bid (RTV) and 400 mg bid (IDV)
Nelfinavir/saquinavir sgc	1250 mg bid (NFV) and 1200 mg bid (SQV sgc) *or* 750 mg tid (NFV) and 800 mg tid (SQV sgc)
Nevirapine/indinavir	200 mg bid (NVP) and 1000 mg every 8 hours (IDV)
Nevirapine/nelfinavir	Standard doses of both
Nevirapine/ritonavir	Standard doses of both
Delavirdine/nelfinavir	Standard doses of both[§]
Efavirenz (EFV)/indinavir[¶]	600 mg qd (EFV) and 1000 mg every 8 hours (IDV)
Efavirenz/saquinavir	Not recommended
Efavirenz/nelfinavir	Standard doses of both

*Most of the dose recommendations in this table are under clinical evaluation and not necessarily recommended for routine clinical use; there are no data to support the use of two NNRTIs concurrently.

[†]Twice-daily indinavir, under evaluation by the manufacturer, does not appear to be as effective at the every-8-hour regimen and is not recommended.

[‡]Of the dual protease inhibitor combinations, long-term clinical data are available for ritonavir plus saquinavir and nelfinavir plus saquinavir.

[¶]Of the NNRTI plus protease inhibitor combinations, long-term data are available for the efavirenz plus indinavir combination.

[§]In small studies, the combination of delavirdine and nelfinavir resulted in neutropenia; close monitoring of the complete blood count is recommended.

Because each protease inhibitor can inhibit the metabolism of certain drugs, serious drug interactions may occur. For example, terfenadine, astemizole, cisapride, midazolam, and triazolam should not be used in combination with any protease inhibitor. Use of protease inhibitors with some antiarrhythmics, anticonvulsants, anticoagulants (coumadin), ergot derivatives, narcotics (including methadone), and estrogens (among others) requires caution. Clinicians should review the package insert of each drug carefully.

Long-Term Complications of Protease Inhibitor Therapy

The long-term safety of protease inhibitors is unknown. In clinical practice, protease inhibitors have been associated with abnormal distributions of body fat.[48] Patients may experience loss of subcutaneous fat tissue in the face and extremities, increased abdominal girth, dorso-cervical fat pad enlargement ("buffalo hump"), and/or breast enlargement.[48–50] The increased abdominal girth is due to an increase in intra-abdominal visceral fat, rather than an increase in subcutaneous fat.[50] The relationship between protease inhibitor therapy and fat accumulation

features and lipodystrophy remains to be determined (see Chapter 17 for more discussion).

Other complications have been associated with protease inhibitor use. These drugs increase fasting triglyceride and cholesterol levels, raising concerns that patients may be at increased risk for premature coronary artery disease. Insulin resistance and diabetes mellitus have also been noted. Increased spontaneous bleeding episodes may occur in hemophiliacs receiving protease inhibitors.

NON-NUCLEOSIDE REVERSE TRANSCRIPTASE INHIBITORS

NNRTIs bind to a pocket adjacent to the active site of the reverse transcriptase enzyme, causing a conformational change in the enzyme that reduces activity. There are currently three NNRTIs available for the treatment of HIV infection (nevirapine, delavirdine, and efavirenz).

In contrast to the nucleoside analogs and protease inhibitors, each NNRTI is unique with regard to chemical structure. Despite this chemical heterogeneity, the NNRTIs have many common characteristics. For example, each drug causes rash. Furthermore, each NNRTI is a substrate of the cytochrome P-450 enzyme (nevirapine and efavirenz tend to induce cytochrome P-450 metabolism, whereas delavirdine tends to inhibit its metabolism). Finally, high-level resistance and cross-resistance may occur with each NNRTI. In general, a single point mutation is sufficient for the development of high-level resistance. Most mutations are localized to a pocket that forms the binding site for the NNRTIs (generally positions near 103 and 181 to 190 of the reverse transcriptase gene). Because each NNRTI binds in the same pocket, resistance to one NNRTI confers broad cross-resistance among all NNRTIs. Therefore, the NNRTIs should only be used in regimens designed to fully suppress viral replication. Suboptimal use of an NNRTI, even for a brief period, will likely select for rapid resistance and therefore eliminate the entire class of drugs from future use.

Nevirapine (Viramune)

Nevirapine was approved by the U.S. Food and Drug Administration in June 1996. Nevirapine is dosed at 200 mg twice daily (with or without food). To prevent the development of rash, the manufacturer recommends dose escalation over the first 2 weeks (200 mg once daily for 2 weeks, then 200 mg twice daily). Based on the drug's pharmacokinetic profile, once-daily dosing may be possible (400 mg once daily).

Nevirapine is an inducer of the hepatic CYP3A system. Therefore, nevirapine may lower the serum concentrations of all currently available protease inhibitors (saquinavir, indinavir, ritonavir, nelfinavir, and amprenavir). When nevirapine is administered with indinavir, the indinavir dose should be increased to 1000 mg three times daily. Dose modification does not appear to be necessary with nelfinavir. Nevirapine reduces saquinavir levels significantly; optimal doses of these two drugs have not been determined. The interaction between nevirapine and either ritonavir or amprenavir remains unclear.

Rash is the most common side effect associated with nevirapine.[51] It usually occurs during the first few weeks of treatment, and is typically a diffuse, maculopapular erythematous eruption involving the trunk, face, and extremities. Severe, life-threatening rashes have been reported. Patients with mild rashes may be treated through the event. Rashes associated with constitutional symptoms, vesicular eruptions, and oral lesions should be managed with drug discontinuation. There have been no consistent laboratory abnormalities associated with nevirapine use, although cases of drug-induced hepatitis have been reported.

Nevirapine is a potent inhibitor of HIV-1 replication in vivo. However, resistance occurs rapidly unless the drug is used optimally.[52] For example, in the ACTG 241 trial, treatment-experienced patients received zidovudine and didanosine in combination with either nevirapine or placebo. After a follow-up period of 48 weeks, there was no difference between the nevirapine and placebo groups in terms of disease progression (there was a small but statistically significant benefit to nevirapine use in terms of CD4+ T-cell levels and plasma HIV RNA levels).[51] In the INCAS trial, the same three drugs (zidovudine, didanosine, and nevirapine) were given to treatment-naïve patients. Durable viral suppression was common (viral load <20 copies/ml through week 48), particularly for patients who adhered to their treatment.[53] Nevirapine (and any NNRTI) should be used with at least two new agents in a regimen designed to fully suppress viral replication.

High-level resistance to nevirapine is commonly associated with mutations at positions 181 and/or 106 (see Table 6–2). Mutations have also been seen at positions 103, 108, 188, and 190.[38] The pattern of resistance changes if nevirapine is given with zidovudine. Cross-resistance between nevirapine and other NNRTIs is likely, particularly if the K103N mutation emerges.

Delavirdine (Rescriptor)

Delavirdine was approved by the U.S. Food and Drug Administration in April 1997. Delavirdine should be taken 400 mg three times daily (with or without food). Antacids appear to decrease delavirdine absorption. Therefore, patients should be encouraged to separate delavirdine and antacid dosing by at least 1 hour. By inhibiting CYP3A activity, delavirdine may increase serum concentrations of some medications, leading to potentially serious drug interactions.

By inhibiting cytochrome P-450 metabolism, delavirdine may increase the serum concentrations of some protease inhibitors, thus allowing reduced dosing. Delavirdine appears to increase the concentrations of saquinavir, indinavir, and ritonavir. The effect of delavirdine on nelfinavir and amprenavir has not been fully reported. Optimal dosing of delavirdine with the protease inhibitors requires further study.

Rash is common with delavirdine therapy. In general, the rash is similar to that observed with nevirapine. Dose escalation to prevent rash (recommended for nevirapine) is not recommended for delavirdine. Severe and potentially life-threatening rashes are rare.

Early clinical studies of delavirdine showed disappointing results. This probably reflected the suboptimal manner in which delavirdine was used; in general, delavirdine was used with only one other agent (zidovudine or didanosine), often in treatment-experienced patients. A recent Phase III study of zidovudine, lamivudine, and delavirdine in treatment-naive patients showed encouraging results. The majority of patients had a durable and potent response.[54] As with nevirapine and efavirenz, delavirdine should be used with two nucleoside analogs in treatment-naîve patients. Delavirdine may have a role in treatment-experienced patients, particularly when combined with a protease inhibitor.

As with other NNRTIs, resistance to delavirdine is associated with mutations at positions 103 and 181 (among others). In addition, delavirdine may select for a unique mutation at position 236. In vitro, this mutation may increase viral susceptibility to nevirapine. The clinical relevance of this observation is unclear.

Efavirenz (Sustiva)

The U.S. Food and Drug Administration approved efavirenz in September 1998. Because of its prolonged serum half-life, efavirenz may be dosed once daily. The typical dose is 600 mg, given before bedtime (with or without food). Efavirenz may be dosed twice daily (200 mg in the morning, 400 mg at night). Like other NNRTIs, efavirenz is metabolized by CYP3A4, and therefore may have significant drug interactions with protease inhibitors. Efavirenz, for example, induces the metabolism of indinavir, necessitating an increase in the indinavir dose to 1000 mg every 8 hours. Although efavirenz may increase serum concentrations of nelfinavir, dose modifications are not recommended.

Central nervous system symptoms (dizziness, light-headedness, a feeling of "disengagement," nightmares) are common but generally resolve after the first few weeks of dosing. Dosing efavirenz before bedtime may limit these side effects. Rash occurs but appears to be less common than that seen with other NNRTIs, and is typically mild to moderate. Based on primate studies, there are concerns that efavirenz may be teratogenetic. Thus, use of efavirenz during pregnancy, or in women attempting to become pregnant, is not recommended.

Efavirenz is a potent inhibitor of HIV-1 in vivo. However, resistance occurs rapidly unless efavirenz is dosed with two nucleoside analogs (in treatment-naïve patients) or with a protease inhibitor (in nucleoside analogue experienced patients). Dupont Study 006 compared zidovudine, lamivudine, and efavirenz with zidovudine, lamivudine, and indinavir. Durable viral suppression was observed in both treatment arms; in fact, a strict analysis of this study suggested that the efavirenz-containing arm performed better and these trends were observed through week 48 of followup.[55] Based largely on this study, protease inhibitor–sparing regimens (i.e., two nucleoside analogs and an NNRTI) are now a valid and recommended alternative to the standard regimen of two nucleoside analogs and a protease inhibitor.

Efavirenz resistance is commonly associated with the K103N mutation, typically in association with at least one other mutation (see Table 6–2). Multiple mutations may be required to confer high-level resistance to efavirenz (>100-fold increase in 50% inhibitory concentration). The K103N mutation confers high-level resistance to nevirapine and delavirdine, suggesting that these latter drugs will have no activity once an efavirenz-based regimen fails.

HYDROXYUREA

Although hydroxyurea has no direct anti-HIV activity, it is increasingly used in the treatment of HIV infection, particularly in combination with didanosine. Hydroxyurea is an inhibitor of ribonucleotide reductase, and decreases the intracellular production of deoxyribonucleotides triphosphates (dNTPs) (the "building blocks" of DNA). By decreasing the level of dATP, the incorporation of an andenosine analog (particularly didanosine) into viral DNA is increased.[56] Based on these in vitro observations, clinical trials were initiated to examine whether hydroxyurea could potentiate the activity of didanosine. In short-term studies, hydroxyurea increased the anti-HIV activity of didanosine, even for patients who have pre-existing didanosine phenotypic resistance.[57,58]

The effect of hydroxyurea on the antiviral activity of other nucleoside analogs is unknown. However, hydroxyurea (and other immunosuppressive agents) may be beneficial in the treatment of HIV infection by suppressing T-cell proliferation and/or activation.[59] Because HIV replication is largely dependent of the presence of activated CD4 T cells, any intervention that decreases the number of these target cells may reduce viral replication. Clinical trials are ongoing to examine the efficacy and safety of hydroxyurea when used to suppress target cell availability.

Hydroxyurea is currently dosed at 500 mg twice daily. In patients with pretherapy baseline CD4 T-cell counts of 200 cells/mm^3 or more, hydroxyurea is generally well tolerated. Mild to moderate anemia and/or neutropenia may occur. The safety of hydroxyurea in patients with more advanced disease remains to be determined. Hydoxyurea tends to blunt the CD4 T-cell increase observed with effective antiretroviral therapy.[57]

KEY CLINICAL QUESTIONS IN HIV THERAPY

Many common and practical questions regarding antiretroviral therapy persist. For reasons outlined below, many of these questions will never be addressed through clinical trials.

When Should Antiretroviral Drug Therapy Be Initiated?

This basic question has generated a surprising amount of controversy. Recently, a consensus has emerged that antiretroviral therapy should be initiated relatively early,[1,2] although how early remains controversial.[3] Current U.S. guidelines recommend therapy as the CD4 T-cell count decreases to 350 to 500 cells/mm^3 or the viral load increases to above 10,000 to 20,000 copies/ml. Therapy is also recommended for all symptomatic patients, regardless of viral load or CD4 T-cell count.[1,2] These recommendations are based on the observation that viral load is a strong independent predictor of disease progression, and that the durability of the virologic response to therapy is greater when therapy is initiated at an earlier stage of HIV disease. Early intervention will also prevent irreversible immunologic damage and the development of multiple viral quasispecies (see the "HIV Pathogenesis" section of this chapter for a summary of these issues).

The potential benefits of early intervention need to be weighed against the potential risks, including nonadherence for patients not ready to commit to a complicated regimen and the potential for long-term toxicities. For otherwise asymptomatic patients, the side effects and inconvenience of early intervention may decrease a patient's quality of life.

It is important to emphasize that these recommendations are based largely on an understanding of HIV pathogenesis, and not on prospective clinical trials. The ideal study to determine when antiretroviral therapy should be initiated will not be performed. Such a study would require placebo-controlled randomization to a wide variety of drug combinations, would need to enroll a large number of previously untreated patients, and would require lengthy follow-up to demonstrate a clinical benefit. It will therefore remain controversial as to whether therapy should be initiated very early (i.e., in all HIV-infected patients),[9] or whether therapy can be safely delayed.[3,60]

In clinical practice, the question of when to begin therapy is based largely on the patient's individual circumstances and motivation. Before initiating a therapy, a detailed discussion between the clinician and the patient is necessary to assess the patient's commitment to therapy. Patients need to be fully informed of the complexities and side effects that may be expected with each regimen. The consequences of poor adherence should be discussed in detail[61] (see Chapter 7 for more discussion). Given the potential for cross-resistance among various antiretroviral therapies, patients should be made aware that failure of an initial regimen will severely limit the efficacy of any subsequent regimen. For patients who lack the ability or motivation to fully adhere to therapy, delaying therapy may be reasonable.[1,2]

Which Drugs Should Be Used as Initial Therapy?

For treatment of established HIV infection, a number of combination regimens have undergone clinical evaluation—many in a preliminary, unpublished fashion. The results of these trials generally indicate that the use of three agents is superior to the use of two agents in suppressing viral replication. Which three- (or four-) drug regimen to use as initial therapy remains unclear, and will probably depend on the patient's individual preference and disease stage.

The specific choice of the best initial antiretroviral treatment should be based on an assessment of the drug combination's potency, expected duration of benefit, resistance, toxicity, potential interactions with other medications, ease of use, and cost. This assessment is largely subjective. Nevertheless, some recommendations have emerged (see Table 6–5).[1–3] Initial therapy should include two nucleoside analogs in combination with a protease inhibitor or NNRTI. Dual nucleoside combinations that have been validated include: zidovudine plus didanosine, zidovudine plus zalcitabine (in treatment-naive patients), zidovudine plus lamivudine, didanosine plus stavudine (in patients with a CD4 T-cell count above 200 cells/mm^3), and stavudine plus lamivudine. The role of abacavir in initial therapy remains to be determined. The combination of stavudine and lamivudine is popular, largely because it is conveniently dosed and well tolerated. Resistance studies suggest a possible benefit from beginning with didanosine or zalcitabine first because the dominant resistance mutation of lamivudine (position 184) may reduce the later effectiveness of these two other drugs. However, this has not been established in vivo. Zidovudine should not be used with stavudine.

There is no clear consensus on the best "third drug." In asymptomatic treatment-naïve patients with CD4 T-cell counts above 200 cells/mm^3, two nucleoside analogs and either a protease inhibitor or NNRTI is reasonable (see Table 6–5). Arguments favoring NNRTI-based regimens over protease inhibitor–based regimens include ease of dosing (resulting in enhanced adherence), lack of long-term protease inhibitor–related toxicities (lipodystrophy), and preservation of second-line "salvage regimens" (i.e., protease inhibitor–based regimens). Arguments favoring protease inhibitor–based regimens as initial therapy include that protease inhibitors may be more potent than NNRTIs and that long-term data are available demonstrating the efficacy of protease inhibitor–based therapies in suppressing viral replication and prolonging life. Because of a perceived benefit in potency/efficacy, many believe that patients with more advanced disease should receive protease inhibitor–based regimens.

Three-drug regimens that spare both protease inhibitors and NNRTIs are undergoing clinical evaluation. Short-term data suggest that such regimens are effective in suppressing viral replication. By using drugs from a single class, second-line (and possibly third-line) options may be preserved. Two possible combinations are zidovudine, lamivudine, and abacavir or stavudine, didanosine, and hydroxyurea.

What Therapies Should Be Used Next?

The overall goal of antiretroviral therapy is to maintain viral suppression for as long as possible. Unfortunately, failure to achieve this goal is common, even with regimens containing two nucleoside analogs and a protease inhibitor. As outlined in Table 6–6, there are multiple risk factors for virologic failure. Given the number of potential patient variables, a simple algorithm for second-line therapy ("salvage therapy") is not possible.

Modifying therapy in the face of virologic failure is complicated, and depends largely on the goal of therapy and the options remaining available to the individual patient. Several guiding principles may be offered.[1,2,62] First, the reason for failure of the current regimen should be established (see Table 6–6). Many factors that lead to failure of an initial regimen may lead to failure of a second regimen. For example, a patient's inability or unwillingness to adhere to therapy is a critical factor that should be addressed prior to initiating salvage therapy. Second, cross-resistance is common within each class of antiretroviral agents. For example, if resistance to an NNRTI has emerged, clinicians should assume that resistance exists to all drugs within that class. Cross-resistance among the nucleoside analogs and protease inhibitors is more complicated and controversial. Third, once the decision is made to switch therapy, and dur-

---

TABLE 6–5. Suggested Antiretroviral Regimens*,†

A: NUCLEOSIDE ANALOGS	B: PROTEASE INHIBITOR OR NNRTI‡
Zidovudine/didanosine	Indinavir
Zidovudine/zalcitabine	Ritonavir
Zidovudine/lamivudine	Nelfinavir
Stavudine/didanosine	Saquinavir sgc
Stavudine/lamivudine	Ritonavir/saquinavir
	Nevirapine
	Delavirdine
	Efavirenz

*These guidelines are based on published guidelines from the U.S. Department of Health and Human Services and the International AIDS Society–USA Panel.[1,2]

†Published guidelines recommend, as initial therapy, combination therapy involving one dual nucleoside analog regimen from column A and one drug from column B. When using ritonavir plus saquinavir, one or two nucleoside analogs should be used. The role of abacavir and amprenavir in initial therapy has not been determined.

‡The role of NNRTI- and protease inhibitor–sparing regimens (i.e., zidovudine, lamivudine, and abacavir or stavudine, didanosine, and hydroxyurea) as initial therapy has not been determined.

TABLE 6–6. Virologic Failure of Combination Therapy: Possible Causes

RISK FACTOR	COMMENT
Advanced disease	Low baseline CD4 T-cell count is a strong independent risk factor for virologic failure[40]; high baseline plasma viral load may also be an independent risk factor
Pre-existing drug resistance	Prior therapy is significant risk factor for subsequent drug failure; presumably this is due to pre-existing drug resistance[62]
Nonadherence	Intermittent adherence may allow viral replication in the face of suboptimal drug exposure; clinical guidelines recommend delaying therapy until patients can commit to long-term adherence[1,2]
Enhanced drug metabolism	Drugs that enhance CYP3A (such as rifampin) may decrease protease inhibitor levels[30]
Poor drug absorption	Factors such as chronic diarrhea and malabsorption may decrease drug absorption
Increased target cell availability	Increased number of activated T cells after initiation of combination therapy may provide a more permissive environment for viral replication[73]
Privileged tissue reservoirs	Some tissue reservoirs (genital tract; central nervous system) may prevent adequate drug distribution[74]
Cellular resistance	Zidovudine may prevent intracellular phosphorylation of stavudine[24]

able viral suppression remains the goal of therapy, then all drugs should be switched simultaneously. If possible, a regimen containing three or more drugs to which the patient is naîve should be initiated. Fourth, if drug failure occurs, and a decision is made to switch, then the switch should occur as soon as possible. Allowing ongoing viral replication in the face of a failing regimen will select for higher levels of resistance and cross-resistance.

When Should HIV Therapy Be Stopped?

The clinical significance of virologic failure (defined as a persistent detectable viral load after at least 16 to 24 weeks of therapy) remains poorly defined. After virologic failure occurs, a persistent CD4 count and clinical benefit is typically observed.[63] Therefore, continued therapy is usually indicated, even if all other options have been used. Still, at some point, patients may develop advanced debilitating disease and request that antiretroviral drugs be discontinued. In general, this request can be honored, as the clinical benefits of such therapy may be limited. Also, many patients will no longer experience an effective viral load or CD4 count effect with combination therapy. Here, too, discontinuation may be reasonable. In general, if therapy needs to be discontinued because of intolerance, it is reasonable to discontinue all antiretroviral medications simultaneously and restart combination therapy at a later date.

Should Antiretroviral Therapy Be Routinely Used as Postexposure Prophylaxis?

The risk of unintended HIV exposure varies widely. While the vast majority (>90%) of recipients of HIV-infected blood transfusions become infected, the risk of a single unprotected sexual exposure is estimated at 1 in approximately 500 or less,[64] and the risk of HIV infection from an accidental needlestick injury ranges from 1 in 200 to 1 in 400.[65] Because of the low absolute risk of isolated sexual and occupational exposure, prospective controlled trials of postexposure prophylaxis are not possible. In a retrospective, case-controlled study, those health care workers who used zidovudine monotherapy following exposure had a significant (more than 75%) reduction in the frequency of subsequent HIV infection.[18] Based on this "proof of principle," early prophylaxis after occupational exposure is strongly recommended. Recommendations for postexposure prophylaxis have been published.[66]

Although controversial, use of combination therapy may be reasonable soon after a high-risk sexual exposure.[67] Public health concerns have been raised that widespread use of postexposure prophylaxis may lead to an increase in unsafe sex, particularly among high-risk populations. The financial costs of postexposure prophylaxis in this setting are also a concern. As with the use of antiretroviral therapy in the setting of occupational exposure, prospective clinical trials evaluating the efficacy of therapy in preventing infection after a high-risk sexual exposure may not be possible.

Should Primary Infection Be Treated with Antiretroviral Therapy?

In patients with primary infection, combination therapy results in dramatic and sustained viral suppression, raising optimism that HIV may be eradicated from an individual if therapy is initiated early. Theoretically, if therapy is initiated early enough, dissemination of HIV within the host is blunted, resulting in decreased viral reservoirs. Given the limited half-life of all cellular reservoirs of HIV infection, sustaining viral suppression until all infected cells die may result in viral eradication. Early models predicted that this goal would be achieved in as little as 3 years for patients who begin therapy during primary infection.[7,68] This optimism has been challenged by reports that a small proportion of resting CD4 memory cells retain integrated, replication-competent HIV-1 proviral DNA, and that the half-life of these cells may be on the order of months to years.[69,70] If this is true, viral eradication with antiretroviral therapy alone may not be feasible.

Although viral eradication may not be possible, early treatment of primary infection may have important long-term immunologic benefits. Immune-mediated suppression of chronic viral infections requires maintenance of virus-specific CD4 and CD8 responses. In HIV-infected adults, these T-cell responses may be lost early, probably as a consequence of HIV-mediated T-cell death. In cross-sectional studies, disease progression is strongly correlated with loss of the virus-specific T-cell response, suggesting that maintenance of the immune response to HIV is clinically beneficial. Because early intervention with antiretroviral therapy may prevent loss of HIV-specific immunity, treatment of primary infection results in long-term viral suppression, perhaps even after antiretroviral therapy is discontinued.[71] This hypothesis is undergoing evaluation in prospective clinical trials.

Although there are compelling reasons to treat primary infection aggressively, concerns persist. For example, are patients being exposed to the long-term toxicities of therapy prematurely? Will early intervention, before a patient is truly able to commit to long-term therapy, result in nonadherence and the potential for drug resistance? Again, answers to these critical questions may never be clear, because randomized trials comparing early treatment to delayed treatment of primary infection are not feasible. For now, aggressive treatment of HIV infection is reasonable and perhaps recommended.[1,2]

Should Pregnant HIV-Infected Women Receive Combination Therapy?

Numerous studies have identified a risk of vertical transmission from an HIV-infected pregnant woman to her newborn child. The ACTG 076 trial found that treating women with zidovudine during the third trimester and treating the newborn after delivery decreased vertical transmission significantly.[17] Based on this study and others, current guidelines recommend that all pregnant HIV-infected women be treated with indicated antiretroviral therapy for their own health and that women should have such therapy recommended in the later stages of pregnancy to decrease the rates of transmission.[1,2,72] The best drug(s) for the prevention of vertical transmission are not known, but such treatment may involve several agents given simultaneously.[72] The treatment of HIV-infected pregnant women, although generally recommended, should be considered in light of the unknown effects of therapy on the developing fetus. Because the risk of transmission during the first trimester is unknown, and because the theoretical risk of teratogenicity is greatest during this period, women in their first trimester of pregnancy may choose to delay therapy until later in the pregnancy[1,2,72] (see Chapter 35 for more discussion).

CONCLUSION

Antiretroviral therapy is a complex, rapidly evolving area of medicine. Advances in our understanding of HIV pathogenesis over the past few years have been dramatic. Novel, sophisticated, and usually expensive technologies to monitor HIV infection are now widely available. Over a dozen effective antiretroviral agents have been approved by the U.S. Food and Drug Administration, and several more are advancing through the later stages of clinical development. Based on this rapid rate of change, it is clear that patients should be cared for by clinicians with expertise in HIV medicine. It is also clear that reviews such as this one quickly become out of date.

The therapeutic advances first presented in 1996 continue to generate widespread optimism that HIV may become a chronic, manageable disease. A large proportion of patients now have evidence of durable viral suppression. Still, many problems persist. The long-term safety of antiretroviral therapy is unknown. Therapy fails in some patients, and many more may experience treatment failure over a longer time frame. Legitimate concerns have been raised that the widespread optimism that HIV may be manageable, if not curable, is now resulting in increased risk taking among at-risk populations. Finally, the advances over the past few years apply only to those with considerable resources. The prognosis remains grim for the millions of individuals infected with HIV in the developing world.

References

1. Department of Health and Human Services and Henry J. Kaiser Family Foundation: Guidelines for the use of antiretroviral agents in HIV infected adults and adolescents. MMWR Morb Mortal Wkly Rep 47(RR-05):43, 1988
2. Carpenter CC, Fischl M, Hammer SM, et al: Antiretroviral therapy for HIV infection in 1998: Updated recommendations of the International AIDS Society–USA Panel. JAMA 280:78, 1998
3. Gazzard B, Moyle G, and the BHIVA Guidelines Writing Committee: 1998 revision to the British HIV Association guidelines for antiretroviral treatment of HIV seropositive individuals. Lancet 352:314, 1998
4. U.S. Department of Health and Human Services: Report of the NIH Panel to Define Principles of Therapy of HIV Infection. Ann Intern Med 128:1057, 1998
5. Ho DD, Neumann AU, Perelson AS, et al: Rapid turnover of plasma virions and CD4 lymphocytes in HIV-1 infection. Nature 373:123, 1995
6. Wei X, Ghosh SK, Taylor ME, et al: Viral dynamics in human immunodeficiency virus type 1 infection. Nature 373:117, 1995
7. Perelson AS, Neumann AU, Markowitz M, et al: HIV-1 dynamics in vivo: Virion clearance rate, infected cell life-span, and viral generation time. Science 271:1582, 1996
8. Coffin JM: HIV population dynamics in vivo: Implications for genetic variation, pathogenesis, and therapy. Science 267:483, 1995
9. Ho DD: Time to hit HIV, early and hard. N Engl J Med 333:450, 1995
10. Hellerstein MK, McCune JM: T cell turnover in HIV-1 disease. Immunity 7:583, 1997
11. Autran B, Carcelain G, Li TS, et al: Positive effects of combination antiretroviral therapy on CD4+ T cell homeostasis and function in advanced HIV disease. Science 277:112, 1997
12. Li TS, Tubiana R, Katlama C, et al: Long lasting recovery of CD4 T-cell function and viral-load reduction after highly active antiretroviral therapy in advanced HIV-1 disease. Lancet 351:1682, 1998
13. Mellors JW, Munoz A, Giorgi JV, et al: Plasma viral load and CD4+ lymphocytes as prognostic markers of HIV-1 infection. Ann Intern Med 126:946, 1997
14. Marschner IC, Collier AC, Coombs RW, et al: Use of changes in plasma levels of human immunodeficiency virus type 1 RNA to assess the clinical benefit of antiretroviral therapy. J Infect Dis 177:40, 1998
15. Katzenstein DA, Hammer SM, Hughes MD, et al: The relation of virologic and immunologic markers to clinical outcomes after nucleoside therapy in HIV-infected adults with 200 to 500 CD4 cells per cubic millimeter. N Engl J Med 335:1091, 1996
16. Price RW: Neurological complications of HIV infection. Lancet 348:445, 1996
17. Connor EM, Sperling RS, Gelber R, et al: Reduction of maternal-infant transmission of human immunodeficiency virus type 1 with zidovudine treatment. N Engl J Med 331:1173, 1994
18. State and Territorial Health Departments, CDC Cooperative Needlestick Surveillance Group: Case-control study of HIV seroconversion in health-care workers after percutaneous exposure to HIV-infected blood—France, United Kingdom, and United States, January 1988–August 1994. MMWR Morb Mortal Wkly Rep 44:929, 1995
19. Volberding PA, Lagakos SW, Koch MA, et al: Zidovudine in asymptomatic human immunodeficiency virus infection. N Engl J Med 322:941, 1990
20. Concorde Coordinating Committee: Concorde: MRC/ANRS randomised double-blind controlled trial of immediate and deferred zidovudine in symptom-free HIV infection. Lancet 343:871, 1994
21. Kahn JO, Lagakos SW, Richman DD, et al: A controlled trial comparing continued zidovudine with didanosine in human immunodeficiency virus infection. N Engl J Med 327:581, 1992
22. Kuritzkes DR, Marschner IC, Johnson VA, et al, and the ACTG 306 Study Team: A randomized, double blind, placebo-controlled trial of lamivudine (3TC) in combination with zidovudine (ZDV), stavudine (d4T), or didanosine (ddI) in treatment naive patients. In: Program and Abstracts of the 5th Conference on Retroviruses and Opportunistic Infections, Chicago, 1998, Abstract 1
23. Hammer SM, Katzentein DA, Hughes MD, et al: A trial comparing nucleoside monotherapy with combination therapy in HIV-infected adults with CD4 cell counts from 200 to 500 per cubic millimeter. N Engl J Med 335:1081, 1996
24. Sommadossi JP, Zhou XJ, Moore J, et al: Impairment of stavudine (d4T) phosphorylation in patients receiving a combination of zidovudine (ZDV) and d4T (ACTG 290). In: Abstracts of the 5th Conference on Retroviruses and Opportunistic Infections, Chicago, 1998, Abstract 3
25. Havlir DV, Friedland G, Pollard R, et al, and the ACTG 290/298 Teams: Combination zidovudine (ZDV) and stavudine (d4T) therapy versus other nucleosides: Report of two randomized trials (ACTG 290 and 298). In: Abstracts of the 5th Conference on Retroviruses and Opportunistic Infections, Chicago, 1998, Abstract 2
26. Larder BA, Kemp SD, Harrigan PR: Potential mechanism for sustained antiretroviral efficacy of AZT-3TC combination therapy. Science 269:696, 1995
27. Eron J, Benoit S, Jemsek J, et al: Treatment with lamivudine, zidovudine or both in HIV-positive patients with 200-500 CD4+ T cells per cubic millimeter. N Engl J Med 333:1662, 1995
28. CAESAR Coordinating Committee: Randomized trial of addition of lamivudine or lamivudine plus loviride to zidovudine-containing regimens for patients with HIV-1 infection: The CAESAR trial. Lancet 349:1413, 1997

29. Dienstag JL, Perrillo RP, Schiff ER, et al: A preliminary trial of lamivudine for chronic hepatitis B infection. N Engl J Med 333:1657, 1995

30. Flexner C: HIV-1 protease inhibitors. N Engl J Med 338:1281, 1998

31. Lalezari J, Haubrich R, Burger HU, et al, and the NV14256 Study Team: Improved survival and decreased progression of HIV in patients infected with saquinavir (Invirase, SQV) plus HIVIV (zalcitabine, ddC). In: Abstracts of the XIth International Conference on AIDS, Vancouver, 1996, Abstract LB.B.6033

32. Mitsuyasu RT, Skolnik RP, Cohen SR, et al: Activity of the soft gelatin formulation of saquinavir in combination therapy in antiretroviral-naive patients. AIDS 12:F103, 1998

33. Roberts NA, Craig JC, Sheldon J: Resistance and cross-resistance with saquinavir and other HIV protease inhibitors: Theory and practice. AIDS 12-453, 1998

34. Para MF, Collier A, Coombs R, et al, for the ACTG 333 Study Team: ACTG 333: Antiviral effects of switching from saquinavir hard capsule (SQVhc) to saquinavir soft gelatin capsule (SQVsgc) vs. switching to indinavir (IDV) after prior saquinavir. In: Program and Abstracts of the 35th Annual Meeting of the Infectious Diseases Society of America, San Francisco, 1997, Abstract 21

35. Cameron DW, Heath-Chiozzi M, Danner S, et al: Prolongation of life and prevention of AIDS complications in a randomized placebo-controlled clinical trial of ritonavir in patients with advanced HIV disease. Lancet 351:543, 1998

36. Cohen C, Revick DA, Nabulsi A, et al, and the Advanced HIV Disease Ritonavir Study Group: A randomized trial of the effect of ritonavir in maintaining quality of life in advanced HIV disease. AIDS 12:1495, 1998

37. Molla A, Korneyeva M, Gao Q, et al: Ordered accumulation of mutations in HIV-1 protease confers resistance to ritonavir. Nat Med 2:760, 1996

38. Schinazi RF, Larder BA, Mellors JW: Mutations in retroviral genes associated with drug resistance. Int Antiviral News 5:129, 1997

39. Gulick R, Mellors J, Havlir D, et al: Simultaneous vs. sequential initiation of therapy with indinavir, zidovudine and lamivudine for HIV-1 infection: 100 week follow-up. JAMA 280:35, 1998

40. Hammer SM, Squires KE, Hughes MD, et al: A controlled trial of two nucleoside analogues plus indinavir in persons with human immunodeficiency virus infections and CD4 cell counts of 200 per cubic millimeter or less. N Engl J Med 337:725, 1997

41. Carpenter CC, Fischl M, Hammer SM, et al, for the International AIDS Society–USA Panel: Antiretroviral therapy for HIV infection in 1997: Updated recommendations of the International AIDS Society–USA Panel. JAMA 277:1962, 1997

42. Condra JH, Holder DJ, Schlief WA, et al: Genetic correlates of in vivo viral resistance to indinavir, a human immunodeficiency virus type 1 protease inhibitor. J Virol 70:8270, 1996

43. Condra JH, Schleif WA, Blahy OM, et al: *In vivo* emergence of HIV-1 variants resistant to multiple protease inhibitors. Nature 374:569, 1995

44. Saag M, Knowles M, Chang Y, et al, for the Viracept Cooperative Study Group: Durable effect of VIRACEPT (nelfinavir mesylate, NFV) in triple combination therapy. In: Program and Abstracts of the 37th International Conference on Antimicrobial Agents and Chemotherapy, Toronto, 1997, Abstract I-101

45. Murphy R, DeGruttola V, Gulick R, et al, for the ACTG 347 Team: 141W94 with or without zidovudine/3TC in patients with no prior protease inhibitor or 3TC therapy—ACTG 347. In: Program and Abstracts of the 5th Conference on Retroviruses and Opportunistic Infections, Chicago, 1998, Abstract 512

46. Cameron DW, Japour A, Mellors J, et al: Antiretroviral safety and durability of ritonavir-saquinavir in protease inhibitor-naive patients in year two of follow-up. In: Program and Abstracts of 5th Conference on Retroviruses and Opportunistic Infections, Chicago, 1998, Abstract 389

47. Posniak A, on behalf of the SPICE Study Team: Study of protease inhibitors in combination in Europe (SPICE). In: Program and Abstracts of the Sixth Annual Conference on Clinical Aspects and Treatment of HIV-Infection, Hamburg, 1997, Abstract 209

48. Carr A, Samaras K, Burton S, et al: A syndrome of peripheral lipodystrophy, hyperlipidaemia and insulin resistance in patients receiving HIV protease inhibitors. AIDS 12:F51, 1998

49. Lo JC, Mulligan K, Tai VW, et al: Buffalo hump in men with HIV-1 infection. Lancet 351:867, 1998

50. Miller KD, Jones E, Yanovsk JA, et al: Visceral abdominal fat accumulation associated with use of indinavir. Lancet 351:871, 1998

51. D'Aquila RT, Hughes MD, Johnson VA, et al, and the NIAID ACTG Protocol 241 Investigators: Nevirapine, zidovudine, and didanosine compared with zidovudine and didanosine in patients with HIV-1 infection. Ann Intern Med 124:1019, 1996

52. Havlir D, McLaughlin MM, Richman DD: A pilot study to evaluate the development of resistance to nevirapine in asymptomatic human immunodeficiency virus-infected patients with CD4 cell counts >500 cells/mm³: AIDS Clinical Trials Group 208. J Infect Dis 172:1379, 1995

53. Montaner JSG, Reiss P, Cooper D, et al, for the INCAS Study Group: A randomized, double-blind trial comparing combinations of nevirapine, didanosine and zidovudine in HIV-infected patients. JAMA 279:930, 1998

54. Green S, Para MF, Day PW, et al: Interim analysis of plasma viral burden reductions and CD4 increases in HIV-1 infected patients with Rescriptor (DLV) + Retrovir (ZDV) + Epivir (3TC). In: Abstracts of the XIIth International Conference on AIDS, Geneva, 1998, Abstract 12219

55. Tashima K, Staszewski S, Stryker R, et al: A Phase III, multicenter, randomized, open-label study to compare the antiretroviral activity and tolerability of efavirenz (EFV) + indinavir (IDV), versus EFV + zidovudine (ZDV) + lamivudine (3TC) versus IDV + ZDV + 3TC at 28 weeks (DMP-266-006). In: 6th Conference on Retroviruses and Opportunistic Infections, Chicago, 1999, Abstract LB16

56. Lori F, Malykh A, Cara A, et al: Hydroxyurea as an inhibitor of human immunodeficiency virus-type 1 replication. Science 266:801, 1994

57. Rutschmann OT, Opravil M, Iten A, et al: A placebo-controlled trial of didanosine plus stavudine, with and without hydroxyurea, for HIV infection. AIDS 12:F71, 1998

58. Montaner JS, Zala C, Conway B, et al: A pilot study of hydroxyurea among patients with advanced human immunodeficiency virus (HIV) disease receiving chronic didanosine therapy: Canadian HIV Trials Network protocol 080. J Infect Dis 175:801, 1997

59. De Boer RJ, Boucher CAB, Perelson AS: Target cell availability and the successful suppression of HIV by hydroxyurea and didanosine. AIDS 12:1567, 1998

60. Levy JA: Caution: Should we be treating HIV infection early? Lancet 352:982, 1998

61. Altice FL, Friedland GH: The era of adherence to HIV therapy. Ann Intern Med 129:503, 1998

62. Hirsch MS, Conway B, D'Aquila RT, et al, for the International AIDS Society–USA Panel: Antiretroviral drug resistance testing in adults with HIV infection: Implications for clinical management. JAMA 279:1984, 1998

63. Kaufmann D, Panteleo G, Sudre P, Telenti A: CD4 T cell count in HIV-1 individuals remaining viremic with highly active antiretroviral therapy (HAART): Swiss HIV Cohort Study [letter]. Lancet 351:723, 1998

64. Padian NS, Shiboski SC, Jewell NP: The effect of number of exposures on the risk of heterosexual HIV transmission. J Infect Dis 161:883, 1990

65. Henderson DK, Fahey BJ, Willy M, et al: Risk for occupational transmission of human immunodeficiency virus type 1 (HIV-1) associated with clinical exposures. Ann Intern Med 113:740, 1990

66. Centers for Disease Control and Prevention: Public health service guidelines for the management of health-care worker exposure to HIV and recommendations for postexposure prophylaxis. MMWR Morb Mortal Wkly Rep 47(RR-7):1, 1998

67. Katz MH, Gerberding JL: The care of persons with recent sexual exposure to HIV. Ann Intern Med 128:306, 1998

68. Perelson A, Essunger Y, Cao Y, et al: Decay characteristics of HIV-1-infected compartments during combination therapy. Nature 387:188, 1997

69. Finzi D, Hermankova MK, Pierson T, et al: Identification of a reservoir for HIV-1 in patients on highly active antiretroviral therapy. Science 278:1295, 1997

70. Wong JK, Hezareh M, Gunthard HR, et al: Recovery of replication-competent HIV despite prolonged suppression of plasma viremia. Science 278:1291, 1997

71. Rosenberg ES, Billingsley JM, Caliendo AM, et al: Vigorous HIV-1-specific CD4+ T cell responses associated with control of viremia. Science 278:1447, 1997

72. Centers for Disease Control and Prevention: Public Health Service Task Force recommendations for the use of antiretroviral drugs in pregnant females infected with HIV-1 for maternal health and for reducing perinatal HIV-1 transmission in the United States. MMWR Morb Mortal Wkly Rep 47(RR-2):1, 1998

73. McClean AR, Nowak MA: Competition between zidovudine-sensitive and zidovudine resistant strains of HIV. AIDS 6:671, 1992

74. Schrager LK, D'Souza MP: Cellular and anatomical reservoirs of HIV-1 in patients receiving potent antiretroviral combination therapy. JAMA 280:67, 1998

7 | Adherence to HIV Therapy

FREDERICK M. HECHT • MARGARET A. CHESNEY

WHY IS ADHERENCE IMPORTANT?

The development of more effective antiretroviral treatments has placed a new emphasis on adherence to treatment. With less effective regimens, viral replication was only partially suppressed, and resistance developed whether or not there was good adherence. Current highly active antiretroviral therapy (HAART) regimens are capable of markedly suppressing HIV replication. This limits the ability of HIV to evolve drug-resistant variants, which requires ongoing replication of virus through which drug-resistant variants develop by chance substitutions in the viral genome (see Fig. 7–1). Missed doses of medication, however, reduce the efficacy of viral suppression, allowing new viral replication and the development of drug-resistant mutations.

Nonadherence to most medical regimens, such as hypertension treatment, reduces the short-term effects of treatment but does not reduce the effectiveness of future treatment. In contrast, nonadherence to HIV antiretroviral treatment is a threat not only to the effectiveness of current treatment but to that of future treatment as well, because drug-resistant mutations can result in a permanent loss of treatment effectiveness. Thus treatment of HIV now parallels that of other infectious diseases such as tuberculosis, which require long-term treatment during which adherence for long periods of time is important to prevent emergence of drug-resistant variants. In HIV treatment, the importance of preventing resistance is compounded by the fact that there is significant cross-resistance between antiretroviral agents within each of the three classes of drugs now available (nucleoside reverse transcriptase inhibitors, non-nucleoside reverse transcriptase inhibitors, and protease inhibitors). This means that developing drug resistance compromises the effectiveness of drugs in the same class as well as the medications to which resistance initially develops. Similar to tuberculosis, recent reports of the transmission of multi-drug-resistant HIV-1[1] underscore the importance of enhancing adherence not only in order to maximize treatment effectiveness in persons taking these regimens, but also as a means of reducing the risk of transmission of drug-resistant HIV-1 to newly infected individuals.

RISK FACTORS FOR NONADHERENCE TO HIV-1 TREATMENT

Demographic variables such as race/ethnicity, sex, occupation, and income have not been shown to be good predictors of adherence in treatment of other diseases. Recent research suggests that these demographic characteristics are similarly poor predictors of adherence in HIV treatment,[2] although one study has suggested that low education levels may be associated with lower adherence.[3] Drug and alcohol use may be associated with nonadherence.[2–4] This link may be exaggerated, however, because of disclosure bias, which can affect studies that rely on self-report measures of adherence: Persons who more readily acknowledge drug and alcohol use may also more readily disclose missed doses of medication.

In a study by the Recruitment, Adherence and Retention Subcommittee of the AIDS Clinical Trials Group, persons who reported missing doses were more likely to work outside the home (85%) compared to those who reported not missing doses (59%).[4] Although this may appear counterintuitive, those who work outside the home may be more likely to miss doses if they forget to carry their medications with them.

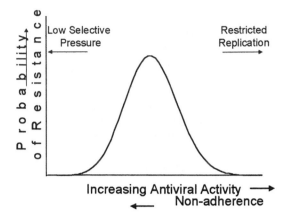

FIGURE 7–1. Antiretroviral activity, adherence, and resistance. Increasing the potency of antiretroviral agents is thought to increase selective pressures favoring the emergence of HIV-1 variants with drug-resistant mutations. This increases the probability of developing drug-resistant variants when regimens with little antiviral activity (left side of curve) are made more potent. Increasing antiviral activity also restricts HIV-1 replication, which decreases the probability of drug-resistant variants emerging because fewer variants are produced. Current regimens are capable of reaching the right-hand side of the figure, where the probability of developing resistance is low because replication is severely restricted. However, nonadherence, through decreasing the antiviral activity of the regimen during periods of low drug levels, can result in shifts to the left on the curve, favoring the emergence of drug-resistant variants.

Although it has received little attention in HIV adherence research, in other conditions, depression has been an important factor associated with nonadherence.[5]

There has been concern about whether the homeless or unstably housed urban poor, a growing segment of the HIV-infected population in the United States, are capable of adhering to HAART regimens. Whereas some have found these more "marginal" patients to be less adherent to the treatments prior to combination therapy,[6,7] others have shown that some patients living in such environments can be adherent, particularly if convinced of treatment efficacy.[8] Early evidence suggests that some of this population can adhere well to HAART regimens.[9] This supports recommendations that, although issues such as stabilizing housing and obtaining treatment for substance abuse and mental health issues may be important prior to starting treatment, decisions about who to start on these regimens need to be individualized, rather than simply based on assuming that these patients cannot adhere to treatment.[10]

Several regimen-related risk factors for nonadherence to treatment of other diseases have been identified. These include increasing the number of times each day that medication needs to be taken, increasing the total number of medications taken, and increasing medication-related side effects. Unfortunately, each of these regimen-related factors applies to current HAART regimens for HIV-1 treatment. HAART regimens require two or more doses daily, the combinations usually consist of at least three medications, other medications may be required for treatment of other HIV-related conditions, and side effects that result in patient symptoms are common.

However, the example of tuberculosis serves as a warning for those who believe that simplifying regimens will solve the problem of adherence to HIV treatment. Despite the availability of regimens that need to be taken only twice weekly, problems with adherence remain one of the biggest challenges in delivering effective treatment and preventing the emergence of drug-resistant tuberculosis. As long as we have treatment regimens for HIV that can suppress viral replication well, but do not rapidly cure infection, achieving good patient adherence to treatment will be a vital component of delivering effective HIV treatment.

HOW IMPORTANT IS ADHERENCE IN ACHIEVING EFFECTIVE SUPPRESSION OF HIV REPLICATION?

Strong theoretical arguments suggest that adherence is key in achieving effective suppression of HIV replication. In clinical practice, there are a series of other factors that may limit the effectiveness of HIV suppression. What is the evidence that adherence really plays a key role in achieving effective control of HIV replication?

Early evidence that adherence would be important came from dose-ranging studies of protease inhibitor treatments, in which different doses of drug were compared to determine optimal drug dosages for clinical practice. For example, in dose ranging of ritonavir, doses of 400 mg or less twice daily were found to achieve very temporary reductions in HIV RNA levels, which quickly rebounded.[11] Raising the dosage to 600 mg twice daily did not achieve the same degree of suppression that starting with the higher dose achieved. Laboratory testing revealed that persons taking the lower dose of ritonavir had developed mutations in the protease gene that appeared to confer resistance to ritonavir. This suggested a sequence of events with implications for treatment adherence: suboptimal levels of drug allowed ongoing replication of virus, resulting in drug-resistant mutations and a loss of long-term treatment effectiveness. This suggests that missed doses of medication might allow drug levels to decline to suboptimal levels, permitting the same process of development of drug resistance and loss of treatment effectiveness.

Evidence is accruing from clinical settings that adherence is a key, although not the only, factor in determining whether HIV replication can be suppressed below the limits of detection on HIV RNA assays. For example, preliminary evidence from a study at San Francisco General Hospital has found that adherence is a key predictor of whether viral replication is suppressed below the limits of detection, after controlling for other factors including prior antiretroviral treatment, type of protease inhibitor used, and CD4 count at the start of treatment.[12]

A recent randomized, controlled trial of an adherence intervention for persons starting protease inhibitor regimens has shown that, when the proportion of persons who took 90% or more of their doses increased from 52% (usual-care group) to 77% (intervention group), this was associated with a decrease from baseline in the log HIV-1 RNA levels in the intervention group of 1.91 log, compared to 0.97 log in the usual-care group ($p = .04$).[13] Looking at patients in both the intervention and usual-care groups, of those taking over 90% of doses, 71% had less than 50 copies of HIV-1 RNA at 24 weeks, compared with 37% of those taking less than 90% of doses.

Taken together, these and other studies suggest that, in current clinical practice, adherence is a key determinant of whether HIV RNA will be suppressed below the limits of detection, and that adherence is not simply a predetermined patient characteristic: steps can be taken to effectively enhance patient adherence to treatment.

HOW GOOD IS ADHERENCE TO HIV TREATMENT?

Since 1990, there have been several studies that have examined adherence among HIV-infected persons. Earlier studies addressed potential or actual barriers to adherence, and with few exceptions focused on zidovudine (AZT). In the studies providing sufficient data on adherence to AZT for an analysis, successful adherence was achieved by 63% of patients in a Veteran's Administration clinic setting using pharmacy refill data to assess adherence[14] and by 67% of patients in a public hospital clinic setting using patient self-report.[7]

More recent studies of adherence to combination antiretroviral therapy suggest that adherence may be better than was achieved with zidovudine alone. For example, a study of clinic patients at San Francisco General Hospital found that 77% were taking 80% or more of their doses by self-report.[12] Although this suggests that adherence to combination HIV treatment is better than might be expected, the levels of adherence that are being obtained still place a significant proportion of patients at risk of developing virologic breakthrough related to nonadherence.

IMPROVING PATIENT ADHERENCE TO HIV TREATMENT

Despite the evidence of the importance of adherence in HIV care, there are few studies evaluating interventions to enhance adherence among HIV-infected persons. Studies of adherence to treatment of other chronic medical illnesses are potentially useful in understanding how to enhance adherence in the outpatient setting.

A review of randomized, controlled adherence intervention trials found studies of 15 interventions that included both measures of adherence and measures of relevant patient outcomes (e.g., changes in blood pressure in studies of adherence to hypertension medications).[15] Seven of these 15 interventions produced documented improvements in adherence, and six showed improvements in patient outcomes. Several conclusions can be drawn from these studies that pertain to improving adherence to HIV medications. First, most of the studies that showed improved adherence and outcomes included several components rather than a single component. The results suggest that adherence is a multifaceted problem that is best addressed with a multistep process. Second, not all interventions that are thought to be useful in improving adherence stand the test of rigorous, randomized controlled trials. Third, the studies that showed improvements in adherence and patient outcomes suggest measures that are likely to be useful in improving adherence to HIV medications when combined together. These include some of the following steps:

- **Educating patients about the importance of adherence**—Although education alone is not sufficient to promote sustained adherence behavior, knowledge of the regimen and the importance of adherence is a necessary component of adherence.[4] Patients should be educated about the importance of adherence in obtaining good clinical results and preventing the development of drug resistance.
- **Clarifying the regimen**—Studies have shown that instructions that providers think are clear to patients are often confusing. For example, a study of patients who were given prescriptions labeled as "take one pill every 8 hours" or "take one pill every 6 hours" found that 77% of patients misunderstood how many times a day they should take the pills, with many patients believing that this meant to take pills at the prescribed intervals during the day, but not to take doses at night while they were asleep.[16] For most patients, it is useful to provide clear, written directions that tell patients exactly what times during the day to take medications, and include other information such as whether to take medications on an empty stomach or with food.
- **Developing an individualized plan for integrating the regimen into daily activities**—Several studies suggest that providing cues from one's daily life that help remind patients to take medications is useful. For example, for patients who brush their teeth every morning when they get up, developing a habit of taking their medications before brushing their teeth can serve as a reminder to take their morning dose of medicine.
- **Asking about adherence**—Asking about adherence during follow-up visits emphasizes the importance of adherence, and offers the opportunity to identify problems the patient is encountering that may be interfering with adherence. How providers do this makes a significant difference in the quality of information obtained. Questions should be specific and nonjudgmental and should give permission to disclose nonadherence. Physicians sometimes ask patients questions like "Are you taking your medicines the way you are supposed to?" This type of question typically fails to elicit accurate information because of the implied message that they are a bad patient if they are "not taking their medicines

the way you are supposed to." When faced with a general question about missing doses that does not specify a time period, patients also tend to round up to the best case scenario.

An example of how to ask about adherence is: "I know how challenging it is to remember to take these medicines, so I want to check in about how taking your HIV medicines is going. Yesterday, how many times did you miss taking a dose of any of your HIV medicines? How about the day before that?" This approach includes a preface that acknowledges that it is common to miss doses, and asks about a specific time period. The accuracy of patient recall of missed doses falls off rapidly after 1 to 2 days, so asking about the last 2 days helps accurately assess nonadherence. For patients who have not missed any doses in the past 1 or 2 days, it may be useful to ask how frequently patients have missed doses in the past week, or when they last missed a dose.

- **Problem solving episodes of nonadherence**—Identifying problems that patients are encountering with adherence offers important opportunities to address these issues. For example, patients who are missing a dose because they are away from home without medicines may need to develop strategies to make sure that, when they go out, they take a dose of medications with them.

Preliminary data now available from one randomized, controlled trial in Spain have demonstrated improvements in adherence and limited improvements in HIV-1 viremia.[13] This trial randomized protease inhibitor–naive participants to receive either usual care or a hospital pharmacist–based adherence intervention. The intervention group received about 1 hour of counseling from a hospital pharmacist after getting their initial prescription. This session educated patients about the importance of adherence, clarified the regimen and instructions for how to take the medication, and developed cues to help participants remember when to take medications. Pharmacists were also available for telephone calls if there were subsequent questions about the regimen. After 24 weeks, 77% of patients in the intervention group were taking over 90% of their doses, compared with 52% of the usual-care group. Plasma HIV-1 RNA levels declined 1.9 log in the intervention group compared with 1.0 log in the usual-care group ($p = .04$). There was no statistically significant difference in the proportion of patients with undetectable HIV-1 RNA, however.

SUMMARY

There is now accumulating evidence that adherence is a key element in achieving effective virologic suppression of HIV-1 and preventing the emergence of drug-resistant virus during combination antiretroviral treatment. This will be an important treatment issue as long as we have potent treatment regimens that are not capable of quickly eradicating virus. The exact level of adherence that is necessary to prevent the emergence of drug-resistant virus is uncertain. This is likely to vary from patient to patient, depending on factors including pretreatment viral load and CD4 count, and prior antiretroviral treatment. However, high levels of adherence appear to be needed, probably in the range of 90% of prescribed doses or higher, to limit the risk of virologic breakthrough on current regimens.

Research on adherence interventions specifically targeted to HIV-infected patients is currently very limited. However, data from studies of adherence in other conditions suggest that providers can enhance patient adherence through a series of steps. These steps include educating patients about the importance of adherence, clarifying regimens, developing cues to remind patients when to take medications, asking about adherence, and troubleshooting problems that arise in taking medicines as prescribed. Carrying out these steps can assist patients in gaining maximal benefit from treatment and help to prevent the emergence of drug-resistant variants.

References

1. Hecht FM, Grant R, Petropoulos C, et al: Sexual transmission of an HIV-1 variant resistant to multiple reverse transcriptase and protease inhibitor. N Engl J Med 323:346, 1998
2. Stone VE, Adelson-Mitty J, Duefield CA, et al: Adherence to protease inhibitor (PI) therapy in clinical practice: Usefulness of demographics, attitudes and knowledge as predictors. In: Abstracts of the XIIth International Conference on AIDS, Geneva, 1998, Abstract 32337
3. Mannheimer S, Hirsch Y, Sadr WE: The impact of the ALR(tm) alarm device on antiretroviral (AR) adherence among HIV-infected outpatients in Harlem. In: Abstracts of the XIIth International Conference on AIDS, Geneva, 1998, Abstract 32325
4. Chesney M, Ickovics J: Adherence to combination therapy in AIDS clinical trials. Paper presented at the Annual Meeting of the AID Clinical Trials Group, Washington, DC, 1997
5. Dunbar-Jacob J: Predictors of patient adherence: Patient characteristics. In Shumaker SA, Schron EB, Ockene J (eds): The Handbook of Health Behavior Change. New York: Springer Publishing Company, 1990, p 349
6. Morse E, Simon P, Coburn M: Determinants of subject compliance with an experimental anti-HIV drug protocol. Soc Sci Med 10:1161, 1991
7. Samet JH, Libman H, Steger KA, et al: Compliance with zidovudine therapy in patients infected with human immunodeficiency virus, type 1: A cross-sectional study in a municipal hospital clinic. Am J Med 92:495, 1992
8. Broers B, Morabia A, Hirschel B: A cohort study of drug users' compliance with zidovudine treatment [see comments]. Arch Intern Med 154:1121, 1994
9. Bangsberg D, Zolopa AR, Charlebois E, et al: Protease inhibitors (PI) are associated with viral load suppression in HIV+ homeless and marginally housed adults. In: Abstracts of the XIIth International Conference on AIDS, Geneva, 1998, Abstract 32390
10. Bangsberg D, Tulsky JP, Hecht FM, Moss AR: Protease inhibitors in the homeless. JAMA 278:63, 1997
11. Korneyeva M, Molla A, Kempf D, et al: Clinical and virological response to ritonavir, an inhibitor of HIV protease. In: Abstracts of the XIth International Conference on AIDS, Vancouver, 1996, Abstract Mo.B.1137
12. Hecht F, Colfax G, Swanson M, Chesney M: Adherence and effectiveness of protease inhibitors in clinical practice. In: Abstracts of the 5th Conference on Retroviruses and Opportunistic Infections, Chicago, 1998, Abstract 151
13. Knobel H, Carmona A, Grau S, et al: Strategies to optimise adherence to highly active antiretroviral treatment. In: Abstracts of the XIIth International Conference on AIDS, Geneva, 1998, Abstract 32322
14. Singh M, Squier C, Sivek C: Determinants of compliance with antiretroviral therapy in patients with human immunodeficiency virus: Prospective assessment with implications for enhancing compliance. AIDS Care 7: 261, 1996
15. Haynes RB, McKibbon KA, Kanani R: Systematic review of randomised trials of interventions to assist patients to follow prescriptions for medications. Lancet 348:383, 1996
16. Hanchak NA, Patel MB, Berlin JA, Strom BL: Patient misunderstanding of dosing instructions. J Gen Intern Med 11:325, 1996

Management of Patients with HIV Infection and Its Complications

8 Primary and Preventive Care for the HIV-Infected Adult

KATHRYN KOCUREK • HARRY HOLLANDER

Caring for people with HIV disease is both rewarding and challenging. New therapies offer prolonged survival and better quality of life, yet have also made the job of the provider more complicated. Recent studies demonstrate that the ability of primary care physicians to diagnose common HIV-related physical findings and provide appropriate management is discouraging, and that diagnostic acumen correlates with the amount of prior HIV experience.[1,2] Therefore, those providing primary care for HIV-infected patients must either develop expertise in the care of HIV patients through frequent review of the literature, continuing medical education courses and national conferences, and caring for many HIV patients, or should refer patients to physicians with HIV expertise for primary care or co-management.

Recent articles have reviewed the data supporting the efficacy of early preventive interventions and therapies in the care of HIV patients.[3-6] Yet, often, patients do not receive all recommended care in a timely fashion.[7-9]

This chapter provides an overview of HIV natural history from a clinical perspective, makes recommendations for the health care maintenance of infected individuals, and reviews the available data about the efficacy of such interventions. Specifically covered are the important elements of the initial evaluation history, physical examination, laboratory tests, and vaccines. Then follows a brief review of the principles of antiretroviral therapy (covered extensively in Chapter 6), recommendations for prophylaxis for opportunistic infections, and approaches to the prevention of wasting. The final section outlines a model for managed HIV care currently in practice at the University of California, San Francisco.

NATURAL HISTORY OF HIV INFECTION

Provision of timely, rational preventive therapy depends upon a detailed understanding of the relationship of clinical events and the degree of immunosuppression. This natural history is now well understood and is reviewed extensively in Chapter 3. The cumulative risk for developing AIDS 10 years into HIV infection ranges from approximately 25% to 50%, depending on the population studied.[10-15] All of these studies suggest a progressively increasing risk of developing AIDS with time since HIV infection.

The best predictor of disease progression is the HIV viral load, quantified by polymerase chain reaction (PCR) or branched-chain DNA (bDNA) methods in copies per microliter of serum (see Chapter 3). High viral titers predict rapid disease progression even for patients with high CD4 cell counts.[16-18] The CD4 cell count and percent remain important for identifying patients at high risk for opportunistic infections but are less reliable than the viral load for predicting disease progression. A study from the National Cancer Institute retrospectively looked at the risk of death as a function of CD4+ cell counts in 55 patients. Of 41 deaths, all but 1 occurred in patients with CD4+ cell counts less than $50/mm^3$. The median survival time of patients whose CD4+ count had fallen below $50/mm^3$ was 1 year.[19] Other laboratory markers for disease progression include anemia and neutropenia.

Multiple clinical predictors of HIV disease progression have been studied. One Italian study found that individuals who were symptomatic with the acute retroviral syndrome were more likely to have rapid progression of disease than asymptomatic seroconverters. The most reliable clinical factors are the development of thrush, persistent fever, unexplained diarrhea, and involuntary weight loss.[13,20–22] Oral hairy leukoplakia and cutaneous herpes zoster also are important clues to disease progression.[10,22] The presence of generalized lymphadenopathy has not been independently associated with a more rapid disease progression. However, the rapid involution of previously persistently enlarged lymph nodes is a poor prognostic sign.[13] Age greater than 35 years is also associated with a worse prognosis.[20]

An Australian study stratified the risk of specific opportunistic infections according to CD4+ cell count. Candidiasis and tuberculosis occurred with CD4+ cell counts of 250 to 500/mm^3; Kaposi's sarcoma, lymphoma, and cryptosporidiosis, with 150 to 200/mm^3; *Pneumocystis carinii* pneumonia (PCP), *Mycobacterium avium* complex (MAC), herpes simplex virus (HSV), toxoplasmosis, cryptococcosis, and esophageal candidiasis with 75 to 125/mm^3; and cytomegalovirus (CMV) retinitis with less than 50/mm^3.[23] Importantly, there is great geographic variability in opportunistic infection incidence and prevalence. As the HIV epidemic becomes entrenched in parts of the world with other endemic infections, these infections may become frequent opportunistic complications in HIV-seropositive people; an example of this is histoplasmosis in the midwestern United States.

HIV infection alters the natural history of some common infections, most notably syphilis, hepatitis B, and hepatitis C (see Chapters 13, 26, and 29).

THE INITIAL EVALUATION OF THE HIV-INFECTED PATIENT

The Office Visit

The initial assessment of the HIV-positive patient is important for establishing a therapeutic relationship with the patient, staging the infection, and planning a preventive strategy of disease management. This requires at least two office visits: the first to complete the history and physical examination and initiate vaccinations and skin testing, and the second to review laboratory data, begin treatment and prophylaxis, and review other preventive interventions as indicated. Furthermore, a visit with a nurse or case manager, or a phone call from the physician, is recommended 1 week into antiretroviral therapy to assess patient understanding and tolerance of the regimen and to emphasize adherence (see Chapter 7). Recommendations for initial evaluation and preventive care interventions are summarized in Table 8–1.

During the initial evaluation, the provider must assess the patient's emotional response to having HIV, understanding of the disease, and social and psychological support networks (see Chapter 15). These will influence the doctor–patient relationship, the patient's ability to cope with a chronic disease, and his or her ability to comply with recommended interventions and therapies. It is important to screen for depression, anxiety, and suicidal ideation, and to know whether the patient's family and friends are aware of his or her HIV status and are supportive. It is often helpful to have a list of emergency contacts in the patient's chart. Sometime early in the doctor–patient relationship, it is critical to assist the patient in establishing a durable power of attorney for health care and advance care directives through discussion and provision of the appropriate forms. These issues are better and more easily handled while the patient is clinically stable and not during a crisis.

Determining the stage of HIV disease has several important implications. From an epidemiologic and surveillance point of view, accurate reporting of individuals with advanced HIV disease allows the tracking of changing trends within the epidemic. More importantly for the individual with HIV infection, accurate staging helps both provider and patient formulate an overall prognosis and therapeutic strategy. Accurate staging is also crucial to individuals trying to obtain medical and other benefits as a result of their HIV disease. A thorough history, including a complete review of systems, may reveal treatable concurrent infections such as sinusitis or sexually transmitted diseases, or constitutional symptoms such as fatigue, weight loss, or night sweats. These may portend a worse prognosis and may indicate underlying opportunistic infections, malignancies, or the need for *P. carinii* prophylaxis.[22] A travel history will reveal patients at higher risk for infection with *Mycobacterium tuberculosis*, *Coccidioides immitis*, and *Histoplasma capsulatum*. It is also important to ask whether the patient is engaging in high-risk behaviors, so that the provider can educate the patient on needle exchange sites, drug treatment programs, and safe sex practices. Additionally, the provider should screen for other health-related habits, including cigarette, alcohol, and drug use, dietary patterns, and ex-

TABLE 8–1. Initial Evaluation and Preventive Care

Psychosocial assessment	• Emotional response to illness • Support networks • Durable power of attorney for health care, advance directives
History	• Illnesses • High-risk behaviors • Travel • Drug allergies • Medications • Cigarette, alcohol, recreational drug use • Review of systems
Physical examination	• Complete physical examination • Cervical Pap smear for women • Consider anal Pap screening for dysplasia
Skin testing and INH prophylaxis	• PPD and baseline CXR • INH for 1 year if + PPD or evidence of old infection on CXR
Vaccines	• Pneumococcal vaccine (early in HIV infection) • Hepatitis A vaccine if HepA IgG negative • Hepatitis B vaccine if seronegative • Flu vaccine if at risk for exposure • Tetanus, MMR, inactivated polio if indicated per usual guidelines
Laboratory data	• CD4 count • HIV viral load by PCR or bDNA • Complete blood count • Electrolytes, creatinine • AST, alkaline phosphatase • Hepatitis A, B, and C serologies • RPR/VDRL, treponemal antibody for positives, lumbar puncture for +RPR • *T. gondii* IgG • G6PD before dapsone • Baseline CXR
Counseling	• Safer sex and birth control • Smoking cessation • Alcohol and drug use • Nutrition and exercise
Referrals	• Registered dietitian with HIV expertise • Ophthalmologist • Dentist • Psychotherapist/drug treatment

Abbreviations: AST, aspartate transaminase; CXR, chest radiograph; G6PD, glucose-6-phosphate dehydrogenase; IgG, immunoglobulin G; INH, isoniazid; MMR, measles-mumps-rubella; PPD, purified protein derivative; RPR, rapid plasma reagin; VDRL, Venereal Disease Research Laboratory.

ercise, all of which may influence the course of HIV disease, or, at the very least, the patient's overall health and sense of well-being.[24–26] Smokers with HIV disease are at higher risk for respiratory infections and anal dysplasia, and should receive counseling on smoking cessation, a referral to a smoking cessation program, and nicotine products or bupropion if needed to quit.[27–29]

Virtually every organ system may be affected during the course of HIV disease, and a careful and thorough physical examination during the initial evaluation may reveal current disease and will provide valuable baseline information. Special attention should be focused on weight and temperature, visual fields, oropharynx, skin, lymph nodes, abdomen, genital, anal, neurologic, and mental status examinations. On subsequent visits, it is prudent to obtain the weight and temperature of the patient and to re-examine the skin, oropharynx, and lymph nodes, in addition to performing an exam directed by the patient's symptoms.[22,30–32]

After the initial visit, both clinical and laboratory reassessment are important. CD4 counts and HIV viral titers should be followed every 3 to 4 months to monitor response to and adequacy of antiretroviral therapy, and to assess whether prophylaxis for opportunistic infections is needed. Once a patient is clinically and virologically stable, office visits for clinical evaluation and reinforcement of adherence to drug regimens every 4 to 6 months are often adequate, but ideal visit frequency must be determined in response to individual patient need and disease stability.

Referrals

Many patients benefit from nutritional assessment and counseling with a registered dietitian who has expertise in HIV. Emphasis in nutritional counseling is placed on avoidance of unsafe foods (e.g., raw and undercooked seafood and meat), the maintenance of lean body mass, the intake of adequate nutrients, and strategies for minimizing symptoms of malabsorption so common with HIV patients.[33,34] Baseline eye and dental examinations are indicated for reasons of general health care maintenance, and because these areas may be especially prone to future disease.

Laboratory Evaluation

Initial labs include measurement of HIV viral load by PCR or bDNA methods twice, 2 weeks apart, to establish a baseline value. CD4 cell counts are drawn at baseline and every 4 months, preferably at the same time of day, calculated by the same laboratory, and repeated in 1 week if major decisions regarding treatment are to be made based on the count.[35,36] Baseline complete blood count and electrolyte, creatinine, aspartate transaminase, and alkaline phosphatase levels are also useful during the initial evaluation to detect HIV-related cytopenias, renal insufficiency, or hepatitis; it is also important to know these values before starting medications that may affect bone marrow, renal, or hepatic function.

Syphilis has a more rapid and aggressive clinical course in HIV disease and, although optimal treatment regimens are not well documented, standard guidelines have been established[36,37] (see Chapter 29). It is recommended that all patients with HIV have annual screening with serum Venereal Disease Research Laboratory (VDRL) or rapid plasma reagin (RPR) tests, with verification of positive results through treponemal antibody testing. Those patients with serologic evidence of latent syphilis infection should undergo lumbar puncture for cerebrospinal fluid VDRL and cell count. Syphilis treatment guidelines are presented in Chapter 29.

Hepatitis B and C share routes of transmission with HIV. Therefore, hepatitis B surface antigen and antibody, and hepatitis C antibody, levels are helpful in identifying patients in need of hepatitis B vaccination or those who are at risk for developing complications from chronic hepatitis. Additionally, checking serum hepatitis A IgG will identify those patients in need of hepatitis A vaccination.

About 97% of the cases of toxoplasmosis in HIV patients occur in those with pre-existing immunoglobulin G (IgG) for *Toxoplasma gondii*, and, before the advent of potent antiretroviral therapy, 25% to 30% of AIDS patients with *T. gondii* antibodies eventual developed active disease.[38] Therefore, obtaining a *T. gondii* antibody level on all patients with HIV identifies those at highest risk for toxoplasmosis; these patients will benefit from prophylaxis when their CD4 counts fall below $100/mm^3$ (see "*Toxoplasma gondii*," below, and Chapter 25).

Cancer Screening

Routine Cancer Screening

Patients with HIV who are well should undergo routine age-specific cancer screening as recommended by the U.S. Preventive Services Task Force.[39]

Screening for Cervical Disease

Invasive cervical cancer in the setting of HIV is AIDS defining.[40] In women with HIV, 50% to 80% have evidence of human papillomavirus (HPV) infection of the cervix, and 30% to 60% have cervical dysplasia.[41–44] Women with HIV also tend to have an increased prevalence of multifocal genital HPV, requiring careful screening of the perineum and anal tissue.[41,45] As HIV disease progresses and CD4 counts fall, the incidence and severity of cervical disease increase.[44–47]

The Centers for Disease Control and Prevention recommends, for HIV-infected women, a Pap smear at baseline and repeated at 6 months, followed by annual Pap smears thereafter if the first two are normal.[36] Women with Pap smear abnormalities should be referred for colposcopy.[48] Other issues in health care maintenance for women, including the issues of fertility, birth control, pregnancy, and gynecologic disease related to HIV, are covered in Chapters 34 and 35.

Screening for Anal Disease

There has been a greater than sevenfold increase in anal cancer in single men in the San Francisco Bay Area over the past two decades,[49] and, whereas the rate of anal cancer in all men in the United States is 0.7/100,000/year, the rate in homosexual men has been estimated at 37/100,000/year.[50] This rise in anal cancer has been attributed to infection with HPV. Furthermore, anal dysplasia and infection with HPV are strongly associated with HIV infection and, in one study, with a history of smoking.[51,52] Among women with HIV, HPV infection associated with cervical and anal disease is common.[45] These data support the need for screening the anal mucosa for precancerous lesions in patients with a history of genital warts, receptive anal intercourse, or cervical dysplasia.

Although anal Pap smears seem a logical means of screening for anal disease, they have been shown to underestimate the extent of disease found at biopsy. In one study, if the anal Pap smears were read as positive when HPV and/or anal intraepithelial neoplasia (AIN) was detected, they had a sensitivity of 88% and specificity of 16%.[53] When a positive reading required both HPV and AIN, the sensitivity dropped to 34% and the specificity rose to 73%. In another study of homosexual men, in the group with anal lesions on colposcopy, the Pap smears revealed 36% with dysplasia, 9% high grade, compared with anal biopsy, which showed 92% with dysplasia, 27% high grade.[54]

Performing an adequate anal Pap smear is made difficult by the redundant anal mucosa, the inability to visualize the anal squamocolumnar junction without using an anoscope, the lower cellularity of the smear compared to cervical samples, the risk of heavy bacterial contamination, and the tendency of the anal Pap specimen to air-dry rapidly, thus creating artifact. However, the anal Pap smear, when done properly and when read as positive with any evidence of atypia, can be up to 70% sensitive (i.e., similar to the cervical Pap smear).[55] The anal Pap smear is performed by inserting a Dacron swab 2 to 5 cm into the anal canal, rotating the swab as it is withdrawn, then rolling the swab on a glass slide and immediately fixing the specimen.[55] For anal colposcopy, a cotton swab with acetic acid is placed in the anal canal through an anoscope and left for a few minutes. Then the canal is visualized with the colposcope. Aceto-white lesions are biopsied.

Unfortunately, missing from the studies on anal HPV and dysplasia are outcome data demonstrating improved quality of life or survival in patients screened and treated for anal disease. These data will probably not be forthcoming given the ethical and logistical difficulties of performing a large multicenter study, randomly assigning patients to anal screening versus not, and then following them for many years. For now, it is logical to assume that the natural history of anal dysplasia will follow that of cervical dysplasia, and therefore it is reasonable to do an annual digital rectal exam and offer screening with an anal Pap smear to all patients with a history of receptive anal intercourse, genital warts, or cervical dysplasia. Abnormalities on digital exam or anal Pap smear should be followed up with anoscopy, colposcopy, and biopsy of internal lesions.

ANTIRETROVIRALS

All patients with HIV infection and a detectable HIV viral load should be offered potent antiretroviral therapy using three or four antiretroviral agents *from the start of therapy*[56] (see Chapter 6 for a complete discussion of antiretroviral therapy). It is no longer standard of care to wait until the CD4 count falls below 500 cells/μL or the patient develops symptomatic disease before offering potent therapy. Antiretroviral drugs should *never* be added in a stepwise fashion, and, in the case of failing therapy, one should *never* add a single new agent, but rather use two or three new drugs the patient has never used in the past. The single most important issue in successful antiretroviral therapy, once a potent regimen has been chosen, is adherence to the multidrug regimen (see Chapter 7). The primary provider must emphasize adherence and follow the patient closely, reinforcing adherence at every visit. Providers who are not expert in choosing and managing antiretrovirals must refer to or co-manage the patient with an expert physician, much as a patient with cancer is referred to an oncologist to choose and administer optimal chemotherapy. Failure to manage antiretroviral therapy correctly can adversely affect the patient's long-term survival.

INFECTIOUS DISEASE SCREENING AND PREVENTION

Skin Testing and Prophylaxis for Tuberculosis

All HIV-infected patients should receive purified protein derivative (PPD) skin testing (5TU, PPD by Mantoux method) at the time of initial evaluation and every year thereafter.[57,58] Anergy panels (commonly using mumps and *Candida* antigens) have been shown to be unreliable in their ability to identify the anergic state or a patient's ability to respond to the PPD after tuberculosis infection, and therefore are no longer recommended.[59] A positive PPD skin test is 5 mm or more induration at 48 to 72 hours after placement and interpreted without regard to prior bacille Calmette-Guérin vaccination. All patients with HIV should have a baseline chest radiograph. Patients with a positive PPD or history of positive PPD and a normal chest radiograph, should receive prophylaxis with isoniazid (INH) 300 mg daily for 1 year. HIV-positive patients with a normal chest radiograph who are exposed to a known active case of tuberculosis should receive prophylaxis with INH for 1 year, or with two drugs in the case of exposure to multidrug-resistant tuberculosis.[60,61] Those patients who have either an abnormal chest radiograph consistent with past or current active tuberculosis, or who have symptoms suggestive of tuberculosis, should undergo three sputum inductions for smear and culture to rule out active disease. If the smears are negative, INH prophylaxis is given for 1 year. If smears are positive, the patient receives four-drug treatment until the drug sensitivities of the organism are available (see Chapter 23).

Vaccinations

The Centers for Disease Control and Prevention currently recommends that HIV-infected adults receive pneumococcal vaccine, influenza vaccine, and hepatitis A and B vaccines for those not previously infected and at risk.[62,63,77,78] Enhanced inactivated polio, diphtheria/tetanus, and measles, mumps, and rubella vaccines are recommended for those patients not previously vaccinated or when clinically indicated.[62,63]

Pneumococcal Vaccine

The same pneumococcal organisms that infect HIV-negative patients also infect HIV patients but with increased frequency and severity such that up to 70% of HIV patients with pneumococcal pneumonia have bacteremia, and they suffer an increased mortality.[64–67] Patients are more likely to develop adequate antibodies to the 23-valent vaccine early in the course of their HIV disease, with asymptomatic patients having up to an 88% response rate.[68,69] Data do not exist on efficacy of the pneumococcal vaccine in HIV, and a substantial rise in HIV viral titers, of unclear clinical consequence, has been reported in response to vaccination.[70] Given the frequency

and severity of pneumococcal disease in HIV patients, and the high potential benefit of vaccination, the pneumococcal vaccine should be considered for HIV patients early in the course of their disease.[63,71]

Influenza Vaccine

Although influenza vaccine is recommended for HIV patients,[72] there is no evidence of an increased attack rate or severity of influenza associated with HIV.[73] Patients who have CD4 counts less than 300/μL have been shown to have no or suboptimal antibody response to the influenza vaccine, whereas individuals with CD4 counts of 300/μL or higher may develop protective levels of antibodies.[74] A recent double-blind, placebo-controlled study of the effect of influenza vaccine on HIV viral titers failed to demonstrate a significant rise in viral load after vaccination compared with placebo.[75] Therefore, patients with high CD4 counts who are at increased risk of exposure to influenza may benefit from influenza vaccination.

Hepatitis A and B Vaccines

Hepatitis A is more prevalent among those at risk for HIV, and, in the setting of chronic hepatitis C infection, acute hepatitis A can be fulminant and fatal.[76] HIV-infected patients should be tested for pre-existing hepatitis A immunity with serum hepatitis A IgG, and those with negative IgG should be offered the hepatitis A vaccine.[77] The clinical efficacy of this relatively new vaccine in people with HIV is not well established; however, one study found that 77% of HIV-infected patients developed protective antibodies to the hepatitis A vaccine.[78]

Hepatitis B and HIV share the same routes of transmission and are often comorbid. HIV patients who are infected with hepatitis B have a higher risk of becoming chronic carriers and of having high hepatitis B viral titers compared with HIV-negative patients.[79] Therefore, hepatitis B vaccine is recommended for all patients with HIV who lack evidence of prior hepatitis B infection or immunity and who may be at risk of infection through high-risk behavior.[62] Response rates to vaccination are in the range of 50% to 60% for asymptomatic patients, with rates falling off as HIV disease progresses.[80] At-risk patients who do not have an adequate antibody response to the initial vaccine may be revaccinated with one to three additional doses.[63]

Diphtheria/Tetanus Vaccine

Diphtheria/tetanus (dT) booster is recommended every 10 years for routine health care maintenance.[62] Antibody responses to tetanus toxoid decrease with worsening immune status in HIV-infected patients.

Prophylaxis for Opportunistic Infections

Prophylaxis for PCP improves survival and lowers health care costs.[81-84] With the advent of PCP prophylaxis, there was a shift in disease patterns associated with HIV such that we saw fewer patients with PCP, and more patients with MAC, wasting syndrome, CMV disease, and esophageal candidiasis.[84] The emergence of these diseases prompted the search for effective preventive interventions. This section briefly reviews the current state of knowledge on prevention of opportunistic diseases, and drug-of-choice recommendations are summarized in Table 8–2. For full information on prevention of PCP, MAC, CMV, fungal infections, and wasting, the reader is referred to Chapters 20, 22, 28, 24, and 18, respectively.

Pneumocystis carinii *Pneumonia*

Prophylaxis for PCP is recommended for patients who have ever had an absolute CD4 count less than 200 cells/μL (roughly correlated with CD4 <14%), in patients with a prior episode of PCP, and in patients with thrush or unexplained fevers regardless of CD4 count.[85,86] Patients with CD4 counts less than 200 cells/μL have about a 20% chance of developing PCP within 12 months.[22]

The mainstays of PCP prophylaxis are trimethoprim-sulfamethoxazole (TMP-SMX), dapsone, atovaquone, and aerosolized pentamidine (see Chapter 20). The drug of choice for PCP prophylaxis is TMP-SMX because of its superior efficacy, low cost, ease of administration, and added protection against bacterial infections and toxoplasmosis.[27,86-90] Every effort should be made to start and maintain PCP prophylaxis with TMP-SMX. Although the standard dosing for prophylaxis is one double-strength tablet TMP-SMX (160 mg/800 mg) daily, the lowest effective dose appears to be one single-strength tablet (80 mg/400 mg) daily, or one double-strength tablet three times per week.[91-93] Alternative regimens with dapsone, atovaquone, or aerosolized pentamidine should not be used unless a patient absolutely cannot tolerate TMP-SMX.

Patients who develop a rash while on high-dose TMP-SMX for treatment of PCP will often tolerate the lower doses used for prophylaxis. The rash is usually dose related and not a true drug allergy; therefore, barring those who developed a life-threatening rash on high-dose TMP-SMX, others can be safely tried on a "desensitization protocol" that spans 8 days, beginning with a very dilute solution and increasing up to one double-strength tablet per day.

Toxoplasma gondii

Before the development of combination antiretroviral therapy, 28% of HIV-infected patients with IgG titers against *T. gondii* developed cerebral toxoplasmosis within 2 years of an AIDS diagnosis.[38] The 1-year incidence of *T. gondii* encephalitis in patients with CD4 counts less than 100/μL and positive *T. gondii* titers was about 25%.[94] Therefore, those patients with CD4 counts <100/μL and positive toxoplasma IgG should receive prophylaxis. TMP-SMX is the drug of choice.[90,92] Dapsone 100 mg daily with

TABLE 8–2. Prophylaxis for Opportunistic Infections*

CD4	ORGANISM	DRUG OF CHOICE	ALTERNATIVES
<200	PCP	TMP-SMX 1 DS qd	• Dapsone 100 mg qd • Atovaquone 1500 mg qd • Aerosolized pentamidine 300 mg q mo
<100	MAC	Azithromycin 1200 mg q wk	• Rifabutin 300 mg qd • Chlarithromycin 500 mg bid
	T. gondii	TMP-SMX 1 DS qd	• Dapsone 100 mg qd + pyrimethamine 50 mg q wk

Abbreviations: CD4, number of CD4+ cells per microliter; DS, double strength; TMP-SMX, trimethoprim-sulfamethoxazole.

*For discussion of controversial prophylaxis for fungal infections and CMV infections, see Chapters 24 and 28, respectively.

pyrimethamine 50 mg weekly is also effective prophylaxis against both PCP and toxoplasmosis, but aerosolized pentamidine offers no protection against toxoplasmosis.[95] Data are lacking on the efficacy of atovaquone for toxoplasmosis prophylaxis.

Herpes Simplex Virus

HSV infections are common and frequently recurrent among patients with HIV, especially as CD4 counts fall (see Chapter 28). Oral acyclovir used as prophylaxis in doses of 400 to 1000 mg daily has been shown to effectively reduce the incidence and duration of HSV recurrences and should be offered to affected patients.

Bacterial Infections

Bacterial infections, including sinusitis, bronchitis, pneumonia, gastroenteritis, and bacteremia, are common among HIV patients.[66] In the setting of HIV, they tend to be more severe than in immunocompetent patients, often relapse after standard treatment, and are therefore a good target for prophylaxis.

Recurrent bacterial pneumonia (more than one episode in a 1-year period) is AIDS defining in HIV infection.[40] It has been found that HIV-infected patients with CD4 counts less than 500/μL are at substantially higher risk for bacterial pneumonia than HIV-negative controls.[27] Injection drug users and patients with CD4 counts less than 200/μL, especially those who smoke, are at highest risk, and mortality was four times higher among patients with an episode of pneumonia than among others in the study. The most common organism isolated from patients with pneumonia is *Streptococcus pneumoniae*, and about 60% of HIV-infected patients with pneumococcal pneumonia are bacteremic.[96]

Over 85% of pneumococcal organisms isolated from patients with HIV are included in the 23-valent vaccine; however, despite reasonable antibody responses to the vaccine, no data are available on its efficacy in HIV-infected adults. Pneumococcal vaccine may be beneficial early in the course of HIV.

TMP-SMX, used for prophylaxis against PCP, has been shown to decrease the incidence of bacterial pneumonia by up to 67%, and is good prophylaxis for PCP, toxoplasmosis, and bacterial infections.[27,88] Azithromycin used for MAC prophylaxis also affords some protection against bacterial infections.[97]

Oral penicillin prophylaxis may be considered in HIV patients with more than one pneu-

mococcal infection in the past year, and for those who are asplenic. Smoking session and avoidance of unsterile needles, undercooked eggs and meats, and unpasteurized milk products are also recommended preventive strategies against bacterial infections.

Mycobacterium avium *Complex*

Before the advent of combination antiretroviral therapy, 40% to 50% of AIDS patients in the United States eventually developed disseminated MAC infection, usually with CD4 counts less than 50/μL and within 2 years of AIDS diagnosis.[98,99] MAC causes fever, sweats, weight loss, and anemia and tremendously reduces the quality of life for end-stage patients. Median survival after MAC diagnosis is about 20 weeks, and MAC appears to reduce overall survival by about 6 months. MAC prophylaxis, given when the CD4 count falls below 100 cells/μL, reduces hospitalization and improves survival.

The drug of choice for MAC prophylaxis is azithromycin 1200 mg as a single dose once weekly. It is more effective than rifabutin 300 mg daily, and less likely than clarithromycin 500 mg bid to select for resistant organisms in cases of breakthrough MAC infection[97,100,101] (see Chapter 22). Before beginning MAC prophylaxis, tuberculosis must be ruled out with skin testing and a chest radiograph, and a blood culture for MAC must be obtained to rule out occult infection.

Fungal Infections

Invasive fungal infections, especially those caused by *Cryptococcus neoformans*, occur in 5% to 10% of patients with AIDS, and esophageal candidiasis occurs in about 20%, making fungal prophylaxis an attractive strategy[84,102,103] (see Chapter 24).

A randomized trial of primary prophylaxis in patients with CD4 counts less than 200/μL compared fluconazole 200 mg daily to 10-mg clotrimazole troches five times daily.[104] Patients on fluconazole were more compliant with therapy and had a significantly lower incidence of cryptococcosis and invasive fungal infections (4.1% vs. 10.9%). For patients with CD4 counts less than 50/μL, the 2-year relative risk of cryptococcosis was 1.6% in the fluconazole group and 9.9% in the clotrimazole group. Although fluconazole was also superior to clotrimazole troches in preventing mucosal disease, 10.6% of patients on fluconazole developed oropharyngeal candidiasis. Unfortunately, resistance data on these breakthrough infections were not collected. Despite the superior efficacy of fluconazole in preventing fungal infections, there was no difference in mortality between the groups. Thus fluconazole for primary prophylaxis does not improve survival, it is costly, and it puts patients at risk for resistant candidal infections requiring treatment with amphotericin. For these reasons, primary fungal prophylaxis with fluconazole has not become the standard of care and is discouraged.[105] However, it remains an excellent drug for treatment in patients with candidal esophagitis and cryptococcal disease, and may be used to treat episodes of mucosal fungal infections that are unresponsive to topical therapy (i.e., thrush and vaginal candidiasis).

Cytomegalovirus

Cytomegalovirus causes severe end-organ disease in up to 45% of patients with AIDS not receiving combination antiretroviral therapy, and is an independent predictor of mortality.[84,106] Patients with CD4 counts less than 100/μL have a 21% 2-year probability of developing CMV disease.[106] It leads to devastating loss of sight, neurologic impairment, and painful gastrointestinal lesions. Treatment with ganciclovir or foscarnet is lifelong, expensive, toxic, and difficult to administer and monitor (see Chapter 28). For these reasons there is great interest in developing CMV prophylaxis.

Although a recent study demonstrated that oral ganciclovir prophylaxis reduced the incidence of CMV disease by about 50%, there was no survival benefit with ganciclovir and there were significant side effects, including neutropenia and anemia requiring granulocyte colony-stimulating factor and erythropoietin.[106a] Efforts are now being directed at identifying subgroups of patients at especially high risk for CMV disease who would have the most to gain from a toxic and very expensive therapy. CMV prophylaxis with oral ganciclovir is not currently recommended.

Patients should be screened with routine eye exams for early detection of peripheral retinal CMV disease. There are no data to support any specific screening interval; however, eye exams every 3 to 6 months in patients with CD4 counts less than 100/μL may be reasonable.

Prevention of Wasting

It has been estimated that 11% to 18% of people with AIDS suffer from wasting syndrome or an involuntary loss of 10% or more of their body weight.[84,107] Wasting in the HIV population is multifactorial, and may be related to altered metabolism, infection, malabsorption, anorexia, and inadequate intake.[108–111] Death has been closely linked to the degree of body cell mass depletion,[112,113] thus prompting the search for preventive strategies.

All patients with HIV infection should have an in-depth nutrition consultation early in the course of their disease, and periodic follow-up with a registered dietitian specialized in HIV nutrition.[33,34] The dietitian will assess the patient's fluid, calorie, protein, and micronutrient intake; weight history; exercise history; and social or economic barriers to adequate nutrition. Anthropometric measurements are used to determine body lean and fat composition. The dietitian will recommend an appropriately balanced diet and supplemental formulas as indicated, based on the patient's gastrointestinal function and nutrient needs.

When evaluating the patient with weight loss, the first step is a careful search for and aggressive treatment of mucosal or systemic infections, malignancy, hypogonadism and bowel pathogens. Once these have been ruled out or treated, every effort should be made to increase oral intake and improve absorption of nutrients. This may require dietary changes (low fat, lactose free, caffeine free); antimotility agents (Diphenoxylate, Loperamide, paregoric, tincture of opium); special oral elemental nutritional formulas (per dietitian); and appetite stimulants (Megestrol acetate, Dronabinol).[114,115] Growth hormone, testosterone, other androgens, and thalidomide are used to prevent and treat wasting and are discussed in detail in Chapter 18.

A MODEL FOR MANAGED HIV CARE

Increasingly, physicians face the challenge of providing high-quality care under the financial restraints of managed care contracts. Models for capitated reimbursement for AIDS care and HIV risk adjustment with distribution of financial risk across broad pools of patients are being proposed in the medical literature and piloted in current contract negotiations.[116,117] Even Medicaid, which covers an estimated 40% of AIDS patients and pays more than twice the proportion of costs of AIDS care as it does for other diseases, is targeted in many states for managed care.[118,119] It is essential to develop a model of case management for HIV that enables the primary provider to deliver high-quality care and reduce costs. This may be especially true for academic medical centers, which, in addition to providing patient care for traditionally underserved and high-acuity populations, have the competing missions of education and research.[120]

At the University of California, San Francisco, we are faced with a very competitive health care market and extremely low, capitated reimbursements for HIV patients in managed care plans. In response, we have built and are expanding an HIV case management system that has decreased costs, admissions, and hospital days; maintained a large pool of primary care providers, including medical residents and nurse practitioners; improved patient and provider satisfaction with the care delivered; and provided a context for faculty and resident education in the area of outpatient HIV care. We have a physician medical director at each outpatient site who oversees the outpatient and inpatient clinical care of HIV patients on managed care plans followed in that group practice. The medical directors review utilization data, costs, home care, and hospitalizations, broken down by patient, physician, ancillary services, and group. This oversight is possible through weekly meetings of the case management team, which consists of the medical directors, the case managers (HIV-experienced nurse, nutritionist, and pharmacist), the administrative nurse from home services, and the overseeing pharmacist for all home infusion services. At meetings, patients who are or have been recently hospitalized, patients receiving home services, and patients who are generally unstable in their disease course or having trouble adhering to their medications, are reviewed. The goals are to optimize adherence, home support services, discharge planning, nutritional status, drug and laboratory regimens, and communication between the various services and providers working with the patient. Information and recommendations from these meetings are given to the primary providers and other involved ancillary services. In addition, every 4 to 6 months, each primary provider meets with the case management team to review his or her patients. Primary providers who are not very experienced in HIV care are strongly encouraged to co-manage their patients with an HIV-expert physician or transfer the patient to such a physician for primary care. The team and provider brainstorm strategies for managing difficult cases, and share information on new studies or expanded access protocols for which the patients may be eligible. The providers also give feedback and suggest changes and improvements in the case management services.

We have developed guidelines for care and quality review criteria, as partially outlined in this chapter, that are similar to those developed by other groups.[4] We have computerized HIV health care maintenance reminders for providers in these various university settings to standardize care. Additionally, through our managed care network, we have been successful in moving infusion services (i.e., ganciclovir induction and maintenance therapy, blood transfusions, intravenous pentamidine and antibiotics) to the outpatient setting.

All HIV patients in the managed care network who require home care services or have been hospitalized meet with a case manager and the nutritionist as part of their intake evaluation. The pharmacist case manager is available to all HIV patients and providers in the system for consultation on adherence with medications, optimal dosing regimens, drug interactions, and alternative drug regimens in the case of intolerance or drug failure. The case managers coordinate communication and services from the primary provider, visiting nurses, nutritionist, physical therapist, respiratory therapist, infusion services, pharmacy, laboratory, hospital, skilled nursing facility, and hospice. In addition, they provide benefits counseling and facilitate access to community services for support groups, meals, transportation, and housing. Most importantly, they serve as patient advocates ensuring timely office visits, medication refills, laboratory follow-up, and early notification of primary providers for medical or psychosocial problems that arise between office visits.

Through this framework of HIV case management, we have been able to provide better continuity of care with less fragmentation between services, improved ease of care for providers through the case managers, and oversight of our group practice in order to improve and standardize care while containing costs. We have also been able to support a wide variety of practice styles and patient choice for providers from the AIDS clinic, general internal medicine, family practice, or an affiliated private community practice. Finally, through the case management network, the resident-attending co-management teams, and monthly primary care AIDS seminars, we have created a system for educating each other in the constantly changing field of HIV care.

References

1. Paauw DS, Wenrich MD, Curtis JR, et al: Ability of primary care physicians to recognize physical findings associated with HIV infection. JAMA 274:1380, 1995

2. Kitahata M, Koepsell T, Deyo R, et al: Physician's experience with the acquired immunodeficiency syndrome as a factor in patients' survival. N Engl J Med 334:701, 1996

3. Branson B: Early intervention for persons infected with human immunodeficiency virus. Clin Infect Dis 20(Suppl 1):S3, 1995

4. Bozzette S, Asch S: Developing quality review criteria from standards of care for HIV disease: A framework. J Acquir Immune Defic Syndr 8(Suppl 1):S45, 1995

5. Jewett J, Hecht F: Preventive health care for adults with HIV infection. JAMA 269:1144,1993

6. Gallant J, Moore R, Chaisson R: Prophylaxis for opportunistic infections in patients with HIV infection. Ann Intern Med 120:932, 1994

7. Curtis J, Paauw D, Wenrich M, et al: Physicians' ability to provide initial primary care to an HIV infected patient. Arch Intern Med 155:1613, 1995

8. Gifford A, McPhee S, Fordham D: Preventive care among HIV-positive patients in a general medicine practice. Am J Prev Med 10:5, 1994

9. Glassroth J, Jordan M, Wallace J, et al: Use of preventive interventions by persons infected with type-1 human immunodeficiency virus. Am J Prev Med 10:259, 1994

10. Blanche S, Rouzioux C, Moscata M-L, et al: A prospective study of infants born to women seropositive for human immunodeficiency virus type 1. N Engl J Med 320:1643, 1989

11. Study EC: Children born to women with HIV-1 infection: Natural history and risk of transmission. Lancet 337:253, 1991

12. Goedert JJ, Kessler CM, Aledort LM, et al: A prospective study of human immunodeficiency virus type 1 infection and the development of AIDS in subjects with hemophilia. N Engl J Med 321:1141, 1989

13. Lifson AR, Rutherford GW, Jaffe HW: The natural history of human immunodeficiency virus infection. J Infect Dis 158:1360, 1988

14. Rutherford GW, Lifson AR, Hessol NA, et al: Course of HIV-1 infection in a cohort of homosexual and bisexual men: An 11 year follow-up study. BMJ 301:1183, 1990

15. Ward JW, Bush TJ, Perkins HA, et al: The natural history of transfusion-associated infection with human immunodeficiency virus: Factors influencing the rate of progression to disease. N Engl J Med 321:947, 1989

16. Mellors JW, Kingsley LA, Rinaldo CR, et al: Quantitation of HIV-1 RNA in plasma predicts outcome after seroconversion. Ann Intern Med 122:573, 1995

17. Mellors J, Munoz A, Giorgi J, et al: Plasma viral load and CD4+ lymphocytes as prognostic markers of HIV-1 infection. Ann Intern Med 126:946, 1997

18. O'Brien T, Blattner W, Waters D, et al: Serum HIV-1 RNA levels and time to development of AIDS in the multicenter hemophilia cohort study. JAMA 276:105, 1996

19. Yarchoan R, Venzon DJ, Pluda JM, et al: CD4 count and the risk for death in patients infected with HIV receiving antiretroviral therapy. Ann Intern Med 115:184, 1991

20. Kaslow RA, Phair JP, Friedman HB: Infection with the human immunodeficiency virus: Clinical manifestations and their relationship to immune deficiency—a report from the Multicenter AIDS Cohort Study. Ann Intern Med 107:474, 1987

21. Melbye R, Biggar R, Ebbesen P, et al: Long-term seropositivity for human T-lymphotrophic virus type III in homosexual men without the acquired immunodeficiency syndrome: Development of immunologic and clinical abnormalities. Ann Intern Med 104:496, 1986

22. Phair J, Munoz A, Detels R, et al: The risk of *Pneumocystis carinii* pneumonia among men infected with human immunodeficiency virus type 1. N Engl J Med 322:161, 1990

23. Crowe SM, Carlin JB, Stewart KI, et al: Predictive value of CD4 lymphocyte numbers for the development of opportunistic infections and malignancies in HIV-infected persons. J Acquir Immune Defic Syndr 4:770, 1991

24. Moseson M, Zeleniuch-Jacquotte A, Belsito D, et al: The potential role of nutritional factors in the induction of immunologic abnormalities in HIV-positive homosexual men. J Acquir Immune Defic Syndr 2:235, 1989

25. Eichner E, Calabrese L: Immunology and exercise: Physiology, pathophysiology, and implications for HIV infection. Med Clin North Am 78:377, 1994

26. MacArthur R, Levine S, Birk T: Supervised exercise training improves cardiopulmonary fitness in HIV-infected persons. Med Sci Sports Exerc 25:684, 1993

27. Hirschtick RE, Glassroth J, Mordan MC, et al: Bacterial pneumonia in persons infected with the human immunodeficiency virus. N Engl J Med 333:845, 1995

28. Chaisson R: Smoking cessation in patients with HIV. JAMA 272:564, 1994

29. Palefsky J, Shiboski S, Moss A: Risk factors for anal human papillomavirus infection and anal cytologic abnormalities in HIV-positive and HIV-negative homosexual men. J Acquir Immune Defic Syndr 7:599, 1994

30. Dover J, Johnson R: Cutaneous manifestations of human immunodeficiency virus infection: Part I. Arch Dermatol 127:1383, 1991

31. Dover J, Johnson R: Cutaneous manifestations of human immunodeficiency virus: Part II. Arch Dermatol 127:1549, 1991

32. Shapiro A, Pincus R: Fine-needle aspiration of diffuse cervical lymphadenopathy in patients with acquired immunodeficiency syndrome. Otolaryngol Head Neck Surg 105:419, 1991

33. McKinley MJ, Goodman-Block J, Lesser ML, Salbe AD: Improved body weight status as a result of nutrition intervention in adult, HIV-positive outpatients. J Am Diet Assoc 94:1014, 1994

34. Task Force on Nutrition Support in AIDS: Guidelines for nutrition support in AIDS. Nutrition 5:39, 1989

35. Hughes M, Stein D, Gundacker H, et al: Within-subject variation in CD4 lymphocyte count in asymptomatic human immunodeficiency virus infection: Implications for patient monitoring. J Infect Dis 169:28, 1994

36. Centers for Disease Control and Prevention: 1993 sexually transmitted diseases treatment guidelines. MMWR Morb Mortal Wkly Rep 42(RR-14):83, 1993

37. Musher D, Hamill R, Baughn R: Effect of human immunodeficiency virus (HIV) infection on the course of syphilis and on the response to treatment. Ann Intern Med 113:872, 1990

38. Grant IH, Gold JWM, Rosenblum M, et al: *Toxoplasma gondii* serology in HIV-infected patients: The development of central nervous system toxoplasmosis in AIDS. AIDS 4:519, 1990

39. U.S. Preventive Services Task Force: Guide to Clinical Preventive Services, 2nd ed. Alexandria, VA, International Medical Publishing, 1996

40. Centers for Disease Control and Prevention: 1993 revised classification system for HIV infection and expanded surveillance case definition for AIDS among adolescents and adults. MMWR Morb Mortal Wkly Rep 41(RR-17):1, 1992

41. Korn AP, Autry M, DeRemer PA, Tan W: Sensitivity of the Papanicolaou smear in human immunodeficiency virus-infected women. Obstet Gynecol 83:401, 1994

42. Feingold AR, Vermund SH, Burk RD, et al: Cervical cytologic abnormalities and papillomavirus in women infected with human immunodeficiency virus. J Acquir Immune Defic Syndr 3:896, 1990

43. Tweddel G, Heller P, Cunnane M, et al: The correlation between HIV seropositivity, cervical dysplasia, and HPV subtypes 6/11, 16/18, 31/33/35. Gynecol Oncol 52:161, 1994

44. Schafer A, Friedman W, Mielke M, et al: The increased frequency of cervical dysplasia-neoplasia in women infected with the human immunodeficiency virus is related to the degree of immunosuppression. Am J Obstet Gynecol 164:593, 1991

45. Williams AB, Darragh TM, Vranizan K, et al: Anal and cervical human papillomavirus infection and risk of anal and cervical epithelial abnormalities in human immunodeficiency virus-infected women. Obstet Gynecol 83:205, 1994

46. Maiman M, Tarricons N, Viera J, et al: Colposcopic evaluation of human immunodeficiency virus seropositive women. Obstet Gynecol 78:84, 1991

47. Fink MJ, Fruchter RG, Maiman M, et al: The adequacy of cytology and colposcopy in diagnosing cervical neoplasia in HIV-seropositive women. Gynecol Oncol 55:133, 1994

48. Minkoff HL, Dehovitz JA: Care of women infected with the human immunodeficiency virus. JAMA 266:2253, 1991

49. Palefsky JM, Holly EA, Gonzales J, et al: Natural history of anal cytologic abnormalities and papillomavirus infection among homosexual men with group IV HIV disease. J Acquir Immune Defic Syndr 5:1258, 1992

50. Daling JR, Weiss NS, Klopfenstein LL, et al: Correlates of homosexual behavior and incidence of anal cancer. JAMA 247:1988, 1982

51. Palefsky JM, Gonzales J, Greenblatt RM, et al: Anal intraepithelial neoplasia and anal papillomavirus infection among homosexual males with group IV HIV disease. JAMA 263:2911, 1990

52. Palefsky JM, Shiboski S, Moss A: Risk factors for anal human papillomavirus infection and anal cytologic abnormalities in HIV-positive and HIV-negative homosexual men. J Acquir Immune Defic Syndr 7:599, 1994

53. de Ruiter A, Carter P, Katz DR, et al: A comparison between cytology and histology to detect anal intraepithelial neoplasia. Genitourin Med 70:22, 1994

54. Surawicz CM, Kirby P, Critchlow C, et al: Anal dysplasia in homosexual men: Role of anoscopy and biopsy. Gastroenterology 105:658, 1993

55. Palefsky JM: Human papilloma infection among HIV-infect individuals. Hematol Oncol Clin North Am 5:357, 1991

56. Carpenter CJ, Fischl MA, Hammer SM, et al: Antiretroviral therapy for HIV infection in 1998: Update recommendations of the International AIDS Society–USA Panel. JAMA 280:78, 1998

57. Centers for Disease Control: Purified protein derivative (PPD)–tuberculin anergy and HIV infection: Guidelines for anergy testing and management of anergic persons at risk of tuberculosis. MMWR Morb Mortal Wkly Rep 40(RR-5):27, 1991

58. Huebner R, Schein M, Barnes S: Delayed-type hypersensitivity anergy in human immunodeficiency virus-infected persons screened for infection with Mycobacterium tuberculosis. Clin Infect Dis 19:26, 1994

59. Chin D, Osmond D, Page-Shafer K, et al: Reliability of anergy skin testing in persons with HIV infection. Am J Respir Crit Care Med 153:1982, 1996

60. Centers for Disease Control: National action plan to combat multidrug-resistant tuberculosis. MMWR Morb Mortal Wkly Rep 41:1, 1992

61. Small P, Shafer R, Hopewell P, et al: Exogenous reinfection with multidrug-resistant *Mycobacterium tuberculosis* in patients with advanced HIV infection. N Engl J Med 328:1137, 1993

62. Centers for Disease Control: Update on adult immunization recommendations of the Immunization Practices Advisory Committee. MMWR Morb Mortal Wkly Rep 40(RR-12):1, 1991

63. Centers for Disease Control and Prevention: Recommendations of the Advisory Committee on Immunization Practices (ACIP): Use of vaccines and immune globulins for persons with altered immunocompetence. MMWR Morb Mortal Wkly Rep 42(RR-4):1, 1993

64. Selwyn P, Feingold A, Hartel D, et al: Increased risk of bacterial pneumonia in HIV-infected intravenous drug users without AIDS. AIDS 2:267, 1988

65. Janoff E, Breiman R, Daley C, Hopewell P: Pneumococcal disease during HIV infection: Epidemiologic, clinical, and immunologic perspectives. Ann Intern Med 117:314, 1992

66. Berger B, Hussain F, Roistacher K: Bacterial infections in HIV-infected patients. Infect Dis Clin North Am 8:449, 1994

67. Falco V, de Sevilla TF, Alegre J, et al: Bacterial pneumonia in HIV-infected patients: A prospective study of 68 episodes. Eur Respir J 7:235, 1994

68. Weiss P, Wallace M, Oldfield E, et al: Response of recent human immunodeficiency virus seroconverters to the pneumococcal polysaccharide vaccine and Haemophilus influenzae type b conjugate vaccine. J Infect Dis 171:1217, 1995

69. Klein R, Selwyn P, Maude D, et al: Response to pneumococcal vaccine among asymptomatic heterosexual partners of persons with AIDS and intravenous drug users infected with human immunodeficiency virus. J Infect Dis 160:826, 1989

70. Janoff EN, Swindells S, Brichacek B, Stevenson M: Increased HIV-1 burden with immune activation following immunization with pneumococcal vaccine. In Abstracts of the 35th Interscience Conference on Antimicrobial Agents and Chemotherapy, 1995, Abstract 1284

71. Centers for Disease Control: Recommendations of the Immunization Practices Advisory Committee: Pneumococcal polysaccharide vaccine. MMWR Morb Mortal Wkly Rep 1989:38, 1989

72. Centers for Disease Control and Prevention: Prevention and control of influenza: Recommendations of the Advisory Committee on Immunization Practices. MMWR Morb Mortal Wkly Rep 46:1, 1997

73. Safrin S, Rush JD, Mills J: Influenza in patients with human immunodeficiency virus infection. Chest 98: 33, 1990

74. Kroon F, van Dissel J, de Jong J, van Furth R: Antibody response to influenza, tetanus and pneumococcal vaccines in HIV-seropositive individuals in relation to the number of CD4 lymphocytes. AIDS 8:469, 1994

75. Glesby M, Hoover D, Farzadegan H, et al: The effect of influenza vaccination on human immunodeficiency viral type 1 load: A randomized, double-blinded, placebo-controlled study. J Infect Dis 174: 1332, 1996

76. Vento S, Garofano T, Renzini C, et al: Fulminant hepatitis associated with hepatitis A virus superinfection in patients with chronic hepatitis C. N Engl J Med 338:286, 1998

77. Centers for Disease Control and Prevention: Prevention of hepatitis A through active or passive immunization. MMWR Morb Mortal Wkly Rep 45:1, 1996

78. Hess G, Clemens R, Bienzle U, et al: Immunogenicity and safety of an inactivated hepatitis A vaccine in anti-HAV positive and negative homosexual men. J Med Virol 46:40, 1995

79. Hadler S, Judson F, O'Malley P, et al: Outcome of hepatitis B virus infection in homosexual men and its relation to prior human immunodeficiency virus infection. J Infect Dis 163:454, 1991

80. Collier AC, Corey L, Murphy VL, et al: Antibody to human immunodeficiency virus and suboptimal response to hepatitis B vaccination. Ann Intern Med 109:101, 1988

81. Chaisson RE, Keruly J, Richman DD, et al: Pneumocystis prophylaxis and survival in patients with advanced human immunodeficiency virus infection treated with zidovudine. Arch Intern Med 152:2009, 1992

82. Fischl M, Dickinson G, LaVoie L: Safety and efficacy of sulfamethoxazole and trimethoprim chemoprophylaxis for Pneumocystis carinii pneumonia in AIDS. JAMA 259:1185, 1988

83. Gallant JE, McAvinue SM, Moore RD, et al: The impact of prophylaxis on outcome and resource utilization in Pneumocystis carinii pneumonia. Chest 107:1018, 1995

84. Hoover DR, Saah AJ, Bacellar H, et al: Clinical manifestations of AIDS in the era of pneumocystic prophylaxis. N Engl J Med 329:1922, 1993

85. 1997 USPHS/IDSA guidelines for the prevention of opportunistic infections in persons infected with human immunodeficiency virus. US Department of Health and Human Services 46:RR12–46, 1997

86. Centers for Disease Control: Recommendations for prophylaxis against Pneumocystis carinii pneumonia for adults and adolescents infected with HIV. MMWR Morb Mortal Wkly Rep 41:1, 1992

87. Bozzette SA, Finkelstein DM, Spector SA, et al: A randomized trial of three antipneumocystis agents in patients with advanced human immunodeficiency virus infection. N Engl J Med 332:693, 1995

88. Hardy WD, Feinber J, Finkelstein DM, et al: A controlled trial of trimethoprim-sulfamethoxazole of aerosolized pentamidine for secondary prophylaxis of Pneumocystis carinii pneumonia in patients with the acquired immunodeficiency syndrome. N Engl J Med 327:1842, 1992

89. Martin MA, Cox PH, Beck K, et al: A comparison of the effectiveness of three regimens in the prevention of Pneumocystis carinii pneumonia in human immunodeficiency virus-infected patients. Arch Intern Med 152:523, 1992

90. Schneider MME, Hoepelman AIM, Schattenkerk JKME, et al: A controlled trial of aerosolized pentamidine or trimethoprim-sulfamethoxazole as primary prophylaxis against Pneumocystis carinii pneumonia in patients with human immunodeficiency virus infection. N Engl J Med 327:1836, 1992

91. Schneider MME, Nielsen TL, Nelsing S, et al: Efficacy and toxicity of two doses of trimethoprim-sulfamethoxazole as primary prophylaxis against Pneumocystis carinii pneumonia in patients with human immunodeficiency virus. J Infect Dis 171:1632, 1995

92. May T, Beuscart C, Reynes J, et al: Trimethoprim-sulfamethoxazole versus aerosolized pentamidine for primary prophylaxis of Pneumocystis carinii pneumonia: A prospective, randomized, controlled trial. J Acquir Immune Defic Syndr 7:457, 1994

93. Stein DS, Stevens RC, Terry D, et al: Use of low-dose trimethoprim-sulfamethoxazole thrice weekly for primary and secondary prophylaxis of Pneumocystis carinii pneumonia in human immunodeficiency virus-infected patients. Antimicrob Agents Chemother 35:1705, 1991

94. Oksenhendler E, Charreau I, Tournerie C, et al: Toxoplasma gondii infection in advanced HIV infection. AIDS 8:483, 1994

95. Girard PM, Landman R, Gaudebout C, et al: Dapsone-pyrimethamine compared with aerosolized pentamidine as primary prophylaxis against Pneumocystis carinii pneumonia and toxoplasmosis in HIV infection. N Engl J Med 328:1514, 1993

96. Janoff EN, Breiman RF, Daley CL, Hopewell PC: Pneumococcal disease during HIV infection: Epidemiologic, clinical, and immunologic perspectives. Ann Intern Med 117:314, 1992

97. Havlir D, Dube M, Sattler F, et al: Prophylaxis against disseminated Mycobacterium avium complex with weekly azithromycin, daily rifabutin, or both. N Engl J Med 335:392, 1996

98. Nightingale S, Byrd L, Southern P, et al: Incidence of Mycobacterium avium-intracellulare complex bacteremia in HIV-positive patients. J Infect Dis 165: 1082, 1992

99. Chaisson RE, Moore RD, Richman DD: Incidence and natural history of Mycobacterium avium-complex infections in patients with advanced human immunodeficiency virus disease treated with zidovudine. Am Rev Respir Dis 146:285, 1992

100. Pierce M, Crampton S, Henry D, et al: A randomized trial of clarithromycin as prophylaxis against disseminated Mycobacterium avium complex infection in patients with advanced acquired immunodeficiency syndrome. N Engl J Med 335:384, 1996

101. Nightingale SD, Camerson DW, Gordin FM, et al: Two controlled trials of rifabutin prophylaxis against Mycobacterium avium complex infection in AIDS. N Engl J Med 329:828, 1993

102. Dismukes WE: Cryptococcal meningitis in patients with AIDS. J Infect Dis 157:624, 1988

103. Chuck SL, Sande MA: Infections with Cryptococcus neoformans in the acquired immunodeficiency syndrome. N Engl J Med 321:794, 1989

104. Powderly WG, Finkelstein DM, Feinberg J, et al: A randomized trial comparing fluconazole with clotrimazole troches for the prevention of fungal infections in patients with advanced human immunodeficiency virus infection. N Engl J Med 332:700, 1995

105. Clumeck N: Primary prophylaxis against opportunistic infections in patients with AIDS [editorial]. N Engl J Med 332:739, 1995

106. Gallant JE, Moore RD, Richman DD, et al: Incidence and natural history of cytomegalovirus disease in patients with advanced human immunodeficiency virus disease treated with zidovudine. J Infect Dis 166:1223, 1992

106a. Spector SA, McKinley GF, Lalezari JP, et al: Oral ganciclovir for the prevention of cytomegalovirus disease in persons with AIDS. Roche Cooperative Oral Ganciclovir Study Group [see comments]. N Engl J Med 334:1491, 1996

107. Nahlen BL, Chu SY, Nwanyanwu OC, et al: HIV wasting syndrome in the United States. AIDS 7:183, 1993

108. Hellerstein MK, Kahn J, Mudie H, Viteri F: Current approach to the treatment of human immunodeficiency virus-associated weight loss: Pathophysiologic considerations and emerging management strategies. Semin Oncol 17(Suppl 9):17, 1990

109. Schwenk A, Burger B, Wessel D, et al: Clinical risk factors for malnutrition in HIV-1-infected patients. AIDS 7:1213, 1993

110. Kotler DP: Malnutrition in HIV infection and AIDS. AIDS 3(Suppl 1):S175, 1989

111. Macallan KC, Noble C, Baldwin C, et al: Energy expenditure and wasting in human immunodeficiency virus infection. N Engl J Med 333:83, 1995

112. Kotler DP, Tierney AR, Wang J, Pierson RN: Magnitude of body-cell-mass depletion and the timing of death from wasting in AIDS. Am J Clin Nutr 50:444, 1989

113. Suttmann U, Ockenga J, Selberg O, et al: Incidence and prognostic value of malnutrition and wasting in human immunodeficiency virus-infected outpatients. J Acquir Immune Defic Syndr 8:239, 1995

114. Von Roenn JH, Armstrong D, Kotler DP, et al: Megestrol acetate in patients with AIDS-related cachexia. Ann Intern Med 121:393, 1994

115. Graham KK, Mikolich DJ, Fisher AE, et al: Pharmacologic evaluation of megestrol acetate oral suspension in cachectic AIDS patients. J Acquir Immune Defic Syndr 7:580, 1994

116. Knowlton D: HIV care: A capitated alternative. J Acquir Immune Defic Syndr 8(Suppl 1):S74, 1995

117. Padgug R: AIDS, risk adjustment, and health care financing in New York State. J Acquir Immune Defic Syndr 8(Suppl 1):S67, 1995

118. Green J, Arno P: The Medicaidization of AIDS. JAMA 264:1261, 1990

119. Aseltyne W, Cloutier M, Smith M: HIV disease and managed care: An overview. J Acquir Immune Defic Syndr 8(Suppl 1):S11, 1995

120. Makadon H, Aseltyne W: HIV and managed care: Implications for academic medicine. J Acquir Immune Defic Synd 8(Suppl 1):S85, 1995

9 The Chest Film in AIDS

PHILIP C. GOODMAN

The variety of opportunistic infections and neoplasms reported in patients with AIDS has not changed much since 1981.[1,2] However, some diseases, such as Legionnaire's pneumonia, are less frequently reported, whereas others, such as aspergillosis and airways disease, are now more common.[3] The chest radiographic features of these entities may overlap, and this has discouraged some from using the chest film as a means of distinguishing among diseases. Nevertheless, some differences in appearance have proven fairly constant and, if recognized, permit diagnoses to be ordered into a sequence of most to least probable.[4] This chapter addresses the chest film abnormalities observed with the more usual opportunistic infections and neoplasms seen in patients with AIDS. Less commentary is given to the infrequently observed diseases associated with the syndrome.

OPPORTUNISTIC INFECTIONS

Pneumocystis carinii Pneumonia

Pneumocystis carinii pneumonia (PCP) is the most common opportunistic pulmonary infection seen in patients with AIDS.[5,6] Chest film abnormalities are frequently present, yet in 10% to 39% of cases, the chest radiograph is normal.[7,8] The diagnosis in such situations is suggested by clinical and laboratory findings such as shortness of breath, lowered concentration of Pvo_2, decreased diffusing capacity, and, occasionally, an abnormal gallium lung scan.[9] Of interest is a recent article showing that lactate dehydrogenase levels did not distinguish between PCP and non-PCP pneumonias.[10] In another study the use of high-resolution computed tomography (CT) scanning reduced the need to perform bronchoalveolar lavage or suggested another diagnosis (chiefly airways disease) rather than PCP.[11] The diagnosis is confirmed by observing *P. carinii* in induced sputum, bronchoalveolar lavage, or lung biopsy samples.

In most patients with PCP, chest films are abnormal and reveal diffuse bilateral and usually fairly symmetric, fine reticular opacities[12-14] (Fig. 9–1). Variations in this pattern occur frequently and include unilateral or focal lung opacities of the same quality, or, rarely, focal alveolar consolidation[15] (Fig. 9–2). Occasionally, the interstitial pattern is medium to coarse, and on rare occasions a miliary pattern is observed (Fig. 9–3). Focal nodules, measuring 1 to 2 cm in diameter, with or without cavitation, have also been attributed to *P. carinii* infection[16,17] (Fig. 9–4). The cavity walls are generally thicker than those observed with pneumatoceles.[18] The outer margins may be irregular or smooth. Cavitary nodules of PCP are usually solitary and fairly pathognomonic. Occasionally, cavitary nodules of *Cryptococcus, Aspergillus, Staphylococcus,* or bronchogenic carcinoma origin may have a similar appearance.

With appropriate therapy, improvement in the radiographic findings is expected within 7 to 10 days. Without therapy, rapid progression to a worsened, diffuse heterogeneous, and in later stages severe bilateral homogeneous, consolidation may occur. Therapy with intravenous trimethoprim-sulfamethoxazole may lead to worsening of the chest film abnormalities within 4 days of beginning treatment. This is most likely caused by pulmonary edema resulting from the large amount of fluid required for intravenous therapy with this antibiotic and does not necessarily indicate worsening of pneumonia.[19] If warranted, diuretic therapy will often result in rapid improvement in the patient's radiographic and clinical state. Eventually, complete resolution of radiographic abnormalities is expected, although in some instances residual interstitial opacities are observed.[20,21] Adjunctive therapy with corticosteroids has been recommended for patients with moderate to severe

139

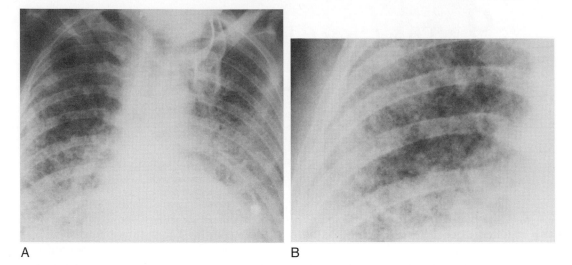

A   B

FIGURE 9–1. *Pneumocystis carinii* pneumonia. *A,* Anteroposterior (AP) chest film demonstrates moderate to severe bilateral reticular heterogeneous opacities. *B,* Close-up of the right midlung demonstrates the fine nature of the reticular opacities seen in PCP. In the peripheral areas of the lung, coalescence of these densities has produced a more homogeneous consolidation, as seen in severe episodes of infection.

PCP.[22,23] Rapid improvement in the chest film findings may be observed after this regimen.[24,25] A complication of steroid use may be an increase in secondary fungal infections.[26]

A few interesting complications of PCP have been recognized with some frequency in the last several years. Spontaneous pneumothorax has been observed in approximately 5% to 10% of patients with PCP[27,28] (Fig. 9–5). The pneumothoraces have varied in size from small to extremely large, and may require tube thoracostomy, chemical pleurodesis, talc poudrage, or surgery.[29–32] Occasionally, in patients too ill to

undergo surgery or for outpatient care, a Heimlich valve has been successful.[33,34] Although somewhat controversial, the timing of the pneumothoraces is probably not related to treatment but apparently is due to infection with *P. carinii* itself.[35,36] Pneumothorax in AIDS patients is virtually pathognomonic of PCP.[37] In some instances, pneumatoceles precede the appearance of pneumothorax (Fig. 9–6). In one series, 10% of patients with PCP were found to have pneumatoceles.[38] These thin-walled air-containing structures are solitary or multiple and may rapidly increase or decrease in size (Fig. 9–7), and

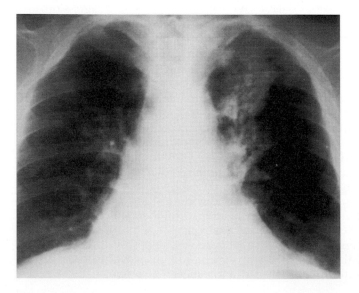

FIGURE 9–2. *Pneumocystis carinii* pneumonia. Posteroanterior (PA) chest film demonstrates a focal area of fairly homogeneous consolidation in the left upper lobe. Air bronchograms are seen in this region of alveolar opacity.

FIGURE 9–3. *Pneumocystis carinii* pneumonia. Close-up of a PA chest film demonstrates a fine to medium nodular or miliary pattern in the right upper and middle lobes.

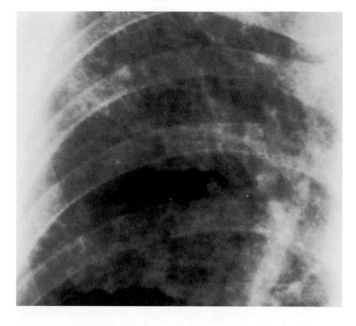

generally resolve in 3 to 6 months. In rare instances, air–fluid levels have been noted within the pneumatoceles. These abnormalities have not been observed in AIDS patients with infections other than PCP. The mechanism for pneumatocele formation in this circumstance is unclear, and, although it may be due to a check valve mechanism, there is little pathologic proof this occurs in these patients.[39] Others suggest that necrosis in subpleural locations of the lung

may result in pneumatoceles and subsequent pneumothorax.[40] Premature formation of bullae seen on CT scans has been described in patients with AIDS.[41]

The distribution of PCP may be altered by prophylactic therapy with inhaled pentamidine. In some patients who have undergone this therapeutic regimen, new cases of PCP may be preferentially located in the upper lobes[42–45] (Fig. 9–8). The reason for this probably is poor cov-

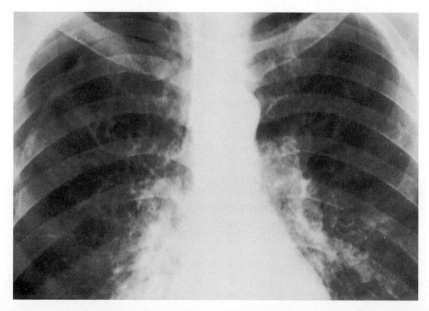

FIGURE 9–4. *Pneumocystis carinii* pneumonia. PA chest film demonstrates a solitary thick-walled cavity in the right upper lobe. PCP may appear in this fashion secondary to ischemic necrosis of affected lung.

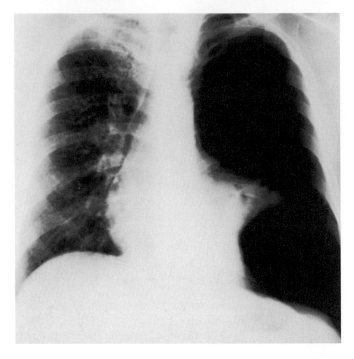

FIGURE 9–5. *Pneumocystis carinii* pneumonia and pneumothorax. PA chest film demonstrates a large left-sided tension pneumothorax. The right lung, particularly the right upper lobe, demonstrates a medium reticulonodular pattern.

erage of the upper lobes by aerosolized pentamidine. These unprotected areas are thus more likely to harbor *P. carinii* and to be selectively involved in pneumonia. Other unusual features of this therapy, including pneumothorax, pneumocystomas, pleural fluid, and lymphadenopathy, have also been reported.[29,46–50,50a] Nevertheless, the presence of pleural fluid or hilar or mediastinal lymphadenopathy should suggest a diagnosis other than PCP.

Mycobacterial Infections

Various mycobacterial species have been responsible for pulmonary infections in patients with AIDS.[14,51–53] Clearly, the majority of infections have been caused by *Mycobacterium tuberculosis* and *Mycobacterium avium* complex (MAC). The overall incidence of tuberculosis in AIDS patients has been reported to be as high as 24%.[54] More recently, in 14% of HIV-seropositive patients with known positive purified protein derivative skin tests, tuberculosis developed within 2 years.[55] Conversely, nearly 30% of adult non-Asian patients with tuberculosis had HIV infection.[56] The radiographic appearance of tuberculosis in this setting depends upon the stage of HIV infection.[57,58,58a] Early in the course of infection, tuberculosis appears as it does in otherwise nonimmunosuppressed individuals; that is, patients with reactivation tuberculosis, considered the most common pathogenesis of tuberculosis in these patients, will

present with heterogeneous nodular and cavitary infiltrates in the superior segments of the lower lobes and apical and posterior segments of the upper lobes (Fig. 9–9). These radiographic findings are not seen later in HIV infection, when diffuse and somewhat coarse interstitial opacities are observed with or without the presence of hilar or mediastinal adenopathy[59] (Fig. 9–10). In patients with CD4+ lymphocyte counts less than 100/mm^3 significantly more adenopathy was seen on chest films.[60] Adenopathy itself may occur with different frequency within different AIDS risk groups. Thus lymphadenopathy was found in a higher percentage (~80%) of injection drug users or Haitian patients with HIV infection and tuberculosis than in HIV-infected homosexual males with tuberculosis (~20%).[61,62] In a study from New York, 84% of patients with AIDS and tuberculosis had low-attenuation mediastinal and hilar nodes on CT scans.[63] Later in the course of HIV infection, tuberculosis may result in cavitation, but at a significantly reduced rate compared to non-HIV-infected patients or those with early-stage HIV infection.[64] Significantly more cavitation was seen on chest films of patients with CD4+ lymphocyte counts of 200/mm^3 or higher.[60] Pleural fluid is seen with varying incidence (9% to 22%) and has been reported to be more common in HIV-positive patients.[59,65,66] The presence of adenopathy, pleural fluid, or a coarse bilateral heterogeneous infiltrate is much more typical of tuberculosis than of PCP.

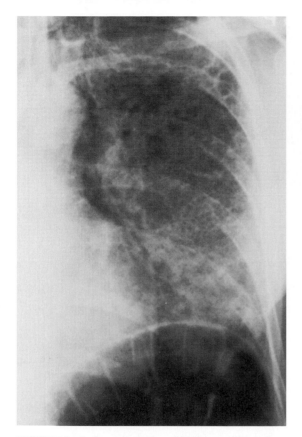

FIGURE 9–6. *Pneumocystis carinii* pneumonia and pneumatoceles. Close-up of a PA chest film demonstrates heterogeneous medium interstitial opacities in the left lung. In the periphery of the left upper lobe, small, thin-walled, air-filled structures representing pneumatoceles are demonstrated. These usually resolve in 3 to 6 months but occasionally lead to pneumothorax.

Antituberculosis therapy should result in chest film improvement that parallels a clinical response by the patient.[67] Within weeks, the radiographic abnormalities seen with this infection should begin to resolve. Worsening of a chest film while a patient is receiving appropriate medication should prompt a work-up for an alternate infection. Recently, an increase in multidrug-resistant tuberculosis cases has been observed; consequently, appropriate individualized drug regimens have been recommended.[68–70]

MAC is typically seen in the lymph nodes, liver, bone marrow, blood, and urine of patients with AIDS. Involvement of pulmonary parenchyma results in diffuse, heterogeneous interstitial patterns with or without lymphadenopathy.[15] No definite features distinguishing this or other species of mycobacterial infection from tuberculosis have been observed on chest films. A comparison of chest films in AIDS patients with tuberculosis or MAC disease revealed that, with the latter infection, approximately 50% had interstitial disease, 11% had adenopathy, and none had pleural fluid.[71] A more recent report suggests that adenopathy and pleural fluid may be noted, but that parenchymal disease caused by nontuberculosis mycobacterial disease is unlikely.[72] Another article supports the unusual occurrence of pulmonary MAC and reports chest films with consolidation, nodular infiltrates, and cavitation.[73]

Mycobacterium kansasii has recently been reported as a cause of predominantly unifocal findings on chest films. Hilar and/or mediastinal adenopathy were seen in 25% of patients. Cav-

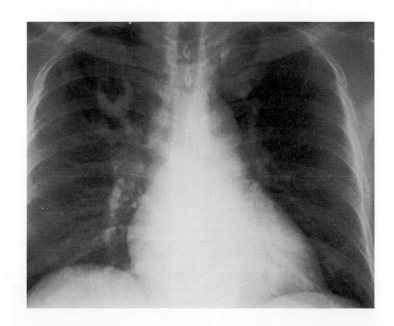

FIGURE 9–7. *Pneumocystis carinii* pneumonia. A PA chest film demonstrates multiple thin-walled pneumatoceles in both lungs. These generally will resolve over months. A pneumothorax is noted in the right hemithorax.

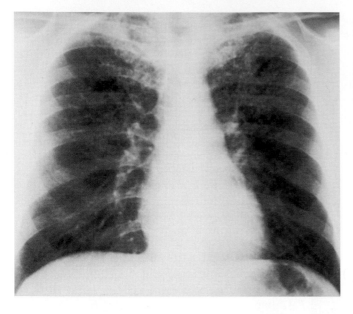

FIGURE 9–8. *Pneumocystis carinii* pneumonia. PA chest film demonstrates predominantly upper lobe medium reticular densities. This distribution of PCP may be the result of prior prophylactic aerosolized pentamidine therapy and mimics the distribution of reactivation tuberculosis.

itation and pleural fluid were less frequent. The majority of patients demonstrated radiographic improvement when tested.[74]

Fungi

A variety of fungal infections have been observed in patients with AIDS. In regions endemic for *Histoplasma capsulatum* and *Coccidioides immitis*, these organisms have been responsible for a number of opportunistic pneumonias in HIV-infected individuals.[75–80,80a] The

radiographic appearance of these pneumonias is similar. Commonly, a diffuse, bilateral, poorly defined nodular infiltrate is noted (Fig. 9–11). Lymphadenopathy is reported with variable incidence with both of these fungal infections. Other manifestations, including cavitation, alveolar consolidation, and pleural fluid, have been reported but are less frequently observed.[81] A recent study of 50 AIDS patients with extrapulmonary histoplasmosis revealed that slightly over 50% had normal chest radiographs. The others demonstrated nodular, linear, or airspace opacities in decreasing frequency, respectively.

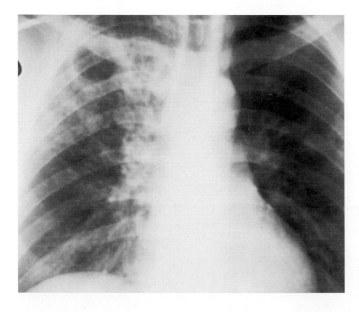

FIGURE 9–9. Tuberculosis. PA chest film demonstrates heterogeneous, medium to coarse reticular opacities in the right upper lobe. A large cavity is seen in this area. Minimal left upper lobe heterogeneous changes are seen. This pattern is typical of reactivation tuberculosis seen in the early stages of HIV infection.

FIGURE 9–10. Tuberculosis. PA chest film demonstrates right paratracheal adenopathy and a diffuse fine to medium reticulonodular infiltrate. This is the pattern seen in patients with late-stage HIV infection and tuberculosis. Because adenopathy is not associated with it, PCP should not be considered a likely cause of disease in this patient.

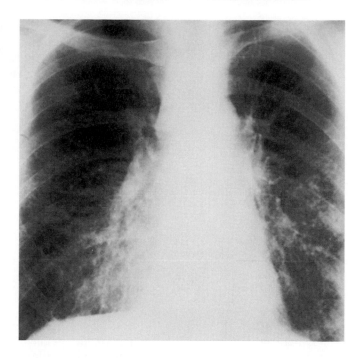

Approximately 20% had small pleural effusions and less than 10% had adenopathy.[82]

Cryptococcal infections of AIDS patients generally affect the central nervous system, but more cases of cryptococcal pneumonia are being reported. The radiographic appearance is variable and includes single or multiple well-defined nodules with or without cavitation, diffuse reticular interstitial infiltrates, pleural fluid, and hilar or mediastinal adenopathy[62,83–85] (Fig. 9–12). A miliary pattern may also be seen with this and other fungal infections.[86,87]

Invasive aspergillosis in AIDS patients has been reported with increasing frequency.[88–91]

Focal infiltrates of the upper lobes with or without cavitation are most commonly noted on chest films.[88,92–94] Occasionally, the focal opacities will remain stable for months. In one series, no air-crescent findings were noted.[95]

Cytomegalovirus

Cytomegalovirus (CMV) pneumonia was one of the initial opportunistic infections seen in patients with AIDS. However, our experience as well as others' suggests that this organism, although frequently observed in patients with

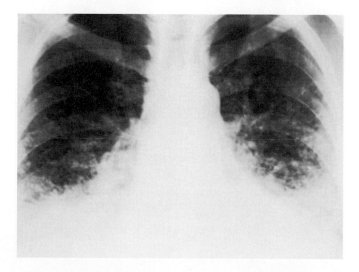

FIGURE 9–11. Histoplasmosis. Diffuse, bilateral, fairly coarse nodular opacities are seen in both lungs. This pattern is commonly reported in patients with disseminated histoplasmosis and coccidioidomycosis. Adenopathy is also associated with these diseases in patients with AIDS.

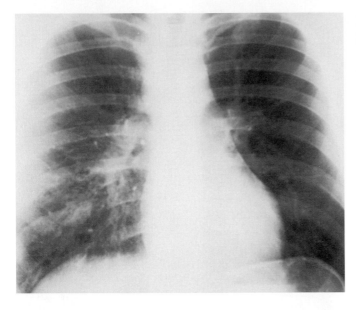

FIGURE 9–12. Cryptococcosis. PA chest film demonstrates right paratracheal and right hilar adenopathy. Occasionally, parenchymal lung nodules and reticular interstitial opacities also are seen in patients with intrathoracic cryptococcosis.

AIDS, may not be responsible for pathologic lung changes.[96] This controversy continues even now.[97,98] It is our policy to emphasize this diagnosis less than the other opportunistic infections. In those patients reported to have CMV pneumonia, a diffuse, fine to medium reticular interstitial pattern has been observed on chest films.[99] However, it is difficult to be certain that the radiographic abnormalities have been caused by this organism because other opportunistic agents frequently coexist. It is extremely rare for CMV to be the sole pathogen responsible for pneumonia.[100,101] However, the incidence of CMV pneumonia may be increasing now that individuals with low CD4 counts are living longer and steroids are being used more frequently.[102,103] A recent assessment of the chest film and CT abnormalities of patients with only CMV pneumonia includes focal and bilateral heterogeneous opacities, lung consolidations and ground-glass opacities, and solitary or multiple well-defined lung nodules.[104] Some reports suggest that patients shedding CMV in respiratory secretions may have a decreased inflammatory response to *P. carinii* and in fact will have a better short-term prognosis.[105]

Pyogenic Infection

Pneumonias caused by pyogenic organisms such as *Streptococcus pneumoniae, Haemophilus in-*

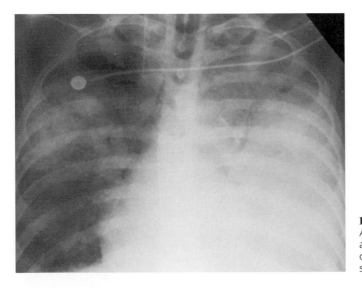

FIGURE 9–13. Pneumococcal pneumonia. AP chest film demonstrates a severe bilateral airspace consolidation, worse on the left than on the right. The findings are typical of severe pyogenic pneumonia.

FIGURE 9–14. Bronchitis. Close-up of the right lower lobe demonstrates thin, linear opacities paralleling the course of segmental bronchi. This finding is called "tram tracking" and has been seen in AIDS patients with clinical bronchitis.

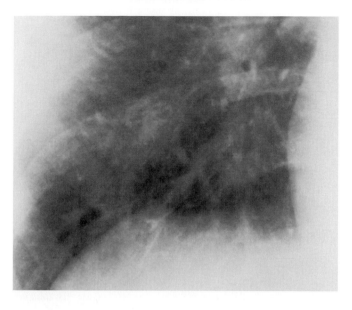

fluenzae, Staphylococcus aureus, and *Pseudomonas aeruginosa* have been reported with increasing frequency in patients with AIDS.[106–109] It has been well established that both T-cell and B-cell immune function is compromised in these patients, thus accounting for the increased frequency of pyogenic infections. The radiographic features are similar to those seen in nonimmunosuppressed individuals.[110,111] Airspace consolidation resulting in homogeneous opacity in a segment or lobe of lung is most frequently observed (Fig. 9–13). Parapneumonic effusions are also seen. Cavitation may occur in patients infected with organisms such as *S. aureus* that can cause necrosis. A different finding has recently been observed in a series from Switzerland in which nearly 50% of patients with bacterial pneumonias had diffuse reticulonodular opacities on chest radiographs.[112] Generally, patients with pyogenic pneumonia do not have concomitant infection with opportunistic organisms such as *P. carinii.* Response to appropriate antibiotics is similar to that of nonimmunosuppressed hosts such that radiographic improvement is seen within 1 to 2 weeks.[113] However, recurrent pneumonia and/or chronic pneumonia may require maintenance therapy.[114] It is important to consider bacterial pneumonias in differential diagnosis lists, because they may have a significant impact on patient morbidity and mortality.[107]

Rhodococcus equi is an unusual organism that has been the cause of lung disease in several HIV-infected patients. The chest films frequently reveal large, moderately thick-walled cavities and empyema.[115–117] In a recent review

of 48 patients, 77% of patients with *R. equi* demonstrated cavitation; 55% also had upper lobe involvement.[118]

Bronchitis caused by pyogenic organisms has also been seen with moderate frequency in patients with AIDS and has been seen with significantly increased incidence in HIV-positive versus HIV-negative patients.[119,120] Radiographically, this is manifested by peribronchial thickening and "tram tracking" (Fig. 9–14). The latter finding is caused by bronchial mucosal edema and peribronchial inflammation and is seen as thin, parallel, linear opacities following the expected course of bronchi. This is not a feature of the pneumonia caused by *P. carinii.* CT is a better modality for detecting airway abnormalities.[121] Bronchiectasis in patients with AIDS has also been identified by CT.[122] Although many of these patients have had recurrent bouts of opportunistic infection, some authors contend that bronchial dilatation may be detected by CT in patients who have not exhibited signs or symptoms of prior infection and is possibly related to HIV infection itself.[123]

NEOPLASMS

Kaposi's Sarcoma

The radiographic features of Kaposi's sarcoma are somewhat distinctive.[7,124–129] Pulmonary parenchymal involvement is manifested by coarse, poorly defined, nodular opacities scattered throughout the lungs (Fig. 9–15). Concomitant

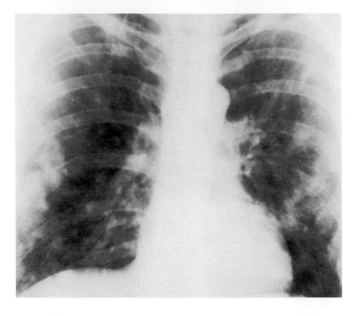

FIGURE 9–15. Kaposi's sarcoma (KS). Scattered, poorly defined nodules are seen in both lungs. This is a classic presentation of pulmonary KS. Other manifestations include pleural fluid and coarse linear interstitial opacities.

coarse, linear opacities usually distributed in a perihilar location are also frequent. Pleural fluid is reported in 35% to 50% of patients with Kaposi's sarcoma and is probably the result of pleural metastases. Kaposi's nodules generally increase slowly in size over several months. Rapid change in size of a suspected Kaposi's sarcoma pulmonary nodule with progression to lung consolidation suggests the possibility of hemorrhage in the region of these highly vascular lesions (Fig. 9–16). Hilar and mediastinal adenopathy may be observed but is uncommon (~8%). CT findings in patients with Kaposi's sarcoma reflect what is seen on chest films, with poorly marginated, nodular, and coarse perihilar opacities being most common.[130,131]

In patients with a background of intravenous drug abuse, differentiating Kaposi's sarcoma nodules from septic emboli may be impossible. However, within a few days, septic emboli will tend to cavitate, whereas Kaposi's sarcoma nodules will not. The use of sequential thallium and gallium scanning has also been proposed as a way to differentiate between pulmonary Kaposi's sarcoma and other pulmonary diseases associated with AIDS.[132] Generally, mucocutaneous Kaposi's sarcoma precedes pulmonary involvement, but occasionally lung disease is the first manifestation.[133]

Non-Hodgkin's Lymphoma

General differences in the lymphomas seen in patients with AIDS as compared to those seen in the general population include a greater stage of involvement at the time of initial discovery, greater aggressiveness of the neoplasm, an almost exclusive tendency for the lymphomas to be the non-Hodgkin's variety, and a decreased frequency of intrathoracic involvement.[134] An early study of AIDS patients with non-Hodgkin's lymphoma revealed that only 10% of patients had chest manifestations.[135] The radiographic features of non-Hodgkin's lymphoma in this setting include unilateral and bilateral pleural effusions in nearly half the patients. Hilar or mediastinal adenopathy is observed in nearly one fourth of chest films (Fig. 9–17). Pulmonary parenchymal involvement is manifest by reticulonodular interstitial infiltrates or alveolar consolidation in nearly one quarter of patients. The appearance of well-defined parenchymal nodules remarkable for their rapidity of growth has been noted in 40% of patients[136] (Fig. 9–18). These nodules do not tend to coalesce as do the poorly defined nodules of Kaposi's sarcoma. Cavitation of these nodules may occur following therapy but is rare.[134] In a recent CT evaluation of 10 patients with non-Hodgkin's lymphoma 90% were found to have pulmonary nodules.[137]

Bronchogenic Carcinoma

There has been speculation and debate about whether HIV infection may be associated with an increased incidence of lung cancer.[120,138,139] Although a definite association has not been

FIGURE 9–16. Kaposi's sarcoma. *A*, PA chest film demonstrates two poorly defined nodules in the right middle lobe and one poorly defined nodule in the left retrocardiac area. These findings are typical of KS. *B*, The same patient 2 weeks later. At this time, more homogeneous consolidation is seen in the lower lobe and right middle lobe. This type of rapid change is most likely due to hemorrhage in the sites of pulmonary KS.

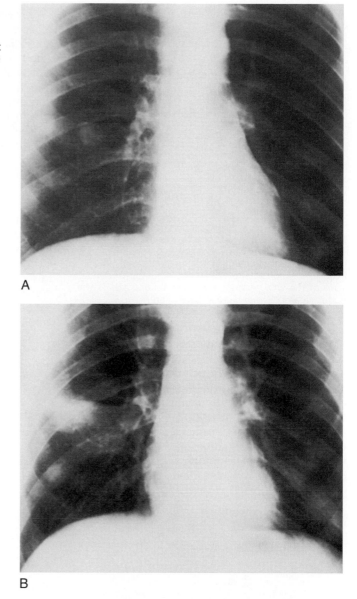

A

B

firmly established, there are numerous reports of bronchogenic carcinoma occurring in patients with HIV infection who are younger than the usual population with cancer. A history of intravenous drug abuse and cigarette smoking is usually elicited in these patients. Survival time in this population is significantly shortened.[140–143] The radiographic abnormalities are similar to those seen in the general population and include focal lung mass, hilar and mediastinal adenopathy, and pleural fluid.[144–147] In patients who have suspected focal PCP or fungal diseases, yet are not responding to appropriate therapy, the possibility of lung neoplasm should be raised. Diagnosis may be forthcoming with sputum cytology, bronchoscopic biopsy, or percutaneous transthoracic needle biopsy.

LYMPHOCYTIC AND NONSPECIFIC INTERSTITIAL PNEUMONITIS

Lymphocytic interstitial pneumonitis is a disease of unknown cause that is characterized by an accumulation of lymphocytes and plasma cells in the pulmonary interstitial space. Although even distribution is usually demonstrated, focal collections of lymphocytes may be

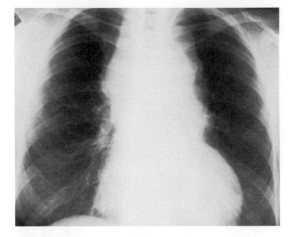

FIGURE 9–17. Non-Hodgkin's lymphoma. PA chest film demonstrates severe mediastinal adenopathy. Intrathoracic involvement in AIDS patients with non-Hodgkin's lymphoma has been observed approximately 10% of the time. Adenopathy, pleural fluid, and nodular parenchymal disease have been noted.

observed.[148,149] This entity has now been recognized as an index diagnosis for AIDS in the pediatric patient. Chest films of these individuals are indistinguishable from those seen in patients with PCP. They typically demonstrate diffuse or focal, fine to medium reticular interstitial infiltrates[150] (Fig. 9–19). Some reports indicate a tendency to small nodular opacities correlating well with pathologic findings.[151] The chest radiographs remain stable initially but worsen over weeks to months. Lymphadenopathy may be seen in the late stages of disease.[152] Cystic lung disease and bronchiectasis may also develop after protracted illness.[153,154] Open lung biopsy is required for definitive diagnosis. Steroid therapy may result in rapid radiographic improvement.

Nonspecific interstitial pneumonitis (NSIP) can be defined pathologically as chronic interalveolar septal inflammation without identifiable cause. In a recent article it was noted that NSIP was the most frequent mimic of PCP both clinically and radiographically.[155] In fact, of all patients thought initially to have PCP, 5% demonstrated NSIP and, of the 67 patients who did not have PCP, 16 had NSIP. Clinically patients with NSIP would be more likely to have higher CD4+ lymphocyte counts than patients with PCP. Their chest radiographs will be less involved with heterogeneous opacities than those patients with PCP; however, clinical and radiographic overlap preclude a definite ability to distinguish between these two entities. The authors of this article did find that NSIP might improve while patients were being treated empirically for PCP.[155]

SUMMARY

The task of interpreting chest radiographs in patients with AIDS will be made easier, it is

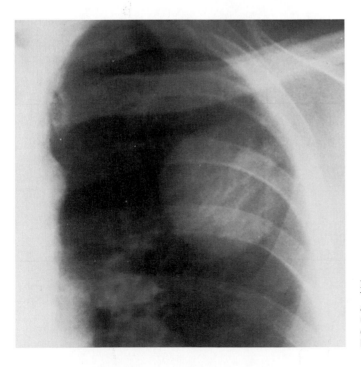

FIGURE 9–18. Non-Hodgkin's lymphoma. This large, well-defined nodule appeared over a period of 6 weeks. A needle biopsy was unrevealing, but an open lung procedure demonstrated a large non-Hodgkin's lymphoma lesion.

FIGURE 9–19. Lymphocytic interstitial pneumonia (LIP). PA chest film demonstrates bibasilar fine to medium reticular interstitial opacities indistinguishable from PCP. An open lung biopsy revealed LIP.

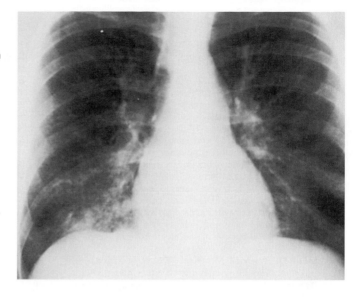

hoped, by applying the information contained in this chapter. Although the various infections and neoplasms seen with this syndrome occasionally have similar appearances on chest films, some patterns should allow construction of a limited differential diagnosis list. Indeed, there are findings that are nearly specific for certain processes. For example, in patients with AIDS, pneumatocele formation is seen exclusively in those with PCP. The finding of poorly defined nodular densities with associated pleural effusions is almost pathognomonic for Kaposi's sarcoma. Conversely, some radiographic findings should dissuade one from considering certain diagnoses. For example, pleural fluid and lymphadenopathy are rarely if ever encountered in patients with PCP alone. Other entities such as non-Hodgkin's lymphoma, tuberculosis, or fungal infection should thus be considered. With experience, clinicians will develop more confidence to *interpret* the chest film, leading to better patient management.

I have emphasized the chest film abnormalities seen in patients with AIDS and have said little about the use of CT. In my experience, CT would not be a cost-beneficial modality. This has recently been confirmed in a study looking at the sensitivity and specificity of chest radiography and CT in the detection of the infections and neoplasms seen in AIDS patients. In this investigation, CT was, as expected, more sensitive to the findings of lung disease, but the authors concluded that, for the majority of patients, chest films were adequate and CT was not indicated.[156]

References

1. Centers for Disease Control: Kaposi's sarcoma and *Pneumocystis* pneumonia among homosexual men: New York City and California. MMWR Morb Mortal Wkly Rep 30:305, 1981
2. Centers for Disease Control: *Pneumocystis* pneumonia—Los Angeles. MMWR Morb Mortal Wkly Rep 30:250, 1981
3. McGuiness G: Changing trends in the pulmonary manifestations of AIDS. Radiol Clin North Am 35: 1029, 1997
4. Boiselle PM, Tocino I, Hooley RJ, et al: Chest radiograph interpretation of *Pneumocystis carinii* pneumonia, bacterial pneumonia, and pulmonary tuberculosis in HIV-positive patients: Accuracy, distinguishing features, and mimics. J Thorac Imaging 12:47, 1997
5. Masur H: Prevention and treatment of *Pneumocystis* pneumonia. N Engl J Med 327:1853, 1992
6. Murray JF, Garay SM, Hopewell PC, et al: Pulmonary complications of the acquired immunodeficiency syndrome: An update. Am Rev Respir Dis 135:504, 1987
7. Goodman PC, Broaddus VC, Hopewell PC: Chest radiographic patterns in the acquired immunodeficiency syndrome. Am Rev Respir Dis 129:26, 1984
8. Opravil M, Marincek B, Fuchs WA, et al: Shortcomings of chest radiography in detecting *Pneumocystis carinii* pneumonia. J Acquir Immune Defic Syndr 7: 39, 1994
9. Kroe DM, Kirsch CM, Jensen WA: Diagnostic strategies for *Pneumocystis carinii* pneumonia. Semin Respir Infect 12:70, 1997
10. Boldt MJ, Bai TR: Utility of lactate dehydrogenase vs radiographic severity in the differential diagnosis of *Pneumocystis carinii* pneumonia. Chest 111:1187, 1997
11. Gruden JF, Huang L, Turner J, et al: High resolution CT in the evaluation of clinically suspected *Pneumocystis carinii* pneumonia in AIDS patients with normal, equivocal, or nonspecific radiographic findings. AJR 169:967, 1997

12. De Lorenzo IJ, Huang CT, Maguire GP, et al: Roentgenographic patterns of *Penumocystis carinii* pneumonia in 104 patients with AIDS. Chest 91:323, 1987

13. Goodman PC: *Pneumocystis carinii* pneumonia. J Thorac Imaging 6:16, 1991

14. Goodman PC, Gamsu G: Radiographic findings in the acquired immunodeficiency syndrome. Postgrad Radiol 7:3, 1987

15. Goodman PC: Pulmonary manifestations of AIDS. Curr Probl Diagn Radiol 17:81, 1988

16. Barrio JL, Suarez M, Rodriguez JL, et al: *Pneumocystis carinii* pneumonia presenting as cavitating and non-cavitating solitary pulmonary nodules in patients with the acquired immunodeficiency syndrome. Am Rev Respir Dis 134:1094, 1986

17. Ferre C, Baguena F, Podzamczer D, et al: Lung cavitation associated with *Pneumocystis carinii* infection in the acquired immunodeficiency syndrome: A report of 6 cases and review of the literature. Eur Respir J 7:134, 1994

18. Klein JS, Warnock M, Webb WR, et al: Cavitating and noncavitating granulomas in AIDS patients with *Pneumocystis* pneumonitis. Am J Roentgenol 152:753, 1989

19. Wharton J, Coleman DL, Wofsy CB, et al: Trimethoprim-sulfamethoxazole or pentamidine for *Pneumocystis carinii* pneumonia in the acquired immunodeficiency syndrome. Ann Intern Med 105:37, 1986

20. Ramaswany G, Jagadha V, Tchnentkoff V: Diffuse alveolar damage and interstitial fibrosis in acquired immunodeficiency syndrome: Patients without concurrent pulmonary infection. Arch Pathol Lab Med 109:408, 1985

21. Wasserman K, Pothoff G, Kirn E, et al: Chronic *Pneumocystis carinii* pneumonia in AIDS. Chest 104:667, 1993

22. Bozzette SA, Satler FR, Chiu J, et al: A controlled trial of early adjunctive treatment with corticosteroids for *Pneumocystis carinii* pneumonia in the acquired immunodeficiency syndrome. N Engl J Med 323:1451, 1990

23. Sleasman JW, Hemenway C, Klein AS, et al: Corticosteroids improve survival of children with AIDS and *Pneumocystis carinii* pneumonia. Am J Dis Child 147:30, 1993

24. Groskin SA, Stadnick ME, Dupont PG: *Pneumocystis carinii* pneumonia: Effect of corticosteroid treatment on radiographic appearance in a patient with AIDS. Radiology 180:423, 1991

25. Rankin JA, Pella JA: Radiographic resolution of *Pneumocystis carinii* pneumonia in response to corticosteroid therapy. Am Rev Respir Dis 136:182, 1987

26. Mahaffey KW, Hippenmeyer CL, Mandel R, et al: Unrecognized coccidioidomycosis complicating *Pneumocystis carinii* pneumonia in patients infected with the human immunodeficiency virus and treated with corticosteroids: A report of two cases. Arch Intern Med 153:1496, 1993

27. Coker RS, Moss F, Peters B, et al: Pneumothorax in patients with AIDS. Respir Med 87:43, 1993

28. Goodman PC, Daley C, Minagi H: Spontaneous pneumothorax in AIDS patients with *Penumocystis carinii* pneumonia. Am J Roentgenol 147:29, 1986

29. Albort JV, Callejas MA, Canalis EA, et al: Surgical management of spontaneous pneumothorax in patients with AIDS. Ann Thorac Surg 55:808, 1993

30. Horowitz MD, Oliva H: Pneumothorax in AIDS patients: Operative management. Am Surg 59:200, 1993

31. Travaline JM, Criner GJ: Persistent bronchopleural fistula in an AIDS patient with *Pneumocystis carinii*

pneumonia: Successful treatment with chemical pleurodesis. Chest 103:991, 1993

32. Wait MA: AIDS-related pneumothorax. Ann Thorac Surg 64:290, 1997

33. Walker WA, Poate JW: AIDS-related bronchopleural fistula. Ann Thorac Surg 55:1048, 1993

34. Trachiotis GD, Vricella LA, Alyono D, et al: Management of AIDS-related pneumothorax. Ann Thorac Surg 62:1608, 1996

35. Scannell KA: Pneumothoraces and *Pneumocystis carinii* pneumonia in two AIDS patients receiving aerosolized pentamidine. Chest 97:479, 1990

36. Toronto Aerosolized Pentamidine Study Group: Aerosolized pentamidine and spontaneous pneumothorax in AIDS patients. Chest 97:510, 1990

37. Sepkowitz KA, Telzak EE, Gold JWM, et al: Pneumothorax in AIDS. Ann Intern Med 103:991, 1993

38. Sandhu JS, Goodman PC: Pulmonary cysts associated with *Pneumocystis carinii* pneumonia in patients with AIDS. Radiology 173:33, 1989

39. Panicek DM: Cystic pulmonary lesions in patients with AIDS. Radiology 173:12, 1989

40. Feuerstein IM, Archer A, Pluda JM, et al: Thin-walled cavities, cysts and pneumothoraces in *Pneumocystis carinii* pneumonia: Further observations with histopathologic correlation. Radiology 174:697, 1990

41. Kuhlman JE, Knowles MC, Fishman EK, et al: Premature bullous pulmonary damage in AIDS: CT diagnosis. Radiology 173:23, 1989

42. Baughman RP, Dohn MN, Shipley R, et al: Increased *Pneumocystis carinii* recovery from the upper lobes in *Pneumocystis* pneumonia: The effect of aerosol pentamidine prophylaxis. Chest 103:426, 1993

43. Case Records of the Massachusetts General Hospital Case 9-1989. N Engl J Med 320:582, 1989

44. Lowery S, Fallat R, Feigal DW, et al: Changing patterns of *Pneumocystis carinii* pneumonia on pentamidine aerosol prophylaxis. In Abstracts of the 4th International Conference on AIDS, 1988, Abstract 1:419

45. Small P, Goodman PC, Montgomery AB: Case 9-1989: AIDS and a cavitary pulmonary lesion [letter]. N Engl J Med 321:395, 1989

46. Albrecht H, Stellbrenk HJ, Fenske S, et al: A novel variety of atypical *Pneumocystis carinii* infection after long-term prophylactic pentamidine inhalation in an AIDS patient: Large lower lobe pneumocystoma. Clin Invest 71:310, 1993

47. Eagar GM, Friedland JA, Sagal SS: Tumefactive *Pneumocystis carinii* infection in AIDS: Report of three cases. Am J Roentgenol 160:1197, 1993

48. Edelstein H, McCabe RE: Atypical presentations of *Pneumocystis carinii* pneumonia in patients receiving inhaled pentamidine prophylaxis. Chest 98:1366, 1990

49. Horowitz ML, Schiff M, Samuels J, et al: *Pneumocystis carinii* pleural effusion: Pathogenesis and pleural fluid analysis. Am Rev Respir Dis 148:232, 1993

50. Mayor B, Schnyder P, Giron J, et al: Mediastinal and hilar lymphadenopathy due to *Pneumocystis carinii* infection in AIDS patients: CT features. J Comput Assist Tomogr 18:408, 1994

50a. Jayes RL, Camerow HN, Hasselquist SM, et al: Disseminated pneumocystosis presenting as a pleural effusion. Chest 103:306, 1993

51. Bamberger DM, Driks MR, Gupta MR, et al: *Mycobacterium kansasii* among patients affected with human immunodeficiency virus in Kansas City. Clin Infect Dis 18:395, 1994

52. Centers for Disease Control: Diagnosis and management of mycobacterial infection and disease in per-

sons with human immunodeficiency virus infection. Ann Intern Med 106:254, 1987

53. Hopewell PC, Luce JM: Pulmonary manifestations of the acquired immunodeficiency syndrome. Clin Immunol Allergy 6:489, 1986

54. Page JW, Liautaud B, Thomas F, et al: Characteristics of the acquired immunodeficiency syndrome (AIDS) in Haiti. N Engl J Med 309:945, 1983

55. Selwin PA, Hartel D, Lewis BA, et al: A prospective study of the risk of tuberculosis in intravenous drug users with human immunodeficiency virus infection. N Engl J Med 320:545, 1989

56. Centers for Disease Control: Advisory committee for elimination of tuberculosis and human immunodeficiency virus infection. MMWR Morb Mortal Wkly Rep 38:236, 1989

57. Hopewell PC: Tuberculosis and human immunodeficiency virus infection. Semin Respir Infect 4:111, 1989

58. Pitchenik AE, Burr J, Suarez M, et al: Human T-cell lymphotropic virus-III (HTLV-III) scropositivity and related disease among 71 consecutive patients in whom tuberculosis was diagnosed. Am Rev Respir Dis 135:875, 1987

58a. Keiper MD, Beumont M, Elshami A, et al: CDR T lymphocyte count and the radiographic presentation of pulmonary tuberculosis. Chest 107:74, 1995

59. Goodman PC: Pulmonary tuberculosis in patients with the acquired immunodeficiency syndrome. J Thorac Imaging 5:38, 1990

60. Perlman DC, El-Sadr WM, Nelson ET, et al: Variation of chest radiographic patterns in pulmonary tuberculosis by degree of human immunodeficiency virus-related immunosuppression: The Terry Beirn Community Programs for Clinical Research on AIDS (CPCRA) and the AIDS Clinical Trials Group (ACTG). Clin Infect Dis 25:242, 1997

61. Chaisson RE, Schecter GF, Theuer CP, et al: Tuberculosis in patients with the acquired immunodeficiency syndrome: Clinical features, response to therapy, and survival. Am Rev Respir Dis 136:570, 1987

62. Suster B, Akerman M. Orenstein M, et al: Pulmonary manifestations of AIDS: Review of 106 episodes. Radiology 161:87, 1986

63. Pastores SM, Naidich DP, Aranda CP, et al: Intrathoracic adenopathy associated with pulmonary tuberculosis in patients with human immunodeficiency virus infection. Chest 103:1433, 1993

64. Goodman PC: Tuberculosis and AIDS. Radiol Clin North Am 33:707, 1995

65. Jones BE, Ryu R, Yang Z, et al: Chest radiographic findings in patients with tuberculosis with recent or remote infection. Am J Respir Crit Care Med 156:1270, 1997

66. Frye MD, Pozsik CJ, Sahn SA: Tuberculous pleurisy is more common in AIDS than in non-AIDS patients with tuberculosis. Chest 12:393, 1997

67. Small P, Hopewell PC, Schecter GF, et al: Evolution of chest radiographs in treated patients with pulmonary tuberculosis and HIV infection. J Thorac Imaging 9:74, 1994

68. American Thoracic Society and Centers for Disease Control: Treatment of tuberculosis and tuberculosis infection in adults and children. Am J Respir Crit Care Med 149:1359, 1994

69. Fischl MA, Daikos GL, Uttanchandani RB, et al: Clinical presentation and outcome of patients with HIV infection and tuberculosis caused by multiple drug-resistant bacilli. Ann Intern Med 117:189, 1992

70. Lessnau K-D, Gorla M, Talavera W: Radiographic findings in HIV-positive patients with sensitive and resistant tuberculosis. Chest 106:687, 1994

71. Modelevsky T, Sattler FR, Barnes PF: Mycobacterial disease in patients with human immunodeficiency virus infection. Arch Intern Med 149:2201, 1989

72. Aronchick JM, Miller WT Jr: Disseminated nontuberculous mycobacterial infections in immunosuppressed patients. Semin Roentgenol 28:150, 1993

73. Kalayjian RC, Toossi Z, Tomashefski JF, et al: Pulmonary disease due to infection by *Mycobacterium avium* complex in patients with AIDS. Clin Infect Dis 20:1186, 1995

74. Fishman JE, Schwartz DS, Sais GJ: *Mycobacterium kansasii* pulmonary infection in patients with AIDS: Spectrum of chest radiographic findings. Radiology 204:171, 1997

75. Abrams DI, Robia M, Blumenfeld W, et al: Disseminated coccidioidomycosis in AIDS. N Engl J Med 310:986, 1984

76. Bonner JR, Alexander WJ, Dismukes WE, et al: Disseminated histoplasmosis in patients with the acquired immune deficiency syndrome. Arch Intern Med 144:2178, 1984

77. Mandell W, Goldberg DM, Neu HC: Histoplasmosis in patients with acquired immune deficiency syndrome. Am J Med 81:974, 1986

78. Stansell JD: Fungal disease in HIV-infected persons: Cryptococcosis, histoplasmosis, and coccidioidomycosis. J Thorac Imaging 6:28, 1991

79. Wheat IJ, Slama TG, Zeckel ML: Histoplasmosis in the acquired immune deficiency syndrome. Am J Med 78:203, 1985

80. Wheat J: Histoplasmosis and coccidioidomycosis in individuals with AIDS: A clinical review. Infect Dis Clin North Am 8:467, 1994

80a. Kovacs A, Forthal DN, Kovacs JA, et al: Disseminated coccidioidomycosis in a patient with acquired immune deficiency syndrome. West J Med 140:447, 1984

81. Marshall BC, Cox JK Jr, Carroll KC, et al: Case report: Histoplasmosis as a cause of pleural effusion in the acquired immunodeficiency syndrome. Am J Med Sci 300:98, 1990

82. Conces DJ Jr, Stockberger SM, Tarver RD, et al: Disseminated histoplasmosis in AIDS: Findings on chest radiographs. Am J Roentgenol 160:15, 1993

83. Chechani V, Camholz SL: Pulmonary manifestations of disseminated cryptococcosis in patients with AIDS. Chest 98:1060, 1990

84. Clark RA, Greer DL, Valaines GT, et al: *Cryptococcus neoformans* pulmonary infection in human immunodeficiency virus-1-infected patients. J Acquir Immune Defic Syndr 3:480, 1990

85. Sider L, Westcott MA: Pulmonary manifestations of cryptococcosis in patients with AIDS: CT features. J Thorac Imaging 9:78, 1994

86. Douketis JD, Kesten S: Miliary cryptococcosis in a patient with the acquired immunodeficiency syndrome. Thorax 48:402, 1993

87. Miller WT Jr, Edelman JM, Miller WT: Cryptococcal pulmonary infection in patients with AIDS: Radiographic appearances. Radiology 175:725, 1990

88. Klapholz A, Salomon N. Perlman DC, et al: Aspergillosis in acquired immunodeficiency syndrome. Chest 100:1614, 1991

89. Lortholary O, Meyokas MC, Dupont B, et al: Invasive aspergillosis in patients with acquired immunodeficiency syndrome: Report of 33 cases. French Coop-

erative Study Group on Aspergillosis in AIDS. Am J Med 95:177, 1993

90. Minamoto GY, Barlam TF, Vander Els NJ: Invasive aspergillosis in patients with AIDS. Clin Infect Dis 14:66, 1992

91. Pursell KJ, Telzak EE, Armstrong D: Aspergillus species colonization and invasive disease in patients with AIDS. Clin Infect Dis 14:141, 1992

92. Fairley CK, Kent SJ, Street A, et al: Invasive aspergillosis in AIDS. Aust N Z J Med 21:747, 1991

93. Morrison DL, Granton JT, Keston S, et al: Cavitary aspergillosis as a complication of AIDS. J Can Assoc Radiol 44:35, 1993

94. Staples CA, Kang EY, Wright JL, et al: Invasive pulmonary aspergillosis in AIDS: Radiographic, CT, and pathologic findings. Radiology 196:409, 1995

95. Miller WT Jr, Sais GJ, Frank I, et al: Pulmonary aspergillosis in patients with AIDS. Chest 105:37, 1994

96. Millar AB, Patou GM, Miller RF, et al: Cytomegalovirus in the lungs of patients with AIDS: Respiratory pathogen or passenger? Am Rev Respir Dis 141:1474, 1990

97. Antoniore M, Chan CK: Determining the pathogenetic significance of cytomegalovirus in patients with AIDS. Chest 110:863, 1996

98. Baughman RP: Cytomegalovirus: The monster in the closet? Am J Respir Crit Care Med 156:1, 1997

99. Stover DE, White DA, Romano PA, et al: Spectrum of pulmonary diseases associated with the acquired immune deficiency syndrome. Am J Med 78:429, 1985

100. Miles PR, Baughman RP, Linnemann CC Jr: Cytomegalovirus in the bronchoalveolar lavage fluid of patients with AIDS. Chest 97:1072, 1990

101. Wallace JM, Hannah J: Cytomegalovirus pneumonitis in patients with AIDS. Chest 92:198, 1987

102. Hoover DR, Saah AJ, Becellar H, et al: Clinical manifestations of AIDS in the era of *Pneumocystis* prophylaxis. N Engl J Med 329:1922, 1993

103. Nelson MR, Erskine D, Hawkins DA, Gazzard BG: Treatment with corticosteroids: A risk factor for the development of clinical cytomegalovirus disease in AIDS. AIDS 7:375, 1993

104. McGuinness G, Scholes JV, Garay SM, et al: Cytomegalovirus pneumonitis: Spectrum of parenchymal CT findings with pathologic correlation in 21 AIDS patients. Radiology 192:451, 1994

105. Bozzette SA, Arcia J, Bartok AE, et al: Impact of *Pneumocystis carinii* and cytomegalovirus on the course and outcome of atypical pneumonia in advanced human immunodeficiency virus disease. J Infect Dis 165:93, 1992

106. Fimberkoff MS, El Sadr W, Schiffman G, et al: *Streptococcus penumoniae* infections and bacteremia in patients with acquired immune deficiency syndrome with report of a pneumococcal vaccine failure. Am Rev Respir Dis 130:1174, 1984

107. Nichols L, Balogh K, Silverman M: Bacterial infections in the acquired immunodeficiency syndrome. Am J Clin Pathol 92:787, 1989

108. Polsky B, Gold JWN, Whimbey E, et al: Bacterial pneumonia in patients with the acquired immunodeficiency syndrome. Ann Intern Med 104:38, 1986

109. Miller RF, Foley NM, Kessel D, Jeffrey AA: Community acquired lobar pneumonia in patients with HIV infection and AIDS. Thorax 49:367, 1994

110. Garcia-Leoni ME, Moreno S, Rodeno P, et al: Pneumococcal pneumonia in adult hospitalized patients infected with the human immunodeficiency virus. Arch Intern Med 152:1808, 1992

111. White S, Tsou E, Waldhorn R, et al: Life threatening bacterial pneumonia in male homosexuals with laboratory features of the acquired immunodeficiency syndrome. Chest 87:486, 1985

112. Magnenat J, Nicod LP, Auckenthaler R, et al: Mode of presentation and diagnosis of bacterial pneumonia in human immunodeficiency virus-infected patients. Am Rev Respir Dis 144:917, 1991

113. Dailey CL: Bacterial pneumonia in HIV-infected patients. Semin Respir Infect 8:104, 1993

114. Baron AD, Hollander H: *Pseudomonas aeruginosa* bronchopulmonary infection in late human immunodeficiency virus disease. Am Rev Respir Dis 148:992, 1993

115. Cury JD, Harrington PT, Hosein IK: Successful medical therapy of *Rhodococcus equi* pneumonia in a patient with HIV infection. Chest 102:1619, 1992

116. Gray BM: Case report: *Rhodococcus equi* pneumonia in a patient infected by the human immunodeficiency virus. Am J Med Sci 303:180, 1992

117. Verville TD, Huycke MM, Greenfield RA, et al: *Rhodococcus equi* infections of humans: Twelve cases and a review of the lieterature. Medicine 73:119, 1994

118. Muntaner L, Leyes M, Payeres A, et al: Radiologic features of *Rhodococcus equi* pneumonia in AIDS. Eur J Radiol 14:66, 1997

119. Wallace JM, Rao V, Glossroth J, et al: Respiratory illness in persons with human immunodeficiency virus infection. Am Rev Respir Dis 148:1523, 1993

120. Chechani V, Allam AA, Smith PR, et al: Bronchitis mimicking opportunistic lung infection in patients with human immunodeficiency virus infection/AIDS. N Y State J Med 92:297, 1992

121. McGuiness G, Gruden JF, Bhalla M, et al: AIDS-related airway disease. AJR 168:67, 1997

122. McGuinness G, Naidich DP, Garay S, et al: AIDS associated bronchiectasis: CT features. J Comput Assist Tomogr 17:260, 1993

123. King MA, Neal DE, St John R, et al: Bronchial dilatation in patients with HIV infection: CT assessment and correlation with pulmonary function tests and findings at bronchoalveolar lavage. AJR 168:1535, 1997

124. Davis SK, Henschke CI, Chamides BK, et al: Intrathoracic Kaposi sarcoma in AIDS patients: Radiographic-pathologic correlation. Radiology 163:495, 1987

125. Garay SM, Belenko M, Fazzini E, et al: Pulmonary manifestations of Kaposi's sarcoma. Chest 91:39, 1987

126. Goodman PC: Kaposi's sarcoma. J Thorac Imaging 6:43, 1991

127. Gruden JF, Huang L, Webb WR, et al: AIDS-related Kaposi sarcoma of the lung: Radiograph, findings and staging system with bronchoscopic correlation. Radiology 195:545, 1995

128. Kaplan L, Hopewell PC, Jaffe H, et al: Kaposi's sarcoma involving the lung in patients with the acquired immunodeficiency syndrome. J AIDS 1:23, 1988

129. Sivit CJ, Schwartz AM, Rockoff SD: Kaposi's sarcoma of the lung in AIDS: Radiologic pathologic analysis. AJR Am J Roentgenol 148:25, 1987

130. Naidich DP, Tarras M, Garay SM, et al: Kaposi's sarcoma: CT radiographic correlation. Chest 96:723, 1989

131. Wolff SD, Kuhlman JE, Fishman EK: Thoracic Kaposi sarcoma in AIDS: CT findings. J Comput Assist Tomogr 17:60, 1993

132. Lee VW, Fuller JD, O'Brien MJ, et al: Pulmonary Kaposi sarcoma in patients with AIDS: Scintigraphic

diagnosis with sequential thallium and gallium scanning. Radiology 180:409, 1991

133. Roux FJ, Bancal C, Dombret MC, et al: Pulmonary Kaposi's sarcoma revealed by a solitary nodule in a patient with acquired immunodeficiency syndrome. Am J Respir Crit Care Med 149:1041, 1994

134. Haskal ZJ, Lindan C, Goodman PC: Lymphoma in the immunocompromised patient. Radiol Clin North Am 28:885, 1990

135. Zieler JL, Beckstead JA, Volberding PA, et al: Non-Hodgkin's lymphoma in 90 homosexual men. N Engl J Med 311:565, 1984

136. Eisner MD, Kaplan LD, Herndier B, et al: The pulmonary manifestations of AIDS-related non-Hodgkin's lymphoma. Chest 110:729, 1996

137. Carignan S, Staples CA, Müller NL: Intrathoracic lymphoproliferative disorders in the immunocompromised patient: CT findings. Radiology 197:53, 1995

138. Chan TK, Aranda CP, Rom WN: Bronchogenic carcinoma in young patients at risk for acquired immunodeficiency syndrome. Chest 103:862, 1993

139. Remick SC: Lung cancer: An HIV-related neoplasm or a coincidental finding? Chest 102:1643, 1992

140. Fraire AE, Awe RJ: Lung cancer in association with human immunodeficiency virus infection. Cancer 70:432, 1992

141. Karp J, Profeta G, Marantz PR, et al: Lung cancer in patients with immunodeficiency syndrome. Chest 103:410, 1993

142. Sridhar KS, Flores MR, Raub WA Jr, et al: Lung cancer in patients with human immunodeficiency virus infection compared with historic control subjects. Chest 102:1704, 1992

143. Vaccher E, Tirelli U, Spina M, et al: Lung cancer in 19 patients with HIV infection: The Italian Cooperative Study Group on AIDS and Tumors. Ann Oncol 4:85, 1993

144. Braun MA, Killam DA, Remick SC, et al: Lung cancer in patients seropositive for human immunodeficiency virus. Radiology 175:341, 1990

145. Fishman JR, Schwartz DS, Sais GJ, et al: Bronchogenic carcinoma in HIV-positive patients: Findings on chest radiographs and CT scans. Am J Roentgenol 164:57, 1995

146. Gruden JF, Klein JS, Webb WR: Percutaneous transthoracic needle biopsy in AIDS: Analysis in 32 patients. Radiology 189:567, 1993

147. White CS, Haramati LB, Elder KH, et al: Carcinoma of the lung in HIV-positive patients: Findings on chest radiographs and CT scans. Am J Roentgenol 164:593, 1995

148. Conces DJ, Tarver RD: Noninfectious and non-malignant pulmonary disease in AIDS. J Thorac Imaging 6:53, 1991

149. Goodman PC: Pulmonary disease in children with AIDS. J Thorac Imaging 6:60, 1991

150. Oldham SAA, Castillo M, Jacobson FL, et al: HIV-associated lymphocytic interstitial pneumonia: Radiologic manifestations and pathologic correlation. Radiology 170:83, 1989

151. Goldman HS, Ziprowski MN, Charytan M, et al: Lymphocytic interstitial pneumonitis in children with AIDS: A perfect radiographic-pathologic correlation [abstract]. Am J Roentgenol 145:868, 1985

152. Haney PJ, Yale-Loehr AJ, Nussbaum AR, et al: Imaging of infants and children with AIDS. Am J Roentgenol 152:1033, 1989

153. Amorosa JK, Miller RW, Laraya-Cuasay L, et al: Bronchiectasis in children with lymphocytic interstitial pneumonia and acquired immune deficiency syndrome: Plain film and CT observations. Pediatr Radiol 22:603, 1992

154. Berdon WE, Mellins RB, Abramson SJ, et al: Pediatric HIV infection in its second decade—the changing pattern of lung involvement: Clinical, plain film, and computed tomographic findings. Radiol Clin North Am 31:453, 1993

155. Sattler F, Nichols L, Hirano L, et al: Nonspecific interstitial pneumonitis mimicking *Pneumocystic carinii* pneumonia. Am J Respir Crit Care Med 156:912, 1997

156. Kang E, Staples CA, McGuinness G, et al: Detection and differential diagnosis of pulmonary infections and tumors in patients with AIDS: Value of chest radiography versus CT. Am J Roentgenol 166:15, 1996

10 | Oral Complications of HIV Infection

JOHN S. GREENSPAN • DEBORAH GREENSPAN

Oral lesions have been recognized as prominent features of AIDS and HIV infection since the beginning of the epidemic.[1,2] Some of these changes are reflections of reduced immune function manifested as oral opportunistic conditions, which are often the earliest clinical features of HIV infection. Some, in the presence of known HIV infection, are highly predictive of the ultimate development of the full syndrome, whereas others represent the oral features of AIDS itself. The particular susceptibility of the mouth to HIV disease is a reflection of a wider phenomenon. Oral opportunistic infections occur in a variety of conditions in which the teeming and varied microflora of the mouth take advantage of local and systemic immunologic and metabolic imbalances. They include oral infections in patients with primary immunodeficiency,[3] leukemia,[4] and diabetes[5] and those patients with immunodeficiency resulting from radiation therapy, cancer chemotherapy, and bone marrow suppression.[6–8] Oral lesions seen in association with HIV infection are classified in Table 10–1, and our general approach to the diagnosis and management of oral HIV disease is summarized in Table 10–2. Standardized definitions and diagnostic criteria for these lesions have been established.[9,10]

In the prospective cohorts of HIV-infected homosexual and bisexual men in San Francisco, hairy leukoplakia is the most common oral lesion (20.4%), and pseudomembranous candidiasis is the next most common (5.8%).[11] These lesions occur at an early stage after seroconversion and are predictors of progression.[12,13] Oral lesions are also common in HIV-infected women[14,15] and children.[16–18] Our clinical impression is that their overall frequency has fallen with the introduction of highly active antiretroviral therapy (HAART). However, they are more common in people who smoke cigarettes.[19] Oth-

ers have shown that a simplified staging system for HIV infection, based on CD4+ cell depletion and oral disease, is more effective than the Walter Reed and other staging classifications.[20]

CANDIDIASIS

The pseudomembranous form of oral candidiasis (thrush) was described in the first group of AIDS patients and is a harbinger of the full-blown syndrome in HIV-seropositive individuals.[21,22] We have shown that both oral candidiasis and hairy leukoplakia predict the development of AIDS in HIV-infected patients independently of CD4 counts.[23] However, it is not well recognized that oral candidiasis can take several forms, some of them with subtle clinical appearances.[2,24] The most common form, pseudomembranous candidiasis, appears as removable white plaques on any oral mucosal surface (Fig. 10–1). These plaques may be as small as 1 to 2 mm or may be extensive and widespread. They can be wiped off, leaving an erythematous or even bleeding mucosal surface.

The erythematous form (Fig. 10–2) is seen as smooth red patches on the hard or soft palate, buccal mucosa, or dorsal surface of the tongue. These lesions may seem insignificant and may be missed unless a thorough oral mucosal examination is performed in good light. Angular cheilitis caused by *Candida* infection produces erythema, cracks, and fissures at the corner of the mouth. We have found that erythematous candidiasis is as serious a prognostic indicator of the development of AIDS as pseudomembranous candidiasis.[24]

Diagnosis of oral candidiasis involves potassium hydroxide preparation of a smear from the lesion (Fig. 10–3). Culture provides information about the species involved.

TABLE 10–1. Oral Lesions in HIV Infection

Fungal	*Viral*
Candidiasis	Herpes simplex
Pseudomembranous	Herpes zoster
Erythematous	Cytomegalovirus ulcers
Angular chelitis	Hairy leukoplakia
Histoplasmosis	Warts
Geotrichosis	
Cryptococcosis	*Neoplastic*
Aspergillosis	Kaposi's sarcoma
	Non-Hodgkin's lymphoma
Bacterial	Squamous cell carcinoma
Linear gingival erythema	(?)
Necrotizing ulcerative	
periodontitis	*Other*
Necrotizing stomatitis	Recurrent aphthous ulcers
Mycobacterium avium	Immune thrombocytopenic
complex	purpura
Klebsiella stomatitis	Salivary gland disease
Bacillary angiomatosis	

Oral candidiasis in patients with HIV infection usually responds[25,26] to topical antifungal agents, including nystatin vaginal tablets (Mycostatin), 100,000 units tid, dissolved slowly in the mouth; nystatin oral pastilles (Mycostatin), 200,000 units, one pastille five times daily; or clotrimazole oral tablets (Mycelex), 10 mg, one tablet five times daily. Amphotericin B (Fungizone) is available in an oral suspension (100 mg/1 ml), and 1 ml should be used as an oral swish and then swallowed four times a day. Efficacy is related to the contact time between the suspension and the mucosa, and so eating or drinking for 20 minutes after use should be discouraged. The effectiveness of topical medications depends on adherence to recommended dosing regimens. Topical tablets, troches, and pastilles need adequate saliva to be effective. For those people with dry mouths, sipping a little water before use and occasionally during use of the medication can be helpful. Some topical medications contain sucrose or dextrose, which have the potential to cause caries, and daily topical fluoride rinses should be used by those taking these medications frequently. For those individuals who find it difficult to use these medications four to five times a day, systemic therapy should be considered. Ketoconazole (Nizoral), available in tablet form, 200 mg once daily, is a systemic antifungal agent that can be used as an alternative. It is effective if absorbed. Fluconazole (Diflucan) is a systemic antifungal agent. The recommended dose is a 100-mg tablet once daily for 14 days. Oral fluconazole is an effective antifungal agent that does not depend on gastric pH for absorption. Side effects include nausea and skin rash. Two 100-mg tablets are used on the first day, followed by one 100-mg tablet daily until the lesions disappear. Fluconazole is also available as an oral suspension (10 mg/ml), and 10 ml is used as a swish and swallow once daily.[27] Antifungal therapy should be continued for 2 weeks, and some patients may need maintenance therapy because of frequent relapse.

In recent years many cases of oral candidiasis resistant to fluconazole have been reported.[28] Factors associated with the development of resistance include CD4 count less than 100 cells/mm^3 previous use of fluconazole, and the emergence of new resistant strains of *Candida albicans* or the emergence of strains such as *C. glabrata, C. tropicalis*, and *C. krusei*, which are inherently less sensitive to fluconazole.[29] However, in most cases fluconazole is an extremely well tolerated and effective antifungal agent.

Itraconazole is a systemic, triazole antifungal agent and is available in 100-mg capsules.[30] Itraconazole, 200 mg/day, is as effective as clotrimazole (10-mg troches five times daily) for the treatment of oral candidiasis. Those using itraconazole responded faster to therapy and had a longer period before relapse. As with ketoconazole, the use of an acidic drink taken with itraconazole improves absorption. Itraconazole oral solution[31,32] has been evaluated in clinical trials as being an effective agent in the treatment of oral candidiasis, and salivary levels of itraconazole persist up to 8 hours after dosing.

For patients who develop oral candidiasis that appears unresponsive to therapy, treatment choices include higher doses of fluconazole, itraconazole 200 to 400 mg/day, ketoconazole 400 mg/day, or amphotericin oral rinse; if none of these is successful, intravenous amphotericin B may be needed. Angular cheilitis usually responds to typical antifungal creams, such as nystatin-triamcinolone (Mycolog II), clotrimazole (Mycelex), or ketoconazole (Nizoral).

Occasionally, other and unusual oral fungal lesions are seen. They include histoplasmosis,[33–35] geotrichosis,[36] aspergillosis,[37] and cryptococcosis.[38–40]

GINGIVITIS AND PERIODONTITIS

Unusual forms of gingivitis and periodontal disease are seen in association with HIV infection. The gingiva may show a fiery red marginal line, known as linear gingival erythema (Fig. 10–4),

TABLE 10–2. Diagnosis and Management of Oral HIV Disease

CONDITION	DIAGNOSIS	MANAGEMENT
Fungal		
Candidiasis	Clinical appearance KOH preparation Culture	Antifungals
Histoplasmosis	Biopsy	Systemic therapy
Geotrichosis	KOH preparation Culture	Polyene antifungals
Cryptococcosis	Culture Biopsy	Systemic therapy
Aspergillosis	Culture Biopsy	Systemic therapy
Bacterial		
Linear gingival erythema	Clinical appearance	Plaque removal, chlorhexidine
Necrotizing ulcerative periodontitis	Clinical appearance	Plaque removal, debridement, povidone-iodine, metronidazole, chlorhexidine
Necrotizing stomatitis	Clinical appearance Culture and biopsy (to exclude other causes) Culture Biopsy	Debridement, povidone-iodine, metronidazole, chlorhexidine
Mycobacterium avium complex	Culture Biopsy	Systemic therapy
Klebsiella stomatitis	Culture	Systemic therapy (based on antibiotic sensitivity testing)
Viral		
Herpes simplex	Clinical appearance Immunofluorescence on smears	Most cases are self-limiting Oral acyclovir for prolonged cases (>10 days)
Herpes zoster	Clinical appearance	Oral or intravenous acyclovir
Cytomegalovirus ulcers	Biopsy, immunohistochemistry for cytomegalovirus	Ganciclovir
Hairy leukoplakia	Clinical appearance Biopsy; in situ hypbridization for Epstein-Barr virus	Not routinely treated Oral acyclovir for severe cases
Warts	Clinical appearance Biopsy	Excision
Neoplastic		
Kaposi's sarcoma	Clinical appearance	Palliative surgical or laser excision for some bulky or unsightly lesions; intralesional chemotherapy or sclerosing agents; radiation therapy; chemotherapy
Non-Hodgkin's lymphoma	Biopsy	Chemotherapy
Squamous cell carcinoma	Biopsy	Excision or radiation therapy or both
Other		
Recurrent aphthous ulcers	History Clinical appearance Biopsy (to exclude other causes)	Topical steroids Thalidomide for most severe cases
Immune thrombocytopenic purpura	Clinical appearance Hematologic work-up	
Salivary gland disease	History, clinical appearance, salivary flow measurements Biopsy (to exclude other causes) Needle or labial salivary gland biopsy	Salivary stimulants or change in systemic medication or both Topical fluorides

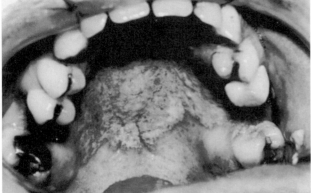

FIGURE 10–1. Pseudomembranous candidiasis.

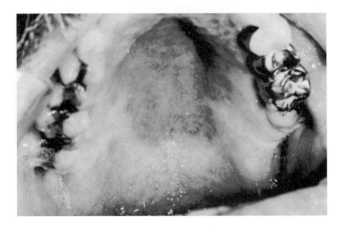

FIGURE 10–2. Erythematous candidiasis.

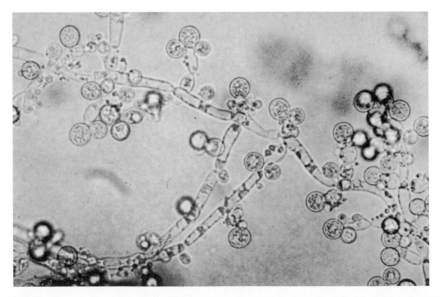

FIGURE 10–3. Potassium hydroxide preparation of oral candidiasis smear showing fungal hyphae and blastospores.

FIGURE 10–4. HIV-associated gingivitis (linear gingival erythema).

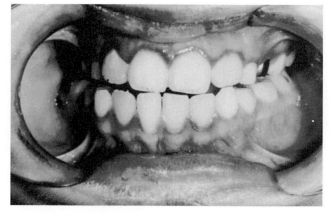

even when there are no significant accumulations of plaque.[41,42] The periodontal disease necrotizing ulcerative periodontitis occurs in approximately 30% to 50% of AIDS clinic patients[43] but is rarely seen in asymptomatic HIV-positive individuals.[44] It resembles, in some respects, acute necrotizing ulcerative gingivitis (ANUG) superimposed on rapidly progressive periodontitis (Fig. 10–5). Thus there may be halitosis in some cases and a history of rapid onset. There is necrosis of the tips of interdental papillae, with the formation of cratered ulcers. However, in contrast to patients with ANUG, these patients complain of spontaneous bleeding and severe, deep-seated pain that is not readily relieved by analgesics. There may be rapid, progressive loss of gingival and periodontal soft tissues and extraordinarily rapid destruction of supporting bone. Teeth may therefore loosen and even exfoliate. The periodontal disease often demonstrates a severity and a rapid rate of progression that were not seen by the majority of practicing dentists and periodontists prior to the AIDS epidemic. Exposure and even sequestration of bone may occur, producing necrotizing stomatitis lesions[45] similar to the noma seen in severely malnourished persons in World War II and more recently in developing countries in association with malnutrition and chronic infection, such as malaria. The pathologic and microbiologic features of these remarkable periodontal lesions are well documented.[46–51]

Standard therapy for gingivitis and periodontitis is ineffective. Instead, the therapeutic regimen that is effective[52,53] involves thorough debridement and curettage, followed by application of a combination of topical antiseptics, notably povidone-iodine (Betadine) irrigation followed with chlorhexidine (Peridex and Periogard) mouthwashes, sometimes supplemented with a 4- to 5-day course of antibiotics, such as metronidazole (Flagyl) 250 mg qid, amoxicillin-clavulanate (Augmentin) 250 mg (1 tab tid), or clindamycin 300 mg tid. Treatment will fail if thorough local removal of bacteria and diseased hard and soft tissue is not achieved during the initial treatment phase and maintained long term.

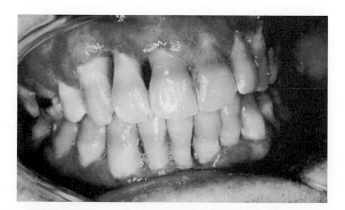

FIGURE 10–5. HIV-associated periodontitis (necrotizing ulcerative periodontitis).

OTHER BACTERIAL LESIONS

A few cases have occurred of oral mucosal lesions associated with unusual bacteria, including *Klebsiella pneumoniae* and *Enterobacter cloacae*.[54-56] These have been diagnosed using aerobic and anaerobic cultures and have responded to antibiotic therapy based on in vitro sensitivity assays. Oral ulcers caused by *Mycobacterium avium* have also been described,[57] as have lesions of bacillary angiomatosis (see Chapter 27).[58]

VIRAL LESIONS

Herpes Simplex

Oral lesions caused by herpes simplex virus (HSV) are a common feature of HIV infection (see Chapter 28). The condition usually occurs as recurrent intraoral lesions with crops of small, painful vesicles that ulcerate. These lesions commonly appear on the palate or gingiva. Smears from the lesions may reveal giant cells, and HSV can be identified using monoclonal antibodies and immunofluorescence. The lesions usually heal, although they may recur. In patients with a history of prolonged bouts (10 days) of such lesions, it may be considered appropriate to treat them with oral acyclovir as soon as symptoms are reported. Usually one 200-mg capsule taken five times a day is effective. Acyclovir-resistant herpes of the lips and perioral structures have been described.[59,60] The lesions responded to foscarnet.

Herpes Zoster

Both chickenpox and herpes zoster (shingles) have occurred in association with HIV infection[61,62] (see Chapter 28). In orofacial zoster, the vesicles and ulcers follow the distribution of one or more branches of the trigeminal nerve on one side. Facial nerve involvement with facial palsy (Ramsay Hunt syndrome) also may occur. Prodromal symptoms may include pain referred to one or more teeth, which often prove to be vital and noncarious. The ulcers usually heal in 2 to 3 weeks, but pain may persist. Oral acyclovir in doses up to 4 gm/day may be used in severe cases, but occasionally patients must be hospitalized to receive intravenous acyclovir therapy.

Cytomegalovirus Ulcers

Oral ulcers caused by cytomegalovirus (CMV) occasionally occur.[63,64] These ulcers can occur on any oral mucosal surface, and diagnosis is made by biopsy and immunohistochemistry. Oral ulcers caused by CMV are usually seen in the presence of disseminated disease, but in some cases the oral ulcer was the first presentation. Whether to treat those ulcers with 3,4-dihydroxyphenylglycol depends on the severity of the viral infection, and full work-up is indicated. Ulcers simultaneously infected by both HSV and CMV also occur.[34,64]

Hairy Leukoplakia

First seen on the tongue in homosexual men,[65] hairy leukoplakia has since been described in several oral mucosal locations, including the buccal mucosa, soft palate, and floor of the mouth, and in all risk groups for AIDS.[11,66-73] Hairy leukoplakia produces white thickening of the oral mucosa, often with vertical folds or corrugations (Fig. 10–6 and Color Plate 1*B*). The lesions range in size from a few millimeters to involvement of the entire dorsal surface of the tongue. The differential diagnosis includes pseudomembranous candidiasis, smoker's leukoplakia, epithelial dysplasia or oral cancer, white sponge nevus, and the plaque form of lichen planus. Biopsy reveals epithelial hyperplasia with a thickened parakeratin layer showing surface irregularities, projections or "hairs," vacuolated prickle cells, and very little inflammation.[65,74,75] Epstein-Barr virus (EBV) can be identified in vacuolated and other prickle cells and in the superficial layers of the epithelium by using cytochemistry, electron microscopy, Southern blotting, and in situ hybridization.[70,74,76-78] For cases in which biopsy is not considered appropriate (e.g., hemophiliacs, children, large-scale epidemiologic studies), we have developed cytospin and filter in situ hybridization techniques.[79] Langerhans' cells are sparse or absent from the lesion.[80] Hairy leukoplakia is not premalignant.[68,70] Indeed, the keratin profile of the lesion suggests reduced, rather than increased, cell turnover.[81,82]

Almost all patients with hairy leukoplakia are HIV seropositive and, without modern antiviral therapy, many subsequently develop AIDS (median time 24 months) and die (median time 44 months).[23,83,84] Patients with tiny or extensive lesions show no difference in this tendency.[75] Rare cases have been described in HIV-negative

FIGURE 10–6. Hairy leukoplakia.

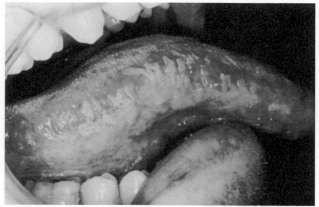

individuals, usually in association with immunosuppression associated with organ transplantation.[85–88] Hairy leukoplakia has not been seen other than on oral mucosal surfaces.[89]

Hairy leukoplakia apparently is an EBV-induced benign epithelial thickening. High doses of oral acyclovir appear to reduce the lesion clinically,[26,90–93] and we have shown that the acyclovir prodrug desciclovir can eliminate both the lesion and the EBV infection present in the epithelial cells.[94] However, these effects are soon reversed after cessation of acyclovir or desciclovir therapy. Hairy leukoplakia occasionally may regress spontaneously, and zidovudine does not appear to increase regression.[95]

It is not clear whether hairy leukoplakia is caused by direct infection or reinfection of maturing epithelial cells by EBV from the saliva, by EBV-infected B cells infiltrating the epithelium, or by latent infection of the basal cell layer.[96–98] EBV variants, unusual EBV types, and even multiple strains of EBV have been found in the lesion.[99–103] Hairy leukoplakia is a fertile model for studies of EBV gene expression.[104,105]

Warts

Oral lesions caused by human papillomavirus (HPV) can occur as single or multiple papilliferous warts with multiple white, spike-like projections, as pink cauliflower-like masses (Fig. 10–7), as single projections, or as flat lesions resembling focal epithelial hyperplasia.[106] In patients with HIV infection, we have seen numerous examples of each type. Southern blot hybridization has not revealed (as would be expected) HPV types 6, 11, 16, and 18, which usually are associated with anogenital warts, but rather HPV type 7, which usually is found in butcher's warts of the skin, or HPV types 13 and 32, previously associated with focal epithelial hyperplasia.[107,108] Novel HPV types are also found.[109]

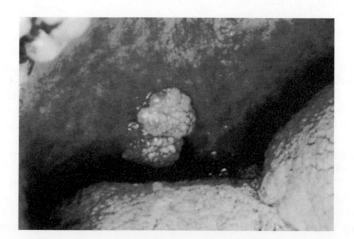

FIGURE 10–7. Wart on the palate.

Venereal transmission thus seems not to be involved in these warts. Instead, they may be attributable to activation of latent HPV infection or perhaps autoinfection from skin and facial lesions. Dysplastic warts caused by novel HPV types also have been described.[109,110]

If large, extensive, or otherwise troublesome, these oral warts can be removed using surgical or laser excision. In some cases, we have seen recurrence after therapy and even extensive spread throughout the mouth. Furthermore, our impression is that the frequency, severity, and response to therapy of oral warts are worse in patients receiving HAART.

NEOPLASTIC DISEASE

Kaposi's Sarcoma

Kaposi's sarcoma (KS) in patients with AIDS produces oral lesions in many cases[111–116] (see Chapter 31). The lesions occur as red or purple macules, papules, or nodules. Occasionally, the lesions are the same color as the adjoining normal mucosa. Although frequently they are asymptomatic, pain may occur because of traumatic ulceration with inflammation and infection. Bulky lesions may be visible or may interfere with speech and mastication. Diagnosis involves biopsy. Lesions at the gingival margin frequently become inflamed and painful because of plaque accumulation. Excision, by surgical means or by laser, is readily performed and can be repeated if the lesion again produces problems. Local radiation therapy has been used to reduce the size of such lesions. Oral lesions usually regress when patients receive chemotherapy for aggressive KS, and individual lesions may respond to local injection of vinblastine[117] or even of sclerosing agents.[118]

Lymphoma

Although not seen as frequently as with oral KS, oral lesions are a common feature of HIV-associated lymphoma[119–122] (see Chapter 31). A biopsy may prove that poorly defined alevolar swellings or discrete oral masses in individuals who are HIV seropositive are non-Hodgkin's lymphoma. No treatment is provided for the oral lesions separate from the systemic chemotherapy regimen that usually is used in such cases.

Carcinoma

Several cases have been seen of oral squamous cell carcinoma, particularly of the tongue, in young homosexual males.[115] It is not clear whether these lesions are related to HIV infection; population-based and cancer registry epidemiologic studies have not produced convincing evidence to support such a link.

OTHER LESIONS

Recurrent aphthous ulcers (RAUs) are a common finding in the normal population. There is an impression,[123–125] not as yet substantiated by prospective studies of incidence, that RAUs are more common among HIV-seropositive individuals. These lesions occur as recurrent crops of small (1- to 2-mm) to large (1-cm) ulcers on the nonkeratinized oral and oropharyngeal mucosa. They can interfere significantly with speech and swallowing and may present considerable problems in diagnosis. When they are large and persistent, biopsy may be indicated to exclude lymphoma. The histopathologic features of RAUs are those of nonspecific inflammation. Treatment with topical steroids often is effective in reducing pain and accelerating healing. Valuable agents include fluocinonide (Lidex), 0.05% ointment, mixed with equal parts of Orabase applied to the lesion up to six times daily; or clobetasol (Temovate), 0.05% mixed with equal parts of Orabase applied three times daily. These are particularly effective treatments for early lesions. Dexamethasone (Decadron) elixir, 0.5 mg/ml used as a rinse and expectorated, is also helpful, particularly when the location of the lesion makes it difficult for the patient to apply fluocinonide. Recently, thalidomide has been found to be useful in the management of steroid-resistant ulcers.[126–130]

Immune thrombocytopenic purpura may produce oral mucosal ecchymoses or small blood-filled lesions.[106] Spontaneous gingival bleeding may occur. Diagnosis by hematologic evaluation is usually straightforward, but, as with any systemic condition presenting as oral lesions, full work-up is indicated.

We have seen several cases of *parotid enlargement* in pediatric AIDS patients[3,16,18,131,132] (Fig. 10–8) and, more recently, among adults who are HIV seropositive.[56,75,85,133–138] HIV-infected children with parotid enlargement progress less rapidly than those without parotid enlargement.[18] No specific cause for HIV-

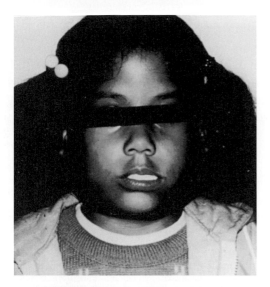

FIGURE 10–8. Parotid enlargement.

associated salivary gland disease has been determined, although viral causes are suspected. Diagnosis to exclude lymphoma, leukemia, and other causes of salivary gland enlargement may involve labial salivary gland biopsy and major salivary gland needle biopsy. Some of these cases show xerostomia. Furthermore, the latter condition may be seen in association with HIV infection in the absence of salivary gland enlargement. The patient may complain of oral dryness, and there may be signs of xerostomia, such as lack of pooled saliva, failure to elicit salivary expression from Stensen's or Wharton's ducts, and obvious mucosal dryness. Tests of salivary function, notably stimulated parotid flow rate determination, show reduced salivary flow. Some of these cases are attributable to side effects of medications that reduce salivation. In such cases, it may be possible to arrange to change the medications or their doses. In other cases, stimulation of salivary flow by use of sugarless candy may alleviate some of the discomfort. Topical fluorides and other preventive dentistry approaches are used to reduce the frequency of caries.

SUMMARY

The oral manifestation of HIV infection occur as a variety of opportunistic infections, neoplasms, and other lesions. Some of them are common, perhaps the most common, features of HIV disease and are highly predictive of the development of AIDS. Clinicians caring for HIV-infected persons should become familiar with the diagnosis and management of this group of conditions.

The oral lesions of HIV infection present challenges of diagnosis and therapy. They also offer unrivaled opportunities to investigate the epidemiology, cause, pathogenesis, and treatment of mucosal diseases. As the epidemic progresses, it can be expected that further lesions will be observed and that additional rational and effective therapeutic approaches will be developed.

References

1. Gottlieb MS, Schroff R, Schantez HM: *Pneumocystis carinii* pneumonia and mucosal candidiasis in previously healthy homosexual men: Evidence of a new acquired cellular immunodeficiency. N Engl J Med 305:1425, 1981
2. Greenspan JS, Greenspan D (eds): Oral Manifestations of HIV Infection. Carol Stream, IL, Quintessence Publishing Co, Inc, 1995
3. Leggott PJ, Robertson PB, Greenspan D, et al: Oral manifestations of primary and acquired immunodeficiency diseases in children. Pediatr Dent 9:89, 1987
4. Barrett AP: Oral changes as initial diagnostic indicators in acute leukemia. J Oral Med 41:234, 1986
5. Glavind L, Lund B, Loe H: The relationship between periodontal state and diabetes duration, insulin dosage and retinal changes. J Periodontol 39:341, 1968
6. Barrett AP: Clinical characteristics and mechanisms involved in chemotherapy-induced oral ulceration. J Oral Med 41:424, 1983
7. DePaola LG, Peterson EE, Overholser DJJ, et al: Dental care for patients receiving chemotherapy. J Am Dent Assoc 112:198, 1986
8. Dreizen S, McCredie KB, Bodey GP, et al: Quantitative analysis of the oral complications of antileukemia chemotherapy. Oral Surg 62:650, 1986
9. EC Clearinghouse on Oral Problems Related to HIV Infection and WHO Collaborating Centre on Oral Manifestations of the Human Immunodeficiency Virus: Classification and diagnostic criteria for oral lesions in HIV infection. J Oral Pathol Med 22:289, 1993
10. Greenspan JS, Barr CE, Sciubba JJ, et al, for the USA Oral AIDS Collaborative Group: Oral manifestations of HIV infection: Definitions, diagnostic criteria and principles of therapy. Oral Surg Oral Med Oral Pathol 73:142, 1992
11. Feigal DW, Katz MH, Greenspan D, et al: The prevalence of oral lesions in HIV-infected homosexual and bisexual men: Three San Francisco epidemiological cohorts. AIDS 5:519, 1991
12. Greenspan JS: Sentinels and signposts: The epidemiology and significance of the oral manifestations of HIV disease. Oral Dis 3(Suppl 1):S13, 1997
13. Hilton JF, Donegan E, Katz MH, et al: Development of oral lesions in human immunodeficiency virus-infected transfusion recipients and hemophiliacs. Am J Epidemiol 145:164, 1997
14. Shiboski CH, Hilton JF, Greenspan D, et al: HIV-related oral manifestations in two cohorts of women

in San Francisco. J Acquir Immune Defic Syndr 7: 964, 1994

15. Shiboski CH, Hilton JF, Neuhaus JM, et al: Human immunodeficiency virus-related oral manifestations and gender: A longitudinal analysis. The University of California, San Francisco Oral AIDS Center Epidemiology Collaborative Group. Arch Intern Med 156:2249, 1996

16. Leggott PJ: Oral manifestations in pediatric HIV infection. In Greenspan JS, Greenspan D (ed): Oral Manifestations of HIV Infection. Carol Stream, II, Quintessence Publishing Co, Inc, 1995, p 234

17. Ramos-Gomez FJ, Hilton JF, Canchola AJ, et al: Risk factors for HIV-related orofacial manifestations in children. Pediatr Dent 18:121, 1996

18. Katz MH, Mastrucci MT, Leggott PJ, et al: Prognostic significance of oral lesions in children with perinatally acquired human immunodeficiency virus infection. Am J Dis Child 147:45, 1993

19. Palacio H, Hilton JF, Canchola AJ, Greenspan D: Effect of cigarette smoking on HIV-related oral lesions. J Acquir Immune Defic Syndr Hum Retrovirol 14: 338, 1997

20. Royce RC, Luckmann RS, Fusaro RE, Winkelstein WJ: The natural history of HIV-1 infection: Staging classifications of disease. AIDS 5:355, 1991.

21. Klein RS, Harris CA, Small CR, et al: Oral candidiasis in high-risk patients as the initial manifestation of the acquired immunodeficiency syndrome. N Engl J Med 311:354, 1984

22. Murray HW, Hillman AD, Rubin BY, et al: Patients at risk for AIDS-related opportunistic infections. N Engl J Med 313:1504, 1985

23. Katz MH, Greenspan D, Westenhouse J, et al: Progression to AIDS in HIV-infected homosexual and bisexual men with hairy leukoplakia and oral candidiasis. AIDS 6:95, 1992

24. Dodd CL, Greenspan D, Katz MH, et al: Oral candidiasis in HIV infection: Pseudomembraneous and erythematous candidiasis show similar rates of progression to AIDS. AIDS 5:1339, 1991

25. Greenspan D: Treatment of oral candidiasis in HIV infection. Oral Surg Oral Med Oral Pathol 78:211, 1994

26. Greenspan D, Shirlaw PJ: Management of the oral mucosal lesions seen in association with HIV infection. Oral Dis 3(Suppl 1):S229, 1997

27. Pons V, Greenspan D, Debruin M: Therapy for oropharyngeal candidiasis in HIV-infected patients: A randomized, prospective multicenter study of oral fluconazole versus clotrimazole troches. The Multicenter Study Group [see comments]. J Acquir Immune Defic Syndr 6:1311, 1993

28. Hitchcock CA, Pye GW, Troke PF, et al: Fluconazole resistance in Candida glabrata. Antimicrob Agents Chemother 37:1962, 1993

29. Heald AE, Cox GM, Schell WA, et al: Oropharyngeal yeast flora and fluconazole resistance in HIV-infected patients receiving long-term continuous versus intermittent fluconazole therapy. AIDS 10:263, 1996

30. Blatchford NR: Treatment of oral candidosis with itraconazole: A review. J Am Acad Dermatol 23(3 Pt 2): 565, 1991

31. Graybill JR, Vasquez J, Darouiche RO, Morhart R: Itraconazole oral solution versus fluconazole treatment of oropharyngeal candidiasis. In Abstracts of the 35th Interscience Conference on Antimicrobial Agents and Chemotherapy, San Francisco. Washington, DC, American Society for Microbiology, 1995, Abstract 1220

32. Levron JC, Reynes J, Bazin C: Bioavailability of itraconazole oral solution during treatment of oropharyngeal candidosis in HIV+ patients. In Abstracts of the 19th International Congress of Chemotherapy, Montreal, 1995, Abstract 2131

33. Heinic G, Greenspan D, MacPhail LA, et al: Oral *Histoplasma capsulatum* in association with HIV infection: A case report. J Oral Pathol Med 21:85, 1992

34. Jones AC, Migliorati CA, Baughman RA: The simultaneous occurrence of oral herpes simplex virus, cytomegalovirus, and histoplasmosis in an HIV-infected patients. Oral Surg Oral Med Oral Pathol 74:334, 1992

35. Liang GS, Diakos GL, Serfling U, et al: An evaluation of oral ulcers in patients with AIDS and AIDS-related complex. J Am Acad Dermatol 29:563, 1993

36. Heinic GS, Greenspan D, MacPhail LA, Greenspan JS: Oral Geotrichum candidum infection in association with HIV infection. Oral Surg Oral Med Oral Pathol 73:726, 1992

37. Shannon MT, Sclaroff A, Colm SJ: Invasive aspergillosis of the maxilla in an immunocompromised patient. Oral Surg Oral Med Oral Pathol 70:425, 1990

38. Kuruvilla A, Humphrey DM, Emko P: Coexistent oral cryptococcosis and Kaposi's sarcoma in acquired immunodeficiency syndrome. Cutis 49:260, 1992

39. Glick M, Cohen SG, Cheney RT, et al: Oral manifestations of disseminated *Cryptococcus neoformans* in a patient with acquired immunodeficiency syndrome. Oral Surg Oral Med Oral Pathol 64:454, 1987

40. Lynch DP, Naftolin LZ: Oral *Cryptococcus neoformans* infection in AIDS. Oral Surg Oral Med Oral Pathol 64:449, 1987

41. Lamster I, Grbic J, Fine J, et al: A critical review of periodontal disease as a manifestation of HIV infection. In Greenspan JS, Greenspan D (eds): Oral Manifestations of HIV Infection: Proceedings of the Second International Workshop. Chicago, Quintessence Publishing Co, 1994, p 247

42. Winkler JR: Pathogenesis of HIV-associated periodontal diseases: What's known and what isn't. In Greenspan JS, Greenspan D (eds): Oral Manifestations of HIV Infection. Carol Stream, IL, Quintessence Publishing Co, Inc, 1995, p 263

43. Masouredis CM, Katz MH, Greenspan D, et al: Prevalence of HIV-associated periodontitis and gingivitis in HIV-infected patients attending an AIDS clinic. J Acquir Immune Defic Syndr 5:479, 1992

44. Winkler JR, Herrera C, Westenhouse J, et al: Periodontal disease in HIV-infected and uninfected homosexual and bisexual men [letter]. AIDS 6:1041, 1992

45. Williams CA, Winkler JR, Grassi M, Murray PA: HIV-associated periodontitis complicated by necrotizing stomatitis. Oral Surg Oral Med Oral Pathol 69: 351, 1990

46. Zambon JJ, Reynolds HS, Genco RJ: Studies of the subgingival microflora in patients with acquired immunodeficiency syndrome. J Periodontol 61:699, 1990

47. Zambon JJ, Reynolds H, Smutko J, et al: Are unique bacterial pathogens involved in HIV-associated periodontal diseases? In Greenspan JS, Greenspan D (eds): Oral Manifestations of HIV Infection: Proceedings of the Second International Workshop. Chicago, Quintessence Publishing Co, 1994, p 257

48. Murray PA, Winkler JR, Peros WJ, et al: DNA probe detection of periodontal pathogens in HIV-associated periodontal lesions. Oral Microbiol Immunol 6:34, 1991

49. Murray PA, Grassi M, Winkler JR: The microbiology of HIV-associated periodontal lesions. J Clin Periodontol 16:636, 1989

50. Murray PA, Winkler JR, Sadkowski L, et al: Microbiology of HIV-associated gingivitis and periodontitis. In Robertson PB, Greenspan JS (eds): Perspectives on Oral Manifestations of AIDS: Diagnosis and Management of HIV-Associated Infections. Littleton, MA, PSG, 1988, p 105

51. Greenspan JS: Periodontal complications of HIV infection. Compend Contin Educ Dent 18S:S694, 1994

52. Grassi M, Williams CA, Winkler JR, Murray PA: Management of HIV-associated periodontal diseases. In Robertson RB, Greenspan JS (eds): Perspectives on Oral Manifestations of AIDS: Diagnosis and Management of HIV-Associated Infections. Littleton, MA, PSG, 1988, p 119

53. Palmer GD: Periodontal therapy for patients with HIV infection. In Greenspan JS, Greenspan D (eds): Oral Manifestations of HIV Infection: Proceedings of the Second International Workshop. Chicago, Quintessence Publishing Co, 1994, p 273

54. Greenspan D, Greenspan JS, Pindborg JJ, Schiodt M: AIDS and the Dental Team. Copenhagen, Munksgaard, 1986

55. Schmidt-Westhausen A, Fehrenbach FJ, Reichart PA: Oral Enterobacteriaceae in patients with HIV infection. J Oral Pathol 19:229, 1990

56. Schiodt MS, Dodd CL, Greenspan D, Greenspan JS: HIV-associated salivary gland disease. In Greenspan JS, Greenspan D (eds): Oral Manifestations of HIV Infection. Carol Stream, IL, Quintessence Publishing Co, Inc, 1995, p 145

57. Volpe F, Schimmer A, Barr C: Oral Manifestations of disseminated Mycobacterium avium-intracellulare in a patient with AIDS. Oral Surg 60:567, 1985

58. Speight PM: Epithelioid angiomatosis affecting the oral cavity as a first sign of HIV infection. Br Dent J 171:367, 1991

59. MacPhail LA, Greenspan D, Schiodt M, et al: Acyclovir-resistant, foscarnet-sensitive oral herpes simplex type 2 lesion in a patient with AIDS. Oral Surg Oral Med Oral Pathol 67:427, 1989

60. Erlich KS, Mills J, Chatis P, et al: Acyclovir-resistant herpes simplex virus infections in patients with the acquired immunodeficiency syndrome. N Engl J Med 320:293, 1989

61. Schiodt M, Rindum J, Bygbert I: Chickenpox with oral manifestations in an AIDS patient. Dan Dent J 91:316, 1987

62. Melbye M, Grossman RJ, Goedert JJ, et al: Risk of AIDS after herpes zoster. Lancet 1:728, 1987

63. Jones AC, Freedman PD, Phelan JA, et al: Cytomegalovirus infections of the oral cavity. Oral Surg Oral Med Oral Pathol 75:76, 1993

64. Heinic GS, Northfelt DW, Greenspan JS, et al: Concurrent oral cytomegalovirus and herpes simplex virus infection in association with HIV infection: A case report. Oral Surg Oral Med Oral Pathol 75:488, 1993

65. Greenspan D, Greenspan JS, Conant M, et al: Oral "hairy" leukoplakia in male homosexuals: Evidence of association with both papillomavirus and a herpesgroup virus. Lancet 2:831, 1984

66. De Maubeuge J, Ledoux M, Feremans W, et al: Oral "hairy" leukoplakia in an African AIDS patient. J Cutan Pathol 13:235, 1986

67. Ficarra G, Barone R, Gaglioti D: Oral hairy leukoplakia among HIV-positive intravenous drug abusers: A clinico-pathologic and ultrastructural study. Oral Surg Oral Med Oral Pathol 65:421, 1988

68. Greenspan D, Greenspan JS: The significance of oral hairy leukoplakia. Oral Surg Oral Med Oral Pathol 73:151, 1992

69. Greenspan D, Hollander H, Friedman-Kien A, et al: Oral hairy leukoplakia in two women, a hemophiliac and a transfusion recipient [letter]. Lancet 2:978, 1986

70. Greenspan JS, Greenspan D, Palefsky JM: Oral hairy leukoplakia after a decade. Epstein-Barr Virus Rep 2: 123, 1995

71. Greenspan JS, Mastrucci T, Leggott P, et al: Hairy leukoplakia in a child. AIDS 2:143, 1988

72. Rindum JL, Schiodt M, Pindborg JJ, Scheibel E: Oral hairy leukoplakia in three hemophiliacs with human immunodeficiency virus infection. Oral Surg Oral Med Oral Pathol 63:437, 1987

73. Kabani S, Greenspan D, de Souza Y, et al: Oral hairy leukoplakia with extensive oral mucosal involvement. Oral Surg Oral Med Oral Pathol 67:411, 1989

74. Greenspan JS, Greenspan D, Lennette ET, et al: Replication of Epstein-Barr virus within the epithelial cells of "hairy" leukoplakia, an AIDS-associated lesion. N Engl J Med 313:1564, 1985

75. Schiodt M, Greenspan D, Daniels TE, Greenspan JS: Clinical and histologic spectrum of oral hairy leukoplakia. Oral Surg Oral Med Oral Pathol 64:716, 1987

76. Belton CM, Eversole LR: Oral hairy leukoplakia: Ultrastructural features. J Oral Pathol 15:493, 1986

77. Loning T, Henke R-P, Reichart P, Becker J: In situ hybridization to detect Epstein-Barr virus DNA in oral tissues of HIV-infected patients. Virchows Arch [A] 412:127, 1987

78. DeSouza YG, Greenspan D, Gelton JR, et al: Localization of Epstein-Barr virus DNA in the epithelial cells of oral hairy leukoplakia using in-situ hybridization on tissue sections [letter]. N Engl J Med 320: 1559, 1989

79. DeSouza YG, Freese UK, Greenspan D, Greenspan JS: Diagnosis of Epstein-Barr virus infection in hairy leukoplakia by using nucleic acid hybridization and noninvasive techniques. J Clin Microbiol 28:2775, 1990

80. Daniels TE, Greenspan D, Greenspan JS, et al: Absence of Langerhans cells in oral hairy leukoplakia, an AIDS-associated lesion. J Invest Dermatol 89:178, 1987

81. Williams DM, Leigh IM, Greenspan D, Greenspan JS: Altered patterns of keratin expression in oral hairy leukoplakia: Prognostic implications. J Oral Pathol Med 20:167, 1991

82. Thomas JA, Felix DH, Wray D, et al: Epstein-Barr virus gene expression and epithelial cell differentiation in oral hairy leukoplakia. Am J Pathol 139:1369, 1991

83. Greenspan D, Greenspan JS, Hearst NG, et al: Oral hairy leukoplakia; human immunodeficiency virus status and risk for development of AIDS. J Infect Dis 155:475, 1987

84. Greenspan D, Greenspan JS, Overby G, et al: Risk factors for rapid progression from hairy leukoplakia to AIDS: A nested case control study. J Acquire Immune Defic Syndr 4:652, 1991

85. Itin P, Rufli I, Rudlinser R, et al: Oral hairy leukoplakia in a HIV-negative renal transplant patient: A marker for immunosuppression. Dermatologica 17: 126, 1988

86. Epstein JB, Sherlock CH, Greenspan JS: Hairy leukoplakia-like lesions following bone marrow transplantation [letter]. AIDS 5:101, 1991

87. Greenspan D, Greenspan JS, DeSouza YG, et al: Oral hairy leukoplakia in an HIV-negative renal transplant recipient. J Oral Pathol Med 18:32, 1989

88. Syrjanen S, Laine P, Happoinen RP, Niemela M: Oral hairy leukoplakia is not a specific sign of HIV infection but related to suppression in general. J Oral Pathol Med 18:28, 1989

89. Hollander H, Greenspan D, Stringari S, et al: Hairy leukoplakia and the acquired immunodeficiency syndrome. Ann Intern Med 104:892, 1986

90. Brockmeyer NH, Kreuzfelder E, Mertins L, et al: Zidovudine therapy of asymptomatic HIV-1-infected patients and combined zidovudine-acyclovir therapy of HIV-1 infected patients with oral hairy leukoplakia. J Invest Dermatol 92:647, 1989

91. Barr C: Treatment of HIV-associated oral diseases. In Greenspan JS, Greenspan D (eds). Oral Manifestations of HIV Infection. Carol Stream, IL, Quintessence Publishing Co, Inc, 1995, p 362

92. Friedman-Kein AL: Viral origin of hairy leukoplakia [letter]. Lancet 2:694, 1986

93. Resnick L, Herbst JHS, Ablashi DV, et al: Regression of oral hairy leukoplakia after orally administered acyclovir therapy. JAMA 259:384, 1988

94. Greenspan D, DeSouza Y, Conant MA, et al: Efficacy of desciclovir in the treatment of Epstein-Barr virus infection in oral hairy leukoplakia. J Acquir Immune Defic Syndr 3:571, 1990

95. Katz MH, Greenspan D, Heinic GS, et al: Resolution of hairy leukoplakia: An observational trial of zidovudine versus no treatment [letter]. J Infect Dis 164:1240, 1991

96. Becker J, Leser U, Marschall M, et al: Expression of proteins encoded by Epstein-Barr virus trans-activator genes depends on the differentiation of epithelial cells in oral hairy leukoplakia. Proc Natl Acad Sci USA 88:8332, 1991

97. Niedobitek G, Young LW, Lau R, et al: Epstein-Barr virus infection in oral hairy leukoplakia: Virus replication in the absence of a detectable latent phase. J Gen Virol 72:3035, 1991

98. Young LS, Lau R, Rowe M, et al: Differentiation-associated expression of the Epstein-Barr virus BZLF1 transactivator protein in oral hairy leukoplakia. J Virol 65:2868, 1991

99. Gilligan K, Rajadurai P, Resnick L, Raab-Traub N: Epstein-Barr virus small nuclear RNAs are not expressed in permissively infected cells in AIDS-associated leukoplakia. Proc Natl Acad Sci USA 87:8790, 1990

100. Patton DF, Shirley P, Raab-Traub N, et al: Defective viral DNA in Epstein-Barr virus-associated oral hairy leukoplakia. J Virol 64:397, 1990

101. Walling DM, Edmiston SN, Sixbey JW, et al: Coinfection with multiple strains of the Epstein-Barr virus in human immunodeficiency virus-associated hairy leukoplakia. Proc Natl Acad Sci USA 89:6560, 1992

102. Sandvej KS, Krenacs L, Hamilton-Dutoit SJ, et al: Epstein-Barr virus latent and replicative gene expression in oral hairy leukoplakia. Histopathology 20:387, 1992

103. Palefsky J, Berline J, Penaranda M-E, et al: Nucleotide sequence heterogeneity of Epstein-Barr virus latent membrane protein 1 gene in oral hairy leukoplakia. In Greenspan JS, Greenspan D (eds): Oral Manifestations of HIV Infection. Carol Stream, IL, Quintessence Publishing Co, Inc, 1995, p 175

104. Palefsky JM, Penaranda ME, Pierik LT, et al: Epstein-Barr virus BMRF-2 and BDLF-3 expression in hairy leukoplakia. Oral Dis 3(Suppl 1):S171, 1997

105. Penaranda ME, Lagenaur LA, Pierik LT, et al: Expression of Epstein-Barr virus BMRF-2 and BDLF-3 genes in hairy leukoplakia. J Gen Virol 78(Pt 12)):3361, 1997

106. Greenspan D, Greenspan JS, Pindborg JJ, Schiodt M: AIDS and the Mouth. Copenhagen, Munksgaard, 1990

107. Syrjanen S, von Krogh G, Kellokoski J, Syrjanen K: Two different human papillomavirus (HPV) types associated with oral mucosal lesions in an HIV-seropositive man. J Oral Pathol Med 18:366, 1989

108. Greenspan JD, de Villiers EM, Greenspan JS, et al: Unusual HPV types in the oral warts in association with HIV infection. J Oral Pathol 17:482, 1988

109. Volter C, He Y, Delius H, et al: Novel HPV types in oral papillomatous lesions from patients with HIV infection. Int J Cancer 66:453, 1996

110. Regezi JA, Greenspan D, Greenspan JS, et al: HPV-associated epithelial atypia in oral warts in HIV+ patients. J Cutan Pathol 21:217, 1994

111. Dodd CL, Greenspan D, Greenspan JS: Oral Kaposi's sarcoma in a woman as a first indication of infection with the human immunodeficiency virus. J Am Dent Assoc 122:61, 1991

112. Regezi JA, MacPhail LA, Daniels TE: Oral Kaposi's sarcoma: A 10-year retrospective histopathologic study. J Oral Pathol Med 22:292, 1993

113. Ficarra G, Person AM, Silverman S, et al: Kaposi's sarcoma of the oral cavity: A study of 134 patients with a review of the pathogenesis, epidemiology, clinical aspects, and treatment. Oral Surg Oral Med Oral Pathol 66:543, 1988

114. Scully C, Laskaris G, Pindborg J, et al: Oral manifestations of HIV infection and their management. I. More common lesions. Oral Surg Oral Med Oral Pathol 71:158, 1991

115. Silverman S, Migliorati CA, Lozada-Nur F, et al: Oral findings in people with or at risk for AIDS: A study of 375 homosexual males. J Am Dent Asoc 112:187, 1986

116. Epstein JB, Scully C: HIV infection: Clinical features and treatment of thirty-three homosexual men with Kaposi's sarcoma. Oral Surg Oral Med Oral Pathol 71:38, 1991

117. Epstein JB, Scully C: Intralesional vinblastine for oral Kaposi's sarcoma in HIV infection. Lancet 2:1100, 1989

118. Lucatoto FM, Sapp JP: Treatment of oral Kaposi's sarcoma with a sclerosing agent in AIDS patients. Oral Surg Oral Med Oral Pathol 75:192, 1993

119. Ziegler JL, Beckstead JA, Volberding PA, et al: Non-Hodgkins lymphoma in 90 homosexual men: Relation to generalized lymphadenopathy and the acquired immunodeficiency syndrome. N Engl J Med 311:565, 1984

120. Dodd CL, Greenspan D, Heinic GS, et al: Multifocal oral non-Hodgkin's lymphoma in an AIDS patient. Br Dent J 175:373, 1993

121. Dodd CL, Greenspan D, Schiodt M, et al: Unusual oral presentation of non-Hodgkin's lymphoma in association with HIV infection. Oral Surg Oral Med Oral Pathol 73:603, 1992

122. Kaugars GE, Burns JC: Non-Hodgkin's lymphoma of the oral cavity associated with AIDS. Oral Surg Oral Med Oral Pathol 67:433, 1989

123. MacPhail LA, Greenspan D, Feigal DW, et al: Recurrent aphthous ulcers in association with HIV infection: Description of ulcer types and analysis of T-cell subsets. Oral Surg Oral Med Oral Pathol 71:678, 1991

124. MacPhail LA, Greenspan D, Greenspan JS: Recurrent aphthous ulcers in association with HIV infection: Diagnosis and treatment. Oral Surg Oral Med Oral Pathol 73:283, 1992

125. MacPhail LA, Greenspan JS: Oral ulceration in HIV infection: Investigation and pathogenesis. Oral Dis 3(Suppl 1):S190, 1997

126. Oldfield ECR: Thalidomide for severe aphthous ulceration in patients with human immunodeficiency virus (HIV) infection. Am J Gastroenterol 89:2276, 1994

127. Paterson DL, Georghiou PR, Allworth AM, Kemp RJ: Thalidomide as treatment of refractory aphthous ulceration related to human immunodeficiency virus infection. Clin Infect Dis 20:250, 1995

128. Youle M, Clarbour J, Farthing C, et al: Treatment of resistant aphthous ulceration with thalidomide in patients positive for HIV antibody. BMJ 298:432, 1989

129. Youle M, Hawkins D, Gazzard B: Thalidomide in hyperalgic pharyngeal ulceration of AIDS [letter]. Lancet 335:1591, 1990

130. Jacobson JM, Greenspan JS, Spritzler J, et al: Thalidomide for the treatment of oral aphthous ulcers in patients with human immunodeficiency virus infection. National Institute of Allergy and Infectious Diseases AIDS Clinical Trials Group. N Engl J Med 336:1487, 1997

131. Leggott PJ, Robertson PB, Culver KW: HIV infection in children. Calif Dent Assoc J 15:56, 1987

132. Leggott PJ: Oral manifestations of HIV infection in children. Oral Surg Oral Med Oral Pathol 73:187, 1992

133. Itescu S, Mathur-Wagh U, Skovron ML, et al: HLA-B35 is associated with accelerated progression to AIDS. J Acquir Immune Defic Syndr 5:37, 1991

134. Itescu S, Dalton J, Zhang HZ, Winchester R: Tissue infiltration in a CD8 lymphocytosis syndrome associated with human immunodeficiency virus-1 infection has the phenotypic appearance of an antigenically driven response. J Clin Invest 91:2216, 1993

135. Finfer MD, Schinella RA, Rothstein SG, Persky MS: Cystic parotid lesions in patients at risk for the acquired immunodeficiency syndrome. Arch Otolaryngol Head Neck Surg 144:1290, 1988

136. Itescu S, Brancato LJ, Buxbaum J, et al: A diffuse infiltrative CD8 lymphocytosis syndrome in human immunodeficiency virus (HIV) infection: A host immune response associated with HLA-DR5. Ann Intern Med 112:3, 1990

137. Itescu S, Brancato LJ, Winchester R: A sicca syndrome in HIV infection: Association with HLA-DR5 and CD8 lymphocytosis [letter]. Lancet 2:466, 1989

138. Schiodt M, Dodd CL, Greenspan D, et al: Natural history of HIV-associated salivary gland disease. Oral Surg Oral Med Oral Pathol 74:326, 1992

11 Ocular Complications of HIV Infection

EMMETT T. CUNNINGHAM, JR.

HIV has infected nearly 1 million people in North America and over 30 million people worldwide.[1,2] More than two thirds of HIV-positive patients eventually develop ocular complications of their infection, most often at advanced stages of illness as their CD4+ T-lymphocyte count falls below 100 cells/μl.[3] Opportunistic infections and unusual neoplasms occur most commonly, although HIV-related hemorrheologic and immunologic abnormalities can cause visual problems as well. This chapter reviews those ocular disorders associated most frequently with HIV disease.[4-7]

THE OCULAR ADNEXA

The ocular adnexa include the eyelids, conjunctiva, and lacrimal drainage system. Disorders affecting these structures occur commonly in HIV-infected patients and can be associated with significant visual morbidity.[8-12]

Herpes Zoster Ophthalmicus

Herpes zoster ophthalmicus (HZO) refers to a varicella-zoster virus (VZV)−associated dermatitis involving the ophthalmic distribution of the trigeminal nerve.[13-18] HZO typically presents as a confluent, vesiculobullous eruption that respects the facial midline. Occasionally, however, relatively few or isolated lesions may develop on the forehead, upper eyelid, or nose. Pain is typically severe, and late postherpetic neuralgia and scarring are common.[14] Approximately 5% to 15% of HIV-positive patients develop HZO.[8-12] Rare HIV-positive patients with bilateral involvement have also been described.[18] More than 50% of patients infected with HIV who develop HZO will develop concurrent or delayed corneal infection (keratitis), scleral infection (scleritis), intraocular inflammation (uveitis), or retinal infection (retinitis), which may be either asymptomatic or heralded by the onset of pain, light sensitivity (photophobia), eye redness, or blurred or decreased visual acuity.[13,15-25] Central nervous system involvement (encephalitis), although uncommon, can also occur and may be fatal. Ocular complications of HZO appear to occur more frequently, and may be more severe, in African cohorts.[26,27]

Traditional treatment of HZO involves acyclovir, given initially as a 1-week course of intravenous therapy (30 mg/kg/day), followed thereafter by oral maintenance therapy (800 mg three to five times a day).[14,28,29] Famciclovir maintenance therapy (500 mg three times a day) can also be used and has the advantage of less frequent daily dosings. Valacyclovir, a prodrug of acyclovir with five times more oral bioavailabilty, appears to be as effective as oral acyclovir or famciclovir, but may be associated with life-threatening thrombocytopenic purpura/hemolytic-uremic syndrome in patents with advanced HIV disease, and should therefore be used with caution in this population of patients. Long-term therapy with oral antiviral medication is often necessary in HIV-infected patients, in whom it has been suggested to reduce the frequency of recurrences and the duration of postherpetic neuralgia. For patients initially unresponsive to acyclovir, or for those patients who show reactivation on oral acyclovir or famciclovir, a trial of intravenous foscarnet should be considered. Postherpetic neuralgia often requires long-term use of capsaicin or anesthetic cream applied to the skin, or oral tricyclic antidepressants. Topical antibiotic ointment may be used to minimize the risk of cutaneous bacterial superinfection.

Kaposi's Sarcoma

Kaposi's sarcoma (KS) is a highly vascularized tumor that involves the skin and mucous membranes.[14] Recent work has implicated a novel member of the herpesvirus family, human herpesvirus-8, in the pathogenesis of these lesions in both HIV-infected and uninfected patients.[30-33] Up to 25% of HIV-positive patients develop KS, which may be the presenting sign of disease[14] (see also Chapter 32). Approximately 5% of HIV-positive patients will develop KS involving the eyelids or the conjunctiva.[4-12,34-37] Periocular cutaneous or conjunctival KS lesions may be flat, slightly raised, or nodular. Eyelid lesions are usually readily visible on gross inspection but may be mistaken for a chalazion. Conjunctival lesions, in contrast, are most commonly concealed under the upper or lower eyelid, where they often resemble benign subconjunctival hemorrhage. Bacillary angiomatosis may produce similar conjunctival or eyelid lesions in HIV-positive patients, and should be considered in the differential diagnosis. Although visual symptoms are uncommon, most patients find facial lesions cosmetically unacceptable.

Local radiation therapy is effective at treating eyelid and conjunctival KS, but is expensive and can be associated with loss of lashes, skin irritation, or conjunctival inflammation, keratinization, or scarring.[38-40] Alternative treatments for isolated lesions of the eyelid or conjunctiva include local cryotherapy and intralesional vinblastine or interferon-α. Excision of eyelid lesions can also be performed but may be complicated by bleeding or difficulties in surgical reconstruction. Conjunctival lesions, in contrast, can usually be excised with ease. Eyelid or conjunctival lesions accompanied by systemic involvement are often best treated with systemic chemotherapy. Recurrences are common regardless of treatment.[14] Prolonged use of combination antiretroviral therapy may lead to spontaneous and sustained remission of KS in HIV-positive patients.[41]

Molluscum Contagiosum

Molluscum contagiosum is a highly contagious papulonodular rash that affects the skin and mucous membranes.[14] Infection is more common, and tends to give rise to larger, more numerous, and more rapidly growing lesions, in patients infected with HIV. Still, less than 5% of HIV-positive patients develop molluscum conta-

giosum involving the ocular adnexa.[42-45] The eyelids are affected most often, typically with multiple, small to medium-size, umbilicated lesions. Conjunctival lesions have also been described but appear to be rare. Patients are usually asymptomatic, although an associated conjunctival inflammation (conjunctivitis) and superficial keratitis may produce mild eye redness, irritation, photophobia, or blurred or decreased vision. Treatment options include cryotherapy, curettage, incision, or excision.

Squamous Cell Carcinoma/ Conjunctival Intraepithelial Neoplasia

Patients infected with HIV appear to be at increased risk for developing conjunctival and eyelid squamous cell carcinoma. Endemic infection with human papillomavirus has been suggested to play a role in many patients, particularly in Africa, where the risk of developing conjunctival or eyelid tumors appears to be greatest.[46-55] Lesions are usually asymptomatic, although large tumors involving the eyelid or cornea can impair vision. Intraocular extension is rare but can occur if tumors are left untreated. Therapy consists of wide excision with frozen-section monitoring of the margins to assure complete resection. A single case of an adnexal basal cell carcinoma has also been reported in an HIV-positive patient,[56] although most believe that HIV-infected patients are not at increased risk for developing such lesions.

Cutaneous/Conjunctival Lymphoma

Non-Hodgkin's lymphoma is more common, and tends to be of higher grade malignancy, in patients infected with HIV.[57] Primary eyelid[58,59] and conjunctival[60] lymphomas have been described in HIV-positive patients but appear to be rare. Vision is typically normal unless lesions are large. Symptoms of mild irritation, foreign-body sensation, or dryness may be present, however. All patients should be evaluated to rule out systemic malignancy. Treatment options include local radiation therapy and interferon-α.

Trichomegaly

Acquired trichomegaly, or hypertrichosis of the eyelashes, has been described in the late stages of HIV infection.[61-69] The cause is unknown, although drug toxicity, poor nutrition, and HIV infection itself have each been suggested to play a role. Vision is unaffected, although excessively long lashes may interfere with the use of spectacles or be cosmetically unacceptable to the patient. The lashes may be trimmed as needed.

Conjunctival Microvasculopathy

More than half of all patients infected with HIV will eventually develop conjunctival microvascular alterations, including segmental vascular dilatation and narrowing, microaneurysm formation, the appearance of comma-shaped vascular fragments, and a visible granularity to the flowing blood column termed *sludging*.[70,71] These changes are most evident at the inferior corneal margin or limbus, but require the use of a slit-lamp biomicroscope to be visualized. Vision is unaffected, although the occurrence of microvascular alterations is highly correlated with the presence of retinal microvasculopathy and advanced HIV disease. The cause of HIV-associated conjunctival microvascular changes is unknown. Theories have included HIV-induced increases in plasma viscosity, HIV-related immune complex deposition, and direct infection of the conjunctival vascular endothelium by HIV. No treatment is indicated.

Conjunctivitis

One of the earliest clinic-based studies, by Holland and colleagues, described a nonspecific, culture-negative conjunctivitis in approximately 10% of patients with AIDS.[72] More recent clinic-based studies have, however, reported a prevalence of less than 1%,[4-7] similar to that of the general population. Whereas redness and irritation are the hallmark features shared by all forms of conjunctivitis, a suppurative discharge with sticking of the lids is more characteristic of an infection, whereas a watery discharge with itching more frequently accompanies allergic disease. Opportunistic organisms uncommonly associated with conjunctivitis in HIV-positive patients have included cytomegalovirus (CMV)[73,74] and *Cryptococcus neoformans*.[75,76] Treatment should be guided by the results of conjunctival Gram's stain and culture. Conjunctival biopsy may be indicated in chronic or unresponsive cases.

Preseptal Cellulitis

Although uncommon, preseptal cellulitis caused by *Staphylococcus aureus* has been reported in patients infected by HIV.[56,77] This is perhaps not unexpected because *S. aureus* is the most common cause of cutaneous and systemic bacterial infections in HIV-positive patients, and because HIV-infected individuals have nearly twice the nasal carriage of *S. aureus* as normal controls.[14] Treatment is the same as for cellulitis in immunocompetent patients, although great care should be taken to rule out postseptal or orbital cellulitis, as suggested by the presence of decreased vision, an afferent pupillary defect, proptosis, conjunctival redness or edema (chemosis), or limited ocular motility.

THE ANTERIOR SEGMENT

The anterior segment includes the cornea, anterior chamber, and iris. Anterior segment disorders occur in more than 50% of HIV-positive patients at some point during their illness.[8-12]

Keratoconjunctivitis Sicca

Keratoconjunctivitis sicca, or dry eye, affects 10% to 20% of HIV-positive patients, usually at advanced stages of disease.[78-87] Patients may be asymptomatic or complain of mild to moderate irritation, foreign-body sensation, photophobia, or blurred or decreased vision. Gross signs of redness or discharge are usually minimal, although rapid tear breakup time, decreased tear meniscus, and interpalpebral rose bengal staining are typically evident on slit-lamp biomicroscopy. Abnormal Schirmer's testing is invariably present. HIV-mediated inflammatory damage to both the lacrimal glands and the conjunctiva have each been suggested to play a role in the pathogenesis of the disorder. Abnormalities in tear composition have also been observed.[82,84,85] Corneal exposure resulting from lagophthalmos and decreased blink rate in the setting of HIV encephalopathy can worsen the condition. Treatment involves combined use of artificial tears and long-acting, lubricating ointments.

Infectious Keratitis

With the exception of VZV keratitis, which is more common in HIV-positive than immunocompetent patients, corneal infections occur at about the same rate in HIV-infected and uninfected individuals.[4-7] When HIV-positive patients do develop keratitis, however, the course tends more often to be severe or protracted, and the organisms seem more likely to be opportunistic.[8-12] Pain, photophobia, and decreased vision are usually present, as are the signs of redness and discharge. Adequate examination requires use of slit-lamp biomicroscopy.

Viral Keratitis

VZV Keratitis

About one third of HIV-positive patients with HZO develop keratitis.[13,15-25] The presence of corneal pseudodendrites, visualized with slit-lamp biomicroscopy following staining with either sodium fluorescein or rose bengal, confirms the diagnosis. Mild anterior chamber inflammation (iridocyclitis) and low-grade conjunctivitis may also be present. Up to 5% of patients develop a chronic form of epithelial infection characterized by severe pain, photophobia, and the presence of persistent pseudodendrites.[13,19,20] VZV keratitis in the absence of skin lesions, a condition termed *herpes zoster sine herpete*, may also occur.[13,19,20,88-90] Decreased corneal sensation, elevated intraocular pressure, and iris heterochromia and/or transillumination defects provide additional clues to the diagnosis. Treatment is the same as for HZO.[28]

Herpes Simplex Virus Keratitis

In contrast to VZV keratitis, herpes simplex virus (HSV) keratitis seems not to be more common but may recur more frequently, and in some cases be more resistant to therapy, in HIV-positive as compared to HIV-negative patients.[91-94] As with VZV keratitis, corneal sensation tends to be decreased and intraocular pressure is often elevated. Corneal dendrites visible on slit-lamp biomicroscopy following the application of sodium fluorescein confirm the diagnosis. Treatment options include 7 to 10 days of (1) oral acyclovir (400 mg five times a day) or famciclovir (500 mg three times daily); or (2) a topical antiviral, such as vidarabine (3% 5 times daily), idoxuridine (0.1% hourly), or trifluridine (1% nine time daily). Debridement of epithelial lesions with a cotton swab moistened with sterile saline has also been suggested to help promote healing.

CMV Keratitis

Asymptomatic corneal endothelial deposits described clinically as linear or stellate, and often forming a reticular pattern, have been reported in up to 80% of eyes with CMV retinitis.[95,96] These findings, which are almost always asymptomatic, are best visualized on the endothelial surface of the inferior cornea using slit-lamp biomicroscopy and retroillumination. Histopathologic analysis suggests that these deposits are composed of fibrin and macrophages, with little evidence of active endothelial infection by the virus. CMV dendritic epithelial keratitis, more characteristic of VZV or HSV infection, has been described in a single HIV-positive patient, although this appears to be rare.[97]

Bacterial and Fungal Keratitis

The prevalence of bacterial and fungal keratitis,[4-12] as well as the composition of conjunctival and lid flora,[98-100] appear to be similar in HIV-positive and HIV-negative patients. When bacterial or fungal keratitis does occur, however, it appears more often to be severe, bilateral, associated with multiple pathogens, and with a higher tendency toward corneal perforation in HIV-infected as compared to uninfected patients.[8-12] Numerous bacterial organisms, including *S. aureus*, *Staphylococcus epidermidis*, *Pseudomonas aeruginosa*, and *Klebsiella oxytoga*, as well as various *Streptococcus, Bacillus, Micrococcus,* and *Capnocytophaga* species, have been identified.[12,100-107] *Candida* species have also been reported and appear particularly common in HIV-positive intravenous drug users.[108] Corneal scraping should be taken for Gram's stain, culture, and sensitivities to help guide therapy. Aggressive treatment with topical and subconjunctival fortified antibiotics is usually indicated, and may preserve vision.

Microsporidial Keratitis

Microsporidia are obligate intracellular protozoan parasites. HIV-positive patients are at increased risk for infection by *Microporidia*, which may cause gastroenteritis, hepatitis, peritonitis, sinusitis, pneumonitis, and urogenital infections.[109] Whereas ocular infection in immunocompetent patients is rare,[110] microsporidiosis involves the eye in 1% to 2% of HIV-infected patients, usually at advanced stages of illness. Symptoms typically include mild irritation, foreign-body sensation, or blurred or decreased vision. Slit-lamp biomicroscopy reveals scattered, punctate, subepithelial opacities, often associated with a mild conjunctivitis.[111-127] The organism is extremely difficult to culture but can be demonstrated within the cytoplasm of corneal or conjunctival epithelial cells on either Gram's or Giemsa stain. Treatment options include oral itraconazole, topical propamidine isethionate, topical fumagillin bicyclohexylammonium salt, and oral albendazole.

Corneal Phospholipidoses

Both antivirals, such as ganciclovir and acyclovir,[128] and atovaquone,[129] used to treat toxoplasmosis, have been associated with the formation of intracellular deposits in the superficial cornea, a condition termed *corneal phospholipidosis*. Patients may be either asymptomatic or complain of mild irritation, foreign-body sensation, photophobia, or blurred or decreased vision. Slit-lamp biomicroscopy reveals a characteristic whirl-like pattern of gray-white opacities at the level of the corneal epithelium, hence the alternative description "vortex keratopathy." The differential diagnosis includes toxic keratopathy, as can occur with overuse of topical medications, and corneal microsporidiosis, as described above. Corneal phospholipidoses resolve slowly as the offending medicine is reduced in dosage or discontinued.

Iridocyclitis

Iridocyclitis, or anterior chamber inflammation, develops in more than 50% of HIV-positive patients at some time during the course of their illness.[8-12] Typical symptoms include pain, photophobia, and blurred or decreased vision, and eye redness is common. Adequate visualization of inflammatory cells in the anterior chamber requires use of high-magnification slit-lamp biomicroscopy, which in severe cases may reveal layering of the white blood cells (hypopyon) or adhesions of the iris to the anterior surface of the lens (posterior synechae). In some patients, HIV infection alone appears capable of causing anterior chamber inflammation.[130,131] Usually, however, iridocyclitis is observed in the setting of viral retinitis, most commonly caused by CMV[132,133] and less frequently by VZV[22-25,134] or HSV.[135,136] Severe iridocyclitis is uncommon in HIV-positive patients but can occur in association with toxoplasmic retinochoroiditis,[137-144] syphilitic chorioretinitis,[145-162] and bacterial or fungal retinitis or endophthalmitis.[163-170] Cases of

isolated iridocyclitis in the absence of retinal infection or endophthalmitis have been described in association with toxoplasmosis,[171] cryptococcosis,[172] syphilis,[157,158] and CMV[173] but are uncommon. Anterior chamber inflammation may also represent endogenous uveitis, such as Reiter's syndrome, which may be more common and appears to be more severe in patients infected with HIV.[174,175] Finally, rifabutin,[176-180] used to treat *Mycobacterium avium* complex, produces iridocyclitis in up to one third of patients, particularly when used at 600 mg/day or in combination with clarithromycin or fluconazole, whereas cidofovir,[181,182] given for CMV disease, can cause severe anterior chamber inflammation in 25% to 44% of patients. Treatment for iridocyclitis should be directed at a specific infectious cause, or at discontinuing or reducing the dose of the offending drug when toxicity is suspected. Topical corticosteroids and cycloplegics are often helpful but should never be used in the setting of infection without appropriate antimicrobial coverage.

Angle-Closure Glaucoma

Acute angle-closure glaucoma has been described in HIV-infected patients resulting from an accumulation of serous fluid in the choroid, located between the sclera and the retina, behind the lens and iris. This condition, termed *choroidal* or *uveal effusion syndrome*, is uncommon, and the cause is unknown.[183-190] Symptoms include pain, photophobia, and blurred or decreased vision. Miotic drops and peripheral iridotomies, which are the treatment of choice for most angle-closure attacks, paradoxically worsen the condition. Intraocular inflammation is minimal or absent, and if significant should raise suspicion of primary choroidal infection or endogenous uveitis. The diagnosis of angle-closure glaucoma requires use of slit-lamp biomicroscopy to examine the anterior chamber angle (gonioscopy), whereas visualization of choroidal or uveal effusions requires use of binocular indirect ophthalmoscopy or ocular ultrasonography. Ocular axial length should be checked in all patients because idiopathic uveal effusions can occur in patients with small eyes (nanophthalmos) unrelated to HIV status. Treatment options for uveal effusion syndrome regardless of cause include cycloplegics, corticosteroids, aqueous suppressants, hyperosmolar agents, and, when necessary, surgical drainage of suprachoroidal fluid.[191]

THE POSTERIOR SEGMENT

The posterior segment of the eye includes the retina, choroid, and optic nerve head. Retinal complications of HIV infection are common, particularly HIV retinopathy and CMV retinitis. Choroidal and optic nerve head disorders, in contrast, occur in only 5% to 10% of HIV-positive patients.[4-7]

Retinal Microvasculopathy

Retinal microvasculopathy, also termed HIV or AIDS retinopathy, occurs in more than half of HIV-positive patients, and is a sign of advanced disease (Color Plate III*A*).[4-7] The most commonly observed manifestations include cotton-wool spots, intraretinal hemorrhages, and microaneurysms,[192,193] all of which are best visualized using either direct or binocular indirect ophthalmoscopy. Symptoms are uncommon and findings are transient, typically lasting from weeks to months. HIV retinopathy may, however, contribute to the progressive optic nerve atrophy,[194,195] electroretinographic abnormalities,[196] and loss of color vision, contrast sensitivity, and visual field[197,198] observed in HIV-infected patients. The role of retinal microvasculopathy in the development of CMV retinitis remains controversial, with some investigators finding no relationship[193] and others suggesting that HIV-associated microvascular damage may provide increased access to circulating CMV-infected lymphocytes.[199] Hypotheses regarding the pathogenesis of retinal microvasculopathy parallel those suggested for conjunctival vascular changes as described above.[70,71] No treatment is necessary.

Infectious Retinitis

CMV Retinitis

CMV retinitis affects 25% to 40% of HIV-positive adults[132,133] and approximately 5% of infected children.[77] CD4+ T-lymphocyte counts are typically below 50 cells/μl, although higher cell counts may be observed following splenectomy or in the setting of successful combination antiretroviral therapy.[200] Any aspect of the retina or the optic nerve head may be affected. Approximately 50% to 75% of patients are symptomatic, typically reporting blind spots (scotomata), visual field loss, flashing lights (phosphens), floaters, or decreased or blurred vi-

sion. Direct or indirect ophthalmoscopy reveals characteristic retinal thickening and opacification, often associated with retinal hemorrhages or retinal vascular sheathing (Color Plate III*B*). Anterior chamber and vitreous inflammation is usually minimal, although may be exacerbated in patients on combination antiretroviral therapy.[201] The most common causes of vision loss include direct infection of the macula or optic nerve head and serous or rhegmatogenous detachment of the macula. Macular edema may also occur, particularly when the retinitis is adjacent to the optic nerve head or macula,[202] or when the accompanying vitreous inflammation is severe in the setting of combination antiretroviral therapy.[203]

Treatment of CMV retinitis is a complicated, rapidly evolving field.[4,132,133,204-208] Currently approved treatments for active retinitis include intravenous ganciclovir, foscarnet, and cidofovir. Any of these medicines, as well as the oral formulation of ganciclovir, can be used for maintenance therapy. Local therapy with intravitreous injection of ganciclovir or foscarnet, or via implantation of a slow-release ganciclovir-containing reservoir, is also possible. Choice of an appropriate antiviral and route of delivery needs to be individualized, and based on the location and extent of ocular and systemic CMV disease, an understanding of potential drug-related side-effects, a complete knowledge of clinical response to past treatments, and the overall health status of the patient. CD4+ T-lymphocyte reconstitution following successful combination antiretroviral therapy can be associated with spontaneous and sustained inactivation of CMV retinitis, and in those patients with inactive disease may allow for judicious discontinuation of anti-CMV therapy.[209-212] Cystoid macular edema often requires local or systemic corticosteroids[202,203] but should only be attempted once the retinitis is inactive. Rhegmatogenous retinal detachments require surgical repair.[132,133]

VZV Retinitis

VZV is the second most common cause of necrotizing retinitis in HIV-infected individuals, affecting 2% to 5% of large cohorts with AIDS.[4-7] Like CMV, VZV produces retinal whitening that may be accompanied by intraretinal hemorrhages or vascular sheathing.[22-25,134] VZV retinitis is usually distinguished, however, by its rapid progression, multifocal nature, and initial involvement of deep retinal layers, a syndrome termed progressive outer retinal necrosis

(PORN; Color Plate III*C*). A concurrent or recent herpes zoster dermatitis provides added circumstantial support for the diagnosis. Visual prognosis is, in general, poor, because of both the rapid rate of progression and the high long-term risk of retinal detachment. Treatment involves use of both intravenous and intravitreous antivirals, typically combination therapy with intravenous acyclovir and foscarnet and intravitreous foscarnet.

HSV Retinitis

HSV is a rare cause of retinitis in patients infected by HIV.[135,136] Initial clinical appearance may mimic either CMV or VZV retinitis. HSV retinitis is usually distinguished from CMV retinitis, however, by abrupt onset of symptoms and rapid progression, in many ways similar to VZV retinitis. Recent or past dermatitis or encephalitis can aid in the diagnosis. Treatment and long-term prognosis are similar to VZV retinitis.

Toxoplasmic Retinochoroiditis

Ocular toxoplasmosis affects less than 1% of patients infected by HIV in North America, although it may be more common in other countries, particularly in South America, Africa, and Southeast Asia.[4-7] Classic toxoplasmic retinochoroiditis is characterized by a focal retinitis accompanied by few intraretinal hemorrhages, a moderate to severe anterior chamber and vitreous inflammation, and adjacent or nearby healed retinochoroidal scars representing areas of prior infection (Color Plate III*D*). Toxoplasmic retinochoroiditis in HIV-infected individuals may, however, be multifocal and bilateral, or with no evidence of prior infection, occasionally making differentiation from other forms of retinitis difficult.[137-144] As with other forms of retinitis, direct or binocular indirect ophthalmoscopy is required to visualize both the active infection and healed scars. Testing should include serology for immunoglobulin G and M toxoplasmic antibodies but may be negative in profoundly immunosuppressed patients. From 30% to 50% of HIV-positive patients with toxoplasmic retinochoroiditis will have central nervous system involvement.[139,140] Initial treatment consists of 4 to 6 weeks of pyrimethamine in combination with a sulfonamide or clindamycin. Long-term or repeated therapy is often necessary. Atovaquone has been used with success to treat toxoplasmic retinochoroiditis in an HIV-positive patient[213]

but is expensive, and has yet to be shown superior to more standard combination therapy.

Bacterial and Fungal Retinitis

Ocular syphilis is the most common intraocular bacterial infection in HIV-positive individuals, affecting up to 2% of patients in most cohorts.[4-7] Patients may present with uveitis, retinitis, or optic nerve involvement.[145-162] Laboratory testing should include both a rapid plasma reagin or Venereal Diseases Research Laboratory test, and a specific treponemal antibody test (FTA-ABS or MHA-TP). Rarely, serologic tests may be negative in HIV-positive individuals despite active intraocular infection.[162] Treatment includes intravenous penicillin G, 24 million units/day for 7 to 10 days. Recurrences can occur following adequate treatment in individuals infected with HIV.

Other bacterial and fungal causes of retinitis or endophthalmitis are uncommon in patients infected by HIV, and may in fact be more related to the use of intravenous drugs than to HIV-induced immunosuppression.[163-170] Retinitis,[214,215] as well as optic nerve edema with a macular star (neuroretinitis),[216,217] have each been reported in the setting of systemic *Bartonella henselae* infection in HIV-positive patients.

Infectious Choroiditis

Infectious choroiditis is uncommon in HIV-infected patients, accounting for less than 1% of all eye findings in most clinic-based series.[4-7] *Pneumocystis carinii* is the most common cause, although other identified organisms have included *C. neoformans*, *M. avium* complex, *Mycobacterium tuberculosis*, *H. capsulatum*, *Candida*, and *Aspergillus fumigatus*.[218,219] Most descriptions of choroiditis in HIV-positive patients have appeared in autopsy series, reflecting the often serious nature of the underlying systemic infections. Up to one third of cases have concurrent CMV retinitis.[218,220]

Intraocular Lymphoma

HIV-infected patients are at increased risk for developing non-Hodgkin's lymphoma.[57] Although uncommon, cases of intraocular lymphoma have been reported in HIV-positive patients.[221-223] Treatment options include radiation and chemotherapy.

Retinal Vein or Artery Occlusion

Large retinal vessel occlusion occurs in less than 1% of patients with AIDS but appears to be more common in severely immunosuppressed individuals.[6] Retinal veins are affected more often than retinal arteries.[6,224] The cause is unknown but might be related to the same hemorheologic and vascular factors that contribute to HIV microvasculopathy.[71] Laser treatment may be required in cases complicated by macular edema or retinal neovascularization.

ORBITAL MANIFESTATIONS OF HIV INFECTION

Orbital complications occur in well under 1% of HIV-positive patients.[4-7] Both orbital lymphoma[56,225-230] or orbital infection or cellulitis[142,231-236] have been reported. Organisms associated with infection of the orbit have included *Aspergillus*,[231-233,237] *Propionibacterium acnes*,[231] *Pseudomonas aeruginosa*,[231,235,236] *S. aureus*,[231] *Treponema pallidum*,[231] *Rhizopus arrhizus*,[238] *Toxoplasma gondii*,[142] and *Pneumocystis carinii*.[231,236] Concurrent infection of the paraorbital sinuses appears to be common.[229,237] Lymphoma is treated with radiation and chemotherapy, whereas orbital cellulitis therapy includes systemic antibiotics and, as needed, surgical debridement.

NEURO-OPHTHALMIC MANIFESTATIONS OF HIV INFECTION

Neuro-ophthalmic manifestations occur in from 10% to 15% of HIV-infected patients.[4-7,239-242] The most common findings include optic nerve head edema related either to increased intracranial pressure (papilledema) or direct optic neuritis, nonspecific optic atrophy, cranial nerve palsies, oculomotor abnormalities such as nystagmus and gaze palsies, and visual field defects. Virtually any infectious or neoplastic process can produce neuro-ophthalmic changes, but meningeal and parenchymal lymphoma or cryptococcal, toxoplasmic, or treponemal infections are most frequent. More diffuse encephalopathies related either to direct HIV effects, so-called HIV encephalopathy, or secondary infection with the polyomavirus JC, termed *progressive multifocal leukoencephalopathy* (PML),[243] may cause similar complications. In most instances evaluation includes magnetic resonance imaging followed by a lumbar puncture for cell count, cytology, culture, and antibody and antigen testing. Treatment includes radiation and chemotherapy in the case of lymphoma, and specific antimicrobial therapy for identified infectious causes. There is currently no treatment for HIV encephalopathy or PML.

References

1. Centers for Disease Control and Prevention: Update: Trends and AIDS incidence, death, prevalence—United States, 1996. MMWR Morb Mortal Wkly Rep 46:165, 1997
2. Joint United Nations Programme on HIV/AIDS: UNAIDS/WHO Report on the Global HIV/AIDS Epidemic. Geneva, World Health Organization, 1997
3. Turner BJ, Hecht FM, Ismail RB: CD4+ T-lymphocyte measures in the treatment of individuals infected with human immunodeficiency virus type 1. Arch Intern Med 154:1561, 1994
4. Cunningham ET Jr, Margolis TP: Ocular manifestations of HIV infection. N Engl J Med 339:236, 1998
5. Sarraf D, Ernest JT: AIDS and the eyes. Lancet 348:525, 1996.
6. Jabs DA: Ocular manifestations of HIV infection. Trans Am Ophthalmol Soc 93:623, 1995
7. Park KL, Smith RE, Rao NA: Ocular manifestations of AIDS. Curr Opin Ophthalmol 6:82, 1995
8. Acharya N, Cunningham ET Jr: Corneal, anterior segment, and adnexal manifestations of HIV infection. Int Ophthalmol Clin 1998 (in press)
9. Ryan-Graham MA, Durand M, Pavan-Langston D: AIDS and the anterior segment. Int Ophthalmol Clin 38:241, 1998
10. Meisler DM, Lowder CY, Holland GN: Corneal and external ocular infections in acquired immunodeficiency syndrome (AIDS). In Krachmer JH, Mannis MJ, Holland EJ (eds): Cornea. Cornea and External Disease: Clinical Diagnosis and Management, Vol II. St Louis, Mosby, 1997, p 1017
11. Akduman L, Pepose JS: Anterior segment manifestations of acquired immunodeficiency syndrome. Semin Ophthalmol 10:111,1995
12. Shuler JD, Engstrom RE, Holland GN: External ocular disease and anterior segment disorders associated with AIDS. Int Ophthalmol Clin 29:98, 1989
13. Margolis TP, Milner MS, Shama A, et al: Herpes zoster ophthalmicus in patients with human immunodeficiency virus infection. Am J Ophthalmol 125:285, 1998
14. Tschachler E, Bergstresser PR, Stingl G: HIV-related skin diseases. Lancet 348:659,1996
15. Karbassi M, Raizman MB, Schuman JS: Herpes zoster ophthalmicus. Surv Ophthalmol 36:395, 1992
16. Sandor EV, Millman A, Croxson TS, et al: Herpes zoster ophthalmicus in patients at risk for AIDS. Am J Ophthalmol 101:153, 1986
17. Cole EL, Meisler DM, Calabrese LH, et al: Herpes zoster ophthalmicus and acquired immune deficiency syndrome. Arch Ophthalmol 102:1027, 1984

18. Yau TH, Butrus SI: Presumed bilateral herpes zoster ophthalmicus in an AIDS patient: A case report. Cornea 15:633, 1996

19. Engstrom RE, Holland GN: Chronic herpes zoster virus keratitis associated with the acquired immunodeficiency syndrome. Am J Ophthalmol 105:556, 1988

20. Chern KC, Conrad D, Holland GN, et al: Chronic varicela zoster virus epithelial keratitis in patients with AIDS. Arch Ophthalmol 1998 (in press)

21. Schwab IR: Herpes zoster sine herpete: A potential cause of iridoplegic granulomatous iridocyclitis. Ophthalmology 104:1421, 1997

22. Foster DJ, Dugel PU, Frangieh GT, et al: Rapidly progressive outer retinal necrosis in the acquired immunodeficiency syndrome. Am J Ophthalmol 110:341, 1990

23. Margolis TP, Lowder CY, Holland GN, et al: Varicella-zoster virus retinitis in patients with acquired immunodeficiency syndrome. Am J Ophthalmol 112:119, 1991

24. Engstrom RE Jr, Holland GN, Margolis TP, et al: The progressive outer retinal necrosis syndrome: A variant of necrotizing herpetic retinopathy in patients with AIDS. Ophthalmology 101:1488, 1994

25. Sellitti TP, Huang AJW, Schiffman J, Davis JL: Association of herpes zoster ophthalmicus with acquired immunodeficiency syndrome and acute retinal necrosis. Am J Ophthalmol. 116:297, 1993

26. Kestelyn P, Stevens AM, Bakkers E, et al: Severe herpes zoster ophthalmicus in young African adults: A marker for HTLV-III seropositivity. Br J Ophthalmol 1987; 71:806, 1987

27. Lewallen S: Herpes zoster ophthalmicus in Malawi. Ophthalmology 101:1801, 1994

28. Pepose JS: The potential impact of the varicella vaccine and new antivirals on ocular disease related to varicella-zoster virus. Am J Ophthalmol 123:243, 1997

29. Seiff SR, Margolis TP, Graham S, O'Donnell J. The use of intravenous acyclovir for treatment of herpes zoster in patients at risk for AIDS. Ophthalmology 20:480, 1988

30. Offermann MK: HHV-8: A new herpesvirus associated with Kaposi's sarcoma. Trends Microbiol 4:383, 1996

31. Foreman K, Friborg J, Kong W, et al: Propagation of a human herpesvirus from AIDS-associated Kaposi's sarcoma. N Engl J Med 336:163, 1996

32. Moore P, Chang Y: Detection of herpesvirus-like DNA sequences in Kaposi's sarcoma in patients with and those without HIV infection. N Engl J Med 332:1181, 1995

33. Chang Y, Cesarman E, Pessin M, et al: Identification of herpesvirus-like DNA sequences in AIDS-associated Kaposi's sarcoma. Science 266:1865, 1994

34. Zuccati G, Tiradriti L, Mastrolorenzo A, et al: AIDS-related Kaposi's sarcoma of the eye. Int J STD AIDS 2:136, 1991

35. Dugel PU, Gill PS, Frangieh GT, Rao NA: Ocular adnexal Kaposi's sarcoma in acquired immunodeficiency syndrome. Am J Ophthalmol 110:500, 1990

36. Shuler JD, Holland GN, Miles SA, et al: Kaposi sarcoma of the conjunctiva and eyelids associated with the acquired immunodeficiency syndrome. Arch Ophthalmol 107:858, 1989

37. Macher AM, Palestine A, Masur H, et al: Multicentric Kaposi's sarcoma of the conjunctiva in a male homosexual with the acquired immune deficiency syndrome. Ophthalmology 90:859, 1983

38. Dugel PU, Gill PS, Frangieh GT, Rao NA: Treatment of ocular adnexal Kaposi's sarcoma in acquired immune deficiency syndrome. Ophthalmology 99:1127, 1992

39. Ghabrial R, Quivey JM, Dunn JP Jr, Char DH: Radiation therapy of acquired immunodeficiency syndrome-related Kaposi's sarcoma of the eyelids and conjunctiva. Arch Ophthalmol 110:1423, 1992

40. Hummer J, Gass JD, Huanga JW: Conjunctival Kaposi's sarcoma treated with interferon alpha-2a. Am J Ophthalmol 116:502, 1990

41. Corey L, Holmes K: Therapy for human immunodeficiency virus infection—what have we learned? N Engl J Med 335:1142, 1996

42. Bardenstein DS, Elmets C: Hyperfocal cryotherapy of multiple molluscum contagiosum lesions in patients with the acquired immune deficiency syndrome. Ophthalmology 102:1031, 1995

43. Charles NC, Friedberg DN: Epibulbar molluscum contagiosum in acquired immune deficiency syndrome: Case report and review of the literature. Ophthalmology 99:1123, 1992

44. Robinson MR, UDell IJ, Garber PF, et al: Molluscum contagiosum of the eyelids in patients with acquired immunodeficiency syndrome. Ophthalmology 99:1745, 1992

45. Kohn SR: Molluscum contagiosum in patients with acquired immunodeficiency syndrome. Arch Ophthalmol 105:458, 1987

46. Winward KE, Curtin VT: Conjunctival squamous cell carcinoma in a patient with human immunodeficiency virus infection. Am J Ophthalmol 107:554, 1989

47. Kim RY, Seiff SR, Howes EL, O'Donnell JJ: Necrotizing scleritis secondary to conjunctival squamous cell carcinoma in acquired immunodeficiency syndrome. Am J Ophthalmol 109:231, 1990

48. Kestelyn PH, Stevens AM, Ndayambaje A, et al: HIV and conjunctival malignancies. Lancet 336:51, 1990

49. Ateenyl-Agaba C: Conjunctival squamous-cell carcinoma associated with HIV infection in Kampala, Uganda. Lancet 345:695, 1995

50. Karp CL, Scott IU, Chang TS, Pflugfelder SC: Conjunctival intraepithelial neoplasia: A possible marker for human immunodeficiency virus infection? Arch Ophthalmol 114:257, 1996

51. Waddell KM, Lewallen S, Lucas SB, et al: Carcinoma of the conjunctiva and HIV infection in Uganda and Malawi. Br J Ophthalmol 80:503, 1996

52. Muccioli C, Belfort R, Burnier M, Rao N: Squamous cell carcinoma of the conjunctiva in a patient with the acquired immune deficiency syndrome. Am J Ophthalmol 121:94, 1996

53. McQueen H, Dhillon B, Ironside J: Squamous cell carcinoma of the eyelid and the acquired immune deficiency syndrome. Am J Ophthalmol 114:219, 1996

54. Lewalen S, Shroyer KR, Keyser RB, Liomba G: Aggressive conjunctival squamous cell carcinoma in three young Africans. Arch Ophthalmol 114:215, 1996

55. Margo CE, Mack W, Guffey JM: Squamous cell carcinoma of the conjunctiva and human immune deficiency virus infection. Arch Ophthalmol 114:349, 1996

56. Mansour AM: Adnexal findings in AIDS. Ophthalmic Plas Reconstr Surg 9:273, 1993

57. Sandler AS, Kaplan L: AIDS lymphoma. Curr Opin Oncol 8:377, 1996

58. Goldberg SH, Fieo AG, Wolz DE: Primary eyelid non-Hodgkin's lymphoma in a patient with acquired

immunodeficiency syndrome. Am J Ophthalmol 113: 216, 1992

59. Tunc M, Simmons ML, Char DH, Herndier B: Non-Hodgkin lymphoma and Kaposi sarcoma in an eyelid of a patient with acquired immunodeficiency syndrome. Multiple viruses in pathogenesis. Arch Ophthalmol 115:1464, 1997

60. Cellini M, Possati GL, Puddu P, Caramazza R: Interferon alpha in the therapy of conjunctival lymphoma in an HIV+ patient. Eur J Ophthalmol 6:475, 1996

61. Janier M, Schwartz C, Dontenwille MN, Civatte J: Hypertrichose des cils au cours du SIDA. Ann Dermatol Venereol 11:1490, 1987

62. Casanova JM, Puig T, Rubio M: Hypertrichosis of the eyelashes in acquired immunodeficiency syndrome. Arch Dermatol 123:1599, 1987

63. Roger D, Vaillant L, Arbeille-Brassart B, et al: Quelle est la cause de l'hypertrichose ciliaire acquise du SIDA? Ann Dermatol Venereol 115:1055, 1988

64. Lopez Dupla JM, Valencia ME, Pintado V, Khamashta MA: Tricomegalia: Una excepcional expression del sindrome de immunodeficiencia adquirida. Med Clin 92:556, 1989

65. Klutman NE, Hinthorn DR: Excessive growth of eyelashes in a patient with AIDS being treated with zidovudine. N Engl J Med 324:1896, 1991

66. Kaplan MH, Sadick NS, Talmor M: Acquired trichomegaly of the eyelashes: A cutaneous marker of acquired immunodeficiency syndrome. J Am Acad Dermatol 25:801, 1991

67. Sahai J, Conway B, Cameron D, Gaber G: Zidovudine-associated hypertrichosis and nail pigmentation in an HIV-infected patient. AIDS 5:1395, 1991

68. Grossman MC, Cohen PR, Grossman ME: Acquired eyelash trichomegaly and alopecia areata in a human immunodeficiency virus-infected patient. Dermatology 193:52, 1996

69. Graham DA, Sires BS: Acquired trichomegaly associated with acquired immunodeficiency syndrome. Arch Ophthalmol 115:557, 1997

70. Teich SA: Conjunctival microvascular changes in AIDS and AIDS-related complex. Am J Ophthalmol 103:332, 1987

71. Engstrom RE, Holland GN, Hardy WD, et al: Hemorheologic abnormalities in patients with human immunodeficiency virus infection and ophthalmic microvasculopathy. Am J Ophthalmol 109:153, 1990

72. Holland GN, Pepose JS, Pettit TH, et al: Acquired immune deficiency syndrome: Ocular manifestations. Ophthalmology 90:859, 1983

73. Brown HH, Glasgow BJ, Holland GN, Foos RY: Cytomegalovirus infection of the conjunctiva in AIDS. Am J Ophthalmol 106:102, 1988

74. Espana-Gregori E, Vera-Sempere FJ, Cano-Parra J, et al: Cytomegalovirus infection of the caruncle in the acquired immunodeficiency syndrome. Am J Ophthalmol 117:406, 1994

75. Balmes R, Bialasiewicz AA, Busse H: Conjunctival cryptococcosis preceding human immunodeficiency virus seroconversion. Am J Ophthalmol 113:719, 1992

76. Muccioli C, Belfort R Jr, Rao N: Limbal and choroidal cryptococcus infection in the acquired immunodeficiency syndrome. Am J Ophthalmol 120:539, 1995

77. Dennehy PJ, Warman R, Flynn JT, et al: Ocular manifestations in pediatric patients with acquired immunodeficiency syndrome. Arch Ophthalmol 107:978, 1989

78. Gordon JJ, Golbus J, Kurtides ES: Chronic lymphadenopathy and Sjögren's syndrome in a homosexual man. N Engl J Med 311:1441, 1984

79. Couderc LJ, D'Agay MF, Danon F, et al: Sicca complex and infection with human immunodeficiency virus. Arch Intern Med 147:898, 1987

80. Pflugfelder SC, Savlsow R, Ullman S: Peripheral corneal ulceration in a patient with AIDS-related complex. Am J Ophthalmol 104:542, 1987

81. Ulirsch RC, Jaffe ES: Sjögren's syndrome-like illness associated with the acquired immunodeficiency syndrome-related complex. Hum Pathol 18:1063, 1987

82. Lucca JA, Farris RL, Bielory L, Caputo AR: Keratoconjunctivitis sicca in male patients infected with human immunodeficiency virus type 1. Ophthalmology 97:1008, 1990

83. Itescu S, Brancato LJ, Buxbaum J, et al: A diffuse infiltrative CD8 lymphocytosis syndrome in human immunodeficiency virus (HIV) infection: A host immune response associated with HLA-DR5. Ann Intern Med 112:3, 1990

84. Meillet D, Hoang PL, Unanue F, et al: Filtration and local synthesis of lacrimal proteins in acquired immunodeficiency syndrome. Eur J Clin Chem Clin Biochem 30:319, 1992

85. Matui R, Nussenblatt R, de Smet MD: Prevalence of tear hyposecretion and vitamin A deficiency in patients with AIDS. Invest Ophthalmol Vis Sci 35:1308, 1994

86. Lucca JA, Kung JS, Farris RL: Keratoconjunctivitis sicca in female patients infected with human immunodeficiency virus. CLAO J 20:49, 1994

87. Lucca JA, Kung JS, Farris RL: Keratoconjunctivitis sicca in HIV-1 infected female patients. Adv Exp Med Biol 350:521, 1994

88. Silverstein BE, Chandler D, Neger R, Margolis TP: Disciform keratitis: A case of herpes zoster sine herpete. Am J Ophthalmol 123:254, 1997

89. Stavrou P, Mitchell SM, Fox JD, et al: Detection of varicella-zoster virus DNA in ocular samples from patients with uveitis but no cutaneous eruption. Eye 8:684, 1999

90. Yamamoto S, Tada R, Shimomura Y, et al: Detecting varicella-zoster virus DNA in iridocyclitis using polymerase chain reaction: A case of zoster sine herpete. Arch Ophthalmol 113:1358, 1995

91. Young TL, Robin JB, Holland GN, et al: Herpes simplex keratitis in patients with acquired immune deficiency syndrome. Ophthalmology 96:1476, 1989

92. McLeish W, Pfulfelder SC, Course C, et al: Interferon treatment of herpetic keratitis in a patient with acquired immunodeficiency syndrome. Am J Ophthalmol 109:93, 1990

93. Rosenwasser GOD, Greene WH: Simultaneous herpes simplex types 1 and 2 keratitis in acquired immunodeficiency syndrome. Am J Ophthalmol 113:102, 1992

94. Hodge WG, Margolis TP: Herpes simplex virus keratitis among patients who are positive or negative for human immunodeficiency virus: An epidemiologic study. Ophthalmology 104:120, 1997

95. Walter K, Coutler V, Palay D, et al: Corneal endothelial deposits in patients with cytomegalovirus retinitis. Am J Ophthalmol 121:391, 1996

96. Drody J, Butrus SI, Laby D, et al: Anterior segment findings in AIDS patients with cytomegalovirus retinitis. Graefe's Arch Clin Exp Ophthalmol 233:374, 1995

97. Wilhelmus KR, Font RL, Lehmann RP, Cernoch PL: Cytomegalovirus keratitis in acquired immunodeficiency syndrome. Arch Ophthalmol 114:869, 1996

98. Gumbel H, Ohroff C, Shah P: The conjunctival flora of HIV-positive patients in an advanced stage. Fortschr Ophthalmol 87:382, 1990
99. De Queiroz Campos MS, de Queiroz Campos L, Rehder JRCL, et al: Anaerobic flora of the conjunctival sac in patients with AIDS and with anophthalmia compared with normal eyes. Acta Ophthalmol (Copenh) 72:242, 1994
100. Gritz DC, Scott TJ, Sedo SF, et al: Ocular flora of patients with AIDS compared with those of HIV-negative patients. Cornea 16:400, 1997
101. Ticho BH, Urban RC JR, Safran MJ, Saggau DD: Capnocytophaga keratitis associated with poor dentition and human immunodeficiency virus infection. Am J Ophthalmol 109:352, 1990
102. Nanda M, Pflugfelder SC, Holland S: Fulminant pseudomonal keratitis and scleritis in human immunodeficiency virus-infected patients. Arch Ophthalmol 109:503, 1991
103. Maguen E, Salz JJ, Nesburn AB: Pseudomonas corneal ulcer associated with rigid, gas-permeable, daily-wear lenses in a patient infected with human immunodeficiency virus. Am J Ophthalmol 113:336, 1992
104. Hemady RK, Griffin N, Aristimuno B: Recurrent corneal infections in a patient with the acquired immunodeficiency syndrome. Cornea 12:266, 1993
105. Aristimuno B, Nirankari VS, Hemady RK, Rodrigues MM: Spontaneous ulcerative keratitis in immunocompromised patients. Am J Ophthalmol 115:202, 1993
106. Santos C, Parker J, Dawson C, Ostler B: Bilateral fungal corneal ulcers in a patient with AIDS-related complex. Am J Ophthalmol 102:118, 1986
107. Parrish CM, O'Day DM, Hoyle TC: Spontaneous fungal corneal ulcer as an ocular manifestation of AIDS. Am J Ophthalmol 104:302, 1987
108. Hemady RK: Microbial keratitis in patients infected with the human immunodeficiency virus. Ophthalmology 102:1026, 1995
109. Bryan RT: Microsporidiosis as an AIDS-related opportunistic infection. Clin Infect Dis 21(Suppl 1):S62, 1995
110. Ashton N, Wirasinha P: Encephalitozoonosi (nosematosis) of the cornea. Br J Ophthalmol 57:669, 1973
111. Lowder CY, Meisler DM, McMahon JT, et al: Microsporidia infection of the cornea in a man seropositive for human immunodeficiency virus. Am J Ophthalmol 109:242, 1990
112. Cali A, Meisler DM, Rutherford I, et al: Corneal microsporidiosis in a patient with AIDS. Am J Trop Med Hyg 44:463, 1991
113. Cali A, Meisler DM, Lowder CY, et al: Corneal microsporidiosis: Characterization and identification. J Protozool 38:215S, 1991
114. Davis RM, Font RL, Keisler MS, Shadduck JA: Corneal microsporidiosis: A case report including ultrastructural observations. Ophthalmology 97:953, 1990
115. Friedberg DN, Stenson SM, Orenstein JM, et al: Microsporidial keratoconjunctivitis in acquired immunodeficiency syndrome. Arch Ophthalmol 108:504, 1990
116. Didier ES, Didier PJ, Friedberg DN, et al: Isolation and characterization of a new human microsporidian, Encephalitozoon hellem (n. sp.), from three AIDS patients with keratoconjunctivitis. J Infect Dis 163:617, 1991
117. Yee RW, Tio FO, Martinez JA, et al: Resolution of microsporidial epithelial keratopathy in a patient with AIDS. Ophthalmology 98:196, 1991
118. Metcalfe TW, Doran RM, Rowlands PL, et al: Microsporidial keratoconjunctivitis in a patient with AIDS. Br J Ophthalmol 76:177, 1992
119. Diesenhouse MC, Wilson LA, Corrent GF, et al: Treatment of microsporidial keratoconjunctivitis with topical fumagillin. Am J Ophthalmol 115:293, 1993
120. McCluskey PJ, Goonan PV, Marriott DJ, Field AS. Microsporidial keratoconjunctivitis in AIDS. Eye 7:80, 1993
121. Schwartz DA, Visvesvara GS, Diesenhouse MC, et al: Pathologic features and immunofluorescent antibody demonstration of ocular microsporidiosis (Encephalitozoon hellem) in seven patients with acquired immunodeficiency syndrome. Am J Ophthalmol 115:285, 1993
122. Rosberger DF, Serdarevic ON, Erlandson RA, et al: Successful treatment of microsporidial keratoconjunctivitis with topical fumagillin in a patient with AIDS. Cornea 12:261, 1993
123. Lowder CY. Ocular microsporidiosis. Int Ophthalmol Clin 33:145, 1993
124. Gunnarsson G, Hurlbut D, DeGirolami PC, et al: Multiorgan microsporidiosis: Report of five cases and review. Clin Infect Dis 21:37, 1995
125. Garvey M, Ambrose P, Ulner J: Topical fumagillin in the treatment of microsporidial keratoconjunctivitis in AIDS. Ann Pharmacother 29:872, 1995
126. Lowder CY, McMahon JT, Meisler DM, et al: Microsporidial keratoconjunctivitis caused by Septata intestinalis in a patient with acquired immunodeficiency syndrome. Am J Ophthalmol 121:715, 1996
127. Shah GK, Pfister D, Probst LE, et al: Diagnosis of microsporidial keratitis by confocal microscopy and the chromatrope stain. Am J Ophthalmol 121:89, 1996
128. Wilhelmus KR, Keener MJ, Jones DB, Font RL: Corneal lipidosis in patients with the acquired immunodeficiency syndrome. Am J Ophthalmol 119:14, 1995
129. Shah GK, Cantrill HL, Holland EJ: Vortex keratopathy associated with atovaquone. Am J Ophthalmol 120:669, 1995
130. Farrell PL, Heinemann M-H, Roberts CW, et al: Response of human immunodeficiency virus-associated uveitis to zidovudine. Am J Ophthalmol 106:7, 1988
131. Rosberger DF, Heinemann M-H, Friedberg DN, Holland GN: Uveitis associated with human immunodeficiency virus infection. Am J Ophthalmol 125:301, 1998
132. Holland GN, Tufail A, Jordan MC: Cytomegalovirus disease. In Pepose JS, Holland GN, Wilhelmus KR (eds). Ocular Infection & Immunity. St Louis, Mosby, 1996, p 1088
133. Dunn JP, Jabs DA: Cytomegalovirus retinitis in AIDS: Natural history, diagnosis, and treatment. Aids Clin Rev 96:99, 1995
134. Short GA, Margolis TP, Kuppermann DB, et al: A PCR based assay for the diagnosis of AIDS associated VZV retinitis. Am J Ophthalmol 123:157, 1997
135. Cunningham ET Jr, Short GA, Irvine AR, et al: AIDS-associated herpes simplex virus retinitis: Clinical description and use of a polymerase chain reaction-based assay as a diagnostic tool. Arch Ophthalmol 114:834, 1996
136. Rummelt V, Rummelt C, Gahn G, et al: Triple retinal infection with human immunodeficiency virus type 1, cytomegalovirus, and herpes simplex type 1: Light and electron microscopy, immunohistochemistry, and in situ hybridization. Ophthalmology 101:270, 1994
137. Holland GN, Engstrom RE, Glasglow BJ, et al: Ocular toxoplasmosis in patients with the acquired im-

munodeficiency syndrome. Am J Ophthalmol 106: 653, 1988

138. Grossniklaus HE, Specht CS, Allaire G, Leavitt JA: Toxoplasma gondii retinochoroiditis and optic neuritis in acquired immune deficiency syndrome. Ophthalmology 97:1342, 1990

139. Gagliuso DJ, Teich SA, Friedman AH, Orellana J: Ocular toxoplasmosis in AIDS patients. Trans Am Ophthalmol Soc 88:63, 1990

140. Cochereau-Massin I, LeHoang P, Lautier-Frau M, et al: Ocular toxoplasmosis in human immunodeficiency virus-infected patients. Am J Ophthalmol 114:130, 1992

141. Berger BB, Egwuagu CE, Freeman WR, Wiley CAA: Miliary toxoplasmic retinitis in acquired immunodeficiency syndrome. Arch Ophthalmol 111:373, 1993

142. Moorthy RS, Smith RE, Rao NA: Progressive ocular toxoplasmosis in patients with acquired immunodeficiency syndrome. Am J Ophthalmol 115:742, 1993

143. Elkins BS, Holland GN, Opremcak EM, et al: Ocular toxoplasmosis misdiagnosed as cytomegalovirus retinopathy in immunocompromised patients. Ophthalmology 101:499, 1994

144. Wei ME, Campbell SH, Taylor C: Precipitous visual loss secondary to optic nerve toxoplasmosis as an unusual presentation of AIDS. Aust N Z J Ophthalmol 24:75, 1996

145. Zaidman GW: Neurosyphilis and retrobulbar neuritis in a patient with AIDS. Ann Ophthalmol 18:260, 1986

146. Johns DR, Tierney M, Felsenstein D: Alteration in the natural history of neurosyphilis by concurrent infection with the human immunodeficiency virus. N Engl J Med 316:1569, 1987

147. Berry CD, Hooton TM, Collier AC, Lukehart SA: Neurologic relapse after benzathine penicillin therapy for syphilis in a patient with HIV infection. N Engl J Med 316:1587, 1987

148. Carter JB, Hamill RJ, Matoba AY: Bilateral syphilitic optic neuritis in a patient with a positive test for HIV. Arch Ophthalmol 105:1485, 1987

149. Kleiner RC, Najarian L, Levenson J, Kaplan HJ: AIDS complicated by syphilis can mimic uveitis and Crohn's disease. Arch Ophthalmol 105:1486, 1987

150. Zambrano W, Perez GM, Smith JL: Acute syphilitic blindness in AIDS. J Clin Neuro-ophthalmol 7:1, 1987

151. Randolf JB, Kaplan RP: Unusual manifestations of secondary syphilis and abnormal humoral immune response to Treponema pallidum antigens in a homosexual man with asymptomatic human immunodeficiency virus infection. J Am Acad Dermatol 18:423, 1988

152. Passo MS, Rosenbaum JT: Ocular syphilis in patients with human immunodeficiency virus infection. Am J Ophthalmol 106:1, 1988

153. Richards BW, Hessburg TJ, Nussbaum JN: Recurrent syphilitic uveitis. N Engl J Med 320:62, 1989

154. Levy JH, Liss RA, Maguire AM: Neurosyphilis and ocular syphilis in patients with concurrent human immunodeficiency virus infection. Retina 9:175, 1989

155. Becerra LI, Ksiazek SM, Savino PJ, et al: Syphilitic uveitis in human immunodeficiency virus-infected and non-infected patients. Ophthalmology 96:1727, 1989

156. Gass JBM, Braunstein RA, Chenoweth RG: Acute syphilitic posterior placoid chorioretinitis. Ophthalmology 97:1288, 1990

157. McLeish WM, Pulido JS, Holland S, et al: The ocular manifestations of syphilis in the human immunodeficiency virus type 1-infected host. Ophthalmology 97: 196, 1990

158. Tamesis RR, Foster CS: Ocular syphilis. Ophthalmology 97:1281, 1990

159. Pillai S, DePaolo F: Bilateral panuveitis, sebopsoriasis, and secondary syphilis in a patient with acquired immunodeficiency syndrome. Am J Ophthalmol 114:773, 1992

160. Halperin LS: Neuroretinitis due to seronegative syphilis associated with human immunodeficiency virus. J Clin Neuro-ophthalmol 12:171, 1992

161. Shalaby IA, Dunn JP, Semba RD, Jabs DA: Syphilitic uveitis in human immunodeficiency virus-infected patients. Arch Ophthalmol 115:469, 1997

162. Kuo IC, Kapusta MA, Rao NA: Vitritis as the primary manifestation of ocular syphilis in patients with HIV infection. Am J Ophthalmol 125:306, 1998

163. Macher A, Rodrigues MM, Kaplan W, et al: Disseminated bilateral chorioretinitis due to *Histoplasma capsulatum* in a patient with the acquired immunodeficiency syndrome. Ophthalmology 92:1159, 1985

164. Kurosawa A, Pollack SC, Collins MP, et al: *Sporothrix schenckii* endophthalmitis in a patient with human immunodeficiency virus infection. Arch Ophthalmol 106:376, 1988

165. Davis JL, Nussenblatt RB, Bachman DM, et al: Endogenous bacterial retinitis in AIDS. Am J Ophthalmol 107:613, 1989

166. Shivaram U, Cash M: Purpura fulminans, metastatic endophthalmitis, and thrombotic thrombocytopenic purpura in an HIV-infected patient. N Y State J Med 92:313, 1992

167. Pavan PR, Margo CE: Endogenous endophthalmitis caused by *Bipolaris hawaiiensis* in a patient with acquired immunodeficiency syndrome. Am J Ophthalmol 116:644, 1993

168. Tufail A, Weisz JM, Holland GN: Endogenous bacterial endophthalmitis as a complication of intravenous therapy for cytomegalovirus retinopathy. Arch Ophthalmol 114:879, 1996

169. Glasgow BJ, Engstrom RE Jr, Holland GN, et al: Bilateral endogenous Fusarium endophthalmitis associated with acquired immunodeficiency syndrome. Arch Ophthalmol 114:873, 1996

170. Walton CR, Wilson J, Chan C-C: Metastatic choroidal abscess in the acquired immunodeficiency syndrome. Arch Ophthalmol 114:880, 1996

171. Rehder JR, Burnier M, Pavesio CE, et al: Acute unilateral toxoplasmic iridocyclitis in an AIDS patient. Am J Ophthalmol 106:740, 1988

172. Charles NC, Boxrud CA, Small EA: Cryptococcosis of the anterior segment in acquired immune deficiency syndrome. Ophthalmology 99:813, 1992

173. Chang M, van der Horst CM, Olney MS, Peiffer RL: Clinicopathologic correlation of ocular and neurologic findings in AIDS: Case report. Ann Ophthalmol 18: 105, 1986

174. Altman EM, Centeno LV, Mahal M, Bielory L: AIDS-associated Reiter's syndrome. Ann Allergy 72:307, 1994

175. Berenbaum F, Duvivier C, Prier A, Kaplan G: Successful treatment of Reiter's syndrome in a patient with AIDS with methotrexate and corticosteroids. Br J Rheumatol 35:295, 1996

176. Siegel F, Eilbott D, Burger H, et al: Dose-limiting toxicity of rifabutin in AIDS-related complex: Syndrome of arthralgia/arthritis. AIDS 4:433, 1990

177. Shafran SD, Deschenes J, Miller M, et al: Uveitis and pseudojaundice during a regimen of clarithromycin,

rifabutin, and ethambutol. N Engl J Med 330:438, 1994

178. Jacobs D, Piliero P, Kuperwaser M, et al: Acute uveitis associated with rifabutin use in patients with human immunodeficiency virus infection. Am J Ophthalmol 118:716, 1994

179. Saran BR, Maguire AM, Nichols C, et al: Hypopyon uveitis in patients with acquired immunodeficiency syndrome treated for systemic Mycobacterium avium complex infection with rifabutin. Arch Ophthalmol 112:1159, 1994

180. Tseng AL, Walmsley SL: Rifabutin-associated uveitis. Ann of Pharmacother 29:1149, 1995

181. Davis JL, Taskintuna I, Freeman WR, et al: Iritis and hypotony after treatment with intravenous cidofovir for cytomegalovirus retinitis. Arch Ophthalmol 115:733, 1997

182. Akler ME, Johnson DW, Burman WJ, Johnson SC: Anterior uveitis and hypotony after intravenous cidofovir for the treatment of cytomegalovirus retinitis. Ophthalology 105:651, 1998

183. Ullman S, Wilson RP, Schwartz L: Bilateral angle-closure glaucoma in association with the acquired immune deficiency syndrome. Am J Ophthalmol 101:419, 1986

184. Williams AS, Williams FC, O'Donnell JJ: AIDS presenting as acute glaucoma. Arch Ophthalmol 106:311, 1988

185. Nash RW, Lindquist TD: Bilateral angle-closure glaucoma associated with uveal effusion: Presenting sign of HIV infection. Surv Ophthalmol 36:255, 1992

186. Joshi N, Constable PH, Margolis TP, et al: Bilateral angle closure glaucoma and accelerated cataract formation in a patient with AIDS. Br J Ophthalmol 78:656, 1994

187. Krzystolik MG, Kuperwasser M, Low RM, Dreyer EB: Anterior-segment ultrasound biomicroscopy in a patient with AIDS and bilateral angle-closure glaucoma secondary to uveal effusions. Arch Ophthalmol 114:878, 1996

188. Zambarakji HJ, Simcock PR: Bilateral angle closure glaucoma in HIV infection. J R Soc Med 89:581, 1996

189. Pimentel L, Booth D, Greenwood J, Browne BJ: Secondary acute angle closure glaucoma: A complication of AIDS. J Emerg Med 15:811, 1997

190. Fineman MS, Emerick G, Dudley D, et al: Bilateral choroidal effusions and angle-closure glaucoma associated with human immunodeficiency virus infection. Retina 17:455, 1997

191. Gass JDM: Uveal effusion syndrome: A new hypothesis concerning pathogenesis and technique of surgical treatment. Retina 3:159, 1983

192. Freeman WR, Chen A, Henderly DE, et al: Prevalence and significance of acquired immunodeficiency syndrome-related retinal microvasculopathy. Am J Ophthalmol 107:229, 1989

193. Glasgow BJ, Weisberger AK: A quantitative and cartographic study of retinal microvasculopathy in acquired immunodeficiency syndrome. Am J Ophthalmol 118:46, 1994

194. Tenhula WN, Xu S, Madigan MC, et al: Morphometric comparisons of optic nerve axon loss in acquired immunodeficiency syndrome. Am J Ophthalmol 113:14, 1992

195. Sadun AA, Pepose JS, Madigan MC, et al: AIDS-related optic neuropathy: A histological, virological and ultrastructural study. Graefes Arch Clin Exp Ophthalmol 233:387, 1995

196. Latkany PA, Holopigian K, Lorenzo-Latkany M, Seiple W: Electroretinographic and psychophysical findings during early and late stages of human immunodeficiency virus infection and cytomegalovirus retinitis. Ophthalmology 104:445, 1997

197. Quiceno JI, Capparelli E, Sadun AA, et al: Visual dysfunction without retinitis in patients with acquired immunodeficiency syndrome. Am J Ophthalmol 113:8, 1992

198. Plummer DJ, Sample PA, Arevalo JF, et al: Visual field loss in HIV-positive patients without infectious retinopathy. Am J Ophthalmol 122:542, 1996

199. Gonzalez CR, Wiley CA, Arevalo JF, et al: Polymerase chain reaction detection of cytomegalovirus and human immunodeficiency virus-1 in the retina of patients with acquired immune deficiency syndrome with and without cotton-wool spots. Retina 16:305, 1996

200. Jacobson MA, Zegans M, Pavan PR, et al: Cytomegalovirus retinitis after initiation of highly active antiretroviral therapy. Lancet 349:1443, 1997

201. Zegans ME, Walton RC, Holland GN, et al: Transient vitreous inflammatory reactions associated with combination antiretroviral therapy in patients with AIDS and cytomegalovirus retinitis. Am J Ophthalmol 125:292, 1998

202. Silverstein BE, Smith JH, Sykes SO, et al: Cystoid macular edema associated with cytomegalovirus retinitis in patients with the acquired immunodeficiency syndrome. Am J Ophthalmol 125:412, 1998

203. Karavellas MP, Lowder CY, Macdonald JC, et al: Immune recovery vitritis associated with inactive cytomegalovirus retinitis. A new syndrome. Arch Ophthalmol 116:169, 1998

204. Jacobson MA: Treatment of cytomegalovirus retinitis in patients with the acquired immunodeficiency syndrome. N Engl J Med 337:105, 1997

205. Cunningham ET Jr: New treatments for CMV retinitis in patients with AIDS. West J Med 166:138, 1997

206. Freeman WR: New developments in the treatment of CMV retinitis. Ophthalmology 103:999, 1996

207. Jabs DA: Treatment of cytomegalovirus retinitis in patients with AIDS. Ann Intern Med 125:144, 1996

208. Engstrom RE Jr, Holland GN: Local therapy for cytomegalovirus retinopathy. Am J Ophthalmol 120:376, 1995

209. Whitcup SM, Fortin E, Nussenblatt RB, et al: Therapeutic effect of combination antiretroviral therapy on cytomegalovirus retinitis. JAMA 277:1519, 1997

210. Reed BJ, Schwab IR, Gordon J, Morse LS: Regression of cytomegalovirus retinitis associated with protease-inhibitor treatment in patients with AIDS. Am J Ophthalmol 124:199, 1997

211. Whitcup SM, Cunningham ET Jr, Polis MA, Fortin E: Spontaneous and sustained resolution of CMV retinitis in patients receiving highly active antiretroviral therapy. Br J Ophthalmol 1998 (in press)

212. Vrabec TR, Baldassano VF, Whitcup SM: Discontinuation of maintenance therapy in patients with quiescent cytomegalovirus retinitis and elevated CD4+ counts. Ophthalmology 105:1259, 1998

213. Lopez JS, de Smet MD, Masur H, et al: Orally administered 566C80 for treatment of ocular toxoplasmosis in a patient with the acquired immunodeficiency syndrome. Am J Ophthalmol 113:331, 1992

214. Jones MR, Cunningham ET Jr: *Bartonella henselae*-associated acute multifocal retinitis in a patient with the acquired immune deficiency syndrome. Retina 17:457, 1997

215. Warren K, Goldstein E, Hung VS, et al: Use of retinal biopsy to diagnose *Bartonella* (formerly *Rochalimaea*) *henselae* retinitis in an HIV-infected patient. Arch Ophthalmol 116:937, 1998

216. Schlossberg D, Morad Y, Krouse TB, et al: Culture-proved disseminated cat-scratch disease in acquired immunodeficiency syndrome. Arch Intern Med 149:1437, 1989

217. Wong MT, Dolan MJ, Lattuada CP Jr, et al: Neuroretinitis, aseptic meningitis, and lymphadenitis associated with *Bartonella (Rochalimaea) henselae* infection in immunocompetent patients and patients infected with human immunodeficiency virus type I. Clin Infect Dis 21:352, 1995

218. Morinelli EN, Dugel PU, Riffenburgh R, Rao NA: Infectious multifocal choroiditis in patients with acquired immune deficiency syndrome. Ophthalmology 100:1014, 1993

219. Rao NA, Zimmerman PL, Boyer D, et al: A clinical, histological, and electron microscopic study of *Pneumocystis carinii* choroiditis. Am J Ophthalmol 107:218, 1989

220. Saran BR, Pomilla PV. Retinal vascular nonperfusion and retinal neovascularization as a consequence of cytomegalovirus retinitis and cryptococcal choroiditis. Retina 16:510, 1996

221. Schanzer MC, Font RL, O'Malley RE: Primary ocular malignant lymphoma associated with the acquired immunodeficiency syndrome. Ophthalmology 98:88, 1991

222. Stanton CA, Sloan DB III, Slusher MM, Greven CM: Acquired immunodeficiency syndrome-related primary intraocular lymphoma. Arch Ophthlmol 110:1614, 1992

223. Matzkin DC, Slamovits TL, Rosenbaum PS: Simultaneous intraocular and orbital non-Hodgkin lymphoma in acquired immune deficiency syndrome. Ophthalmology 101:850, 1994

224. Park KL, Marx JL, Lopez PF, Rao NA: Noninfectious branch retinal vein occlusion in HIV-positive patients. Retina 17:162, 1997

225. Fujikawa LS, Schwartz LK, Rosenbaum EH: Acquired immunodeficiency syndrome associated with Burkitt's lymphoma presenting with ocular findings. Ophthalmology 90(Suppl):50, 1983

226. Tien DR: Large cell lymphoma in AIDS. Ophthalmology 98:412, 1991

227. Antle CM, White VA, Horsman De, Rootman J: Large cell orbital lymphoma in a patient with acquired immune deficiency syndrome. Case report and review. Ophthalmology 97:1484, 1990

228. Mansour AM: Orbital findings in acquired immunodeficiency syndrome. Am J Ophthalmol 110:706, 1990

229. Brooks HL Jr, Downing J, McClure JA, Engel HM: Orbital Burkitt's lymphoma in a homosexual man with acquired immune deficiency. Arch Ophthalmol 102:1533, 1984

230. Font RL, Laucirica R, Patrimely JR: Immunoblastic B-cell malignant lymphoma involving the orbit and maxillary sinus in a patient with acquired immune deficiency syndrome. Ophthalmology 100:966, 1993

231. Kronish JW, Johnson TE, Gilberg SM, et al: Orbital infections in patients with human immunodeficiency syndrome. Ophthalmology 103:1483, 1996

232. Vitale AT, Spaide RF, Warren FA, et al: Orbital aspergillosis in an immunocompromised host. Am J Ophthalmol 113:725, 1992

233. Cahill KV, Hogan CD, Koletar SL, Gersman M: Intraorbital injection of amphotericin B for palliative treatment of Aspergillus orbital abscess. Ophthalmic Plast Reconstr Surg 10:276, 1994

234. Friedberg DN, Warren FA, Lee MH, et al: *Pneumocystis carinii* of the orbit. Am J Ophthalmol 113:595, 1992

235. Cano-Parra J, Espana E, Esteban M, et al: Pseudomonas conjunctival ulcer and secondary orbital cellulitis in a patient with AIDS. Br J Ophthalmol 78:72, 1994

236. Cheung SW, Lee KC, Cha I: Orbitocerebral complications of pseudomonas sinusitis. Laryngoscope 102:1385, 1992

237. Meyer RD, Gaultier CR, Yamashita JT, et al: Fungal sinusitis in patients with AIDS: Report of 4 cases and review of the literature. Medicine 73:69, 1994

238. Blatt SP, Lucey DR, DeHoff D, Zellmer RB: Rhinocerebral zygomycosis in a patient with AIDS. J Infect Dis 164:215, 1991

239. Currie J: AIDS and neuro-ophthalmology. Curr Opin Ophthalmol 6:34, 1995

240. Miller NR: Viruses and viral diseases. In: Walsh and Hoyt's Clinical Neuro-Ophthalmology, 4th ed, Vol Five, Part Two. Baltimore, Williams & Wilkins, 1995, p 4107

241. Keane JR: Neuro-ophthalmologic signs of AIDS. Neurology 41:841, 1991

242. Friedman DI: Neuro-ophthalmic manifestations of human immunodeficiency virus infection. Neurol Clin 9:55, 1991

243. Ormerod LD, Rhodes RH, Gross SA, et al: Ophthalmic manifestations of acquired immune deficiency syndrome-associated progressive multifocal leukoencephalopathy. Ophthalmology 103:889, 1996

12 | Dermatologic Care of the AIDS Patient

TIMOTHY G. BERGER

Skin disease is an extremely common complication of HIV infection, affecting up to 90% of seropositive persons.[1] Some of the skin conditions are commonly seen in uninfected persons (e.g., seborrheic dermatitis) but are of increased severity in those infected with HIV. Other skin diseases are relatively unique to HIV infection (e.g., Kaposi's sarcoma [KS]). The average HIV-infected patient has at least two and often more different skin conditions simultaneously. It is useful to classify the cutaneous disorders seen with HIV disease as either infectious disorders, hypersensitivity disorders and drug reactions, or neoplasms. The treatment of these conditions is summarized in Table 12–1.

The type of skin disease seen in the course of HIV disease relates to the patient's immune status. In general, in persons with early HIV disease (CD4 count > 500 cells mm[3]), only skin disease typical of the risk factors for HIV disease are seen (e.g., genital herpes simplex virus [HSV], genital warts). At this stage human papillomavirus (HPV) infection (warts) is resistant to therapy. KS may appear at this stage. Less common are thrush, oral hairy leukoplakia, and herpes zoster. During the early symptomatic phase (CD4 count 200 to 500/mm[3]; formerly called AIDS-related complex), disorders of subtle immune imbalance occur: candidiasis, oral hairy leukoplakia, herpes zoster, psoriasis, seborrheic dermatitis, and atopic dermatitis. Response to treatment is normal. Once the CD4 count is less than 200/mm[3] (AIDS), skin disease becomes somewhat different. Opportunistic infections such as cryptococcosis and histoplasmosis may occur on the skin, and skin infections become chronic.

Patients with advanced HIV disease appear anergic as a result of progressive infections with viruses, fungi, and intracellular parasites (e.g., *Leishmania*). However, this anergy is only in part analogous to iatrogenic immunosuppression caused by chemotherapy and corticosteroid treatments. Psoriasis, for example, disappears during chemotherapy but is increased in patients with advanced HIV disease. In fact, the skin of patients with advanced HIV disease is actually hyperreactive. This hyperreactivity may be manifested by the appearance of pruritic and nonpruritic inflammatory skin diseases. Drug reactions, insect bite hypersensitivity, and itchy folliculitis are all manifestations of the enhanced cutaneous reactivity.

Once the CD4 count is less than 50/mm[3], bizarre patterns of skin disease occur. Biopsies are frequently required to confirm diagnoses. Treatment failures, drug resistance, and chronicity are the hallmark of this stage of HIV disease.

Highly active antiretroviral therapy (HAART) has changed the pattern of skin diseases seen in patients with HIV infection. As expected, with reduction in viral load and improvement in CD4 counts, certain infectious diseases that used to be seen in patients with advanced immunosuppression either resolve or do not occur. Molluscum contagiosum is the best example; refractory cases spontaneously resolve after 4 to 6 months of effective HAART. However, pruritic skin disorders and drug eruptions do not seem to be less frequent, and in some cases appear to be induced by HAART.

INFECTIOUS CUTANEOUS DISORDERS

Bacterial Infections

Staphylococcus aureus is the most common cutaneous bacterial pathogen.[2] The following patterns of staph infection may be seen: folliculitis,

TABLE 12–1. Diagnosis and Treatment of Skin Conditions Commonly Seen with HIV Infection

CONDITION	MORPHOLOGY	LOCATION	TREATMENT	DURATION
Staphylococcal folliculitis	Erythematous follicular pustules or papules; may be pruritic	Face, trunk, groin	Dicloxacillin, 500 mg PO qid, or other penicillinase-resistant antistaphylococcal antibiotic	7–21 days
			Refractory: add rifampin, 600 mg qd to above	First 5 days antibiotic therapy with above
Bacillary angiomatosis	Friable, vascular papules, cellulitic plaques, subcutaneous nodules	Skin, bone, liver, spleen, lymph node	Erythromycin, 500 mg qid or Doxycycline, 100 mg bid	Skin: 8 weeks Visceral: unknown, but consider 16 weeks
Herpes zoster (shingles)	Grouped vesicles on erythematous bases	Dermatomal distribution; may spill onto adjacent dermatomes	Acute: acyclovir, 800 mg PO 5 times per day Dissemination, severe immunosuppression, or involvement of ophthalmic branch of trigeminal nerve: acyclovir, 10 mg/kg IV q8h (corrected for creatinine clearance)	7–10 days Give IV until no new blisters for 72 h, then finish orally as above
Herpes simplex	Grouped vesicles on erythematous bases, rapidly evolving into superficial mucocutaneous ulcerations or fissures; necrotizing ulcers may be seen when chronic	Face, hand, or anogenital area	Acute: acyclovir, 200–400 mg PO 5 times per day Oral acyclovir failure or dissemination: acyclovir, 5 mg/kg IV q8h (corrected for creatinine clearance) Maintenance: acyclovir, 200 mg PO tid or 400 mg PO bid Acyclovir resistance: foscarnet	7–10 days or until ulcers healed Indefinitely
Molluscum contagiosum	2- to 5-mm pearly, flesh-colored papules, often with central umbilication	Face, anogenital area	Cryotherapy or electrosurgery or curettage	For all treatments: repeat at 2- to 3-week intervals until resolved
Insect bite reactions	Erythematous, urticarial papules	Scabies: axillae, groin, finger webs	Scabies: lindane 1% lotion for 12 hr: permethrin (Elimite) 5% lotion for 12 hr	Twice, 1 week apart
		Fleas: lower legs Mosquitoes: upper and lower extremities	Fleas, mosquitoes: 1. Insect repellants 2. Antihistamines 3. Insecticide spray of environment (fleas)	Constant, regular use
Photosensitivity	Eczematous eruption	Face (tip of nose), extensor forearms, neck	1. Sun protection, sunscreens 2. Discontinuation of photosensitizing medications 3. Topical steroids	Continuous for *1* and *2*; as needed for *3*
Eosinophilic folliculitis	Urticarial follicular papules	Trunk, face	Astemizole, 10 mg qd itraconazole 200–400 mg daily *and* topical steroids, *or* ultraviolet light	Constant treatment
Seborrheic dermatitis	Fine, white scaling without erythema (dandruff) to patches and plaques of erythema with indistinct margins and yellowish, greasy scale	Scalp, central face, eyebrows, nasolabial and retroauricular folds, chest, upper back, axillae, groin	Hydrocortisone 2.5% cream and ketoconazole 2% cream applied bid Maintenance: Hydrocortisone 1% cream and ketoconazole 2% cream applied bid	Until lesions resolve Indefinitely
Psoriasis and Reiter's syndrome	Sharply marginated plaques with a silvery scale	Elbows, knees, lumbosacral area	Triamcinolone acetonide 0.1% cream tid	Indefinitely

bullous impetigo, ecthyma, abscesses, hidradenitis suppurativa–like plaques, and cellulitis. The effect of HAART on the prevalence and pattern of HIV-associated staphylococcal infections is unknown.

Folliculitis is the most common form of staphylococcal infection seen in HIV-infected persons (Fig. 12–1). The central trunk, groin, and face are the most common sites of infection. The primary lesion is a follicular pustule, but lesions may be almost urticarial. Many HIV-infected patients with staphylococcal folliculitis of the trunk have severe pruritus, and this represents one of the more treatable pruritic eruptions seen in HIV disease.[2] Often many of the lesions have been excoriated, and the patient must be carefully examined for a primary lesion adequate for culture. Bullous impetigo is quite common in the groin and axillae, presenting as flaccid blisters that quickly rupture, leaving small superficial erosions with a peripheral scale. The lesions are usually asymptomatic and occur more commonly during hot, humid weather. Ecthyma is a punched-out ulcer with a sharp border. The base may be purulent or covered with a thick, adherent crust (Fig. 12–2). Lesions are most common on the lower legs, commonly overlying a pre-existing dermatitis. Violaceous tender cystic plaques and nodules in the axillae

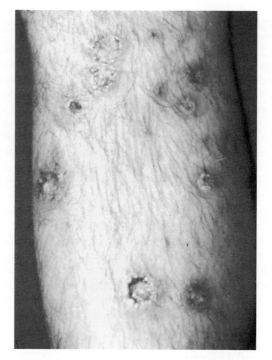

FIGURE 12–2. Ecthyma showing punched-out staphylococcal ulcers of the lower leg.

and groin may be due to *S. aureus* alone, as are virtually all suppurative abscesses. All of the above patterns may be accompanied by an associated cellulitis (Color Plate II*A*).

The treatment of cultaneous staphylococcal infections is determined by the severity of the infection and the presence of systemic symptoms. Patients with chills, fever, large abscesses, or cellulitis are usually admitted for intravenous therapy. Abscesses should be incised and drained. Localized infection may be treated on an outpatient basis with oral agents once cultures are obtained. Patients are re-examined after 3 to 5 days to be sure the appropriate antibiotic was chosen and that there is improvement. A penicillinase-resistant penicillin or first-generation cephalosporin is the first choice for therapy. Because nasal carriage approaches 50% in these patients, rifampin 600 mg in a single daily dose for at least 5 days or intranasal mupirocin may be added in refractory or relapsing cases. Benzoyl peroxide washes or antibacterial soaps may be help prevent relapses, but should be accompanied by vigorous lubrication because dry skin is so common. Antibiotic prophylaxis with clindamycin reduces the frequency of staphylococcal infections; however, any patient using a macrolide for mycobacterial prophylaxis will have erythromycin-resistant staphylococcal

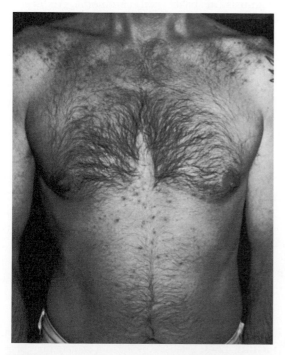

FIGURE 12–1. Pruritic bacterial folliculitis of the trunk. *Staphylococcus aureus* was cultured from a lesion; the condition cleared with oral antibiotics.

infection, which precludes the use of erythromycin or azithromycin for skin infections.

Helicobacter cinaedi is a hard-to-culture organism frequently carried in the gastrointestinal tracts of homosexual men. It is an uncommon cause of bacteremia in these patients. In about one third of patients with bacteremia, there is a coexistent multicentric chronic cellulitis that most commonly occurs on the lower legs and presents as tender red plaques but is subacute, growing gradually over days to weeks. Multiple lesions are common. Gastrointestinal symptoms are frequently absent in patients with the cellulitis, although a monoarticular arthritis may also occur. Antibiotic sensitivity profiles are not predictable, and, because the organism is frequently not recovered by routine methods, treatment is difficult. In addition, 6 weeks or more of treatment may be required to clear the infection. Clarithromycin, ciprofloxacin, and doxycycline are all possible initial treatments.[3]

Viral Infections

Primary HIV infection (symptomatic seroconversion) may be associated with a skin eruption.[4] This eruption may be quite subtle or florid. It tends to occur in patients who are most symptomatic during seroconversion; its frequency is unknown. In patients sick enough to seek medical attention, skin lesions occur in up to 75%. In those with less severe symptoms, the frequency may be much lower. The eruption typically consists of oval, slightly scaly plaques on the upper chest. The lesions may have focal petechiae. The eruption is asymptomatic but may be accompanied by oral and genital ulcerations.

Herpesvirus

The herpesviruses are common cutaneous viral pathogens, with HSV and varicella-zoster viruses frequently causing skin disease. Herpes zoster occurs in up to 8% of HIV-infected persons, and the average CD4 count for the initial episode is 315/mm.[3,5] Any person, especially under the age of 65, who develops shingles should be queried about risk factors for HIV infection. Usually, the course of herpes zoster is uneventful, although persistent postherpetic neuralgia may occur. In patients with more advanced HIV disease, herpes zoster may be very painful, severe, and prolonged. Dissemination may occur but is usually limited to skin. Disseminated herpetic lesions are almost always due to varicella-

zoster, disseminated herpes simplex is rare in HIV disease. In advanced HIV infection, chronic lesions of varicella-zoster may be verrucous and resemble warts or psoriasis.

Herpes simplex infections occur in the genital, digital, and orofacial areas. Once the CD4 count is less than 200/mm³, herpetic lesions present as persistent nonhealing ulcers. It is not unusual for lesions to be secondarily infected, so cultures may yield *S. aureus* or other pathogens. A viral culture should be obtained or a fluorescent antibody examination performed. If either is negative, a biopsy of the edge of the ulcer should be considered. It is sometimes impossible to clinically diagnose chronic ulcerations in HIV-infected persons, and multiple cultures and skin biopsy may be required.

Molluscum Contagiosum

Molluscum contagiosum is extremely common in patients with AIDS whose CD4 count is less than 100/mm³. Lesions present as umbilicated, pearly, 2- to 5-mm papules on the face and genital area and scattered on the trunk. There is a particular predilection for lesions to occur on the eyelids. Lesions may number from one to hundreds. Occasional lesions may exceed 1 cm (giant molluscum) (Fig. 12–3). Their pearly borders and telangiectasias may lead to the misdiagnosis of basal cell carcinoma. Extensive molluscum of more than one anatomic region

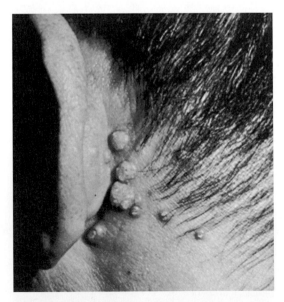

FIGURE 12–3. Extensive molluscum contagiosum of the head and neck, an almost certain indication of advanced HIV disease with a helper T-cell count of less than 200/mm³.

(e.g., face and groin) is highly suggestive of a CD4 count less than 50/mm^3. We and others have seen disseminated cryptococcosis, penicilliosis, and herpetic folliculitis mimic molluscum contagiosum.[6]

Complete eradication of molluscum contagiosum is extremely difficult, unless the patient's immune status is improved. Dramatic resolution of molluscum is seen approximately 6 months after effective HAART is instituted and the patient responds. This observation, as in KS, has made optimizing HAART the most important aspect of managing AIDS-associated molluscum contagiosum. Lesions are usually treated with destructive modalities (cryotherapy with liquid nitrogen, light electrocautery, or curettage). Topical retinoic acid (Retin A) applied once nightly to the face may slow down the rate at which lesions appear but, unless applied to the point of severe irritation, does little for established lesions, nor can it be used on the eyelids or genitalia. Studies on the use of imiquimod have not been published, and, given the limited effect of systemic interferon on AIDS-associated molluscum, confirmatory data of its efficacy is needed before it can be recommended routinely. Systemic and topical treatment with cidofovir, a nucleotide analog with activity against many DNA viruses, has been reported to be effective in recalcitrant molluscum in AIDS patients.[7] However, the patients were also put on HAART within 6 months prior to assessing the response, which clearly presents a confounding effect. Compounded 3% cidofovir cream is costly. Studies on the efficacy of 1% cream have concluded but the data are not yet available.

Human Papillomavirus

HPVs induce a variety of squamous papillomas that we recognize as "warts." Warts of all types are very common in patients with HIV infection. The most common and difficult patterns are genital warts, common warts, plantar warts, and flat warts. Unlike molluscum, improved immunity does not have much effect on the warts, at least in the short term (up to 1 year). Complete eradication is often impossible, and simple control offering wart-free and symptom-free periods is a reasonable expectation until better treatments are available.

Seventy-five percent of the sexually active population in the United States has evidence of current or prior genital HPV infection, and over 90% of homosexual men have been infected. For HIV-infected patients, standard treatments are recommended and are effective, but to a lesser degree. Topical podophyllotoxin, cryotherapy, and trichloracetic acid may all be used. Simple surgical removal and electrosurgery are most effective but may need to be repeated at regular intervals. Topical cidofovir may eventually be of value.

Atypical, hyperpigmented, or flat lesions should be biopsied because they may demonstrate high-grade squamous intraepithelial lesions (the new name for high-grade dysplasia). The risk of cancer from these lesions is highest in the anal canal and on the glans penis of uncircumcised men.

Common and plantar warts are managed by standard methods (cryotherapy, topical salicyclic acid). In refractory cases, intralesional bleomycin, pulse-dye laser treatment, heat therapy, and eventually surgical eradication are effective, but recurrences are common.

Flat warts are most common on the face. They are difficult to treat and may be quite extensive. Retin A cream nightly, cryotherapy, and light electrosurgery may all reduce or eliminate lesions.

Parasitic Infections

Acanthamebiasis is a rare form of encephalitis that may occur in immunocompetent and immunosuppressed hosts. Acanthamebiasis may occur in advanced AIDS (CD4 count <50/mm^3).[8] In AIDS patients, skin lesions are the most common presentation (75% of cases), and may precede evidence of involvement of other tissues by weeks to months. Lesions occur as deep-seated nodules that suppurate, crust, or weep serosanguinous fluid. They occur most commonly on the extremities but, with time, trunk and visceral disease may occur. Sinusitis is commonly present, and the palate or nasal septum may be perforated. The diagnosis is established by biopsy of an ulcer, which will show suppurative and granulomatous inflammation with vasculitis. The vasculitis is uncommon in other infectious granulomas and should alert the pathologist to search for acanthameba. The organisms are hard to identify on routine histologic material because they resemble macrophages. Special stains are not very useful; therefore, the clinician must notify the pathologist that acanthameba is a possible diagnosis. Most patients die, despite multidrug therapy with imidazole, pentamidine, and topical chlorhexidine.

HYPERSENSITIVITY DISORDERS

Drug Reactions

It has long been recognized that, in approximately 50% of persons treated with trimethoprim-sulfamethoxazole (TMP-SMX) for *Pneumocystis* pneumonia, a widespread morbilliform eruption will develop[9] (Color Plate II*B*). This simple eruption is most common in persons with a CD4 count between 25 and 200/mm[3]. HAART may induce this or more severe reactions in patients who have tolerated TMP-SMX for long periods. The rash may resolve with continued treatment but often persists or progresses. Therapy may be continued if symptoms are not too severe. Progression of a simple TMP-SMX rash to a life-threatening reaction has not been reported during a single course of treatment. Reexposure later may lead to a more severe reaction. Similar reactions are seen as a result of virtually all other medications but seem to be most common to antibiotics, especially the penicillins, and sulfa drugs. Cutaneous reactions are rare with certain frequently used medications, especially acyclovir and the antiretrovirals. Nevirapine may uncommonly cause skin eruptions.

Some patients develop adverse reactions to many chemically unrelated medications, and may have increasingly severe reactions with each medication exposure. They may eventually develop erythema multiforme major. In addition to morbilliform reactions, erythema multiforme and fixed drug eruptions are seen with dramatically increased frequency in HIV-infected individuals. In some patients, the erythema multiforme may have quite a severe appearance, as Stevens-Johnson syndrome or toxic epidermal necrolysis (Fig. 12–4). These severe reactions are most commonly due to sulfa drugs and anticonvulsants used to treat central nervous system toxoplasmosis or *Pneumocystis* pneumonia.[10] Any HIV-infected person with a widespread eruption should be carefully evaluated for the possibility of its being medication induced.

If a morbilliform eruption occurs in response to TMP-SMX, the drug may be continued because the eruption may resolve even with treatment. Introduction of TMP-SMX gradually, with progressively increasing doses, reduces the likelihood of initial and recurrent eruptions.[11] This is not true "densensitization," but may relate to drug metabolism rather than immunologic alteration. Rechallenge is not recommended in patients who have had major skin reactions.

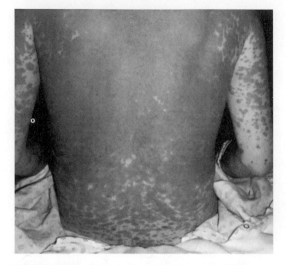

FIGURE 12–4. Drug-induced erythema multiforme major.

Insect Bite Reactions

Scabies, flea bites, and mosquito bites may all be extremely florid in patients with HIV disease. These eruptions present as nonfollicular papules to cellulitic plaques with marked pruritus. The nature of the offending arthropod is determined by the distribution of the eruption and the biting insects in the patient's environment. In San Francisco, fleas are a common cause of lower leg pruritic papules, nodules, and blisters, whereas in Miami, mosquitoes are the most important cause.[12] In all patients, the fingerwebs, genitalia, axillae, and feet should be carefully examined for lesions. When lesions are found in these areas, they should be scraped to search for scabetic mites. Scabies is spread by close personal contact, so the affected person must also be examined for sexually transmitted diseases. Treatment of scabies is with lindane or permethrin applied to the whole body once for 12 hours and repeated 1 week later. Extensive, crusted scabies (Norwegian scabies) may occur in patients with advanced HIV disease. It may be nonpruritic and mimics psoriasis. Daily sequential applications of permethrin (Elimite), crotamiton (Eurax), or 6% sulfur in petrolatum are recommended (permethrin one day and crotamiton or sulfur on the six other days comprising 1 week of therapy). This should be repeated for several weeks until the patient is cured. Ivermectin as a single 12-mg oral dose may be used for refractory cases.[13]

Other insect bite reactions are treated by three steps: (1) eliminate the biting insects from the patient's environment with insecticides, (2) make the patient less attractive to the insect with insect repellents (products containing diethyltoluamide [DEET]), and (3) block the patient's reaction to the bite with potent antihistamines taken regularly—not "as needed." At least a generous nightly dose should be given (e.g., hydroxyzine 50–75 mg), with additional doses during the day if this is inadequate. Cetirizine 10 mg once daily appears to be more effective for insect bite reactions than are other antihistamines. Persistent pruritic papules are treated with medium- to high-potency topical steroids until they resolve.

Photosensitivity

The presence of HIV disease alone, or the medications that HIV-infected patients take, may lead to cutaneous eruptions predominantly in sun-exposed areas—that is, photodermatitis.[14] These eruptions initially may resemble a heightened sunburn, but may progress to or initially appear as pruritic scaly patches. They are frequently excoriated, become thickened, and often cause increase or loss of skin pigment (Fig. 12–5), especially in persons of color. With time, the eruption may extend to unexposed skin. Short-wave ultraviolet irradiation (UVB) is the usual precipitating spectrum. Photodermatitis is managed by (1) discontinuing potential photosensitizers (sulfa drugs, nonsteroidal anti-inflammatory drugs); (2) protecting the patient from the sun with sunscreens, hats and clothing, and sun avoidance; and (3) applying a medium- to high-potency topical steroid to the lesions. In my experience, this is relatively easy to manage if the pattern is recognized. If the condition is allowed to persist, the patient may progress to a state of heightened photosensitivity that will not respond to these simple measures. Black men with a CD4 count less than 50/mm³ are at particular risk for severe photodermatitis.

PRURITIC FOLLICULITIS

Eosinophilic folliculitis is the most common nonstaphylococcal folliculitis in HIV-infected persons. It occurs in patients with CD4 counts less than 200/mm³. Characteristically, it is a chronic, waxing and waning eruption with mod-

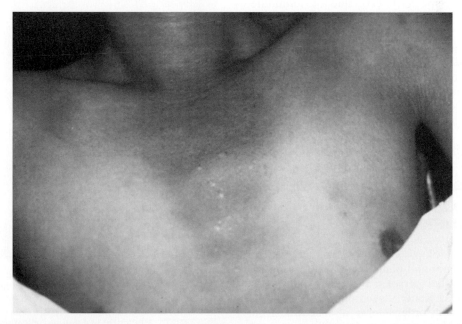

FIGURE 12–5. Hyperpigmentation and dermatitis exclusively in sun-exposed areas may be induced by certain medications (sulfa drugs, nonsteroidal anti-inflammatory drugs) or may be due to HIV infection alone.

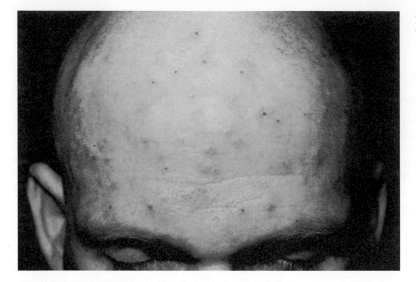

FIGURE 12–6. Eosinophilic folliculitis of the forehead.

erate to severe pruritus.[15,16] The primary lesion is an edematous papule up to 1 cm in size with a tiny central pustule. The lesions are scattered on the upper trunk, head (especially forehead), neck, and proximal upper extremities (Fig. 12–6); 90% of lesions are above a line drawn across the nipples. Culture results for bacteria are uniformly negative, and patients do not respond to antibiotics effective against *S. aureus*. Skin biopsy reveals inflammation-containing eosinophils surrounding and involving the hair follicle. In my experience, chronic use of antihistamines, especially cetirizine or loratidine, and potent topical steroids are partially effective. Phototherapy with UVB or psoralen plus ultraviolet A (PUVA) may be beneficial. Itraconazole in a dose of 200 to 400 mg/day may cause improvement in about 60% of patients with eosinophilic folliculitis. Prolonged (4- to 6-week) topical therapy chronically every other day with 5% permethrin cream or Sulfacet-R may lead to a more sustained remission. Accutane (isotretinoin) in a dose of about 0.75 to 1.0 mg/kg/day may also be of benefit.[16]

PAPULOSQUAMOUS DISORDERS

Three dermatologic disorders characterized by scaling patches and plaques are seen commonly in HIV-infected persons: seborrheic dermatitis, psoriasis, and Reiter's syndrome.[1] These papulosquamous disorders form a spectrum from mild and skin only (seborrheic dermatitis), to moderate or severe and skin only (psoriasis), to severe with systemic findings (severe psoriasis

or Reiter's syndrome).[17,18] There is considerable overlap, and a mild form may progress to a more severe form.

Seborrheic dermatitis is extremely common, affecting, to varying degrees, most persons with

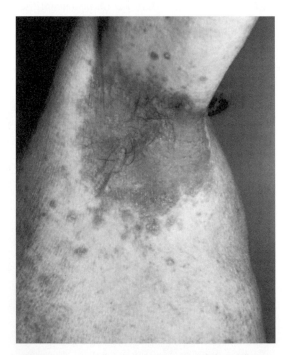

FIGURE 12–7. Seborrheic dermatitis of the axilla in a patient with AIDS. Seborrheic dermatitis commonly is accentuated in the axillae and groin in HIV-infected persons and is distinguished from cutaneous candidiasis by a negative potassium hydroxide scraping. The patient was treated successfully with a mild topical steroid and an imidazole cream mixed together and applied twice daily.

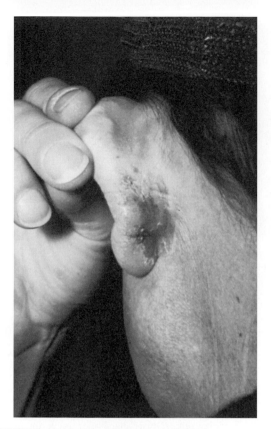

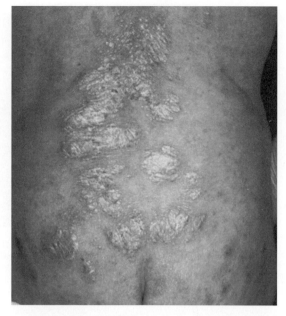

FIGURE 12–9. Typical plaque-like psoriasis that began in the sixth decade in this HIV-infected man. Pruritus was severe.

FIGURE 12–8. Seborrheic dermatitis in the retroauricular area. Erosion, weeping, and secondary staphylococcal infection are common in this location.

symptomatic HIV disease. Lesions are usually located in the hairy areas of the central face, scalp, chest, back, and groin (Figs. 12–7 and 12–8). The lesions are mildly erythematous with a yellowish greasy scale. When limited to the face, lesions are usually asymptomatic, but scalp and trunk lesions are often pruritic. Therapy for the scalp includes the regular use of a dandruff shampoo containing ketoconazole (Nizoral), selenium sulfide (e.g., Selsun Blue), zinc pyrithione (e.g., Head and Shoulders, Danex, Zincon), or sulfur and salicylic acid (e.g., Van Seb, Sebulex). In addition, a medium-potency steroid solution (triamcinolone 0.1%) may be applied. For facial, trunk, and groin lesions a topical imidazole cream (ketoconazole 2%, clotrimazole 1%), plus a low-potency topical steroid (hydrocortisone 1% to 2.5%) may be applied twice daily. For refractory trunk lesions, the strength of the topical steroid may be increased.

Psoriasis often begins after HIV infection, although pre-existing psoriasis may also flare up following infection. The initial lesions frequently begin like seborrheic dermatitis but extend to the axillae and groin, and finally involve the elbows, knees, and lumbosacral areas (Fig. 12–9). The lesions of psoriasis and seborrheic dermatitis in the axillae and groin are identical. When psoriasis involves the trunk, it tends to form more fixed, less easily treatable lesions with a thicker scale. Psoriasis of the palms and soles often begins as superficial pustules that evolve into hyperkeratotic papules identical to the keratoderma blenorrhagicum of Reiter's syndrome (Fig. 12–10). Arthritis may be present with psoriasis alone or as a part of Reiter's syndrome.

Mild to moderate psoriasis is managed with topical steroids, tar, and calcipotriene. Patients with severe psoriasis and HIV disease may note a significant improvement of their skin lesions with HAART.[19] This response correlates with the overall response of the HIV disease. HAART is most effective in patients in whom the psoriasis began after the HIV infection. Etretinate or acetretin, vitamin A analogs, are frequently beneficial, nonimmunosuppressive, and well tolerated in HIV-infected persons. The initial dose is 25 mg/day, and rarely needs to exceed 50 mg daily. Response is delayed, taking 6 to 8 weeks and reaching maximum benefit at 6 months.

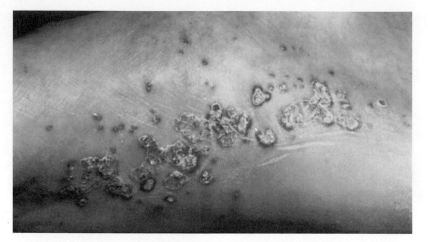

FIGURE 12–10. Pustules evolving into keratotic plaques on the sole. This was the initial manifestation of psoriasis in this HIV-infected person. Although the lesions were identical to those of Reiter's syndrome, this patient had no other characteristic stigmata.

References

1. Coldiron BM, Bergstresser PR: Prevalence and clinical spectrum of skin diease in patients infected with human immunodeficiency virus. Arch Dermatol 125:357, 1989
2. Duvic M: Staphylococcal infections and the pruritus of AIDS-related complex. Arch Dermatol 123:1599, 1987
3. Kiehlbauch JA, Tauxe RV, Baker CN, Wachsmuth IK: Helicobacter cinaedi-associated bacteremia and cellulitis in immunocompromised patients. Ann Intern Med 121:90, 1994
4. Kinloch-de Loës S, de Saussure P, Saurat JH, et al: Symptomatic primary infection due to HIV type 1: Review of 31 cases. Clin Infect Dis 17:59, 1993
5. Buchbinder SP, Katz MH, Hessol NA, et al: Herpes zoster and human immunodeficiency virus infection. J Infect Dis 166:1153, 166
6. Concus AP, Helfand RF, Imber MJ, et al: Cutaneous cryptococcosis mimicking molluscum contagiosum in a patient with AIDS. J Infect Dis 158:897, 1988
7. Meadows, KP, Tyring SK, Pavia AT, Rallis TM: Resolution of recalcitrant molluscum contagiosum virus lesions in HIV-infected patients treated with cidofovir. Arch Dermatol 133:987, 1997
8. Murakawa GJ, McCalmont T, Altman J, et al: Disseminated acanthamebiasis in patients with AIDS. Arch Dermatol 131:1291, 1995
9. Gordin FM, Simon GL, Wofsy CB, et al: Adverse reactions to trimethoprim-sulfamethoxazole in patients with the acquired immunodeficiency syndrome. Ann Intern Med 100:495, 1984
10. Porteous DM, Berger TG: Severe cutaneous drug reactions (Stevens-Johnson syndrome and toxic epidermal necrolysis) in human immunodeficiency virus infection. Arch Dermatol 127:740, 1991
11. Caumes E, Guermonprez G, Lecomte C, et al: Efficiency and safety of desensitization with sulfamethoxazole and trimethoprim in 48 previously hypersensitive patients infected with HIV. Arch Dermatol 133:465, 1997
12. Penneys NS, Nayar JK, Bernstein H, et al: Chronic pruritic eruption in patients with acquired immunodeficiency syndrome associated with increased antibody tiers of mosquito salivary gland antigens. J Am Acad Dermatol 21:421, 1989
13. Taplin D, Meinking TL: Treatment of HIV-related scabies with emphasis on the efficacy of ivermectin. Semin Cutan Med Surg 16:235, 1997
14. Pappert A, Grossman M, DeLeo V: Photosensitivity as the presenting illness in four patients with human immunodeficiency viral infection. Arch Dermatol 130:618, 1994
15. Rosenthal D, LeBoit PE, Klumpp L, et al: HIV-associated eosinophilic folliculitis: A unique dermatosis associated with advanced HIV infection. Arch Dermatol 127:206, 1991
16. Otley CC, Avram MR, Johnson RA: Isotretinoin treatment of human immunodeficiency virus-associated eosinophilic folliculitis: Results of an open, pilot trial. Arch Dermatol 131:1047, 1995
17. Reveille JD, Conant MA, Duvic M: Human immunodeficiency virus-associated psoriasis, psoriatic arthritis, and Reiter's syndrome: A disease continuum? Arthritis Rheum 33:1574, 1990
18. Winchester R, Bernstein DH, Fischer HD, et al: The co-occurence of Reiter's syndrome and acquired immunodeficiency. Ann Intern Med 106:19, 1987
19. Kaplan MH, Sadick NS, Wieder J, et al: Antipsoriatic effects of zidovudine in human immunodeficiency virus-associated psoriasis. J Am Acad Dermatol 20:76, 1989

13 Gastrointestinal and Hepatic Manifestations of HIV Infection

ANDREW H. TALAL • DOUGLAS T. DIETERICH

IMPORTANCE OF THE GASTROINTESTINAL TRACT IN HIV INFECTION

The gastrointestinal tract plays a pre-eminent role in many aspects of HIV infection. Anoreceptive sexual intercourse is the primary route of infection in men who have sex with men.[1] Because the gastrointestinal tract contains approximately 50% of the lymphoid mass in the entire body and HIV is known to concentrate in the lymphoid tissue,[2,3] the gut-associated lymphoid tissue (GALT) may be an important site of HIV replication. Additionally, the behavior of HIV in the unique immunologic environment of the intestinal mucosa may differ from that observed in the periphery. HIV replicates most efficiently in activated CD4+ memory cells.[4] From their chronic exposure to antigen in the gastrointestinal lumen, the vast majority of intestinal lamina propria lymphocytes (LPL) express the memory phenotype CD45RO.[5] When analyzed by flow cytometry, 15% of freshly isolated intestinal LPL express the activation marker CD25, compared to less than 3% of lymphocyte isolated from other body compartments. Higher levels of major histocompatibility complex class II antigens and other T-cell activation markers are also expressed by LPL when compared to lymphocytes from other body compartments.[6] The gastrointestinal mucosa, through the application of a mucosal vaccine, may play an important part in protection against HIV infection.[7]

Dramatic decreases in HIV-attributable mortality have been associated with the implementation of highly active antiretroviral therapy (HAART).[8] Prior to these recent developments, 18% to 50% of HIV-infected individuals in industrialized countries and 90% of HIV-infected individuals in developing countries were afflicted with diarrhea at some point during the course of their disease.[9] With the implementation of HAART, the incidence of opportunistic infections in HIV-infected individuals has declined precipitously. However, many of the agents that comprise HAART are associated with adverse effects on the gastrointestinal tract and liver.[10] These adverse effects may be precipitated by coexisting hepatic disease. For example, although not an officially recognized opportunistic infection, viral hepatitis can progress more rapidly and exacerbate hepatotoxicity associated with the use of the protease inhibitors.[11]

Basics of Mucosal Immunology of GALT

The mucosal immune system consists of the gastrointestinal tract, the genitourinary tract, the nasobronchial tree, the inner ear, the tonsils, the mesenteric lymph nodes, and the appendix. The mucosal lymphocytes have homing and circulatory patterns that differ from those in the systemic circulation. The GALT can be divided into an afferent limb and an efferent limb. The afferent limb consists of organized lymphoid aggregates (including the Peyer's patches) that are found distributed throughout the intestinal mucosa; the efferent limb is composed of lymphocytes scattered diffusely in the epithelium and in the lamina propria.[12] Intraepithelial lymphocytes consist primarily of CD8+ cells whose function is thought to include sampling of the contents of the gastrointestinal lumen. Seventy to 80% of intraepithelial lymphocytes express the CD8 phenotype.[13] The lamina propria contains a diffuse collection of T and B lymphocytes, plasma cells, eosinophils, and neutrophils. The LPL have a CD4/CD8 ratio similar to that of the peripheral blood.[14] Although HIV can bind to and fuse with both quiescent and activated CD4+ T cells, only activated CD4+ T cells will preferentially result in productive infection.[15] Activated CD4+ LPL serve as the primary site of HIV infection, and are preferentially depleted in this body compartment prior to other organs in both humans and rhesus macaques.[16,17] The early depletion of virally infected CD4+ lymphocytes from the gastrointestinal tract may account for the reason why, after 1 year of combination antiretroviral therapy, the HIV RNA level in the cells of the gastrointestinal tract decreases below the level of detection in the majority of individuals.[18]

Within the small intestine, organized mucosal structures, the Peyer's patches, consist of a germinal center surrounded by follicular-associated epithelium (FAE). The FAE continually samples luminal contents. Because the regions overlying the Peyer's patches contain a range of class II–positive cells, they may be involved in antigen presentation. The M cells form part of the FAE.[19]

Transmission of HIV at Mucosal Sites

Several hypotheses have been proposed to explain the migration of HIV from the lumen of the gastrointestinal tract through the mucosa to the bloodstream. Initial reports suggested that disruption of the mucosal lining of the gastrointestinal tract was necessary for transmission of HIV. However, subsequent investigation demonstrated that HIV could gain entry through intact mucosa. Other investigators determined that HIV could bind to galactosylceramide receptors, which are present on the surface of intestinal epithelial cells.[20] It was hypothesized that, once HIV was bound to the receptors, it could use the cellular mechanism to traverse the cell to gain access to the bloodstream. Other hypotheses include trafficking of the virus through M cells, as has been demonstrated with other viruses. Recently, transcytosis through the epithelial cell has been proposed as a possible mechanism of viral transmission.[21] Currently, an in vivo model is being used to determine if the same method is applicable to the human gastrointestinal tract.

GASTROINTESTINAL DISORDERS ASSOCIATED WITH HIV

Esophageal Disorders

Prior to the advent of HAART, one third of AIDS patients had esophageal opportunistic infections.[22] Odynophagia and dysphagia are common symptoms of esophageal disease in this patient population. Uncommon symptoms include retrosternal chest pain, coughing, hiccups, and aspiration that are usually due to esophageal inflammation or acid reflux. Scarring may occur after esophageal ulcers heal, resulting in the formation of esophageal strictures.

Pathogenesis

Table 13–1 presents common causes of infectious esophagitis as a consequence of infection with HIV-1. Most fungal esophagitis is caused by *Candida albicans*, which characteristically causes whitish plaques adherent to the wall of the esophagus.[23] The plaques may coalesce to cover large portions of the esophageal wall with invasion into the epithelial layer and the submucosa.[24–26] Noncandidal fungal species not sensitive to fluconazole can also cause esophagitis.

The most common viral causes of esophagitis are cytomegalovirus (CMV) and herpes simplex virus (HSV). The clinical presentation of CMV in the gastrointestinal tract is largely dependent on the site of infection. Esophageal disease usually presents with odynophagia or dysphagia. CMV most commonly causes ulcers at the lower esophageal sphincter, but can cause diffuse esophagitis, ulcers higher in the esophagus, gastritis, gastric ulcers, duodenitis, duodenal ulcers, and enteritis.[27] Unusual viral causes of esophagitis include Epstein-Barr virus and human herpes virus 6.[23]

In the era of HAART, the incidence of viral esophagitis has decreased. However, the emergence of resistance to azole drugs, which are used in the prophylaxis against fungal esophagitis, is increasing as a result of their continued use. *Mycobacterium tuberculosis* and *Mycobacterium avium* complex (MAC) have both been identified as causes of esophageal disease in HIV-infected individuals. Lymphomatoid granulomatosis,[28] papovavirus,[29] mucormycosis,[30] cryptosporidia,[31] *Pneumocystis carinii*,[32] *Nocardia*,[33,34] *Leishmania donovani*,[35,36] and *Actino-*

TABLE 13–1. Esophageal Diseases in HIV-1–Infected Individuals

ORGANISM	SYMPTOMS	COMPLICATIONS	ENDOSCOPY	RADIOLOGY	HISTOLOGY	DIAGNOSIS	TREATMENT
CMV	Odynophagia Dysphagia	Stricture Bacterial superinfection	Ulcers >1 cm "Heaped up" appearance 58% multiple ulcers	Superficial erosion Granular mucosa Ulcer—shallow to deep	Cytoplasmic inclusion Intranuclear inclusions	IHC ISH Viral culture PCR	Foscarnet 90 mg/ kg IV bid Ganciclovir 5 mg/ kg IV bid Cidofovir 5 mg/kg q wk
HSV	Odynophagia Dysphagia Chest pain Fever Nausea Vomiting Hematemesis Extraesophageal HSV	Mucosal necrosis Bacterial superinfection Hemorrhage Strictures HSV pneumonia TEF Perforation Disseminated HSV Siglinus (hiccups)	Vesicles 1–3 mm Discrete, superficial stellate ulcers Plaques, cobblestones or ulceration similar to *Candida* "Volcano ulcer" Biopsy most specific if obtained from ulcer edge			IHC ISH Viral culture PCR	Acyclovir 15–30 mg/kg/d
Candida	Dysphagia Odynophagia		Creamy whitish-yellow adherent plaques Erythematous mucosa	Plaque-like lesions Submucosal edema Cobblestone Thickened folds	Hyphae Pseudohyphae Budding yeast	H & E stain Silver stain PAS Gram's stain	Fluconazole 200 mg PO qd Ketoconazole 200 mg PO qd
Idiopathic ulcers	Odynophagia		Similar to other fungal esophagitis Single or multiple ulcers in mid to distal esophagus Mucosal bridging				Prednisone 40 mg qd × 1 mo Thalidomide 200 mg qd × 2 wk
Aspergillus	Recurrent esophagitis				Septate hyphae Conidiophores		
Aphthous ulcers	Odynophagia Substernal chest pain	Fistula, sinus tract Sitophobia Weight loss					Prednisone 40 mg qd × 1 mo Thalidomide 200 mg qhs × 2 wk
MAC/MTb	Pulmonary symptoms Cough Chest infiltrate Adenopathy Fever, weight loss Malaise	Esophagoesophageal fistula Esophagobronchial fistula Double-channel esophagus	Transmural inflammation Ulcers Thickened folds Fistula	Diffuse irregularity of mucosa Ulcer Sinus tract			Multiple drug regimen similar to mycobacterial disease at other sites

Abbreviations: CMV, cytomegalovirus; H&E, hematoxylin and eosin; HSV, herpes simplex virus; IHC, immunohistochemistry; ISH, in situ hybridization; MAC, *Mycobacterium avium* complex; MTb, *Mycobacterium tuberculosis*; PAS, periodic acid–Schiff; PCR, polymerase chain reaction; TEF, tracheoesophageal fistula.

myces[37] are unusual causes of esophageal disease in HIV-infected individuals.

Idiopathic ulcers that are frequently found in infected individuals are thought to be caused by HIV. Kotler et al. used in situ hybridization to document the presence of HIV at the ulcer base in two patients with solitary ulcers of the esophagus.[38] Smith et al. used in situ hybridization to detect HIV-1 mRNA in lamina propria macrophages. The prevalence of these cells in AIDS patients with esophageal symptoms was 0.059 ± 0.01%, whereas none of these cells were found in AIDS patients without esophageal symptoms.[39]

Noninfectious processes can also cause esophageal symptoms in HIV-infected individuals. Although neoplasms of the esophagus are generally considered rare in HIV-infected individuals, both Kaposi's sarcoma (KS) and lymphoma can occur. KS usually occurs as an incidental finding visualized during endoscopy or on a barium esophagram.[22] It usually occurs in association with cutaneous or palatal disease.[40,41] Lymphoma of the esophagus can have an aggressive course.[42]

Pill-induced esophagitis can occur in the HIV-infected individual secondary to the large number of medications typically ingested and to an underlying motility disorder that may occur in HIV infection.[43] In addition to the typical causes of pill-induced esophagitis (i.e., potassium supplements, iron, quinidine, nonsteroidal anti-inflammatory agents, doxycycline) in the HIV-negative individual,[44] zidovudine and zalcitabine have been reported to cause esophageal ulceration.[45]

Gastroesophageal reflux disease is uncommon in HIV-infected individuals.[41] Decreased acid production was reported in HIV-infected individuals in one early report,[47] but in several later reports HIV has not been associated with hypochlorhydria.[48,49]

Aphthous ulcers have been noted to occur more frequently in the HIV-infected individual compared to individuals who do not have HIV. These are defined as ulcers with no identifiable cause despite a thorough histopathologic examination of tissue.[50] Clinical symptoms, diagnostic criteria, and microscopic characteristics typically associated with aphthous ulcers are listed in Table 13–1.

The role of HIV as a cause of either idiopathic or aphthous ulcers of the esophagus has not been definitively established. HIV RNA and p24 antigen have been detected from ulcers using in situ hybridization and immunoperoxidase staining.[52] However, HIV RNA has not been

identified in epithelial cells.[53] Particles 120 to 160 nm in diameter with bar-shaped nucleoids have been identified by electron microscopy in biopsies obtained from idiopathic ulcers.[54,55] HIV can also be cultured from biopsy specimens obtained from these ulcers.

Treatment Approach to the HIV-Infected Individual with Esophageal Disease

Oral fluconazole is the treatment of choice for *Candida* esophagitis in patients with HIV. In patients already taking fluconazole, a higher dose may be necessary or substitution of amphotericin B may be required. One week's treatment with an azole for presumptive *Candida* esophagitis should be followed by an endoscopy with biopsy if there is no relief of symptoms.[23] Although topical agents may be effective for treatment of oropharnygeal candidiasis, esophageal disease requires systemic therapy. Low-dose maintenance antifungal therapy with either ketoconazole or itraconazole may prevent a recurrence of *Candida* esophagitis.

For CMV esophagitis, either ganciclovir or foscarnet can be used as initial therapy and should be administered for a period of 3 to 4 weeks depending on the severity of the infection. When a CMV esophageal ulcer recurs following monotherapy with either foscarnet or ganciclovir, combination therapy with the standard medication dosages should be proscribed for the treatment and maintenance of CMV infection.[56] Esophagitis caused by HSV should be treated with intravenous acyclovir. If acyclovir fails secondary to drug resistance, foscarnet may be effective.[57]

If no pathogen is found on multiple adequate biopsies of an esophageal ulcer and after thorough review by an experienced pathologist, the patient could be treated with prednisone 40 mg by mouth daily until symptoms improve. The corticosteroid dose should then be tapered by 10 mg each week. Thalidomide, which inhibits the cytokine tumor necrosis factor-α, and corticosteroids, which inhibit arachidonic acid metabolites, both appear to be effective in the treatment of esophageal aphthous ulcers.[50,51] Recently, thalidomide has also been shown to improve idiopathic esophageal ulcers.[58,59]

Gastric Disease

Many of the pathogens that cause disease in the esophagus, including CMV, HSV, *Mycobacteria*, *Toxoplasma*, lymphoma, and KS, can also cause gastric abnormalities. *Helicobacter pylori* has been shown to be a major risk factor for the development of peptic ulcer disease.[60] However, the prevalence of this organism is much lower in HIV-infected individuals than in uninfected individuals until profound immunodeficiency develops.[61] In one study, individuals with CD4 counts below 200 cells/mm^3 had a higher prevalence of peptic ulcer disease secondary to *H. pylori* than individuals with higher CD4 cell counts.[62]

Opportunistic Infections of the Small and Large Intestine

Diarrhea and wasting frequently occur as a consequence of infection with HIV. Prior to the widespread use of HAART, diarrhea secondary to opportunistic pathogens was a very common problem in HIV-infected individuals. It was more common in developing countries, where approximately 90% of HIV-infected than in developed individuals were afflicted with the symptom at some point during the course of their disease.[27,63-66] Severe diarrhea (for more than 1 month) and weight loss of at least 10% are AIDS-defining conditions.[67] Furthermore, morbidity and mortality are increased in AIDS patients with chronic diarrhea secondary to opportunistic infections,[68] and chronic diarrhea is an independent marker of a poor prognosis.[69,70] Individuals with diarrhea have annual health costs that are 50% higher than individuals without diarrhea.[71]

Two recent studies have focused on the etiology and outcome of gastrointestinal bleeding in patients with AIDS. Among 58 HIV-infected individuals presenting with acute upper gastrointestinal bleeding, esophagogastric varices, gastric ulcer, and gastric malignancy were the most frequent etiologies. The number of units of blood transfused, the need for surgery, the length of hospital stay, and the mortality rate did not differ between the HIV-infected individuals and the controls.[72] Lower gastrointestinal bleeding is uncommon in HIV-infected individuals, occurring in only 2.6% of patients referred for gastrointestinal consultation. The most common causes of lower gastrointestinal bleeding in 18 patients with AIDS were CMV colonic disease (39%), idiopathic colonic ulcers (28%), and hemorrhoids (17%).[73] In 78% of the individuals, the bleeding stopped spontaneously. Other causes of lower gastrointestinal bleeding in AIDS patients include lymphoma,[74,75] colonic KS,[76] ileal CMV,[77] colonic histoplasmosis,[78] and pneumatosis intestinalis.[79]

Cytomegalovirus

Viruses, bacteria, protozoa, and fungi can cause diarrhea in AIDS patients. Of the viruses, CMV is the most common and the most serious organism affecting the intestine of HIV-infected individuals.[80,81] Symptoms of CMV gastrointestinal disease include intermittent or persistent diarrhea with crampy lower abdominal pain, tenesmus, rebound tenderness, fever, anorexia, malaise, and weight loss.[82] The endoscopic appearance of CMV colitis is variable. Most commonly CMV appears as a diffusely erythematous and friable mucosa with submucosal hemorrhage and mucosal ulcerations. The most common site of infection with CMV is the colon. In one study, 41% of the patients had patchy colitis, 39% had disease limited to the cecum, and 50% had disease in the left colon. Up to 25% of patients with CMV colitis can have normal-appearing mucosa, signifying the need for mucosal biopsies even in the absence of grossly visible abnormalities. Cytomegalovirus-infected cells were found in the cecum and right colon in 68%, in the transverse colon in 37%, and in the left colon and rectosigmoid in 42% of cases.[82,83]

CMV can resemble either Crohn's disease or ulcerative colitis, with either diffuse ulcerations or aphthous ulcerations and "skip areas."[84] Given the predominance of CMV in the cecum and ascending colon and the possibility of uninvolved segments of the intestinal mucosa, a colonoscopic examination has been advocated as being an important component of the evaluation of diarrhea in HIV-infected individuals. In order to assure adequate sensitivity to detect CMV, 10 to 12 biopsy samples should be obtained from the ascending, transverse, descending, and sigmoid colon. Samples should also be obtained from endoscopically normal-appearing mucosa since CMV may not cause visible mucosal abnormalities.

Complications of CMV colitis include vasculitis leading to thrombosis, occlusion, and ischemia. The full thickness of the bowel wall may be involved, causing ulceration and ultimately perforation.[85,86] Other complications of CMV colitis include hemorrhage, obstruction, and toxic megacolon.[87] The prognosis of AIDS patients with CMV colitis is poor. Individuals with more profound immunodeficiency are at higher risk for the disease, and a diagnosis of CMV infection is an independent predictor of death.[88]

Treatment of AIDS patients with CMV disease most frequently consists of ganciclovir (5 mg/kg twice daily) or foscarnet (60 to 90 mg/

kg intravenously three times daily) for an induction period of 3 to 6 weeks.[89,90] One study showed a trend toward better control of CMV disease with maintenance foscarnet therapy compared to induction therapy alone.[91] In the era of HAART, maintenance with intravenous antiviral agents is impractical and probably unnecessary. In the case of relapse, however, maintenance therapy should be considered.[92] Maintenance should be attempted with 3 to 6 gm of oral ganciclovir prior to the use of intravenous medications. If monotherapy fails, the combination of intravenous foscarnet and intravenous ganciclovir may be effective. Adverse reactions to ganciclovir include neutropenia in 25% to 40% and thrombocytopenia in 9% to 19% of patients.[93,94] Adverse effects of foscarnet include elevation of serum creatinine and renal wasting of magnesium, calcium, and phosphate in 10% to 23% of patients.[95] Individuals with CMV gastrointestinal disease should undergo regular ophthalmologic screening for CMV retinitis.

Herpes Simplex Virus

The other principle cause of viral esophagitis, HSV, usually causes proctitis or distal colitis as a pathogen in the intestine. Symptoms of HSV intestinal disease include anorectal pain, tenesmus, hematochezia, mild diarrhea, and occasionally constipation. Because of neural involvement, patients may have dysuria or sacral paresthesias.

Endoscopically, the infection may first appear as small vesicles that may rupture to form small, round ulcers. Histologic examination of biopsy specimens, with the appearance of typical Cowdry type A intranuclear inclusions in multinucleated giant cells, is important to differentiate HSV from CMV.

Acyclovir at a dose of 5 mg/kg every 8 hours intravenously for 7 days, or at a dose of 400 mg every 8 hours orally for 14 to 21 days, is indicated for the treatment of colonic or anorectal HSV. For acyclovir-resistant virus strains, intravenous foscarnet at a dose of 90 mg/kg intravenously twice each day is effective.[96,97]

Adenovirus

Adenovirus has been isolated from immunocompromised individuals as well as children with diarrhea, but the role of adenovirus as a cause of diarrhea remains controversial because only one half of patients with the virus actually have symptoms.[98,99] Colonic cells infected with adenovirus have vacuolated and mucin-filled cy-

toplasm with intranuclear inclusions.[100] A monoclonal antibody directed against adenovirus and electron microscopy can be used to aid in the detection of adenovirus.[101]

Fungal Infections

Esophagitis secondary to fungal infections is much more common than diarrhea caused by these organisms. *Candida albicans* and *Histoplasma capsulatum* are the two most common fungal causes of colitis. *Candida* has been identified in a colonic biopsy specimen in a patient suffering from watery diarrhea and abdominal pain.[102] Although *Candida* has been implicated as a cause of colonic ulcers, the significance of the organism as a cause of diarrhea has not been conclusively determined. Infection with the organism usually responds to a course of oral nystatin. In refractory cases, systemic therapy with amphotericin B, intraconazole, or fluconazole can be used.

Histoplasma capsulatum infection usually occurs as a result of reactivation of latent infection in the setting of depressed cell-mediated immunity. Up to 75% of patients with disseminated disease may have gastrointestinal involvement.[103,104]

Protozoa

Microsporida and cryptosporidia have both been demonstrated to cause diarrhea in HIV-infected individuals. *Cryptosporidium parvum* causes a transient infection in immunocompetent adults.[105] Paromomycin,[105–107] letrazuril,[108] and azithromycin[105] have limited efficacy against cryptosporidial infection.

Over 90% of intestinal microsporidiosis is caused by *Enterocytozoon bieneusi*; the other 10% is caused by *Encephalitozoon intestinalis*. Microsporidiosis has been reported most commonly from immunocompromised individuals (i.e., HIV infected or treated with steroids posttransplant). One report noted that African children from an area with a low prevalence of HIV had a high prevalence of *E. bieneusi*.[109] Atovaquone has limited efficacy against microsporidiosis,[110] while albendazole has adequate efficacy against *E. intestinalis*.[27,111]

Bacteria

MAC is the most common systemic bacterial infection in HIV-infected individuals, especially in those with CD4 cell counts below 50 cells/mm^3.[112,113] MAC usually causes a protracted diarrheal illness that is accompanied by abdominal pain, fever, anemia, weight loss, and night sweats. Although the organism can readily be cultured from the blood or the bone marrow, the diagnosis of gastrointestinal MAC usually necessitates gastrointestinal endoscopy. Although the mucosa may appear normal, MAC characteristically causes granular white nodules measuring 1 to 4 mm in diameter with a surrounding rim of erythema. On biopsy, Ziehl-Neelsen staining will demonstrate the organism within foamy marcophages. Bacterial culture of biopsy specimens can also aid in the diagnosis. Complications of MAC infection include intestinal obstruction, perforation, fistula formation, and gastrointestinal bleeding. Current recommendations of the U.S. Public Health Service Task Force include treatment of MAC with at least two agents, including azithromycin or clarithromycin in combination with clofazimine (100 mg/day), ethambutol (15 mg/kg/day), ciprofloxacin (1500 mg/day), rifabutin (300 mg/day), rifampin (600 mg/day), or amikacin (500 mg intravenously for 6 weeks).[114]

Salmonella species, *Shigella flexneri, Campylobacter jejuni,* and *Clostridium difficile* are all pathogenic in HIV-infected individuals. *Salmonella* and *Campylobacter* are usually diagnosed in individuals with more advanced disease, whereas *Shigella* occurs in the early stages of HIV.[115] Typical symptoms associated with these organisms include abdominal cramping, tenesmus, bloating, and nausea. Long-term colonization may result from failure of both humoral and cytotoxic immune responses to clear these organisms despite treatment with antibiotics.[116] However, the incidence of *Salmonella* bacteremia has declined with the use of trimethoprim-sulfamethoxazole prophylaxis and antiretroviral therapy.[117] Complications of infection with these organisms include toxic megacolon and pseudomembranous colitis.

Recently there has been an increase in the incidence of enteroadherent *Escherichia coli* associated with diarrhea in AIDS.[118,119] These organisms are most frequently localized to the right colon, and the diagnosis can usually be made through stool culture. Characteristically, light microscopy will reveal clusters of the organism adherent to the small bowel or colonic mucosa brush border.

Clostridium difficile can also cause diarrhea in this patient population whether or not they have recently been treated with antibiotics.[120] The organism typically produces a bloody, mucoid diarrhea with abdominal pain and fever. The infection should be treated with metroni-

dazole (250 mg four times per day) or oral vancomycin (125 to 500 mg four times daily). As an adjunctive agent, cholestyramine can be used to bind the cytotoxin produced by the organism, thereby preventing toxin absorption.

HIV Enteropathy

HIV has been isolated from epithelial cells from both the small and large intestine in vitro and in vivo.[121,122] In the absence of enteric pathogens, p24 antigen expression has been described in colonic mucosa associated with an inflammatory disease.[123] Pathogen-negative diarrhea in HIV-infected individuals can also be caused by bacterial overgrowth,[124] decreased mucosal immune function,[125] and abnormal enteric neural and endocrine function.[126]

Drug-Related Diarrhea

Many of the agents that comprise HAART have been associated with diarrhea. Table 13–2 demonstrates the major gastrointestinal adverse effects of the drugs that are used to treat HIV infection. Pancreatitis is the most serious gastrointestinal side effect associated with the reverse transcriptase inhibitors. Gastrointestinal side effects (i.e., nausea, vomiting, and diarrhea) are the major adverse effects associated with the protease inhibitors. Currently, the four most commonly prescribed protease inhibitors are nelfinavir, indinavir, saquinavir, and ritonavir. Nelfinavir has been associated with the worst gastrointestinal side effects, which have led to drug discontinuation in approximately 4% of individuals. The use of ritonavir and saquinavir results in milder diarrhea than does nelfinavir.

Antidiarrheal agents are effective in the majority of individuals for symptomatic treatment of diarrhea. Three categories of antidiarrheal agents exist: luminal agents, antimotility agents, and hormones. Luminal agents, such as cholestyramine or fiber, can bind diarrheagenic substances (i.e., bile acids) or can add bulk to the stool. Antimotility agents, such as loperamide (Imodium) or diphenoxylate plus atropine (Lomotil), reduce diarrhea by decreasing intestinal motility and increasing intestinal absorption by increasing the amount of time luminal contents are in contact with the mucosal surface. More potent remedies include the opiates: codeine, morphine, methadone, paregoric, and deodorized tincture of opium. As a third line of treatment, hormone therapy can be tried. Octreotide, the synthetic version of natural somatostatin, slows intestinal transit time, de-

TABLE 13–2. Gastrointestinal Adverse Effects of Antiretroviral Medications (in Percentages)*

MEDICATION	DIARRHEA	NAUSEA	VOMITING	ABD PAIN	CONSTIPATION	REGURG	FLATULENCE	PANCREATITIS	ULCER[†]
Indinavir	4.6	11.7	4.1	8.7		10	3		10
Nelfinavir	5	5		4					
Ritonavir	12	23	1.2	3			1		
Saquinavir	15	13		10	3		10	<2	
ddI	20–28	6–10	6–10	6–10	16				
ddC	7	7	7	7	<1			0	
AZT	5–25	61	5–25	5–25	5–25				8–17

Abbreviations: Abd, abdominal; AZT, zidovudine; ddC, zalcitabine; ddI, didanosine; Regurg, regurgitation.
*Data from American Hospital Formulary Service: Antiretroviral agents. In McEvoy GK (ed): Information. Bethesda, MD, American Hospital Formulary Society, 1998, p 539.
[†]Oral and esophageal ulcer can occur in patients who take ddC or AZT without fluid while in a recumbent position.

creases active intestinal secretion, and inhibits all gastrointestinal hormones.

Evaluation of Diarrhea in HIV-Infected Individuals

There is controversy regarding what the best diagnostic approach to use in HIV-infected individuals with diarrhea. The initial history should ascertain any recent travel, diarrheogenic medications, or dietary practices that may contribute to diarrhea (i.e., lactose or gluten intolerance). Symptoms associated with diarrhea can also indicate whether the small or large bowel is the primary site of involvement. Small-bowel diarrhea is characterized by nocturnal, large volume, infrequent fecal movements. Frequent bloody stools accompanied by abdominal pain and rebound tenderness are more frequently associated with colonic infection.

A recent technical review prepared by the American Gastrointestinal Association recommended the diagnostic evaluation demonstrated in Table 13–3.[127] For patients with symptoms of small bowel involvement, upper gastrointestinal endoscopy with small bowel biopsies should be included as part of the initial evaluation. The diagnostic yield is likely to be higher in patients with more profound immunodeficiency (CD4 count <100 cells/mm^3).[127] For patients with symptoms that suggest a colonic infection, whether the initial evaluation should be a flexible sigmoidoscopy or a colonoscopy remains controversial. Most investigators believe that flexible sigmoidoscopy has a sufficient diagnostic yield and that colonoscopy should be reserved for patients with more refractory conditions. However, one recent study concluded that 30% of infectious etiologies and 75% of lymphomas would have been missed if full colonoscopy had not been performed.[82,128] Given the predominance of CMV in the right colon and its occurrence in normal-appearing mucosa, colonoscopy with biopsies of normal-appearing mucosa is recommended. Staining of sections with hematoxylin and eosin may reveal the charac-

teristic changes resulting from CMV, including cell enlargement and basophilic intranuclear inclusion surrounded by a clear halo. Using Wright-Giemsa stain, smaller intracytoplasmic inclusions may be visualized. In order to avoid having to perform two separate tests to evaluate the lower gastrointestinal tract, colonoscopy may be the initial procedure of choice, particularly for patients who are at an increased risk for CMV gastrointestinal disease. However, the decision as to which procedure to perform should be made individually for each patient after considering the patient-reported symptoms, the history of opportunistic infections, the stage of HIV infection, and the local availability of diagnostic procedures. For patient comfort, it is important to remember that both the upper and lower gastrointestinal endoscopic procedures can be performed during the same visit.

HEPATIC DISEASE IN HIV INFECTION

Prior to the use of HAART, intrahepatic opportunistic infections and malignancies were seen in an estimated 33% to 78% of patients with AIDS at autopsy.[81,129–131] The histologic pattern of liver injury in HIV-infected individuals can be divided into five different categories: hepatitis, granulomatous lesions, mass lesions, vascular lesions and lesions related to the use of hepatotoxic medications. Each of the histologic entities is discussed below in more detail.

Hepatitis

Viral hepatitis, primarily caused by hepatitis B virus (HBV) and hepatitis C virus (HCV), is a common coincident infection in HIV-infected individuals because of the epidemiologic risk factors of intravenous drug use and sexual contact. Up to 95% of AIDS patients have serologic markers of past HBV infection (anti-HBs or anti-HBC positive), and 10% to 15% are chronic carriers (hepatitis B surface antigen [HBsAg] positive).[132–134] The effect of HIV infection increases the severity of the course of chronic hepatitis and can result in a loss of HBsAg and a reappearance of hepatitis Be antigen (HBeAg). The reactivation of the disease is thought to be due to a progressive decline in humoral and cell-mediated immunity.[135] In rare cases, reactivation can be fulminant, resulting in death.[136] However, in most cases, the increased activity of HBV

TABLE 13–3. Diagnostic Evaluation of Chronic Diarrhea in HIV-Infected Individuals

1. Fecal culture
2. Ova and parasite examination
3. *Clostridium difficile* toxin (if recent history of antibiotic use)
4. Empiric trial of antidiarrheal agents
5. Flexible sigmoidoscopy with mucosal biopsies
6. Upper endoscopy with duodenal biposies

does not result in decreased survival.[137] Clearance of HBV is inversely associated with the degree of immunosuppression, with CD4+ lymphocytes playing the central role in the clearance of infected hepatocytes. With increasing HBV titers, an increased proportion of the cells infiltrate the liver and trigger CD8+ lymphocyte cytotoxic activity, resulting in hepatocellular necrosis.[138] As cell-mediated immunity wanes as a result of progressive HIV infection, less immunologic damage to infected hepatocytes may occur, hepatic inflammation is minimized, and progression to cirrhosis is unusual.

As the morbidity and mortality secondary to HIV have decreased as a result of the use of HIV-1 protease inhibitors, treatment of viral hepatitis, which frequently accompanies HIV infection, has become an option in these individuals. Every attempt should be made to vaccinate individuals at risk for HBV despite the questionable success of inducing an immune response.[139]

HCV, an RNA virus, is a member of the flavivirus family. In contrast to HBV, HCV is cytopathic to the liver. Current estimates suggest that approximately 5 million individuals are infected with HCV in the United States (see Chapter 27). The reported prevalence of HCV in HIV-infected individuals ranges from 9% to 40%. The virus is most commonly transmitted parenterally, either through blood transfusions or intravenous drug use. Sexual and transplacental transmission are much less effective routes of viral dissemination. Several studies have documented that liver-related mortality is higher in those patients coinfected with HCV and HIV than in those with HCV infection alone.[140–143] Factors implicated as determining the rate of progression to liver failure include the degree of impaired cell-mediated immunity (i.e., CD4 cell count), the age of the individual at the time of infection, and the timing of HCV infection in relation to HIV infection.[144] In a 3-year prospective study of hemophiliacs, liver failure was only observed in the patients with more pronounced immune deficiency (CD4 cell count <200 × 10^9/L).[145] In another study, 12% of HIV–HCV coinfected patients progressed to liver cirrhosis over a 15-year period, compared to 5% of individuals infected with only HCV.[146] HIV infection has also been shown to increase HCV RNA levels dramatically, and the HCV RNA levels inversely correlate with CD4 cell counts.[141,147] Treatment of HIV-1 with protease inhibitors can also increase the HCV RNA level in coinfected individuals.[11] As the prognosis for individuals with HIV improves with the use of combination antiretroviral therapy, treatment of HCV in coinfected individuals has become an important consideration.

The diagnosis of HCV relies on screening with a second-generation antibody with confirmation with a recombinant immunoblot assay to improve specificity. However, immunosuppressed patients may have indeterminate assay results from diminished reactivity to HCV antigens.[148] Supplementation of the immunologic assays with quantitative assays that directly measure the viral load will determine active viremia and will provide an additional variable to monitor a response to therapy. (Chapter 26 provides a more detailed discussion of HCV and its management.)

CMV is the most common viral opportunistic infection of the liver.[149] In the majority of cases, the disease is asymptomatic. A patient with CMV is more likely to come to medical attention if the biliary tree is involved. Other viruses that involve the liver include Epstein-Barr virus, adenovirus, varicella-zoster virus, and human herpesvirus type 6.[150–152]

Granulomatous Lesions

Granulomatous lesions of the liver are the most common histologic finding in liver biopsies from HIV-infected individuals, present in 37.2% of 501 biopsy specimens in one study.[150] The most common hepatic infection is MAC, which is found in 10% to 30% of liver biopsy specimens in AIDS patients and most commonly results in granulomatous inflammation.[132,133,148,153,154] Clinically, hepatic MAC infection of the liver usually results in an elevation of alkaline phosphatase that should be differentiated from AIDS cholangiopathy. Features that favor MAC infection of the liver as opposed to AIDS cholangiopathy include marked hepatomegaly, malaise, pancytopenia, and prolonged, high, spiking fever.[155] Elevation of alkaline phosphatase may result from infiltration of the hepatic parenchyma with granulomata, resulting in obstruction of the terminal branches of the biliary tree.[129]

Mycobacterium tuberculosis can also cause hepatic granulomas and hepatic abscesses in HIV-infected individuals. Seven percent of individuals with extrapulmonary tuberculosis have hepatic involvement.[156] Other mycobacteria implicated in hepatic disease in HIV-infected individuals include *M. xenopi, M. genavense,* and *M. kansasii.*[157]

Mass Lesions

The most common cause of mass lesions of the liver in HIV-infected individuals is neoplasia, most commonly KS and non-Hodgkin's lymphoma (NHL). Up to one third of individuals with cutaneous KS will also have liver involvement, although KS may be limited to the liver.[129,158-160] The most common presenting symptoms are abdominal pain, hepatosplenomegaly, elevated alkaline phosphatase, and hyperechoic areas visualized on ultrasonographic examination of the liver. KS lesions are hypoattenuated on a noncontrast computed tomography (CT) scan but enhance after a bolus of contrast material.[161] On biopsy, the lesion originates in the capsular, hilar, and portal areas and subsequently invades the parenchyma.

Biopsy of an affected mass will reveal characteristic irregular, purple-brown soft nodules deep to the liver capsule. KS can also be characterized by vascular endothelial cell proliferation associated with spindle-cell proliferation, extravasated erythrocytes, and vascular lakes. Immunohistochemical evaluation for Factor VIII can increase the sensitivity of finding an abnormality. Vascular complications of the tumor include hemorrhage and central necrosis; obstructive complications include obstructive jaundice and cholangitis.

NHL is frequently a high-grade B-cell malignancy in AIDS patients. The liver is the most frequently involved abdominal solid organ in NHL, a disease that is associated with a high incidence of extranodal involvement. Symptoms commonly associated with NHL include weight loss, fever, night sweats, right upper quadrant (RUQ) abdominal pain, hepatomegaly, and jaundice. Laboratory evaluation typically reveals mild elevation of liver function test values, predominantly alkaline phosphatase. Ultrasound may reveal low-attenuated and hypoechoic cystic masses with septations.[162,163] CT may reveal masses that are less dense than the surrounding hepatic parenchyma and may be surrounded by a thin enhancing rim.[164]

Vascular Lesions

Common causes of hepatic vascular lesions include KS, peliosis hepatis, and sinusoidal dilation and congestion. Peliosis hepatis may be due to *Bartonella henselae*, which has been implicated as a cause of bacillary angiomatosis. Symptoms of liver involvement include fever, weight loss, abdominal pain, and hepatosplenomegaly. Laboratory evaluation typically reveals mild to moderate elevations of aminotransferase levels and moderate to severe elevation of alkaline phosphatase levels. Radiographic evaluation reveals multiple, small, low-attenuated lesions throughout the hepatic parenchyma.[165] Histologic evaluation, either wedge resection or parenchymal biopsy, characteristically reveals cystic blood-filled spaces that are often associated with fibromyxoid stroma containing few inflammatory cells, capillaries, and clumps of bacilli.[166] The causative agent can be identified within sinusoidal endothelial cells and extracellularly by Warthin-Starry stain or by electron microscopy.[167] Indirect immunofluorescent antibody testing, polymerase chain reaction, or enzyme immunoassay can all provide supplemental support for the diagnosis. Complications of peliosis hepatis include transfusion-unresponsive anemia, thrombocytopenia, and a consumptive coagulopathy.[168]

Hepatotoxic Medications

The use of hepatotoxic medications is very common in HIV-infected individuals. Previous studies have reported that up to 90% of AIDS patients are treated with at least one drug associated with hepatotoxicity, often necessitating dosage reduction or drug discontinuation.[169] Hepatotoxic drug reactions can result in a hepatocellular, cholestatic, or mixed pattern. Table 13-4 demonstrates the hepatotoxic adverse events that occur as a result of the use of antiretroviral medications. (Chapter 6 discusses drug interactions in greater detail.)

Nucleoside analogs are commonly used in the treatment of HIV-infected individuals as a component of HAART therapy. These medications have been reported as a cause of fatty liver (steatohepatitis) and lactic acidosis. Steatohepatitis has been reported in at least 11 patients treated with zidovudine. Therefore, individuals with a history of steatohepatitis or those with risk factors for steatohepatitis (i.e., female, obesity, diabetes mellitus) should be closely followed while receiving zidovudine.[170] Severe hepatotoxicity and death can occur as a result of treatment with nucleoside analogs, as occurred with fialuridine in a trial of the treatment of hepatitis B.[171] Although this adverse event is a rare complication of therapy with this class of compounds, all patients with hepatomegaly and elevated liver-associated enzymes should be carefully monitored. Abnormal liver function test results may occur in individuals who re-

TABLE 13–4. Hepatic Adverse Effects of Antiretroviral Medications (in Percentages)*

MEDICATION	ELEV AST	ELEV ALT	ELEV ALK PHOS	ELEV TB	ELEV GGT	HEPATITIS	JAUNDICE	CIRRHOSIS	HEPATIC FAILURE
Indinavir	<1–7	<1–7		2–10			<2%	<2%	
Nelfinavir	3	3	<2%		<2				
Ritonavir	6	5	1	1		<2%			
Saquinavir	1–6	1–6		1.6	6–7	<2	<2		
ddI	2–10	2–10	2–10	10					
ddC	10	10	10						
AZT†						<1	<1		0.2

Abbreviations: Alk Phos, alkaline phosphatase; ALT, alanine transaminase; AST, aspartate transaminase; AZT, zidovudine; ddC, zalcitabine; ddI, didanosine; Elev, elevated; GGT, γ-glutamyltranspeptidase; TB, total bilirubin.

*Data from American Hospital Formulary Service: Antiretroviral agents. In McEvoy GK (ed): Information. Bethesda, MD, American Hospital Formulary Society, 1998, p 539.

†Syndrome of hepatic steatosis and potentially fatal lactic acidosis manifest by fever, malaise, weakness, nausea, vomiting, diarrhea, epigastric pain, and increasing serum transaminase concentration has been reported with the use of this medication.[221]

ceive didanosine or zalcitabine. In rare cases, didanosine may be associated with liver failure. Adefovir dipivoxil, an adenine nucleoside analog, has also been noted to cause reversible elevated liver enzymes.

Recently the HIV-1 protease inhibitors have been recognized as an important cause of hepatic abnormalities in HIV-infected individuals. Several case reports have highlighted the problems associated with their use. Indinavir has been associated with a mixed hepatocellular and cholestatic pattern of liver-associated enzyme abnormalities and has been reported to cause severe hepatitis.[172] The medication has also been associated with asymptomatic hyperbilirubinemia (total bilirubin >2.5 mg/dl) in 10% of treated individuals (Crixivan package insert). During Phase I/II clinical trials, elevated liver enzymes and bilirubin were observed in fewer than 5% of patients receiving 400 mg four times daily. Among indinavir-treated individuals in New York City, the prevalence of clinically significant hepatic complications was approximately 1%. Eight out of 10 individuals with significant hepatic disease had serologic evidence of hepatitis, and all were being treated concomitantly with additional potentially hepatotoxic medications.[173] Ritonavir has been associated with hepatocellular dysfunction resulting in elevated serum triglyceride levels and steatohepatitis.

BILIARY TRACT DISEASE

Pathogenesis

Cryptosporidiosis[174] and CMV[175] were the first etiologic agents to be identified as causes of AIDS-related cholangitis. Subsequently, distinctive cholangiographic patterns were identified in HIV-infected individuals.[176] *Enterocytozoon bieneusi*[177] has been identified as a cause of cholangitis, and *Isospora belli*[178] as a cause of acalculous cholecystitis. MAC, lymphoma, and KS are uncommon causes of AIDS-related cholangitis.[179,180] Prior to HAART, cryptosporidiosis was the most commonly identified cause of cholangitis in AIDS patients. After an outbreak of intestinal cryptosporidiosis in Milwaukee in 1993,[181] cryptosporidiosis of the biliary tract was noted in 29% of the HIV-infected individuals who had intestinal cryptosporidiosis.[105] CMV is the second most common cause of biliary tract disease in HIV-infected individuals[182] (Color Plate II*C*). Coinfection of the biliary tract by both CMV and *Cryptosporidium* can occur in a large percentage of patients with profound immunodeficiency (CD4 counts <50 cells/mm³).[183] *Cryptosporidium* infection of the biliary ducts is associated with an interstitial inflammatory cell infiltrate composed primarily of small and intermediate-sized lymphocytes with occasional plasma cells and macrophages. Interstitial edema, microabscesses secondary to a neutrophilic infiltrate, and cuboidal transition of the biliary epithelium can occur in response to cryptosporidium infection.

Diagnosis, Therapy, and Complications

AIDS-related cholangitis typically occurs in individuals with advanced disease with a CD4 count less than 100 cells/mm³.[184] Common presenting symptoms (RUQ abdominal pain, fever, and cholestasis) associated with AIDS cholangiopathy are similar to those of other pathogenic processes that can occur in the biliary tract unrelated to HIV infection. However, pruritis is uncommon, and jaundice is less common than in individuals who are not infected with HIV.[184,185] Symptoms are similar regardless of which organism is the cause of the biliary tract disease. Nausea, vomiting, weight loss, and diarrhea all occur frequently.[105,180,185] Anicteric cholestasis with a mean bilirubin of 1.4 mg/dl, a mean alkaline phosphatase of 744 mg/dl, and a mild elevation of transaminases were the most common laboratory abnormalities in one series.[179]

Abdominal ultrasound and CT are typically the initial imaging modalities in the investigation of individuals with fever, RUQ abdominal pain, and elevated alkaline phosphatase. Ultrasound is useful for visualizing extrahepatic bile ducts, and approximately 75% of individuals with typical symptoms will have an abnormal abdominal ultrasound.[179,183,185] Imaging may also show thickening of the gallbladder wall and the common bile duct. CT can identify intrahepatic duct dilitation.[186] However, endoscopic retrograde cholangiopancreatography (ERCP) is the gold standard for the diagnosis of AIDS-related cholangitis.[187] The procedure can be both diagnostic and therapeutic: (1) the biliary tract can be radiographically visualized, (2) biopsies of the biliary epithelium can be obtained through the endoscope, (3) brushings for cytologic staining can also be obtained, (4) bile can be aspirated and sent for ova and parasite examination, and (5) sphincterotomy, a potentially therapeutic

TABLE 13–5. Cholangiopathic Patterns in AIDS Cholangiopathy

DISEASE	GENERAL CHARACTERISTICS	RADIOGRAPHIC PATTERN	FREQUENCY	CHARACTERISTICS
AIDS cholangiopathy	1) CBD—beaded or scalloped appearance 2) Left IHD dilated > right IHD 3) CBD with polypoid filling defect in 25%	Papillary stenosis	15–20%	Bile duct >8 mm with smooth tapering and delayed emptying
		Sclerosing cholangitis	20%	Focal strictures and dilatation of intra- and extrahepatic ducts
		Mixed papillary and sclerosing cholangitis	50%	
		Extrahepatic bile duct stricture	15%	1- to 2-cm idiopathic stricture
PSC	1) Rare CBD dilitation 2) Paucity of IHD 3) Stricturing and dilitation of IHD 4) Rare intraductal debris			

Abbreviations: CBD, common bile duct; IHD, intrahepatic duct; PSC, primary sclerosing cholangitis.

procedure, can be performed. Common cholangiographic patterns associated with AIDS cholangiopathy, as well as important features that differentiate AIDS cholangiopathy from primary sclerosing cholangitis, are presented in Table 13–5.

Biopsy of the duodenum, ampulla, or liver may reveal circumstantial evidence of an organism that may be the cause of biliary tract disease. Liver biopsies have demonstrated cryptosporidium, CMV, MAC, and microsporidia as causes of AIDS-related cholangitis.[188,189] Additionally, the suspect organism may be isolated from the feces (as is almost always the case in the diagnosis of AIDS-related cholangiopathy secondary to cryptosporidium).

Fifty-four percent of individuals with biliary cryptosporidiosis reported a partial response to paromomycin.[105] Although intestinal infection caused by *Encephalitozoon intestinalis* responds to treatment with albendazole, there has not been a trial of this medication in the treatment of *E. intestinalis* biliary tract disease. For patients with biliary tract disease secondary to CMV, a therapeutic trial of ganciclovir or foscarnet may be appropriate. Sphincterotomy has successfully alleviated pain secondary to extrahepatic biliary tract disease in the 70% of patients with AIDS cholangiopathy who have papillary stenosis.[176,183,185,190] However, 50% of patients may have progression of intrahepatic disease after the procedure.[176] Individuals with long extrahepatic biliary strictures may benefit

from placement of endoscopic stents. Ursodeoxycholic acid has been proposed as salvage therapy in individuals whose symptoms failed to improve after sphincterotomy.[191]

Complications of AIDS cholangiopathy can occur as a result of ERCP, of the pathogenic process, or of therapeutic maneuvers (i.e., sphincterotomy) performed during ERCP. In one series, complications occurred in 10% of individuals who underwent sphincterotomy, and 0.4% had fatal complications.[192] Pancreatitis and hemorrhage were the two most frequent complications, occurring in 5.4% and 2.0% of patients, respectively. Ascending cholangitis and biliary sepsis can also occur as a complication of ERCP or underlying infection.[179,185] For these reasons, very solid indications should exist before performing an ERCP in HIV-infected patients just as in immunocompetent individuals.

PANCREATIC DISEASE IN HIV-INFECTED INDIVIDUALS

Pathogenesis

The incidence of acute pancreatitis associated with HIV infection ranges from 4% to 46%.[193] Pancreatic disease in HIV-infected individuals has been divided into three broad categories: (1) that associated with the use of medications, (2) that associated with opportunistic infections,

TABLE 13–6. Causes of Pancreatic Disease in HIV-Infected Individuals

MEDICATIONS	INFECTIONS	NEOPLASMS	GENERAL
Didanosine	*Mycobacterium avium* complex	Kaposi's sarcoma	Alcohol
Zalcitabine	*Mycobacterium tuberculosis*	Non-Hodgkin's lymphoma	Gallstone disease
Trimethoprim-sulfamethoxazole	Cytomegalovirus	Adenocarcinoma	Hypercalcemia
Octreotide	*Toxoplasma gondii*		Hypertriglyceridemia
Pentamidine	*Candida albicans*		Salivary gland disease
	Herpes simplex virus		Macroamylasemia
	Cryptosporidium parvum		Renal failure
	Cryptococcus neoformans		Congenital anomalies
			Duct strictures

and (3) that associated with neoplastic conditions[194–196] (Table 13–6). In one series, acute pancreatitis occurred much more frequently in HIV-infected individuals evaluated during a 1-year period at a community hospital than in the general population.[197]

Acute pancreatitis is characterized by abdominal pain, nausea, vomiting, and anorexia. Laboratory evaluation characteristically reveals elevated serum amylase and lipase levels. Imaging of the pancreas by CT scan or ultrasonography is indicated to verify the diagnosis and will characteristically reveal pancreatic inflammation, pancreatic edema, and peripancreatic fluid.

Medication-Associated Pancreatic Disease

Pancreatitis occurs at an increased frequency in individuals treated with antiretroviral medications. The nucleoside analogs didanosine and zalcitabine have both been associated with a high incidence of pancreatitis.[198,199] Seventeen percent of the patients treated in Phase I/II clinical trials of didanosine reported a dose-related risk of pancreatitis. The risk of pancreatitis is increased in individuals with a history of pancreatitis.

Pentamidine, used primarily in HIV-infected individuals as an agent against *P. carinii*, may have a cytolytic effect on pancreatic β cells and on pancreatic acinar cells. In patients who have received at least 1 gm of the drug,[200] pancreatic injury leading to release of insulin and hypoglycemia can occur. In late stages, hypoglycemia occurs in combination with low serum C-peptide levels.[201] Histologically, the pancreas may manifest injury by spotty acinar necrosis, steatonecrosis, focal hemorrhage, inflammation, and inspissated ductular secretions.[202] Pancreatitis has not been associated with the use of aerosolized pentamidine.[197]

Mass Lesions—Infections and Neoplastic Conditions

Masses visualized on imaging of the pancreas can result from intrinsic lesions, peripancreatic lymph nodes, or neoplastic processes. Characteristically, these lesions appear solid and must be differentiated from cystic lesions that can be caused by pseudocysts, cystic tumors, or infections. The most common infectious causes of pancreatic or peripancreatic abscesses are *M. tuberculosis* and MAC.[203] CMV, toxoplasmosis, *Cryptococcus*, *Cryptosporidium*, HSV, and disseminated *P. carinii* infection can also cause pancreatic infection that may appear as mass lesions on radiographic evaluation. Although rare, NHL and KS can also cause pancreatic mass lesions.

Evaluation of pancreatic mass lesions requires biopsy, usually under CT or ultrasound guidance. Endoscopic ultrasound and laparotomy are additional procedures that can be utilized when diagnosis is difficult. Endoscopic ultrasound has enhanced sensitivity over traditional methods for the evaluation of mass lesions of the pancreas and has the advantage that biopsies can be easily obtained from small lesions.[204] Samples should be sent for cytologic analysis, histologic evaluation, and viral, bacterial, and fungal cultures. The HIV serostatus of an individual does not affect the treatment of pancreatitis, which is identical in HIV-infected individuals and in HIV-seronegative individuals. Treatment is largely supportive, with withholding of oral intake, supplementation with fluid, and analgesics. Endocrine and exocrine pancreatic failure requires supplementation with insulin and pancreatic enzymes.

RECENT CHANGES IN THE INCIDENCE OF OPPORTUNISTIC INFECTIONS AFTER HAART

Several new classes of compounds have been developed to combat HIV infection, including the protease inhibitors, nucleoside analogs, and non-nucleosides.[205] With the use of these agents in combination, coupled with their use as early in HIV infection as possible,[206] the production of new infectious viral particles is prevented. This has led to the first decrease in the incidence of AIDS cases (first noticed in 1996) since the recognition of the epidemic.[8] Several other studies have subsequently reported that HAART induces a decrease in the HIV viral load, an increase in absolute CD4 count, improved survival, and a decrease in the number of AIDS-related opportunistic infections.[8,207–210] Because the number of individuals on combination antiretroviral therapy is expected to increase, physicians should be familiar with the potential adverse effects of these medications.[211] (See Chapter 6.)

Prevention of Gastrointestinal AIDS-Related Opportunistic Infections

Prophylaxis against AIDS-related opportunistic infections has been an important component of the treatment of HIV-infected individuals. As the CD4 cell count declines, prophylaxis is initiated against various opportunistic organisms. HIV infection induces random depletions within the CD4+ T-cell receptor that can result in substantial defects in immune function at the level of receptor repertoire. Although there are substantial increases in the number of CD4+ T cells induced by antiretroviral and immune-based therapy, the diversity of the T-cell receptor is not immediately restored. The loss of CD4+ T cells with specificity for particular antigens and their failure to be restored in response to antiretroviral therapy may be an important event in the development or relapse of opportunistic infections in the HAART era.[212,213] Because there is incomplete restoration of the immune system in response to antiretroviral therapy, prophylaxis against AIDS related opportunistic infections may still be necessary. Revised guidelines for prophylaxis against AIDS-related opportunistic infections in the era of HAART have recently been released.[214]

In clinical practice, the incidence of the first episode of CMV disease has decreased from 18.7 first episodes per 100 person-years prior to HAART to 5.0 first episodes per 100 person-years in the HAART era.[215] However, several reports have demonstrated that CMV disease can develop after initiation of HAART in individuals with CD4+ cell counts greater than 100 cells/mm^3. Jacobson et al. described five patients who developed CMV retinitis within 4 to 7 weeks of the initiation of HAART.[216] Gilquin et al. reported 10 cases of acute CMV infection that developed after the initiation of HAART.[217] Four patients developed CMV infection with CD4+ cell counts below 50 cells/mm^3 and six patients had CD4+ cells above 100 cells/mm^3.

Several studies have reported an improvement in AIDS-related opportunistic infections in response to combination antiretroviral medication. Neither cryptosporidia nor microsporidia could be detected on fecal or intestinal biopsy examinations in nine patients with a history of these pathogens who were treated with combination antiretroviral therapy including an HIV-1 protease inhibitor.[218] Neither infection was eradicated based on the persistent macrophage infiltrate and the rapid reappearance of the infection with a falling CD4 cell count, and the patients remained stable for as long as the HAART-induced immunologic improvements were sustained. However, improved immunologic status may complicate the clinical course in patients who are coinfected with HIV and HBV. A HBV-seropositive patient with HBsAg and HBeAg+ who began HAART therapy had worsening of hepatitis B, with nausea, vomiting, hepatomegaly, and abnormalities of hepatic enzymes. Eventually, the patient had a decrease in HBV DNA to below detectable levels and an increase in the serologic response to hepatitis B.[219]

Besides the significant decrease in the incidence of gastrointestinal opportunistic infections in HIV-infected individuals, protease inhibitors have significantly improved the treatment of diarrhea in individuals with an identified pathogen.[220] In the era of HAART, gastrointestinal symptoms are more likely to be due to adverse reactions from antiretroviral medications than to opportunistic infections. However, physicians must not cease in their vigilance in detecting and treating opportunistic infections. Underlying viral hepatitis (HBV and HCV) are likely causes of increased protease inhibitor and possibly reverse transcriptase inhibitor toxicity. The treatment of viral hepatitis in coinfected individuals is likely to decrease the potential antiretroviral-associated hepatotoxicity.

References

1. Winkelstein W Jr, Lyman DM, Padian N, et al: Sexual practices and risk of infection by the human immunodeficiency virus: The San Francisco Men's Health Study. JAMA 257:321, 1987
2. Embretson J, Zupancic M, Ribas JL, et al: Massive covert infection of helper T lymphocytes and macrophages by HIV during the incubation period of AIDS. Nature 362:359, 1993
3. Pantaleo G, Graziosi C, Demarest JF, et al: HIV infection is active and progressive in lymphoid tissue during the clinically latent stage of disease. Nature 362:355, 1993
4. Schnittman SM, Lane HC, Greenhouse J, et al: Preferential infection of CD4+ memory T cells by human immunodeficiency virus type 1: Evidence for a role in the selective T-cell functional defects observed in infected individuals. Proc Natl Acad Sci USA 87: 6058, 1990
5. Schieferdecker H, Ullrich L, Hirseland H, Zeitz M: T cell differentiation antigens on lymphocytes in the human intestinal lamina propria. J Immunol 149:2816, 1992
6. James SP, Zeitz M: Human gastrointestinal mucosal T cells. In Ogra PL, Lamm ME (eds): Handbook of Mucosal Immunology, 4th ed. New York, Academic Press, 1994, p 275
7. Mestecky J, Jackson S: Reassessment of impact of mucosal immunity in infection with the human immunodeficiency virus (HIV) and design of relevant vaccines. J Clin Immunol 14:259, 1994
8. Centers for Disease Control and Prevention: Update: Trends in AIDS incidence, deaths, and prevalence—United States, 1996. MMWR Morb Mortal Wkly Rep 46:165, 1997
9. Smith PD, Mai UEH: Immunopathophysiology of gastrointestinal disease in HIV infection. Gastroenterol Clin North Am 21:331, 1992
10. Flexner C: HIV-protease inhibitors. N Engl J Med 338:1281, 1998
11. Rutschmann OT, Negro F, Hirschel B, et al: Impact of treatment with human immunodeficiency virus (HIV) protease inhibitors on hepatitis C viremia in patients coinfected with HIV. J Infect Dis 177:783, 1998
12. Clayton F, Snow G, Reka S, Kotler DP: Selective depletion of rectal lamina propria rather than lymphoid aggregate CD4 lymphocytes in HIV infection. Clin Exp Immunol 197:288, 1997
13. Cerf-Bensussan N, Schneeberger EE, Bhan AK: Immunohistologic and immunoelectron microscopic characterization of the mucosal lymphocytes of the human small intestine by the use of monoclonal antibodies. J Immunol 130:261, 1983
14. Selby WS, Janossy G, Bofill M, et al: Intestinal lymphocytes subpopulations inflammatory bowel disease: An analysis by immunohistological and cell isolation techniques. Gut 25:32, 1984
15. Chun TW, Chadwick K, Margolick J, Siliciano RF: Differential susceptibility of naive and memory CD4+ T cells to the cytopathic effects of infection with human immunodeficiency virus type 1 strain LAI. J Virol 71:4436, 1997
16. Veazey RS, DeMaria MA, Chalifoux LV, et al: Gastrointestinal tract as a major site of CD4+ T cell depletion and viral replication in SIV infection. Science 280:427, 1998
17. Schneider T, Jahn H-U, Schmidt W, et al: Loss of CD4 T lymphocytes in patients infected with human immunodeficiency virus type 1 is more pronounced in the duodenal mucosa than in the peripheral blood. Gut 37:524, 1995
18. Talal A, Vesanen M, Cao Y, et al: Gut associated lymphoid tissue sampling to determine response to antiretroviral therapy. In Abstracts of the Symposium on HIV-1 Infection, Mucosal Immunity and Pathogenesis, National Institutes of Health, Bethesda, MD, 1997, Abstract 99
19. Owen RL, Jones AL: Epithelial cell specialization within human Peyer's patches: An ultrastructural study of intestinal lymphoid follicles. Gastroenterology 66:189, 1974
20. Fantini J, Yahi N, Chermann JC: Human immunodeficiency virus can infect the apical and basolateral surfaces of human colonic epithelial cells. Proc Natl Acad Sci USA 88:9297, 1991
21. Bomsel M: Transcytosis of infectious human immunodeficiency virus across a tight human epithelial cell line barrier. Nature Med 3:42, 1997
22. Wilcox CM: Esophageal disease in the acquired immunodeficiency syndrome: Etiology, diagnosis and management. Am J Med 92:412, 1992
23. Dieterich DT, Wilcox CM: Diagnosis and treatment of esophageal diseases associated with HIV infection. Am J Gastroenterol 91:2265, 1996
24. Andersen LI, Frederiksen H-J, Appleyard M: Prevalence of esophageal Candida colonization in a Danish population: Special reference to esophageal symptoms, benign esophageal disorders, and pulmonary disease. J Infect Dis 165:389, 1992
25. Baehr PH, McDonald GB: Esophageal infections, risk factors, presentation, diagnosis, and treatment. Gastroenterology 106:509, 1994
26. Walsh TJ, Pizzo PA: Nosocomial fungal infections. Annu Rev Microbiol 42:517, 1988
27. Dieterich DT, Lew EA, Kotler DP, et al: Treatment with albendazole for intestinal disease due to Enterocytozoon bieneusi in patients with AIDS. J Infect Dis 169:178, 1994
28. Lin-Greenberg A, Villacin A, Moussa G: Lymphomatoid granulomatosis presenting as ulcerodestructive gastrointestinal tract lesions in patients with human immunodeficiency virus infection: A new association. Arch Intern Med 150:2581, 1990
29. Schechter M, Pannain VLN, de Oliveira AV: Papovavirus-associated esophageal ulceration in a patient with AIDS. AIDS 5:238, 1991
30. Margolis PS, Epstein A: Mucormycosis esophagitis in a patient with the acquired immunodeficiency syndrome. Am J Gastroenterol 89:1900, 1994
31. Kazlow P, Shah K, Benkov K, et al: Esophageal cryptosporidiosis in a child with acquired immunodeficiency syndrome. Gastroenterology 91:1301, 1986
32. Grimes MM, LaPook JD, Bar MH, et al: Disseminated Pneumocystis carinii infection in a patient with acquired immunodeficiency syndrome. Hum Pathol 18:307, 1987
33. Kim J, Minamoto GY, Grieco MH: Nocardial infection as a complication of AIDS: Report of six cases and review. Rev Infect Dis 13:624, 1991
34. Stoopack PM, de Silva R, Raufman JP: Inflammatory double-barreled esophagus in two patients with AIDS. Gastrointest Endosc 36:394, 1990

35. Gradon JD, Timpone JG, Schnittman SM: Emergence of unusual opportunistic pathogens in AIDS: A review. Clin Infect Dis 15:134, 1992

36. Villaneuva JL, Torre-Cisneros J, Jurado R, et al: Leishmania esophagitis in an AIDS patient: An unusual form of visceral leishmaniasis. Am J Gastroenterol 89:273, 1994

37. Poles MA, McMeeking AA, Scholes JV, et al: Actinomyccs infcction of a cytomegalovirus esophageal ulcer in two patients with acquired immunodeficiency syndrome. Am J Gastroenterol 89:1569, 1994

38. Kotler DP, Wilson CS, Haroutiounian G, et al: Detection of human immunodeficiency virus-1 by ^{35}S-RNA in situ hybridization in solitary esophageal ulcers in two patients with the acquired immunodeficiency syndrome. Am J Gastroenterol 84:313, 1989

39. Smith PD, Fox CH, Masur H, et al: Quantitative analysis of mononuclear cells expressing human immunodeficiency virus type 1 RNA in esophageal mucosa. J Exp Med 180:1541, 1994

40. Barrison IG, Foster S, Harris JW, et al: Upper gastrointestinal Kaposi's sarcoma in patients positive for HIV antibody without cutaneous disease. Br Med J 2: 92, 1988

41. Connolly GM, Hawkins D, Harcourt-Webster JN, et al: Oesophageal symptoms, their causes, treatment and prognosis in patients with the acquired immunodeficiency syndrome. Gut 30:1033, 1989

42. Bernal A, del Juncod GW: Endoscopic and pathologic features of esophageal lymphoma: A report of four cases in patients with the acquired immunodeficiency syndrome. Gastrointest Endosc 32:96, 1986

43. Fried RL, Brandt LJ, Kauvar D, et al: Esophageal motility in AIDS patients with symptomatic opportunistic infections of the esophagus. Am J Gastroenterol 89:2003, 1994

44. Kikendall JW, Friedman AC, Oyewolfe MA, et al: Pill-induced esophageal injury: Case reports and review of the medical literature. Dig Dis Sci 28:174, 1983

45. Edwards P, Turner J, Gold J, et al: Esophageal ulceration induced by zidovudine. Ann Intern Med 112:65, 1990

46. Indorf AS, Pegram PS: Esophageal ulceration related to zalcitabine (ddC). Ann Intern Med 117:133, 1992

47. Lake-Bakaar G, Quadros E, Baidas S, et al: Gastric secretory failure in patients with the acquired immune deficiency syndrome. Ann Intern Med 109:502, 1988

48. Shaffer RT, LaHatte LJ, Kelly JW, et al: Gastric acid secretion in HIV-1 infection. Am J Gastroenterol 87: 1777, 1992

49. Belitsos PC, Greenson JK, Yardley JH, Sisler JR, Bartlett JG: Association of gastric hypoacidity with opportunistic enteric infections in patients with AIDS. J Infect Dis 166:277, 1992

50. Wilcox CM, Schwartz DA: A pilot study of oral corticosteroid therapy for idiopathic esophageal ulcerations associated with human immunodeficiency virus infection. Am J Med 93:131, 1992

51. Moreria A, Sampaio E, Zmuidzinas A, et al: Thalidomide exerts its inhibitory action on tumor necrosis factor a by enhancing mRNA degradation. J Exp Med 177:1675, 1993

52. Kotler DP, Reka S, Orenstein JM, et al: Chronic idiopathic esophageal ulceration in the acquired immunodeficiency syndrome: Characterization and treatment with corticosteroids. J Clin Gastroenterol 15: 284, 1992

53. Smith PD, Eisner MS, Manischewitz JF, et al: Esophageal disease in AIDS is associated with pathogenic

54. Rabeneck L, Boyko WJ, McLean DM, et al: Unusual esophageal ulcers containing enveloped viruslike particles in homosexual men. Gastroenterology 90:1882, 1986

55. Rabeneck L, Popovic M, Gartner S, et al: Acute HIV infection presenting with painful swallowing and esophageal ulcers. JAMA 263:2318, 1990

56. Dieterich DT, Poles M, Lew EA: Gastrointestinal manifestations of HIV disease. In Broder S, Merigan TC Jr, Bolognesi D (eds): Textbook of AIDS Medicine. Baltimore, Williams & Wilkins, 1994, p 541

57. Oberg B: Antiviral effects of phosphonoformate. Pharmacol Ther 490:213, 1989

58. Youle M, Clarbour J, Farthing C, et al: Treatment of resistant aphthous ulceration with thalidomide in patients positive for HIV antibody. BMJ 298:432, 1989

59. Patterson DL, Georghou PR, Allwoth AM, Kemp RJ: Thalidomide as treatment of refractory aphthous ulceration related to human immunodeficiency virus infection. Clin Infect Dis 20:250, 1995

60. NIH Consensus Conference: Helicobacter pylori in peptic ulcer disease. JAMA 272:65, 1994

61. Marano BJ Jr, Smith F, Bonanno CA: Helicobacter pylori prevalence in acquired immunodeficiency syndrome. Am J Gastroenterol 88:687, 1993

62. Cacciarelli AG, Marano BJ, Gualtieri NM, et al: Helicobacter pylori infection and peptic ulcer disease prevalence in patients with AIDS and suppressed CD4 counts. Am J Gastroenterol 91:1783, 1996

63. Bartlett JG, Belitsos PC, Sears CL: AIDS enteropathy. Clin Infect Dis 15:726, 1992

64. Colebunders R, Francis H, Mann JM, et al: Persistent diarrhea strongly associated with HIV infection in Kinshasa, Zaire. Am J Gastroenterol 82:859, 1987

65. Gazzard B, Blanshard C: Diarrhea in AIDS and other immunodeficiency states. Baillieres Clin Gastroenterol 7:387, 1993

66. Grohman GS, Glass RI, Pereira HG, et al: Enteric viruses and diarrhea in HIV-infected patients. N Engl J Med 329:12, 1993

67. Centers for Disease Control: Revision of the CDC survelliance case definition for acquired immunodeficiency syndrome. MMWR Morb Mortal Wkly Rep 36(Suppl 1):1S, 1987

68. Greenson JK, Belitsos PC, Yardley JH, et al: AIDS enteropathy: Occult enteric infections and duodenal mucosal alterations in chronic diarrhea. Ann Intern Med 114:366, 1991

69. Justice AC, Feinstein AR, Wells CK: A new prognostic staging system for the acquired immunodeficiency syndrome. N Engl J Med 320:1388, 1989

70. Lindan CP, Allen S, Serufilira A, et al: Predictors of mortality among HIV-infected women in Kigali, Rwanda. Ann Intern Med 116:320, 1988

71. Lubeck DP, Bennett CL, Mazonson PD, et al: Quality of life and health service use among HIV-infected patients with chronic diarrhea. J Acquir Immune Defic Syndr 6:478, 1993

72. Hernandez EJ, Jain R, Burdick JS, et al: HIV does not affect outcome in acute upper gastrointestinal hemorrhage [Abstract G4069]. Gastroenterology 114: A993, 1998

73. Chalasani N, Wilcox CM: Etiology and outcome of lower gastrointestinal bleeding in patients with AIDS. Am J Gastroenterol 93:175, 1998

74. Patel NR, Oliva PJ, McCoy S, et al: Massive lower gastrointestinal hemorrhage in an AIDS patient: First

case report of ulcerated lymphoma in a Meckel's diverticulum. Am J Gastroenterol 89:133, 1994

75. Sharma VS, Valji K, Bookstein JJ: Gastrointestinal hemorrhage in AIDS: Arteriographic diagnosis and transcatheter treatment. Radiology 185:447, 1992

76. Lew EA, Poles MA, Dieterich DT: Diarrheal diseases associated with HIV infection. Gastroenterol Clin North Am 26:259, 1997

77. Evans JD, Robertson CS, Clague MB, et al: Severe lower gastrointestinal hemorrhage from cytomegalovirus ulceration of the terminal ileum in a patient with AIDS. Eur J Surg 159:373, 1993

78. Becherer PR, Sokol-Anderson M, Joist JH, Milligan T: Gastrointestinal histoplasmosis presenting as hematochezia in human immunodeficiency virus-infected hemophilic patients. Am J Hematol 47:229, 1994

79. Balbi HJ, McAbee G, Annuziato GM, et al: Fatal gastrointestinal tract hemorrhage in a child with AIDS [letter] JAMA 262:1470, 1989

80. Mintz L, Drew WL, Miner RC, et al: Cytomegalovirus infections in homosexual men: An epidemiologic study. Ann Intern Med 99:326, 1983

81. Reichert CM, O'Leary TJ, Levens DL, et al: Autopsy pathology in the acquired immunedeficiency syndrome. Am J Pathol 357:11A, 1983

82. Dieterich DT, Rahmin M: Cytomegalovirus colitis in AIDS: presentation in 44 patients and a review of the literature. J Acquir Immune Defic Syndr 4(Suppl 1): S29, 1991

83. Fleming SC, Kapembwa MS, McDonald TT, et al: Direct in vitro infection of human intestine with HIV-1. AIDS 6:1099, 1992

84. Frager DH, Frager JD, Wolf EL, et al: Cytomegalovirus colitis in acquired immunodeficiency syndrome: Radiologic spectrum. Radiology 11:241, 1986

85. Ferguson CM: Surgical complications of acquired immunodeficiency virus infection. Am Surg J 54:4, 1988

86. Wilson SE, Robinson G, Williams RA, et al: Acquired immune deficiency syndrome (AIDS): Indications for abdominal surgery, pathology, and outcome. Ann Surg 210:428, 1989

87. Beaugerie L, Ngo Y, Goujard F, et al: Etiology and management of toxic megacolon in patients with human immunodeficiency virus infection. Gastroenterology 107:358, 1994

88. Gallant J, Moore RD, Richman DD, et al: Incidence and natural history of cytomegalovirus disease in patients with advanced human immunodeficiency virus disease treated with zidovudine. J Infect Dis 166:1223, 1992

89. Dieterich DT, Kotler DP, Busch DF, et al: Ganciclovir treatment of cytomegalovirus colitis in AIDS: A randomized, double-blind, placebo-controlled multicenter study. J Infect Dis 167:278, 1993

90. Blanshard C, Benhamou Y, Dohin E, et al: Treatment of AIDS-associated gastrointestinal cytomegalovirus infection with foscarnet and ganciclovir: A randomized comparison. J Infect Dis 172:622, 1995

91. Martin-Munley S, Dieterich DT: Efficacy of intravenous foscarnet for cytomegalorvirus gastrointestinal disease in human immunodeficiency virus-infected individuals. (submitted)

92. Whitley RJ, Jacobson MA, Friedberg DN, et al: Guidelines for the treatment of cytomegalovirus diseases in patients with AIDS in the era of potent antiretroviral therapy: Recommendations of an international panel. Arch Intern Med 158:957, 1998

93. Buhles WC Jr, Mastre BJ, Tinker AJ, et al, for The Syntex Collaborative Ganciclovir Treatment Study group: Ganciclovir treatment of life- or sight-threatening cytomegalovirus infection: Experience in 314 immunocompromised patients. Rev Infect Dis 10(Suppl 3):S495, 1988

94. Drew WL: Cytomegalovirus infection in patients with AIDS. J Infect Dis 158:449, 1988

95. Decay G, Martinez F, Katlama C, et al: Foscarnet nephrotoxicity: Mechanism, incidence and prevention. Am J Nephrol 9:31, 1989

96. Safrin S, Crumpacker C, Chatis P, et al: A controlled trial comparing foscarnet with vidarabine for acyclovir-resistant mucocutaneous herpes simplex in the acquired immunodeficiency syndrome. N Engl J Med 325:551, 1991

97. Safrin S, Kemmerly S, Plotkin B, et al: Foscarnet-resistant herpes simplex virus infection in patients with AIDS. J Infect Dis 169:193, 1994

98. Khoo SH, Bailey AS, de Jong JC, et al: Adenovirus infections in human immunodeficiency virus-positive patients: Clinical features and molecular epidemiology. J Infect Dis 172:629, 1995

99. Kaljot KT, Ling JP, Gold JWM, et al: Prevalence of enteric viral pathogens in acquired immunodeficiency syndrome patients with diarrhea. Gastroenterology 97:1031, 1989

100. Maddox A, Moss FJ, Blanshard C, et al: Adenovirus infection of the large bowel in HIV positive patients. J Clin Pathol 45:684, 1992

101. McGowan I, Allason-Jones E: Symptomatic management of HIV associated gastrointestinal disease. Cancer Surv 21:157, 1994

102. Jayagopal S, Cervia JS: Colitis due to Candida albicans in a patient with AIDS. Clin Infect Dis 15:555, 1992

103. Driks M, Gupta MR, McKinsey DS, et al: Gastrointestinal histoplasmosis in patients with the acquired immunodeficiency syndrome. In Abstracts of the 30th Interscience Conference on Antimicrobial Agents and Chemotherapy. Washington, DC, American Society for Microbiology, 1990

104. Haggerty CM, Britton MC, Dorman JM, et al: Gastrointestinal histoplasmosis in suspected acquired immunodeficiency syndrome. West J Med 143:244, 1985

105. Vakil NB, Schwartz FN, Buggy BP, et al: Biliary cryptosporidiosis in HIV infected people after the waterborne outbreak cryptosporidiosis in Milwaukee. N Engl J Med 334:19, 1996

106. White AC, Chappell CL, Hayat CS, et al: Paromomycin for cryptosporidiosis in AIDS: A prospective double blind trial. J Infect Dis 170:419, 1994

107. Bissuel F, Cotte L, Rabodonirina M, et al: Paromomycin: An effective treatment for cryptosporidial diarrhoea in patients with AIDS. Clin Infect Dis 18:447, 1994

108. Harris M, Deutsch G, MacLean D, Tsoukas CM: A Phase I study of letrazuril in AIDS-related cryptosporidiosis. AIDS 8:1109, 1994

109. Weber R, Bryan RT: Microsporidial infections in immunodeficient and immunocompetent patients. Clin Infect Dis 19:517, 1994

110. Anwar-Bruni DM, Hogan SE, Schwartz DA, et al: Atovaquone is effective treatment for the symptoms of gastrointestinal microsporidiosis in HIV-1 infected patients. AIDS 10:619, 1996

111. Molina J-M, Chastang C, Gouguel J, et al: Albendazole for treatment and prophylaxis of microsporidiosis due to Encephalitozoon intestinalis in patients with AIDS: A randomized double-blind controlled trial. J Infect Dis 177:1373, 1998

112. Horsburgh CR: *Mycobacterium avium* complex infection in the acquired immunodeficiency syndrome. N Engl J Med 324:1332, 1991

113. Rotterdam H, Tsang P: Gastrointestinal disease in the immunocompromised patient. Hum Pathol 25:1123, 1994

114. Masur H: Recommendations on prophylaxis and therapy for disseminated Mycobacterium avium complex disease in patients with human immunodeficiency virus. N Engl J Med 329:893, 1993

115. Nelson MR, Shanson DC, Hawkins DA, et al: *Salmonella, Campylobacter,* and *Shigella* in HIV-seropositive patients. AIDS 6:1495, 1992

116. Blaser MJ, Hale TL, Formal SB: Recurrent shigellosis complicating human immunodeficiency virus infection: Failure of pre-existing antibodies to confer protection. Am J Med 86:105, 1989

117. Salmon D, Detruchis P, Leport C, et al: Efficacy of zidovudine in preventing relapses of Salmonella bacteremia in AIDS. J Infect Dis 163:415, 1991

118. Mayer HB, Wanke C: Enteroaggregative Escherichia coli as a possible cause of diarrhea in an HIV-infected patient. N Engl J Med 332:273, 1995

119. Orenstein JM, Kotler DP: Diarrheogenic bacterial enteritis in acquired immunedeficiency syndrome: A light and electron microscopic study of 52 cases. Hum Pathol 26:481, 1995

120. Cappell MS, Clark P: *Clostridium difficile* infection as a treatable cause of diarrhea in patients with advanced human immunodeficiency virus infection: A study of seven consecutive patients admitted from 1986 to 1992 to a university teaching hospital. Am J Gastroenterol 88:891, 1993

121. Heise C, Dandekar S, Kumar P, et al: Human immunodeficiency virus infection of enterocytes and mononuclear cells in human jejunal mucosa. Gastroenterology 100:1521, 1991

122. Fleming SC, Kapembwa MS, McDonald TT, et al: Direct in vitro infection of human intestine with HIV-1 AIDS 6:1099, 1992

123. Kotler DP, Reka S, Clayton F: Intestinal mucosal inflammation associated with human immunodeficiency virus infection. Dig Dis Sci 38:105, 1989

124. Belitsos PC, Greenson JK, Yearley JH, et al: Association of gastric hypoacidity with opportunistic enteric infections in patients with AIDS. J Infect Dis 166:277, 1992

125. Keating J, Bjarnason I, Somasundaram S, et al: Intestinal absorptive capacity, intestinal permeability and jejunal histology in HIV and their relation to diarrhoea. Gut 37:623, 1995

126. Sharkey KA, Sutherland LR, Davison JS, et al: Peptides in the gastrointestinal tract in human immunodeficiency virus infection. Gastroenterology 103:18, 1992

127. Wilcox CM, Rabeneck L, Friedman S: Malnutrition and cachexia, chronic diarrhea and hepatobiliary disease in patients with human immunodeficiency virus infection. Gastroenterology 111:1724, 1996

128. Bini EJ, Weinshel EH: Endoscopic evaluation of chronic human immunodeficiency virus-related diarrhea: Is colonoscopy superior to flexible sigmoidoscopy? Am J Gastroenterol 93:56, 1998

129. Glasgow BJ, Anders K, Layfield LJ, et al: Clinical and pathologic findings of the liver in the acquired immunedeficiency syndrome (AIDS). Am J Clin Pathol 83:582, 1985

130. Guarda LA, Luna MA, Smith J, et al: Acquired immunedeficiency syndrome: Post-mortum findings. Am J Clin Pathol 81:549, 1984

131. Welch K, Finkbeiner W, Alpers CE, et al: Autopsy findings in the acquired immunedeficiency syndrome. JAMA 252:1152, 1994

132. Gordon SC, Reddy KR, Gould EE, et al: The spectrum of liver disease in the acquired immunodeficiency syndrome. J Hepatol 2:475, 1986

133. Lebovics E, Dworkin BM, Heier SK, et al: The hepatobiliary manifestations of human immunodeficiency virus infection. Am J Gastroenterol 83:1, 1988

134. Lebovics E, Thung SN, Schaffner F, et al: The liver in the acquired immunodeficiency syndrome: A clinical and histologic study. Hepatology 5:293, 1985

135. Vandercam B, Cornu C, Gala JL, et al: Reactivation of hepatitis B virus in a previously immune patient with human immunodeficiency virus infection. Eur J Clin Microbiol Infect Dis 9:701, 1990

136. Boue F, Goujard C, Lazzizi Y, et al: Fatal fulminant hepatitis linked to HBV reactivation in AIDS patient. In Programs and Abstracts of the IXth International Conference on AIDS, Berlin, 1993, Abstract PO-B08-1351

137. Housset C, Pol S, Carnot F, et al: Interactions between human immunodeficiency virus-1, hepatitis delta virus and hepatitis B virus infections in 260 chronic carriers of hepatitis B virus. Hepatology 15:578, 1992

138. Pham BN, Mosnier JF, Walker F, et al: Flow cytometry CD4+/CD8+ ratio of liver-derived lymphocytes correlates with viral replication in chronic hepatitis B. Clin Exp Immunol 97:403, 1994

139. Collier AC, Corey L, Murphy VL, et al: Antibody to human immunodeficiency virus (HIV): A suboptimal response to hepatitis B vaccination. Ann Intern Med 109:101, 1988

140. Eyster ME, Diamondstone LS, Lien JM, et al: Natural history of hepatitis C virus infection in multitransfused hemophiliacs: Effect of co-infection with human immunodeficiency virus. J Acquir Immune Defic Syndr 6:602, 1993

141. Eyster ME, Fried MW, Diseglie AM, et al: Increasing hepatitis C virus RNA in hemophiliacs: Relationship to HIV infection and liver disease. Blood 84:1020, 1994

142. Thomas DL, Shih JW, Alter HJ, et al: Effect of HIV on hepatitis C virus infection among injecting drug users, J Infect Dis 174:690, 1996

143. Tefler P, Sabin C, Devereux H, et al: The progression of HCV-associated liver disease in a cohort of haemophiliac patients. Br J Haemotol 94:746, 1994

144. Collier J, Heathcote J: Hepatitis C viral infection in the immunosuppressed patient. Hepatology 27:2, 1998

145. Rockstroh JK, Spengler U, Sudhop T, et al: Immunosuppression may lead to progression of hepatitis C virus-associated liver disease in haemophiliacs coinfected with HIV. Am J Gastroenterol 91:2563, 1996

146. Soto B, Sanchez-Quijano A, Rodrigo L, et al: Human immunodeficiency virus infection modifies the natural history of chronic parenterally-acquired hepatitis C with an unusually rapid progression to cirrhosis. J Hepatol 26:1, 1997

147. Ghany MG, Leissinger C, Laiger R, et al: Effect of human immunodeficiency virus infection on hepatitis C virus infection in hemophiliacs. Dig Dis Sci 141:1265, 1996

148. Marcellin P, Martinot-Peignoux M, Elias M, et al: Hepatitis C virus (HCV) viremia in human immunodeficiency virus-seronegative and seropositive patients with indeterminate HCV recombinant immunoblot assay. J Infect Dis 170:433, 1994

149. Waisman J, Rotterdam H, Niedt GN, et al: AIDS: An overview of the pathology. Pathol Res Pract 182:729, 1987

150. Poles MA, Dieterich DT, Schwarz ED, et al: Liver biopsy findings in 501 patients infected with human immunodeficiency virus (HIV). J Acquir Immune Defic Syndr Hum Retrovirol 11:170, 1996

151. Knox KK, Carrigan DR: Disseminated active HHV-6 infections in patients with AIDS. Lancet 343:577, 1994

152. Soriano V, Bru F, Gonzalez-Lahoz J: Fatal varicella hepatitis in a patient with AIDS. J Infect 25:107, 1992

153. Kahn SA, Saltzman BR, Klein RS, et al: Hepatic disorders in the acquired immunodeficiency syndrome: A clinical and pathological study. Am J Gastroenterol 81:1145, 1986

154. Hawkins CC, Gold JW, Whimbey E, et al: Mycobacterium avium complex infections in patients with the acquired immunodeficiency syndrome. Ann Intern Med 105:184, 1986

155. Cappell MS: Hepatobiliary manifestations of the acquired immunodeficiency syndrome. Am J Gastroenterol 86:1, 1991

156. Chaisson RE, Schecter GF, Theuer CP, et al: Tuberculosis in patients with the acquired immunodeficiency syndrome: Clinical features, responses of therapy and survival. Am Rev Respir Dis 136:570, 1987

157. Maschek H, Georgii A, Schmidt RE, et al: Mycobacterium genavense autopsy findings in three patients. Am J Clin Pathol 101:95, 1994

158. Hasan FA, Jeffers LJ, Welsh SW, et al: Hepatic involvement as the primary manifestation of Kaposi's sarcoma in the acquired immunodeficiency syndrome. Am J Gastroenterol 84:1449, 1989

159. Nakanuma Y, Liew CT, Peters RL, et al: Pathologic features of the liver in acquired immune deficiency syndrome (AIDS). Liver 6:158, 1986

160. Schneiderman DJ, Arenson DM, Cello JP, et al: Hepatic disease in patients with the acquired immune deficiency syndrome (AIDS). Hepatology 7:925, 1987

161. Luburich P, Bru C, Ayuso MC, et al: Hepatic Kaposi sarcoma in AIDS: US and CT findings. Radiology 175:172, 1990

162. Soyer P, Van Beers B, Teillet-Thiebaud F, et al: Hodgkin's and non-Hodgkin's hepatic lymphoma: Sonographic finding. Abdom Imaging 18:339, 1993

163. Townsend RR, Laing FC, Jeffrey RB Jr, et al: Abdominal lymphoma in AIDS: Evaluation with US. Radiology 171:719, 1989

164. Radin DR, Esplin JA, Levine AM, et al: AIDS-related non-Hodgkin's lymphoma: Abdominal CT findings in 112 patients. Am J Roentgerol 160:1133, 1993

165. Wyatt SH, Fishman EK: Hepatic bacillary angiomatosis in a patient with AIDS. Abdom Imaging 18:336, 1993

166. Perkocha LA, Geaghan SM, Yen TS, et al: Clinical and pathological features of bacillary peliosis hepatitis in association with human immunodeficiency virus infection. N Engl J Med 323:1581, 1990

167. Leong SS, Cazen RA, Yu GS, et al: Abdominal visceral peliosis associated with bacillary angiomatosis: Ultrastructural evidence of endothelial destruction by bacilli. Arch Pathol Lab Med 116:866, 1992

168. Garcia-Tsao G, Panzini L, Yoselevitz M, et al: Bacillary peliosis hepatis as a cause of acute anemia in a patient with the acquired immunodeficiency syndrome. Gastroenterology 102:1065, 1992

169. Dworkin BM, Stahl RE, Giardina MA, et al: The liver in the acquired immunodeficiency syndrome: Empha-sis on patients with intravenous drug abuse. Am J Gastroenterol 82:231, 1987

170. Schuman P, Kinsey J, Merlino N: Fatty infiltration of the liver associated with lactic acidosis in 3 women with HIV infection. In Program and Abstracts of the 33nd Interscience Conference on Antimicrobial Agents and Chemotherapy. Washington, DC, American Society for Microbiology, 1992, Abstract 1085

171. McKenzie R, Fried MW, Sallie R, et al: Hepatic failure and lactic acidosis due to fialuridine (FIAU), an investigational nucleoside analogue for chronic hepatitis B, N Engl J Med 333:1099, 1995

172. Brau N, Leaf KL, Wieczorek RL, Margolis DM: Severe hepatitis in three AIDS patients treated with Indinavir [letter]. Lancet 349:924, 1997

173. Kravetz JD, Lee C, Stein JJ, et al: Hepatic complications in HIV-infected individuals treated with indinavir. Am J Gastroenterol (submitted)

174. Pitlick S, Fainstein V, Rios A, et al: Cryptosporidial cholecystitis. N Engl J Med 308:967, 1983

175. Blumberg RS, Kelsey P, Perrone T, et al: Cytomegalovirus and cryptosporidium associated acalculus gangrenous cholecystitis. Am J Med 76:1118, 1984

176. Cello JP, Chan MF: Long-term follow-up of endoscopic retrograde cholangiopancreatography sphincterotomy for patients with acquired immunodeficiency syndrome papillary stenosis. Am J Med 99:600, 1995

177. Pol S, Romana C, Richard S, et al: *Enterocytozoon bieneusi* infection in acquired immunodeficiency syndrome related sclerosing cholangitis. Gastroenterology 102:1178, 1992

178. Benator DA, French AL, Beaudet LM, et al: Isospora belli infection associated with acalculous cholecystitis in a patient with AIDS. Ann Intern Med 121:663, 1994

179. Cello JP: Acquired immunodeficiency syndrome cholangiopathy: Spectrum of disease. Am J Med 86:539, 1989

180. Farman J, Brunetti J, Baer JW, et al: AIDS-related cholangiopancreatographic changes. Abdom Imaging 19:417, 1994

181. MacKenzie WR, Hoxie NJ, Proctor ME, et al: A massive outbreak in Milwaukee of cryptosporidium infection transmitted through the public water supply. N Engl J Med 331:1035, 1994

182. Forbes A, Blanshard C, Gazzard B: Natural history of AIDS-related sclerosing cholangitis: A study of 20 cases. Gut 34:116, 1993

183. Benhamou Y, Caumes E, Gerosa Y, et al: AIDS-related cholangiopathy critical analysis of a perspective series of 26 patients. Dig Dis Sci 38:1113, 1993

184. Cello JP: Human immunodeficiency virus associated biliary tract disease. Semin Liver Dis 12:213, 1992

185. Bouche H, Housset C, Dumont JL: AIDS related cholangitis: Diagnostic features in course of 15 patients. J Hepatol 17:34, 1993

186. Dolmatch BL, Laing FC, Federle MP, et al: AIDS-related cholangitis radiographic findings in nine patients. Radiology 163:313, 1987

187. Nash JA, Cohen SA: Gallbladder and biliary tract disease in AIDS. Gastroenterol Clin North Am 26:323, 1997

188. Texidor HS, Goodwin TA, Ramirez EA: Cryptosporidiosis with a biliary tract in AIDS. Radiology 180:51, 1991

189. Pol S, Romana C, Richard S, et al: Microsporidiosis infection in patients with human immunodeficiency virus and unexplained cholangitis. N Engl J Med 328:95, 1993

190. Lynche KD, Savides TJ, Weiner KJ: AIDS cholangi-opathy: The role of therapeutic ERCP. Gastrointest Endosc 40:A117, 1994

191. Chan MF, Koch J, Cello JP: Ursodeoxycholic acid for symptomatic AIDS associated cholangiopathy. Gastrointest Endosc 40:A108, 1994

192. Freeman ML, Nelson DB, Sheriman S, et al: Complications of endoscopic biliary sphincterotomy. N Engl J Med 335:909, 1996

193. Dowell SF, Moore GW, Hutchins GM: The spectrum of pancreatic pathology in patients with AIDS. Mod Pathol 3:49, 1990

194. Cappell MS, Hassan T: Pancreatic disease in AIDS: A review. J Clin Gastroenterol 17:254, 1993

195. Bonacini M: Pancreatic involvement in human immunodeficiency virus infection. J Clin Gastroenterol 13:58, 1991

196. Kumar S, Schnadig VJ, MacGregor MG: Fatal acute pancreatitis associated with pentamidine therapy. Am J Gastroenterol 84:451, 1989

197. Dutta SK, Ting CD, Lai LL: Study of prevalence, severity, and etiological factors associated with acute pancreatitis in patients infected with human immunodeficiency virus. Am J Gastroenterol 92:2044, 1997

198. Seidlin M, Lambert JS, Dolin R, et al: Pancreatitis and pancreatic dysfunction in patients taking dideoxyinosine. AIDS 6:831, 1992

199. Maxson CJ, Greenfield SM, Turner JL: Acute pancreatitis as a common complication of 2'3'-dideoxyinosine therapy in the acquired immunodeficiency syndrome. Am J Gastroenterol 87:708, 1992

200. O'Neil MG, Selub SE, Hak LJ: Pancreatitis during pentamidine therapy in a patient with AIDS. Clin Pharm 10:56, 1991

201. Perrone C, Bricaire F, Leport C, et al: Hypoglycemia and diabetes mellitus following parenteral pentamidine mesylate treatment in AIDS patients. Diabet Med 6:831, 1992

202. Klatt EC: Pathology of pentamidine-induced pancreatitis. Arch Pathol Lab Med 116:162, 1992

203. Jaber B, Gleckman R: Tuberculous pancreatic abscess as an initial AIDS-defining disorder in a patient infected with the human immunodeficiency virus: Case report and review. Clin Infect Dis 20:890, 1995

204. Meier H, Friebel H: Ultrasound and endoscopic ultrasound in the diagnosis of pancreatic tumors. In Malfertheiner P, Dominguez-Munoz J, Schultz H, Lippert H (eds): Diagnostic Procedures in Pancreatic Disease. Berlin, Springer Verlag, 1997, p 343

205. Deeks SG, Smith M, Holodniy M, Kahn JO: HIV-1 protease inhibitors. JAMA 277:145, 1997

206. Ho DD: Time to hit HIV, early and hard. N Engl J Med 333:451, 1995

207. Perelson AS, Essunger P, Cao Y, et al: Decay characteristics of long-lived HIV-1 infected compartments: A minimal estimate of the treatment time needed for eradication of HIV. Nature 387:188, 1997

208. Hirsch M, Melbohm A, Rawlins S, Leavitt R: Indinavir in combination with zidovudine (ZDV) and lamivudine in ZDV-experienced patients with CD4 counts <50 cells/mm^3. In Program and Abstracts of the 4th Conference on Retroviruses and Opportunistic Infections. Washington, DC, Foundation for Retrovirology and Human Health, 1997, Abstract LB7

209. Cameron B, Heath-Chiozzi M, Kravcik S, et al: Prolongation of life and prevention of AIDS in advanced HIV immunodeficiency with ritonavir. In Program and Abstracts of the 3rd Conference on Retroviruses and Opportunistic Infections. Washington, DC, Foundation for Retrovirology and Human Health, 1996, Abstract LB6a

210. Palella F, Moorman A, Delaney K, et al: Declining morbidity and mortality in an ambulatory HIV-infected population [abstract I-17]. In Program and Abstracts of the 37th Interscience Conference on Antimicrobial Agents and Chemotherapy. Washington, DC, American Society for Microbiology, 1997, p 245

211. Carpenter CC, Fischl MA, Hammer SM, et al: Antiretroviral therapy for HIV infection in 1997: Updated recommendations of the International AIDS Society–USA panel. JAMA 277:1962, 1997

212. Connors M, Kovacs JA, Krevath S, et al: HIV infection induces changes in CD4+ T cell phenotype and depletions within the CD4+ T cell repertoire that are not immediately restored by antiviral or immune based therapies. Nature Med 3:533, 1997

213. Kelleher AD, Carr A, Zaunders J, Cooper DA: Alterations in the immune response of human immunodeficiency virus (HIV)-infected subjects treated with an HIV-specific protease inhibitor, ritonavir. J Infect Dis 173:321, 1996

214. USPHS/IDSA Prevention of Opportunistic Infections Working Group: 1997 USPHS/IDSA guidelines for the prevention of opportunistic infections in persons infected with human immunodeficiency virus: Disease-specific recommendations. Clin Infect Dis 25(Suppl 3): S313, 1997

215. Baril L, Jouan M, Caumes E, et al: The impact of highly active antiretroviral therapy on the incidence of CMV disease in AIDS patients [abstract I-31]. In Program and Abstracts of the 37th Interscience Conference on Antimicrobial Agents and Chemotherapy. Washington, DC, American Society for Microbiology, 1997, p 248

216. Jacobson MA, Zegans M, Pavan PR, et al: Cytomegalovirus retinitis after initiation of highly active antiretroviral therapy. Lancet 349:1443, 1997

217. Gilquin J, Piketty C, Thomas V, et al: Acute cytomegalovirus infection in AIDS patients with CD4 counts above 100×10^6 cells/l following combination antiretroviral therapy including protease inhibitors. AIDS 11:1659, 1997

218. Carr A, Marriott D, Field A, et al: Treatment of HIV-1-associated microsporidiosis and cryptosporidiosis with combination antiretroviral therapy. Lancet 351: 256, 1998

219. Carr A, Cooper DA: Restoration of immunity to chronic hepatitis B infection in HIV-infected patient on protease inhibitors. Lancet 349:996, 1997

220. Bini EJ, Cohen J: effect of protease inhibitors on the outcome of therapy for chronic HIV-related diarrhea [abstract G3822]. Gastroenterology 114:A933, 1998

14 | Management of the Neurologic Complications of HIV-1 Infection and AIDS

RICHARD W. PRICE

HIV-1 infection, and particularly its late phase, AIDS, is complicated by a variety of central nervous system (CNS) and peripheral nervous system (PNS) disorders (for general reviews, see Price,[1] Berger and Levy[2] and Gendelman[3]). Classification of these disorders according to their underlying pathogenetic processes provides a rational framework for comprehending and managing the spectrum of conditions to which these patients are susceptible (Table 14–1) and also allows one to deal systematically with new or unusual conditions as they are encountered.

The most important determinant of pathogenetic susceptibility is the stage of systemic HIV-1 infection, and particularly the resultant degree of immunosuppression. The underlying immune status exerts a predominating effect on disease vulnerability and therefore strongly influences the probabilities of differential diagnosis. This consideration continues to be paramount in the era of highly active antiretroviral therapy (HAART), in which immune function may be preserved or partially restored, thereby preventing or forestalling some of the most severe complications of infection. For this reason, in the following discussion the neurologic aspects of HIV-1 infection are first segregated according to the phase of systemic infection in which they develop, and the conditions that occur in early HIV-1 infection are considered before the more common conditions that complicate the late, severely immunocompromised phase of infection.

Discussion of the complications of late HIV-1 infection then uses a classification based upon neuroanatomic localization. This is founded upon the predilection of different pathologic processes to select certain parts of the CNS and

PNS, which provides a practical starting point for differential diagnosis.

NERVOUS SYSTEM INVOLVEMENT EARLY IN HIV-1 INFECTION

Major clinical attention has focused on the common neurologic sequelae of later HIV-1 infection because of their frequency, but the earlier phases of systemic HIV-1 infection can, although less commonly, be accompanied by clinically important neurologic disorders. This includes both the phase of acute infection with seroconversion and the middle "asymptomatic" period of "clinical latency." During these phases, the principal pathogenetic mechanisms appear to involve immunopathology, either through triggering autoimmune reactions or resulting from host responses to ongoing HIV-1 infection. Additionally, a number of observations indicate that the CNS is exposed to HIV-1 early in the course of systemic infection and likely throughout its course, and that this infection can trigger local host responses, although these are most commonly asymptomatic.

Early Neurologic Complications of Acute HIV-1 Infection

A variety of CNS disorders have been described in the period after initial HIV-1 infection; these have been reviewed by Brew and Tindall.[4] Their reported frequency ranges from 8% for encephalopathies and neuropathies to as high as 45% for less specific manifestations such as head-

TABLE 14-1. Classification of the Most Common Neurologic Complications of HIV-1 Infection According to Underlying Pathophysiologic and Pathogenetic Categories

UNDERLYING PROCESS	EXAMPLES
Opportunistic infections	Cerebral toxoplasmosis Cryptococcal meningitis Progressive multifocal leukoencephalopathy (PML) Cytomegalovirus (CMV) encephalitis, polyradiculopathy, and mononeuritis multiplex
Opportunistic neoplasms	Primary CNS lymphoma Metastatic lymphoma
Metabolic, toxic, and other complications of systemic disease	Hypoxic encephalopathy Sepsis Stroke
Functional (psychiatric) disorders	Anxiety disorder Psychotic depression
Unique conditions (?) related to a primary effect of HIV-1 itself	AIDS dementia complex (ADC) Distal sensory polyneuropathy (DSPN)
Autoimmune disorders	Guillain-Barré syndrome Chronic inflammatory demyelinating polyneuropathy (CIDP)

ache.[5-16] They may begin at the time of or within several weeks after the seroconversion-related illness that resembles mononucleosis or, less often, in the absence of overt systemic illness. They may evolve acutely or subacutely and may take the form of focal or diffuse encephalitis or leukoencephalopathy, meningitis, ataxia, or myelopathy, either alone or together with PNS abnormalities, which include cranial neuropathy, brachial plexopathy, or neuropathy, which may be presenting features. They are characteristically monophasic, and most patients appear to recover within a number of weeks, although cognitive deficits may persist in some patients with encephalitis. The cerebrospinal fluid (CSF) usually shows a minor lymphocyte-predominant pleocytosis with a modest rise in protein, although this might not distinguish them from individuals with asymptomatic CSF abnormalities (see below). Results of neuroimaging using computed tomography (CT) have been normal, but experience with magnetic resonance imaging (MRI) is very limited. The electroencephalogram may be focally or diffusely slow. Although these early syndromes apparently are uncommon, it is possible that their incidence is underappreciated.

Neurologic Complications During the "Asymptomatic" Phase of Systemic HIV-1 Infection

Most common among the neurologic complications manifesting during the "asymptomatic"

or clinically latent phase of HIV-1 infection are demyelinating neuropathies.[17] These resemble the subacute Guillain-Barré syndrome or chronic inflammatory demyelinating polyneuropathy seen in other contexts, with the exception that the CSF often exhibits uncharacteristic, albeit mild, pleocytosis.[18,19] The pathophysiology of HIV-1–related demyelinating neuropathies probably parallels that of demyelinating neuropathies in other settings and has an autoimmune basis. Indeed, these disorders provide evidence that HIV-1 infection is accompanied by disordered immune regulation and not simply impaired host defenses; during this middle phase of infection, autoimmunity is more important than opportunistic infections that dominate the late phase. Patients with these demyelinating neuropathies appear to respond favorably to corticosteroids, plasma exchange, and intravenous immunoglobulin, with the latter two treatments currently preferred. The prognosis of demyelinating neuropathies in this setting may not be as good as that in the non-HIV-1–infected patient.[20,21]

Two other, less common, types of polyneuropathy have been described early in HIV-1 infection. Moulignier and colleagues have characterized a painful polyneuropathy associated with the diffuse infiltrative lymphocytosis syndrome, a disorder usually presenting with Sjögren's syndrome–like picture and multivisceral infiltrates of CD8+ T lymphocytes.[22-24] It also can involve peripheral nerves and manifest with symmetrical or asymmetrical painful neuropathy. Both anti–HIV-1 treatment and corticosteroids have been reported to be beneficial. Bradley and Verma reported another cause of painful neuropathy in the transitional phase of infection.[25] This was associated with a vasculitis that responded to prednisone therapy. Although this may be related to the benign form of mononeuritis multiplex discussed below, its presentation with more symmetrical symptoms suggesting polyneuropathy is noteworthy.

A rare but intriguing multiple sclerosis-like illness also has been reported in HIV-1–infected patients in the latent phase of infection.[26–28] The presentation is in the setting of preserved CD4+ T-lymphocyte counts and may include remissions and exacerbations, along with corticosteroid responsiveness. Although these cases may represent the concurrence of two diseases, more likely, as with the demyelinating neuropathies, they relate to an autoimmune process triggered by HIV-1 infection with clinical (and perhaps pathogenetic) features similar to those of multiple sclerosis.

Asymptomatic HIV-1 Infection of the CNS

Although clinically overt nervous system involvement may rarely present early in the course of HIV-1 infection, neurologically asymptomatic infection is the rule. Studies of CSF in clinically well patients have shown: (1) abnormalities of routine studies, including cell count, total protein, and immunoglobulin; (2) local, intrablood–brain barrier synthesis of anti–HIV-1 antibody; and (3) culture isolation of virus or detection of viral nucleic acid after polymerase chain reaction (PCR) amplification.[7,29–40] These abnormalities have been noted in fully functional, asymptomatic patients who have remained well during follow-up care for a year or more. Presumably they relate to traffic of infected blood cells into the CSF, where these cells then release virus without clinical sequelae other than eliciting a local host response. Clinically, these incidental abnormal levels in cell count, protein, immunoglobulin, oligoclonal bands, and HIV-1 detection must be taken into account when interpreting CSF results obtained for other diagnostic purposes or in following therapy.

These CSF findings and rare demonstration of HIV-1 in the brain following initial infection[41] imply that entry into the nervous system is an intrinsic part of the ecology of the virus in the human host throughout the course of infection.

They also indicate that HIV-1 can be relatively nonpathogenic for the CNS, underscoring the critical question of what leads to the subsequent conversion of this asymptomatic state in some patients to either aseptic meningitis or parenchymal encephalitis.[42–44]

LATE NERVOUS SYSTEM INVOLVEMENT BY HIV-1

In the late stages of HIV-1 infection, when immune defenses have been severely compromised and systemic complications begin to accumulate, the nervous system becomes highly susceptible to a wide array of disorders. These may involve all levels of the neuraxis, including meninges, brain, spinal cord, peripheral nerve, and muscle.

Meningitis and Headache

Several disorders involving the leptomeninges may afflict patients with advanced HIV-1 disease (Table 14–2), with symptoms ranging from frontal mild headache to severe disability with hydrocephalus, cranial nerve palsies, and death. Additionally, a number of conditions can mimic meningitis or cause headache.[45,46] For example, parenchymal brain diseases, such as toxoplasmosis (Chapter 25) and primary CNS lymphoma (Chapter 30), may initially manifest with headache as an important symptom without clear focal brain dysfunction.

Headache also may occur with no accompanying meningeal reaction. In some patients, this occurs as a complication of systemic illness. For example, patients with *Pneumocystis carinii* pneumonia (PCP) may have headache as an earlier and more prominent symptom than shortness of breath or cough. The headache may then

---

TABLE 14–2. Meningitides Complicating HIV-1 Infection

Common
Asymptomatic (HIV-1) meningeal reaction
Aseptic (HIV-1) meningitis
Cryptococcal meningitis

Uncommon
Tuberculous meningitis (*Mycobacterium tuberculosis*)
Syphilitic meningitis
Histoplasmosis
Coccidioidomycosis
Lymphomatous meningitis (metastatic)
Listeria monocytogenes

resolve with treatment of the PCP. In other patients, however, a precipitating opportunistic infection is not identified; the term *HIV headache* has been used to describe this condition, which may be severe and protracted.[47,48] It is speculated that circulating vasoactive cytokines may be involved in the pathogenesis of this headache. Although some of these patients seem to be helped by tricyclic antidepressants, others are not and may even require narcotic analgesics.

Among the true meningitides, a syndrome of aseptic meningitis, presumably relating to direct HIV-1 infection of the meninges, can occur acutely in the setting of seroconversion as described previously, but is more common in patients with advanced HIV-1 infection.[49,50] Clinically this may segregate into two types: an acute form and a chronic form. Both occur in late HIV-1 infection, usually in the transitional phase (CD4+ T-lymphocyte count >200 to 300/mm^3) or, somewhat less frequently, in the phase of overt AIDS (CD4+ cell count <200/mm^3). Both are accompanied by meningeal symptoms (e.g., headache and photophobia), although meningeal signs (e.g., nuchal rigidity) are more characteristic of the acute group. Cranial nerve palsies can complicate the course, affecting cranial nerves V, VII, and VIII, with Bell's palsy sometimes recurring. The CSF shows mild mononuclear pleocytosis, usually with normal glucose and mildly elevated protein levels. The presumption that this condition is due to direct HIV-1 infection of the meninges relates to two observations: the virus can be isolated from the CSF of some, and no other cause has been identified. However, whether HIV-1 infection is the sole or even major cause of the disorder can be questioned, because other causes of aseptic meningitis might be expected to provoke an influx of HIV-1–infected lymphocytes and monocytes into the CSF, thereby increasing the likelihood of viral isolation. Additionally, because of the high prevalence of abnormalities in the CSF of HIV-1–infected individuals described earlier, the definition of aseptic meningitis becomes less certain, and difficulties arise when one tries to distinguish HIV-1–related aseptic meningitis from the HIV headache discussed previously. Although the degree of pleocytosis might be used as a guide, presuming that the cellular reaction is involved in the genesis of symptoms, asymptomatic pleocytosis can vary widely, making it difficult to define a threshold CSF white blood cell count. Whatever its limits and cause, the syndrome of aseptic meningitis is benign but may imply a poor prognosis in relation to impending progression to AIDS in some patients. Although there have been no reports on the effects of antiretroviral therapy on this disorder, my colleagues and I have observed remarkable resolution of asymptomatic pleocytosis following HAART (unpublished observation).

The most important meningeal infection in AIDS patients is caused by *Cryptococcus neoformans*, also the most common CNS fungal infection in these patients[51–58] (Chapter 24). This infection usually presents as subacute meningitis or meningoencephalitis with headache, nausea, vomiting, and confusion, just as in non-AIDS patients. However, in many AIDS patients symptoms are remarkably mild, and the CSF formula may, likewise, contain few or no cells and little or no perturbation in glucose or protein levels. Hence, it is imperative that in such patients cryptococcal antigen is assessed and fungal cultures are obtained. An India ink study of the CSF may be helpful to visualize the organism's capsule, especially if the CSF cryptococcal antigen is not immediately available. Of note, the serum cryptococcal antigen is almost always positive, thereby serving as a screen for patients in whom the diagnostic suspicion is low or lumbar puncture is more risky. Therapeutic management of cryptococcal meningitis is reviewed in Chapter 24.

Meningitis appears to be an uncommon complication of tuberculosis in HIV-1–infected patients, and, in the absence of drug resistence, there is no evidence that the clinical presentation and response to therapy differs compared to other settings in which subacute or chronic meningitis manifests with neck stiffness, cranial nerve palsies, hydrocephalus, and vascular occlusions.[59,60] Differentiation from cryptococcal meningitis is aided by the tendency of tuberculous meningitis to occur with higher CD4+ lymphocyte counts and in patients from lower socioeconomic circumstances, to induce a partial polymorphonuclear cell response in the CSF, and to be accompanied by evidence of systemic infection. Other diagnostic and treatment aspects of *Mycobacterium tuberculosis* are discussed in Chapter 23.

Meningeal involvement by syphilis in HIV-1–infected individuals may take the form of acute meningitis or meningovascular syphilis.[61] Although the extent to which underlying HIV-1 infection alters the presentation, clinical course, or response to therapy of CNS syphilis is not fully settled, there is some evidence suggesting that meningovascular syphilis may occur both more commonly and earlier in those with HIV-1 infection. This and other aspects of neurosyphilis are discussed in detail in Chapter 29. The previously discussed CSF abnormalities common in asymptomatic seropositive patients, including elevated protein and cell counts, render interpretation of such findings in patients with positive syphilis serologies or those undergoing treatment more difficult.

Systemic lymphoma complicating HIV-1 infection may spread secondarily to the CNS, involving the meninges.[62-65] Clinical manifestations may be cryptic but often include cranial nerve palsies, headaches, or increased intracranial pressure. Other fungal infections, including coccidioidomycosis[66-69] and histoplasmosis,[69,70] may cause chronic meningitis in patients with endemic exposure (see Chapter 24).

Other causes of meningitis are uncommon in AIDS patients. Pyogenic meningitis is usually a complication of systemic sepsis, at times related to iatrogenic manipulations, including indwelling venous catheters, systemic antibiotics, and other predisposing factors. *Listeria monocytogenes* meningitis has been identified but seems to be rare. In these cases, as in the more common causes of meningitis discussed earlier, specific therapy should be combined with management of secondary sequelae such as elevated intracranial pressure caused by CSF outflow obstruction. This often can be remedied with repeated lumbar punctures, but some patients may also require a ventricular or lumbar shunt.

Diffuse Brain Disease and Dementia

Affliction of the brain parenchyma in AIDS can be usefully divided into conditions that cause predominantly focal symptoms and signs and those accompanied by more diffuse dysfunction (Table 14–3). Although there is some overlap in these disorders (e.g., cerebral toxoplasmosis may have both an "encephalitic" and the more common focal clinical picture), this division is

---

TABLE 14–3. Diffuse Brain Disease Complicating HIV-1 Infection

With Concomitant Depression of Alertness
Metabolic/toxic encephalopathies (alone or as an exacerbating influence on AIDS dementia complex)
Toxoplasmosis—"encephalitic" form
Cytomegalovirus encephalitis
Secondary to fungal, bacterial, or mycobacterial meningitis (as in Table 14–2)
Herpes simplex encephalitis

With Preservation of Alertness
AIDS dementia complex

---

generally valuable as the first step in differential diagnosis. The nonfocal disorders can, in turn, be subdivided into (1) those with parallel impairment of both alertness and cognition and (2) a disorder, the AIDS dementia complex (ADC), in which alertness is characteristically spared but cognition, motor function, and behavior are impaired.

Diffuse Encephalopathies

The various meningitides discussed earlier may cause diffuse brain dysfunction. Additionally, the metabolic or toxic encephalopathies developing as sequelae to the systemic non-neurologic diseases suffered by AIDS patients, such as pneumonias with hypoxia and systemic sepsis, may cause generalized encephalopathy. Clinicians should be alert to the development of Wernicke's encephalopathy, which may complicate AIDS, usually in the setting of severe systemic disease.[71,72] CNS-active drugs, including sedatives and narcotic analgesics, may cloud mentation or alertness just as in non-AIDS patients; these effects can occur alone but also may manifest as an exacerbating or unmasking influence on the ADC, resulting in a mixture of the two conditions and exaggerating medication effects. It has been suggested that HIV-1–infected patients may be more sensitive to neuroleptics and thereby manifest parkinsonism or other movement disorders at comparatively lower doses.[73]

Certain brain infections also can produce diffuse brain dysfunction. CNS toxoplasmosis, which usually causes focal neurologic symptoms and signs, may present as a generalized encephalopathy with clouding of consciousness and diffuse cerebral dysfunction.[74,75] This may be a particularly fulminating illness and relates to the presence of abundant toxoplasmic microabscesses, which may be poorly imaged by CT scan or MRI. Similarly, CNS lymphoma can infiltrate deep structures and impair cognition, alertness, and motor function without prominent focal symptoms or signs.

Although the overall clinical importance of cytomegalovirus (CMV) encephalitis remains imprecisely defined, CMV encephalitis is the most important infection in the differential diagnosis in patients with more severe ADC. Systemic CMV infection is very common in AIDS patients, and the brain is frequently infected. Thus evidence of mild brain infection is a frequent finding at autopsy. In perhaps one quarter of patients dying of AIDS, CMV infection is marked by scattered microglial nodules with occasional characteristic intranuclear inclusion bodies noted by routine histologic examination or by CMV antigens and nucleic acid when immunocytochemical or in situ hybridization techniques are used. However, clinical-pathologic correlation suggests that this type of CMV infection plays a minor role in causing overt CNS.[76-80] However, it is also clear that some patients manifest more severe CMV encephalitis, with subacute clouding of consciousness, brain stem signs, or seizures.[81-83] The clinical diagnosis in such patients is often difficult. A few features of more severe CMV encephalitis may be helpful in raising suspicion.[81,82,84-88] These include lethargy or somnolence, or focal features including nystagmus, ataxia, or cranial neuropathies. Neuroimaging features may be more distinct in some patients and include periventricular signal change or enhancement related to ependymal infection.[89] Although the CSF of CMV encephalitis is usually indistinguishable from that of ADC, some patients have a polymorphonuclear pleocytosis. Hyponatremia may also develop. When these clinical and laboratory findings are not present, diagnosis using routine studies is difficult. Fortunately, CSF PCR or bDNA detection of CMV sequences appears to provide a useful adjunct and likely is both sensitive and specific.[90-92] Because of the treatment implications (see Chapter 28), CMV PCR of the CSF should be performed when any of the above features are present or if there are other atypical features of patients being evaluated for ADC.

Encephalitis related to herpes simplex virus types 1 (HSV-1) and 2 (HSV-2) also occurs in AIDS patients and may present as a subacute nonfocal or focal encephalopathy, although neither the frequency nor the core of the clinical presentation is clearly defined.[93,94]

AIDS Dementia Complex

ADC is characterized by a triad of cognitive, motor, and behavioral dysfunction.[76,95-98] It is perhaps the most common CNS complication of HIV-1 infection and, if its mild form is included, may eventually afflict the majority of untreated AIDS patients. It is generally a late complication of HIV-1 infection and characteristically manifests during the same phase as the major opportunistic infections and neoplasms that define systemic AIDS, although patients can present with this syndrome before these major systemic complications.[99] Results of larger cohort studies indicate that this syndrome is uncommon in patients who are systemically

well.[100-105] It was the impression of our group that, prior to the widespread use of zidovudine and other antiretroviral treatments, the majority of patients with very low CD4+ T-lymphocyte counts eventually exhibited mild to severe ADC, while an additional number suffered subclinically. Early and widespread use of zidovudine and other antiretrovirals appears to have reduced the prevalence of ADC.[106-108]

TERMINOLOGY AND CLASSIFICATION. The term *AIDS dementia complex* was introduced to describe a cohesive constellation of symptoms and signs rather than an established disease entity of uniform etiopathogenesis.[42,95,96,109,110] Each of the three component terms was included for a defined reason. *AIDS* was included because the morbidity and prognosis of the condition are comparable to those of other clinical AIDS-defining complications of HIV-1 infection. *Dementia* was included because of the acquired and persistent cognitive decline, marked by prominent mental slowing and inattention. The dementia is characteristically unaccompanied by alterations in the level of alertness. The third component, *complex*, was added because the syndrome also, importantly, includes impaired motor performance and, at times, characteristic behavioral changes. Myelopathy and organic psychosis were encompassed within this term, but neither neuropathy nor functional psychiatric disturbance is included.

We have used a five-part staging system for describing the severity of ADC based on functional and motor status for adult patients.[110,111] It provides a common descriptive vocabulary for both clinical and investigative purposes. Although the World Health Organization (WHO) and the American Academy of Neurology (AAN) have introduced new terminologies with certain useful features, including segregation of myelopathy and dementia,[112,113] we have continued to use the AIDS dementia staging scheme in our own studies and clinical practice because of its simplicity and parsimony.

The ADC scheme and the WHO/AAN classification can be cross-translated as outlined in Table 14-4. The WHO/AAN classification introduced the term *HIV-1–associated cognitive/ motor complex* to encompass the full constellation of ADC and added subcategories to refer to patients with predominantly cognitive (HIV-1 associated dementia) or myelopathic (HIV-1– associated myelopathy) presentations of sufficient severity to interfere with work or activities of daily living (hence severe enough to qualify as stage 2 or greater in ADC staging). The term *HIV-associated minor cognitive/motor disorder*

TABLE 14–4. Comparison of AIDS Dementia Complex Staging and WHO/AAN Classifications

AIDS DEMENTIA COMPLEX STAGING	WHO/AAN CLASSIFICATION: HIV-ASSOCIATED COGNITIVE-MOTOR COMPLEX
Stage 0: Normal	
Stage 0.5: Subclinical or Equivocal Minimal or equivocal symptoms Mild (soft) neurologic signs No impairment of work or activities of daily living (ADL)	No corresponding designation
Stage 1: Mild Unequivocal intellectual or motor impairment Able to do all but the more demanding work or ADL	**HIV-1–Associated Minor Cognitive-Motor Disorder** Symptoms: Two of five types in cognitive, motor, behavioral spheres Examination: neurologic or neuropsychological abnormalities Mild impairment of work or ADL
	HIV-Associated Dementia and HIV-Associated Myelopathy
Stage 2: Moderate Cannot work or perform demanding ADL Capable of self-care Ambulatory but may need a single prop	*Mild* Impaired work and ADL Capable of basic self-care Ambulatory but may need a single prop
Stage 3: Severe Major intellectual disability or Cannot walk unassisted	*Moderate* Unable to work or function unassisted or Cannot walk unassisted
Stage 4: End Stage Nearly vegetative Rudimentary cognition Para- or quadriplegic	*Severe* Unable to perform ADL unassisted Confined to bed or wheelchair

was introduced to designate patients with mild symptoms and signs and only minimal functional impairment of work or activities of daily living (stage 1 ADC).

CLINICAL PRESENTATION. The clinical features of ADC are summarized briefly in Table 14–5. Patients' earliest symptoms usually consist of difficulties with concentration and memory. They begin to lose track of their train of thought or conversation. Many complain of "slowness" in thinking. Complex tasks become more difficult and take longer to complete, and memory impairment or difficulty in concentration leads to missed appointments and the need to keep lists of daily chores.

Despite these complaints, early in the evolution of the illness the relatively insensitive bedside mental status examination may be within normal limits; responses may be correct, although they are characteristically slowed. As the condition progresses, however, patients begin to perform poorly on tasks requiring concentration and attention, such as word and digit reversals and subtracting serial 7s. With further worsening a larger array of mental status tests becomes abnormal. Nonetheless, the core difficulty of

slowing, poor attention and concentration remains most prominent. Afflicted individuals also may appear apathetic, with poor insight and indifference to their illness.

Symptoms of motor dysfunction usually lag behind those of intellectual impairment. When

TABLE 14–5. Major Clinical Manifestations of the AIDS Dementia Complex, A Subcortical Dementia Affecting Cognition, Motor Performance, and Behavior

EARLY	LATE
Cognition Inattention Reduced concentration Forgetfulness	Global dementia
Motor Performance Slowed fine and repetitive movements Clumsiness Ataxia	Paraplegia
Behavior Apathy Altered personality (Agitation)	Mutism

present, complaints most often include poor balance or incoordination. Gait difficulty can result in more frequent tripping or falling or a perceived need to exercise new care in walking. Similarly, patients may drop things more frequently or become slower and less precise with normal hand activities, such as eating or writing. However, even when such symptoms are lacking, motor abnormalities can almost always be detected on examination early in the course of the disease. These include slowing of rapid successive and alternating movements of the extremities (e.g., attempts at rapid opposition of index finger and thumb or foot tapping) and impaired ocular smooth pursuits and saccadic eye movements. Abnormal reflexes also may be present, with generalized hyper-reflexia and the development of release signs, such as snout, glabellar, and, less commonly, grasp responses. As the disease evolves, spastic ataxia and, subsequently, leg weakness may limit walking. Patients with an early or predominating spastic-ataxic gait usually have vacuolar myelopathy pathologically. Bladder and bowel incontinence may develop in the later stages of the condition but is uncommon early. At the end stage of ADC, patients are nearly vegetative, lying in bed with a vacant stare, seemingly unaware of their surroundings, unable to ambulate, and incontinent. However, unless intercurrent illness develops, the level of arousal is usually preserved so that they appear awake.

Psychological depression is surprisingly infrequent in these patients, despite the prominence of psychomotor slowing. Patients appear uninterested and lack initiative but are without dysphoria. In a minority, a more agitated organic psychosis may be the presenting or predominant aspect of the illness.[114] Such patients are irritable and hyperactive and may be overtly manic; however, there is always an element of confusion and when their hyperactive state comes under control, the underlying cognitive impairment is evident.

In children, the disorder has the same general features, although the course may vary somewhat and occur in either a progressive or static form.[115-118] The progressive form is characterized by the gradual loss of previously acquired motor skills in conjunction with the evolution of motor abnormalities ranging from spastic paraparesis to quadriplegia with pseudobulbar palsy and rigidity. Acquired microcephaly is almost universal.

NEUROPSYCHOLOGICAL TEST PROFILE. Formal neuropsychological studies quantitatively support the clinical findings of ADC and are, at times, helpful in confirming both the presence and characteristic profile of its cognitive impairment. They are perhaps most useful in longitudinally following the course of disease or response to therapy. In general, the neuropsychological tests most sensitive to ADC include some or all of the following characteristics: performance under time pressure, motor speed, and alternation between two performance rules or stimulus sets.[100,102,111,119,120]

NEUROIMAGING STUDIES. Neuroimaging procedures and CSF examination usually are essential to the evaluation of AIDS patients with CNS dysfunction, including those with ADC. Imaging may be needed to exclude other neurologic conditions that can present with overlapping symptoms and signs, and also shows characteristic, although often unspecific, abnormalities (Table 14−6). These include the nearly universal finding of cerebral atrophy with widened cortical sulci and enlarged ventricles noted on either CT scanning or MRI.[95,121-125] Basal ganglia are also reduced in volume.[126] Additionally, some patients have patchy or diffuse T_2-weighted abnormalities on MRI in the hemispheric white matter and, less commonly, the basal ganglia or thalamus.[122,127-130] Children with AIDS-related dementia often have basal ganglion calcification and atrophy.[131]

CSF. Examination of the CSF in patients with ADC reveals abnormalities in both routine and more specialized tests. However, routine analysis is confounded by the CSF abnormalities described earlier in patients with asymptomatic HIV-1 infection, including HIV-1 isolation or detection of amplified nucleic acid CSF. The likelihood of detecting HIV-1 p24 core antigen in the CSF increases with ADC severity, although free antigen is still a relatively infrequent finding and thus of lower sensitivity diagnostically.[132,133] Among patients with low CD4+ counts, correlation of CSF HIV-1 RNA (detected by quantitative amplification methods) with ADC stage has been reported.[134-136] However, because comparable CSF HIV-1 RNA can also be found in non-ADC patients, including those with higher CD4+ cell counts in which correlation is with the blood RNA level rather than ADC, this measurement is not diagnostically useful in most individual patients. Earlier studies suggested that other CSF surrogate markers that reflect immune activation, including CSF β_2-microglobulin and neopterin, might have some utility. Their concentrations correlate with the presence and severity of ADC, although they are also elevated by opportunistic infections and other CNS diseases.[137-140] These mark-

TABLE 14–6. Some Comparative Features of Major CNS Processes in AIDS

	CLINICAL FEATURES				NEUROIMAGING FEATURES		
	Temporal Profile	Level of Alertness	Fever	No. of Lesions	Type of Lesions	Location of Lesions
Cerebral toxoplasmosis	Days	Reduced	Common	Multiple	Mass effect; spherical ring enhancing; eccentric target sign	Basal ganglia, cortex
Primary CNS lymphoma	Days to weeks	Variable	Absent	One or few	Mass effect; irregular; weakly enhancing	Often periventricular with subependymal spread, white matter
Progressive multifocal leukoencephalopathy (PML)	Weeks	Preserved	Absent	Multiple	No mass effect; nonenhancing; white on T_2, black on T_1 MRI	White matter, usually subcortical involving U-fibers
AIDS dementia complex	Weeks to months	Preserved	Absent	None, diffuse, or multiple	Cerebral atrophy; fluffy or diffuse T_2 signal, no mass effect or enhancement	Central white matter (sparing U-fibers), basal ganglia
CMV encephalitis	Days to weeks	Reduced	Common	Few	Small; T_2 signal enhancement	Ventricular ependyma, small cortical
Cryptococcal meningitis	Days	Variable	Common	Variable	Dilated perivascular spaces	Basal ganglia

ers may be helpful in cases where there is the need to distinguish mild ADC from psychiatric disease. Although it assesses a "parallel compartment" rather than the brain itself, quantitative assessment of CSF HIV-1 RNA may eventually have a role in evaluating the virologic response in the CNS.[141]

NEUROPATHOLOGY. Histologic abnormalities in demented AIDS patients are most prominent in the subcortical structures, and the findings on routine examination can be segregated into three seemingly discontinuous but overlapping sets: (1) gliosis and diffuse white matter pallor, (2) multinucleated-cell encephalitis, and (3) vacuolar myelopathy. A less common additional finding is diffuse or focal spongiform change of the cerebral white matter.[76,77,142–144] The most common of these abnormalities is the central gliosis (including astrocytosis and microgliocytosis) and accompanying diffuse white matter pallor that, in isolation, correlate with milder ADC. Inflammation is otherwise scant, consisting of a few perivascular lymphocytes and brown-pigmented macrophages. The blood–brain barrier is also abnormal in many of these brains.[130]

Multinucleated cells characteristically are found in patients with more severe clinical disease.[76,145] The multinucleated cells derive from fusion of HIV-1–infected macrophages and microglia and are accompanied by neighboring macrophage and microglial reaction, along with local edema and white matter rarefaction. They are concentrated most often in the white matter and deep gray structures. It is in these severe cases that neuronal changes have most frequently been detected, including both selected loss of cortical neurons and alterations in their dendritic structures.[146]

Although inflammation with multinucleated cells also may occur in the spinal cord, in our experience, vacuolar myelopathy is more common.[147] The latter pathologically resembles subacute combined degeneration resulting from vitamin B_{12} deficiency, but levels of this vitamin generally are normal in serum. Although there is a general correlation between the incidence of vacuolar myelopathy and the other pathologic abnormalities found in the brain, the myelopathy can occur in the absence of the multinucleated cells and, indeed, does not appear to correlate with local productive HIV-1 infection.[148–151]

ETIOLOGY AND PATHOGENESIS. Evidence from a variety of studies supports a primary role for HIV-1 in ADC.[3,42,152,153] There is also near-consensus that macrophages and microglia, along with multinucleated cells derived from these two cell types, are the principal participants in *productive* infection. Recent observations using combined PCR amplification in concert with in situ localization and other techniques to detect expression of nonstructural viral gene products suggest that other cell types in the brain, including particularly astrocytes and vascular endothelial cells and, less securely, neurons, may also be infected, although without the capacity to produce progeny virus.[154–156] This is consistent with cell culture studies that have demonstrated low-level infection of astrocytic and other neuroectodermal cells and cell lines, usually involving a non-CD4 virus–cell interaction. The recently characterized group of secondary cell receptors, members of the chemokine receptor family, may be important in infection of these cells.

Because brain infection alone does not readily explain brain injury, leading hypotheses regarding the links between infection and ADC center on an intermediary role for cytokines and endogenous neurotoxic pathways (for reviews, see Gendelman et al.,[3] Price,[43] Lipton and Gendelman,[153] and Wesselingh et al.[157]). This linkage is supported by studies of CSF, autopsied brain and cell culture model systems. These studies have identified a number of viral gene products that might act as signal molecules initiating pathology. Most attention in this regard has centered on the viral envelope glycoprotein gp120 as the predominant molecule, although there have also been studies implicating gp41 and the viral *tat* and *nef* gene products. Putative intermediates in the pathway have included tumor necrosis factor-α, nitric oxide, and quinolinic acid, among others. The *N*-methyl-D-aspartate glutamine receptor and its effect on intracellular calcium metabolism may provide a common neuropathogenic pathway. The potential importance of understanding these mechanisms is that they may provide targets for therapeutic intervention, so-called adjuvant therapies.[96] In fact, this strategy is currently being pursued in clinical trials.

Variation in the genetic and phenotypic character of the infecting virus has received most attention as a possible explanation of why individual patients do or do not develop ADC. A number of studies have established that virus isolates (identified by culture or by PCR amplification and direct cloning) share the biologic property of "macrophage tropism" and more recently of CCR5 chemokine receptor utilization; studies also indicate that brain infection in ADC patients may be compartmentalized, with genetically different predominant populations found in brain (and CSF) compared to blood.[158–164] What was initially hypothesized as neurotropism (enhanced capacity to infect the nervous system) involves as a minimum the capacity to infect macrophages and microglia, which, in turn, relates to chemokine receptor utilization. Whether or not there are other properties that more specifically define neurotropism, neurovirulence (capacity to damage the nervous system), or neurotoxicity (elaboration of directly or indirectly toxic gene products) is currently less clear but under study both in patients and in animal models, including the primate models of simian immunodeficiency virus.[165]

TREATMENT. Although the adjuvant strategies mentioned above aimed at inhibiting secondary neurotoxic pathways are theoretically attractive, there is no established evidence of an effective intervention of this type. Rather, the main approach to treatment is antiviral therapy. Unfortunately, the optimum regimen for ADC is not established, largely because this issue has not been directly addressed with respect to contemporary combination therapy. In fact, evidence of antiviral efficacy derives principally from earlier experience with zidovudine monotherapy, which has been shown in a number of adult and pediatric studies to prevent and reverse clinically symptomatic ADC and also to reduce the incidence of brain infection.[166–173] However, in the absence of direct testing, it seems reasonable to extrapolate to the likelihood that combination therapy would be even more effective in treating ADC than monotherapy. This inference is now supported by uncontrolled studies and anecdotal observations.[108,174]

An additional issue relates to the antiviral drug penetration into the brain, across the blood–brain barrier. At present the necessity of such penetration is not known. Although it seems reasonable that antiviral drugs should reach the site of brain infection, there are reports of neurologic improvement of patients treated with protease inhibitors, which penetrate the blood–brain barrier poorly.[108] Given this uncertainty as well as the limited information on penetration of some of the antiviral drugs, I have recommended the following empirical approach: (1) ADC patients should be treated with aggressive antiretroviral therapy; (2) combinations of three, four, or more drugs should usually be used, (3) these drugs should be chosen first on the basis of whether they are likely to be effective in suppressing systemic infection in the individual patient (particularly that the patient's predominating viral quasispecies is un-

likely to be resistant to the component drugs) and second that they also will be practically tolerated by the patient, and (4) to include, if possible, two drugs with appreciable penetration of the blood–brain barrier. Among the nucleoside reverse transcriptase inhibitors, zidovudine, stavudine, and abacavir likely have the best penetration, and lamivudine penetrates to a lesser extent.[175–177] Nevirapine, a non-nucleoside reverse transcriptase inhibitor, also has favorable penetration. Among the protease inhibitors, only indinavir has been reported to appreciably penetrate into CSF.[178] More precise definition of the penetration of these and other drugs is likely to be available in the near future.

FOCAL BRAIN DISEASES

A number of focal brain disorders can afflict AIDS patients (Table 14–7). Evaluation of these conditions begins with the recognition of their focal nature along with associated background systemic symptoms and signs (e.g., fever, headache). Because these disorders have a high frequency, initial evaluation most often focuses on distinguishing the three most common causes of focal brain disease: cerebral toxoplasmosis, primary CNS lymphoma, and progressive multifocal leukoencephalopathy (PML) (see Chapter 25 for discussion of some of these). The diagnostic approach includes neuroradiologic characterization, analysis of CSF in some cases, therapeutic trial in others, and brain biopsy in the remaining few.

The temporal profile of the onset and evolution of these focal brain disorders is an important aspect of their clinical presentation and both guides the approach and influences the proba-

---

TABLE 14–7. Focal Brain Disease Complicating HIV-1 Disease

Acute
Vascular disorders
Seizures*

Subacute
Cerebral toxoplasmosis
Primary CNS lymphoma (PCNSL)
Progressive multifocal leukoencephalopathy (PML)
Tuberculous brain abscess (*Mycobacterium tuberculosis*)
Cryptococcoma
Varicella-zoster virus encephalitis
Herpes encephalitis

---

*Secondary to subacute focal (macroscopic) disorders or to nonfocal (microscopic or toxic-metabolic) processes.

bilities of different diagnoses. An abrupt onset suggests either a vascular cause or seizure. AIDS patients may suffer transient ischemia or even stroke, leaving residual brain injury.[179-181] Fortunately, most have a benign outcome. Seizures may be related to HIV-1 infection (ADC) or to focal opportunistic infections and neoplasms. Careful clinical and neuroimaging investigations are warranted to evaluate such patients for underlying focal diseases.[182-186]

However, the three most common focal disorders all characteristically have a subacute or more indolent onset and evolve over days or, at times, weeks. Of these, cerebral toxoplasmosis characteristically progresses most rapidly (days) and PML most slowly (weeks), whereas primary CNS lymphoma lies somewhere between. A comparison of some of the major clinical and neuroradiologic features of the common CNS complications of AIDS is outlined in Table 14-6. However, although these group differences in the associated findings help to distinguish the three major focal disorders, each may cause similar neurologic deficits, and the presentations of individual cases overlap clinically. Patients with toxoplasmosis commonly present with a combination of focal deficits and a generalized encephalopathy that includes confusion or clouding of consciousness[75,187] (Chapter 25). This contrasts with the patient with PML, at least at the onset, in whom focal neurologic deficits are unaccompanied by either diffuse brain dysfunction or evidence of a systemic toxic state. Primary CNS lymphoma, when accompanied by significant mass effect or when located deep in the frontal or periventricular region, can cause more global mental dysfunction. Cryptococcoma is usually a complication of cryptococcal meningitis, albeit a rare one, but may also occur in isolation, making diagnosis difficult.[52,188] We have encountered several patients with an unusual focally invasive encephalitis presenting with seizures and focal hemispheric dysfunction in the setting of treated cryptococcal meningitis in which the cryptococcal antigen in the CSF was low.[189]

In patients with focal disease, neuroimaging, particularly MRI, is critical both to confirm the presence of macroscopic focal disease and to determine the morphology and character of the "lesion." Of the three most common diseases, two—toxoplasmosis and lymphoma—cause mass lesions with local edema and variable contrast enhancement, whereas the third, PML, does not induce mass effect. Multiple lesions involving the cortex or deep brain nuclei (thalamus, basal ganglia) with mass effect and surrounded by edema strongly favor cerebral toxoplasmosis. Toxoplasmic abscesses characteristically exhibit "ring-like" contrast enhancement on CT scans or MRI, and they may have what is called an "eccentric target sign"—a small, contrast-enhancing spot that is off-center and may touch the surrounding ring. However, rarely, either homogeneously enhancing or nonenhancing hypodense lesions may be noted. In general, MRI is the preferred modality for more clearly detecting and defining the multiple spherical lesions characteristic of the disease. Only rarely is the CT scan normal in the face of fulminant microscopic encephalitis.[75,190]

Primary CNS lymphomas of B-cell origin are opportunistic neoplasms that complicated the course of AIDS in approximately 5% of patients earlier in the epidemic[62,105,191-196] (see Chapter 30). Patients with primary brain lymphomas present with progressive focal or multifocal neurologic deficits similar to those seen with toxoplasmosis, although the tempo of disease evolution is often slower. Neuroradiologic studies are usually sensitive in detecting primary brain lymphomas, and attention to their appearance may be helpful in suggesting this diagnosis over toxoplasmosis. Characteristically, these tumors are multicentric at autopsy but often show only one or two lesions on CT or MRI. Their location is usually deep in the brain in proximity to the lateral ventricles, where they show a characteristic spread under the ependymal lining. Likewise, they occur more often in the white rather than gray matter and may extend into the corpus callosum. On CT they may enhance only weakly after contrast administration; again, MRI is more sensitive and more often shows contrast uptake. Functional neuroimaging using single-photon emission CT or positron emission tomography to examine blood flow or glucose utilization has been shown to distinguish primary CNS lymphoma ("hot" with local isotope uptake by the lesion) from toxoplasmosis lesions ("cold" on these tests) in many patients; however, because these studies provide only a small extra margin of diagnostic information and, in the case of lymphoma, do not substitute for pathologic or etiologic diagnosis, I suspect that their utility will remain limited, although this is not the opinion of a number of investigators.[197-200]

Nonimaging studies and individual background risk are also important diagnostic variables. Toxoplasma serology is particularly helpful in distinguishing among causes of focal brain lesions with mass effect. Because cerebral toxoplasmosis almost always results from reactivation of previously acquired and dormant infection, patients with cerebral toxoplasmosis characteristically have positive serum immunoglobulin G antibodies.[75,187,201] Although group analysis may show higher risk of toxoplasmosis in those patients with higher levels of serum antibodies, it is also important to appreciate that individual patients with cerebral toxoplasmosis can manifest low titers (occasionally, an apparently negative titer will be positive when a more concentrated specimen such as a 1:4 dilution is tested). Moreover, antibody titers usually do not rise during the early course of the illness. Thus a positive titer indicates susceptibility, and a true negative titer casts doubt on the diagnosis and points to the likelihood of another condition.

More recently, PCR amplification of nucleic acid in CSF has shown utility in diagnosis of focal CNS lesions. Initial studies suggest that detection of Epstein-Barr virus (EBV) sequences in CSF may be particularly helpful in diagnosis of primary CNS lymphoma. Detection of EBV nucleic acid has been reported to exhibit excellent specificity and sensitivity in this setting.[202] If this is borne out by broader, community-based experience, this approach will likely obviate the necessity for brain biopsy in many cases.

Earlier in the AIDS epidemic, cerebral toxoplasmosis was the most common cause of focal brain disease in the developed world, manifesting eventually in 5% to 15% of AIDS patients, and the one that was considered "most treatable." This reason, in concert with the rapid response to therapy, underlay the general policy of subjecting all patients with cerebral focal mass lesions (and some without mass effect) to a trial of antitoxoplasma therapy. However, the diminishing relative frequency of cerebral toxoplasmosis following the widespread use of trimethoprim-sulfamethoxazole prophylaxis and, more particularly, refinements of diagnosis have reduced the justification of this treatment as a universal approach. When applied indiscriminately, this approach results in a delay in treatment of CNS lymphoma that likely compromises outcome. These considerations indicate that the initial management of cerebral mass lesions should be more selective, and we now advocate consideration of early biopsy in some patients without a preceding trial of antitoxoplasma therapy. Candidates for early biopsy include patients with negative antitoxoplasma blood serology results and those with MRI abnormalities highly suggestive of lymphoma as described above. A history of adherence to trimethoprim-sulfamethoxazole prophylaxis also raises the probability of another diagnosis. Moreover, in some patients biopsy may not be needed for diagnosis of lymphoma at a level of certainty justifying radiation therapy; if EBV PCR in the CSF proves to be sufficiently specific for this diagnosis, it may replace biopsy in many patients. These issues are addressed in detail along with supporting data by Antinori and colleagues.[202]

In those patients who undergo a diagnostic trial of antitoxoplasma therapy, corticosteroids should be avoided when possible. Because primary CNS lymphoma may respond symptomatically to corticosteroids alone, clinical or neuroimaging improvement on a combination antibiotic–steroid treatment is difficult to interpret. More generally, corticosteroids intensify the impairment of immune defenses in AIDS patients, potentially worsening not only toxoplasmosis but also other systemic opportunistic infections. However, if cerebral edema threatens to result in brain herniation, judicious short-term corticosteroid therapy may be instituted along with appropriate specific therapy and subsequently tapered rapidly once the patient improves.

PML can usually be distinguished from cerebral toxoplasmosis and lymphoma by neuroimaging. This is an opportunistic infection caused by a human papovavirus, JC virus.[203–206] Before effective antiretroviral therapy, it developed in approximately 4% of AIDS patients, and in some was the presenting illness. The incidence is likely lower now, although the condition certainly has not disappeared. Pathologically, it is distinguished by selective white matter destruction. Clinical evolution usually is more protracted than that of either toxoplasmosis or CNS lymphoma, and altered consciousness related to brain swelling is not a usual feature. Until recently, definitive diagnosis required brain biopsy or autopsy. However, the combination of "hard" focal clinical deficits with corresponding white matter lesions (white on T_2- and black on T_1-weighted images) without mass effect and usually without contrast enhancement on MRI is often sufficient to make the diagnosis with reasonable certainty (Table 14–6). More definitive diagnosis can be established either by PCR amplification of JC virus DNA in CSF, or brain biopsy, with the former obviously being less invasive although only about 85% sensitive.[202,207–209] There is no proven effective therapy for the disease. Although anecdotal experience had suggested that cytosine arabinoside might be helpful in some patients,[210] this was not supported by a controlled trial.[211]

Spontaneous remission of PML in AIDS patients had been clearly documented before the advent of HAART[212]and likely is more common in the face of this treatment of HIV-1.[213-217] Berger and colleagues have recently reviewed the natural history and prognostic factors influencing the course of PML in patients with HIV-1 infection.[218,219] Experimental therapies now under study include cidofovir and topotecan and are supported by in vitro observations and scattered anecdotal reports.

Although unusual, varicella-zoster virus (VZV) and, to a lesser extent, HSV-1 and HSV-2 have been reported as causes of brain disease in AIDS patients. VZV infections are of at least three types, and are sometimes admixed[220]: (1) multifocal direct brain infection affecting principally the white matter and partially mimicking PML[221-223]; (2) cerebral vasculitis, which characteristically follows ophthalmic herpes zoster and causes contralateral hemiplegia, but may occur after zoster in other locations and be more widespread in the brain[224,225]; and (3) myelopathy complicating herpes zoster with both vasculitic and parenchymal elements.[226] These may occur temporally remote from or in the absence of cutaneous herpes zoster. Both HSV-1 and HSV-2 have been identified in the brains of some AIDS patients,[93,94] but the clinical correlates of these infections in AIDS patients have not been wholly delineated.

MYELOPATHIES

Myelopathies complicating HIV-1–infected individuals can be classified into segmental and diffuse forms (Table 14–8). The segmental forms tend to follow an acute or subacute time course and are relatively rare. VZV, toxoplasmosis, and spinal epidural or intradural lymphoma may all give a clinical picture of partial or complete transverse myelitis.[226-230] In addition, CMV polyradiculopathy may also involve the spinal cord in a segmental manner, typically evolving over a number of weeks.[231,232] Combined CMV and HSV infection of the spinal cord has been described, although antemortem recognition may be exceptionally difficult.[233]

The more slowly progressive vacuolar myelopathy is far more common.[147,148,151] Usually, it is accompanied by varying degrees of cognitive and upper extremity affliction, and has therefore been included under the umbrella of ADC, discussed previously. In some patients, however, it occurs in relative isolation or with a marked preponderance. These patients exhibit progressive, painless gait disturbance with ataxia and spasticity. Bladder and bowel difficulties usually become significant only after considerable gait symptoms appear, and sensory disturbance is less conspicuous unless there is concomitant neuropathy. Patients do not usually manifest a distinct sensory or motor level as in patients with transverse myelopathy. Even in those patients with seemingly isolated lower extremity symptoms, examination usually reveals some evidence of disturbance higher in the neuraxis, including, most often, slowed rapid alternating finger movements and hyperactive deep tendon reflexes, including the jaw jerk. In typical cases, we do not recommend either spinal MRI or myelography, because both are usually negative in vacuolar myelopathy. These studies are needed only if there is question of another type of myelopathy, usually one with segmental features.

Human T-cell lymphotropic virus types I and II (HTLV-I, HTLV-II) can also cause "diffuse" myelopathy in the same population that is at high risk for HIV-1 infection.[234,235] This relates principally to the convergent epidemiologies of these viruses, which can be spread by intravenous drug use and sexual contact. Clinically, these myelopathies are similar to vacuolar myelopathy in not exhibiting a distinct segmental level, although spasticity may be more prominent. Diagnosis is suspected when positive HTLV-I/II serology is present.[236-240]

TABLE 14–8. Myelopathies Complicating HIV-1 Infection

Segmental (Focal), Acute or Subacute

Transverse Myelitis
Varicella-zoster virus (herpes zoster) myelopathy
Spinal epidural or intradural lymphoma
Toxoplasmosis

With Polyradiculopathy
Cytomegalovirus (CMV)

Subacute or Chronic, Progressive, and Diffuse Form
Vacuolar myelopathy (part of ADC)
HTLV-I–associated myelopathies

PERIPHERAL NEUROPATHIES

Peripheral neuropathies of several types can complicate the various stages of HIV-1 infection (Table 14–9) (for reviews, see Simpson and Tagliati,[17] Cornblath,[19] Fuller et al.,[241] and Griffin et al.[242]). Those occurring in the acute and

TABLE 14–9. Peripheral Neuropathies Complicating HIV-1 Infection

Acute or Seroconversion Phase of Systemic HIV-1 Infection
Mononeuritides, brachial plexopathy
Acute demyelinating polyneuropathy

Clinical Latent ("Asymptomatic") and Transitional Phases (CD4+ T Lymphocytes >200/mm³)
Herpes zoster neuropathy
Acute demyelinating polyneuropathy (Guillain-Barré syndrome)
Chronic inflammatory demyelinating polyneuropathy (CIDP)
Mononeuritis multiplex, "benign" type
Diffuse infiltrative lymphocytosis syndrom (DILS)–associated neuropathy

Late Phase (<200 CD4+ Cells)
Predominantly sensory polyneuropathy
Nucleoside (ddC, ddI, d4T) toxicity
Autonomic neuropathy
CMV polyradiculopathy
CMV mononeuritis multiplex, severe type
Cranial mononeuropathies associated with aseptic meningitis
Mononeuropathies-radiculopathies secondary to lymphomatous meningitis

latent phases of infection have been discussed previously. The latter can also manifest in those with more advanced disease as the CD4 cell counts fall to the 200 cells/mm³ range. Other neuropathies during the transitional phase include herpes zoster, usually readily diagnosed by the rash, although sometimes after a delay of several days, and one type of mononeuritis multiplex that, although unusual, is important to recognize.[243,244] It appears to have a benign outcome and may have an autoimmune, vasculitic pathogenesis. It is distinguished from the more severe mononeuritis multiplex by the stage of systemic infection and involvement of only a few nerves. It appears to remit spontaneously; whether or not intravenous immunoglobulin, plasma exchange, or other measures speed recovery is uncertain.

The second form of mononeuritis multiplex occurs later in the course of systemic HIV-1 infection when CD4+ counts are lower and is more aggressive, leading to progressive paralysis and death in some patients. It is caused by multifocal CMV nerve infection.[21,84,243–245] Because definitive diagnosis is difficult, suspicion of this neuropathy should lead to empirical anti-CMV therapy unless another etiology is proven (Chapter 28). CMV also causes another unusual but also therapeutically very important neuro-

pathic syndrome—severe ascending polyradiculopathy. This usually begins with painful involvement of lumbosacral roots and progresses rostrally with loss of sensory, motor, and autonomic functions.[231,246,247] The characteristic polymorphonuclear CSF pleocytosis is helpful in diagnosis because this type of cell reaction is unusual in any other AIDS-related complication, particularly with this clinical presentation. Thickened spinal roots can be seen by myelography or spinal MRI, which also shows contrast enhancement of the roots. Although CMV can be cultured from the CSF of these patients, this usually takes several days and should not delay therapy. PCR detection of CMV DNA in CSF may accelerate diagnosis but also often takes a few days. As a result, clinical diagnosis should lead to rapid institution of anti-CMV therapy.

The most common neuropathy in AIDS patients is a distal, predominantly sensory polyneuropathy (DSPN) which may eventually afflict a majority.[18,105,248–250] This is an axonal neuropathy, and, although suspected to relate in some fundamental way to HIV-1, its etiology and pathogenesis remain unknown. HIV-1 infection has only occasionally been identified in peripheral nerves, and then only in macrophages.[48,250–252] The most favored explanation of pathogenesis parallels that proposed for ADC and involves cytokine-mediated neurotoxicity.[249] Afflicted patients complain of burning or painful dysesthesia of the feet. Most often this is mild and tolerable, but in a minority the pain is severe enough to preclude walking. Pain and paresthesias usually begin on the underside of the toes or ball of the foot and ascend symmetrically in a circumferential, "stocking" distribution. When they extend to or above the ankle, similar sensations may also manifest in the fingers. Sensory symptoms usually far exceed either sensory or motor dysfunction, and thus walking is altered because of discomfort rather than by sensory ataxia. Although this has not been addressed since the advent of HAART, this neuropathy does not appear to improve with treatment of HIV-1 infection. As a result, therapy now relies on symptom management. The mainstays of pain suppression are tricyclic antidepressants and gabapentin, with judicious use of narcotic analgesics in severe cases.

A second type of sensory neuropathy that may be difficult to distinguish from this HIV-1–associated DSPN is the toxic axonal neuropathy caused by some of the antiretroviral nucleosides, including (in order of incidence) zalcitabine (ddC), didanosine (ddI), and stavudine (d4T)—the so-called "d" drugs.[253–259] These dose-related axonal neuropathies may present initially with either "aching" or "bruise-like" discomfort of the feet or the more typical dysesthesias described above. They are thought to relate to a toxic effect of these drugs on neuronal mitochondrion DNA polymerase. Unfortunately, laboratory tests, including electromyography, are not usually helpful in distinguishing this from HIV-related DSPN, and the clinician must rely on the clinical setting, including onset within weeks or a few months of starting the drugs and remission when the drugs are stopped. If recognized early, the toxic neuropathies are reversible; however, improvement may not begin for several weeks.

Autonomic neuropathy of varying severity has also been reported in AIDS patients.[21,260,261] This may accompany sensory neuropathy, suggesting a common pathogenesis, but in some cases the severity of autonomic and sensory dysfunction diverges. The clinical features of the former range from mild positional hypotension to cardiovascular collapse during invasive procedures. In addition, autonomic neuropathy may contribute to chronic diarrhea in some HIV-1–infected individuals.[262]

MYOPATHIES

Myopathies can occur at several stages of HIV-1 infection (Table 14–10) but are less common and less well characterized than the neuropathies.[17,251,263–267] A wide range of presentations, from asymptomatic creatine kinase elevation to progressive severe proximal weakness, has been reported. A polymyositis- or dermatomyositis-like illness has been described in AIDS patients, and, although the pathogenesis is not proven, local HIV-1 infection or autoimmunity has been suspected. Although HIV-1 antigens have been reported in the inflammatory cells, these are usually scant and have not been detected in myocytes.[264]

Zidovudine therapy can also cause myopathy affecting proximal muscles, especially of the legs.[17,265,268–271] In many of these patients, abnormalities of mitochondria are found in muscle

biopsy specimens. Because it is dose-related, this syndrome now seems much less common than several years ago. When zidovudine therapy is discontinued, there is clinical and laboratory improvement.

CONCLUSION

As with other aspects of AIDS, precise diagnosis is important in patients with neurologic symptoms or signs, because an increasing number of these disorders can be treated, resulting in relief of morbidity or prevention of death. Too often, we have seen physicians give up prematurely on patients because of their despair over reversing neurologic impairment before this is objectively justified by an established diagnosis and prognosis, particularly when patients have not had the full benefit of antiretroviral therapy. The approach to diagnosis and management of the neurologic complications of HIV-1 infection and AIDS follows that used in general neurologic practice, but with an important difference that relates to the altered probabilities of differential diagnosis in this group of patients, whose vulnerabilities to opportunistic and HIV-1–related neurologic diseases far overshadow the background incidence of ordinary neurologic diseases. With the diagnosis of underlying HIV-1 infection and an understanding of its systemic state, the neurologic history establishes the temporal profile of the neurologic disease and usually provides an initial impression of anatomic localization. The neurologic examination refines this localization and uncovers additional, including asymptomatic, abnormalities. Neuroimaging studies using CT or MRI and, less commonly, angiography add further precision to anatomic localization and narrow the range of possible underlying pathologic processes. Electrodiagnosis using electromyography can be helpful in delineating and localizing physiologic nerve or muscle dysfunction. Examination of CSF provides a direct view of inflammatory reactions in the meninges and, with the expansion of PCR testing, can now be used for definitive diagnosis of some of the major organisms or neoplasms afflicting the CNS. Therapeutic trial and tissue biopsy may be needed for exact diagnosis in some instances. These evaluations, pursued with a background understanding of the spectrum of neurologic disorders affecting these patients, allow accurate neurologic diagnosis in the great majority of patients.

TABLE 14–10. Myopathies Complicating HIV-1 Infection

Inflammatory myopathy (polymyositis)
Noninflammatory myopathies
Toxic myopathy: zidovudine therapy

References

1. Price R: Neurological complications of HIV infection. Lancet 348:445, 1996
2. Berger JR, Levy RM. (eds): AIDS & the Nervous System, 2nd ed. Philadelphia, Lippincott-Raven, 1997
3. Gendelman HE, Lipton SA, Epstein L, Swindells S: The Neurology of AIDS. New York, Chapman & Hall, 1998
4. Brew B, Tindall B: Neurological manifestations of primary human immunodeficiency virus-1 infection. In Berger J, Levy R (eds): AIDS and the Nervous System, 2nd ed. Philadelphia, Lippincott-Raven, 1997, p 517
5. Tindall B, Cooper D: Primary HIV infection: Host responses and intervention strategies. AIDS 5:1, 1991
6. Brew B, Perdices M, Darveniza P, et al: The neurological features of early and 'latent' human immunodeficiency virus infection. Aust N Z J Med 19:700, 1989
7. Ho D, Sarngadhara M, Resnick L, et al: Primary human T lymphotropic virus type III infection. Ann Intern Med 103:880, 1985
8. Denning D, Anderson J, Rudge P, et al: Acute myelopathy associated with primary infection with human immunodeficiency virus. Br Med J 294:143, 1987
9. Piette A, Tusseau F, Vignon D, et al: Letter to the editor. Acute neuropathy coincident with seroconversion for anti-LAV/HTLV-III. Lancet 1:852, 1986
10. Wiselka M, Nicholson K, Ward S, Flower A: Acute infection with human immunodeficiency virus associated with facial nerve palsy and neuralgia. J Infect 15:189, 1987
11. Hagberg L, Malmval B, Svennerholm L, et al: Guillain-Barre syndrome as an early manifestation of HIV central nervous system infection. Scand J Infect Dis 18:591, 1987
12. Carne C, Smith A, Elkington S, et al: Acute encephalopathy coincident with seroconversion for anti HTLV-III. Lancet 2:1206, 1985
13. Calabrese L, Proffitt M, Levin K, et al: Acute infection with the human immunodeficiency virus (HIV) associated with acute brachial neuritis and exanthematous rash. Ann Intern Med 107:849, 1987
14. Clark SJ, Saag MS, Decker WD, et al: High titers of cytopathic virus in plasma of patients with symptomatic primary HIV-1 infection. N Engl J of Med 324:954, 1991
15. Gaines H, von Sydow M, Pehrson PO, Lundbergh P: Clinical picture of primary HIV-1 infection presenting as a glandular-fever-like illness. Lancet 297:1363, 1988
16. Rabeneck L, Popovic M, Gartner S, et al: Acute HIV-1 infection presenting with painful swallowing and esophageal ulcers. JAMA 263:2318, 1990
17. Simpson D, Tagliati M: Neuromuscular syndromes in human immunodeficiency virus disease. In Berger J, Levy R (eds): AIDS and the Nervous System, 2nd ed. Philadelphia, Lippincott-Raven, 1997, p 189
18. Cornblath D, McArthur J: Predominantly sensory neuropathy in patients with AIDS and AIDS-related complex. Neurology 38:794, 1988
19. Cornblath D: Treatment of the neuromuscular complications of human immunodeficiency virus infection. Ann Neurol 23(Suppl):S88, 1988
20. Cornblath D, Chaudhry V, Griffin J: Treatment of chronic inflammatory demyelinating polyneuropathy with intravenous immunoglobin. Ann Neurol 30:104, 1991
21. Simpson DM, Olney RK: Peripheral neuropathies associated with human immunodeficiency virus infection [review]. Neurol Clin 10:685, 1992
22. Moulignier A, Authier FJ, Baudrimont M, et al: Peripheral neuropathy in human immunodeficiency virus-infected patients with the diffuse infiltrative lymphocytosis syndrome. Ann Neurol 41:438, 1997
23. Gherardi RK, Chraetien F, Delfau-Larue MH, et al: Neuropathy in diffuse infiltrative lymphocytosis syndrome: An HIV neuropathy, not a lymphoma [see comments]. Neurology 50:1041, 1998
24. Price R: Commentary: Neuropathy complicating diffuse infiltrative lymphocytosis. Lancet 352:592, 1998
25. Bradley WG, Verma A: Painful vasculitic neuropathy in HIV-1 infection: Relief of pain with prednisone therapy. Neurology 47:1446, 1996
26. Berger J, Sheremata W, Resnick L, et al: Multiple sclerosis-like leukoencephalopathy revealing human immunodeficiency virus infection. Neurology 39:324, 1989
27. Gray F, Chimelli L, Mohr M, et al: Fulminating multiple sclerosis-like leukoencephalopathy revealing human immunodeficiency virus infection. Neurology 41:105, 1991
28. Berger JR, Tornatore C, Major EO, et al: Relapsing and remitting human immunodeficiency virus-associated leukoencephalomyelopathy. Ann Neurol 31:34, 1992
29. Resnick L, diMarzo-Veronese F, Schupbach J, et al: Intra-blood-brain-barrier synthesis of HTLV-III-specific IgG in patients with neurologic symptoms associated with AIDS or AIDS-related complex. N Engl J Med 313:1498, 1985
30. Resnick L, Berger J, Shapshak P, Tourtellotte W: Early penetration of the blood-brain-barrier by HIV. Neurology 38:9, 1988
31. Goudsmit J, Wolters E, Bakker M, et al: Intrathecal synthesis of antibodies to HTLV-III in patients without AIDS or AIDS related complex. Br Med J 292:1231, 1986
32. Appleman M, Marshall D, Brey R, et al: Cerebrospinal fluid abnormalities in patients without AIDS who are seropositive for the human immunodeficiency virus. J Infect Dis 158:193, 1988
33. Marshall D, Brey R, Cahill W, et al: Spectrum of cerebrospinal fluid findings in various stages of human immunodeficiency virus infection. Arch Neurol 45:954, 1988
34. McArthur J, Cohen B, Farzadegan H, et al: Cerebrospinal fluid abnormalities in homosexual men with and without neuropsychiatric findings. Ann Neurol 23(Suppl):S34, 1988
35. Elovaara I, Nykyri E, Poutiainen E, et al: CSF follow-up in HIV-1 infection: Intrathecal production of HIV-specific and unspecific IGG, and beta-2-microglobulin increase with duration of HIV-1 infection. Acta Neurol Scand 87:388, 1993
36. Van Wielink G, McArthur JC, Moench T, et al: Intrathecal synthesis of anti-HIV IgG: Correlation with increasing duration of HIV-1 infection. Neurology 40:816, 1990
37. Rolfs A, Schumacher HC: Early findings in the cerebrospinal fluid of patients with HIV-1 infection of the central nervous system [letter]. N Engl J Med 323:418, 1990
38. Ellis RJ, Hsia K, Spector SA, et al: Cerebrospinal fluid human immunodeficiency virus type 1 RNA levels are elevated in neurocognitively impaired individuals with acquired immunodeficiency syndrome: HIV

Neurobehavioral Research Center Group [see comments]. Ann Neurol 42:679, 1997

39. McArthur JC, McClernon DR, Cronin MF, et al: Relationship between human immunodeficiency virus-associated dementia and viral load in cerebrospinal fluid and brain [see comments]. Ann Neurol 42:689, 1997

40. Conrad A, Schmid P, Syndulko K, et al: Quantifying HIV-1 RNA using the polymerase chain reaction on cerebrospinal fluid and serum of seropositive individuals with and without neurologic abnormalities. J Acquir Immune Defic Syndr Hum Retrovirol 10:425, 1995

41. Davis LE, Hjelle BL, Miller VE, et al: Early viral brain invasion in iatrogenic human immunodeficiency virus infection. Neurology 42:1736, 1992

42. Price R, Brew B, Sidtis J, et al: The brain in AIDS: Central nervous system HIV-1 infection and AIDS dementia complex. Science 239:586, 1988

43. Price R: The cellular basis of central nervous system HIV-1 infection and the AIDS dementia complex: Introduction. J Neuro-AIDS 1:1, 1995

44. Price RW, Staprans S: Measuring the "viral load" in cerebrospinal fluid in human immunodeficiency virus infection: Window into brain infection? [editorial; comment]. Ann Neurol 42:675, 1997

45. Goldstein J: Headache and acquired immunodeficiency syndrome. Neurol Clin 8:947, 1990

46. Lipton RB, Feraru ER, Weiss G, et al: Headache in HIV-1-related disorders. Headache 31:518, 1991

47. Brew BJ, Miller J: Human immunodeficiency virus-related headache. Neurology 43:1098, 1993

48. Holloway RG, Kieburtz KD: Headache and the human immunodeficiency virus type 1 infection. Headache 35:245, 1995

49. Hollander H, Stringari S: Human immunodeficiency virus-associated meningitis: Clinical course and correlations. Am J Med 83:813, 1987

50. Hollander H, McGuire D, Burack JH: Diagnostic lumbar puncture in HIV-infected patients: Analysis of 138 cases. Am J Med 96:223, 1994

51. Saag MS: Cryptococcosis and other fungal infections (histoplasmosis coccidioidomycosis): In Sande M, Volberding P (eds): The Medical Management of AIDS, 6th ed. Philadelphia, WB Saunders, 1999

52. Andreula CF, Burdi N, Carella A: CNS cryptococcosis in AIDS: Spectrum of MR findings. J Comput Assist Tomogr 17:438, 1993

53. Dismukes WE: Management of cryptococcosis [review]. Clin Infect Dis 17:S507, 1993

54. Powderly WG: Cryptococcal meningitis and AIDS [review]. Clin Infect Dis 17:837, 1993

55. Saag MS, Powderly WG, Cloud GA, et al: Comparison of amphotericin B with fluconazole in the treatment of acute AIDS-associated cryptococcal meningitis: The NIAID Mycoses Study Group and the AIDS Clinical Trials Group [see comments]. N Engl J Med 326:83, 1992

56. Sugar AM: Overview: Cryptococcosis in the patient with AIDS [review]. Mycopathologia 114:153, 1991

57. Chuck S, Sande M: Infections with *Cryptococcus neoformans* in the acquired immunodeficiency syndrome. N Engl J Med 321:794, 1989

58. Powderly WG, Finkelstein D, Feinberg J, et al: A randomized trial comparing fluconazole with clotrimazole troches for the prevention of fungal infections in patients with advanced human immunodeficiency virus infection: NIAID AIDS Clinical Trials Group [see comments]. N Engl J Med 332:700, 1995

59. Dube MP, Holtom PD, Larsen RA: Tuberculous meningitis in patients with and without human immunodeficiency virus infection. Am J Med 93:520, 1992

60. Berenguer J, Moreno S, Laguna F, et al: Tuberculous meningitis in patients infected with the human immunodeficiency virus [see comments]. N Engl J Med 326:668, 1992

61. Marra C: Syphilis, human immunodeficiency virus, and the nervous system. In Berger J, Levy R (eds): AIDS and the Nervous System, 2nd ed. Philadelphia, Lippincott-Raven, 1997, p. 677

62. Formenti SC, Gill PS, Lean E, et al: Primary central nervous system lymphoma in AIDS: Results of radiation therapy. Cancer 63:1101, 1989

63. Berger JR, Flaster M, Schatz N, et al: Cranial neuropathy heralding otherwise occult AIDS-related large cell lymphoma. J Clin Neuro-Ophthalmol 13:113, 1993

64. Bomfim da Paz R, Kolmel HW: Meningitis with Burkitt like B-cell lymphoma in HIV infection. J Neurooncol 13:73, 1992

65. Enting RH, Esselink RA, Portegies P: Lymphomatous meningitis in AIDS-related systemic non-Hodgkin's lymphoma: A report of eight cases. J Neurol Neurosurg Psychiatry 57:150, 1994

66. Singh VR, Smith DK, Lawerence J, et al: Coccidioidomycosis in patients infected with human immunodeficiency virus: Review of 91 cases at a single institution. Clin Infect Dis 23:563, 1996

67. Jones JL, Fleming PL, Ciesielski CA, et al: Coccidioidomycosis among persons with AIDS in the United States. J Infect Dis 171:961, 1995

68. Mischel PS, Vinters HV: Coccidioidomycosis of the central nervous system: Neuropathological and vasculopathic manifestations and clinical correlates. Clin Infect Dis 20:400, 1995

69. Wheat J: Histoplasmosis and coccidioidomycosis in individuals with AIDS. A clinical review. Infect Dis Clin North Ame 8:467, 1994

70. Anaissie E, Fainstein V, Samo T, et al: Central nervous system histoplasmosis: An unappreciated complication of the acquired immunodeficiency syndrome. Am J Med 84:215, 1988

71. Boldorini R, Vago L, Lechi A, et al: Wernicke's encephalopathy: Occurrence and pathological aspects in a series of 400 AIDS patients. Acta Bio-Med Ateneo Parmense 63(1-2):43, 1992

72. Butterworth RF, Gaudreau C, Vincelette J, et al: Thiamine deficiency and Wernicke's encephalopathy in AIDS. Metab Brain Dis 6:207, 1991

73. Hollander H, Golden J, Mendelson T, Cortland D: Extrapyramidal symptoms in AIDS patients given low dose metoclopramide or chlorpromazine. Lancet 2:1186, 1985

74. Gray F, Gherardi R, Wingate E, et al: Diffuse "encephalitic" cerebral toxoplasmosis in AIDS: Report of four cases. J Neurol 236:273, 1989

75. Navia B, Petito C, Gold J, et al: Cerebral toxoplasmosis complicating the acquired immune deficiency syndrome: Clinical and neuropathological findings in 27 patients. Ann Neurol 19:224, 1986

76. Navia B, Cho E-W, Petito C, Price R: The AIDS dementia complex: II. Neuropathology. Ann Neurol 19:525, 1986

77. Petito C, Cho E-S, Lemann W, et al: Neuropathology of acquired immunodeficiency syndrome (AIDS): An autopsy review. J Neuropathol Exp Neurol 45:635, 1986

78. Vinters H, Kwok M, Ho H, et al: Cytomegalovirus in the nervous system of patients with the acquired immuno deficiency syndrome. Brain 112:245, 1989
79. Wiley CA, Nelson JA: Role of human immunodeficiency virus and cytomegalovirus in AIDS encephalitis. Am J Pathol 133:73, 1988
80. Morgello S, Cho E, Neilsen S, et al: Cytomegalovirus encephalitis in patients with acquired immunodeficiency syndrome. Hum Pathol 18:289, 1987
81. Kalayjian RC, Cohen ML, Bonomo RA, Flanigan TP: Cytomegalovirus ventriculoencephalitis in AIDS. A syndrome with distinct clinical and pathologic features [review]. Medicine 72:67, 1993
82. Holland NR, Power C, Mathews VP et al: Cytomegalovirus encephalitis in acquired immunodeficiency syndrome (AIDS). Neurology 44(3 Pt 1):507, 1994
83. Berman SM, Kim RC: The development of cytomegalovirus encephalitis in AIDS patients receiving ganciclovir. Am J Med 96:415, 1994
84. Fuller GN: Cytomegalovirus and the peripheral nervous system in AIDS [review]. J Acquir Immunc Defic Syndr 5:S33, 1992
85. Cohen B, Dix R: Cytomegalovirus and other herpesviruses. In Berger J, Levy R (eds): AIDS and the Nervous System, 2nd ed. Philadelphia, Lippincott-Raven, 1997, p 595
86. McCutchan JA: Clinical impact of cytomegalovirus infections of the nervous system in patients with AIDS. Clin Infect Dis 21(Suppl 2):S196, 1995
87. Setinek U, Wondrusch E, Jellinger K, et al: Cytomegalovirus infection of the brain in AIDS: A clinicopathological study. Acta Neuropathol 90:511, 1995
88. Salazar A, Podzamczer D, Reane R, et al: Cytomegalovirus ventriculoencephalitis in AIDS patients. Scand J Infect Dis 27:165, 1995
89. Clifford DB, Arribas JR, Storch GA, et al: Magnetic resonance brain imaging lacks sensitivity for AIDS associated cytomegalovirus encephalitis. J Neurovirol 2:397, 1996
90. Gozlan J, el Amrani M, Baudrimont M, et al: A prospective evaluation of clinical criteria and polymerase chain reaction assay of cerebrospinal fluid for the diagnosis of cytomegalovirus-related neurological diseases during AIDS. AIDS 9:253, 1995
91. Arribas JR, Clifford DB, Fichtenbaum CJ, et al: Level of cytomegalovirus CMV DNA in cerebrospinal fluid of subjects with AIDS and CMV infection of the central nervous system. J Infect Dis 172:527, 1995
92. Cinque P, Vago L, Dahl H, et al: Polymerase chain reaction on cerebrospinal fluid for diagnosis of virus-associated opportunistic diseases of the central nervous system in HIV-infected patients. AIDS 10:951, 1996
93. Levy RM, Bredesen DE, Rosenblum ML: Neurological manifestations of the acquired immunodeficiency syndrome (AIDS): Experience at UCSF and review of the literature [review]. J Neurosurg 62:475, 1985
94. Rhodes R: Histopathology of the central nervous system in the acquired immunodeficiency syndrome. Hum Pathol 18:636, 1987
95. Navia B, Jordan B, Price R: The AIDS dementia complex: I. Clinical features. Ann Neurol 119:517, 1986
96. Price R: Management of AIDS dementia complex and HIV-1 infection of the nervous system. AIDS 9(Supment A):S221, 1995
97. Price RW: Understanding the AIDS dementia complex (ADC): The challenge of HIV and its effects on the central nervous system [review]. Res Publ Assoc Nerv Ment Dis 72:1, 1994
98. Price RW: The AIDS dementia complex and human immunodeficiency virus type 1 infection of the central nervous system. In Aminoff M (ed): Handbook of Clinical Neurology, Part III: Systemic Diseases. Amsterdam, Elsevier Science Publishers, 1998, in press
99. Navia B, Price R: The acquired immunodeficiency syndrome dementia complex as the presenting or sole manifestation of human immunodeficiency virus infection. Arch Neurol 44:65, 1987
100. Selnes O, Miller E, McArthur J, et al: No evidence of cognitive decline during the asymptomatic stages. Neurology 40:204, 1990
101. Selnes OA, Galai N, Bacellar H, et al: Cognitive performance after progression to AIDS: A longitudinal study from the Multicenter AIDS Cohort Study. Neurology 45:267, 1995
102. Miller E, Selnes O, McArthur J, et al: Neuropsychological performance in HIV-1-infected homosexual men: The Multi-center AIDS Cohort Study (MACS). Neurology 40:197, 1990
103. McArthur JC, Hoover DR, Bacellar H, et al: Dementia in AIDS patients: Incidence and risk factors. Multicenter AIDS Cohort Study. Neurology 43:2245, 1993
104. Neaton J, Wentworth D, Rhame F, et al: Methods of studying interventions. Considerations in choice of a clinical endpoint for AIDS clinical trials. Stat Med 13:2107, 1994
105. Bacellar H, Munoz A, Miller EN, et al: Temporal trends in the incidence of HIV-1-related neurologic diseases: Multicenter AIDS Cohort Study, 1985–1992. Neurology 44:1892, 1994
106. Portegies P, de Gans J, Derix M, et al: Declining incidence of AIDS dementia complex after introduction of zidovudine treatment. Br Med J 299:819, 1989
107. Portegies P, Enting RH, de Gans J, et al: Presentation and course of AIDS dementia complex: 10 years of follow-up in Amsterdam, The Netherlands. AIDS 7:669, 1993
108. Sacktor N, Skolasky R, Esposito D, et al: Combination antiretroviral therapy including protease inhibitors improves psychomotor speed performance in HIV infection. Neurology 50(Suppl 4):A248, 1998
109. Price RW, Sidtis JJ, Brew BJ: AIDS dementia complex and HIV-1 infection: A view from the clinic [review]. Brain Pathol 1:155, 1991
110. Price R, Brew B: The AIDS dementia complex. J Infect Dis 158:1079, 1988
111. Sidtis JJ, Price RW: Early HIV-1 infection and the AIDS dementia complex [comment]. Neurology 40:323, 1990
112. Nomenclature and research case definitions for neurologic manifestations of human immunodeficiency virus-type 1 (HIV-1) infection. Report of a Working Group of the American Academy of Neurology AIDS Task Force [review]. Neurology 41:778, 1991
113. World Health Organization consultation on the neuropsychiatric aspects of HIV-1 infection. AIDS 4:935, 1990
114. Harris MJ, Jeste DV, Gleghorn A, Sewell DD: New-onset psychosis in HIV-infected patients [review]; [see comments]. J Clin Psychiatry 52:369, 1991
115. Belman A, Ultmann M, Horoupian D, et al: Neurological complications in infants and children with acquired immune deficiency syndrome. Ann Neurol 18:560, 1985
116. Belman AL: HIV-1-associated CNS disease in infants and children. [review]. Res Publ Assoc Res Nerv Ment Dis 72:289, 1994
117. Belman AL: Infants, children and adolescents. In Berger JR, Levy RM (eds): AIDS and the Nervous Sys-

tem, 2nd ed. Philadelphia, Lippincott-Raven, 1997, p 223

118. Mintz M: Clinical features of HIV infection in children. In Gendelman H, Lipton S, Epstein L, Swindells S (eds): The Neurology of AIDS. New York, Chapman & Hall, 1998, p 385

119. Tross S, Price R, Navia B, et al: Neuropsychological characterization of the AIDS dementia complex: A preliminary report. AIDS 2:81, 1988

120. Sidtis JJ: Evaluation of the AIDS dementia complex in adults [review]. Res Publ Assoc Res Nerv Ment Dis 72:273, 1994

121. Post MJ, Berger JR, Quencer RM: Asymptomatic and neurologically symptomatic HIV-seropositive individuals: Prospective evaluation with cranial MR imaging [see comments]. Radiology 178:131, 1991

122. Post M, Tate L, Quencer R, et al: CT, MR, and pathology in HIV encephalitis and meningitis. AJR 151: 373, 1988

123. Petty RK: Recent advances in the neurology of HIV infection [review]. Postgrad Med J 70:393, 1994

124. Dal Pan GJ, McArthur JH, Aylward E, et al: Patterns of cerebral atrophy in HIV-1-infected individuals: Results of a quantitative MRI analysis. Neurology 42: 2125, 1992

125. Gelman B, Guinto FJ: Morphometry, histopathology, and tomography of cerebral atrophy in the acquired immunodeficiency syndrome. Ann Neurol 31:32, 1992

126. Aylward EH, Henderer JD, McArthur JC, et al: Reduced basal ganglia volume in HIV-1-associated dementia: Results from quantitative neuroimaging. Neurology 43:2099, 1993

127. Jakobsen J, Gyldensted C, Brun B, et al: Cerebral ventricular enlargement relates to neuropsychological measures in unselected AIDS patients. Acta Neurol Scand 79:59, 1989

128. Moeller AA, Backmund HC: Ventricle brain ratio in the clinical course of HIV infection. Acta Neurol Scand 81:512, 1990

129. Jarvik J, Hesselink J, Kennedy C, et al: Acquired immunodeficiency syndrome: Magnetic resonance patterns of brain involvement with pathologic correlation. Neurology 45:731, 1988

130. Power C, Kong PA, Crawford TO, et al: Cerebral white matter changes in acquired immunodeficiency syndrome dementia: Alterations of the blood-brain barrier. Ann Neurol 34:339, 1993

131. Belman AL, Lantos G, Horoupian D, et al: AIDS: Calcification of the basal ganglia in infants and children. Neurology 36:1192, 1986

132. Brew BJ, Paul MO, Nakajima G, et al: Cerebrospinal fluid HIV-1 p24 antigen and culture: Sensitivity and specificity for AIDS-dementia complex. J Neurol Neurosurg Psychiatry 57:784, 1994

133. Portegies P, Epstein L, Hung S, et al: Human immunodeficiency virus type 1 antigen in cerebrospinal fluid: Correlation with clinical neurological status. Arch Neurol 46:261, 1989

134. Brew B, Pemberton L, Cunningham P, Law M: Levels of human immunodeficiency virus type 1 RNA in cerebrospinal fluid correlate with AIDS dementia stage. J Infect Dis 175:963, 1997

135. Ellis R, Hsia K, Spector S, et al: CSF HIV-1 RNA levels are elevated in neurocognitively impaired individuals. Ann Neurol 42:679, 1997

136. McArthur J, McClernon D, Cronin M, et al: Relationship between HIV-associated dementia and viral load in CSF and brain. Ann Neurology 42:689, 1997

137. Brew B, Bhalla R, Paul M, et al: Cerebrospinal fluid neopterin in human immunodeficiency virus type 1 infection. Ann Neurol 28:556, 1990

138. Brew B, Bhalla R, Fleisher M, et al: Cerebrospinal fluid B2 microglobulin in patients infected with human immunodeficiency virus. Neurology 39:830, 1989

139. Brew BJ, Bhalla RB, Paul M, et al: Cerebrospinal fluid beta 2-microglobulin in patients with AIDS dementia complex: An expanded series including response to zidovudine treatment. AIDS 6:461, 1992

140. Griffin DE, McArthur JC, Cornblath DR: Neopterin and interferon-gamma in serum and cerebrospinal fluid of patients with HIV-associated neurologic disease. Neurology 41:69, 1991

141. Price R, Staprans S: Measuring the viral load in cerebrospinal fluid in human immunodeficiency virus infection: Window into brain infection? Ann Neuol 42: 675, 1997

142. Budka H: Neuropathology of human immunodeficiency virus infection [review]. Brain Pathol 1:163, 1991

143. Rosenblum M: Infection of the central nervous system by the human immunodeficiency virus type 1: Morphology and relation to syndromes of progressive encephalopathy and myelopathy in patients with AIDS. Pathol Ann 25:117, 1990

144. Gray F, Haug H, Chimelli L, et al: Prominent cortical atrophy with neuronal loss as correlate of human immunodeficiency virus encephalopathy. Acta Neuropathol 82:229, 1991

145. Brew B, Rosenblum M, Cronin K, Price R: The AIDS dementia complex and HIV-1 brain infection: Clinical-virological correlations. Ann Neurol 38:563, 1995

146. Masliah E, Achim CL, Ge N, et al: Cellular neuropathology in HIV encephalitis [review]. Res Publ Assoc Res Nerv Ment Dis 72:119, 1994

147. Petito C, Navia B, Cho E, et al: Vacuolar myelopathy pathologically resembling subacute combined degeneration in patients with acquired immunodeficiency syndrome (AIDS). N Engl J Med 312:874, 1985

148. Dal Pan GJ, Glass JD, McArthur JC: Clinicopathologic correlations of HIV-1-associated vacuolar myelopathy: An autopsy-based case-control study. Neurology 44:2159, 1994

149. Petito CK, Vecchio D, Chen YT: HIV antigen and DNA in AIDS spinal cords correlate with macrophage infiltration but not with vacuolar myelopathy. J Neuropathol Exp Neurol 53:86, 1994

150. Rosenblum M, Scheck A, Cronin K, et al: Dissociation of AIDS-related vacuolar myelopathy and productive human immunodeficiency virus type 1 (HIV-1) infection of the spinal cord. Neurology 39:892, 1989

151. Tan SV, Guiloff RJ, Scaravilli F: AIDS-associated vacuolar myelopathy: A morphometric study. Brain 118:1247, 1995

152. Price R: AIDS dementia complex and HIV-1 brain infection: A pathogenetic framework for treatment and evaluation. Curr Top Microbiol Immunol 202:33, 1995

153. Lipton SA, Gendelman HE: Seminars in medicine of the Beth Israel Hospital, Boston: Dementia associated with the acquired immunodeficiency syndrome [review]. N Engl J Med 332:934, 1995

154. Nuovo G, Gallery F, MacConnell P, Braun A: In situ detection of polymerase chain reaction-amplified HIV-1 nucleic acids and tumor necrosis factor-alpha

RNA in the central nervous system. Am J Pathol 144: 659, 1994

155. Tornatore C, Chandra R, Berger JR, Major EO: HIV-1 infection of subcortical astrocytes in the pediatric central nervous system. Neurology 44(3 Pt 1):481, 1994

156. Saito Y, Sharer L, Epstein L, et al: Overexpression of nef as a marker for restricted HIV-1 infection of astrocytes in postmortem pediatric central nervous system tissues. Neurology 44:474, 1994

157. Wesselingh SL, Glass J, McArthur JC, et al: Cytokine dysregulation in HIV-associated neurological disease [review]. Adv Neuroimmunol 4:199, 1994

158. Koyangi Y, Miles S, Mitsuyasu R, et al: Dual infection of the central nervous system by AIDS viruses with distinct cellular tropisms. Science 236:819, 1987

159. Li Y, Hui H, Burgess CJ, et al: Complete nucleotide sequence, genome organization, and biological properties of human immunodeficiency virus type 1 in vivo: Evidence for limited defectiveness and complementation. J Virol 66:6587, 1992

160. Li Y, Kappes JC, Conway JA, et al: Molecular characterization of human immunodeficiency virus type 1 cloned directly from uncultured human brain tissue: Identification of replication-competent and -defective viral genomes. J Virol 65:3973, 1991

161. O'Brien W: Genetic and biologic basis of HIV-1 neurotropism. In Price R, Perry S (eds): HIV, AIDS and the Brain. New York, Raven Press, 1994, p 47

162. He J, Chen Y, Farzan M, et al: CCR3 and CCR5 are co-receptors for HIV-1 infection of microglia. Nature 385:645, 1997

163. Lavi E, Strizki JM, Ulrich AM, et al: CXCR-4 Fusin, a co-receptor for the type 1 human immunodeficiency virus HIV-1, is expressed in the human brain in a variety of cell types, including microglia and neurons. Am J Pathol 151:1035, 1997

164. Vallat AV, De Girolami U, He J, et al: Localization of HIV-1 co-receptors CCR5 and CXCR4 in the brain of children with AIDS. Am J Pathol 152:167, 1998

165. Sasseville VG, Smith MM, Mackay CR, et al: Chemokine expression in simian immunodeficiency virus-induced AIDS encephalitis. Am J Pathol 149:1459, 1996

166. Schmitt F, Bigleg J, McKinnis R, et al: Neuropsychological outcome of azidothymidine (AZT) in the treatment of AIDS and AIDS-related complex: A double blind, placebo-controlled trial. N Engl J Med 319: 1573, 1988

167. Sidtis JJ, Gatsonis C, Price RW, et al: Zidovudine treatment of the AIDS dementia complex: Results of a placebo-controlled trial. AIDS Clinical Trials Group. Ann Neurol 33:343, 1993

168. Brouwers P, Moss H, Wolters P, et al: Effect of continuous-infusion zidovudine therapy on neuropsychologic functioning in children with symptomatic human immunodeficiency virus infection. J Pediatr 116:980, 1990

169. Gray F, Belec L, Keohane C, et al: Zidovudine therapy and HIV encephalitis: A 10-year neuropathological survey. AIDS 8:489, 1994

170. Galgani S, Balestra P, Narciso P, et al: Nimodipine plus zidovudine versus zidovudine alone in the treatment of HIV-1-associated cognitive deficits [letter]. AIDS 11:1520, 1997

171. Chiesi A, Vella S, Dally LG, et al: Epidemiology of AIDS dementia complex in Europe: AIDS in Europe Study Group. J Acquir Immune Defic Syndr Hum Retrovirol 11:39, 1996

172. Baldeweg T, Catalan J, Lovett E, et al: Long-term zidovudine reduces neurocognitive deficits in HIV-1 infection. AIDS 9:589, 1995

173. Portegies P: Review of antiretroviral therapy in the prevention of HIV-related AIDS dementia complex ADC. Drugs 49(Suppl 1):25, 1995

174. Filippi CG, Sze G, Farber SJ, et al: Regression of HIV encephalopathy and basal ganglia signal intensity abnormality at MR imaging in patients with AIDS after the initiation of protease inhibitor therapy. Radiology 206:491, 1998

175. Burger D, Kraaijeveld C, Meenhorst P, et al: Penetration of zidovudine into the cerebrospinal fluid of patients infected with HIV. AIDS 7:1581, 1993

176. Foudraine N, Hoetelmans R, Lange J, et al: Cerebrospinal-fluid HIV-1 RNA and drug concentrations after treatment with lamivudine plus zidovudine or stavudine. Lancet 351:1547, 1998

177. Aweeka F, Sheiner L, Bellibas S, et al: Pharmacokinetics of abacavir (1592U89) in cerebrospinal fluid (CSF) using multiple lumbar punctures in few subjects and sparse sampling techniques. In: Abstracts of the XIIth International Conference on AIDS, Geneva, 1998, Abstract 42271

178. Collier A, Marra C, Coombs R: Cerebrospinal fluid (CSF) HIV RNA levels in patients on chronic indinavir therapy. In: Abstracts of the 35th Annual Meeting of the Infectious Diseases Society of America, San Francisco, 1997, Abstract 22

179. Engstrom JW, Lowenstein DH, Bredesen DE: Cerebral infarctions and transient neurologic deficits associated with acquired immunodeficiency syndrome. Am J Med 86:528, 1989

180. Moriarty DM, Haller JO, Loh JP, Fikrig S: Cerebral infarction in pediatric acquired immunodeficiency syndrome. Pediatr Radiol 24:611, 1994

181. Philippet P, Blanche S, Sebag G, et al: Stroke and cerebral infarcts in children infected with human immunodeficiency virus. Arch Pediatr Adolesc Med 148: 965, 1994

182. So Y, Holtzman D, Abrams D, Olnery R: Peripheral neuropathy associated with acquired immunodeficiency syndrome: Prevalence and clinical features from a population based survey. Arch Neurol 45:945, 1988

183. Bartolomei F, Pellegrino P, Dhiver C, et al: [Epilepsy seizures in HIV infection: 52 cases (review)]. Presse Med 20:2135, 1991

184. Holtzman D, Kaku D, So Y: New onset seizures associated with human immunodeficiency virus infection: Causation and clinical features in 100 cases. Am J Med 87:173, 1989

185. Van Paesschen W, Bodian C, Maker H: Metabolic abnormalities and new-onset seizures in human immunodeficiency virus-seropositive patients. Epilepsia 36: 146, 1995

186. Wong M, Suite N, Labar D: Seizures in human immunodeficiency virus infection. Arch Neurol 47:640, 1990

187. Luft BJ, Hafner R, Korzun AH, et al: Toxoplasmic encephalitis in patients with the acquired immunodeficiency syndrome. Members of the ACTG 077p/ANRS 009 Study Team. N Engl J Med 329:995, 1993

188. Kovacs J, Kovacs A, Polis M, et al: Cryptococcosis in the acquired immunodeficiency syndrome. Ann Intern Med 103:533, 1985

189. McGuire D, Bromley E, Aberg J, et al: Focal posterior hemisphere invasive cryptococcal encephalitis: A distinct neuroimaging entity complicating cryptococcal

meningitis in AIDS [abstract]. Ann Neurol 41:467, 1997

190. Falangola MF, Reichler BS, Petito CK: Histopathology of cerebral toxoplasmosis in human immunodeficiency virus infection: A comparison between patients with early-onset and late-onset acquired immunodeficiency syndrome. Hum Pathol 25:1091, 1994

191. So Y, Beckstead J, Davis R: Primary central nervous system lymphoma in acquired immune deficiency syndrome: A clinical and pathological study. Ann Neurol 20:566, 1986

192. Levine AM: Non-Hodgkin's lymphomas and other malignancies in the acquired immune deficiency syndrome [review]. Semin Oncol 14(Suppl 3):34, 1987

193. Meeker TC, Shiramizu B, Kaplan L, et al: Evidence for molecular subtypes of HIV-associated lymphoma: Division into peripheral monoclonal, polyclonal and central nervous system lymphoma. AIDS 5:669, 1991

194. Baumgartner JE, Rachlin JR, Beckstead JH, et al: Primary central nervous system lymphomas: Natural history and response to radiation therapy in 55 patients with acquired immunodeficiency syndrome. J Neurosurg 73:206, 1990

195. Remick S, Diamond C, Migliozzi J, et al: Primary central nervous system lymphoma in patients with and without the acquired immune deficiency syndrome: A retrospective analysis and review of the literature. Medicine 69:345, 1990

196. DeAngelis L: Primary CNS lymphoma: A new clinical challenge. Neurology 41:619, 1991

197. Brightbill TC, Post MJ, Hensley GT, Ruiz A: MR of *Toxoplasma* encephalitis: Signal characteristics on T2-weighted images and pathologic correlation. J Comput Assist Tomogr 20:417, 1996

198. Lorberboym M, Estok L, Machac J, et al: Rapid differential diagnosis of cerebral toxoplasmosis and primary central nervous system lymphoma by thallium-201 SPECT. J Nucl Med 37:1150, 1996

199. Hoffman JM, Waskin HA, Schifter T, et al: FDG-PET in differentiating lymphoma from nonmalignant central nervous system lesions in patients with AIDS. J Nucl Med 34:567, 1993

200. Ruiz A, Ganz WI, Post MJ, et al: Use of thallium-201 brain SPECT to differentiate cerebral lymphoma from toxoplasma encephalitis in AIDS patients [see comments]. AJNR Am J Neuroradiol 15:1885, 1994

201. Grant I, Gold J, Rosemblum M, et al: *Toxoplasma gondii* serology in HIV-infected patients: The development of central nervous system toxoplasmosis in AIDS. AIDS 4:519, 1990

202. Antinori A, Ammassari A, De Luca A, et al: Diagnosis of AIDS-related focal brain lesions: A decision-making analysis based on clinical and neuroradiologic characteristics combined with polymerase chain reaction assays in CSF. Neurology 48:687, 1997

203. Richardson E: Progressive multifocal leukoencephalopathy. In Vinken P, Bruyn G (eds): Handbook of Clinical Neurology. Amsterdam, Elsevier, 1978, p 307

204. Houff S, Major E, Katz D, et al: Involvement of JC virus-infected mononuclear cells from the bone marrow and spleen in the pathogenesis of progressive multifocal leukoencephalopathy. N Engl J Med 318:301, 1988

205. Schmidbauer M, Budka H, Shah K: Progressive multifocal leukoencephalopathy (PML) in AIDS and in the pre-AIDS era. Acto Neuropathol 80:375, 1990

206. Berger J, Kaszovitz B, Donovan Post M, Dickinson G: Progressive multifocal leukoencephalopathy in association with human deficiency virus infection: A review of the literature with a report of sixteen cases. Ann Intern Med 107:78, 1987

207. Weber T, Turner RW, Frye S, et al: Specific diagnosis of progressive multifocal leukoencephalopathy by polymerase chain reaction. J Infect Dis 169:1138, 1994

208. Weber T, Turner RW, Frye S, et al: Progressive multifocal leukoencephalopathy diagnosed by amplification of JC virus-specific DNA from cerebrospinal fluid. AIDS 8:49, 1994

209. McGuire D, Barhite S, Hollander H, Miles M: JC virus DNA in cerebrospinal fluid of human immunodeficiency virus-infected patients: Predictive value for progressive multifocal leukoencephalopathy. Ann Neurol 37:395, 1995

210. Portegies P, Algra P, Hollak C, et al: Response to cytarabine in progressive multifocal leukoencephalopathy in AIDS. Lancet 1:680, 1991

211. Hall CD, Dafni U, Simpson D, et al: Failure of cytarabine in progressive multifocal leukoencephalopathy associated with human immunodeficiency virus infection. AIDS Clinical Trials Group 243 Team [see comments]. N Engl J Med 338:1345, 1998

212. Berger J, Mucke L: Prolonged survival and partial recovery in AIDS-associated progressive multifocal leukoencephalopathy. Neurology 38:1060, 1988

213. Garrels K, Kucharczyk W, Wortzman G, Shandling M: Progressive multifocal leukoencephalopathy: Clinical and MR response to treatment. AJNR Am J Neuroradiol 17:597, 1996

214. Berger JR, Concha M: Progressive multifocal leukoencephalopathy: The evolution of a disease once considered rare. J Neurovirol 1:5, 1995

215. Domingo P, Guardiola JM, Iranzo A, Margall N: Remission of progressive multifocal leucoencephalopathy after antiretroviral therapy [letter; comment]. Lancet 349:1554, 1997

216. Baldeweg T, Catalan J: Remission of progressive multifocal leucoencephalopathy after antiretroviral therapy [letter; comment]. Lancet 349:1554, 1997

217. Elliot B, Aromin I, Gold R, et al: 2.5 year remission of AIDS-associated progressive multifocal leukoencephalopathy with combined antiretroviral therapy [letter] [see comments]. Lancet 349:850, 1997

218. Berger J, Levy R, Flomenhhoft D, Dobbs M: Predictive factors for prolonged survival in acquired immunodeficiency syndrome-associated progressive multifocal leukoencephalopathy. Neurology 44:341, 1998

219. Berger J, Lorraine P, Lanska D, Whiteman M: Progressive multifocal leukoencephalopathy in patients with HIV infection. J Neurovirol 4:59, 1998

220. Gray F, Belec L, Lescs MC, et al: Varicella-zoster virus infection of the central nervous system in the acquired immune deficiency syndrome [review]. Brain 117(Pt 5):987, 1994

221. Horten B, Price R, Jimenez D: Multifocal varicella-zoster virus leukoencephalitis temporally remote from herpes zoster. Ann Neurol 9:251, 1981

222. Ryder JW, Croen K, Kleinschmidt-DeMasters BK: Progressive encephalitis three months after resolution of cutaneous zoster in a patient with AIDS. Ann Neurol 19:182, 1986

223. Morgello S, Block G, Price R, et al: Varicella-zoster virus leukoencephalitis and cerebral vasculopathy. Arch Pathol Lab Med 112:173, 1988

224. Hilt D, Bucholz D, Krumholz A, et al: Herpes zoster ophthalmicus and delayed contralateral hemiparesis

caused by cerebral angiitis: Diagnosis and management approaches. Ann Neurol 14:543, 1983

225. Eidelberg D, Sotrel A, Horopian D, et al: Thrombotic cerebral vasculopathy associated with herpes zoster. Ann Neurol 19:7, 1986

226. Devinsky O, Cho E, Petito C, Price R: Herpes zoster myelitis. Brain 114:1181, 1991

227. Mehren M, Burns PJ, Mamani F, et al: Toxoplasmic myelitis mimicking intramedullary spinal cord tumor. Neurology 38:1648, 1988

228. Harris TM, Smith RR, Bognanno JR, Edwards MK: Toxoplasmic myelities in AIDS: gadolinium-enhanced MR. J Comput Assist Tomogr 15:809, 1990

229. Gilden DH, Kleinschmidt-DeMasters BK, Wellish M, et al: Varicella zoster virus, a cause of waxing and waning vasculitis: The New England Journal of Medicine case 5-1995 revisited. Neurology 47:1441, 1996

230. Kenyon LC, Dulaney E, Montone KT, et al: Varicella-zoster ventriculo-encephalitis and spinal cord infarction in a patient with AIDS. Acta Neuropathol 92:202, 1996

231. Miller R, Parry G, Lang W, et al: AIDS-related inflammatory polyradiculoneuropathy: Successful treatment with plasma exchange [abstract]. Neurology 36: 206, 1986

232. So YT, Olney RK: Acute lumbosacral polyradiculopathy in acquired immunodeficiency syndrome: Experience with 23 patients. Ann Neurol 35:53, 1994

233. Tucker T, Dix RD, Katzen C, et al: Cytomegalovirus and herpes simplex virus ascending myelitis in a patient with acquired immune deficiency syndrome. Ann Neurol 18:74, 1985

234. Aboulafia DM, Saxton EH, Koga H, et al: A patient with progressive myelopathy and antibodies to human T-cell leukemia virus type I and human immunodeficiency virus type I in serum and cerebrospinal fluid. Arch Neurol 47:477, 1990

235. Rosenblum M, Brew B, Hahn B, et al: Human T-lymphotropic virus type I associated myelopathy in patients with the acquired immune deficiency syndrome. Hum Pathol 23:513, 1992

236. Izumo S, Umehara F, Kashio N, et al: Neuropathology of HTLV-1-associated myelopathy HAM/TSP. Leukemia 11(Suppl 3):82, 1997

237. Kitze B, Brady JN: Human T cell lymphotropic retroviruses: Association with diseases of the nervous system. Intervirology 40:132, 1997

238. Lehky TJ, Flerlage N, Katz D, et al: Human T-cell lymphotropic virus type II-associated myelopathy: Clinical and immunologic profiles. Ann Neurol 40: 714, 1996

239. Nakagawa M, Nakahara K, Maruyama Y, et al: Therapeutic trials in 200 patients with HTLV-I-associated myelopathy/tropical spastic paraparesis. J Neurovirol 2:345, 1996

240. Nakagawa M, Izumo S, Ijichi S, et al: HTLV-I-associated myelopathy: Analysis of 213 patients based on clinical features and laboratory findings. J Neurovirol 1:50, 1995

241. Fuller GN, Jacobs JM, Guiloff RJ: Nature and incidence of peripheral nerve syndromes in HIV infection. J Neurol Neurosurg Psychiatry 56:372, 1993

242. Griffin JW, Wesselingh SL, Griffin DE, et al: Peripheral nerve disorders in HIV infection. Similarities and contrasts with CNS disorders [review]. Res Publ Assoc Res Nerv Ment Dis 72:159, 1994

243. Said G, Lacroix C, Chemouilli P, et al: CMV neuropathy in AIDS: A clinical and pathological study. Ann Neurol 29:139, 1991

244. So Y, Olney R: The natural history of mononeuropathy multiplex and simplex in patients with HIV infection [abstract]. Neurology 41(Suppl):374, 1991

245. Roullet E, Assuerus V, Gozlan J, et al: Cytomegalovirus multifocal neuropathy in AIDS: Analysis of 15 consecutive cases. Neurology 44:2174, 1994

246. Eidelberg D, Sotrel A, Vogel H, et al: Progressive polyradiculopathy in acquired immune deficiency syndrome. Neurology 36:912, 1986

247. Fuller G, Gill S, Guilloff R, et al: Ganciclovir treatment of lumbosacral polyradiculopathy in AIDS. Lancet 335:48, 1990

248. Miller R, Parry G, Pfaeffl W, et al: The spectrum of peripheral neuropathy associated with ARC and AIDS. Muscle Nerve 11:857, 1988

249. Tyor W, Wesselingh S, Griffin J, et al: Unifying hypothesis for the pathogenesis of HIV-associated dementia complex, vacuolar myelopathy, and sensory neuropathy. J Acquir Immune Defic Syndr Hum Retrovirol 9:379, 1995

250. Rizzuto N, Cavallaro T, Monaco S, et al: Role of HIV in the pathogenesis of distal symmetrical peripheral neuropathy. Acta Neuropathol 90:244, 1995

251. Dalakas MC, Pezeshkpour GH: Neuromuscular diseases associated with human immunodeficiency virus infection [review]. Ann Neurol 23:S38, 1988

252. Chaunu MP, Ratinahirana H, Raphael M, et al: The spectrum of changes on 20 nerve biopsies in patients with HIV infection. Muscle Nerve 12:452, 1989

253. Berger AR, Arezzo JC, Schaumburg HH, et al: 2',3'-dideoxycytidine (ddC) toxic neuropathy: A study of 52 patients. Neurology 43:358, 1993

254. Fischl MA, Richman DD, Saag M, et al: Safety and antiviral activity of combination therapy with zidovudine, zalcitabine, and two doses of interferon-alpha2a in patients with HIV: AIDS Clinical Trials Group Study 197. J Acquir Immune Defic Syndr Hum Retrovirol 16:247, 1997

255. Rana KZ, Dudley MN: Clinical pharmacokinetics of stavudine. Clin Pharmacokinet 33:276, 1997

256. Adkins JC, Peters DH, Faulds D: Zalcitabine: An update of its pharmacodynamic and pharmacokinetic properties and clinical efficacy in the management of HIV infection. Drugs 53:1054, 1997

257. Blum AS, Dal Pan GJ, Feinberg J, et al: Low-dose zalcitabine-related toxic neuropathy: Frequency, natural history, and risk factors. Neurology 46:999, 1996

258. Fichtenbaum CJ, Clifford DB, Powderly WG: Risk factors for dideoxynucleoside-induced toxic neuropathy in patients with the human immunodeficiency virus infection. J Acquir Immune Defic Syndr Hum Retrovirol 10:169, 1995

259. Simpson DM, Tagliati M: Nucleoside analogue-associated peripheral neuropathy in human immunodeficiency virus infection. J Acquir Immune Defic Syndr Hum Retrovirol 9:153, 1995

260. Craddock C, Pasvol G, Bull R, et al: Cardiorespiratory arrest and automatic neuropathy in AIDS. Lancet 2: 16, 1987

261. Welby SB, Rogerson SJ, Beeching NJ: Autonomic neuropathy is common in human immunodeficiency virus infection. J Infect 23:123, 1991

262. Batman P, Miller A, Sedgewick P, Griffin G: Autonomic denervation in jejunal mucosa of homosexual men infected with HIV. AIDS 5:1247, 1991

263. Bailey RO, Turok DI, Jaufmann BP, Singh JK: Myositis and acquired immunodeficiency syndrome. Hum Pathol 18:749, 1987

264. Illa I, Nath A, Dalakas M: Immunocytochemical and virological characteristics of HIV-associated inflam-

matory myopathies: Similarities with seronegative polymyositis. Ann Neurol 29:474, 1991

265. Simpson DM, Citak KA, Godfrey E, et al: Myopathies associated with human immunodeficiency virus and zidovudine: Can their effects be distinguished? Neurology 43:971, 1993

266. Gherardi RK: Skeletal muscle involvement in HIV-infected patients [review]. Neuropathol Appl Neurobiol 20:232, 1994

267. Manji H, Harrison MJ, Round JM, et al: Muscle disease, HIV and zidovudine: The spectrum of muscle disease in HIV-infected individuals treated with zidovudine. J Neurol 240:479, 1993

268. Chalmers A, Greco C, Miller R: Prognosis in AZT myopathy. Neurology 41:1181, 1991

269. Dalakas MC, Leon-Monzon ME, Bernardini I, et al: Zidovudine-induced mitochondrial myopathy is associated with muscle carnitine deficiency and lipid storage. Ann Neurol 35:482, 1994

270. Damati G, Lewis W: Zidovudine causes early increases in mitochondrial ribonucleic acid abundance and induces ultrastructural changes in cultured mouse muscle cells. Lab Invest 71:879, 1994

271. Peters BS, Winer J, Landon DN, et al: Mitochondrial myopathy associated with chronic zidovudine therapy in AIDS. Q J Med 86:5, 1993

15 Psychosocial Issues and Psychiatric Complications of HIV Disease

LISA CAPALDINI

People with HIV disease are confronted with multiple psychosocial stressors at all stages of their illness. Sometimes, these stressors are life changes that are brought on by disease and require accommodations, such as dealing with finances, preparing a will, or transferring to a residential housing unit. Increasingly, patients must balance the frustration of living with cumulative chronic symptoms, such as fatigue and neuropathy, with the more hopeful overall prognoses of HIV disease in the highly active antiretroviral therapy (HAART) era. Patients' ability to cope with these challenges depends on their pre-HIV psychological status, their social and psychological support network, and their stage of HIV disease.

HIV-infected patients, like all patients with chronic medical disorders, are at increased risk for specific psychiatric disorders: depression, anxiety, delirium, organic brain disease (OBD), mania, and psychosis. Many of the psychosocial complications of HIV disease—including social isolation, personal distress, and specific psychiatric syndromes such as depression and panic disorder—are treatable. For this reason, all HIV caregivers should learn to recognize patients with these conditions and either *treat* such patients *or refer* them for treatment. For example, depression is one of the most common and treatable complications of advanced HIV disease. Even in patients with advanced AIDS, effective treatment of depression may result in fewer physical symptoms, better sleep, and overall improvement in quality of life.

The optimal treatment of the psychosocial sequelae of HIV disease requires communication between the primary medical provider and mental health and social work consultants. The role of primary care providers includes

- Familiarizing themselves with drug side effects that may cause complications, such as anxiety, depression, delirium, and mania
- Identifying patients' coping styles and social resources
- Referring patients when distress results in decreased compliance with medical treatment, significant psychological problems, or decreased quality of life

Because primary care providers are usually the first practitioners to witness these complications, they need to be familiar with the full range of medical and psychotherapeutic resources available to their patients. Finally, medical practitioners need to develop a referral network for mental health consultation or management if and when their patients develop a psychiatric syndrome that requires special management by mental health professionals.

By the same token, mental health professionals need to recognize that many HIV psychiatric syndromes mimicking pure functional disorders are likely to be of organic etiology. They need to be aware not only of medication side effects that result in psychiatric symptoms but also of the spectrum and natural history of HIV disease. In this way, primary caregivers and mental health professionals play complementary roles in counseling patients and their loved ones.

This chapter has two major sections. The first is a review of the major psychiatric syndromes seen with HIV disease: depression, dementia/OBD, anxiety/panic disorder, delirium, mania, and psychosis. The second is a summary of the issues that patients coping with HIV disease must face, with emphasis on caregivers' ability to help patients address multiple losses, helplessness, and role and lifestyle adjustments. This section reviews such topics as ethical/legal issues, pain control, fatigue, bereavement, and caregiver coping issues.

MAJOR PSYCHIATRIC SYNDROMES

Like other life-threatening and chronic diseases, AIDS may be complicated by psychiatric symptoms. In some cases, these may be precipitated by discrete biologic or psychosocial stressors.[1] In other cases, substance abuse or mood disorder may predate actual HIV infection.[2,3] Diagnosis of psychiatric syndromes may be complicated by the significant overlap between symptoms of HIV disease per se (fatigue, weight loss, sleep disorder, decreased libido, concentration impairment) and symptoms of depression. Finally, organic HIV disease may mimic a purely functional syndrome. For instance, HIV OBD may cause symptoms indistinguishable from functional psychosis.[4,5]

Classification of HIV disease has been modified several times over the last half-decade. Older studies using terms such as *AIDS-related complex* and *AIDS* are difficult to compare to more recent studies that use such characteristics as T-cell count, viral load, or Centers for Disease Control and Prevention stages. With the recognition that there is wide variability in the functional status of HIV-infected people within given T-cell subsets and with specific complications of HIV disease (e.g., Kaposi's sarcoma), it has been increasingly difficult to compare patient cohorts between studies with any assurance of equivalent patient subgroups.

HIV-related neuropsychological impairment can precede a diagnosis of otherwise asymptomatic HIV disease.[6] In a review of organic mental disorders caused by HIV, Perry[7] identified six observations suggesting that organic mental changes caused by HIV could precede other symptoms of HIV infection.

The actual prevalence of neuropsychiatric disorders among HIV-infected people is not known with precision. The incidence of HIV infection in psychiatric outpatients and inpatients has not been well defined either. One study[8] demonstrated that 7% of inpatients admitted to a voluntary psychiatric facility were HIV positive. HIV dementia, which may be the sole manifestation of HIV disease in some patients, may in turn be complicated by personality changes or organic psychosis. A study of 29 patients with AIDS dementia found that 11 had concomitant

personality changes and 2 had a concomitant organic psychosis.[6]

Two investigators have suggested that psychiatric disorders may be seen with increased prevalence in people at risk for HIV but who are not necessarily HIV positive. A study of 56 ambulatory gay men, some of whom were HIV positive, found an increased lifetime rate of alcohol or nonopiate drug abuse, generalized anxiety disorder, and major depression, which often preceded symptomatic HIV disease or knowledge of HIV status, compared to 22 healthy heterosexual controls.[2] In another study, 207 physically asymptomatic adults who were attending a center for serologic testing for the HIV virus had relatively higher lifetime rates of mood and substance abuse disorders, but did not show evidence of current *Diagnostic and Statistical Manual of Mental Disorders*, *Third Edition*, Axis I psychopathology.[3] These findings did not support the conclusion that individuals at risk for AIDS are a psychiatrically morbid population.

Patients with psychiatric disease require specific preventative interventions to reduce the likelihood of HIV infection.[9-12] Although the bulk of observational studies do not suggest a link between HIV infection and any psychiatric disorders other than substance use, all psychiatric patients are at risk for HIV infection. Mental health specialists should address HIV-related issues with their clients and identify factors that may interfere with medical care or medication adherence.[13-15]

Psychiatric syndromes may complicate any of the stages of HIV disease.[16-18] Even individuals who have not been tested and individuals who are known to be HIV negative may experience HIV-related psychological distress. Some experience anxiety about being tested, and even those who receive negative test results may still develop anxiety,[19] depression, or even delusional disorders related to AIDS fears.[20]

Patients who recently have tested seropositive may experience transient anxiety and depression, adjustment disorder (i.e., a maladaptive reaction that interferes with functioning occurring within 3 months of testing and resolving within 6 months), anxiety disorder, major depression, or even brief reactive psychosis.[21] Shortly after testing, HIV-positive people are at increased risk of suicide. A study of active-duty Air Force members who were HIV positive and attempted suicide showed that 46.7% attempted suicide within 3 months of learning they were seropositive, and four of the seven suicide attempts occurred within the first week after notification.[22]

More recent studies have shown a risk for suicide in patients with HIV disease at all phases of HIV infection.[23,24]

Focused psychoeducational interventions may help reduce the distress of patients who learn they are HIV seropositive.[25] At this time, counselors can also assist patients with medical referrals and address patients' questions about safe sex, confidentiality, and partner notification.

Many patients with HIV disease develop an emotional crisis at the time they first recognize HIV-related symptoms. The psychological meaning of even ostensibly mild symptoms may be overwhelming to patients. The first physical symptom is a concrete reminder that they are infected with a previously dormant virus that usually is lethal and that their life expectancy is, therefore, limited. It is at this time that many HIV-infected people may first seek medical care.

The initial care provider should assess the patient's physical status and, equally important, assess the impact and meaning of the patient's physical symptoms on his or her emotional well-being. Patients may need guidance about coping with disease progression. This may include developing a personal and social support system, voicing fears about disability, learning about financial support in the event of progressive disability, and even discussing options about life-sustaining treatment in the event of rapid disease progression.[26] Non–mental health specialists can provide patients with brief psychotherapeutic interventions during regular office appointments.[27]

The importance of all caregivers helping their clients develop coping strategies cannot be overestimated.[28–31] Isolation, fear, anxiety, and marginalization are common psychosocial complications of chronic or disabling diseases. In a groundbreaking study, a psychosocial intervention was found to significantly improve the life expectancy of women with systemic advanced breast cancer.[32] Others[33–38] have elucidated a connection between immunologic function and stressors and have suggested that immunocompetence in HIV-infected people may be related to primary neuropsychiatric parameters, such as depression and distress.[36,39] One study of upwardly mobile gay men noted that psychological resilience correlated with long-term survival.[40] Taylor et al.[41] noted that psychological optimism correlated with a psychologically adaptive response to being HIV infected. Folkman et al.[42] noted that coping styles correlated well with the presence or absence of high-risk sexual behavior. Coping style may of itself affect the social support the patient may seek in an effort to adapt to HIV disease.[28,43] To date, no controlled, randomized studies definitively prove that psychosocial intervention can favorably alter the history of HIV disease[44–46] or prevent morbid psychiatric outcomes, such as substance abuse or suicide. Given the established prevalence and profound psychosocial and physical impact of these psychiatric complications, however, an active effort toward recognition, prevention, and treatment of psychiatric disease is warranted.

Six major neuropsychiatric syndromes have been identified as complications of HIV disease. They are depression, dementia/OBD, anxiety/panic disorder, delirium, mania, and psychosis. Each complication is addressed here separately, although many of these conditions may overlap in any given patient (e.g., patients with OBD with prominent cognitive defects may also have features of depression or psychosis).

Wolcott et al.[20] outlined five general principles of assessment of suspected neuropsychiatric disorders in patients with HIV disease:

- All new psychiatric disorders should be considered secondary to a neuropsychiatric complication of HIV disease until thorough evaluation indicates otherwise.
- Organic mental disorder may appear weeks to months before an underlying primary central nervous system (CNS) disease becomes apparent.
- Neurodiagnostic tests may be normal or nondiagnostic in patients with HIV-related organic mental disease, underlying primary CNS disease, or both.
- Careful preventive screening is crucial to the early diagnosis of organic mental disease because mental status changes are often the first clinical sign of primary CNS changes, many of which are treatable.
- Primary care physicians and practitioners should consider early patient referral when HIV-related neuropsychiatric disorder is suspected.

Depression

Depression may be especially prevalent and difficult to diagnose in medically ill patients.[47,48] This is particularly true of HIV disease, wherein life stressors, premorbid psychiatric predispositions, specific organic complications, and centrally acting medications may all predispose to depression. Several studies have established that depression is more common in medical outpatients, patients with cancer, and especially patients with diseases affecting the CNS.[49-54] Other studies have established that, in both specialty and primary care settings, practitioners tend to under-recognize and misdiagnose depression.[55,56] Finally, studies of patients with depression and comorbid medical illnesses have demonstrated that depression and chronic medical conditions have additive, even synergistic effects on physical and social functioning[57-60] and that failure to identify and treat even milder forms of depression may result in increased social morbidity.[61,62]

Early reports of depression and HIV disease suggested that depression was a widespread syndrome in HIV disease. These studies, however, were not well controlled and essentially relied on self-reporting. More recent studies using standardized depression rating scales suggest that the current prevalence of depression is between 4% and 14% in non-drug-using HIV-positive people, compared to a prevalence rate of 5% in the general population.[63]

The relationship between HIV disease progression, stressors, and depressive symptoms is complex. While one study has documented a correlation between stressors and HIV disease progression,[64] other studies have shown a complex relationship between symptoms of HIV disease and depression.[65-68]

Etiology

The causes of depression in HIV-positive patients are multiple. All patients with HIV disease, regardless of physical health status, face fundamental questions regarding the quality and length of their lives. Specific stressors experienced by HIV-positive people may include prolonged periods of physical discomfort, disability, and dependence; lifestyle disruption; loss of work and reduced socioeconomic status; disruption of support networks, including family supports; decreased self-esteem; and sustained periods of loss of personal autonomy.[20,69] Also, some medications used to treat HIV disease may themselves cause depression, including zidovudine (Retrovir or AZT),[60,70] acyclovir,[71] anticonvulsants,[71] corticosteroids,[71,72] dapsone,[71] histamine-2 (H_2)-receptor antagonists,[71] interferon-α,[71] isoniazid,[71] metoclopramide,[71] nonsteroidal anti-inflammatory drugs,[71] and sulfonamides.[71] In evaluation of HIV-positive patients with symptoms of depression, it is critical to rule out intercurrent primary CNS complications, such as meningitis, encephalitis, or space-occupying CNS lesions. All of these complications are extremely rare in patients with CD4 (helper) cell counts greater than $200/mm^3$. HIV-positive patients with depressive symptoms also need to be carefully screened for substance abuse because chronic substance abuse also can cause depressive symptoms.

Although medical and social advances may help people with HIV disease live longer, these long-term survivors often must cope with more physical limitations (fatigue, pain, medication side effects), emotional stressors (loss of many friends to AIDS, isolation, fear of overtaxing caregivers), and spiritual struggles (struggling with the meaning of suffering, when/if to "give up").[73] Long-term survivors of HIV disease, although often temperamentally very psychologically hardy, are at high risk for depression as they cope with survivor's guilt, uncertainty about their ultimate prognosis, or multiple medical problems.

Diagnosis

The psychiatric diagnosis of major depression as currently defined cannot be made unless the patient exhibits five of the nine following symptoms during a 2-week period. In addition, either one of the first two symptoms must be present. The symptoms are

1. Depressed mood
2. Markedly diminished pleasure in all activities
3. Significant and unintentional weight loss or gain
4. Insomnia or oversleeping
5. Fidgetiness or slowed movement or speech (psychomotor agitation or slowing)
6. Fatigue or loss of energy
7. Feelings of worthlessness or excessive inappropriate guilt
8. Diminished ability to think or concentrate
9. Recurrent suicidal thoughts

Clearly, many of these symptoms are also symptoms of primary HIV disease, specifically weight loss, increased sleeping or difficulty sleeping, psychomotor slowing (which may be a symptom of primary HIV dementia), fatigue, and diminished ability to think or concentrate. Thus, *there is a significant overlap between common organic complications of HIV disease and the screening symptoms for depression.*[74,75] Noting this diagnostic and methodologic difficulty, Fernandez and Levy[76] recommend screening for depression in a diagnostically inclusive way. With this method, all symptoms consistent with either depression or primary physical disease are included as possible symptoms of depression until proven otherwise. In patients with psychological symptoms that improve after treatment of a primary disease, it can be safely concluded that the neuropsychiatric syndrome was indeed secondary to primary organic physical disease. Without such an inclusive approach to diagnosis, depression will go unrecognized in most patients with HIV disease because all their symptoms can be "accounted for" by the progression of their disease.

Another methodologic problem in diagnosing depression in patients with HIV disease is the significant overlap between symptoms of depression and symptoms of *encephalopathy/OBD*.[77] Like the geriatric population,[78] HIV-positive patients are at risk for both depression and dementia. Many of the symptoms of these two diseases overlap, such as forgetfulness, decreased concentration, sleep disturbance, behavioral abnormalities, and depressed mood. Early signs of HIV OBD, such as forgetfulness, loss of interest in work, decreased libido, blunted affect, withdrawal, and poor concentration, can be easily misdiagnosed as a primary depressive problem.[1] Although surrogate markers for HIV disease, such as T-cell testing and viral load testing, are clearly not adequately sensitive to rule out OBD in HIV-positive patients with high T-cell counts and low or undetectable viral loads, the presence of cognitive symptoms in patients with relatively good physical health and good surrogate marker parameters is more consistent with a depressive reaction than a demential disorder. Researchers have developed special geriatric depression scales to help differentiate the expected physical symptoms of aging, such as sleep disorder and concern about health status, from specific symptoms of depression, determinable by responses to such questions as "Do you often get bored?" and "Are you in good spirits most of the time?"[78] At this time, no specific depression screening scales like these have been used in the HIV-positive population. Clearly, they would be a useful diagnostic instrument to help clinicians differentiate core physical symptoms of HIV disease from affective complications of OBD and both of these from cognitive complications of OBD.

Hypogonadism is extremely common in men and women with advanced HIV disease and can also be present in patients with less advanced disease.[79-81] The symptoms of hypogonadism (e.g., fatigue, decreased libido, weight loss and appetite problems, concentration, and mood impairment) are very similar to the symptoms of depression,[82,83] and patients may have both hypogonadism and depression. Hypogonadism in men with HIV disease is relatively easy to diagnose and treat. Importantly, many men will have clinical symptoms when their total testosterone level is in the low-normal range (e.g., 350 ng/dl; normal range 300 to 1100 ng/dl). In these cases, the free testosterone level is usually low. All men with suspected hypogonadism should be treated with a trial of testosterone replacement therapy. These replacement doses are not associated with the behavioral side effects seen with the supraphysiologic doses used by athletes.

Hypogonadism in women—loss of both androgens and estrogens—is more difficult to diagnose and treat. Anecdotal experience to date has shown that most women can receive low-dose testosterone (1.25 to 2.5 mg methyltestosterone orally daily) without virilization side effects. Oxandrolone, a pure anabolic agent, can be given to women in full doses (10 mg orally twice a day) without virilization.

Finally, depression is often overlooked as a comorbid complication of medical disease because it may seem situationally appropriate: "I'd be depressed, too, if I had AIDS." Although clinical depression is more frequent in the medically ill, it is never a normal finding in people with HIV disease, any more than mechanical falls are normal in the elderly. Even when depression is a sequela of life-threatening, multisystem diseases such as AIDS or cancer, it can be effectively diagnosed and treated.[48,59,84-86]

Treatment

Depression can be safely and effectively treated by non–mental health professionals if the primary care practitioner is able to direct the time and attention to the recognition and management of this disorder.[87,88] In the Western industrialized world, the majority of patients with depression are treated in the primary care setting by general practitioners, family practitioners, and general internists. The principles of treating depression in HIV-positive patients are quite similar to those of treating depression in the general population and in medically ill patients. Some specific caveats in this setting are that HIV-positive patients may be especially prone to cognitive and functional deterioration if they take anticholinergic agents, such as sedating tricyclic antidepressants (TCAs), especially if the patient has a pre-existing cognitive impairment.[89] Second, patients with AIDS seem to be more prone to drug side effects and incomplete therapeutic responses than are seronegative patients.[76] Third, as noted below, stimulants may be a particularly effective treatment for depression in physically fatigued or cognitively impaired HIV-positive patients with depressive symptoms.[89]

Non–mental health professionals may be understandably reluctant to treat depression because it is a complication outside of their usual range of practice. Nonetheless, it is important to recognize that many physicians who treat HIV-positive patients have learned in effect to practice subspecialty care (i.e., in diagnosing and treating complex infections and dermatologic, neurologic, and hematologic complications of HIV disease). It is important for primary practitioners treating HIV-positive patients to familiarize themselves with the recognition and, ideally, the treatment of depression because many HIV-positive patients may not have the personal resources to obtain specific mental health care or may be unwilling to be treated in a mental health setting. More importantly, the primary care practitioner, being aware of the full spectrum of the patient's medical diagnoses, is in the ideal situation to help select medical therapy when pharmacologic intervention is appropriate for the treatment of depression.

As with seronegative patients who manifest depression, *the consideration governing the choice of an antidepressant is not so much to optimize efficacy as to avoid or exploit medication side effects*.[74,76,90–95] Parallels can be drawn between the treatment of depression in HIV-positive patients with symptomatic complications of HIV disease and, for example, common management of hypertension in patients with other medical disorders. For example, in treating hypertension in the elderly patient with postural hypertension, a physician would avoid drugs likely to aggravate orthostatic hypotension, such as centrally acting agents or α-adrenergic blockers. Similarly, a physician treating a patient with hypertension and angina would tend to use a β-blocker or calcium channel blocker because it would ameliorate both medical conditions. Similarly, in the case of depression, physicians should pick a medication that does not exacerbate prior symptoms and has the potential of ameliorating other symptoms of HIV disease (Table 15–1). For example, some patients with HIV disease have a syndrome of dry mouth similar to Sjögren's syndrome. In these patients, it is best to avoid TCAs with significant anticholinergic side effects because these are likely to aggravate the dry mouth condition. In patients with cognitive disorder along with depression, drugs with significant anticholinergic side effects should be avoided because they can aggravate cognitive impairment. Conversely, patients with HIV-related dermatitis and pruritus, whether caused by underlying dry skin or idiopathic, may benefit from taking an antidepressant with significant antihistamine effects, such as doxepin, at bedtime. In this case, the clinician would have to weigh the benefits of reducing nighttime itching against the benefits and risks of inducing sedation and anticholinergic side effects.

With the advent of the newer antidepressants, such as selective serotonin reuptake inhibitors (SSRIs) and bupropion (Wellbutrin), the clinician has a good range of well-tolerated antidepressants from which to choose.

In the case of TCAs, medications fall along a spectrum in which the most sedating medications tend also to have the most anticholinergic side effects. The prototype of this type of TCA is amitriptyline (Elavil). Low doses of amitriptyline may help to induce sleep but may leave patients with morning somnolence or confusion. Low doses of amitriptyline occasionally are very helpful for chronic pain syndromes, but the same caveats regarding somnolence apply. In general, most consultants treating HIV-positive patients for depression recommend using less sedating medicines with fewer anticholinergic effects.[75] Dosing guidelines need to be based on the patient's overall physical and psychological health. For example, in patients with advanced AIDS, who often have compromised hepatic and renal function and whose physiology may approximate that of geriatric patients, antidepressants should be begun with lower than standard dosages and be titrated upward very slowly until the desired clinical result is achieved. Patients receiving potent cytochrome P-450 enzyme suppressors such as ritonavir and delavirdine should be treated with especially low doses of P-450-metabolized antidepressants, and antidepressants that can cause cardiac arrhythmias (TCAs) and seizures (TCAs, bupropion) should be avoided with these drugs. In HIV-positive patients in good physical health, standard doses of antidepressants may be safely initiated. In general, the optimal TCA for people with HIV-related depression is either nortriptyline, which has the fewest anticholinergic side effects of all TCAs, beginning at a dosage of 25 mg/day; or desipramine, which has the least sedating effect of the TCAs, beginning at 50 mg/day.

The advent of *SSRIs* has provided physicians with four new and very helpful alternatives to

TABLE 15–1. Antidepressants

NAME (TRADE NAME)	STARTING DOSE	THERAPEUTIC DOSE (ORAL)	COMMENTS
Tricyclic Antidepressants (TCA)			
Amitriptyline (Elavil)	10–25 mg qhs	125–250 mg	Very sedating, very anticholinergic
Doxepin (Sinequan)	10–25 mg qhs	150–300 mg	Very sedating, an excellent antihistamine (can treat itching with 10 mg bid)
Nortriptyline (Aventyl, Pamelor)	25–50 mg qhs	75–200 mg	Has the least anticholinergic effects of tricyclics; established efficacy in neuropathy pain palliation
Desipramine (Norpramin)	25–50 mg	150–300 mg	The least sedating of tricyclics; good choice for treating peripheral neuropathy pain
Selective Serotonin Reuptake Inhibitors (SSRIs)*			
Fluoxetine (Prozac)	10 mg qAM	20–80 mg	Has longest half-life of SSRIs and most prone to cause stimulant symptoms initially
Sertraline (Zoloft)	25 mg qAM	50–200 mg	Occasionally causes diarrhea
Paroxetine (Paxil)	10 mg qAM	25–50 mg	If daytime drowsiness occurs, take qhs
Fluvoxamine (Luvox)	50 mg qhs	100–150 mg qhs	
Atypical Agents			
Venlafaxine (Effexor)	37.5 mg SR† tid	75–150 mg SR qd	
Bupropion (Wellbutrin)	150 mg SR qAM	150 mg SR bid	Least likely to cause sexual dysfunction; contraindicated in patients with unstable seizure disorders
Nefazodone (Serzone)	50 mg	150–200 mg bid	Good in anxious patients, patients with insomnia
Stimulants			
Methylphenidate (Ritalin)	5 mg qAM, early afternoon (bid)	10–20 mg bid	Can be used to augment other antidepressants, especially in patients with refractory fatigue
Dextroamphetamine (Dexadrine)	5 mg qAM	5–20 mg bid	
Monoamine Oxidase Inhibitors	Contraindicated		

*Note: SSRIs as a class are more prone to cause sexual dysfunction than other antidepressants
†SR, sustained release.

TCAs. These new medications are paroxetine (Paxil), sertraline (Zoloft), fluoxetine (Prozac), and fluvoxamine (Luvox). In general, SSRIs have minimal anticholinergic side effects and rarely cause sustained sedation, although sedation occasionally may be a side effect in the induction phase of medication, particularly with paroxetine. These medications also tend not to exacerbate functional gastrointestinal and genitourinary symptoms, such as decreased gastric emptying and incomplete bladder emptying, which are commonly seen to complicate HIV disease.

The two main disadvantages of SSRIs are that they initially can have a stimulant effect, which patients with pre-existing anxiety may find intolerable, and that they tend to cause sexual dysfunction, which may not recede with continued use of the medication. It is important to advise a patient of both of these potential side effects of SSRIs. In general, the initial stimulant effect tends to diminish with continued use of the medication, whereas symptoms of sexual dysfunction (e.g., decreased libido, decreased arousal, inability to reach orgasm) tend to be chronic. If the latter symptoms persist, an alternative medication may be indicated.

Unlike initial doses of TCAs, which are generally one third to one quarter of the final therapeutic dose, the initial starting dose of SSRIs as generally recommended may be also the final therapeutic dose. In patients who need to avoid the initial stimulant effect, it can be helpful to start at half-dose therapy.

A significant benefit of the SSRIs is that they pose less risk of suicide in the overdose setting.

The potential disadvantages are that, to date, SSRIs have not been shown in randomized controlled studies to ameliorate peripheral neuropathy, as have some of the TCAs, such as nortriptyline (Pamelor), amitriptyline (Elavil), and desipramine. Additionally, these tricyclics have been shown to ameliorate chronic pain, which is a common symptom of depression in advanced HIV disease. An important area of future research addressing the treatment of depression in the setting of HIV disease is these other potential benefits of antidepressant therapy. The SSRIs with short half-lives (sertraline, paroxetine, fluvoxamine) must be *tapered* when stopped. If stopped abruptly, a benign but dysphoric constellation of serotonin withdrawal symptoms (headache, disorientation, visual disorders) may occur.

Bupropion (Wellbutrin) is another newer antidepressant that is nonsedating and may be especially helpful in fatigued patients. Bupropion is contraindicated in patients with unstable seizure disorders. Seizures have been noted in patients receiving over 400 mg/day of medication. It is known that advanced HIV disease may be complicated by seizures in the absence of known primary CNS disease. In patients with advanced HIV disease, higher doses of bupropion (400 mg/day) should be used cautiously because of the possibility of inducing seizures. To date, this specific complication has not been reported in HIV-positive patients.

Nefazodone (Serzone) is reported to be especially useful in anxious depressed patients, and is a good choice for patients with severe insomnia.

Venlafaxine (Effexor) is a novel antidepressant that inhibits reuptake of both serotonin and norepinephrine. Although most widely used to treat patients who have been refractory to other antidepressants,[96] it is also a well-tolerated first-line agent. Venlafaxine should be started at low doses to avoid severe agitation or anxiety that can occur with too-rapid drug initiation. Venlafaxine (Effexor) is an SSRI-like medication at lower doses and has more stimulating effects at higher doses. Like other SSRIs with short half-lives, it should be tapered slowly. Among the newer antidepressants, it is one of the least likely to have interactions with HIV antivirals.

Monoamine oxidase (MAO) *inhibitors* have been used for decades in the treatment of depression. Although highly effective, they are extremely risky to use in patients with cognitive deficits because patients using MAO inhibitors must be very careful about their diet and concomitant medication intake. Because patients with HIV disease generally take multiple medications and may be prone to dementia, MAO inhibitors should not be used in the treatment of affective disorders associated with HIV disease. If it is considered, MAO therapy should be initiated and monitored by a psychiatric consultant.

Stimulants such as methylphenidate (Ritalin) and dextroamphetamine have been used in the treatment of depression in the medically ill with good success. Stimulants tend to be more rapidly effective than standard antidepressants and are well tolerated in the medically ill.[89,97–102] Fernandez et al.[103,104] have used stimulants in treating cognitive impairment caused by AIDS-related OBD as well as cognitive impairment with attendant affective dysfunction. In their series, 90% of patients showed at least moderate response to stimulants, and no adverse effects were encountered. The maximum dose of methylphenidate used was 90 mg/day in divided doses. In the case of dextroamphetamine, 60 mg/day in divided doses was used.

Stimulants are an excellent adjunctive treatment for HIV-associated fatigue, or depressogenic fatigue.[86] Stimulants may also be especially effective for patients with acute despondency related to acute medical disease. In this situation, stimulants may allow patients to mobilize their emotional resources to cope with the losses attendant with their disease and may enhance compliance with the therapeutic regimen. The standard initial dose of dextroamphetamine is 5 to 10 mg every morning with an optional supplemental dose at noon. Some patients experience a dysphoric stimulatory effect that they describe as being "wired." In these patients, stimulants are ineffective and should be discontinued. Although stimulants in general are not appropriate treatment for depression unrelated to medical illness, partly because tachyphylaxis is commonly seen, stimulants may be effective short- to moderate-term therapy for patients with advanced medical illness secondary to HIV disease. Stimulants are contraindicated in patients with a prior history of psychostimulant abuse.

Once an antidepressant is chosen, antidepressant therapy should be continued for 6 to 8 weeks to assess the patient's response to a specific dose. In cases in which rapid amelioration of depression is necessary, dosages may be escalated more quickly with the understanding that they may need to be adjusted downward if and when medication side effects ensue. Once an effective dosage is found, it should be continued for 6 to 12 months unless the patient develops a medication side effect or requires a dosage increase because of intercurrent stressors or drug malabsorption.

Depression, like hypertension, is a physiologically and biochemically heterogeneous disorder. The only medical information that can help predict medication efficacy in a given patient is a family history of favorable medication response to a particular medication. One advantage of tricyclic therapy is that serum levels may be obtained for some tricyclics to confirm that the patient is taking the medication and that the serum levels are in the therapeutic range. Mental health experts disagree as to the necessity and appropriateness of monitoring serum levels, with many arguing that, in the absence of side effects and in the presence of a good clinical response, serum level determinations are not necessary. Serum levels are not obtainable in clinical practice for non-TCA antidepressants. Medication titration in that setting is based on presence or absence of side effects and clinical response to the medication.

Anecdotal reports suggest that insomnia with early morning awakening may be a specific neuropsychiatric complication of HIV disease apart from any associated primary psychiatric disease, such as depression.[105] In this case, a low dose of a relatively sedating antidepressant such as doxepin or amitriptyline may be appropriate. In low doses (e.g., 50 mg), trazodone is also a useful sedating antidepressant but must be used with caution in men because it can cause priapism.

Psychotherapy and psychopharmacology play complementary roles in the treatment of HIV-associated depression.[106,107] Although medication often relieves many of the physical and mood symptoms of depression, most patients can benefit from an opportunity to share their fears and suffering with a skilled therapist and/or within a support group. Traditional "open-ended" psychotherapeutic approaches are often inappropriate for people with HIV disease, especially those with advanced disease. Therapeutic flexibility is especially important for these patients, whose needs may rapidly change from session to session.[32,108]

Treatment Failure

Patients who do not respond to one or two antidepressants should be referred for psychiatric consultation. Causes of treatment resistance include comorbid psychiatric conditions, comorbid medical illness, and family issues.[109]

All patients with depression should be screened carefully for suicidality, bipolar dis-

ease, and substance use. Actively suicidal patients (i.e., the patient has a specific plan and actively intends to implement it) require emergency psychiatric hospitalization, while suicidal thoughts and fantasies ("I sometimes wish I just didn't wake up") are a normal symptom of depression. Patients with suicidal fantasies need reassurance about their symptoms. Inquiring about suicidal thoughts does not aggravate or cause suicidality in depressed patients. Instead, most patients are relieved to have the opportunity to discuss these symptoms with their clinician.[110,111]

Manic–depressive patients who receive only antidepressants (without mood stabilizers) may escalate into "manic" episodes. When taking a history for mania, the clinician should also inquire about family history of bipolar disease.

"Dual-diagnosed" patients with both depression and active substance use problems are commonly seen in the general medical and HIV-care populations. In some cases, the substance use may be due to the patient self-treating his or her mood disorders; in other cases, the substance may be depressogenic. Whenever possible, these challenging patients should receive their care through a well-integrated mental health team. Even moderate alcohol intake may precipitate mood disorders and/or interfere with antidepressant treatment in some cases.[112] Smoking cessation may also precipitate depressive symptomatology.

Summary

Depression is extremely common in patients with chronic medical disorders, life-threatening diseases, and diseases affecting the CNS, all characteristic of HIV disease. Depression is associated with significant morbidity, and is often partly if not fully reversible with appropriate intervention. Clinicians can best treat depression by screening *all* their patients with HIV disease for depression and by regularly assessing their patients for depression, just as they might regularly assess a patient's tuberculin status or safe-sex practices.

Dementia/Organic Brain Disease

Several studies have established that AIDS dementia complex (ADC) or OBD is a common complication of AIDS and one that is quite variable in its presentation and severity.[1,7,20,113–117] The precise prevalence of ADC depends both on the overall stage of HIV disease of any given patient population and on the neuropsychiatric testing and criteria used to make the diagnosis. Researchers have reached conflicting conclusions about the prevalence of subtle neuropsychiatric impairment in functionally and clinically asymptomatic seropositive patients.[7,118] Overall, possibly 10% of people with AIDS have a comorbid neurologic disorder at the time of their index diagnosis, with 70% experiencing OBD during the course of their illness, 66% experiencing moderate to severe impairment, and 33% having mild or subclinical symptoms. Autopsy studies show evidence of HIV-related CNS abnormalities in approximately 90% of patients with AIDS.[10,114]

Although on some level the subcortical dementia of HIV disease is technically a neurologic complication of AIDS, its clinical manifestations are often behavioral, cognitive, or psychiatric.[1,114] For example, in some patients with organic brain impairment, the primary presenting symptom may be psychomotor agitation, impaired social or occupational functioning, impairment of judgment, personality changes, mood and cognitive symptoms suggestive of depression, and even psychosis.[6,114,116] The overlap between these cognitive, affective, and functional symptoms may make accurate diagnosis difficult. Although neurocognitive examination may be helpful in identifying clinically occult cognitive impairment, standard neuropsychiatric examinations, including the standard mental status examinations, may not identify abnormalities in substantial numbers of patients with mild OBD.[7] Moreover, the type and severity of symptoms a patient manifests may vary greatly with the clinical situation (e.g., a scheduled routine office visit versus hospitalization for an acute febrile illness), and with other confounding intercurrent factors, such as medication use, substance abuse, and intercurrent psychosocial stressors. Studies of patients with HIV-associated depression, mania, and delirium have established that many of these patients have comorbid OBD, and that in many instances the actual etiology of these neuropsychiatric symptoms may indeed be OBD.[7,20] Thus clinicians caring for patients manifesting any neuropsychiatric symptoms should screen the patient carefully for associated OBD. This screening should consist of administering standard basic mental status examinations as well as taking a careful history from family, friends, or coworkers who can provide useful information about the patient's functional status. Often, the first clue to function-threatening OBD may be inability to complete ordinary work tasks in a prompt manner or problems managing routine household responsibilities. In the case of children, OBD may be manifested by developmental abnormalities even in the absence of other symptoms of HIV disease.[7,119]

Clinicians treating HIV-associated dementia need to consider aggressive antiretroviral therapy for potential reversal or slowing of the dementia process,[113,120] providing optimal milieu management for the patient, and providing appropriate practical and psychosocial support for the patient's loved ones. Two published studies[120,121] and several anecdotal reports[26] suggest that treatment with zidovudine may ameliorate the symptoms and natural history of HIV dementia. Some patients with even relatively severe cognitive impairments have been known to exhibit remarkable behavioral and cognitive improvement after receiving zidovudine therapy in supervised settings. Of note, the patients described in these anecdotal reports have taken doses of zidovudine larger than those now generally used, usually in the 800-mg/day range.[122] It is unknown whether other antiretrovirals with good CNS penetration (didanosine, stavudine, nevirapine, indinavir) are effective against HIV dementia. When HIV-associated OBD is complicated by symptoms of depression, the optimal treatment may not be standard antidepressive therapy but stimulant therapy.[103,104] Studies of stimulant therapy for patients with AIDS-related cognitive impairment and associated organic affective disorders have demonstrated that stimulants may improve both the cognitive status and mood of the patient and are safe even in patients with advanced AIDS. Symptoms of depression in patients with dementia may not take the form of standard mood changes but instead may be reflected in the patient's neglect of personal needs, such as hygiene and nutrition, or the patient's indifference to the environment, the disease, and medical treatments.[114,123] In patients with dementia, TCAs should be used with caution because those antidepressants with high anticholinergic receptor affinities are apt to increase confusion.[20]

Depression commonly complicates all dementias, including HIV dementia. Because the symptoms of depression and dementia overlap, *depression is the most under-recognized and undertreated complication of dementia.* Most demented patients should receive a trial of antidepressants to treat any undiagnosed depressive symptoms.

Milieu management involves carefully assessing a patient's neurocognitive status (motor function, orientation, and memory) and adjusting the environment accordingly to maximize the patient's autonomy and to minimize the patient's risk.[26,124] The patient's need for supervision must be assessed carefully as well, be it by a health professional or by family members.[114] A home safety assessment should be conducted by a home nurse or social worker. The person making this assessment should check for the presence of reality-orientation cues, such as calendars and clocks, and ensure that hallways and living areas are brightly lit; that walkways are clear and free of electrical wires or unstable furniture; and that potentially dangerous items, such as sharp objects, chemicals and poisons, and power tools, are safely stored away. In addition, knobs should be removed from stoves to ensure that a confused patient will not inadvertently burn himself or herself or set fire to the home.

Milieu management extends to the patient's milieu on a communication level. Patients and their caregivers often find that communication difficulties are the most frustrating and heart-wrenching complications of OBD. Many caregivers may feel inadequate in the face of an unpredictably angry, agitated, or incommunicative loved one despite their best efforts at compassionate and "36-hour-per-day" care. Helpful communication techniques include

- Asking the patient simple yes-or-no questions, and avoiding lengthy explanations and instead giving short, pragmatic answers
- Remembering that long-term memory is often intact and, thus, sharing remote reminiscences might be soothing; by contrast, immediate memory is likely to be quite impaired and, thus, immediate recall efforts may be frustrating for the patient
- Speaking in a low-pitched, even tone of voice

Caregivers need to be instructed in these techniques as well as in specific techniques to help confused, agitated patients.

It is also critical for medical caregivers to assess the well-being of the patient's family and other caregivers. As brain disease advances, the patient may become less communicative. The caregiver may in effect lose his or her loved one before the patient's actual physical death. Some caregivers may respond to this loss by inappropriately increasing the time and intensity of their practical home efforts. Families and caregivers of patients with OBD need to be encouraged to take regular respites and to voice their needs. They, too, need to be monitored for signs of burnout or depression.[114] Over 30% of spousal caregivers of Alzheimer's patients meet criteria for major depression.[119]

The patient's home-based caregivers are much more likely to cope well and respond appropriately to the patient's increasing disability if they have some sense of understanding of the course of the disease and the types of measures they can take when problems arise. Simple instruction in basic techniques such as managing patient transfers, dealing with incontinence, responding to agitation, and dealing with unpredictable behavior can enhance caregivers' coping abilities and help them play a more practical and meaningful role in their loved one's care.[97,125]

Wolcott et al.[20] summarized the principles of management of patients with OBD as follows. First, clinicians should minimize drugs with CNS toxicity and recognize that some drugs used to treat HIV disease may in themselves cause or aggravate symptoms of ADC. Second, psychosocial treatment should begin early in the treatment of OBD. With appropriate intervention, a patient may develop "compensatory prostheses" to compensate for impaired cognitive function. In addition, at the time of recognition of OBD, early arrangements should be made for assessment of terminal care wishes and to arrange legal matters, such as wills and power of attorney. Social treatment also involves initiating appropriate home care services and, as importantly, appropriate respite services for home-based caregivers.

Wolcott et al. also outlined several principles of pharmacologic treatment of patients with OBD. First, medically ill patients with OBD should initially receive low doses of antidepressants or stimulants or medium to low doses of neuroleptics, with doses gradually adjusted to minimize CNS complications. Second, cognitively impaired patients manifesting depression may respond better to stimulants than to antidepressants, and psychotic syndromes, be they organic or functional, should be treated with the lowest effective dose of neuroleptics[20,89] (Table 15–2). In some cases, non-neuroleptic medications such as carbamazepine or buspirone may reduce agitation and other behavioral problems.[126,127]

Clearly, dementia is one of the most heartbreaking and medically challenging complications of HIV disease. Effective disease recognition by the clinician requires a high index of suspicion of dementia whenever the patient manifests neurocognitive symptoms. Effective treatment of dementia in the AIDS setting requires a thorough understanding of the patient's

TABLE 15–2. Neuroleptic/Antipsychotic Medications

RELATIVE POTENCY (TRADE NAME)	STARTING ADULT DOSE (ORAL)	THERAPEUTIC ADULT DAILY DOSE	COMMENTS
Low potency (Thorazine, Mellaril)	25–50 mg q8–12h	50–800 mg	Very sedating/anticholinergic, low risk for extrapyramidal symptoms (EPS)
Midpotency (Trilafon)	4 mg q8–12h	12–64 mg	Medium-range risk for sedation/anticholinergic/EPS side effects
High potency (Haldol)	1–2 mg q6–8h	2–10 mg	Low risk for sedation, anticholinergic side effects; high risk for EPS; case reports in AIDS patients of neuroleptic malignant syndrome
Atypical: Risperidone (Risperdal)	1 mg bid	2–5 mg bid	Low risk for EPS, tardive dyskinesia

medical status as well as his or her home situation and support network. Finally, patients with HIV-related dementia who remain at home need a well-coordinated interdisciplinary approach to make their home-based care safe, comprehensive, and humane.

Anxiety/Panic Disorder

Anxiety is commonly experienced by HIV-positive patients. When it is chronic and global, it is described as a generalized anxiety disorder. Manifestations of this disorder may include trouble falling asleep, impaired concentration, psychomotor agitation, and fatigue. Anxiety also may be a complication of medications, including anticonvulsants, corticosteroids, ganciclovir, nonsteroidal anti-inflammatory drugs, and sulfonamides.[71] Anxiety also may be due to drug withdrawal, and all patients with new symptoms of anxiety should be carefully screened for drug withdrawal or substance use. Discrete episodes of anxiety characterized by physiologic flight-or-fight symptoms, such as palpitations, shortness of breath, dizziness, headache, paresthesias, derealization, and depersonalization, are called panic attacks. Panic attacks are seen with increased frequency in the HIV primary care setting relative to the population in general.[128] Panic disorder is also commonly seen with major depression, alcohol abuse, and post-traumatic stress disorders.[128]

In choosing therapy for anxiety or panic disorder, the clinician and patient must decide whether to use quick and short-acting medicines (e.g., alprazolam [Xanax] or lorazepam [Ativan]) to ameliorate intermittent symptoms or whether to use long-acting round-the-clock antianxiety medications (e.g., clonazepam [Klonopin]) to prevent chronic anxiety (Table 15–3). In general, patients with relatively infrequent and predictable anxiety, such as before an office visit, can be managed well with small doses of quick and short-acting antianxiety medicines. Conversely, patients with chronic anxiety are best managed with scheduled doses of long-acting antianxiety medicines to prevent breakthrough anxiety or anxiety secondary to withdrawal from anxiolytic agents. In these cases of chronic anxiety, buspirone (BuSpar) may be quite useful. Although it may take up to 2 to 3 weeks for buspirone to be fully effective as an anxiolytic, it has the great advantages of being

TABLE 15–3. Anxiolytics

NAME (TRADE NAME)	STARTING DOSE	THERAPEUTIC DOSE	COMMENTS
Clonazepam (Klonopin)	0.5 mg bid	0.5–2 mg bid	Excellent long-acting, round-the-clock anxiolytic; onset of action slow
Lorazepam (Ativan)	0.5–1 mg q8h prn	0.5–2 mg q8h prn	Rapid onset of action, no active metabolites
Alprazolam (Xanax)	0.5–1 mg q8h prn	0.5–2 mg q8h prn	Rapid onset of action
Buspirone (BuSpar)	10 mg tid	10–15 mg tid	Nonsedating, nonaddictive; not useful for acute anxiety; suitable for patients with chronic anxiety

nonaddictive and of not causing respiratory depression.[129] Buspirone has been shown in one study to help reduce anxiety and drug use in drug users with AIDS or AIDS-related complex.[130] Buspirone is not effective for treatment of acute anxiety. In cases in which a long-acting anxiolytic is indicated, clonazepam can be titrated between 0.5 and 2 mg orally twice a day. Because many comorbid psychiatric conditions, such as substance abuse, can be seen with anxiety, patients need to be carefully screened for concomitant psychiatric conditions before anxiolytic therapy is undertaken.

Panic attacks, in particular, may mimic physiologic symptoms of HIV complications, such as shortness of breath or dizziness. Certain clues suggest that the symptoms stem from a panic attack rather than a primary organic complication of HIV disease. A panic attack is suspected if the physical symptoms are situational (e.g., occurring before an important laboratory study or on the anniversary of the death of a loved one) or if the symptoms produce significant apprehension out of proportion to the fear the patient experiences with analogous physical symptoms. Patients with panic disorder typically have multiple symptoms involving multiple organ systems during panic attacks. Panic attacks may last from minutes to hours and are often self-limited. Panic disorder is commonly complicated by agoraphobia. Clues to the presence of panic disorder include a previous patient history of depression or a family history of either panic disorder or depression.

Long-term therapy of panic disorder generally is best achieved with antidepressant medications. TCAs have historically been the mainstay in treatment of panic disorder. However, the newer agents, such as SSRIs and venlafaxine, are effective against panic disorders and are generally better tolerated than TCAs. It is important to recognize that, although patients with panic disorder may not be overtly depressed, they are at high risk for suicide. Although there are no published reports of HIV-positive people with panic disorder committing suicide, it is clear that, in the general population, patients with panic disorder are at significant risk for suicide and need to be monitored accordingly.

Patients receiving short-acting benzodiazepines need to be counseled about the possibility of drug withdrawal when these medicines are discontinued. In general, these medicines should be tapered rather than abruptly stopped. In the case of longer acting benzodiazepines, tapering is partly achieved by the long-acting nature of the medicine, but a short taper period should be considered when patients have been on long-acting benzodiazepines for a considerable period of time.

Obsessive-compulsive disorder (OCD) is commonly misdiagnosed as simple anxiety, or missed altogether. OCD is treated with high-dose SSRIs, and cases of comorbid OCD/HIV disease have been reported.[131]

Delirium

Delirium is a serious complication of any illness, and HIV disease is no exception. The causes of delirium can include primary CNS opportunistic infections, drug side effects, systemic illness, and primary functional disease related to disorientation and confusion. Patients with delirium have a very guarded medical prognosis and should be managed accordingly, with an inclusive diagnostic approach that incorporates frequent re-evaluation by the caregiver in a monitored setting.

Important specific causes of delirium in the medically ill HIV-positive patient include hypoglycemia or hypotension resulting from intravenous pentamidine therapy, hyperkalemia secondary to high-dose trimethoprim-sulfamethoxazole (Septra) therapy, severe agitation caused by high-dose corticosteroid therapy, electrolyte disorders caused by renal tubular dysfunction secondary to foscarnet or amphotericin therapy, hypoxemia secondary to respiratory illness, hyponatremia secondary to the syndrome of inappropriate antidiuretic hormone secretion or hypotonic fluid administration, acute disinhibitory states resulting from use of benzodiazepines or other sedatives, and use of or withdrawal from recreational drugs.[76]

The general principles of treating delirium in HIV-positive patients are the same as those of patients in general.[12,20,73,89,132,133] General treatment measures include providing orienting information, minimizing disruption of the sleep/wake cycle, avoiding medications with CNS side effects, and treating agitation with appropriate pharmacologic intervention.[20]

Early studies of delirious AIDS patients suggested that AIDS patients were at risk for neuroleptic malignant syndrome and/or extrapyramidal symptoms when treated with high-potency neuroleptics such as haloperidol.[14,17,64,134–136] However, more recent studies have demonstrated that neuroleptics are more effective and better tolerated than benzodiazepines, and failed to show any efficacy/toxicity differential between high- and low-potency neuroleptics.[137]

Because of haloperidol's IV/IM/PO route flexibility, it is the initial best treatment for most agitated patients. Anecdotal reports suggest that the newer atypical agents such as risperidone (Risperdal) are also effective and well tolerated in patients able to take oral medications.[135,138,139]

Patients with delirium need to be managed in a setting where regular, thorough neuropsychiatric assessments are undertaken by appropriate personnel. Drugs that can cause delirium include amphotericin, anticonvulsants, ciprofloxacin, corticosteroids, ganciclovir, α-interferon, and metoclopramide.[71]

Mania

Mania is characterized by persistently elevated expansive or irritable mood associated with less need for sleep, pressured speech, distractibility, flight of ideas, psychomotor agitation or increase in goal-directed activity, inflated self-esteem or grandiosity, and excessive involvement in pleasurable activities that have a high potential for painful consequences. Mania may occur as an initial manifestation of HIV disease; as a mood disorder superimposed on previously known advanced HIV disease, as hypomania, as a complication of corticosteroids, narcotics, or other medications; or as a first manifestation of an opportunistic or systemic illness. In most cases, mania seems to be a complication of HIV-related OBD because it tends to occur late in the course of disease and to be commonly correlated with cognitive defects that often may not resolve when the manic episode recedes.[140,141] From the evidence of current case report studies, mania in AIDS carries a poor prognosis. In one study, over one quarter of the patients died within 6 months of their psychiatric presentation.[140]

Although patients with HIV disease are generally responsive to standard antimania medicines (Table 15–4),[142,143] their response may be incomplete, and they may be prone to more significant side effects.[140] Medications known to precipitate mania include anticonvulsants, bupropion, buspirone, corticosteroids, dapsone, H_2-receptor antagonists, metoclopramide, and zidovudine.[71] Lithium has generally been the mainstay of treatment of mania. However, lithium therapy poses many potential problems in patients with advanced HIV disease. Because these patients often take medicines that may alter renal function or affect tubular salt clearance, lithium dosing may be very difficult. Additionally, patients with HIV disease are prone to dehydration. They commonly experience protracted episodes of vomiting or diarrhea or both, placing them at increased risk for dehydration and thus lithium toxicity. Because of these potential problems, other agents, such as neuroleptics and anticonvulsants, should be considered for management of patients with both acute and chronic HIV-associated mania.

HIV-related mania should be treated as follows. First, potential offending medicines as noted above should be decreased or stopped as soon as is medically feasible. Initial therapy may consist of a neuroleptic. Although low-potency neuroleptics are theoretically appealing because of their sedative effects, their usefulness is limited by their tendency to cause confusion even at low dosages (this probably reflects the underlying OBD that predisposes patients with HIV disease to mania).[89] Anticonvulsants, such as carbamazepine and valproic acid, also have been used to stabilize mood in patients with HIV-associated mania. Newer anticonvulsants (gabapentin, lamotrigine) are also being used as

TABLE 15–4. Antimania Drugs

NAME (TRADE NAME)	STARTING ADULT DOSE (ORAL)	THERAPEUTIC ADULT DAILY DOSE	COMMENTS
Lithium	(Onset 7–10 days) 300 mg tid (to start maintenance)	Acute: 1200–2400 mg/day Maintenance: 900–1500 mg/day	Avoid in patients with unstable volume status, fluctuating renal status, those receiving nephrotoxic drugs
Carbamazepine (Tegretol)	200 mg bid	400 mg bid	An increased risk of bone marrow effects has not been reported in AIDS patients; monitor liver function tests, CBC, drug levels
Valproic acid (Depakote)	250 mg bid	250 mg tid	Nausea is the main side effect limiting therapy

mood stabilizers. In the setting of HIV disease, mania is commonly associated with depressive disease and cognitive impairment, and all patients with HIV-associated mania should be carefully screened for both of these comorbid conditions. Hypomanic patients, although not at immediate risk regarding their medical health, may have a poor overall prognosis because of inability to comply with medical plans or treatment protocols as a result of unrealistic assessments about their health. These patients should receive aggressive treatment to enhance cooperation with the treatment program. When subject to intercurrent stressors, these hypomanic patients may develop symptoms consistent with full-blown mania and thus need to be carefully monitored.

Psychosis

Patients with HIV disease may present with organically based psychoses that are phenomenologically indistinguishable from functional psychoses.[5] All patients with a new psychosis disorder should therefore be carefully screened for risk factors for HIV disease, and appropriate work-up should be undertaken for HIV-related problems when indicated. Medications that may cause psychosis and hallucinations include anabolic steroids, amphotericin, anticonvulsants, ciprofloxacin, buspirone, corticosteroids, dapsone, ganciclovir, H_2-receptor antagonists, interferon-α, isoniazid, ketoconazole, nonsteroidal anti-inflammatory agents, metronidazole (Flagyl), salicylates, sulfonamides, and zidovudine.[71] The same primary medical conditions noted previously as causes of mania and depression can precipitate psychosis. For this reason, the clinician should conduct a thorough medical evaluation and medication review to rule out a primary medical basis for any psychotic episode. Substance abuse should be carefully ruled out. Acute antipsychotic medications are reviewed in the delirium section. All patients with schizophrenia or who require ongoing neuroleptic medications should be evaluated by a psychiatric consultant.

PSYCHOSOCIAL ISSUES

Ethical/Legal Issues

All patients with life-threatening illnesses, particularly those likely to affect CNS function and, therefore, legal competence,[144] need to make difficult decisions regarding their medical treatment in the last stages of their disease. These issues are best discussed when the patient is relaxed and cognitively intact, and the discussion is best initiated by the primary care provider with the broadest understanding of the patient's psychosocial circumstances and the tempo of his or her HIV disease.[145] Proactively broaching issues, such as designating a power of attorney and making a will, is especially important in patients who have nontraditional families (e.g., gay male couples) or in situations where the stress of the patient's illness has resulted in significant intrafamily conflict.[145,146] Studies of persons with AIDS show that most of them wish to discuss their preferences for life-sustaining measures with their physicians, and few actually have been given the opportunity.[147] Some patients, on initially learning of their HIV positivity, immediately have concerns about their ability to remain independent and autonomous if and when their disease progresses. These patients may wish to discuss this issue on the initial visit with their caregiver. Primary care practitioners need to be prepared for these discussions. It is important to reassure patients that they will not be abandoned as their condition progresses and that their wishes regarding life-sustaining treatment and palliative treatment will be respected should that time come.

Some patients with HIV disease want to discuss the option of rational suicide with their primary caregiver.[25,125,148-151] In one uncontrolled survey of HIV-infected patients, 67% of the respondents indicated that they had considered rational suicide as an option for themselves. In these respondents, suicidal feelings and depression were not necessarily related. Some reported that the ability to discuss this in an open setting, such as a support group, helped them normalize their feelings and manage their suicidal thoughts.[151]

Rational suicide and euthanasia are extremely controversial issues within the medical profession.[150,152-154] Nonetheless, practitioners must realize that many HIV-positive patients have at least considered suicide as an option for themselves. Thus it is important for practitioners to examine their feelings about this issue because they are likely to be approached about it by their patients. In some cases, a candid and empathic discussion about terminal and palliative care issues may help relieve the patient's concerns about intractable physical or emotional suffering. In these discussions, it is appropriate for the clinician to carefully screen the patient for a reactive depression, especially one that is inappropriate to disease stage (e.g., a patient with no symptoms of HIV disease who is considering rational suicide).[151,155]

Estate planning and designation of power of attorney are important issues best mediated through professional legal counsel. These discussions are ideally undertaken during periods of relative good health between acute illnesses, but occasionally may need to be undertaken in a hospital setting. Social workers may be an appropriate source of referral for legal assistance in cases in which legal planning is deferred until relatively late. The attorney preparing legal documents in the acute medical setting needs to verify that the patient is legally competent to make or amend a will. Essentially, legal competence means the patient is aware of his or her setting and is aware of the changes or designations he or she is making in the will. Clinicians can help evaluate the patient's competency to assist legal counsel in the timing of legal planning. In the setting of even the intensive care unit, where patients typically have multiorgan complications, clinical and formal assessments of cognition can be made to document a patient's cognitive status.[156] Because hospitalized and terminally ill patients with HIV disease are especially prone to delirium, it is critical that clinicians document a patient's mental status when legal documents are prepared or modified. Jones et al.[157] developed a straightforward bedside test

of cognition for patients with HIV disease, the results of which correlated well with more complex instruments such as the formal Mini-Mental State Examination and the Trail Making Tests.

Fatigue

Many patients with HIV disease, even those with "good" T cell counts and low viral loads, are profoundly limited and frustrated by fatigue. In some cases, the fatigue takes the form of an unpredictable cyclic disorder; for example, the patient may get easily exhausted with simple tasks for 2 days, then be able to go without a nap and even take a long walk the third day, only to be exhausted again for the next few days. In other cases, patients may, on a daily basis, wake up with good energy only to find they must rest after minor activities.

The psychological impact of either cyclical or unremitting fatigue is extensive. Patients may be isolated, fail to shop or eat, have difficulty with medication compliance, and become demoralized. *Fatigue is the most under-reported symptom of HIV disease*, and is often undertreated by clinicians.[158] Patients with fatigue should be aggressively evaluated (see Table 15–5), and their symptoms should be recorded in the medical chart to corroborate their disability. Even in cases in which fatigue is idiopathic, it can often

TABLE 15–5. Fatigue in HIV Disease

CAUSE	CLUES	DIAGNOSTIC TESTS	TREATMENT
Hypogonadism	Decreased libido	Testosterone level	*Men*: • testosterone cypionate 400 mg IM q2wk • Androderm patch (5 mg qd) • Testoderm ITS (5 mg qd) *Women/Men*: • oxandrolone (10 mg po bid) *Women*: • methyltestosterone 1.25–2.5 mg po bid
Adrenal insufficiency	Postural dizziness, fevers	Cortrosyn stimulation test	Hydrocortisone 20 mg qAM, 10 mg midday
Methemoglobinemia	Dapsone-treated patient	Methemaglobin level	Stop dapsone
Anemia	Headaches, dizziness	Complete blood count	Erythropoietin; discontinue myelosuppressive medications if able
Depression	Fatigue present on wakening; prior family history of depression	None	Antidepressants; stimulants
Malnutrition (decreased lean body mass)	Muscle wasting; decreased body mass index	Check for hypogonadism	Androgens, anabolics; appetite stimulants; human growth hormone

be palliated. Appropriate exercise usually helps rather than worsens fatigue.

Pain Control

Chronic and acute pain are common complications of HIV disease. These pain syndromes may include acute pain, such as that from a surgical incision or central line placement in the thorax, or chronic pain, such as peripheral neuropathy, chronic sinusitis, or chronic myalgias. The principles of pain management in HIV-positive patients are similar to those in other medically ill patients.[159-161] Pain is underreported and undertreated in HIV patients, as it is in many medically ill populations.[136,162-165] Minority group members, women, and substance users are at highest risk for undiagnosed pain.[136,162,166,167] Pain in HIV disease adversely affects quality of life. Although most patients have a specific cause(s) of their pain, about 10% will have no specific diagnosis to account for their pain syndrome.[168-170] It can be helpful in both the inpatient and outpatient setting to take "pain vital signs" to assess the patient's degree of pain and his or her response to the current analgesic program.[165] In general, short-acting narcotics are best used for unpredictable or breakthrough pain, and longer acting narcotics (e.g., sustained-release morphine [MS Contin], sustained-release oxycodone [Oxycontin] are best used for chronic pain. Newer narcotic medicine delivery systems include Roxanol, a liquid morphine solution that can be absorbed sublingually; fentanyl patches, a cutaneous delivery system that provides round-the-clock analgesia for 2 to 3 days; and portable patient-controlled analgesia units that deliver both constant and bolus infusions of parenteral narcotic medication. In addition, antidepressant therapy may be a very useful analgesia adjunct in patients with chronic pain, particularly neuropathic pain.

Peripheral neuropathy may respond to low-dose (10 to 100 mg every h.s.) TCA therapy alone. Other antidepressants, such as SSRIs, may palliate chronic pain.[134,171] Neuroleptic medications (carbamazepine, valproic acid, gabapentin, lamotrigine) often help chronic nerve pain.[172] Lancinating or shooting neuropathic pain seems to respond best to carbamazepine therapy. Nontraditional pain control interventions, such as body work, acupuncture, herbal therapy, and massage, may have very effective analgesic and psychosocial effects for some patients (see Chapter 38). Patients with advanced HIV disease receiving centrally acting medications, including narcotic therapy, should be closely monitored because these patients are particularly susceptible to confusion or delirium after receiving these agents. Postherpetic neuralgia may be palliated with TCAs. Postherpetic neuralgia has not been shown to be prevented by treating acute herpes zoster with high-dose acyclovir therapy.

Bereavement

HIV disease, like all progressive, chronic illnesses, is characterized by cumulative losses: loss of physical function, loss of work, loss of identity, loss of dreams, and loss of control. All people with HIV disease benefit from discussing these losses with their clinician. In some cases, simply sharing the pain and frustration of these losses is helpful for the patient.[61,173-178] Most patients develop a psychospiritual coping system in the face of life's challenges. The resources and strength patients bring to their disease are as relevant to their care as are their limitations.[174,179,180]

In addition to grieving about their own multiple losses, many HIV-infected patients have lost friends, family, and lovers to HIV disease. Distinguishing "appropriate bereavement" from depression or from complicated grief disorders is very, very difficult in this context.[181-183] Because some patients with apparent recurrent simple bereavement do have depressive disorders, a depressive diagnosis with mental health referral or careful empiric antidepressant treatment should be considered in all patients with atypical bereavement symptoms.

Caregiver Issues

Practitioners caring for HIV-positive patients need to recognize the psychiatric morbidity seen in HIV-negative caregivers of people with HIV disease. This morbidity may take the form of caregiver stress. Often, a fully employed spouse or partner may attempt to act as a primary practical caregiver to a loved one. Caregivers in this situation are extremely prone to burnout and depression and need active support from the primary practitioner. The primary medical practitioner should arrange for respite care and practical support at home to allow the home caregiver to focus on emotional and psychological support rather than practical caregiving. The primary care practitioner can also provide invaluable support to HIV-negative caregivers by validating their difficult role and helping them manage priorities. HIV-negative caregivers may experience survivor guilt and in some cases may develop frank adjustment disorders or major depression. In addition, primary care practitioners can help families share the burden of a family member's illness by encouraging them to seek help when they are feeling overwhelmed.

Ironically, within many families and communities, the primary home-based caregiver of an HIV-positive patient is also HIV positive. In these situations, the practical difficulties involved in caregiving for an HIV-positive person may be compounded by the caregiver's understandable fears of future illness. It is natural for the caregiver to anticipate his or her illness, projecting his or her future course from the patient's present medical course. Additionally, in some communities, particularly the gay male community, many people with HIV disease and their caregivers have suffered multiple losses of friends, family, and even other caregivers. Standard models of coping with grief have emphasized a somewhat closed model of bereavement followed by resolution of grief. However, many HIV-positive people and their caregivers are in chronic mourning and never have the opportunity to fully resolve their grief from one loss before they must face yet another ill companion or friend.[184] No simple psychotherapeutic model has been developed to address these seemingly impossible psychological burdens. Intuitively, however, it appears that simply giving patients and their loved ones an opportunity to air their difficulties and to receive emotional support may not only provide solace but also bond the relationship among the physician, the patient, and loved ones.

As importantly, caregivers and people with HIV disease need to find support in the community. These meaningful connections can include participating in public rituals, such as the AIDS Quilt and memorial services, belonging to a support group, receiving pastoral counseling, and participating in a religious congregation or other spiritual practices.[179,180] Because of the stigmas associated with AIDS, especially the stigmas of intravenous drug use and nontraditional lifestyles, many people with AIDS-related grief may be reluctant to seek solace from their pastors. Social workers should identify sensitive and knowledgeable pastoral counselors in the community who can provide solace and guidance to these individuals and families.

Medical caregivers, too, need to recognize their high risk for burnout.[176,185,186] Caregivers may be confronted with fears of contagion or negative attitudes toward various populations at risk for HIV disease. Caregivers also may be in chronic mourning and may have suffered the cumulative loss of many patients and even colleagues. Medical caregivers generally are not well prepared by their training programs to treat patients with progressive terminal illnesses. Instead, training programs tend to emphasize curative therapies rather than palliative therapies, which does not prepare trainees for the psychologic dilemmas and spiritual stress involved in caring for people with life-threatening or terminal illnesses.[187–191] Program administrators and clinic leaders can help their staffs cope with the psychological and spiritual stress of working with people with HIV disease by setting up regular inservices for didactic training addressing the management of end-stage symptoms; by setting up informal group sessions to share feelings about difficult or beloved patients; and by ensuring regular respite from stressful care in the form of short work weeks, regular vacations, and regular mental health days.

Practitioners in solo practice settings need to ensure that they are well trained in all aspects of palliative care and have at least rudimentary training in assessment of the major psychiatric syndromes. Regular exercise, regular respites, and strict time off from work can physically and spiritually replenish medical caregivers, preparing them to provide optimal care for their patients.

Return to Work, Disability Issues, and Living with HIV

Previously, the psychosocial challenge of HIV disease was coping with early death and a relentless progressive disease. In the HAART era, HIV-infected women, men, and children must cope with a still potentially terminal disease with a much more favorable prognosis. Many of the patients who prepared to die of HIV disease are now struggling with the practical (work, education, mortgage, long-term financial planning) and psychospiritual challenges of living with HIV disease. While many HIV-infected patients feel much better, and some are even asymptomatic, many patients continue to have "outlier" symptoms such as cognitive impairment, muscle wasting, neuropathy, fatigue, sexual dysfunction, chronic diarrhea, and arthralgias that may not improve despite substantial improvements in T-cell/viral load indices. Other patients who cannot tolerate or who do not respond to

HAART may feel especially isolated or abandoned in this era of higher expectations.

Clinicians should regularly check in with patients with regard to these functional and psychological issues. Stopping *or* returning to work are complex decisions that require active teamwork between patients, clinicians, and benefits counselors.

CONCLUSION

A psychosocial approach to the care of HIV-positive patients involves a global, inclusive approach to the patient's life and to the patient's illness. Stoeckle et al.[192] have characterized this type of global perspective as "the work of care." This work includes the standard information-gathering work and physical examination work involved in the standard history and physical examination, but also involves emotional work (eliciting psychologic information), biographic work (understanding and knowing the patient), comfort work (personal support of patients in all stages of disease), negotiation and interpretive work (helping the patient understand the course of the disease), educational work (helping the patient prevent disease complications), brokering work (helping the patient negotiate the health care system), moral and ethical work (including eliciting preferences), collaborative colleague work (helping provide personal care in multispecialty settings), and self-reflective work (optimizing interpersonal relations among the patient, the family, and the practitioner).[192]

This inclusive model of the work of care is an excellent approximation to the ideal primary care model. Although mental health complications as discussed may have been managed traditionally by consultants, primary care practitioners, given their comprehensive approach to the patient and the emphasis on continuity and coordination of care, are in an optimal position to assess and treat the neuropsychiatric complications of AIDS.[193] The actual impact of psychological intervention in the care of HIV-positive patients has not been established.[194] However, actively investigating and compassionately treating the psychosocial complications of HIV disease will likely result in improved medical outcomes for the patient, better allocation of medical resources, increased comfort for patients and their loved ones, and increased satisfaction for the providers who can give comprehensive and compassionate care.

In an era in which the benefits of "HIV specialists" have been documented, it is critical that all clinicians caring for HIV patients integrate the best features of generalist care (viewing the patient as a whole person, palliative care, integrating multisystem treatments)[195,196] with the demonstrated benefits of specialty care.

References

1. Holland J, Tross S: The psychosocial and neuropsychiatric sequelae of the acquired immunodeficiency syndrome and related disorders. Ann Intern Med 103:760, 1985
2. Atkinson J, Grant I, Kennedy C, et al: Prevalence of psychiatric disorders among men infected with human immunodeficiency virus. Arch Gen Psychiatry 45:859, 1988
3. Perry S, Jacobsberg L, Fishman B, et al: Psychiatric diagnosis before serological testing for the human immunodeficiency virus. Am J Psychiatry 147:89, 1990
4. Buhrich N, Cooper D, Freed E: HIV infection associated with symptoms indistinguishable from functional psychosis. Br J Psychiatry 152:649, 1988
5. Sewell D, Jeste D, Atkinson JH, Heaton R: HIV-associated psychosis: A study of 20 cases. Am J Psychiatry 151:237, 1994
6. Navia B, Price R: The acquired immunodeficiency syndrome dementia complex as the presenting sole manifestation of human immunodeficiency virus infection. Arch Neurol 44:65, 1987
7. Perry S: Organic mental disorders caused by HIV: Update on early diagnosis and treatment. Am J Psychiatry 147:696, 1990
8. Sacks M, Dermatis H, Looser-Ott S, Perry S: Seroprevalence of HIV and risk factors for AIDS in psychiatric inpatients. Hosp Community Psychiatry 43:736, 1992
9. Cournes F, Herman R, Kaplan M, et al: AIDS prevention for people with severe mental illness. J Pract Psychiatry Behav Health 3:285, 1997
10. Ferrando S: Substance use disorders and HIV illness. AIDS Reader Mar/Apr:57, 1997
11. Johnson J, Williams J, Goetz R, et al: Personality disorders predict onset of Axis I disorders and impaired functioning among homosexual men with and at risk of HIV infection. Arch Gen Psychiatry 53:350, 1996
12. Susser E, Colson P, Jandorf L, et al: HIV infection among young adults with psychotic disorders. Am J Psychiatry 154:864, 1997
13. Bialer P, Wallack J, Prenziauer S, et al: Psychiatric comorbidity among hospitalized AIDS patients vs. non-AIDS patients referred for psychiatric consultation. Psychosomatics 37:469, 1996
14. Johnson J, Williams J, Rabkin J: Axis I psychiatric symptoms associated with HIV infection and personality disorder. Am J Psychiatry 152:551, 1995
15. Roland M: Antiviral adherence dilemmas. Focus 13(3):1, 1998
16. Atkinson J, Grant I: Natural history of neuropsychiatric manifestations of HIV disease. Psychiatr Clin North Am 17:17, 1994
17. Baldeweg T, Catalan J, Pugh K, et al: Neurophysiological changes associated with psychiatric symptoms in HIV-infected individuals without AIDS. Biol Psychiatry 41:478, 1997

18. Levy J, Fernandez F: Neuropsychiatric aspects of HIV infection of the central nervous system. In Hales R, Yudofsky S (eds): The American Psychiatric Press Synopsis of Psychiatry. Washington, DC, American Psychiatric Press, 1996, p 663

19. Craven D, Steger K, La Chapelle R, et al: Factitious HIV infection: The importance of documenting infection. Ann Intern Med 121:763, 1994

20. Wolcott D, Fawzy F, Namir S: Clinical management of psychiatric disorders in HIV spectrum disease. Psychiatr Med 7:107, 1989

21. Soloway B: Preparing for disability and death. AIDS Clin Care 3:76, 1991

22. Rundell J, Kyle K, Brown G, Thomason J: Risk factors for suicide attempts in a human immunodeficiency virus screening program. Psychosomatics 33: 24, 1992

23. Dannenberg A, McNeil J, Brundage J, et al: Suicide and HIV infection. JAMA 276:1743, 1996

24. Marzuk P, Tardiff K, Leon A, et al: HIV seroprevalence among suicide victims in New York City, 1991–1993. Am J Psychiatry 154:1720, 1997

25. Perry S, Fishman B, Jacobsberg L, et al: Effectiveness of psychoeducational interventions in reducing emotional distress after human immunodeficiency virus antibody testing. Arch Gen Psychiatry 48:143, 1991

26. Carlson D, Fleming K, Smith G, Evans J: Management of dementia-related behavioral disturbances: A nonpharmacologic approach. Mayo Clin Proc 70: 1108, 1995

27. Eisendrath S: Brief psychotherapy in medical practice: Keys to success. West J Med 158:376, 1993

28. Carson V, Soekn K, Shanty J, et al: Hope and spiritual well-being: Essentials for living with AIDS. Perspect Psychiatr Care 26:28, 1990

29. Grossman G: Psychotherapy with HIV-infected gay men. In Kato PM, Mann T (eds): Handbook of Diversity Issues in Health Psychology. New York, Plenum Press, 1996, p 237

30. Hays R, Turner H, Coates T: Social support, AIDS-related symptoms, and depression among gay men. J Consult Clin Psychol 60:463, 1992

31. Lackner J, Joseph J, Ostrow D, et al: A longitudinal study of psychological distress in a cohort of gay men. J Nerv Ment Dis 181:4, 1993

32. McCormick TR, Conley BJ: Patients' perspectives on dying and on the care of dying patients. In Caring for Patients at the End of Life (Special Issue). West J Med 163:236, 1995

33. Calabrese J, Kling M, Gold P: Alterations in immunocompetence during stress, bereavement and depression: Focus on neuroendocrine regulation. Am J Psychiatry 144:1123, 1987

34. Cavanaugh S: Depression in the medically ill. Psychosomatics 36:48, 1995

35. Evans D, Folds J, Petitto J, et al: Circulating natural killer cell phenotypes in men and women with major depression: Relation to cytotoxic activity and severity of depression. Arch Gen Psychiatry 49:388, 1992

36. Irwin M, Daniels M, Bloom E, et al: Life events, depressive symptoms, and immune function. Am J Psychiatry 144:437, 1987

37. Post R: Transduction of psychosocial stress into the neurobiology of recurrent affective disorder. Am J Psychiatry 149:999, 1992

38. Zorilla E, McKay J, Luborosky L, et al: Relation of stressors and depressive symptoms to clinical progression of viral illness. Am J Psychiatry 153:626, 1996

39. Rabkin J, Williams J, Remien R, et al: Depression, distress, lymphocyte subsets, and human immunodeficiency virus symptoms on two occasions in HIV-positive homosexual men. Arch Gen Psychiatry 48: 111, 1991

40. Rabkin J, Remien R, Katoff L, et al: Resilience in adversity among long-term survivors of AIDS. Hosp Community Psychiatry 44:162, 1993

41. Taylor S, Kemeny M, Aspinwall L, et al: Optimism, coping, psychological distress, and high-risk sexual behavior among men at risk for acquired immunodeficiency syndrome (AIDS). J Pers Soc Psychol 63: 460, 1992

42. Folkman S, Chesney M, Pollack L, et al: Stress, coping, and high-risk sexual behavior. Health Psychol 11: 218, 1992

43. Wolf T, Balson P, Morse E, et al: Relationship of coping style to affective state and perceived social support in asymptomatic and symptomatic HIV-infected persons: Implications for clinical management. J Clin Psychiatry 52:171, 1991

44. Burack J, Barrett D, Stall R, et al: Depressive symptoms and CD4 lymphocytes decline among HIV-infected men. JAMA 270:2568, 1993

45. Lyketsos C, Hoover D, Guccione M, et al: Depressive symptoms as predictors of medical outcome in HIV infection. JAMA 270:1563, 1993

46. Perry S, Fishman B: Depression and HIV: How does one affect the other? JAMA 270:2609, 1993

47. Cassem E: Depressive disorders in the medically ill. Psychosomatics 36:S2, 1995

48. Petty F: Depression and medical/surgical illness: "Who wouldn't be depressed?" Prim Care 14:669, 1987

49. Cassem E: Anxiety and depression as secondary phenomena. Psychiatr Clin North Am 13:597, 1990

50. Jones B, Reifler B: Depression coexisting with dementia. Med Clin North Am 78:823, 1994

51. Feinstein A: Multiple sclerosis, depression, and suicide. BMJ 315:691, 1997

52. Katon W: Depression: Relationship to somatization and chronic medical illness. Clin Psychiatry 45:4, 1984

53. McCann R, Hall W, Groth-Junctier A: Comfort care for terminally ill patients. JAMA 272:1263, 1994

54. Migliorelli R, Tesón A, Sabe L, et al: Prevalence and correlates of dysthymia and major depression among patients with Alzheimer's disease. Am J Psychiatry 152:37, 1995

55. Gerber P, Barrett J, Barrett J, et al: Recognition of depression by internists in primary care: A comparison of internist and "gold standard" psychiatric assessments. J Gen Intern Med 4:7, 1989

56. Perez-Stable E, Miranda J, Munoz R, et al: Depression in medical outpatients: Underrecognition and misdiagnosis. Arch Intern Med 50:1083, 1990

57. Borson S, McDonald G, Gayle T, et al: Improvement in mood, physical symptoms, and function with nortriptyline for depression in patients with chronic obstructive pulmonary disease. Psychosomatics 33:190, 1992

58. Bruera E, Miller J, Macmillan K, Kuehn N: Neuropsychological effects of methylphenidate in patients receiving a continuous infusion of narcotics for cancer pain. Pain 48:163, 1992

59. Evans D, McCartney C, Haggerty J, et al: Treatment of depression in cancer patients is associated with better life adaptation: A pilot study. Psychosom Med 50: 72, 1988

60. Wells K, Stewart A, Hays R, et al: The functioning and well-being of depressed patients. JAMA 262:914, 1989

61. Broadhead WE, Blazer DG, George LK, Tse CK: Depression, disability days, and days lost from work in a prospective epidemiologic survey. JAMA 264:2524, 1990

62. Brody D, Larson D: The role of primary care physicians in managing depression. J Gen Intern Med 7: 243, 1992

63. Rabkin J, Gewirtz G: Depression and HIV. GMHC Treatment Issues 6:1, 1992

64. Evans D, Leserman J, Perkins D, et al: Severe life stress as a predictor of early disease progression in HIV infection. Am J Psychiatry 154:630, 1997

65. Fell M, Newman S, Herns M, et al: Mood and psychiatric disturbance in HIV and AIDS: Changes over time. Br J Psychiatry 162:604, 1993

66. Mayne T, Vittinghoff E, Chesney M, et al: Depressive affect and survival among gay and bisexual men infected with HIV. Arch Intern Med 156:2233, 1996

67. Perkins D, Laserman J, Stern R, et al: Somatic symptoms and HIV infection: Relationship to depressive symptoms and indicators of HIV disease. Am J Psychiatry 152:1776, 1995

68. Rabkin J, Goetz R, Remein R: Stability of mood despite HIV illness progression in a group of homosexual men. Am J Psychiatry 154:231, 1997

69. Chesney M, Folkman S: Psychological impact of HIV disease and implications for intervention. Psychiatr Clin North Am 17:163, 1994

70. Drugs for AIDS and associated infections. Med Lett 35:79, 1993

71. Drugs that cause psychiatric symptoms. Med Lett 35: 65, 1993

72. Mitchell A, O'Keane V: Steroids and depression. BMJ 316:244, 1998

73. Adams F: Emergency intravenous sedation of the delirious, medically ill patient. J Clin Psychiatry 49(Suppl):22, 1988

74. Hintz S, Kuck J, Peterhin J: Depression in the context of HIV infection: Implications for treatment. J Clin Psychiatry 51:497, 1990

75. Ostrow D, Grant I, Atkinson H: Assessment and management of the AIDS patient with neuropsychiatric disturbances. J Clin Psychiatry 49:14, 1988

76. Fernandez F, Levy J: Psychopharmacology in HIV spectrum disorders. Psychiatr Clin North Am 17:135, 1994

77. Grant I, Olshen R, Atkinson JH, et al: Depressed mood does not explain neuropsychological deficits in HIV-infected persons. Neuropsychology 7:53, 1993

78. Yesavage J: Differential diagnosis between depression and dementia. Am J Med 94(Suppl 5A):23S, 1993

79. Grinspoon S, Corcoran C, Askari H, et al: Effects of androgen administration in men with the AIDS wasting syndrome. Ann Intern Med 129:18, 1998

80. Poretsky L, Cass S, Zumoff B: Testicular dysfunction in HIV-infected men. Metabolism 44:946, 1995

81. Rabkin J, Rabkin R: Testosterone therapy for HIV-infected men. AIDS Reader, July/Aug:136, 1995

82. Rubinow D, Schmidt P: Androgens, brain, and behavior. Am J Psychiatry 153:974, 1996

83. Wang C, Alexander G, Berman N, et al: Testosterone replacement therapy improves mood in hypogonadal men—a clinical research study center. J Clin Endocrinol Metab 81:3578, 1996

84. El-Mallakh R: Mania in AIDS: Clinical significance and theoretical considerations. Int J Psychiatry Med 21:383, 1991

85. Ferrando S, Goldman J, Charness A: Selective serotonin reuptake inhibitor treatment of depression in symptomatic HIV infection and AIDS. Gen Hosp Psychiatry 19:89, 1997

86. Wagner G, Rabkin J, Rabkin R: Dextroamphetimine as a treatment for depression and low energy in AIDS patients: A pilot study. J Psychosom Res 42:407, 1997

87. Eisenberg L: Treating depression and anxiety in primary care: Closing the gap between knowledge and practice. N Engl J Med 326:1080, 1992

88. Sherbourne C, Wells K, Hays R, et al: Subthreshold depression and depressive disorder: Clinical characteristics of general medical and mental health specialty outpatients. Am J Psychiatry 151:1777, 1994

89. Fernandez F, Levy J: Psychopharmacology of psychiatric syndromes in asymptomatic and symptomatic HIV infection. Psychiatr Med 9:377, 1991

90. Choice of an antidepressant. Med Lett Drugs Ther 35: 25, 1993

91. Feiger A, Kiev A, Shrivastava R, et al: Nefazadone versus sertraline in outpatients with major depression: Focus on efficacy, tolerability, and effects on sexual function and satisfaction. J Clin Psychiatry 57(Suppl 2):53, 1996

92. Feighner J, Gardner E, Johnston J, et al: Double-blind comparison of bupropion and fluoxetine in depressed outpatients. J Clin Psychiatry 52:329, 1991

93. Lader M: Tolerability and safety: Essentials in antidepressant pharmacotherapy. J Clin Psychiatry 57:39, 1996

94. Preskhorn S: Comparison of the tolerability of bupropion, fluoxetine, imipramine, nefazadone, paroxetine, sertraline, and venlafaxine. J Clin Psychiatry 56: 12, 1995

95. St. John's wort. Med Lett 39:107, 1997

96. Novack D, Suchman A, Clark W, et al: Calibrating the physician: Personal awareness and effective patient care. JAMA 278:502, 1997

97. Bascom P, Tolle S: Care of the family when the patient is dying. West J Med 163:292, 1995

98. Frierson RL, Wey JJ, Tabler JB: Psychostimulants for depression in the medically ill. Am Fam Physician 43: 163, 1991

99. Kaufmann M, Murray G, Cassem N: Use of psychostimulants in medically ill depressed patients. Psychosomatics 23:817, 1982

100. Olin J, Masand P: Psychostimulants for depression in hospitalized cancer patients. Psychosomatics 37:57, 1996

101. Schmitt F, Bigley J, McKinnis R, et al: Neuropsychological outcome of zidovudine (AZT) treatment of patients with AIDS and AIDS-related complex. N Engl J Med 319:1573, 1988

102. Woods S, Tesar G, Murray G, et al: Psychostimulant treatment of depressive disorders secondary to medical illness. Clin Psychiatry 47:12, 1986

103. Fernandez F, Adams F, Levy J, et al: Cognitive impairment due to AIDS-related complex and its response to psychostimulants. Psychosomatics 29:38, 1988

104. Holmes V, Fernandez F, Levey J: Psychostimulant response in AIDS-related complex patients. J Clin Psychiatry 50:5, 1989

105. White J, Darko D, Brown S, et al: Early central nervous system response to HIV infection: Sleep distortion and cognitive-motor decrements. AIDS 9:1043, 1995

106. Markowitz J: Treating HIV-associated depression with psychotherapy. AIDS Reader May/June:95, 1995

107. Markowitz JC, Rabkin JG, Perry SW: Treating depression in HIV-positive patients. AIDS 8:403, 1994

108. Zegans L, Gerhard A, Coates T: Psychotherapies for the person with HIV disease. Psychiatr Clin North Am 17:149, 1994

109. Dunbar H, Mueller C, Medina C, et al: Psychological and spiritual growth in women living with HIV. Social Work 43:144, 1998

110. Breitbart W: Suicide risk in cancer and AIDS patients. In Chapman C-R, Foley K (eds): Current and Emerging Issues in Cancer Pain Research and Practice: The Bristol-Myers Squibb Symposium on Pain Research. New York, Raven Press, 1993

111. Hirschfield R, Russell J: Assessment and treatment of suicidal patients. N Engl J Med 337:910, 1997

112. Casteneda R, Sussman N, Weistreich L, et al: A review of the effects of moderate alcohol intake on the treatment of anxiety and mood disorders. J Clin Psychiatry 57:207, 1996

113. Boccellari A, Dilley J, Shore M: Neuropsychiatric aspects of AIDS dementia complex: A report on a clinical series. Neurotoxicology 9:381, 1988

114. Donnell M: Nursing care of the patient with dementia. In Martin J, Hughes A, Franks P (eds): AIDS Home Care and Hospice Manual, 2nd ed. San Francisco, Visiting Nurses and Hospice of San Francisco, 1990, p 103

115. Katz A: AIDS dementia complex. J Palliat Care 10: 46, 1994

116. Navia B, Jordan B, Price R: The AIDS dementia complex: I. Clinical features. Ann Neurol 19:517, 1986

117. Portegies P: AIDS dementia complex: A review. J Acquir Immune Defic Syndr 7(Suppl 2):S38, 1994

118. Newman S, Lunn S, Harrison M: Do asymptomatic HIV-seropositive individuals show cognitive deficit? AIDS 9:1211, 1995

119. Zeifert P, Leary M, Borcellari A: Treatment of cognitive impairment. Focus 11:1, 1996

120. Burger D, Kraaijeveld CL, Meenhorst PL, et al: Penetration of zidovudine into the cerebrospinal fluid of patients infected with HIV. AIDS 7:1581, 1994

121. Baldeweg T, Catalan J, Lovett E: Long-term zidovudine reduces neurocognitive deficits in HIV-1 infection. AIDS 9:589, 1995

122. Price R, Brew B: The AIDS dementia complex. J Infect Dis 158:1079, 1988

123. MacKenzie T, Robiner W, Knopman D: Differences between patient and family assessments of depression in Alzheimer's disease. Am J Psychiatry 146:1174, 1989

124. Boccellari A, Zeifert P: Management of neurobehavioral impairment in HIV-1 infection. Psychiatr Clin North Am 17:183, 1994

125. Garfield C: Sometimes My Heart Goes Numb: Love and Caring in a Time of AIDS. San Francisco, Jossey-Bass, 1995, p 261

126. Bostwick J, Masterson B: Psychopharmacological treatment of delirium to restore mental capacity. Psychosomatics 39:112, 1998

127. Schneider L, Sobin P: Non-neuroleptic treatment of behavioral symptoms and agitation in Alzheimer's disease and other dementia. Psychopharmacol Bull 28:71, 1992

128. Katon W: Panic disorder: Epidemiology, diagnosis, and treatment in primary care. J Clin Psychiatry 47: 21, 1986

129. Drugs for psychiatric disorders. Med Lett 33:43, 1991

130. Batki S: Buspirone in drug users with AIDS or AIDS-related complex. J Clin Psychopharmacol 10(Suppl): 111S, 1993

131. McDaniel J, Johnson K: Obsessive-compulsive disorder in HIV disease: Response to fluoxetine. Psychosomatics 36:147, 1995

132. Fish N: Treatment of delirium in the critically ill patient. Clin Pharm 110:456, 1991

133. Gelfand S, Indelicato J, Benjamin J: Using intravenous haloperidol to control delirium. Hosp Community Psychiatry 43:215, 1992

134. Jung A, Staiger T, Sullivan M: The efficacy of selective serotonin reuptake inhibitors for the management of chronic pain. J Gen Intern Med 12:384, 1997

135. Kane J: The new antipsychotics. J Pract Psychiatry Behav Health 12:343, 1997

136. McCormack J, Li R, Zarowny D, et al: Inadequate treatment of pain in ambulatory HIV patients. Clin J Pain 9:279, 1993

137. Breitbart W, Marotta R, Platt M, et al: A double-blind trial of haloperidol, chlorpromazine, and lorazepam in the treatment of delirium in hospitalized AIDS patients. Am J Psychiatry 153:231, 1996

138. Amadio P, Cross A, Amadio P: New drugs for schizophrenia: An update for family physicians. Am Fam Physician 56:1149, 1997

139. Singh A, Catalan J: Respidodone in HIV-related manic psychosis [letter]. Lancet 344:1029, 1994

140. Elliot A, Uldall K, Bergam K, et al: Randomized, placebo-controlled trial of paroxetine versus imipramine in depressed HIV-positive patients. Psychiatry 155:367, 1998

141. Kieburtz K, Zettelmaier A, Ketonen L: Manic syndrome in AIDS. Am J Psychiatry 148:1068, 1991

142. Gerner R: Treatment of acute mania. Psychiatr Clin North Am 16:443, 1993

143. Kahn D: New strategies in bipolar disorder: Part II treatment. J Pract Psychiatr Behav Health 1:148, 1995

144. Mahler J, Perry S: Assessing competency in the physically ill: Guidelines for psychiatric consultants. Hosp Community Psychiatry 39:856, 1988

145. Davis D: Rich cases: The ethics of thick description. Hastings Center Rep July/August:12, 1991

146. Zuger A: Ethical decision making in AIDS. AIDS Clin Care 2:49, 1990

147. Haas J, Weissman J, Cleary P, et al: Discussion of preferences for life-sustaining care by persons with AIDS: Predictors of failure in patient-physician communication. Arch Intern Med 153:1241, 1993

148. Bindels P, Krol A, Ameijian E, et al: Euthanasia and physician-assisted suicide in homosexual men with AIDS. Lancet 347:499, 1996

149. Breitbart W, Rosenfeld B, Passik S: Interest in physician-assisted suicide among ambulatory HIV-infected patients. Am J Psychiatry 153:238, 1996

150. Cooke M, Gourlay L, Collette L, et al: Informal caregivers and the intention to hasten death. Arch Intern Med 158:69, 1998

151. Jones J, Dilley J: Rational suicide and HIV disease. Focus 1993, 5

152. Block S, Billings A: Patient requests to hasten death. Arch Intern Med 154:2039, 1994

153. Emanuel E, Daniels E, Fairclough D, et al: The practice of euthanasia and physician-assisted suicide in the United States: Adherence to proposed safeguards and effects on physicians. JAMA 280:507, 1998

154. Heilig S, Brody R, Marcus F, et al: Physician-hastened death: Advisory guidelines for the San Francisco Bay Area from the Bay Area Network of Ethics Committees. West J Med 166:370, 1997

155. Block S, Billings JA: Patient requests for euthanasia and assisted suicide in terminal illness. Psychosomatics 36:445, 1995

156. Coates T: Counseling patients seropositive for human immunodeficiency virus: An approach for medical practice. West J Med 153:629, 1990
157. Jones B, Teng E, Folstein M, et al: A new bedside test of cognition for patients with HIV infection. Ann Intern Med 119:1001, 1993
158. Breitbart W, McDonald M, Rosenfeld B, et al: Fatigue in ambulatory AIDS patients. J Pain Symptom Manage 15:150, 1998
159. Breitbart W: Psychiatric management of cancer pain. Cancer 63(Suppl):2336, 1989
160. Breitbart W: Pharmacotherapy of pain in AIDS. In Wormser G (ed): A Clinical Guide to AIDS and HIV. New York, Lippincott-Raven, 1996, p 359
161. O'Neill W, Sherrard J: Pain in human immunodeficiency disease: A review. Pain 54:3, 1993
162. Breitbart W, Rosenfeld B, Passik S, et al: The under treatment of pain in ambulatory AIDS patients. Pain 65:243, 1996
163. Breitbart W, Rosenfeld B, Passik S, et al: A comparison of pain report and adequacy of analgesic therapy in ambulatory AIDS patients with and without a history of substance abuse. Pain 72:235, 1997
164. Larue F, Fontaine A, Colleau S: Under estimation and under treatment of pain in HIV disease: Multi-centre study. BMJ 314:23, 1997
165. Lebovits A, Lefkowitz M, McCarthy D, et al: The prevalence and management of pain in patients with AIDS: A review of 134 cases. Clin J Pain 5:245, 1989
166. Cleeland C, Gonin R, Baez L, et al: Pain and treatment of pain in minority patients with cancer. Ann Intern Med 127:813, 1997
167. Portenoy R, Dole U, Joseph H, et al: Pain management and chemical dependency. JAMA 278:592, 1997
168. Breitbart W, McDonald M, Rosenfeld B, et al: Pain in ambulatory AIDS patients: Pain chaaracteristics and medical correlates. Pain 68:315, 1996
169. Hewitt D, McDonald M, Portenoy R, et al: Pain syndromes and etiologies in ambulatory AIDS patients. Pain 70:117, 1997
170. Rosenfeld B, Breitbart W, McDonald M, et al: Pain in ambulatory AIDS patients: Impact of pain on psychological functioning and quality of life. Pain 68:323, 1996
171. McQuay H: Antidepressants and chronic pain. BMJ 314:763, 1997
172. McQuay H, Carroll D, Jahad A, et al: Anticonvulsant drugs for management of pain: A systematic review. BMJ 311:1047, 1995
173. Coulehan J: The word is an instrument of healing. Lit Med 10:111, 1991
174. Fox E: Predominance of the curative model in medical care. JAMA 278:761, 1997
175. Jackson S: The listening healer in the history of psychological healing. Am J Psychiatry 149:1623, 1992
176. Nierenberg A, Feighner J, Rudolph R, et al: Venlafaxine for treatment-resistant unipolar depression. J Clin Psychopharmacol 14:419, 1994
177. Quill T, Lo B, Brock D: Palliative options of last resort. JAMA 278:2099, 1997
178. Zinn W: The empathetic physician. Arch Intern Med 153:306, 1993
179. Dubovsky S, Thomas M: Approaches to the treatment of refractory depression. J Pract Psychiatr Behav Health 2:14, 1996
180. Hardy R (ed): Loving Men: Gay Male Partners, Spirituality and AIDS. Idyllwild, CA, Continuum Press, 1998
181. Horowitz M, Siegal B, Holen A, et al: Diagnostic criteria for complicated grief disorder. Am J Psychiatry 154:904, 1997
182. Neugebauer R, Rabkin J, Williams J, et al: Bereavement reactions among homosexual men experiencing multiple losses in the AIDS epidemic. Am J Psychiatry 149:1374, 1992
183. Sheldon F: Bereavement. BMJ 316:456, 1998
184. Markowitz JC, Klerman G, Perry S: Interpersonal psychotherapy of depressed HIV-positive outpatients. Hosp Community Psychiatry 43:885, 1992
185. Creagan E: Stress among medical oncologists: The phenomenon of burnout and a call to action. Mayo Clin Proc 68:614, 1993
186. Fernandez F, Holmes V, Levy J, et al: Consultation-liaison psychiatry and HIV-related disorders. Hosp Community Psychiatry 40:146, 1989
187. Burckhardt C: Coping strategies of the chronically ill. Nurs Clin North Am 22:543, 1987
188. MacDonald N: Suffering and dying in cancer patients: Research issues in controlling confusion, cachexia, dyspnea. In Caring for Patients at the End of Life (Special Issue). West J Med 163:278, 1995
189. Muldoon M, King N: Spirituality, health care, and bioethics. J Religion Health 34:329, 1995
190. Remen R: Spirit: Resource for healing. Noetic Sci Rev Autumn:5, 1988
191. Remen R: Working in the gray zone: The dilemma of the private practitioner. Adv J Mind-Body Health 7:36, 1991
192. Stoeckle J, Ronan L, Ehrlich C, et al: The uses of shadowing the doctor and patient: On seeing and hearing their work of care. J Gen Intern Med 8:561, 1993
193. Smith M: Primary care and HIV disease. J Gen Intern Med 6(Suppl):S56, 1991
194. Jewett J, Hecht F: Preventive health care for adults with HIV infection. JAMA 269:1144, 1993
195. Donohue M: Comparing generalist and specialty care. Arch Intern Med 158:1596, 1998
196. Johnson W: Comparing apples with oranges. Arch Intern Med 158:1591, 1998

16 | Hematologic Complications of HIV Infection

JULIE HAMBLETON

Infection with HIV is associated with a wide spectrum of hematologic abnormalities. These abnormalities may be found at all stages of HIV disease and involve the bone marrow, cellular elements of the peripheral blood, and coagulation pathways. The cause of these abnormalities is multifactorial. A direct suppressive effect of HIV infection, ineffective hematopoiesis, infiltrative disease of the bone marrow, nutritional deficiencies, peripheral consumption secondary to splenomegaly or immune dysregulation, and drug effect all contribute to the variety of hematologic findings in these patients. Specific abnormalities in the bone marrow, peripheral blood cell lines, and coagulation complex are reviewed here in turn.

BONE MARROW

Hematologic abnormalities in patients with HIV infection are very common.[1,2] Ineffective hematopoiesis resulting from direct suppression by HIV infection,[3,4] infiltrative disease (infectious or neoplastic), nutritional deficiencies, and drug effect have all been described.

Morphologic Features

The common morphologic features of bone marrow findings in patients with AIDS have been described.[2,5,6] Bone marrow biopsies are frequently performed to evaluate peripheral cytopenias or persistent fevers in this patient population. Most patients demonstrate normocellular marrow elements, although dysplasia has been noted, without the progression to acute leukemia. Increased numbers of plasma cells and lymphoid aggregates composed of benign-appearing, well-differentiated lymphocytes have

also been noted.[4-6] The myeloid-to-erythroid (M:E) ratio is generally normal in patients undergoing bone marrow biopsy. Reticulin fiber staining often reveals increased reticulin fibrosis. Abnormalities in maturation with dysmyelopoiesis (dysplasia),[7] megaloblastosis, and hemophagocytosis have also been described, whereas myeloproliferative syndromes and leukemia are not more prevalent in this patient population.[4,5]

Infiltrative disease of the bone marrow commonly contributes to the hematologic abnormalities seen in these patients. Infectious causes of infiltrative diseases include mycobacterial disease (both *Mycobacterium avium* complex and *M. tuberculosis*), fungal disease (*Histoplasma, Cryptococcus*, and *Coccidioides*), and rarely parasitic disease (*Pneumocystis* and *Leishmania*). Neoplastic infiltration is due primarily to lymphoma. Infiltration of the bone marrow by *M. avium* complex usually results in isolated anemia, whereas infiltrative disease of other causes typically manifests as pancytopenia.

Nutritional Effects

Nutritional deficiencies are not common causes of hematologic abnormalities in HIV-infected patients, although disorders of iron metabolism or iron deficiency and occult vitamin B_{12} deficiency have been described. Folate deficiency is not more prevalent in this patient population. Variable reports of increased to absent iron stores have been published. Most patients have ineffective incorporation of iron into erythroid precursors, the so-called *anemia of chronic disease*. This leads to normal or increased iron stores on Prussian blue iron staining of the bone marrow biopsy. Conversely, chronic blood loss from the gastrointestinal tract secondary to neoplastic infiltration or invasive infectious enteropathies may lead to an iron-deficient state.

The prevalence of vitamin B_{12} deficiency secondary to gastrointestinal malabsorption has been increasingly described in patients with AIDS. Low serum vitamin B_{12} levels associated with altered cobalamin transport proteins or abnormal absorption of vitamin B_{12} secondary to chronic diarrhea have been described.[4,8–10] Occult vitamin B_{12} deficiency may worsen the anemia associated with zidovudine therapy.[11] Therefore, it is prudent to monitor vitamin B_{12} levels periodically in patients with chronic gastrointestinal dysfunction, especially in those patients receiving zidovudine therapy.

Diagnostic Utility of Bone Marrow Biopsy

For the most part, the marrow changes in asymptomatic HIV-infected patients appear nonspecific and offer little to the clinician as a diagnostic or prognostic tool. There are, however, certain conditions for which performing bone marrow aspiration, culture, and biopsy is indicated.

HIV-infected patients with both non-Hodgkin's and Hodgkin's lymphoma frequently have marrow involvement. Marrow examination is useful not only for staging but also to assess the myeloid reserves before the initiation of cytotoxic chemotherapy. Patients with thrombocytopenia in the absence of anemia or leukopenia warrant bone marrow evaluation to assure adequate megakaryocytes. In rare instances, diagnoses other than immune thrombocytopenic purpura may be established.

Occasionally a patient has constitutional symptoms associated with anemia and/or other cytopenias. In the absence of a revealing workup, bone marrow examination may be indicated to rule out lymphoma or underlying opportunistic infection. Evidence of Kaposi's sarcoma does not characteristically appear in the bone marrow aspirate or biopsy specimen; however, lymphomatous involvement may be found. Granulomatous disease with a positive acid-fast bacillus strain suggests *M. avium* complex or *M. tuberculosis* infection, although well-formed granulomas may not be apparent.

In a retrospective review of patients with known or suspected HIV infection, 387 bone marrow biopsy examinations were performed to evaluate the presence of opportunistic pathogens or lymphoma.[12] Disseminated fungal infections occurred in less than 5% of patients studied, with bone marrow examination leading to the most rapid and accurate diagnosis. Mycobacterial infection was diagnosed in 16% of patients studied. Bone marrow culture was found to be equally sensitive for the diagnosis of disseminated mycobacterial disease as blood culture (86% vs. 77% sensitivity, respectively; $p > .05$). No previously undiagnosed case of lymphoma was found by bone marrow examination for cytopenias and constitutional symptoms; however, bone marrow biopsies were routinely performed for staging lymphoma.

PERIPHERAL CELL LINES

Peripheral cytopenias are common in HIV-infected individuals, and are due to either decreased production in the bone marrow or accelerated destruction in the peripheral circulation. In general, the cytopenias increase in frequency as HIV disease progresses. Anemia, granulocytopenia, and thrombocytopenia occur in 17%, 8%, and 13%, respectively, of asymptomatic HIV-infected individuals.[13] These percentages all increase with advancing HIV disease.

Erythrocytes

Review of the peripheral blood smear in patients with HIV infection often reveals nonspecific abnormalities. Anisopoikilocytosis, often with ovalocytes and rouleaux formation, is a common finding, and increased vacuolization of peripheral monocytes may be seen.[14] Anemia is the most common hematologic abnormality noted in patients with HIV disease[15] (Table 16–1). In patients with persistent lymphadenopathy, the development of anemia often antedates the evolution to overt AIDS. In patients with overt AIDS, anemia occurs in 66% to 85%.[4,13] The majority have chronic disease–type anemia, with low reticulocyte counts and low erythropoietin levels.[15] In such states, adequate iron stores are demonstrated in the reticuloendothelial system, but the inability to incorporate this stored iron into erythroid precursors results in a normocytic, normochromic anemia. The etiology of anemia in these patients is multifactorial and complex. Ineffective erythropoiesis may be a consequence of actual HIV infection of erythroid precursors or result from inappropriate tumor necrosis factor release, which is an inhibitor of red blood cell (RBC) production in vitro.[15,16]

TABLE 16–1. Special Considerations for the Differential Diagnosis of Anemia in HIV-Infected Individuals

Normocytic Anemia

A. Isolated anemia, with hemoglobin level >10 gm/dl and patient exhibits no unexplained constitutional symptoms; consider anemia of chronic disease secondary to HIV infection. Continued observation is advised. If isolated anemia is severe and protracted, consider parvoviral infection.

B. Bi- or trilineage cytopenia accompanying anemia, hemoglobin level >10 gm/dl, and the patient exhibits unexplained constitutional symptoms; consider bone marrow infiltrative process.

Differential Diagnosis
- Infectious
  Acid-fast bacillus—*M. avium* complex of *M. tuberculosis*
  Fungal—cryptococcosis, histoplasmosis, coccidioidomycosis
  Parvovirus
- Neoplastic
  Lymphoma
  Rarely Kaposi's sarcoma

Evaluation
- Blood culture for *M. avium* complex and fungus
- Cryptococcal antigen testing
- Giemsa stain of peripheral blood for histoplasmosis
- Purified protein derivative and *Coccidioides* skin testing
- Tissue biopsy: liver, lymph node (if clinically indicated)
- Bone marrow biopsy, special stains and culture

Macrocytosis

Differential Diagnosis
- Vitamin B_{12} or folate deficiency secondary to enteropathy with malabsorption
- Hemolysis with reticulocytosis
  Drugs: dapsone, sulfa
  Autoimmunity
  Thrombotic microangiopathy* if concomitant thrombocytopenia present
- Zidovudine antiretroviral drug therapy

Evaluation
If patient is receiving zidovudine therapy:
- Check endogenous erythropoietin (EPO) level; consider therapy with recombinant EPO if endogenous level <500 mU/dl
- Evaluate vitamin B_{12} level and treat if low

Microcytosis
Evaluate gastrointestinal tract for involvement with Kaposi's sarcoma, lymphoma, or infectious enteropathy (e.g., cytomegalovirus colitis) causing iron deficiency secondary to chronic blood loss

*Thrombotic thrombocytopenic purpura, hemolytic–uremic syndrome, or disseminated intravascular coagulation.

Iron deficiency with a microcytic, hypochromic anemia may result from chronic blood loss, which can result from Kaposi's sarcoma or lymphomatous involvement of the gastrointestinal tract. Thrombocytopenia with resultant occult bleeding may lead to iron deficiency.

Infiltrative disease of the bone marrow caused by *M. avium* complex is a common cause of isolated anemia, usually without concomitant decrement in the other cell lines.[17] Some of the most profound anemias, with hematocrit concentrations in the 15% to 20% range, occur in patients with mycobacterial disease. Similarly, patients with lymphoma may develop profound anemia, often with concomitant cytopenias of the other cell lines.

Infection with B19 parvovirus is increasingly recognized as a cause of intractable anemia in patients with HIV disease. Classically associated with transient aplastic crises in patients with underlying hemolytic diseases or with erythroblastosis fetalis, parvovirus selectively infects actively replicating erythroid precursors, resulting in RBC lysis and erythroid hypoplasia. Clearance of this infection is mediated by an intact humoral response. Immunocompromised patients, however, may fail to clear the infection[18,19] or maintain an adequate immunoglobulin G antibody response.[20] Diagnosis of B19 parvovirus infection is made by serologic studies, or by bone marrow examination noting giant, abnormal pronormoblasts and in situ hybridization using sequence-specific DNA probes. A course of intravenous or intramuscular immunoglobulin is the therapy of choice. Profound or symptomatic anemia should be corrected with packed RBC transfusions.

Despite the prevalance of RBC autoantibodies, antibody-mediated hemolysis is not a common cause of anemia in this patient population. Upward of 20% to 43% of AIDS patients have a positive direct antiglobulin test (direct Coombs'), but frank hemolysis is rare.[21,22] Conversely, drug-induced anemia is commonly noted. Dapsone therapy for the treatment of *Pneumocystis carinii* pneumonia or other infections can induce methemaglobinemia or hemolysis in patients with glucose-6-phosphate dehydrogenase deficiency, and zidovudine antiretroviral therapy results in a transfusion-dependent anemia in approximately 20% of patients.[11]

Leukocytes

HIV infection affects the lymphocyte, neutrophil, and macrophage-monocyte cell lines. Despite the hypergammaglobulinemia noted in these patients, they suffer complications from both defective cellular immunity and dysregulated humoral immunity. The hallmark of HIV infection is the progressive depletion of CD4+ lymphocytes. This decrement presumably occurs through direct viral invasion of these cells. Early in HIV infection, one may see an initial increase in the CD8+ population before a decline in the number of CD4+ cells is noted. Infection of macrophages and monocytes and the triggering of an autoimmune response are two other mechanisms by which lymphocyte depletion may occur. Normally, activated T lymphocytes and monocytes produce cytokines or growth factors necessary for stem cell growth and differentiation. Decreased production of these cytokines results from HIV invasion of these cells. For a review of the immunopathogenic mechanisms of HIV infection, the reader is referred to the paper by Fauci et al.[16]

Granulocytopenia independent of drug use has been described in patients with AIDS. The most common cause appears to be ineffective granulopoiesis.[23] Anti-neutrophilic antibodies have been described as a possible cause of peripheral neutropenia; however, their clinical significance remains elusive.[3,4,24,25] Defects in qualitative functions of the monocyte-macrophage and granulocyte line have also been described. Defective polymorphonuclear leukocyte chemotaxis, deficient degranulating responses, in-

TABLE 16–2. Drugs Commonly Used in Treating Patients with HIV Infection That Cause Myelosuppression

Antiretroviral nucleotide analogs (primarily zidovudine)
Antiviral agents (e.g., ganciclovir, foscarnet)
Antifungal agents (e.g., flucytosine, amphotericin)
Sulfonamides
Dihydrofolate reductase inhibitors (e.g., trimethoprim, pyrimethamine)
Pentamidine
Antineoplastic therapy
α-Interferon

hibition of leukocyte migration, and ineffective killing have all been reported.[26,27] Similarly, monocytes exhibit a marked reduction in chemotaxis in response to stimuli.[28]

Drug-induced neutropenia is common in the HIV-infected individual.[11,23] Medications used to treat infections such as *P. carinii* pneumonia, toxoplasmosis, and cytomegaloviral retinitis or colitis cause neutropenia. Similarly, zidovudine is also implicated as a cause of neutropenia, often necessitating dose reduction or cessation of therapy. Other dideoxynucleosides (e.g., lamivudine [3TC], zalcitabine [ddC], and didanosine [ddI]) and protease inhibitors are associated with less bone marrow toxicity (Table 16–2 lists the more commonly used drugs that cause neutropenia). Moreover, patients receiving chemotherapy for treatment of HIV-associated malignancies typically develop neutropenia. Irrespective of the cause of neutropenia, severe neutropenia complicated by a febrile episode should be evaluated aggressively for development of bacteremia, as in the non-HIV-infected population.[29]

Platelets

The most common platelet abnormality found in HIV-infected patients is thrombocytopenia. In patients with HIV-related immune thrombocytopenia (ITP), platelet-associated immunoglobulin is present.[30] Other causes of HIV-related thrombocytopenia include circulating immune complexes that precipitate on the platelet surface, resulting in clearance by the reticuloendothelial system[30]; cross-reactive antibodies to platelet surface glycoproteins[31]; and direct retroviral infection of megakaryocytes.[32–34]

Most patients with HIV-related ITP have only minor submucosal bleeding, characterized by petechiae, ecchymoses, and occasional epistaxis. Rare patients have gastrointestinal blood loss. The majority, however, have not had life-threatening bleeding episodes. Unlike non-AIDS-related immune thrombocytopenia, mild splenomegaly may occur, especially in patients with generalized lymphadenopathy.

Laboratory findings typically reveal isolated thrombocytopenia, with a dearth of platelets seen on review of the peripheral blood smear. An increased number of megakaryocytes typical of peripheral platelet consumption may be noted on examination of the bone marrow aspirate and biopsy.

Management of HIV-Related Thrombocytopenia

As with non-HIV-infected persons, thrombocytopenic patients with HIV infection should be evaluated for a secondary cause of their thrombocytopenia, and medications known to cause thrombocytopenia should be discontinued. For autoimmune-mediated thrombocytopenia (ITP), steroid and immunoglobulin therapy can be initiated for those patients needing immediate restoration of their platelet counts. This may include patients who are experiencing bleeding, who will be undergoing a splenectomy procedure, or in whom the platelet count is dangerously low and the treating physician wishes to raise the count immediately. The response of patients with HIV-related ITP to steroid therapy is variable because the platelet count oftentimes falls as the steroid dose is tapered, and the risk of further immune suppression is real. Splenectomy has been a successful therapeutic intervention for patients who fail to respond to steroid therapy, and is generally not associated with greater morbidity or mortality than in patients with non-HIV-associated ITP.[35,36]

Intravenous gammaglobulin (400 mg/kg qd for 4 to 5 days) may be used to raise the platelet count rapidly, although transiently, lasting 2 to 3 weeks.[37] The mechanism probably is blockade of the reticuloendothelial system. The high cost and transient nature of immunoglobulin therapy limit its use to situations in which acute bleeding is occurring or as a preoperative intervention for patients undergoing splenectomy when rapid elevation of the platelet count is necessary. Although platelet transfusions generally are not indicated in patients with thrombocytopenia of immune origin, treatment with intravenous gammaglobulin before transfusion in emergency situations may improve platelet elevation.

For those patients who do not require an immediate increase in their platelet counts, the institution of antiretroviral therapy, if the patient is not yet on such therapy, may be warranted.

Normalization and partial responses of platelet counts have been noted when zidovudine therapy is instituted.[38,39] Currently, little is known about the efficacy of using triple antiretroviral therapy to treat HIV-related thrombocytopenia. Early studies examined monotherapy with zidovudine because that was the standard of care. In the last several years, overwhelming evidence supports the use of triple therapy, but this approach has not been studied with respect to thrombocytopenia. Anecdotal reports suggest that patients' thrombocytopenia may relapse when zidovudine is substituted for ddI. Whether this will hold up for all nonzidovudine regimens is, as yet, unknown. α-Interferon has also been shown to be efficacious in treating patients with HIV-associated ITP in several small studies, yet may be more beneficial to those patients with less advanced HIV disease.[40-42] Partial responses appear to be more common than complete normalization of platelet counts, and the drug is relatively well tolerated at doses of 3 million units subcutaneously three times a week. Intravenous or intramuscular administration of anti-D immunoglobulin has been shown to benefit some Rh-positive patients who have not had a splenectomy.[43-45] The presumed mechanism of this therapy is Fc receptor blockade by antibody-coated RBCs substituting for the antibody-coated platelets. Clinically significant hemolysis does not appear to complicate this approach in patients without significant anemia.[43]

The nonandrogenizing testosterone danazol, initially thought to be efficacious in reversing HIV-related thrombocytopenia, has not proved to be efficacious in large-scale clinical trials, and less widely accepted interventions include vincristine and plasmapheresis.

Patients with isolated ITP associated with HIV infection are generally the most healthy in the spectrum of HIV-infected individuals. Clinical bleeding is minimal, responses to therapeutic interventions are variable, and spontaneous remissions do occur. Thus a viable alternative is to simply observe the patient closely and refrain from giving therapies directed at correcting the thrombocytopenia until necessary. For those patients with evidence of CD4+ lymphocyte depletion, antiretroviral therapy may be beneficial.

HIV-ASSOCIATED COAGULOPATHIES

In patients with a variety of disease states such as systemic lupus erythematosus or AIDS, who are intravenous drug users, who receive certain drug therapy (i.e., chlorpromazine), and who have lymphoproliferative malignancies, a circulating inhibitor of coagulation may be noted. These so-called *lupus anticoagulants* are acquired antibodies, either immunoglobulin G or M, that are directed against proteins that bind phospholipids.[46] The presence of such an inhibitor is established by the use of phospholipid-dependent coagulation assays, such as the activated partial thromboplastin time (aPTT) or Russell viper venom time (RVV), or is confirmed on enzyme-linked immunosorbent assay, depending on the nature of the antibody.[46] Paradoxically, this "anticoagulant" is associated with in vitro prolongation of the aPTT or RVV, but clinically is associated with increased thrombosis in the non-HIV-infected individual. In patients with HIV infection, the presence of a lupus anticoagulant does not appear to be associated with an increased incidence of thrombosis.[47] The anticoagulant may manifest during HIV-related infections and often disappears with treatment of the infection.[4,13] If a patient has a prolonged aPTT with no history of bleeding, presence of the lupus anticoagulant should be suspected. Invasive procedures may be performed in the presence of the lupus anticoagulant without increased bleeding risk.[47]

Several reports describe thrombotic thrombocytopenic purpura (TTP) in the HIV-infected population.[48-50] TTP is a relatively rare disease that includes fever, neurologic abnormalities, renal abnormalities, purpura, microangiopathic hemolysis, and thrombocytopenia. The exact pathogenesis of this disease is unknown, but TTP seems to arise from vascular injury caused by immune complexes, endotoxin, or other causes of endothelial injury. The disorder has been associated with increased platelet agglutination and abnormally large circulating von Willebrand factor complexes.

At present, it is unclear whether the occurrence of TTP in HIV-infected individuals is related to circulating immune complexes or immunoglobulin dysregulation associated with HIV disease. The mortality of this disease is high, as in the non-HIV-infected population, and therapy should include plasmapheresis and plasma transfusion.

Patients with concomitant coagulation defects and HIV infection may warrant additional monitoring. The HIV epidemic has devastated the hemophilia community, as upward of 50% of patients with hemophilia using plasma-derived Factor VIII and IX products in the 1980s seroconverted to HIV. HIV-infected patients with hemophilia may experience complications of

HIV infection unique from patients without hemophilia. First, up to 100% of patients with hemophilia were also exposed to hepatitis C via plasma-derived products in the 1980s, and 60% to 80% of these patients are now chronic carriers for hepatitis C. Subsequently, many of these patients have hepatosplenomegaly and resultant thrombocytopenia or pancytopenia. The degree of cytopenias may limit zidovudine use, and the complications of long-term protease inhibitor therapy in patients with chronic liver disease are unknown. Moreover, early reports gathered by the Centers for Disease Control and Prevention noted an increased rate of spontaneous bleeding and decreased efficacy of factor infusion therapy in persons with hemophilia and concomitant HIV infection who were begun on protease inhibitor therapy. Several small studies to date have been unable to recapitulate these early reports or identify an additional defect in hemostasis in these patients. Finally, HIV-infected patients on warfarin therapy for thrombosis also pose a unique challenge to the practitioner. These patients often require higher doses of warfarin when protease inhibitor therapy is instituted, presumably on the basis of increased drug clearance.

HEMATOLOGIC CONSEQUENCES OF ANTI-HIV THERAPY

Many therapeutic interventions contribute to HIV-related hematologic disorders. Zidovudine, a thymidine analog and the most widely used drug in the care of these patients, greatly affects all three hematopoietic cell lines, and in vitro studies have demonstrated its toxicity toward myeloid and erythroid precursors.[51] As a thymidine analog, the primary action of zidovudine is termination of reverse transcriptase activity of the HIV virus. Zidovudine may also inhibit DNA polymerases, thus impairing normal hematopoiesis in the host.[4,11] Other nucleotide analogs used for antiretroviral therapy (e.g., ddC, ddI, stavudine, and 3TC) and the protease inhibitors are associated with less bone marrow toxicity. In a large-scale collaborative study, all three hematopoietic cell lines were affected by zidovudine therapy: significant anemia developed in 34% of patients, and blood transfusions were required in 21%; neutropenia developed in 16% of patients; and thrombocytopenia developed in 12%.[11] Advanced HIV disease, preexisting cytopenias, and low vitamin B_{12} levels were associated with a greater risk of zidovudine-induced hematologic toxicities. Although zidovudine increases the mean corpuscular volume in most patients, bone marrow examination usually reveals hypoplasia, aplasia, or maturation arrest.[4,11,52,53] Overt megaloblastic changes are not always noted.

In general, the myelosuppression seen with zidovudine therapy is reversed by discontinuing the drug,[11,53] but close observation with monitoring of blood counts is necessary. Drug trials have documented the efficacy of lower dose zidovudine therapy, which results in fewer side effects. Other drugs commonly used in treating HIV infections, including gancyclovir, foscarnet, sulfa derivatives (used to treat toxoplasmosis or *Pneumocystis* infections), and pentamidine, also cause myelosuppression.

COLONY-STIMULATING FACTORS IN HIV DISEASE

Colony-stimulating factors (CSFs) now play an integral role in the treatment of HIV-related cytopenias[54,55] (Table 16–3). Theoretically, these agents could increase the number of target cells for HIV replication or enhance viral replication within target cells, leading to HIV disease progression.[56] In vitro studies have documented increased viral production in the presence of macrophage CSF (M-CSF), granulocyte-macrophage CSF (GM-CSF), and interleukin-3 but not granulocyte CSF (G-CSF).[23] Clinical studies, however, have not documented an acceleration of HIV disease caused by the use of CSFs.[56,57]

In several trials, neutropenic patients with AIDS responded to GM-CSF with a rapid increase in neutrophils and their precursors in conjunction with improved qualitative neutrophil functions,[58,59] and many chemotherapeutic trials now involve the administration of CSFs.

Human recombinant erythropoietin is oftentimes administered to HIV-infected patients with anemia secondary to zidovudine therapy. The best response is seen in patients whose endogenous erythropoietin levels are less than 500 mU/dl.[4,58] Individual patients with elevated erythropoietin levels may respond to such therapy, but this should be addressed on a case-by-case basis.[60] The concomitant administration of G-CSF or GM-CSF and erythropoietin may limit the hematologic toxicities of zidovudine therapy,[61] making it easier to maintain a therapeutic dose of this antiretroviral drug despite its bone marrow–suppressive effects. Future cytokine therapy may include agents that promote thrombocytopoiesis, such as thrombopoietin and recombinant interleukin-11, and other agents such as stem cell factor that will improve our ability to administer anti-HIV therapeutic medications while controlling their hematologic toxicities.

TABLE 16–3. Guidelines for Use of Colony-Stimulating Factors

Erythropoietin (EPO)
Indications: Symptomatic anemia, zidovudine therapy, and EPO level <500 mU/dl
Dosing
    Initial dose, 100 mcg/kg/day SQ three times a week
    Obtain pretreatment EPO level, reticulocyte count, and ferritin level
    Follow reticulocyte count; decrease EPO dose if possible
    Administer iron replacement therapy if reticulocyte count and ferritin level decrease

Granulocyte Colony-Stimulating Factor (CSF)
Indications
    Chemotherapy (per protocol guidelines)
    Neutropenia (absolute neutrophil count [ANC] <500) secondary to HIV infection of anti-HIV therapeutics
    Granulocyte-macrophage CSF less commonly used secondary to its side effect profile
Dosing
    Initial dose, 5 mcg/kg/day SQ
    Titration
      • For neutropenia unresponsive to initial dose after 1 week of therapy, increase dose to 7.5 mcg/kg/day
      • If unresponsive to 7.5 mcg/kg/day after 1 week, increase to 10 mcg/kg/day
      • If unresponsive to 10 mcg/kg/day after 1 week, discontinue CSF therapy
    Discontinue therapy for unresponsive neutropenia or ANC >500
    Common side effects, such as viral-like prodrome, fever, and myalgias, are typically associated with granulocyte-macrophage CSF therapy

References

1. Doweiko J: Hematologic aspects of HIV infection. AIDS 7:753, 1993
2. Perkocha L, Rodgers G: Hematologic aspects of human immunodeficiency virus infection: Laboratory and clinical considerations. Am J Hematol 29:94, 1988
3. Donahue R, Johnson M, Zon L: Suppression of in vitro haematopoiesis following human immunodeficiency virus infection. Nature 326:200, 1987
4. Scadden D, Zon L, Groopman J: Pathophysiology and management of HIV-associated hematologic disorders. Blood 74:1455, 1989
5. Abrams D, Chinn E, Lewis B: Hematologic manifestations in homosexual men with Kaposi's sarcoma. Am J Clin Pathol 81:13, 1984
6. Castella A, Croxson T, Mildvan D: The bone marrow in AIDS: A histologic, hematologic, and microbiologic study. Am J Clin Pathol 84:425, 1985
7. Goasguen J, Bennett J: Classification and morphologic features of the myelodysplastic syndromes. Semin Oncol 19:4, 1992
8. Ehrenpreis E, Carlson S, Boorstein H, Craig R: Malabsorption and deficiency of vitamin B12 in HIV-infected patients with chronic diarrhea. Dig Dis Sci 39: 2159, 1994
9. Harriman G, Smith P, Horne M: Vitamin B12 malabsorption in patients with acquired immunodeficiency syndrome. Arch Intern Med 149:2039, 1989
10. Paltiel O, Falutz J, Veilleux M, et al: Clinical correlates of subnormal vitamin B12 levels in patients infected with the human immunodeficiency virus. Am J Hematol 49:318, 1995
11. Richman D: AZT Collaborative Working Group: The toxicity of azidothymidine in the treatment of patients with AIDS and AIDS-related complex. N Engl J Med 317:192, 1987
12. Northfelt D, Mayer A, Kaplan L: The usefulness of diagnostic bone marrow examination in patients with human immunodeficiency virus (HIV) infection. J Acquir Immune Defic Syndr 4:659, 1991
13. Zon L, Groopman J: Hematologic manifestations of the human immune deficiency virus. Semin Hematol 25: 208, 1988
14. Treacy M, Lai L, Costello C, Clark A: Peripheral blood and bone marrow abnormalities in patients with HIV related disease. Br J Haematol 65:289, 1987
15. Spivak J, Barnes D, Buchs E, Quinn T: Serum immunoreactive erythropoietin in HIV-infected patients. JAMA 261:3104, 1989
16. Fauci A, Schnittman S, Polii G: Immunopathogenic mechanisms in human immunodeficiency virus (HIV) infection. Ann Intern Med 114:678, 1991
17. Gascom P, Sathe S, Rameshwar P: Impaired erythropoiesis in the acquired immunodeficiency syndrome with disseminated *Mycobacterium avium* complex. Am J Med 94:41, 1993
18. Frickhofen N, Abkowitz J, Safford M, et al: Persistent B19 parvovirus infection in patients infected with HIV type 1: A treatable cause of anemia in AIDS. Ann Intern Med 113:926, 1990
19. Naides S, Howard E, Swack N, et al: Parvovirus B19 infection in HIV type 1-infected persons failing or intolerant to zidovudine therapy. J Infect Dis 168:101, 1993
20. Bremner J, Beard B, Cohen A: Secondary infection with parvovirus B19 in an HIV-positive patient. AIDS 7:1131, 1993
21. McGinniss M, Macher A, Rook A, Alter H: Red cell autoantibodies in patients withi acquired immune deficiency syndrome. Transfusion 26:405, 1986
22. Toy P, Reid M, Burns M: Positive direct antiglobulin test associated with hyperglobulinemia in acquired immunodeficiency syndrome. Am J Hematol 19:145, 1985
23. Israel D, Plaisance K: Neutropenia in patients infected with human immunodeficiency virus. Clin Pharm 10: 268, 1991
24. Leiderman I, Greenberg M, Adelsberg B, Siegal F: A glycoprotein inhibitor of in vitro granulopoiesis associated with AIDS. Blood 70:1267, 1987
25. Murphy P, Lane C, Fauci A, Gallin J: Impairment of neutrophil bactericidal capacity in patients with AIDS. J Infect Dis 158:627, 1988
26. Murphy M, Metcalfe P, Waters A: Incidence and mechanism of neutropenia and thrombocytopenia in patients with human immunodeficiency virus infection. Br J Haematol 66:337, 1987
27. Valone F, Payan D, Abrams D, Goetzl E: Defective polymorphonuclear leukocyte chemotaxis in homosexual men with persistent lymph node syndrome. J Infect Dis 150;267, 1984
28. Brizzi M, Porcu P, Porteri A, Pegoraro L: Haematologic abnormalities in the acquired immunodeficiency syndrome. Haematologica 75:454, 1990
29. Hambleton J, Aragon T, Modin G, et al: Outcome for hospitalized patients with fever and neutropenia who are infected with the human immunodeficiency virus. Clin Infect Dis 20:363, 1995
30. Karpatkin S: Immunologic thrombocytopenic purpura in HIV-seropositive homosexuals, narcotic addicts and hemophiliacs. Semin Hematol 25:219, 1988
31. Battaieb A, Fromont P, Louache F, et al: Presence of cross-reactive antibody between HIV and platelet glycoproteins in HIV-related immune thrombocytopenic purpura. Blood 80:162, 1992
32. Louche F, Bettaieb A, Henri A, et al: Infection of megakaryocytes by HIV in seropositive patients with immune thrombocytopenic purpura. Blood 78:1697, 1991
33. Zucker-Franklin D, Termin C, Cooper M: Structural changes in the megakaryocytes of patients infected with HIV-1. Am J Pathol 134:1295, 1989
34. Zucker-Franklin D, Seremetius S, Zheng Z: Internalization of HIV-type 1 and other retroviruses by megakaryocytes and platelets. Blood 75:1920, 1990
35. Oksenhendler E, Bierling P, Chevret S, et al: Splenectomy is safe and effective in HIV-related immune thrombocytopenia. Blood 82:29, 1993
36. Schneider P, Abrams D, Rayner A, Hohn D: Immunodeficiency-associated thrombocytopenic purpura. Response to splenectomy. Arch Surg 122:1175, 1987
37. Perret B, Baumgartner C: Workshop on immunoglobulin therapy of lymphoproliferative syndromes, mainly AIDS-related complex, and AIDS. Vox Sang 52:1, 1986
38. Oksenhendler E, Bierling P, Ferchal F: Zidovudine for thrombocytopenic purpura related to human immunodeficiency virus infection. Ann Intern Med 110:365, 1989
39. Zidovudine for the treatment of thrombocytopenia associated with human immunodeficiency virus (HIV): A prospective study. The Swis Group for Clinical Studies on the Acquired Immunodeficiency Syndrome (AIDS). Ann Intern Med 109:718, 1988
40. Fabris F, Sgarabotto D, Zanon E, et al: The effect of a single course of alpha-2B-interferon in patients with HIV-related and chronic idiopathic immune thrombocytopenia. Autoimmunity 14:175, 1993

41. Stellini R, Rossi G, Paraninfo G: Interferon therapy in intravenous drug users with HIV-associated idiopathic thrombocytopenic purpura. Haematologica 77:418, 1992

42. Vianelli N, Cantai L, Gugliotta L: Recombinant alpha interferon 2b in the therapy of HIV-related thrombocytopenia. AIDS 7:823, 1993

43. Bussel J, Graziano J, Kimberly RP, et al: Intravenous anti-D treatment of immune thrombocytopenic purpura: Analysis of efficacy, toxicity, and mechanism of effect. Blood 77:1884, 1991

44. Gringeri A, Cattaneo M, Santagostino E, Mannucci P: Intramuscular anti-D immunoglobulins for home treatment of chronic immune thrombocytopenic purpura. Br J Haematol 80:337, 1992

45. Rossi E, Damasio E, Terragna A: HIV-related thrombocytopenia: A therapeutical update. Haematologica 76:141, 1991

46. Roubey RAS: Autoantibodies to phospholipid-binding plasma proteins: A new view of lupus anticoagulants and other "antiphospholipid" autoantibodies. Blood 84:2854, 1994

47. Bloom E, Abrams D, Rodgers G: Lupus anticoagulant in the acquired immunodeficiency syndrome. JAMA 256:491, 1986

48. Leaf A, Laubenstein L, Raphael B: Thrombotic thrombocytopenic purpura associated with human immunodeficiency virus type 1 infection. Ann Intern Med 109:194, 1988

49. Nair J, Bellevue R, Bertoni M, Dosik H: Thrombotic thrombocytopenic purpura in patients with the acquired immunodeficiency syndrome-related complex. Ann Intern Med 109:209, 1988

50. Thompson C, Damon L, Ries C, Linker C: Thrombotic microangiopathies in the 1980s: Clinical features, response to treatment, and the impact of the HIV epidemic. Blood 80:1890, 1992

51. Groopman J: Zidovudine intolerance. Rev Infect Dis 12(Suppl 5):S500, 1990

52. Gill P, Rarick M, Brynes R: Azidothymidine associated with bone marrow failure in the acquired immunodeficiency syndrome. Ann Intern Med 107:502, 1987

53. Walker R, Parker R, Kovacs J: Anemia and erythropoiesis in patients with the acquired immunodeficiency syndrome and Kaposi sarcoma treated with zidovudine. Ann Intern Med 108:372, 1988

54. Groopman J, Feder D: Hematopoietic growth factors in AIDS. Semin Oncol 19:408, 1992

55. Miles S: Hematopoietic growth factors as adjuncts to antiretroviral therapy. AIDS Res Hum Retroviruses 8:1073, 1992

56. Miles S: The use of hematopoietic growth factors in HIV infection and AIDS-related malignancies. Cancer Invest 9:229, 1991

57. Groopman J: Management of the hematologic complications of human immunodeficiency virus infection. Rev Infect Dis 12:931, 1990

58. Baldwin C, Gasson J, Quan S: Granulocyte-macrophage colony-stimulating factor enhances neutrophil function in acquired immunodeficiency syndrome patients. Proc Natl Acad Sci USA 85:2763, 1988

59. Groopman J, Mitsuyasu R, DeLeo M: Effect of recombinant human granulocyte-macrophage colony-stimulating factor on myelopoiesis in the acquired immunodeficiency syndrome. N Engl J Med 317:593, 1987

60. DaCosta N, Hultin M: Effective therapy of human immunodeficiency virus-associated anemia with recombinant human erythropoietin despite high endogenous erythropoietin. Am J Hematol 36:71, 1991

61. Henry D, Beall G, Benson C: Recombinant human erythropoietin in the therapy of anemia associated with HIV infection and zidovudine therapy: Overview of four clinical trials. Ann Intern Med 117:739, 1992

17 Cardiovascular Complications of HIV Infection

MELVIN D. CHEITLIN

The most important pandemic at the close of the 20th century is that of AIDS. By the beginning of the 21st century, it is estimated that there will be 20 million HIV-infected people.[1] In the United States, moreover, 1 million people are HIV positive and almost half a million have been diagnosed with AIDS.[2,3] Although cardiovascular involvement in patients with AIDS was recognized early in the epidemic, the incidence of cardiovascular disease specifically related to the AIDS infection is low. Pericarditis and pulmonary hypertension are well-recognized problems that require specific treatment, and these are certainly the most frequently seen clinical problems. Myocardial involvement with AIDs is clinically unusual, but, despite this, much has been written about the incidence, significance, and approach to therapy in patients who have been demonstrated to have left ventricular dysfunction.

With the introduction of protease inhibitor drugs, patients have developed abnormalities of lipid metabolism resulting in hypertriglyceridemia and hypercholesterolemia.[4] With patients living longer, we might expect to see an increase in the incidence of clinical coronary artery disease, even in relatively young patients.

This chapter reviews the approach to treatment of cardiovascular disease present in patients with AIDS, both related and incidental to the AIDS infection.

CARDIOVASCULAR INVOLVEMENT IN PATIENTS WITH AIDS

Disease of the cardiovascular system can be related to the AIDS infection itself or be present in patients with AIDS and unrelated to the primary disease. Thus pericarditis and pulmonary hypertension are probably related to the HIV disease, either via direct involvement by the HIV organism or because the patient's autoimmune defenses against opportunistic infection are weakened by the HIV disease. Conversely, infective endocarditis in intravenous drug abusers is common in patients both with and without HIV disease. Furthermore, coronary artery disease and congenital heart disease may be incidentally found in patients who are HIV positive. Nevertheless, the treatment of the nonrelated disease is affected by the presence of the HIV disease.

The most important clinical problems seen in patients with HIV infection are the following:

- Pericarditis—in my experience, this is the most frequently encountered cardiovascular clinical problem in patients with HIV disease, both with and without tamponade.
- Pulmonary hypertension—this is seen mostly in patients with multiple pulmonary infections, usually *Pneumocystis carinii*, but occasionally is seen in patients without preceding pulmonary infection.
- Myocardial involvement—the incidence of myocardial involvement depends on the way in which myocardial involvement is diagnosed.
  - In autopsy studies on consecutive patients dying with AIDS, the incidence of myocardial involvement is 15% to 50%. For the most part, this involvement is that of focal myocarditis.
  - If echocardiography is used, the incidence of abnormal wall motion varies from 12% to 41%.
  - In both autopsy and echocardiographic series, the abnormalities are found in patients

who have no clinical findings of heart disease.

- Clinical involvement of the cardiovascular system as myocarditis or cardiomyopathy is distinctly unusual.
- Valvular abnormalities—this includes infective endocarditis, marantic endocarditis, and mitral valve prolapse.
- Arrhythmias.
- Venous thrombosis and pulmonary embolism.
- Hyperlipidemia and hypercholesterolemia.

Clinical cardiovascular disease is unusual in AIDS patients. In large autopsy series, cardiovascular disease as a cause of death is rare. Most patients die of opportunistic infection, central nervous system involvement, neoplasms, or gastrointestinal involvement.[5-7] The prevalence of cardiovascular disease reported in AIDS patients varies depending on whether diagnosis is based on clinical findings or more sensitive techniques, such as echocardiography or microscopic examination of the heart at autopsy. The incidence of cardiovascular disease also depends on the population of AIDS patients reported. In a series reported from New York City, where 40% to 50% of the IV drug abusers are HIV positive, the incidence of clinical cardiovascular disease, especially infective endocarditis, is higher than in series reported from San Francisco, where the HIV risk factor is overwhelmingly homosexuality.[8]

It is also important to recognize that reports from hospitals that do primary care for HIV-positive patients will have a lower incidence of clinical cardiovascular disease than reports from tertiary care facilities, where problem cases are referred. For these reasons, in autopsy reports of cardiovascular involvement from primary care centers, the prevalence of cardiovascular involvement is 5% to 20%.[5,6] When echocardiography and microscopic evidence of lymphocytic infiltration of the myocardium are used as an indicator for cardiovascular involvement, the prevalence of cardiovascular involvement in AIDS patients is closer to 50%.[9]

CLINICAL DIAGNOSIS AND WORK-UP

The only patients with AIDs who require specific cardiovascular diagnostic evaluation are those with clinically evident cardiovascular problems. There is no therapeutic advantage to identifying patients with subclinical cardiovascular involvement and, therefore, no justification for screening of patients with electrocardiograms (ECGs) or more expensive techniques, such as echocardiography.

Symptoms of cardiovascular disease are nonspecific, and many, such as dyspnea, commonly are due to pulmonary involvement rather than cardiovascular disease. Specific signs of cardiovascular involvement, such as the presence of an enlarged cardiac silhouette on chest radiograph, the development of a pericardial friction rub, the clinical picture of congestive heart failure with S_3 gallop, pulmonary edema, or the development of a pathologic systolic or diastolic murmur, are all findings that should necessitate a cardiovascular diagnostic work-up. The coincidental occurrence of coronary artery disease, hypertensive cardiovascular disease, congenital heart disease, and myocardial disease caused by use of illicit drugs, such as cocaine, should also be considered.[10]

The most helpful laboratory studies are the chest radiograph, an ECG, and two-dimensional transthoracic echocardiography. In patients on protease inhibitors, a lipid profile including total cholesterol, serum triglycerides, low-density lipoproteins (LDLs), and high-density lipoproteins should be done after the patient has taken the drug for 4 to 6 weeks. To evaluate valvular function or diastolic left ventricular function, Doppler echocardiography is the most useful. Whenever a question of pulmonary hypertension arises, the use of Doppler in detecting tricuspid regurgitation, found in a high proportion of normal hearts, makes it possible to estimate the pulmonary artery systolic pressure. By knowing the velocity of the regurgitant jet by the modified Bernoulli equation, the clinician can calculate the systolic pressure gradient between the right ventricle and the right atrium across the tricuspid valve. By adding this pressure to the clinically estimated central venous pressure, the systolic pressure of the pulmonary artery can be estimated with a fair degree of accuracy.[11]

For almost all patients with suspected cardiovascular involvement, these simple, noninvasive tests should suffice. Proceeding to invasive studies, such as cardiac catheterization or angiography, is rarely necessary unless indicated by the need to work up incidental problems, such as coronary heart disease.

The value of doing pericardial and myocardial biopsy to find treatable etiologies in patients with pericardial or myocardial disease is controversial. In general, the incidence of finding treatable etiologies of pericardial or myocardial disease is very low. However, if such a problem that is treatable with special therapy is found, it is obviously important.

WORK-UP AND THERAPY OF SPECIFIC CARDIOVASCULAR PROBLEMS

Pericarditis and Pericardial Effusion

In autopsy series, the prevalence of pericardial involvement varies from 3%[12] to almost 37%.[13] In the experience at San Francisco General Hospital, pericardial effusion is found in about 30% of patients who have had an echocardiogram ordered for suspicion of cardiovascular involvement. This prevalence by echocardiography is similar to that reported by Corallo et al., 38% of whose patients studied by echocardiography had pericardial effusion.[14]

Although clinical presentation of pericarditis with pleuritic-type chest pain and pericardial friction rub is seen, asymptomatic pericardial effusion is more common. The initial suspicion of cardiovascular disease frequently is made on finding a large cardiac silhouette on chest radiograph. Dyspnea resulting from compression of the lung by a large pericardial effusion is another common presentation of pericardial effusion.

Cardiac tamponade manifested by an enlarged cardiac silhouette, elevation of central venous pressure, pulsus paradoxus, and later tachycardia and hypotension is not uncommon. Deaths from tamponade have been reported occasionally.[15] In the experience at San Francisco General Hospital, cardiac tamponade is seen in about one third of patients with pericardial effusion,[16] which is similar to the report by Monsuez et al. of 28% already having or developing cardiac tamponade.[17]

The etiology of the pericardial effusion can be heart failure or pericarditis caused by specific organisms, such as *Mycobacterium tuberculosis*, or by unknown pathogens, either viral infections or the HIV organism itself. Another important etiology for pericardial effusion is tumor involvement by Kaposi's sarcoma or lymphoma. Reynolds et al. reported 14 AIDS patients with pericarditis among whom *M. tuberculosis* was found to be the etiology in 37%.[18] Other organisms, such as *Mycobacterium avium-intracellulare*,[19] and other pathogens, such as staphylococcus, pneumococcus, and fungi, have been reported.

Treatment

An asymptomatic small pericardial effusion needs no therapy. If the patient has a large effusion compressing the lung or has signs of tamponade, such as an elevated central venous pressure, pericardiocentesis is indicated, with removal of fluid to reverse the hemodynamic compromise and to examine the fluid by culture and microscopic examination for possible treatable etiologies, such as *M. tuberculosis* or lymphoma. Waiting for diastolic collapse of the right atrium by echocardiography before doing a pericardiocentesis is not necessary. With large effusion, a catheter can be introduced percutaneously into the pericardial cavity and connected to closed-drainage suction for 24 to 48 hours. Usually, there is no recurrence. If the patient has clinical pericarditis with pain and fever with a small effusion, examination of the pericardial fluid and pericardial tissue looking for a treatable etiology is possible by drainage through an open pericardiotomy, usually from a subxiphoid approach.

At San Francisco General Hospital, in 10 of 25 patients with clinical pericardial effusion, pericarditis, or both, no specific etiology was found on examination of the pericardial effusion and pericardial tissue.[16] Some of the patients had lymphoma, and the pericardial effusion was thought to be related to the tumor, but in none in whom tissue or fluid was examined could evidence of a tumor be found.

The presence of pericardial effusion is probably a sign of poor prognosis. We have done a prospective study of 195 HIV-positive patients recruited as outpatients and followed with serial echocardiograms every 4 months for 3 years at San Francisco General Hospital.[20] We found an incidence of pericardial effusion of 4% per year for all infected patients and 11% per year for AIDS patients. The presence of pericardial effusion was a sign of poor prognosis, since these patients had a 6-month mortality of 64% versus 7% for similar AIDS patients without effusion. It is doubtful that the pericardial effusion is the cause of the poor prognosis, since it is rare for patients to die from pericardial tamponade.

Flum and colleagues[21] have also noted the grave prognostic significance of the presence of pericardial effusion in patients with AIDS. In their study, they also did surgical "pericardial windows," with histologic examination and culture of fluid and tissue. In 94% of the cases there was no change in clinical management based on the results of biopsy or culture because either the patient was already on appropriate therapy or therapy could not be instituted because of the underlying illness. They concluded that pericardial windows were of little practical use for diagnosis and were justified only to relieve pericardial tamponade.[21]

Pulmonary Hypertension

Early in the epidemic, patients were seen with ECG evidence of right ventricular hypertrophy. At autopsy, dilatation of the right ventricle and a normal left ventricle were described in about 15% of cases.[5,22] Himelman et al.[23] reported six patients with severe pulmonary hypertension who had increased pulmonary vascular resistance on catheterization. The majority of these patients had multiple pulmonary infections, mostly *P. carinii*, although one of their patients had had no previous pneumonias. Patients with primary pulmonary hypertension have been reported.[24] At autopsy, no evidence for HIV infection in the pulmonary vascular endothelium was found by polymerase chain reaction or in situ hybridization. There were electron-microscopic changes in the endothelial cells similar to those seen in patients with lupus erythematosus, and these authors postulated a sequence of injury to the endothelial cell by paracrine cytokines releasing vasoactive substances or growth factors, resulting in increased pulmonary vascular resistance.[24] With multiple pulmonary infections, interstitial fibrosis and destruction of the capillary bed are possible causes of increased pulmonary vascular resistance. With the development of pulmonary hypertension, increased afterload on the right ventricle, right ventricular hypertrophy and dilatation, and eventually right heart failure result.

Treatment

If the patient's pulmonary hypertension and its consequences are the most important clinical problem, normalization of blood gases and treatment of underlying pulmonary infection are most important. Hypoxia, respiratory acidosis, and to a lesser degree hypercarbia are powerful causes of pulmonary vasoconstriction. If hypoxia persists, supplemental low-flow oxygen can be helpful. If these measures are not successful, an empiric trial of a variety of vasodilators is indicated in an attempt to find one that will reduce pulmonary vascular resistance and increase to normal or maintain cardiac output without dropping systemic vascular resistance to the point where systemic arterial pressure drops.

To do this safely, the patient must be hospitalized, and the cardiac output, pulmonary artery pressure, pulmonary vascular resistance, and systemic arterial pressure must be monitored invasively.[25] When a pulmonary arterial catheter is in place, I have used the following vasodilators sequentially: 100% oxygen, nitroglycerin, hydralazine, nifedipine, lisinopril, converting enzyme inhibitors, and prostaglandin E_1. If an appropriate drug is found, it can be continued chronically. If arterial blood pressure drops, the drug must be discontinued.

Barst and colleagues have reported longterm success in decreasing pulmonary vascular resistance and pulmonary artery pressure without a drop in systemic arterial pressure in patients with primary pulmonary hypertension using a continuous infusion of prostacyclin.[26] This will be worth investigating, especially if an orally active form of prostacyclin becomes available. In my experience, finding a drug that is effective chronically is rare, and the patient with pulmonary hypertension has a very poor prognosis.

Myocardial Involvement

This is the most controversial topic concerning cardiovascular disease in AIDS patients. The prevalence of myocardial involvement in patients with HIV disease depends on the definition. Clinical cardiomyopathy, that is, myocardial disease causing signs and symptoms including heart failure, is unusual. Myocardial involvement defined as microscopic inflammatory cell myocarditis with or without any evidence of myocardial cell necrosis is found more commonly. Focal myocarditis is seen in 15% to 50% of cases in serial autopsy.[5,6,8,22] What is being described is usually focal collections of inflammatory cells with or without adjacent myocardial cell necrosis. Rarely is the myocarditis diffuse. Rarely was there clinical evidence of myocardial involvement before death. When searched for diligently, pathogenic organisms, both fungal and parasitic, such as *Toxoplasma*, *Candida albicans*, and *Coccidioides*, can be found about a quarter to a third of the time. It is probable that opportunistic viral infections known to cause myocarditis also could be responsible for these findings. These might include Coxsackie B virus and cytomegalic inclusion disease.

Myocarditis is rarely the cause of death in these patients. Myocarditis is said to occur in the late stages of the disease in patients with a low CD4 count. When the diagnosis of myocardial involvement is made by echocardiography, where decreased left ventricular function or dilated left ventricle is seen, the prevalence is also high. Himelman et al.[27] reported 71 patients with AIDS who had been sent for echocardiography. There were eight patients who had left ventricular dilatation, decreased contractility, or both, four of whom had clinical congestive heart failure. Corallo et al.[14] performed echocardiograms on 102 consecutive patients with AIDS, none with congestive heart failure, and found 41% with left ventricular hypokinesia.

Prospective studies by echocardiography are beginning to be reported. Blanchard et al.[28] followed 50 patients with AIDS and found that 7 (14%) developed echocardiographic evidence of left ventricular dysfunction. When repeat echocardiograms were done, three had improved left ventricular function and four did not. All four who did not improve died within 1 year. Herskowitz et al.[29] followed 59 AIDS patients with normal initial echocardiograms for 11 months and performed serial echocardiograms. Eleven developed left ventricular dysfunction over 725 months of follow-up, a rate of 1.5 patients per 100 patient-months. DeCastro and colleagues[30] followed 136 HIV-positive patients prospectively with serial echocardiograms over a follow-up time of 415 ± 220 days. Three quarters of their patients were intravenous drug users. Seven patients, all with AIDS, developed clinical and echocardiographic findings of acute global left ventricular dysfunction. Six patients died and five had autopsies. Of those with postmortem examination, three had acute lymphocytic myocarditis, one had cryptococcal myocarditis, and one had interstitial edema and fibrosis.

At San Francisco General Hospital, my colleagues and I have conducted a 4-year prospective study using serial quantitative echocardiographic Doppler techniques. All patients were recruited as outpatients. There were 74 AIDS patients followed for a mean of 16.5 ± 12 months. The control populations were HIV-positive patients without disease, HIV-positive patients with AIDS-related complex, and HIV-negative gay men. Over the follow-up period, there were no differences in systolic left ventricular function (end-diastolic volume, end-systolic volume, or ejection fraction) within or among any of the groups. There were no differences between groups in the numbers of patients whose ejection fraction changed more than 2 standard deviations over the time of follow-up. Most of the patients with reduced left ventric-

ular function on echocardiogram had no clinical evidence of cardiac disease, and the etiology of these changes is not obvious.

Currie and colleagues[31] reported 296 HIV-positive patients recruited prospectively. By echocardiogram 44 had cardiac dysfunction. Thirteen had left ventricular dysfunction, 19 had borderline left ventricular dysfunction, and 12 had isolated right ventricular dysfunction. In a 4-year follow-up period, the incidence of left ventricular dysfunction was 13/296 or 1.1% of HIV-positive patients per year. If only AIDS patients were included, the incidence would be 3.25% per year. Survival was significantly reduced in patients with cardiomyopathy compared to those with normal hearts on echocardiography. Median survival in those patients whose deaths were related to AIDS was 101 days in those with cardiomyopathy compared to 472 days in those with normal hearts on echocardiography. Death in cardiomyopathy patients was most often due to AIDS-related causes rather than to congestive heart failure.

In summarizing most series of patients, the number of AIDS patients seen with clinically important cardiomyopathy not explained by known agents, such as alcohol, toxoplasmosis, hypertrophic cardiomyopathy, cocaine use, acute myocardial infarction, or drug toxicity, is small. Clinical cardiomyopathy is seen in 1% to 3% of AIDS patients.

The etiology of the changes in left ventricular function is as yet undetermined. Obviously, HIV infection (myocarditis) is a leading contender. The fact that the myocardial cell lacks the CD4 receptor is against the possibility of direct HIV invasion of the myocardial cell. By in situ hybridization, polymerase chain reaction, and culture,[32-35] the HIV organism has been located in or near the myocardial cell. These findings have been sparse, with the HIV organism not proved to be within the myocardial cell rather than in a macrophage or endothelial cell and frequently being found in tissue from patients without clinical or microscopic evidence of myocarditis. It is possible that the myocardial cell is injured by some other mechanism, allowing entrance of the HIV organism. Epstein-Barr virus has been demonstrated to facilitate entry and replication of HIV into CD4 receptor-negative B cells.[36]

Opportunistic infections can cause myocarditis and even clinical congestive heart failure and death. Toxoplasmosis has been reported as well as myocarditis caused by cytomegalovirus and Epstein-Barr virus.[37,38] Niedt and Schinella,[39] in a study of 56 AIDS patients, found that 77% had been infected with cytomegalovirus, 4 of whom had clinical cardiac involvement (ECG changes, arrhythmias, or congestive heart failure) and demonstrated inclusion bodies and myocarditis.

Myocardial damage can result from cytokine release from HIV-infected monocytes and lymphocytes. The cytokine acts as a paracrine substance, and the adjacent myocardial cells are affected. Ho et al.[40] reported this mechanism as the etiology of neuroglial cell dysfunction in patients with AIDS. If cytokines are released into the circulation by infected macrophages and monocytes, myocardial cell dysfunction could result.[41] Circulating cytokines have been demonstrated in patients with advanced HIV infection.[42-44]

Another postulated mechanism for myocardial cell dysfunction is autoimmune myocarditis, which could be initiated by a change in some myocardial cell component, inducing autoimmune antibodies. Such cardiac autoantibodies have been demonstrated in AIDS patients with cardiomyopathy by Herskowitz et al.,[45] but it is not clear whether the cardiac autoantibodies are the cause or the result of myocardial injury.

Although other etiologies for cardiac myocardial dysfunction, such as nutritional deficiency of both calories[46] and such microelements as selenium,[47] have been reported, the effects of both therapeutic and illicit drugs are the most likely etiology of myocardial dysfunction. Most patients with HIV infection are taking multiple drugs, some of which are known to be cardiotoxic. Reversible cardiomyopathy has been described in patients taking interleukin-2,[48] α_2-interferon,[49] and Adriamycin. More recently, foscarnet[50] and high-dose ifosfamide[51] have been reported to cause severe reversible cardiomyopathy.

Herskowitz et al.[52] reported decreases in left ventricular function by echocardiography in AIDS patients taking zidovudine. On withdrawal of zidovudine, there was improvement of left ventricular dysfunction in some of the patients. Other drugs to which patients with HIV disease are exposed, such as cocaine and alcohol, have regularly been reported to cause cardiomyopathy.[53]

Treatment of Myocarditis, Cardiomyopathy, and Congestive Heart Failure

There is no evidence that a patient with HIV disease without clinical evidence of cardiac involvement benefits from screening with ECG, chest radiograph, or more expensive techniques, such as echocardiography or Doppler. Any abnormality found would not justify any specific treatment at that point in the patient's HIV disease.

In the patient with symptoms, cardiac involvement must be suspected and differentiated from symptoms caused by pulmonary or renal disease. The most effective way of doing this is by echocardiography. There are two reasons why echocardiography is essential in patients with congestive heart failure: (1) the etiology of the congestive heart failure may be apparent, that is, the patient may have valve disease, arteriosclerotic heart disease, or congenital heart disease; and (2) the echocardiogram allows identification of the pathophysiologic type of congestive heart failure. Most patients with heart failure have a dilated left ventricle and decreased systolic function. Some patients, especially elderly, hypertensive patients, have good left ventricular function, with diastolic dysfunction as the cause of the congestive heart failure.[54] This occurs in up to one third of cases. In these patients, the treatment is different from that of systolic dysfunction heart failure; inotropic agents and afterload reduction should be avoided and there should be judicious use of nitrates, diuretics, β-blockage, and calcium channel blockers.

Patients with clinical congestive heart failure manifested by an S_3 gallop or pulmonary edema, or an elevated central venous pressure, should have an echocardiogram. Pericardial effusion resulting in tamponade can occur as right heart failure and is treatable by pericardiocentesis. Occasionally, other reasons for congestive heart failure are found, such as a hypertrophic cardiomyopathy or cocaine or alcohol abuse, and withdrawal of these substances is essential. When the patient has clinical cardiomyopathy, Herskowitz et al. have suggested a drug-free trial, with the removal of all drugs not absolutely essential.[52] The echocardiogram should be repeated in 2 weeks. If improvement has occurred, the suspected drug should be eliminated. Patients with clinical congestive heart failure are treated in the conventional way with rest, diuretics, digoxin, and afterload reduction, preferably by angiotensin-converting enzyme inhibition.

The value of myocardial biopsy is still under debate. The most impressive argument for myocardial biopsy was that, if microscopic myocarditis was found, a steroid and/or antimetabolite therapy would be indicated. However, Mason and colleagues[55] have shown that steroid or antimetabolite therapy in myocarditis has no advantage over conventional management. Some authorities believe that the rare finding of a treatable cause of myocarditis is a justifiable reason for recommending myocardial biopsy in patients with congestive heart failure. However, it is difficult even at autopsy, when the entire heart is available for examination, to find organisms that are treatable, so that the few pieces of tissue obtainable by myocardial biopsy would likely miss such organisms.

The stage of HIV disease in the patient is an important factor. Patients who are late in their course of HIV disease and who develop congestive heart failure should be treated for their congestive heart failure without invasive studies. If congestive heart failure is found earlier in the course of the HIV infection and does not respond to a drug-free trial, it is clinically justifiable to attempt to find a treatable etiology by myocardial biopsy even though the chances of discovering such a treatable cause are very low.

Myocardial involvement by neoplasm is usually an incidental finding and not the cause of congestive heart failure. Kaposi's sarcoma was one of the first neoplasms to be described involving the heart.[56] At present, lymphoma, especially non-Hodgkin's lymphoma, is seen most often, and pericardial effusion is the most frequent clinical condition.[57] The tumor can invade the myocardium, causing arrhythmias, heart block, and even obstruction to blood flow requiring surgical excision.[57–59] When the tumor is found, specific treatment is required.

VALVULAR ABNORMALITIES

Most valvular abnormalities in patients with AIDS are coincidental rather than related to the HIV infection. Patients with marantic endocarditis usually are found by virtue of the fact that they have suffered a systemic embolization. Occasionally, a marantic thrombus is found incidentally on echocardiography. In these instances, the treatment is anticoagulation as long as no absolute contraindication to anticoagulation exists. Although it is conceivable that such a large, mobile vegetation could be found and surgical removal would be indicated, I have never seen such a case.

Patients with valvular insufficiency resulting from infective endocarditis, frequently with the usual streptococcal or staphylococcal organism, should be treated in the same way as in HIV-negative patients. In my experience, infective endocarditis occurs almost exclusively in intravenous drug users and is rare in other HIV-

positive patients.[60] Obviously, clinical judgment should be used when infective endocarditis is the last tragedy in the late course of a patient's HIV disease. In this instance, surgery should be avoided, since the outcome in the near future will be determined by the HIV disease and not by the endocarditis.

Patients with mitral valve prolapse have been described who had HIV disease. These patients are usually cachectic, and the mitral valve prolapse may be secondary to the decrease in volume of the left ventricle, resulting in systolic prolapse of the mitral valve into the left atrium. In these patients, unless the mitral regurgitation is severe, no treatment is necessary. If mitral regurgitation is severe, the patient should be treated as would an HIV-negative patient unless the patient is late in the course of disease.

ARRHYTHMIAS AND OTHER CARDIOVASCULAR INVOLVEMENT

Arrhythmias can be seen as a result of myocarditis, pulmonary hypertension, congestive heart failure, or drug therapy. Torsade de pointes has been reported to result from both intravenous and inhaled pentamidine.[61,62]

Venous thrombosis[63] and pulmonary embolism[4] have been described in patients with AIDS. They can be a cause of pulmonary hypertension and are treated by anticoagulation.[64] AIDS patients have prothrombotic abnormalities, such as increased anticardiolipin immunoglobulin G (IgG) activity[65] and low protein S and protein C levels.[66] To evaluate patients with venous thrombosis and pulmonary embolism, a search for low protein C and protein S levels and elevated anticardiolipin IgG should be carried out, and a duplex Doppler examination for deep venous thrombosis should be performed. The treatment for venous thrombosis is anticoagulation.

HYPERLIPIDEMIA AND CORONARY ATHEROSCLEROSIS

A recent problem termed *lipodystrophy* has been described[67] in patients on protease inhibitor drugs, including indinavir, ritonavir, and saquinavir.[68] An abnormal distribution of fat deposits in the abdominal wall, posterior neck, and upper back characterize this problem. It can be accompanied by an increase in triglycerides of at times over 1000 mg/dl, usually seen within weeks of starting the drug.[69] The development of new-onset type II diabetes mellitus and insulin resistance has also been reported with some protease inhibitors.[70] In some patients elevation of serum cholesterol and LDLs is seen, and there have been increasing reports of young patients developing angina pectoris and myocardial infarction with coronary artery disease on angiography.[71]

The pathogenesis of the protease inhibitor–associated hypertriglyceridemia is not known but could involve impaired clearance as well as increased synthesis of circulating triglyceride-rich lipoproteins. Reduced insulin release or increased peripheral insulin resistance may also be involved.

Protein and genomic sequence library analysis has found the 12 amino acids spanning the catalytic site of HIV protease to have a 70% homology with LDL receptor–like protein, hepatic scavenger of circulating lipids.[69] As HIV-infected patients live longer, it is probable that an increased incidence of coronary atherosclerosis and acute ischemic syndromes, and possibly cerebrovascular and peripheral vascular disease, will be seen.[34]

Treatment of hypertriglyceridemia involves a low-fat diet and fibric acid drugs such as gemfibrozil. If LDL is elevated, HMG-CoA reductase inhibitors should be used. An added concern is that the HMG-CoA reductase inhibitors and protease inhibitors are both metabolized through the hepatic cytochrome P-450 system.

INVASIVE CARDIOVASCULAR PROCEDURES IN THE PATIENT WITH AIDS

In the work-up and treatment of the patient with HIV infection, it is necessary occasionally to consider a catheterization or cardiovascular surgery. Usually, the need for invasive techniques arises because of diseases that are occurring incidentally in the HIV-positive patient, such as congenital heart disease, coronary artery disease, or valve disease. Because health care workers fear HIV infection, there is a hesitancy to do invasive procedures where there would be no question with a similar indication in an HIV-negative patient.

The incidence of HIV infection in health care workers with no other risk factors for AIDS is very small. As of 1992, there have been 100

such health care workers who seroconverted after accidental exposure, usually needlestick or knife wound, who were known to be HIV negative before the incident. Combining 14 prospective studies of the risk of HIV-1 infection to health care workers, there were 2042 parenteral exposures in 1948 patients.[72] The chance of seroconversion was 0.29% per exposure (95% confidence intervals, 0.13% to 0.7%). There were no seroconversions from mucous membrane exposures in 688 people with 1061 mucous membrane exposures. The risk, therefore, of developing an HIV seroconversion from work exposure is very low, approximately 1 infection in 300 documented parenteral exposures to HIV-positive blood. The risk of HIV infection after percutaneous exposure with a needle used for an HIV-positive patient increases with a larger volume of blood injected and probably with a higher titer of HIV in the blood of the infected patient.[73]

Even though the risk is low, if it happens, it is a tragedy to that person, and so it is necessary to maintain vigorous discipline in performing invasive procedures in these patients. Judgment is necessary in deciding when the small risk of infection is justified by the value of the procedure to the patient. Patients in the late stages of HIV infection who have problems that ordinarily would justify catheterization or open heart surgery will not be benefited by such surgery if the prognosis is determined by the HIV disease. It is therefore unlikely that coronary or valve surgery can be justified if the goal is to prolong life when 70% of patients with AIDS die within 3 to 4 years of the diagnosis.[43] However, if patients with AIDS are on maximal medical management and still are incapacitated by the coronary or the valve disease, surgery is justifiable.

More commonly, the question arises in patients with HIV infection but no defining diagnosis of AIDS. Such patients may live 10 to 15 years before they develop the disease, which ultimately will be fatal, and they deserve evaluation and therapy, including invasive procedures, for the same indications as would be the case in an HIV-negative person.

CONCLUSION

Patients with HIV infection have serious problems with opportunistic infections, central nervous system involvement, and gastrointestinal disorders. Clinical cardiovascular involvement is unusual. The most important and treatable cardiovascular involvement is pericarditis and tamponade. The unusual patient with clinical cardiomyopathy should be recognized, evaluated by echocardiography, and treated with conventional treatment for congestive heart failure. It is rare that invasive techniques such as catheterization or myocardial biopsy are useful, although in the patient early in the HIV disease, where clinical cardiomyopathy is the major problem, a vigorous search for treatable etiologies is justified.

References

1. World Health Organization, Office of Information: Press release WHO/101, December 10, 1993. Geneva, World Health Organization
2. Centers for Disease Control and Prevention: HIV/AIDS Surveill Rep 6(2):7, 1994
3. Steele FR: A moving target: CDC still trying to estimate HIV-1 prevalence. J NIH Res 6:25, 1994
4. Becker DM, Saunders TJ, Wispelwey B, Schain DC: Venous thromboembolism in AIDS: Case report. Am J Med Sci 303:395, 1992
5. Lewis W: AIDS: Cardiac findings from 115 autopsies. Prog Cardiovasc Dis 32:207, 1989
6. Magno J, Margaretten W, Cheitlin M: Myocardial involvement in acquired immunodeficiency syndrome: Incidence in a large autopsy study [abstract]. Circulation 78(Suppl II):II-C459, 1988
7. Moskowitz L, Hensley GT, Chan JC, Adams K: Immediate causes of death in acquired immunodeficiency syndrome. Arch Pathol Lab Med 109:735, 1985
8. Francis CK: Cardiac involvement in AIDS. Curr Probl Cardiol 15:575, 1990
9. Levy WS, Simon GL, Ross JC, Ross AM: Prevalence of cardiac abnormalities in human immunodeficiency virus infection. Am J Cardiol 63:86, 1989
10. Brown J, King A, Francis CK: Cardiovascular effects of alcohol, cocaine, and acquired immune deficiency. Cardiovasc Clin 21:341, 1991
11. Yock PG, Popp RL: Noninvasive estimation of right ventricular systolic pressure by Doppler ultrasound in patients with tricuspid regurgitation. Circulation 70: 657, 1984
12. Wilkes MS, Fortin AH, Felix JC, et al: Value of necropsy in acquired immunodeficiency syndrome. Lancet 2:85, 1988
13. Marche C, Trophilme D, Mayorga R, et al: Cardiac involvement in AIDS: A pathological study. In: Abstracts of the 4th International Conference on AIDS, Stockholm, 1988, Abstract 7103
14. Corallo S, Mutinelli MR, Moroni M, et al: Echocardiography detects myocardial damage in AIDS: Prospective study in 102 patients. Eur Heart J 9:887, 1988
15. Steigman CK, Anderson DW, Macher AM, et al: Fatal cardiac tamponade in acquired immunodeficiency syndrome with epicardial Kaposi's sarcoma. Am Heart J 116:1105, 1988
16. Galli FC, Cheitlin MD: Pericardial disease in AIDS: Frequency of tamponade and therapeutic and diagnostic use of pericardiocentesis. J Am Coll Cardiol 19: 226A, 1992
17. Monsuez JJ, Kinney EL, Vittecoq D, et al: Comparison among acquired immune deficiency syndrome patients with and without clinical evidence of cardiac disease. Am J Cardiol 62:1311, 1988
18. Reynolds M, Berger M, Hecht S, et al: Large pericardial effusions associated with the acquired immune deficiency syndrome (AIDS) [abstract]. J Am Coll Cardiol 17:221A, 1991
19. Woods GL, Goldsmith JC: Fatal pericarditis due to *Mycobacterium avium-intracellulare* in acquired immunodeficiency syndrome. Chest 95:1355, 1989
20. Heidenreich PA, Eisenberg MJ, Kee LL, et al: Pericardial effusion in AIDS: Incidence and survival. Circulation 92:3229, 1995
21. Flum DR, McGinn JT, Tyras DH: The role of the "pericardial window" in AIDS. Chest 107:1522, 1995
22. Anderson DW, Virmani R, Reilly JM, et al: Prevalent myocarditis at necropsy in the acquired immunodeficiency syndrome. J Am Coll Cardiol 11:792, 1988
23. Himelman RB, Dohrmann M, Goodman P, et al: Severe pulmonary hypertension and cor pulmonale in the acquired immunodeficiency syndrome. Am J Cardiol 64: 1396, 1989
24. Mette SA, Palevsky HI, Pietra GG: Primary pulmonary hypertension in association with human immunodeficiency virus infection: A possible viral etiology for some forms of hypertensive disease. Am Rev Respir Dis 145:1196, 1992
25. Rich S: Primary pulmonary hypertension. Prog Cardiovasc Dis 31:205, 1988
26. Barst RJ, Rubin LJ, Long WA, et al: A comparison of continuous intravenous epoprostenol (prostacyclin) with conventional therapy for primary pulmonary hypertension. N Engl J Med 334:296, 1996
27. Himelman RB, Chung WS, Chernoff DN, et al: Cardiac manifestations of human immunodeficiency virus infection: A two-dimensional echocardiographic study. J Am Coll Cardiol 13:1030, 1989
28. Blanchard DG, Hagenhoff C, Clow LC, et al: Reversibility of cardiac abnormalities in human immunodeficiency virus (HIV)-infected individuals: A serial echocardiographic study. J Am Coll Cardiol 17:1270, 1991
29. Herskowitz A, Vlahor D, Willoughby S, et al: Prevalence and incidence of left ventricular dysfunction in patients with human immunodeficiency virus infection. Am J Cardiol 71:955, 1993
30. DeCastro S, D'Amati G, Gallo P, et al: Frequency of development of acute global left ventricular dysfunction in human immunodeficiency virus infection. J Am Coll Cardiol 24:1018, 1994
31. Currie PF, Jacob AJ, Foreman AR, et al: Heart muscle disease related to HIV infection: Prognostic implications. BMJ 309:1605, 1994
32. Calabrese LH, Proffitt MR, Yen-Lieberman B, et al: Congestive cardiomyopathy and illness related to the acquired immunodeficiency syndrome (AIDS) associated with isolation of retrovirus from myocardium. Ann Intern Med 107:691, 1987
33. Cenacchi G, Re MC, Furlini G, et al: Human immunodeficiency virus type 1 antigen detection in endomyocardial biopsy: An immunomorphological study. Microbiologica 13:145, 1990
34. Grody WW, Cheng L, Lewis W: Infection of the heart by the human immunodeficiency virus. Am J Cardiol 66:203, 1990
35. Lipshultz SE, Fox CH, Perez-Atayde AR, et al: Identification of human immunodeficiency virus-1 RNA and DNA in the heart of a child with cardiovascular abnormalities and congenital acquired immune deficiency syndrome: Case report. Am J Cardiol 66:246, 1990

36. Goldblum N, Daefler S, Llana T, et al: Susceptibility to HIV-1 infection of a human B-lymphoblastoid cell line, DG75, transfected with subgenomic DNA fragments of Epstein-Barr virus. Dev Biol Stand 72:309, 1990

37. Acierno LJ: Cardiac complications in acquired immunodeficiency syndrome (AIDS): A review. J Am Coll Cardiol 13:1144, 1989

38. Hofman P, Drici M-D, Gibelin P, et al: Prevalance of toxoplasma myocarditis in patients with acquired immunodeficiency syndrome. B Heart J 70:376, 1993

39. Niedt GW, Schinella RA: Acquired immunodeficiency syndrome: Clincopathologic study of 56 autopsies. Arch Pathol Lab Med 109:727, 1985

40. Ho DD, Pomerantz RJ, Kaplan JC: Pathogenesis of infection with human immunodeficiency virus. N Engl J Med 317:278, 1987

41. Parrillo JE, Burch C, Shelhamer JH, et al: A circulating myocardial depressant substance in humans with septic shock: Septic shock patients with a reduced ejection fraction have a circulating factor that depresses in vitro myocardial cell performance. J Clin Invest 76:1539, 1985

42. Lähdevirta J, Maury CPJ, Teppo AM, Repo H: Elevated levels of circulating cachectin/tumor necrosis factor in patients with acquired immunodeficiency syndrome. Am J Med 85:289, 1988

43. Centers for Disease Control: Acquired immunodeficiency syndrome—UnitedStates update. MMWR Morb Mortal Wkly Rep 35:17, 1986

44. Matsuyama T, Kobayashi N, Yamamoto N: Cytokines and HIV infection: Is AIDS a tumor necrosis factor disease? AIDS 5:1405, 1991

45. Herskowitz A, Ansari AA, Neumann DA, et al: Cardiomyopathy in acquired immunodeficiency syndrome: Evidence for autoimmunity [abstract]. Circulation 80(Suppl II):II-322, 1989

46. Goldberg SJ, Comerci GD, Feldman L: Cardiac output and regional myocardial contraction in anorexia nervosa. J Adolescent Health Care 9:15, 1988

47. Kavanaugh-McHugh AL, Ruff A, Perlman E, et al: Selenium deficiency and cardiomyopathy in acquired immunodeficiency syndrome. J Parenter Enter Nutr 15:347, 1991

48. Samlowski WE, Ward JH, Craven CM, Freedman RA: Severe myocarditis following high-dose interleukin-2 administration. Arch Pathol Lab Med 113:838, 1989

49. Deyton LR, Walker RE, Kovacs JA, et al: Reversible cardiac dysfunction associated with interferon alfa therapy in AIDS patients with Kaposi's sarcoma. N Engl J Med 321:1246, 1989

50. Brown DL, Sather S, Cheitlin MD: Reversible cardiac dysfunction association with foscarnet therapy for cytomegalovirus esophagitis in an AIDS patient. Am Heart J 125:1439, 1993

51. Quezado ZM, Wilson WH, Cunnion RE, et al: High-dose ifosfamide is associated with severe, reversible cardiac dysfunction. Ann Intern Med 118:31, 1993

52. Herskowitz A, Willoughby SB, Baughman KL, et al: Cardiomyopathy associated with antiretroviral therapy in patients with HIV infection: A report of six cases. Ann Intern Med 116:311, 1992

53. Chokshi SK, Moore R, Pandian NG, Isner JM: Reversible cardiomyopathy associated with cocaine intoxication. Ann Intern Med 111:1039, 1989

54. Shah PM, Pai RG: Diastolic heart failure. Curr Probl Cardiol 17:787, 1992

55. Mason JW, O'Connell JD, Herskowitz A, et al: A clinical trial of immunosuppressive therapy for myocarditis: The Myocarditis Treatment Trial Investigation. N Engl J Med 333:269, 1995

56. Welch K, Finkbeiner W, Alpers CE, et al: Autopsy findings in the acquired immune deficiency syndrome. JAMA 252:1152, 1984

57. Goldfarb A, King CL, Rosenzweig BP, et al: Cardiac lymphoma in the acquired immunodeficiency syndrome. Am Heart J 118:1340, 1989

58. Horowitz MD, Cox MM, Neibart RM, et al: Resection of right atrial lymphoma in patients with AIDS. Int J Cardiol 34:139, 1992

59. Kelsey RC, Saker A, Morgan M: Cardiac lymphoma in a patient with AIDS. Ann Intern Med 115:370, 1991

60. Currie PF, Sutherland GR, Jacob AJ, et al: A review of endocarditis in acquired immunodeficiency syndrome and human immunodeficiency virus infection. Eur Heart J 16(Suppl B):15, 1995

61. Engrav MB, Coodley G, Magnusson AR: Torsade de pointes after inhaled pentamidine. Ann Emerg Med 21:1403, 1992

62. Wharton JM, Demopulos PA, Goldschlager N: Torsades de pointes during administration of pentamidine isethionate. Am J Med 83:571, 1987

63. Cohen JR, Lackner R, Wenig P, Pillari G: Deep venous thrombosis in patients with AIDS. NY State J Med 90:159, 1990

64. Maliakkal R, Friedman SA. Sridhar S: Progressive pulmonary thromboembolism in association with HIV disease. NY State J Med 92:403, 1992

65. Stimmler MM, Quismorio FP Jr, McGehee WG, et al: Anticardiolipin antibodies in acquired immunodeficiency syndrome. Arch Intern Med 149:1833, 1989

66. Lafeuillade A, Alessi MC, Poizot-Martin I, et al: Protein S deficiency and HIV infection [letter]. N Engl J Med 324:1220, 1991

67. Miller KD, Jones E, Yanovaski JA, et al: Visceral abdominal-fat accumulation associated with use of indinavir. Lancet 351:871, 1995

68. Sullivan AK, Nelson MR: Marked hyperlipidemia on ritonavir therapy. AIDS 11:938, 1997

69. Carr A, Sanaras K, Burton S, et al: A syndrome of peripheral lipodystrophy (LD), hyperlipidemia, and insulin resistance due to HIV protease inhibitors (PIs). In: Program and Abstract of the 5th National Conference on Retroviruses and Opportunistic Infections, Chicago, 1998, Abstract 410

70. Eastone JA, Decker CF: New-onset diabetes mellitus associated with use of protease inhibitors. Ann Intern Med 127:948, 1997

71. Henry K, Melroe H, Heubsch J, et al: Severe premature coronary artery disease with protease inhibitors [research letter]. Lancet 351:1328, 1998

72. Henderson DK, Fahey BJ, Willy M, et al: Risk for occupational transmission of human immunodeficiency virus type I (HIV-1) associated with clinical exposures: A prospective evaluation. Ann Intern Med 113:740, 1990

73. Kardo DM, Culver DN, Ciesielski CA, et al: A case-controlled study of HIV seroconversion in health care workers after percutaneous exposure. N Engl J Med 337:1485, 1997

18 Endocrinologic Manifestations of HIV Infection

MORRIS SCHAMBELAN • DEBORAH E. SELLMEYER •
CARL GRUNFELD

Endocrine dysfunction can result from HIV infection, from its associated opportunistic infections and malignancies, or as a complication of drugs used in the treatment of these disorders. As in any severe illness, HIV infection and its complications can also be accompanied by changes in the rate of hormone secretion and/or clearance without overt clinical manifestations. In this chapter we attempt to distinguish those abnormalities of endocrine function that require further evaluation and possible treatment from those that merely represent the body's normal response to severe illness.

HYPOTHALAMIC–PITUITARY AXIS

Studies that have systematically evaluated pituitary functional reserve in patients with HIV infection (e.g., using gonadatropin- or thyrotropin-stimulating hormones) have generally not found evidence for anterior pituitary dysfunction.[1–3] These findings contrast with the relatively high incidence of pathologic findings at autopsy: In 49 patients with AIDS in whom the pituitary was specifically examined, direct infectious involvement was noted in six adenohypophyses (five by cytomegalovirus [CMV] and one by *Pneumocystis carinii*) and three neurohypophyses (two by CMV and one by *Toxoplasma gondii*).[4] A single patient has been described who had well-documented panhypopituitarism in association with cerebral toxoplasmosis; a large necrotic pituitary was noted

at autopsy, and toxoplasma was demonstrated in cerebral abscesses, although not in the pituitary per se.[5] Another patient with cerebral CMV infection developed hypopituitarism on a hypothalamic basis.[6]

Although attenuation of the normal circadian pattern of growth hormone (GH) secretion was noted when samples were obtained every 4 hours for a 24-hour period in HIV-infected adults,[7] no differences in peak number, amplitude, length, or interval were noted between asymptomatic HIV-infected patients, those with an AIDS-defining illness, and normal control subjects when more elaborate studies of GH secretion were done using samples obtained every 10 minutes for 24 hours.[8] Similarly, insulin-like growth factor I (IGF-I) as well as IGF-binding protein 3 levels did not differ between groups, leading these latter authors to conclude that the GH–IGF-I axis is normal in clinically stable adults with HIV infection.

Growth failure occurs in some children with HIV infection, but GH deficiency does not appear to be common. In three boys with hemophilia, HIV infection, and short stature, peak GH levels were normal but two had low IGF-I levels.[9] Similarly, GH response to glucagon stimulation was normal and IGF-I levels were subnormal in 14 HIV-positive children with failure to thrive.[10] However, another group found a subnormal IGF-I level only in one malnourished child, while eight others who were less ill had normal levels.[11] A fourth study reported no differences in IGF-I levels between control, asymptomatic HIV-positive, and symptomatic HIV-positive children; however, they found resistance to GH, IGF, and insulin stimulation of erythroid precursor colony formation in symptomatic HIV-infected children, suggesting a syndrome of hormone resistance.[12] A subnormal

This work was supported in part by grant R90SF211 from the Universitywide AIDS Research Program and by grants DK40990, DK45833, DK49448, and T32-DK07418 from the National Institutes of Health.

IGF-I level, in the face of an apparently normal GH level, is a common occurrence in malnutrition.[13] Thus growth failure in children with HIV infection may be due to malnutrition rather than hypothalamic–pituitary dysfunction.

In adults, low levels of IGF-I were found in malnourished patients with HIV infection.[14] In contrast, two cohorts of AIDS patients with significant previous weight loss had normal levels of IGF-I.[15,16] When these patients were given pharmacologic doses of GH, IGF-I levels were increased, although not quite to the same extent as in patients without HIV, suggesting GH resistance.

Three groups have found normal prolactin levels in patients with AIDS.[1,2,17] However, small but statistically significant[18] or moderate[19] elevations in prolactin levels have been noted in some patients with AIDS. Concomitant drug treatment (e.g., with opiates or phenothiazines) may have contributed to the hyperprolactinemia in some cases.[19] Whether the perturbation in prolactin levels could contribute to gonadal dysfunction (see below) has not been determined.

Hyponatremia occurs commonly in patients with AIDS: At the time of admission to the hospital, one third to one half of patients with AIDS have a low serum sodium level.[20–22] In one report, two thirds of the hyponatremic patients were judged to be euvolemic on the basis of clinical assessment and their serum sodium level remained subnormal despite saline administration.[20] In these patients, arginine vasopressin levels were noted to be inappropriately high for the serum osmolality, a finding that is compatible with a diagnosis of the syndrome of inappropriate antidiuretic hormone secretion (SIADH). However, since more than half of this group were being treated with trimethoprim, which could have impaired sodium conservation during saline replacement,[23] it is possible that pathogenetic mechanisms other than SIADH may have contributed to the hyponatremia.

ADRENAL

Adrenal pathology, particularly CMV infection, is found commonly in patients who have died from AIDS.[24–33] In at least one such postmortem study, the degree of CMV involvement correlated with the degree of adrenal necrosis.[33] In most reports, the estimated loss of functioning tissue was below the level required to produce adrenal insufficiency. However, two other case reports have appeared describing adrenal insufficiency in patients with CMV and very exten-

sive adrenalitis.[24,25] Other pathologic lesions that have been noted frequently include hemorrhage; infection with *Toxoplasma*, *Cryptococcus*, *Mycobacterium tuberculosis*, and *Mycobacterium avium* complex; and infiltration with Kaposi's sarcoma and lymphoma.[26,33]

Glucocorticoid Hormones

Although a few initial reports of adrenal insufficiency in patients with AIDS[34,35] implied an important clinical consequence for the frequently observed adrenal pathology, subsequent prospective studies in larger groups of patients indicate that glucocorticoid (cortisol) deficiency is relatively rare in this setting.[1–3,11,36–38] Perhaps this is not surprising in view of the functional reserve of this organ: It is generally thought that more than 90% of adrenal tissue must be destroyed before clinically significant cortisol deficiency occurs. In the most detailed examination of adrenal function in patients with HIV infection, Membreno et al.[37] noted that basal levels of cortisol, rather than being low, were actually significantly greater in hospitalized patients with AIDS than in normal control subjects and that only 4 patients out of 74 had impaired glucocorticoid secretion. Notably, among the patients with impaired glucocorticoid secretion, adrenocorticotropin (ACTH) levels were not elevated, suggesting an abnormality in the hypothalamic–pituitary axis rather than a primary adrenal lesion as the cause of their impaired glucocorticoid secretion. Another study reported similar increases in basal cortisol, but also ACTH levels, in 63 HIV-infected patients, 23 of whom had AIDS[38]; with one exception, these patients responded normally to stimulation with ACTH. Many other studies report normal[1,3,39] or elevated[36–38,40,41] basal cortisol levels.

Elevations in circulating levels of cortisol are seen frequently during severe illness, including infection.[42,43] These changes are likely due to cytokines, such as interleukin-1 (IL-1), interleukin-6 (IL-6), and tumor necrosis factor (TNF), that have been shown to directly stimulate both cortisol and ACTH secretion.[44] When cortisol secretion is increased under conditions of severe illness, the response to dynamic tests of adrenal functional reserve (using ACTH or insulin) may not be normal, yet such individuals may have normal adrenal function after recuperation.[45] Recovery from adrenal insufficiency induced by both meningococcus and blastomycosis has also been reported.[46,47]

Although clinically significant glucocorticoid deficiency is relatively infrequent, subtle abnormalities of adrenal biosynthesis may be quite common in patients with HIV infection. For example, plasma concentrations of the products of the 17-deoxysteroid pathway (corticosterone, deoxycorticosterone, and 18-OH-deoxycorticosterone) were substantially reduced in comparison to controls both before and after ACTH stimulation, whereas cortisol (17-hydroxy pathway) secretion was normal.[37] A diminished response of 17-deoxysteroids with normal cortisol levels was also noted in children with HIV infection who underwent acute stimulation with ACTH.[48] Because the 17-deoxysteroid products are probably not functionally important at normal plasma concentrations, these findings cannot be taken as evidence of clinically significant adrenal functional impairment. Whether this altered biosynthetic pattern could represent a harbinger of subsequent impaired adrenal capacity in patients with AIDS[37] or an adaptive mechanism that preserves cortisol secretion at the expense of reduced secretion of steroids that do not appear to have biologic significance remains to be determined.

The concept of shunting of adrenal biosynthetic products toward glucocorticoids was also suggested by Villette et al.,[49] who noted that levels of adrenal androgen were decreased while cortisol was increased in HIV-infected men undergoing studies of hormonal circadian variation. Because ACTH levels were significantly reduced in those patients, these authors further suggested that cortisol levels might be maintained by a nonpituitary factor. The finding of high cortisol levels with normal levels of ACTH may be due to the effects of a cytokine such as IL-1 or TNF, which directly stimulate cortisol production and could result in a secondary inhibition of ACTH secretion.[50] However, IL-1 and IL-6 may also affect the hypothalamic–pituitary axis by directly stimulating the release of corticotropin-releasing hormone by the hypothalamus or ACTH by pituitary cells.[51,52]

Several drugs that are used commonly in the treatment of patients with AIDS are known to alter adrenal function or steroid hormone metabolism. For example, ketoconazole inhibits cortisol synthesis[53] and could lead to adrenal insufficiency, particularly in patients with limited adrenal reserve. Rifampin enhances cortisol metabolism, which can result in adrenal insufficiency in patients with Addison's disease who are on maintenance glucocorticoid therapy,[54] and which could also produce adrenal failure in patients with limited adrenal reserve.[55] Megestrol acetate can reduce plasma cortisol levels, perhaps as a result of its intrinsic cortisol-like activity at the high doses (400 to 1200 mg/day) used to stimulate appetite.[56]

Even if relatively uncommon, the prevalence of glucocorticoid insufficiency in patients with AIDS is clearly greater than that in the general population, in which Addison's disease has been estimated to occur in 60 cases per million.[57] Patients with CMV retinitis or CMV antigenemia[58] may be at particular risk. It seems reasonable, therefore, to test adrenal function in those patients with AIDS who have symptoms or signs consistent with the diagnosis of adrenal insufficiency. Patients with low baseline cortisol levels who fail to respond to stimulation with ACTH clearly require glucocorticoid maintenance therapy. It is more difficult to propose the appropriate treatment for those individuals with the more common finding of a normal or high basal cortisol level with minimal or no further increase in response to acute ACTH stimulation,[59] since the majority of such individuals will have a normal cortisol response to 3 days of continuous ACTH stimulation.[37] These results suggest that patients with "borderline" stimulated cortisol values may not require routine glucocorticoid maintenance therapy. However, some clinicians would give glucocorticoids to such patients at times of stress, provided that treatment is limited in duration, so that the adverse effects of prolonged steroid therapy can be avoided.

Mineralocorticoid Hormones

Mineralocorticoid hormone deficiency results in renal sodium wasting, hypotension, hyperkalemia, metabolic acidosis, and elevated levels of plasma renin activity. Despite the frequency of hyponatremia and hyperkalemia in patients with AIDS, specific studies of mineralocorticoid hormone secretion and of the functional integrity of the renin–angiotensin system in such patients are quite limited. One patient who presented with hyponatremia, hyperkalemia, and normal cortisol levels may have had an isolated deficiency of aldosterone secretion, because aldosterone levels were low normal despite hyperreninemia.[60] His cortisol reserve appeared to be subnormal in response to ACTH stimulation, however, and the apparent benefit of treatment with a mineralocorticoid (fludrocortisone) may have been due in part to concomitant administration of a glucocorticoid (hydrocortisone). However, in a more systematic study, no abnormalities in circulating renin or aldosterone levels were noted in 63 HIV-infected patients, 23 of whom had AIDS.[38] Similarly, no abnormalities in aldosterone or renin levels were reported in 74 patients with AIDS and 19 with AIDS-related complex who underwent an extensive evaluation of adrenal function, including direct stimulation of aldosterone secretion by the angiotensin peptide des-asp$_1$-angiotensin II.[37]

The finding of low renin and aldosterone values that failed to increase normally in response to intravenously administered furosemide and assumption of an upright posture suggested the diagnosis of so-called hyporeninemic hypoaldosteronism in four patients with AIDS and unexplained hyperkalemia.[61] It should be noted, however, that these patients were taking trimethoprim-sulfamethoxazole at the time they were studied. Sulfonamides can cause interstitial nephritis,[62] a disorder associated with hyporeninemic hypoaldosteronism.[63] Alternatively, abnormalities of potassium homeostasis in patients taking trimethoprim-sulfamethoxazole may be due to the trimethoprim, which, in the large doses frequently employed in the treatment of *P. carinii* pneumonia, can block amiloride-sensitive luminal sodium channels and secondarily limit potassium secretion in distal nephron segments.[23] Transient hyperkalemia has also been reported to occur during treatment with pentamidine, a finding that was reversed on discontinuation of the agent and that was attributed to nephrotoxicity.[64]

THYROID

Autopsy series in patients dying of AIDS have reported both opportunistic infections and AIDS-related neoplasms in the thyroid gland. The relationship between these lesions and clinical abnormalities is not clear, because CMV inclusion bodies have been found in the thyroid even in the absence of significant thyroid dysfunction.[65] Inflammatory thyroiditis caused by *P. carinii* has been reported in at least 12 patients.[66-74] Seven patients had hypothyroidism, three had hyperthyroidism, and one had normal thyroid function. Antibodies were negative when tested, and thyroid gland visualization with radionucleotide scanning was decreased. Treatment of pneumocystis reversed hyperthyroidism in two patients. Invasion of the thyroid with Kaposi's sarcoma[32,75,76] has been reported; in one case, destruction of the thyroid by Kaposi's sarcoma with resulting primary hypothyroidism has been described.[76] The thyroid can also be infected during disseminated fungal

infections such as *Cryptococcus neoformans* and *Aspergillus fumigatus*.[77,78]

It is important to distinguish between abnormalities of thyroid function that are secondary to destruction of the thyroid or pituitary and those that are the result of severe illness. With thyroid/pituitary destruction, levels of thyroxine (T$_4$) decrease dramatically, while triiodothyronine (T$_3$) levels may be low or in the low normal range. With thyroidal destruction, thyroid-stimulating hormone (TSH) levels increase dramatically, whereas with pituitary disruption, TSH levels may be low or low normal. During severe systemic nonthyroidal illness, the conversion of T$_4$ to T$_3$ is impaired, resulting in decreased circulating levels of T$_3$ and variable levels of T$_4$. These changes are usually accompanied by increases in reverse T$_3$ (rT$_3$) levels. A variable but usually small increase in TSH levels may occur during the recovery from nonthyroidal illness. Such changes in thyroid hormone homeostasis are commonly referred to as the "euthyroid-sick syndrome."[79,80] Experiments studying caloric deprivation, which is accompanied by a decrease in T$_3$, demonstrate that replacement therapy with T$_3$ accelerates negative nitrogen balance.[81,82] As a consequence, it is thought that decreases in T$_3$ during severe illness limit both protein catabolism and energy expenditure.[79,80]

Patients with AIDS show abnormalities of thyroid function tests that are similar in many respects to those in other acute and chronic illnesses; however, true hypothyroidism is rare. There are many studies of thyroid hormone levels in patients with AIDS but, whereas some studies have found decreased T$_3$ levels, others have not.[1-3,83-88] As a consequence, the question has been raised as to whether the failure to decrease T$_3$ in AIDS is inappropriate and could therefore contribute to weight loss and/or negative nitrogen balance.[87] Review of these studies indicates that, in the presence of severe illness, patients with AIDS show the appropriate decrease in serum T$_3$ levels.[84] For example, those patients who have active weight loss show decreased T$_3$ levels, whereas patients with stable weight have higher levels and show significantly decreased rT$_3$ levels.[84] Many of these patients with decreased T$_3$ levels have acute secondary infection. Indeed, when patients with *P. carinii* pneumonia and other infections are studied, serum T$_3$ levels are consistently depressed.[83,84,86-88] Serum T$_3$ levels serve as a marker for the severity of illness; patients who die during admissions for those illnesses have a higher prevalence of low T$_3$ levels.[2,87,88]

Some changes in thyroid hormone homeostasis occur in AIDS that are not commonly found in the euthyroid-sick syndrome. The clinical importance of these changes is not yet understood, but they may influence interpretation of thyroid function. For example, the serum protein that binds thyroid hormone, thyroid-binding globulin (TBG), is increased early in the course of HIV infection and AIDS.[84,86,87,89–91] As a consequence, total T_3 levels may underestimate the decrease in free (or active) T_3 levels. In contrast, during severe nonthyroid illness TBG can be decreased.

In patients with AIDS, particularly in the absence of secondary infection, TSH levels are elevated and TSH secretion in response to thyroid-releasing hormone is exaggerated.[10,84,90,91] Thus patients with AIDS who are not infected and whose weight is stable may have a compensated hypothyroid state. In contrast, TSH is not elevated during the acute course of most other nonthyroidal illnesses, although there are some exceptions.[79,80]

Levels of rT_3 consistently decrease early in the course of HIV infection and AIDS even in the absence of decreased T_3 levels.[84,86,87] In contrast, during other nonthyroidal illnesses, serum rT_3 levels usually increase when conversion of T_4 to T_3 is decreased. Severely ill patients with AIDS, particularly those who are terminal, may show such increases in rT_3.[87] The functional significance of rT_3 is unknown.

Rifampin increases thyroid clearance by inducing hepatic microsomal enzymes similar to the effects on hepatic steroid metabolism. As a consequence, patients on L-thyroxine replacement treated with rifampin may require higher doses, and rifampin may precipitate hypothyroidism in patients with limited pituitary or thyroid reserve.[92]

GONADS

Testicular atrophy and infections are frequent findings in patients with AIDS. In men with AIDS in whom testes were examined at autopsy, marked decrease in spermatogenesis, thickening of the tunica propria, mild to moderate interstitial infiltrate, and/or fibrosis have been reported.[93–95] Opportunistic infections, predominantly CMV, have been noted in 25% to 31% of testes examined in the larger series reported.[93,95] Expression of HIV protein is found in the interstitium of the testes, as well as in lymphocytes in the seminiferous tubules.[95,96] Furthermore, HIV RNA can be found in testicular spermatogonia by in situ polymerase chain reaction hybridization.[97]

Although it is difficult to interpret the functional significance of decreased testicular volume and spermatogenesis in autopsy specimens, symptomatic hypogonadism clearly occurs in patients with HIV infection.[1,3,19,41,49,98,99] Dobs et al.[1] found that 28 of 42 patients with AIDS had decreased libido and 14 were impotent. Free testosterone levels were subnormal in 45% of the patients with AIDS yet, in the majority, luteinizing hormone (LH) and follicle-stimulating hormone (FSH) levels were not elevated and the response to stimulation with gonadotropin-releasing hormone was normal in all but one. These findings and similar results by Raffi et al.[3] suggest that the hypogonadism is due to a functional disorder of the hypothalamus. Croxson et al.,[19] who also found lower total testosterone levels in patients with AIDS, did not observe inappropriately low LH or FSH values, implying primary testicular failure rather than hypogonadotrophic hypogonadism in their patients. The discrepancy in these findings may be explained in part by the absence, within their population, of intravenous drug abusers, who were included in the patient population studied by Dobs et al.[1] Opiate abuse per se is known to cause hypogonadotropic hypogonadism.[100]

Drugs that are used commonly in the treatment of patients with AIDS may affect gonadal function. Ketoconazole is associated with decreased levels of total and free testosterone leading to oligospermia, azospermia, and gynecomastia.[53] Chemotherapy for lymphoma also commonly results in infertility.

In summary, men with AIDS tend to have an increased incidence of impotence and low testosterone levels. In women with advanced AIDS, particularly in those with severe wasting, ovarian failure, manifested clinically by amenorrhea, is commonly noted.[101]

Menstrual irregularities are considerably less frequent in patients with earlier stages of infection.[102] Estradiol levels are lower in amenorrheic than eumenorrheic women, but estradiol levels do not correlate with body composition.[103] Interestingly, women with wasting have decreased levels of free testosterone and dehydroepiandrosterone sulfate that do correlate with decreased muscle mass, suggesting that androgen deficiency may contribute to the loss of lean tissue in this population.[103]

PANCREAS

When the euglycemic hyperinsulinemic clamp technique was used, patients with clinically stable HIV infection demonstrated similar rates of glucose uptake despite lower steady-state insulin concentrations and increased rates of insulin clearance, as compared with HIV-negative controls.[104] These results suggest that HIV infection is associated with increased insulin sensitivity, unlike other infectious states that generally lead to insulin resistance.[105] Furthermore, the observed increase in insulin sensitivity reflects the true effect of insulin on peripheral glucose uptake and not merely changes in non-insulin-mediated glucose uptake.[106]

In contrast to these results, there have been several recent reports of hyperglycemia in patients receiving protease inhibitors, suggesting that these agents may adversely affect glucose regulation.[107–109] Hyperglycemia has been reported with all of the currently available protease inhibitors (indinavir, ritonavir, saquinavir, nelfinavir), and typically occurs within 8 months of initiating therapy. Presentations range from mild diet-controlled diabetes to severe hyperglycemia requiring insulin therapy, but ketoacidosis is uncommon. Although a clear causal relationship with protease inhibitor therapy has not yet been established, available data support the postulated mechanism of acquired insulin resistance.[110]

When administered intravenously in the large doses employed in the treatment of *P. carinii* infections, pentamidine commonly causes pancreatic β-cell toxicity, resulting in acute hypoglycemia caused by increased insulin secretion. If the injury to the β-cell is of sufficient magnitude, the hypoglycemic phase may be followed by β-cell death and the development of diabetes mellitus.[111–114] Both hypoglycemia and diabetes mellitus may also occur during treatment with inhaled pentamidine.[115,116]

Megestrol acetate is used widely as an appetite stimulant in the treatment of anorexia and cachexia in AIDS. It has recently been reported that the drug can induce diabetes mellitus,[117] although the prevalence of hyperglycemia in controlled trials is low and may not exceed that seen in the placebo group. Whether this side effect is secondary to increased caloric intake or another effect of the drug (such as its intrinsic cortisol-like activity) is not yet known.

MINERAL HOMEOSTASIS

Foscarnet, which is used in the treatment of refractory CMV retinitis and mucocutaneous herpes simplex virus infections, has been reported to cause hypocalcemia, possibly by forming a complex with ionized calcium.[118] The hypocalcemia can result in potentially serious clinical sequelae. Fatal hypocalcemia has been reported when foscarnet was given together with parenteral pentamidine.[119] Hypomagnesemia, hyperphosphatemia, and hypokalemia can also occur with foscarnet treatment,[120] as can nephrogenic diabetes insipidus.[121]

Hypercalcemia has been reported in patients with both AIDS- and non-AIDS-associated lymphoma[122] as well as in one patient with *P. carinii* pneumonia.[123] In both of these settings hypercalcemia was associated with increased levels of 1,25-dihydroxyvitamin D.

LIPID METABOLISM

Plasma cholesterol levels decrease early in the course of HIV infection, a finding that is sustained through the development of AIDS.[124–127] High-density lipoprotein levels appear to decrease first and remain at the same level. Low-density lipoprotein (LDL) levels progressively decrease but, in the later stages of AIDS, very-low-density lipoprotein cholesterol levels increase slightly. The LDL particles are abnormally dense.[128] The causes of hypocholesterolemia have not yet been defined. In particular, the role of gastrointestinal disturbances and malabsorption is unknown.

With progression from asymptomatic HIV infection to AIDS, plasma triglyceride levels increase.[125,127,129,130] In Centers for Disease Control and Prevention (CDC) stage IV AIDS, triglycerides average twice normal. However, a subset of patients may have higher plasma triglyceride levels (>500 mg/dl), which puts them at risk for triglyceride-induced pancreatitis. The latter syndrome is of particular concern in patients taking antiretroviral therapy that also predisposes to pancreatitis (i.e., didanosine and zalcitabine). Patients with the higher levels of triglycerides may have underlying genetic defects in addition to the abnormalities induced by HIV infection. However, antiretroviral therapy of previously untreated patients with AIDS lowers both interferon-α and triglyceride levels.[130]

Several changes in triglyceride metabolism have been reported in AIDS that contribute to hypertriglyceridemia. First, lipoprotein lipase, the enzyme responsible for triglyceride clearance, is decreased.[125] The actual clearance of triglycerides is even more dramatically slowed.[125] Finally, the hepatic synthesis of fatty acids from other substrates is increased in patients with

HIV infection and AIDS, with consequent increase in newly synthesized fatty acids in the circulation.[131]

The increase in plasma triglyceride levels is highly correlated with circulating levels of interferon-α, a cytokine that appears in circulation with the onset of CDC stage IV AIDS.[125] An even stronger correlation is found between interferon-α levels and both the decreases in triglyceride clearance and the increase in fasting levels of newly synthesized fatty acids.[125,131]

Recently, some patients receiving protease inhibitor therapy, particularly those on ritonavir,[132] have developed striking elevations in plasma triglyceride levels. Increases in LDL cholesterol have also been noted, raising the possibility that such patients may be at increased risk for atherogenic complications.

THE WASTING SYNDROME IN AIDS

A variety of metabolic disturbances have been described in AIDS that could theoretically contribute to the wasting syndrome. However, recent studies indicate that such metabolic disturbances alone cannot account for the wasting syndrome. For example, an early theory linked weight loss to abnormalities in triglyceride metabolism. However, there is no correlation between the presence of hypertriglyceridemia and wasting in AIDS.[129] AIDS patients with elevated triglyceride levels frequently maintain body weight for extended periods of time.[125]

Increased resting energy expenditure (REE) is a common indication of hypermetabolism, a phenomenon that occurs in patients with sepsis and burns and was thought to cause the wasting syndrome (for review, see the paper by Grunfeld and Feingold[133]). It was therefore of interest to find striking elevations in REE in patients with HIV infection and AIDS.[16,85,133–137] REE increases very early in HIV infection even before CD4 cell counts drop,[135] presumably reflecting the host response to the virus; these findings suggest that HIV is not latent but rather contained. REE increases further with the development of AIDS, but such increases may reflect the presence of secondary infections.[134,136] Surprisingly, there was no correlation between the increase seen in REE and weight loss.[85,134]

In contrast, studies on the mechanism of wasting suggested that patients with AIDS who have active secondary infections universally show rapid weight loss, averaging 5% of body weight in 4 weeks.[134] Such patients have striking decreases in caloric intake that correlate with weight loss.[134,138] However, it should be pointed out that patients with AIDS and secondary infection maintain a high REE in the face of decreased caloric intake. These findings should be contrasted to those in non-HIV-infected patients who develop compensatory decreases in REE that limit weight loss during decreased caloric intake.[133] Patients with rapid weight loss have decreased total energy expenditure (TEE), and hence in a sense are hypometabolic, but their decrease in caloric intake leaves them with a large relative energy deficit.[138] Thus, the rapid weight loss seen in AIDS with secondary infection is a product of a failed homeostatic mechanism and is a function of both decreased food intake and increased REE.

Prospective studies have confirmed that rapid weight loss is a harbinger of infection. Rapid weight loss episodes (>4 kg in <4 months) were accompanied by secondary infection 82% of the time.[139] When patients with slower weight loss (>4 kg in >4 months) were analyzed, 65% had gastrointestinal disease. Patients with slow weight loss may also have elevated REE, slightly lower TEE, and reduced caloric intake.[138] On the basis of these studies, it is strongly recommended that the weight for each patient with HIV infection and AIDS be plotted on a graph in the patient's chart; weight loss should then prompt the clinician to look for appropriate causes.[140]

The first line of treatment for patients with AIDS and active weight loss is to find the underlying causes and treat them. However, recovery from weight loss is frequently only partial, resulting in long-term wasting.[139] As a consequence, direct therapies of the wasting syndrome are being sought. Two agents that stimulate appetite have been approved: dronabinol for AIDS-related anorexia, and megestrol acetate for AIDS-related weight loss. Megestrol acetate (at doses of 800 mg/day) leads to more weight gain, fewer significant side effects, and less dropout from therapy. Use of these agents should be considered in patients with significant weight loss (<90% of ideal body weight), especially in the presence of anorexia. However, both agents lead to increases in weight that primarily consist of fat. Other therapies are being studied for their ability to form lean body mass, particularly muscle; these include GH,[16] IGF-1,[15] and anabolic steroids. Recently, GH has been approved for the treatment of AIDS wasting.

SYNDROMES OF ABNORMAL FAT DISTRIBUTION

A number of abnormal body fat changes have been reported in HIV-infected patients on antiretroviral therapy, and concerns have been raised that these alterations may be therapy related. The syndromes that have been reported broadly relate to fat accumulation or loss: dorsocervical fat pad enlargement (buffalo hump), benign symmetrical lipomatosis, abdominal girth enlargement, breast hypertrophy, and lipodystrophy. Whether these changes are separate clinical entities or represent different manifestations of the same syndrome is not yet understood.

Of the more than 25 published cases of dorsocervical fat pad enlargement in patients with HIV infection,[141–145] approximately three fourths have occurred in patients receiving protease inhibitor therapy. However, clear examples of this syndrome have been reported in patients who have not received this therapy.[141] The current estimated prevalence of buffalo hump among patients treated with protease inhibitors is less than 2%.[143] Cushing's syndrome, which is classically associated with dorsocervical fat pad enlargement, has been excluded in all reported cases. Hypertriglyceridemia is also a common presenting sign in affected patients, and some have experienced increased neck size, neck fat deposition, abdominal enlargement, and fat loss in the extremities, suggesting that the body fat changes may be systemic in nature. Benign symmetrical lipomatosis, a related phenomenon, has also been observed in HIV-infected patients,[146] but, unlike buffalo hump, symmetrical lipomatosis has only been reported in patients taking protease inhibitors. These patients have a marked accumulation of subcutaneous fat in the neck and shoulder region, often accompanied by dorsocervical fat pad enlargement.

Increased abdominal girth (frequently referred to as *protease paunch* or *Crix belly*) has also been reported primarily, but not exclusively, in patients on protease inhibitor therapy.[142,145,147] Individuals with this syndrome generally complain of bloating and dyspepsia and, in some, loss of adipose tissue in their extremities. The cause of this syndrome is currently unclear, although computed tomography findings in men on indinavir therapy suggest that an increase in visceral adiposity accounts for the increased girth.[147] Women on protease inhibitor therapy have also experienced increases in abdominal girth, although they may be undergoing additional body habitus changes that are gender specific. Of note, many women on protease inhibitor therapy have developed breast enlargement, frequently in association with increased abdominal girth, weight gain, peripheral and gluteal wasting, and dorsocervical fat pad enlargement.[148] All of these observations in both men and women should be considered in light of recent data suggesting that the pattern of decreased peripheral and increased central fat redistribution was evident before the existence of combination antiretroviral or protease inhibitor therapy.[149]

Several recent reports of protease inhibitor–associated lipodystrophy occurring in patients with HIV infection have raised the possibility that these drugs may also promote regional fat loss.[110,150] Subcutaneous fat wasting in the face and/or extremities, with relative preservation of abdominal fat, has been observed in patients receiving indinavir, ritonavir, nelfinavir, or saquinavir.[110] These findings have been associated with insulin resistance and hypertriglyceridemia. However, the prevalence of lipodystrophy varies widely among patients receiving protease inhibitor therapy and may reflect the use of different diagnostic criteria or potential selection bias. Furthermore, a uniform case definition has yet to be established. The term *lipodystrophy* is, unfortunately, being used by many clinicians to describe fat accumulation features in HIV-infected patients. This has led to confusion in the medical community as well as divergence from historical case descriptions in seronegative individuals.[151]

References

1. Dobs AS, Dempsy MA, Ladenson PW, Polk F: Endocrine disorders in men infected with HIV. Am J Med 84:611, 1988
2. Merenich JA, McDermott MT, Asp AA, et al: Evidence of endocrine involvement early in the course of human immunodeficiency virus infection. J Clin Endocrinol Metab 70:566, 1990
3. Raffi F, Brisseau J-M, Plachon B, et al: Endocrine function in 98 HIV-infected patients: A prospective study. AIDS 5:729, 1991
4. Sano T, Kovacs K, Scheithauer BW, et al: Pituitary pathology in acquired immunodeficiency syndrome. Arch Pathol Lab Med 113:1066, 1989
5. Milligan SA, Katz MS, Craven PC, et al: Toxoplasmosis presenting as panhypopituitarism in a patient with AIDS. Am J Med 77:760, 1984
6. Sullivan WM, Kelley GG, O'Connor PG, et al: Hypopituitarism associated with a hypothalamic CMV infection in a patient with AIDS. Am J Med 92:221, 1992
7. Rondanelli M, Solerte SB, Fioravanti M, et al: Circadian secretory pattern of growth hormone, insulin-

like growth factor type I, cortisol, adrenocorticotropic hormone, thyroid-stimulating hormone, and prolactin during HIV infection. AIDS Res Hum Retroviruses 13:1243, 1997

8. Heijligenberg R, Sauerwein HP, Brabant G, et al: Circadian growth hormone secretion in asymptomatic human immune deficiency virus infection and acquired immunodeficiency syndrome. J Clin Endocrinol Metab 81:4028, 1996

9. Kaufman FR, Gomperts ED: Growth failure in boys with hemophilia and HIV infection. Am J Pediatr Hematol Oncol 11:292, 1989

10. Schwartz LJ, St. Louis Y, Wu R, et al: Endocrine function in children with human immunodeficiency virus infection. Am J Dis Child 145:330, 1991

11. Laue L, Pizzo PA, Butler K, Cutler GB: Growth and neuroendocrine dysfunction in children with AIDS. J Pediatr 117:541, 1990

12. Geffner ME, Yeh DY, Landaw EM, et al: In vitro insulin-like growth factor-1, growth hormone, and insulin resistance in symptomatic human immunodeficiency virus infected children. Pediatr Res 34:66, 1993

13. Hintz RL, Suskind R, Amatayakul K, et al: Plasma somatomedin and growth hormone values in children with protein-calorie malnutrition. J Pediatr 92:153, 1978

14. Salbe AD, Kotler DP, Wang J, et al: Predictive value of IGF1 concentration in HIV-infected patients. Clin Res 39:385A, 1991

15. Lieberman SA, Buttefield GE, Harrison D, Hoffman AR: Anabolic effects of recombinant insulin-like growth factor-I in cachectic patients with the acquired immunodeficiency syndrome. J Clin Endocrinol Metab 78:404, 1994

16. Mulligan K, Grunfeld C, Hellerstein MK, et al: Anabolic effects of recombinant human growth hormone in patients with wasting associated with human immunodeficiency virus infection. J Clin Endocrinol Metab 77:956, 1993

17. Gorman JM, Warne PA, Begg MD, et al: Serum prolactin levels in homosexual men and bisexual men with HIV infection. Am J Psychiatry 149:367, 1992

18. Graef AS, Gonzalez SS, Baca VR, et al: High serum prolactin levels in asymptomatic HIV-infected patients and in patients with acquired immunodeficiency syndrome. Clin Immunol Immunopathol 72:390, 1994

19. Croxson TS, Chapman WE, Miller LK, et al: Changes in the hypothalamic-pituitary-gonadal axis in human immunodeficiency virus infected homosexual men. J Clin Endocrinol Metab 68:317, 1989

20. Agarwal A, Soni A, Ciechanowsky M, et al: Hyponatremia in patients with acquired immunodeficiency syndrome. Nephron 53:317, 1989

21. Cusano AJ, Thies HL, Siegal FP, et al: Hyponatremia in patients with acquired immunodeficiency syndrome. J Acquir Immune Defic Syndr 3:949, 1990

22. Tang WW, Kaptein EM, Feinstein EI, Massry SG: Hyponatremia in hospitalized patients with the acquired immunodeficiency syndrome (AIDS) and the AIDS-related complex. Am J Med 94:169, 1993

23. Choi MJ, Fernandez PC, Patnaik A, et al: Brief report: Trimethoprim-induced hyperkalemia in a patient with AIDS. N Engl J Med 328:703, 1993

24. Angulo JC, Lopez JI, Flores N: Lethal cytomegalovirus adrenalitis in a case of AIDS. Scand J Urol Nephrol 28:105, 1994

25. Bleiweis IJ, Pervez NK, Hammer GS, et al: Cytomegalovirus-induced adrenal insufficiency and asso-

ciated renal cell carcinoma in AIDS. Mt Sinai J Med 53:676, 1986

26. Bricaire F, Marche C, Zoubi D, et al: Adrenocortical lesions and AIDS. Lancet 1:881, 1988

27. Drew WL: Cytomegalovirus infection in patients with AIDS. J Infect Dis 158:449, 1988

28. Klatt EC, Shibata D: Cytomegalovirus infection in the acquired immunodeficiency syndrome. Arch Pathol Lab Med 112:540, 1988

29. Laulund S, Visfeldt J, Klunken L: Patho-anatomical studies of patients dying of AIDS. Acta Pathol Microbiol Immunol Scand 94:201, 1986

30. Pillay D, Lipman MCI, Lee CA, et al: A clinico-pathological audit of opportunistic viral infections in HIV-infected patients. AIDS 7:969, 1993

31. Pulakhandam U, Dincsoy HP: Cytomegaloviral adrenalitis and insufficiency in AIDS. Am J Clin Pathol 93:651, 1990

32. Welch K, Finkbeiner W, Alpers CE, et al: Autopsy findings in the acquired immune deficiency syndrome. JAMA 252:1152, 1984

33. Glasgow BJ, Steinsapir KD, Anders K, Layfield LJ: Adrenal pathology in AIDS. Am J Clin Pathol 84:594, 1985

34. Greene LW, Cole W, Greene JB, et al: Adrenal insufficiency as a complication of AIDS. Ann Intern Med 101:497, 1984

35. Guenther EE, Rabinowe SL, Van Niel A, et al: Primary Addison's disease in a patient with AIDS. Ann Intern Med 100:847, 1984

36. Hilton CW, Harrington PT, Prasad C, Svec F: Adrenal insufficiency in AIDS. South Med J 81:1493, 1988

37. Membreno L, Irony I, Dere W, et al: Adrenocortical function in AIDS. J Clin Endocrinol Metab 65:482, 1987

38. Verges B, Chavanet P, Desgres J, et al: Adrenal function in HIV infected patients. Acta Endocrinol 121:633, 1989

39. Findling JW, Buggy BP, Gilson IH, et al: Longitudinal evaluation of adrenocortical function in patients infected with the human immunodeficiency virus. J Clin Endocrinol Metab 79:1091, 1994

40. Biglino A, Limone P, Forno B, et al: Altered adrenocorticotropin and cortisol response to corticotropin-releasing hormone in HIV-1 infection. Eur J Endocrinol 133:173, 1995

41. Christeff N, Gharakhanian S, Thoble N, et al: Evidence for changes in adrenal and testicular steroids during HIV infection. J Acquir Immune Defic Syndr 5:841, 1992

42. Beisel WR: Metabolic response to infection. In Sanford JB, Luby JP (eds): The Science and Practice of Clinical Medicine. New York, Grune & Stratton, 1981

43. Edgehl RH, Meguid MM, Aun F: The importance of the endocrine and metabolic responses to shock and trauma. Crit Care Med 5:257, 1977

44. Grunfeld C, Feingold KR: The metabolic effects of tumor necrosis factor and other cytokines. Biotherapy 3:148, 1991

45. Sibbald WJ, Short A, Cohen MP, Wilson RF: Variations in adrenocortical responsiveness during severe bacterial infections. Ann Surg 186:29, 1977

46. Bosworth DC: Reversible adrenocortical insufficiency in fulminant meningococcemia. Arch Intern Med 139:823, 1979

47. Osa SR, Peterson RE, Roberts RB: Recovery of adrenal reserve following treatment of disseminated South American blastomycosis. Am J Med 71:298, 1981

48. Oberfield SE, Kairam R, Bakshi S, et al: Steroid response to adrenocorticotropin stimulation in children with human immunodeficiency virus infection. J Clin Endocrinol Metab 70:578, 1990

49. Villette JM, Bourin P, Doinel C, et al: Circadian variations in plasma levels of hypophyseal, adrenocortical and testicular hormones in men infected with human immunodeficiency virus. J Clin Endocrinol Metab 70:572, 1990

50. Darling G, Goldstein DS, Stull R, et al: Tumor necrosis factor: Immune endocrine interaction. Surgery 106:1155, 1989

51. Sapolsky R, Rivier C, Yamamoto G, et al: Interleukin-1 stimulates the secretion of hypothalamic corticotropin releasing factor. Science 238:522, 1987

52. Woloski BMRNJ, Smith EM, Meyer WJ III, et al: Corticotropin-releasing activity of monokines. Science 230:1035, 1985

53. Pont A, Graybill JR, Craven PC, et al: High dose ketoconazole therapy and adrenal and testicular function in humans. Arch Intern Med 144:2150, 1984

54. Kyriazopoulou V, Parparousi O, Vagenakis AG: Rifampicin-induced adrenal crisis in addisonian patients receiving corticosteroid replacement therapy. J Clin Endocrinol Metab 59:1204, 1984

55. Ediger SK, Isley WL: Rifampicin-induced adrenal insufficiency in the acquired immunodeficiency syndrome: Difficulties in diagnosis and treatment. Postgrad Med J 64:405, 1988

56. Loprinzi CL, Jensen MD, Jiang N-S, Schaid DJ: Effect of megestrol acetate on the human pituitary-adrenal axis. Mayo Clin Proc 67:1160, 1992

57. Nerup J: Addison's disease — a review of some clinical, pathological and immunological features. Dan Med Bull 21:201, 1974

58. Hoshino Y, Nagata Y, Gatanaga H, et al: Cytomegalovirus (CMV) retinitis and CMV antigenemia as a clue to impaired adrenocortical function in patients with AIDS. AIDS 11:1719, 1997

59. May ME, Carey RM: Rapid adrenocorticotropic hormone test in practice. Am J Med 79:679, 1985

60. Guy RJC, Turberg Y, Davidson RN, et al: Mineralocorticoid deficiency in HIV infection. BMJ 298:496, 1989

61. Kalin MF, Poretsky L, Seres DS, Zumoff B: Hyporeninemic hypoaldosteronism associated with AIDS. Am J Med 82:1035, 1987

62. Appel GB, Neu HC: The nephrotoxicity of antimicrobial agents (third of three parts). N Engl J Med 296:784, 1977

63. Schambelan M, Sebastian A, Biglieri EG: Prevalance, pathogenesis, and functional significance of aldosterone deficiency in hyperkalemic patients with chronic renal insufficiency. Kidney Int 17:89, 1980

64. Lachaal M, Venuto RC: Nephrotoxicity and hyperkalemia in patients with acquired immunodeficiency syndrome treated with pentamidine. Am J Med 87:260, 1989

65. Frank TS, Livolsi VA, Connor AM: Cytomegalovirus infection of the thyroid in immunocompromised adults. Yale J Biol Med 60:1, 1987

66. Battan R, Mariuz P, Raviglione MC, et al: *Pneumocystis carinii* infection of the thyroid in a hypothyroid patient with AIDS: Diagnosis by fine needle aspiration biopsy. J Clin Endocrinol Metab 72:724, 1991

67. Drucker D, Bailey D, Rotstein L: Thyroiditis as the presenting manifestation of disseminated extrapulmonary *Pneumocystis carinii* infection. J Clin Endocrinol Metab 71:1663, 1990

68. Gallant JE, Enriquez RE, Cohen KL, Hammers LW: *Pneumocystis carinii* thyroiditis. Am J Med 84:303, 1988

69. Guttler R, Singer P: *Pneumocystis carinii* thyroiditis: Case report and review of the literature. Arch Intern Med 153:393, 1993

70. McCarthy M, Coker R, Claydon E: Case report: Disseminated *Pneumocystis carinii* infection in a patient with the acquired immunodeficiency syndrome causing thyroid gland calcification and hypothyroidism. Clin Radiol 45:209, 1992

71. Patel A, Snowden D, Kemp R, et al: Pneumocystis thyroiditis. Med J Aust 156:136, 1992

72. Ragni MV, Dekker A, De Rubertis FR, et al: *Pneumocystis carinii* infection presenting as necrotizing thyroiditis and hypothyroidism. Am J Clin Pathol 95:489, 1991

73. Spitzer RD, Chan JC, Marks JB, et al: Case report: Hypothyroidism due to *Pneumocystis carinii* thyroiditis in a patient with acquired immunodeficiency syndrome. Am J Med Sci 302:98, 1991

74. Vijayakumar V, Bekerman C, Blend MJ, et al: Role of Ga-67 citrate in imaging extrapulmonary pneumocystis in HIV positive patients. Clin Nucl Med 18:337, 1993

75. Krauth PH, Katz JF: Kaposi's sarcoma involving the thyroid in a patient with AIDS. Clin Nucl Med 12:848, 1987

76. Mollison LC, Mijch A, McBride G, Dwyer B: Hypothyroidism due to destruction of the thyroid by Kaposi's sarcoma. Rev Infect Dis 13:826, 1991

77. Mahac J, Mejatheim M, Goldsmith SJ: Gallium-67 citrate uptake in cryptococcal thyroiditis in a homosexual male. J Nucl Med Allied Sci 29:283, 1985

78. Martinez-Ocana JC, Romen J, Llatjos M, et al: Goiter as a manifestation of disseminated aspergillosis in a patient with AIDS. Clin Infect Dis 17:953, 1993

79. Cavalieri RR: The effects of nonthyroid disease and drugs on thyroid function tests. Med Clin North Am 75:27, 1991

80. Wartofsky L, Burman KD: Alterations in thyroid function in patients with systemic illness: The "euthyroid sick syndrome." Endocr Rev 3:164, 1982

81. Burman KD, Wartofsky L, Dinterman RE, et al: The effect of T3 and reverse T3 administration on muscle protein catabolism during fasting as measured by 3-methylhistidine excretion. Metabolism 8:805, 1979

82. Gardner DF, Kaplan MM, Stanley CA, Utiger RD: Effect of triiodothyronine replacement on the metabolic and pituitary response to starvation. N Engl J Med 300:579, 1979

83. Fried JC, LoPresti JS, Micon M, et al: Serum triiodothyronine values: Prognostic indicators of acute mortality due to *Pneumocystis carinii* pneumonia associated with the acquired immunodeficiency syndrome. Arch Intern Med 150:406, 1990

84. Grunfeld C, Pang M, Doerrler W, et al: Indices of thyroid function and weight loss in human immunodeficiency virus infection and the acquired immunodeficiency syndrome. Metabolism 42:1270, 1993

85. Hommes MJT, Romijn JA, Godfried MH, et al: Increased resting energy expenditure in HIV-infected men. Metabolism 39:1186, 1990

86. Lambert M, Zech F, De Mayer P, et al: Elevation of serum thyroxine-binding globulin (but not of cortisol-binding globulin and sex hormone-binding globulin) associated with the progression of human immunodeficiency virus infection. Am J Med 89:748, 1990

87. Lopresti JS, Fried JC, Spencer CA, Nicolof JT: Unique alterations of thyroid hormone indices in AIDS. Ann Intern Med 110:970, 1989

88. Tang WW, Kaptein EM: Thyroid hormone levels in AIDS or ARC. West J Med 151:627, 1989

89. Bourdoux PR, DeWitt SA, Servais GM, et al: Biochemical thyroid profile in patients infected with the human immunodeficiency virus. Thyroid 1:147, 1991

90. Hommes MJT, Romijn J, Endert E, et al: Hypothyroid-like regulation of the pituitary-thyroid axis in stable human immunodeficiency virus infection. Metabolism 42:556, 1993

91. Olivieri A, Sorcini M, Fazzini C, et al: Thyroid hypofunction related with the progression of human immunodeficiency virus infection. J Endocrinol Invest 16:407, 1993

92. Isley WL: Effect of rifampin therapy on the thyroid function tests in a hypothyroid patient on replacement L-thyroxine. Ann Intern Med 107:517, 1987

93. Chabon AB, Stenger RJ, Grabstald H: Histopathology of testis in acquired immunodeficiency syndrome. Urology 29:658, 1987

94. Da Silva M, Schevchuk MM, Cronin WJ, et al: Detection of HIV-related protein in testes and prostates of patients with AIDS. Am J Clin Pathol 93:196, 1990

95. De Paepe ME, Waxman M: Testicular atrophy in AIDS: A study of 57 autopsy cases. Hum Pathol 20: 210, 1989

96. Pudney J, Anderson D: Orchitis and human immunodeficiency virus type 1 infected cells in reproductive tissues from men with the acquired immunodeficiency syndrome. Am J Pathol 139:149, 1991

97. Nuovo GJ, Becker J, Simsir A, et al: HIV-1 nucleic acids localize to the spermatogonia and their progeny: A study by polymerase chain reaction in situ hybridization. Am J Pathol 144:1142, 1994

98. Lefrere JJ, Laplance JL, Vittecoq D, et al: Hypogonadism in AIDS. AIDS 2:135, 1988

99. Wagner G, Rabkin JG, Rabkin R: Illness stage, concurrent medications, and other correlates of low testosterone in men with HIV illness. J Acquir Immune Defic Syndr Hum Retrovirol 8:204, 1995

100. Smith CG, Asch RH: Drug abuse and reproduction. Fertil Steril 48:355, 1987

101. Widy-Wirski R, Berkely S, Downing R, et al: Evaluation of the WHO clinical case definition of AIDS in Uganda. JAMA 260:3186, 1985

102. Shah PN, Smith JR, Wells C, et al: Menstrual symptoms in women infected by the human immunodeficiency virus. Obstet Gynecol 83:397, 1994

103. Grinspoon S, Corcoran C, Miller K, et al: Body composition and endocrine function in women with acquired immunodeficiency syndrome wasting. J Clin Endocrinol Metab 82:1332, 1997

104. Hommes MJT, Romijn JA, Endert E, et al: Insulin sensitivity and insulin clearance in human immunodeficiency virus-infected men. Metabolism 40:651, 1991

105. Yki-Jarvinen H, Sammalkorpi K, Koivisto VA, et al: Severity, duration, and mechanisms of insulin resistance during acute infections. J Clin Endocrinol Metab 69:317, 1989

106. Heyligenberg R, Romijn JA, Hommes MJT, et al: Non-insulin-mediated glucose uptake in human immunodeficiency virus-infected men. Clin Sci 84:209, 1993

107. Dube MP, Johnson DL, Currier JS, et al: Protease inhibitor-associated hyperglycaemia. Lancet 350:713, 1997

108. Eastone JA, Decker CF: New-onset diabetes mellitus associated with use of protease inhibitor. Ann Intern Med 127:948, 1997

109. Visnegarwala F, Krause KL, Musher DM: Severe diabetes associated with protease inhibitor therapy. Ann Intern Med 127:947, 1997

110. Carr A, Samaras K, Burton S, et al: A syndrome of peripheral lipodystrophy, hyperlipidaemia and insulin resistance in patients receiving HIV protease inhibitors. AIDS 12:F51, 1998

111. Bouchard PH, Sal P, Reach G, et al: Diabetes mellitus following pentamidine induced hypoglycemia in humans. Diabetes 31:40, 1982

112. Osei K, Falko JM, Nelson KP, Stephens R: Diabetogenic effect of pentamidine: In vitro and in vivo studies in a patient with malignant insulinoma. Am J Med 77:41, 1984

113. Stahl-Bayliss CM, Kalman CM, Laskin OL: Pentamidine induced hypoglycemia in patients with the acquired immunodeficiency syndrome. Clin Pharmacol Ther 39:271, 1986

114. Waskin H, Stehr-Green JK, Helmick CG, Sattler FR: Risk factors for hypoglycemia associated with pentamidine therapy for Pneumocystis pneumonia. JAMA 260:345, 1988

115. Chen JP, Braham RL, Squires KE: Diabetes after aerosolized pentamidine. Ann Intern Med 114:913, 1991

116. Karboski JA, Godley PJ: Inhaled pentamidine and hypoglycemia. Ann Intern Med 108:490, 1988

117. Henry K, Rathgaber S, Sullivan C, McCabe K: Diabetes mellitus induced by megestrol acetate in a patient with AIDS and cachexia. Ann Intern Med 116: 53, 1992

118. Jacobson MA, Gambertoglio JG, Aweeka FT, et al: Foscarnet-induced hypocalcaemia and effects of foscarnet on calcium metabolism. J Clin Endocrinol Metab 72:1130, 1991

119. Youle MS, Clarbour J, Gazzard B: Severe hypocalcaemia in AIDS patients treated with foscarnet and pentamidine. Lancet 1:1455, 1988

120. Gearhart MO, Sorg TB: Foscarnet-induced severe hypomagnesemia and other electrolyte disorders. Ann Pharmacother 27:285, 1993

121. Farese RV, Schambelan M, Hollander H, et al: Nephrogenic diabetes insipidus associated with foscarnet treatment of cytomegalovirus retinitis. Ann Intern Med 112:955, 1990

122. Adams JS, Fernandez M, Gacad MA, et al: Vitamin D metabolite-mediated hypercalcemia and hypercalciuria patients with AIDS and non-AIDS lymphoma. Blood 73:235, 1989

123. Ahmed B, Jaspan JB: Case report: Hypercalcemia in a patient with AIDS and Pneumocystis carinii pneumonia. Am J Med Sci 306:313, 1993

124. Constans J, Pellegrin JL, Peuchant E, et al: Plasma lipids in HIV-infected patients: A prospective study in 95 patients. Eur J Clin Invest 24:416, 1994

125. Grunfeld C, Pang M, Doerrler W, et al: Lipids, lipoproteins, triglyceride clearance and cytokines in human immunodeficiency virus infection and the acquired immunodeficiency syndrome. J Clin Endocrinol Metab 74:1045, 1992

126. Shor-Posner G, Basit A, Lu Y, et al: Hypocholesterolemia is associated with immune dysfunction in early human immunodeficiency virus-1 infection. Am J Med 94:515, 1993

127. Zangerle R, Sarcletti M, Gallati H, et al: Decreased plasma concentrations of HDL cholesterol in HIV-

infected individuals are associated with immune activation. J Acquir Immune Defic Syndr 7:1149, 1994

128. Feingold KR, Krauss RM, Pang M, et al: The hypertriglyceridemia of acquired immunodeficiency syndrome is associated with an increased prevalence of low density lipoprotein subclass pattern B. J Clin Endocrinol Metab 76:1423, 1993

129. Grunfeld C, Kotler DP, Hamadeh R, et al: Hypertriglyceridemia in the acquired immunodeficiency syndrome. Am J Med 86:27, 1989

130. Mildvan D, Machado SG, Wilets I, Grossberg SE: Endogenous interferon and triglyceride concentrations to assess response to zidovudine in AIDS and advanced AIDS-related complex. Lancet 339:453, 1992

131. Hellerstein MK, Grunfeld C, Wu K, et al: Increased de novo hepatic lipogenesis in HIV-infected humans. J Clin Endocrinol Metab 76:559, 1993

132. Sullivan AK, Nelson MR: Marked hyperlipidaemia on ritonavir therapy. AIDS 11:938, 1997

133. Grunfeld C, Feingold KR: Metabolic disturbances and wasting in the acquired immunodeficiency syndrome. N Engl J Med 327:329, 1992

134. Grunfeld C, Pang M, Shimizu L, et al: Resting energy expenditure, caloric intake and short term weight change in human immunodeficiency virus infection and the acquired immunodeficiency syndrome. Am J Clin Nutr 55:455, 1992

135. Hommes MJT, Romijn JA, Endert E, Sauerwein HP: Resting energy expenditure and substrate oxidation in human immunodeficiency virus (HIV)-infected asymptomatic men: HIV affects host metabolism in the early asymptomatic stage. Am J Clin Nutr 54:311, 1991

136. Melchior JC, Raguin G, Boulier A, et al: Resting energy expenditure in human immunodeficiency virus-infected patients: Comparison between patients with and without secondary infections. Am J Clin Nutr 57:614, 1993

137. Melchior JC, Salmon D, Rigaud D, et al: Resting energy expenditure is increased in stable, malnourished HIV-infected patients. Am J Clin Nutr 53:437, 1991

138. Macallan DC, Noble C, Baldwin C, et al: Energy expenditure and wasting in human immunodeficiency virus infection. N Engl J Med 333:83, 1995

139. Macallan DC, Noble C, Baldwin C, et al: Prospective

analysis of patterns of weight change in stage IV human immunodeficiency virus infection. Am J Clin Nutr 58:417, 1993

140. Grunfeld C, Feingold KR: Body weight as essential data in the management of patients with human immunodeficiency virus infection and the acquired immunodeficiency syndrome. Am J Clin Nutr 58:317, 1993

141. Lo JC, Mulligan K, Tai VW, et al: "Buffalo hump" in men with HIV-1 infection. Lancet 351:867, 1998

142. Lo JC, Mulligan K, Tai VW, et al: Body shape changes in HIV-infected patients. J Acquir Immune Defic Syndr Hum Retrovirol 19:307, 1998

143. Roth VR, Kravcik S, Angel JB: Development of cervical fat pads following therapy with human immunodeficiency virus type 1 protease inhibitors. Clin Infect Dis 27:65, 1998

144. Miller KK, Daly PA, Sentochnik D, et al: Pseudo-Cushing's syndrome in human immunodeficiency virus-infected patients. Clin Infect Dis 27:68, 1998

145. Striker R, Conlin D, Marx M, et al: Localized adipose tissue hypertrophy in patients receiving human immunodeficiency virus protease inhibitors. Clin Infect Dis 27:218, 1998

146. Hengel RL, Watts NB, Lennox JL: Benign symmetric lipomatosis associated with protease inhibitors. Lancet 350:1596, 1997

147. Miller KD, Jones E, Yanovski JA, et al: Visceral abdominal-fat accumulation associated with use of indinavir. Lancet 351:871, 1998

148. Dong K, Flynn MM, Dickinson BT, et al: Changes in body habitus in HIV(+) women after initiation of protease inhibitor therapy. In: Abstracts of the XIIth International Conference on AIDS, Geneva, 1998, Abstract 177-12373

149. Engelson ES, Kotler DP, Tan YX, et al: Altered body fat distribution in HIV infection: Regional body composition measurements by whole body MRI and DXA scans. In: Abstracts of the XIIth International Conference on AIDS, Geneva, 1998, Abstract 32181

150. Viraben R, Aquilina C: Indinavir-associated lipodystrophy. AIDS 12:F37, 1998

151. Senior B, Gellis SS: The syndromes of total lipodystrophy and of partial lipodystrophy. Pediatrics 33:593, 1964

19 Renal Complications of HIV Infection

RUDOLPH A. RODRIGUEZ • MICHAEL H. HUMPHREYS

The renal manifestations of HIV infection occur commonly during all stages of infection. Fluid, electrolyte, and acid–base abnormalities, as well as acute renal failure, have been observed frequently in HIV-infected patients, mainly as a consequence of drug toxicity or opportunistic infections. The most clinically relevant disorder is chronic renal failure progressing to end-stage renal disease (ESRD), which has also been observed with a high frequency in some centers.

FLUID, ELECTROLYTE, AND ACID–BASE ABNORMALITIES

Hyponatremia

The most common electrolyte disturbance in HIV-infected patients is hyponatremia. It has been reported in as many as 20% to 56% of hospitalized patients with AIDS and has also been identified in outpatients.[1-5] The basis for the hyponatremia is variable. The largest single cause is volume depletion resulting from extrarenal fluid losses, usually from diarrhea. In most of these cases, when normal extracellular fluid volume is restored, the hyponatremia is corrected.[2-5] A smaller number of patients develop hyponatremia in the absence of any evidence of hypovolemia. These patients have the characteristic findings of the syndrome of inappropriate secretion of antidiuretic hormone (SIADH). Plasma antidiuretic hormone (ADH) concentration, when measured in some of these patients, has been inappropriately elevated for the degree of hyponatremia and hypo-osmolality, lending strong support for this being the mechanism underlying the hyponatremia.[3] Patients with symptomatic AIDS frequently present with opportunistic infections of the lungs and central nervous system. Such infections are known to stimulate excessive release of ADH to produce SIADH. In a few patients, evidence of adrenal insufficiency has accompanied the hyponatremia, and treatment with glucocorticoid hormone has improved the serum sodium concentration.[3-5] AIDS patients have a high incidence of adrenal abnormalities (see Chapter 18). Whatever its cause, the development of hyponatremia in an HIV-infected patient is a sign of poor prognosis, because survival time is much shorter compared with patients who are not hyponatremic.[2,4,5]

Potassium Disorders

Both hypokalemia and hyperkalemia commonly develop in HIV-infected patients. Hypokalemia usually occurs as a result of gastrointestinal losses incurred with diarrheal illness. However, hyperkalemia may occur as a result of the effects of high doses of either trimethoprim or intravenous pentamidine; the mechanism seems to be inhibition of distal nephron sodium transport leading to decreased distal potassium secretion.[6,7] Trimethoprim shares structural similarity with the potassium-sparing diuretic triamterene.

Adrenal abnormalities may be responsible for the hyperkalemia in some patients. Adrenal insufficiency and the syndrome of hyporeninemic hypoaldosteronism have been described in some patients with hyperkalemia and hyponatremia.[8,9] Severe acute or chronic renal insufficiency may also contribute to the development of hyperkalemia. Treatment of hyperkalemia should be guided by the cause and severity; it should respond to cessation of offending drugs, or to treatment with loop diuretics or with fludrocortisone for adrenal causes.[8]

Metabolic Acidosis

Patients with HIV infection may present with a variety of simple and mixed acid–base disorders. As a result of pulmonary and central nervous system infections, patients may present with respiratory alkalosis or acidosis. Both high and normal anion gap metabolic acidosis are also seen in HIV-infected patients. Stool base losses, adrenal insufficiency, the syndrome of hyporeninemic hypoaldosteronism, or amphotericin-B–related renal tubular acidosis all may cause a normal anion gap metabolic acidosis.[8–10] In addition to the expected causes of high anion gap acidosis, such as sepsis and chronic renal failure, type B lactic acidosis has been described in this patient population.[11,12] One well-documented case suggested that the cause of the excess lactate production was a "mitochondrial myopathy" caused by interruption of normal mitochondrial respiration in skeletal muscle by zidovudine.[12] However, not all case reports have been of patients who received this drug.[11] Recognition of this entity rests with a severe metabolic acidosis with an increased anion gap; blood lactate levels, when measured, have been greater than 5, and frequently greater than 10, mmol/L.[11,12] No form of treatment has been uniformly successful, and survival is shortened in these patients.[11]

ACUTE RENAL FAILURE

Mild acute renal failure, as defined by a serum creatinine level greater than 2.0 mg/dl, occurs in 20% of hospitalized HIV-infected patients.[13] Patients with acute renal failure on admission to the hospital are likely to have a prerenal cause related to hypovolemia. In patients who develop acute renal failure during the hospitalization, the likely cause is acute tubular necrosis from hypotension or drug nephrotoxicity (Table 19–1).[13,14] Urinalysis is extremely helpful in the differential diagnosis of acute renal failure in HIV-infected patients. The urine sediment should be normal in prerenal patients, whereas patients with acute tubular necrosis will have muddy brown, granular casts and/or renal tubular cells and casts. Urinalysis in cases of acute interstitial nephritis will predominately show white blood cells, white blood cell casts, and a small amount of proteinuria and hematuria.

The common causes of acute renal failure, including a list of some potentially nephrotoxic agents used in HIV-infected patients, are presented in Table 19–1. Note that patients on sulfadiazine or indinavir are at risk for acute renal failure from drug crystal–induced obstruction.[15–18] These patients should be evaluated immediately with ultrasound to exclude large drug stones as the cause of obstruction, which would necessitate emergent urologic intervention. However, the renal failure may be caused by intratubular obstruction, which will not be seen on ultrasound. This diagnosis is made when the urine sediment shows the typical indinavir or sulfadiazine crystals in the urine along with microscopic hematuria. Renal function generally is restored once rigorous hydration is administered and the inciting agent is discontinued.

The prognosis of patients with acute renal failure depends on the underlying illness. In HIV-infected patients hospitalized for a reversible illness accompanied with acute renal failure, dialysis should be offered when indicated because the overall prognosis is favorable.[19]

CHRONIC RENAL DISEASE

The two main types of glomerular involvement leading to proteinuria and renal insufficiency are HIV-associated nephropathy (HIVAN) and HIV-associated immune-mediated renal disease.[20–22] HIV-associated immune-mediated renal disease is the most common glomerular disease found on renal biopsy in series reported from Italy and France.[23,24] Immune complex deposition in glomeruli leads to a proliferative glomerulonephritis and renal insufficiency. The direct role of the HIV in immune complex formation was described in four patients in whom circulating immune complexes containing HIV antigen were present. Renal biopsy revealed proliferative glomerulonephritis, and eluates of biopsy tissue revealed the same types of complexes in renal tissue after polymerase chain reaction amplification.[22] The role of HIV as a stimulus for immune complex formation in immunoglobulin A nephropathy and other forms of HIV-associated immune-mediated renal disease was also suggested in a study showing circulating immune complexes with HIV antigens and eluates of renal biopsy tissue revealing the presence of HIV Gag and Env sequences.[20,22] Thus deposition in glomeruli of immune complexes containing HIV antigens may result in proliferative glomerulonephritis. These complexes may arise from trapping of circulating complexes or from in situ complex formation to viral antigens in renal tissue. Another form of HIV-associated immune-mediated renal disease is hepatitis C vi-

TABLE 19–1. Causes of Acute Renal Failure in HIV-Infected Patients

PRERENAL	RENAL	POSTRENAL/OBSTRUCTION
Dehydration	Acute tubular necrosis	Drugs
Sepsis	Amphotericin B	Sulfadiazine
NSAIDs	Aminoglycosides	Indinavir
	Pentamidine	Acyclovir
	Foscarnet	Malignancy
	Acyclovir	
	Cidofovir	
	Hypotension	
	Radiocontrast	
	Acute interstitial nephritis	
	Sulfamethoxazole	
	Dapsone	
	NSAIDs	
	Rifampin	
	Glomerular diseases	
	HIVAN	
	HCV-MPGN	
	Microangiopathic hemolytic anemia	

Abbreviations: HCV-MPGN, hepatitis C virus–mediated membranoproliferative glomerulonephritis; HIVAN, HIV-associated nephropathy; NSAIDs, nonsteroidal anti-inflammatory drugs.

rus (HCV)-associated cryoglobulinemic glomerulonephritis.[25] HCV infection is almost universal in HIV-infected patients with a history of intravenous drug use.[26,27] (see Chapter 26).

HIV-associated immune-mediated renal disease usually presents with mild to no renal insufficiency, low-grade proteinuria, and hematuria. Patients rarely progress to ESRD. The exception is HCV cryoglobulinemic glomerulonephritis, which can present with nephrotic syndrome, hypertension, and rapidly progressive renal insufficiency. Patients with HCV cryoglobulinemic glomerulonephritis may respond to treatment with interferon-α, but there is little experience with this agent in patients coinfected with HIV.[25,28]

In contrast to the HIV-associated immune-mediated renal diseases, HIVAN has a poor prognosis, with most patients progressing quickly to ESRD. The U.S. Renal Data System reported that 1336 adult HIV-infected patients developed ESRD between 1989 and 1993, and the majority probably had HIVAN. The histologic characteristics of HIVAN are those of focal and segmental glomerulosclerosis (FSGS) with interstitial inflammation and fibrosis, tubular dilatation and atrophy, and tubular reticular inclusion bodies in endothelial cells seen with electron microscopy; indeed, these characteristics have been regarded as so distinctive as to comprise a specific pathologic entity.[21,29] HIVAN has been reported primarily from centers in urban areas of the east and west coasts of the United States; worldwide, over 90% of

reported cases have occurred in people of African descent, with a high preponderance of males.[30,31] Clinically, it is characterized by high-grade proteinuria, usually in the nephrotic range (>3.5 gm/day), normal or large kidneys with increased echodensity on diagnostic ultrasound, and renal insufficiency that rapidly progresses in weeks to months to ESRD; noteworthy is the rarity of hypertension and peripheral edema in these patients despite the severity of the renal failure and proteinuria.[30,31] Although usually diagnosed in patients with AIDS, HIVAN has been the initial manifestation of HIV infection in a small number of cases. It was thought to be highly associated with injection drug use, but this mode of HIV transmission is involved in fewer than half the cases, and the occurrence of this lesion in infants and children with AIDS from vertical HIV transmission indicates that drug use is not necessary for its development.[32,33]

The pathogenesis of this form of renal involvement in HIV infection is unclear, but human and animal studies suggest that a direct effect of HIV gene expression in the kidney rather than the systemic effects of HIV infection may cause HIVAN. HIV DNA has been demonstrated in tubular epithelium, glomerular endothelial cells, and mesangial cells by a variety of techniques in vitro and in renal biopsy tissue of HIV-infected patients.[34–37] Although these studies were initially thought to provide evidence for the role of viral DNA in the pathogenesis of HIVAN, HIV DNA has also been identified in the tissue of HIV-infected patients without any renal disease.[35] Mice transgenic for a noninfective HIV construct express viral DNA in kidney tissue, and also develop FSGS.[38] A preliminary report indicates that HIV is a potent stimulator of transforming growth factor-β,[39] a cytokine strongly implicated in the development of fibrosis.[40] The transgenic mouse model suggests that activation of this cytokine could well be the basis for the extensive interstitial fibrosis and glomerular sclerosis that are the hallmarks of HIVAN.[41] This same model suggests that viral gene products expressed in the kidney, and not some systemic consequence of HIV infection, leads to HIVAN. Kidneys were transplanted between normal and transgenic mice, and HIVAN developed in the transgenic kidneys transplanted into the nontransgenic littermates. However, the normal kidneys transplanted into the transgenic littermates remained normal.[42]

At the present time, there is no proven therapy for HIVAN. However, because there is a 20% to 40% response rate to corticosteroid therapy in non-HIV or idiopathic FSGS, and because serendipitous treatment of HIVAN with corticosteroids resulted in renal improvement in HIV-infected patients actually treated for *Pneumocystis carinii* pneumonia, corticosteroids have now been studied in a small series of patients with HIVAN.[43-46] One study of 20 patients had no control group, and the duration of therapy was individualized depending on initial response.[43] However, acknowledging the rapid course of HIVAN, the study did show that prednisone at a dose of 60 mg/day for 2 to 11 weeks leads to a significant reduction in serum creatinine and 24-hour urine protein excretion.[43] The improvement in renal function may be a result of a reversal of interstitial inflammation by the corticosteroids.[47]

Because of the possible direct role of HIV in the pathogenesis of HIVAN, antiretroviral therapy would be expected to have beneficial effects on the renal disease. However, there are few data on the role of antiretroviral therapy in HIVAN. Retrospective studies and case reports suggest that monotherapy with zidovudine may slow or even reverse the rapid deterioration associated with HIVAN.[48-52] However, most of these studies provide only anecdotal evidence to support the beneficial effect of zidovudine on HIVAN. The renal effects of combination antiretroviral therapy have not yet been studied, but our clinical experience at San Francisco General Hospital seems to support the beneficial effects of antiretroviral therapy on HIVAN.[53]

Angiotensin-converting enzyme inhibitors are effective in slowing the progression of renal insufficiency in a variety of chronic renal diseases, and they may be beneficial in HIVAN by blocking the angiotensin II-driven increase in cellular synthesis of transforming growth factor-β. Although not resulting in dramatic renal improvements, angiotensin-converting enzyme inhibitors have been shown to slow down progression in both humans and HIV-transgenic mice.[54-56]

Decisions about dialysis treatment must be made on an individual basis. Initial reports indicated that AIDS patients treated with hemodialysis had a very short survival time, an observation that raised the question of whether dialysis should even be offered.[14] However, overall improvement in AIDS management, and earlier diagnosis of HIV-associated renal disease, has led to an improvement in the poor initial results, and some patients will do well on continuous ambulatory peritoneal dialysis.[57,58]

References

1. Glassock R, Cohan A, Danovitch G, et al: Human immunodeficiency virus infection and the kidney. Ann Intern Med 112:35, 1990
2. Tang W, Kaptein E, Feinstein E: Hyponatremia in hospitalized patients with acquired immunodeficiency syndrome and the AIDS-related complex. Am J Med 94:169, 1993
3. Agarwal A, Soni A, Ciechanowsky M, et al: Hyponatremia in patients with the acquired immunodeficiency syndrome. Nephron 53:317, 1989
4. Cusano A, Thies H, Siegal F: Hyponatremia in patients with acquired immune deficiency syndrome. J Acquir Immune Defic Syndr 3:949, 1990
5. Vitting K, Gardenswart M, Zabetakis P: Frequency of hyponatremia and nonosmolar vasopressin release in the acquired immunodeficiency syndrome. JAMA 263:973, 1990
6. Kleyman T, Roberts C, Ling B: A mechanism for pentamidine-induced hyperkalemia: Inhibition of distal nephron sodium transport. Ann Intern Med 122:103, 1995
7. Velazquez H, Perazella M, Wright F, et al: Renal mechanism of trimethoprim-induced hyperkalemia. Ann Intern Med 119:296, 1993
8. Kalin M, Poretsky L, Seres D, et al: Hyporeninemic hypoaldosteronism associated with acquired immune deficiency syndrome. Am J Med 82:1035, 1987
9. Marks J: Endocrine manifestations of human immunodeficiency virus infection. Am J Med Sci 302:110, 1991
10. Berns J, Cohen R, Stumacher R, et al: Renal aspects of therapy for human immunodeficiency virus and associated opportunistic infections. J Am Soc Nephrol 1:1061, 1991
11. Chattha G, Arieff A, Cummings C, et al: Lactic acidosis complicating the acquired immunodeficiency syndrome. Ann Intern Med 118:37, 1993

12. Gopinath R, Hutcheon M, Cheema-Dhadli S, et al: Chronic lactic acidosis in a patient with acquired immunodeficiency syndrome and mitochondrial myopathy: Biochemical studies. J Am Soc Nephrol 3:1212, 1992

13. Valeri A, Neusy A: Acute and chronic renal disease in hospitalized AIDS patients. Clin Nephrol 33:110, 1991

14. Rao T, Friedman E, Nicastri A: The types of renal disease in the acquired immunodeficiency syndrome. N Engl J Med 316:1062, 1987

15. Carbone L, Bendixen B, Appel G: Sulfadiazine-associated obstructive nephropathy occurring in a patient with the acquired immunodeficiency syndrome. Am J Kidney Dis 12:72, 1988

16. Simon D, Brosius F, Rothstein D: Sulfadiazine crystalluria revisited: The treatment of Toxoplasma encephalitis in patients with acquired immunodeficiency syndrome. Arch Intern Med 150:2379, 1990

17. Tashima K, Horowitz J, Rosen S: Indinavir nephropathy. N Engl J Med 336:138, 1997

18. Kopp J, Miller K, Mican J, et al: Crystalluria and urinary tract abnormalities associated with indinavir. Ann Intern Med 127:119, 1997

19. Rao TKS, Friedman EA: Outcome of severe acute renal failure in patients with acquired immunodeficiency syndrome. Am J Kidney Dis 25:390, 1995

20. Kimmel P, Phillips T, Garrett C: HIV associated immune-mediated renal disease. Kidney Int 44:1327, 1993

21. Cohen A, Nast C: HIV-associated nephropathy. A unique combined glomerular, tubular, and interstitial lesion. Mod Pathol 1:87, 1988

22. Kimmel P, Phillips T, Ferreira-Centeno A, et al: Brief report: Idiotypic IgA nephropathy in patients with human immunodeficiency virus infection. N Engl J Med 327:702, 1992

23. Casanova S, Mazzucco G, di Belgiojoso B, et al: Pattern of glomerular involvement in human immunodeficiency virus-infected patients: An Italian study. Am J Kidney Dis 26:446, 1995

24. Nochy D, Glotz D, Dosquet P, et al: Renal disease associated with HIV infection: A multicentric study of 60 patients from Paris hospitals. Nephrol Dial Transplant 8:11, 1993

25. Stokes M, Chawla H, Brody R: Immune complex glomerulonephritis in patients coinfected with human immunodeficiency virus and hepatitis C virus. Am J Kidney Dis 29:514, 1997

26. Rall C, Dienstag J: Epidemiology of hepatitis C virus infection. Semin Gastrointest Dis 6:3, 1995

27. Mendel I, Clotteau L, Lambert S, et al: Hepatitis C virus infection in an HIV-positive population in Normandy: Antibodies, HCV RNA and genotype prevalence. J Med Virol 47:231, 1995

28. Johnson R, Gretch D, Couser W, et al: Hepatitis C virus-associated glomerulonephritis. Effect of α-interferon therapy. Kidney Int 46:1700, 1994

29. D'Agati V, Suh J, Carbone L, et al: The pathology of HIV-nephropathy: A detailed morphologic and comparative study. Kidney Int 35:1358, 1989

30. Humphreys M: Human immunodeficiency virus-associated glomerulosclerosis. Kidney Int 48:311, 1995

31. D'Agati V, Appel G: HIV infection and the kidney. J Am Soc Nephrol 8:138, 1997

32. Strauss J, Abitbol C, Zilleruelo G: Renal disease in children with the acquired immunodeficiency syndrome. N Engl J Med 321:625, 1989

33. Bourgoignie J, Pardo V: The nephropathology in human immunodeficiency virus (HIV-1) infection. Kidney Int 40:S19, 1991

34. Cohen A, Sun N, Imagawa D: Demonstration of human immunodeficiency virus in renal epithelium in HIV-associated nephropathy. Mod Pathology 2:125, 1989

35. Kimmel P, Ferreira-Centeno A, Farkas-Szallasi T, et al: Viral DNA in microdissected renal biopsy tissue from HIV infected patients with nephrotic syndrome. Kidney Int 43:1347, 1993

36. Green D, Resnick L, Bourgoignie J: HIV infects glomerular endothelial and mesangial but not epithelial cells in vitro. Kidney Int 41:956, 1992

37. Alpers C, McClure J, Bursten S: Human mesangial cells are resistant to productive infection by multiple strains of human immunodeficiency virus types 1 and 2. Am J Kidney Dis 19:126, 1992

38. Kopp J, Klotman M, Adler S: Progressive glomerulosclerosis and enhanced renal accumulation of basement membrane components in mice transgenic for HIV-1 genes. Proc Natl Acad Sci USA 89:1577, 1992

39. Shukla RR, Kumar A, Kimmel PL: Transforming growth factor beta increases the expression of HIV-1 gene in transfected human mesangial cells. Kidney Int 44:1022, 1993

40. Sharma K, Ziyadeh FN: The emerging role of transforming growth factor-β in kidney diseases. Am J Physiol 266:F829, 1994

41. Kopp J, McCune B, Notkins A, et al: Increased expression of transforming growth factor beta in HIV-transgenic mouse kidney. [abstract]. J Am Soc Nephrol 3:600, 1992

42. Bruggerman L, Dikman S, Meng C: Nephropathy in human immunodeficiency virus-1 transgenic mice is due to renal transgene expression. J Clin Invest 100:84, 1997

43. Smith M, Austen J, Carey J, et al: Prednisone improves renal function and proteinuria in human immunodeficiency virus-associated nephropathy. Am J Med 101:41, 1996

44. Korbet S, Schwartz M, Lewis E: Primary focal segmental glomerulosclerosis: clinical course and response to therapy. Am J Kidney Dis 23:773, 1994

45. Smith M, Pawar R, Carey J, et al: Effect of corticosteroid therapy on human immunodeficiency virus-associated nephropathy. Am J Med 97:145, 1994

46. Appel R, Neill J: A steroid-responsive nephrotic syndrome in a patient with human immunodeficiency virus (HIV) infection. Ann Intern Med 113:892, 1990

47. Briggs W, Tanawattanacharoen S, Choi M, et al: Clinicopathologic correlates of prednisone treatment of human immunodeficiency virus-associated nephropathy. Am J Kidney Dis 28:618, 1996

48. Ifudu O, Rao T, Tan C, et al: Zidovudine is beneficial in human immunodeficiency virus associated nephropathy. Am J Nephrol 15:217, 1995

49. Cook P, Appel R: Prolonged clinical improvement in HIV-associated nephropathy with zidovudine therapy. J Am Soc Nephrol 1:842, 1990

50. Lam M, Park M: HIV-associated nephropathy—beneficial effect of zidovudine therapy. N Engl J Med 323:1775, 1990

51. Michel C, Dosquet P, Ronco P, et al: Nephropathy associated with infection by human immunodeficiency virus: A report on 11 cases including 6 treated with zidovudine. Nephron 62:434, 1992

52. Babut-Gay M, Echard M: Zidovudine and nephropathy with human immunodefiency virus (HIV) infection. Ann Intern Med 111:856, 1989

53. Rodriguez R, Johansen K, Balkovetz D, et al: Clinical characteristics and renal biopsy findings in human im-

munodeficiency virus (HIV) infected outpatients with renal disease. [abstract]. J Am Soc Nephrol 7:1342, 1996

54. Kimmel P, Mishkin M, Umana W: Captopril and renal survival in patients with human immunodeficiency virus nephropathy. Am J Kidney Dis 28:202, 1996

55. Bird J, Durham S, Giancarli M, et al: Captopril ameliorates nephropathy in HIV-transgenic mice. [abstract]. J Am Soc Nephrol 7:1850, 1996

56. Burns G, Paul S, Sivak S, et al: Beneficial effect of angiotensin-converting enzyme inhibition in human immunodeficiency virus-associated nephropathy. [abstract]. J Am Soc Nephrol 7:1329, 1996

57. Kimmel P, Umana W, Simmens S: Continuous ambulatory peritoneal dialysis and survival of HIV infected patients with end-stage renal disease. Kidney Int 44:373, 1993

58. Tebben J, Rigsby O, Selwyn A: Outcome of HIV infected patients on continuous ambulatory peritoneal dialysis. Kidney Int 44:191, 1993

Specific Infections and Malignancies in HIV Disease

20 | *Pneumocystis carinii* Pneumonia

LAURENCE HUANG • JOHN D. STANSELL

Pneumocystis carinii increasingly has become recognized as a cause of disease among immunocompromised populations since its discovery nearly 90 years ago.[1] An organism of relatively low virulence, *P. carinii* poses no significant health threat to immunocompetent persons. However, *P. carinii* is a major source of suffering and death in persons with impaired host immunity resulting from malnutrition, neoplasia, organ transplant, or HIV infection. Prior to the 1980s, the number of *P. carinii* pneumonia cases diagnosed in the United States each year was small. Since 1981, this number has exploded, paralleling the rise of symptomatic HIV infection. Indeed, the occurrence of *P. carinii* pneumonia in clusters of homosexual men and injection drug users in 1981 was the harbinger of the current AIDS epidemic.[2,3] Although *P. carinii* pneumonia accounted for nearly two thirds of AIDS-index diagnoses early in the epidemic,[4] recent data suggest a reduction in this proportion as a result of widespread primary *P. carinii* prophylaxis use.[5,6] Moreover, improved management of acute *P. carinii* pneumonia and routine use of secondary *P. carinii* prophylaxis have resulted in improved treatment outcomes and longer life expectancy for those persons at risk for the disease.

Although many gaps in our knowledge of *P. carinii* persist, we have gained significant knowledge about susceptibility, diagnosis, treatment, and prevention of this disease over the nearly twenty years of the AIDS epidemic. This chapter focuses upon the current state of knowledge and emerging concepts about *P. carinii* pneumonia in HIV-infected persons.

MICROBIOLOGY

The inability to culture *P. carinii* outside of immunocompromised animal models has severely hampered our understanding of this organism. The lack of a reliable in vitro culture method has made drug development and epidemiologic study difficult. Furthermore, a definitive environmental reservoir for the organism has never been identified, and the inability to observe the life cycle of the organism has led to much misunderstanding.

In 1909, Chagas described *P. carinii* in the lungs of trypanosome-infected guinea pigs and believed it to be a new trypanosome.[1] Despite recognition as being unique from trypanosomes, the misconception that *P. carinii* was a protozoan persisted for 80 years after its discovery based on the organism's morphology, inability to grow on fungal media, and susceptibility to antiprotozoal agents. In 1970, ultrastructural studies noting that *P. carinii* lacked organelles characteristic of protozoa while possessing features suggestive of fungi began to cast doubt upon the protozoal classification.[7]

In 1988, two independent groups presented evidence from 18S ribosomal RNA homology studies that strongly indicated the organism was a fungus.[8,9] Since these first reports, a watershed of studies have corroborated the assignment of *P. carinii* to the fungal kingdom. Sequence analysis of genes encoding dihydrofolate reductase,[10] thymidylate synthase,[11] actin,[12] tubulin,[13] and ATPase,[14] as well as mitochondrial gene sequences,[15] all incontrovertibly link *P. carinii* to the fungi. Although the exact phylogenetic lineage is still undetermined, recent reviews place *P. carinii* among the ascomycetes.[16]

Pneumocystis carinii is a unicellular eukaryote that reproduces by both sexual and asexual means and has several distinct stages to its life cycle.[17] The trophozoite, the predominant intrapulmonary form, is 3 to 5 μm in size and avidly adheres to type 1 pneumocytes. This adhesion may facilitate absorption of nutrients directly through the alveolar-capillary membrane. Large trophozoites likely undergo asexual binary fission to produce small, haploid trophs that subsequently mature to large, diploid trophozoites. The fusion of two haploid trophs, or gametic cells, may initiate the sexual reproduction of the organism, sporogenesis, or encystment. The parent cell, which resembles a large trophozoite, becomes round and smooth and develops a thick cell wall. Within the mature cyst, eight haploid intracytoplasmic bodies or spores develop. These spores, which are indistinguishable from trophozoites, are released from a rupture in the cell wall. The collapsed cysts, which resemble crescents, are readily observed on silver-stained clinical specimens from *P. carinii*-infected persons (Color Plate IC).

EPIDEMIOLOGY AND TRANSMISSION

Pneumocystis carinii can be found in the lungs of many mammalian species, including human, mouse, rat, ferret, pig, horse, and rabbit. Morphologically, these organisms are indistinguishable and, based on the widespread presence of the organism among commonly encountered animals, it might be tempting to consider human *P. carinii* infection a zoonosis. However, evidence is clear from immunologic and genetic studies that these organisms are not identical. Examination of DNA homology of highly conserved portions of the gene encoding mitochondrial ribosomal RNA has demonstrated significant divergence among all species.[18,19] Examination of the chromosomes from each mammalian species reveals unique species karyotypes.[20] Analysis of genetic divergence of the gene coding for the major surface glycoprotein of *P. carinii* suggests organisms infecting different mammalian species are genetically distinct and that *P. carinii* is host-species specific.[21] Transmission studies further document this species specificity. Although transmission of *P. carinii* can be achieved between animals of the same species,[22] attempts to transmit *P. carinii* infection between separate, distinct species have failed.[21] Thus it is unlikely that animals are the environmental reservoir for *P. carinii* transmittal to humans.

Transmittal of *P. carinii* is likely to require inhalation of the infectious unit. Studies by Hughes documented that immunocompromised germ-free rats maintained in sterile environments did not develop *P. carinii* pneumonia.[23] Similarly, immunocompromised animals maintained in isolators and fed unsterilized food and water or lung tissue from infected animals did not develop the disease.[22] Conversely, even limited exposure of germ-free severe combined immunodeficiency (SCID) mice to ambient air or infected animals resulted in disease transmission.[24] These studies indicate that de novo infection results from inhalation of airborne organisms. Moreover, air samples obtained from both laboratory and rural settings have demonstrated human *P. carinii* genetic material when subjected to polymerase chain reaction (PCR).[21,25]

Several serologic studies have demonstrated that most humans develop an antibody response to specific *P. carinii* antigens by 4 years of age.[26-28] This seroconversion occurs worldwide, attesting to the ubiquitous nature of *Pneumocystis*.[29] It also attests to the asymptomatic nature of primary infection in immunocompetent persons. Because of the widespread exposure to *P. carinii* and subsequent development of disease only in the setting of immunocompromise, it has been theorized that *P. carinii* organisms lay dormant in the immunocompetent host and *P. carinii* pneumonia occurs as a result of reactivation at a time of progressive immunocompromise. However, recent studies involving sensitive molecular probes failed to identify resident *P. carinii* genetic material in the lungs of immunocompetent persons. Peters and colleagues searched with PCR probes for *P. carinii* genetic material in the homogenized postmortem lungs of 15 immunocompetent persons, with negative results.[30] Similarly, others failed to identify *P. carinii* in immunocompetent persons by monoclonal antibody staining of fixed lung specimens[31] or by PCR probes of bronchoalveolar lavage fluid.[32]

The situation is quite different in immunocompromised persons, however. Several studies have now identified *P. carinii* genetic material in sputum, bronchoalveolar lavage fluid, and blood of persons with immunocompromising conditions, specifically organ transplantation or HIV infection.[33-37] Despite the presence of *P. carinii* in these immunocompromised individuals, many of them did not have clinical symptoms that would suggest pneumonia, nor did they progress to clinical *P. carinii* pneumonia thereafter.[35] This suggests that long periods of asymptomatic colonization may precede recognizable respiratory disease in immunocompromised persons. In addition, the clearance of *Pneumocystis* organisms from the lungs of immunocompromised persons who have been treated for *P. carinii* pneumonia may be slow or may not occur at all. Vargas et al.[38] have looked at the persistence of organisms in the lungs of steroid-treated rats after specific treatment for the infection and subsequent withdrawal of immunocompromising drugs. These investigators found organisms persisting for 1 year in a significant number of study animals.[38] It is conceivable that, in the face of progressive immunologic decline, AIDS patients, even with clinical resolution of respiratory illness and subsequent use of secondary *P. carinii* prophylaxis, may not have *P. carinii* completely eradicated from their lungs. These findings beg the question of whether person-to-person transmission of *P. carinii* occurs. Early reports of disease caused by *P. carinii* were clusters of pneumonia among malnourished children[39] or among children hospitalized for treatment of malignant disease.[40,41] *Pneumocystis carinii* colonization in a seemingly immunocompetent person exposed to *P. carinii*–infected animals has been described.[42] In a multicenter, observational study of the pulmonary complications of HIV infection, two HIV-seronegative control subjects who had exposure to patients with *P. carinii* pneumonia were subsequently found to harbor *P. carinii* in induced sputum and bronchoalveolar lavage fluid specimens. Neither of these subjects had clinical evidence of pulmonary disease at the time of discovery or over the course of the study (J.D. Stansell, unpublished observations). Finally, serum titers of antibodies directed against *P. carinii* have been found to be elevated among health care workers who care for AIDS patients.[43] These results call into question whether infection control measures, especially respiratory isolation, are warranted for persons with *P. carinii* pneumonia. Recommendations await further research.

HOST DEFENSES

The natural host defenses and immunologic responses that both protect humans from *P. carinii* and modify the expression of disease in immunocompromised persons are incompletely understood. Although cell-mediated immunity appears to play the decisive role in protection from *P. carinii*, studies indicate that humoral immunity also appears to be important in the host's ability to avoid infection or recover from *P. carinii* pneumonia. Patients with seemingly pure B-lymphocyte dysfunction or pure T-lymphocyte dysfunction, or both, are at risk for developing *P. carinii* pneumonia.

Early studies indicated that immunization and significant serum antibody titers against *P. carinii* were inadequate to protect rats subjected to

corticosteroid immunosuppression from *P. carinii* pneumonia. One study, however, demonstrates near-complete protection of mice immunized against *P. carinii*, subsequently inoculated with intratracheal organisms and then selectively depleted of their CD4 lymphocytes by administration of monoclonal antibodies directed against CD4 or Thy-1 epitopes.[44] Not only were *P. carinii* organisms absent on microscopy at days 10 and 19 of the study, but they were undetectable by PCR probe as well. This study suggests a major role for humoral immunity in protection from *P. carinii* infection.

Studies illustrate that passively administered antibodies to *P. carinii* can modulate the burden of organisms in immunodeficient animal models with *P. carinii* pneumonia.[45] Analogously, B cells, in addition to T cells, are necessary for resolution of *P. carinii* pneumonia in immunodeficient rodents.[46] Similar results are obtained using SCID mice that spontaneously develop *P. carinii* infection.[47] This study also documented an improvement in survival by greater than threefold in mice treated with hyperimmune serum. How humoral immunity exerts its effect upon *P. carinii* pneumonia is uncertain, but opsonization, complement-mediated organism lysis, and interference with cell adhesion have all been postulated as possible mechanisms. Confirmation awaits further research.

Cell-mediated immunity appears to occupy the pivotal role in prevention and control of *P. carinii* infection. Shellito and colleagues demonstrated that conventional BALB/c rats could be rendered susceptible to *P. carinii* pneumonia by administration of monoclonal antibodies directed against CD4 lymphocytes.[48] SCID mice, which develop *P. carinii* pneumonia spontaneously from their environment, can be protected from *P. carinii* by administration of CD4 lymphocytes from immunocompetent donors.[49] Moreover, administration of anti-CD4 monoclonal antibody to these mice eliminates the protective effect. Similar studies in SCID mice have shown that CD4 lymphocytes, but not CD8 lymphocytes, play a vital role in control of *P. carinii*.[50] One study suggests a role for the major surface glycoprotein in eliciting the cellular immune response. In this study, CD4 lymphocytes incubated with the glycoprotein had a salutary effect upon *P. carinii* pneumonia in rats.[51] Although CD4 lymphocytes are clearly essential for the control of *P. carinii*, the manner in which these cells exert their effect and their interaction with other effector cells are largely unknown. The CD4 lymphocyte, through secretion of cytokines (particularly interferon-γ and interleukin-2), orchestrates much of cell-mediated immunity and, possibly, humoral immunity. CD4 lymphopenia and disruption of cytokine activity are hallmarks of HIV disease.

PATHOPHYSIOLOGY

Overwhelmingly, *P. carinii* infection is a pulmonary process. Once inhaled, the infective form of *P. carinii*, the precise identity of which is unknown, establishes residence in the alveolus. There, the organism attaches itself to alveolar type 1 cells through bridges of cellular fibronectin and surface glycoproteins.[52,53] Although the organism tightly interdigitates with the type 1 cell, there is no fusion of the cellular membranes. Attachment may facilitate nutrient access directly from the alveolar-capillary bed and appears necessary for organism replication.

It is clear from the prolonged immunosuppression required to induce *P. carinii* pneumonia in animal models and the indolent onset of respiratory symptoms in AIDS patients that *P. carinii* replicates at a relatively slow pace. Eventually, however, large numbers of organisms inhabit the alveoli and alveolar-capillary permeability increases abnormally. Microscopic examination of lung tissue at this time will reveal alveoli filled with foamy, vacuolated, eosinophilic exudates. This exudate consists of *P. carinii* organisms, degenerative cell membranes, surfactant, and host proteins.[54,55] There is a paucity of inflammatory cells present. There is a disruption of surfactant production by type II cells, with a fall in phospholipid production.[54] Rarely, organisms may invade the interstitium, and interstitial fibrosis may follow successful treatment of severe cases. Subsequently, the alveolar epithelial surface degenerates. Subepithelial blebs form, filled with fluid that has traversed the alveolar-capillary membrane as a result of disrupted permeability. Ultimately, the epithelial cells are lost, with denudation of the basement membrane. This presents a clinical picture not unlike the diffuse alveolar damage seen with adult respiratory distress syndrome (ARDS). Lung volumes, lung compliance, and the diffusing capacity for carbon monoxide (DL_{CO}) are severely reduced. The resulting functional abnormality in patients with *P. carinii* pneumonia is impairment of gas exchange. Poor distribution of inspired air into alveoli that are partially or completely filled with organisms and inflammatory debris leads to ventilation–perfusion mismatch or frank right-to-left shunt.

The result is progressive dyspnea and hypoxemia and, ultimately, respiratory failure.

INCIDENCE

The incidence of *P. carinii* pneumonia has undergone dramatic declines during the course of the epidemic. Both the use of *P. carinii* prophylaxis and, more recently, the use of potent combinations of antiretroviral regimens have contributed to this decline. Yet despite these therapies, *P. carinii* pneumonia remains the most common AIDS-defining opportunistic infection in the United States.[56] In 1992, the last year prior to the inclusion of a CD4 lymphocyte count less than 200 cells/μl or a CD4 percentage less than 14 as an AIDS-defining condition, *P. carinii* pneumonia was the AIDS-defining diagnosis in 42% of that year's more than 46,000 AIDS cases.[57] In 1996 and 1997, when excluding those persons diagnosed with AIDS solely on the basis of a CD4 lymphocyte count, *P. carinii* pneumonia was the AIDS-defining diagnosis in 39% of those years' cases.[56,58] Thus, it appears that the recent decline in *P. carinii* pneumonia has paralleled the decline in AIDS cases.

At San Francisco General Hospital (SFGH), we have seen a dramatic decline in the number of cases of *P. carinii* pneumonia. Early in the epidemic, *P. carinii* pneumonia accounted for the vast majority of pneumonias seen among hospitalized HIV-infected persons at our institution. This remained the case until 1995, when community-acquired pneumonia became the most frequent pulmonary cause of hospitalization at our institution, with *P. carinii* pneumonia a distant second.

RISK FACTORS FOR *PNEUMOCYSTIS CARINII* PNEUMONIA

Risk factors for *P. carinii* pneumonia include a CD4 lymphocyte count of 200 cells/μl or less, previous *P. carinii* pneumonia irrespective of CD4 lymphocyte count, and unexplained fevers or oral candidiasis. The Multicenter AIDS Cohort Study (MACS) found a markedly increased risk for *P. carinii* pneumonia among HIV-infected participants with a CD4 lymphocyte count of 200 cells/μl or less at study entry.[59] These subjects had a nearly fivefold greater risk of developing *P. carinii* pneumonia compared to subjects who had a CD4 lymphocyte count over 200 cells/μl at study entry (relative risk [RR] = 4.9, 95% confidence interval [CI] = 3.1 to 8.0). The presence of fever and oral thrush also independently influenced the risk of progression to *P. carinii* pneumonia (RR = 2.15, 95% CI = 1.02 to 4.54 and RR = 1.86, 95% CI = 1.13 to 3.06, respectively). The results of this study led directly to the publication of the Centers for Disease Control and Prevention recommendations for the use of prophylaxis against *P. carinii* in HIV-infected persons.[60] Unfortunately, a number of factors limited the generalizability of the MACS data: (1) the cohort was composed entirely of homosexual and bisexual men; (2) there was often a broad interval between CD4 lymphocyte count determination and *P. carinii* pneumonia diagnosis; (3) data were censored for any AIDS-defining illness; and (4) subjects receiving *P. carinii* prophylaxis were excluded.

In contrast, the Pulmonary Complications of HIV Infection Study (PCHIS) was specifically designed to define the types, frequency, and outcomes of lung disorders in HIV-infected persons. The PCHIS cohort closely approximated the demographics of the AIDS epidemic in 1990 and included homosexual or bisexual men (71%), injection drug–using men and women (25%), and women who acquired HIV infection through heterosexual contact (4%).[61] The cohort was followed for a mean of 52 months and CD4 lymphocyte counts were obtained at each scheduled visit (3 or 6 months). As a result, the median time from last CD4 lymphocyte count determination to *P. carinii* pneumonia diagnosis was 26 days.[62] Data were censored only after subjects developed an episode of *P. carinii* pneumonia or died; the development of other opportunistic infections or malignancies did not preclude inclusion, nor did the use of *P. carinii* prophylaxis. In fact, 79% of the subjects with a CD4 lymphocyte count of 200 cells/μl or less reported receiving primary prophylaxis. Overall, 95% of *P. carinii* pneumonia cases occurred in subjects with a CD4 lymphocyte count of 200 cells/μl or less, and 79% had a CD4 lymphocyte count of 100 cells/μl or less. The median CD4 lymphocyte count at the time of *P. carinii* pneumonia diagnosis was 29 cells/μl. Overall, the rate of *P. carinii* pneumonia among persons with a baseline CD4 lymphocyte count of 200 cells/μl or less was 8.08 cases per 100 person-years, irrespective of the use of *P. carinii* prophylaxis. However, this rate was not uniform throughout CD4 lymphocyte count ranges. Persons with baseline CD4 lymphocyte counts of 101 to 200 cells/μl had a rate of 5.95 cases per 100 person-

years; this increased dramatically to 11.13 cases per 100 person-years for persons with baseline CD4 lymphocyte counts of 100 cells/μl or less.

CLINICAL PRESENTATION

Data from the PCHIS confirm that *P. carinii* pneumonia rarely presents without respiratory symptoms. In this study, subjects underwent a complete history and physical examination, laboratory testing including CD4/CD8 lymphocyte count measurement, chest radiography, and pulmonary function testing at 3- to 6-month intervals in order to identify subclinical opportunistic infections.[61] Despite this intensive effort, no diagnoses of *P. carinii* pneumonia were established in asymptomatic subjects.[63–65] Respiratory illnesses, including *P. carinii* pneumonia, were preceded by respiratory symptoms—cough and/or shortness of breath. Nonspecific constitutional symptoms such as fever, night sweats, fatigue, or weight loss, while associated with increased risk for developing *P. carinii* pneumonia, were not associated with identifiable lung diseases in the absence of respiratory symptoms.

Unlike persons immunocompromised for reasons other than HIV, HIV-infected persons usually have a prolonged prodromal illness associated with *P. carinii* pneumonia. One study found nearly 1 month of constitutional symptoms prior to presentation in most HIV-infected patients.[66] However, the tempo of the illness varies from one patient to the next. Moreover, in assessing the HIV-infected patient with respiratory complaints, an understanding of that patient's baseline status is important. In the PCHIS, 90% of the subjects had respiratory complaints at some time during the study, and over two thirds had complained of a cough during a study visit. For many of these subjects, their respiratory symptoms were secondary to chronic conditions rather than acute infection.

Characteristically, *P. carinii* pneumonia presents with fever, slowly progressive dyspnea on exertion, and a dry, nonproductive cough. Profound fatigue usually presents in concert with these symptoms. Pleuritic chest pain can accompany either *P. carinii* or pyogenic bacterial pneumonia. The rapid onset of spiking fevers, chills, or rigors is uncommon and distinguishes *P. carinii* from bacterial infection. A cough productive of purulent sputum indicates a pyogenic infection or co-infection. Persons at risk for *P. carinii* presenting with a cough productive of purulent sputum should undergo an evaluation for an alternate etiology, receive several days of antibacterial therapy, and then be reassessed. If the suspicion for *P. carinii* pneumonia remains significant after antibacterial treatment, then an evaluation for *P. carinii* pneumonia should be undertaken.

On physical examination, a temperature greater than 38.5°C, tachypnea, and the stigmata of immunosuppression, such as thrush or oral hairy leukoplakia, are frequently encountered. Auscultation and percussion of the lungs is often normal. Occasionally, fine basilar inspiratory rales may be encountered on auscultation. Findings of focal lung consolidation are unusual for *P. carinii* pneumonia, are more suggestive of a bacterial pneumonia, and should prompt an evaluation for an alternate or at least a coexisting etiology.

Laboratory data reflect the underlying HIV infection rather than infection with *P. carinii*. One laboratory test frequently elevated in patients with *P. carinii* pneumonia is the serum lactate dehydrogenase (LDH). Published studies report the sensitivity of an elevated serum LDH for *P. carinii* pneumonia to be in the range of 83% to 100%.[67-74] Proper interpretation, however, requires consideration of a number of factors. First, the serum LDH is nonspecific for *P. carinii* pneumonia, and elevations result from many pulmonary and nonpulmonary etiologies. Next, patients with *P. carinii* pneumonia may have a normal or minimally elevated serum LDH, and there is significant overlap between the serum LDH values in patients with *P. carinii* pneumonia and in those with other pulmonary diseases. Third, most of the published studies consisted of hospitalized patients with *P. carinii* pneumonia, some of who had respiratory failure from *P. carinii* pneumonia. The study that reported the lowest sensitivity of an elevated serum LDH for *P. carinii* pneumonia (83%) consisted of ambulatory outpatients presenting to an urgent care clinic,[71] suggesting that severity of disease and the patient population studied affect the sensitivity of this test for *P. carinii* pneumonia. Finally, many of the studies occurred at a time when *P. carinii* prophylaxis was not in routine use, and perhaps the presentation of disease was more severe. One study that measured the serum LDH in patients who developed *P. carinii* pneumonia despite receiving aerosolized pentamidine prophylaxis reported a sensitivity of an elevated serum LDH for *P. carinii* pneumonia of 82%.[75]

Despite these diagnostic limitations, the serum LDH often has value in assessing prognosis and response to therapy. Multiple studies have shown a strong correlation between the degree of serum LDH elevation and survival.[67,70,72,74,76,77] A high or a rising value while on *P. carinii* treatment correlates with a worse prognosis, a failure of therapy, and increased mortality, whereas a low or a declining value on *P. carinii* treatment correlates with a better prognosis, a response to therapy, and decreased mortality.

The chest radiograph is the cornerstone of the evaluation of an HIV-infected patient with suspected *P. carinii* pneumonia. Similar to the serum LDH, however, the degree of radiographic abnormality seen depends on the severity of disease and the population studied. Classically, *P. carinii* pneumonia presents with diffuse bilateral, symmetrical reticular or granular opacities.[78-81] Thin-walled cysts or pneumatoceles are a common finding[82] and seem to be associated with prolonged, indolent disease and perhaps choice of prophylaxis (Fig. 20–1). Pneumatoceles may be present at the time of

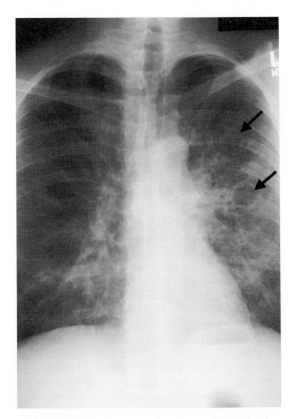

FIGURE 20–1. Posteroanterior chest radiograph of an HIV-infected patient with *P. carinii* pneumonia revealing the characteristic bilateral reticular and granular infiltrates as well as two pneumatoceles (*arrows*). (From Huang L, Stansell JD: AIDS and the lung. Med Clin North Am 80:775, 1996, with permission.)

diagnosis, may develop while a patient is on therapy, and may persist despite successful therapy. The pneumatoceles may be single or multiple in number and small or large in size (Fig. 20–2), and may predispose patients to pneumothorax (Fig. 20–3). However, pneumothorax may also occur spontaneously in the absence of demonstrable pneumatoceles on chest radiographs.[83,84] Focal infiltrates, lobar/segmental consolidation, or nodules with or without cavitation are occasionally seen.[85] Apical disease mimicking tuberculosis has been associated with aerosolized pentamidine prophylaxis,[86,87] although a similar presentation also occurs in patients receiving other forms of *P. carinii* prophylaxis or no preventive therapy. Intrathoracic adenopathy and pleural effusions are rarely due to *P. carinii* pneumonia. These radiographic findings should prompt a search for an alternate or at least a coexisting process such as bacterial pneumonia, tuberculosis, fungal pneumonia, or pulmonary Kaposi's sarcoma.

P. carinii pneumonia may present with a normal chest radiograph. Published studies report the incidence of this to be in the range of 0% to 39%.[78–81,88] In our experience, *P. carinii* pneu-

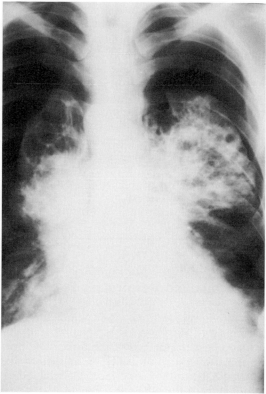

FIGURE 20–3. Posteroanterior chest radiograph of an HIV-infected patient with *P. carinii* pneumonia presenting with bilateral pneumothoraces.

monia presents with a normal chest radiograph in fewer than 10% of cases.

Unfortunately, there are few studies on the resolution or diminution of respiratory signs/symptoms and chest radiographic abnormalities in successfully treated *P. carinii* pneumonia. In our experience, just as the onset of *P. carinii* pneumonia may be gradual, the resolution from disease may be slow. Fever, tachypnea, and oxygen requirements may persist for several days to a week or more, even with successful therapy. Often the first indication of therapeutic success is the patient's subjective feeling of recovery and the observation that the patient can take a deeper breath. The pace of weaning from supplemental oxygen is dependent not only on the severity of disease but also on the antecedent pulmonary function. Persons with severe disease or disease superimposed on underlying chronic lung disease will experience a protracted requirement for supplemental oxygen.

The chest radiograph may worsen during the first week of treatment despite clinical improvement and eventual successful therapy. Usually, radiographic abnormalities improve over the

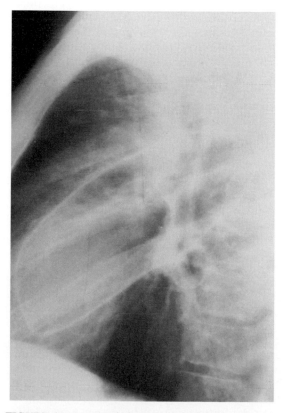

FIGURE 20–2. Lateral chest radiograph of an HIV-infected patient demonstrating a large pneumatocele.

course of a week to several weeks. However, occasionally radiographic abnormalities will persistent for weeks to months after successful therapy. Similarly, the single-breath DL_{CO} usually improves to a plateau over several weeks but rarely returns to predisease values. Occasionally, severe inflammation with resulting fibrosis produces a clinical picture similar to advanced restrictive lung disease with markedly reduced lung volumes, decreased lung compliance, and severe reductions in the DL_{CO}. Unfortunately, patients with these conditions may remain pulmonary cripples throughout the remainder of their lives.

COMPLICATIONS

Hypoxemia and Respiratory Failure

Moderate to severe *P. carinii* pneumonia is characterized by disruption of the alveolar epithelial surface and perturbation of the forces that govern the movement of gases and fluids across the alveolar-capillary interface. Cellular debris sloughed from the alveolar epithelium and fluid leaked across the denuded alveolar-capillary membrane accumulate in the alveolar space as a consequence of *P. carinii* infection. Gas exchange is impaired, pulmonary shunt fraction increases, and hypoxemia results. In severe cases of *P. carinii* pneumonia, this pathophysiologic process is similar to ARDS. Even less fulminant cases are often accompanied by a "treatment effect." In these cases, the initiation of therapy is accompanied by a deterioration in gas exchange and worsening hypoxemia 3 to 5 days into therapy. One hypothesis for this deterioration is that the dead or dying *P. carinii* organisms elicit an inflammatory reaction that furthers the injury to the alveolar-capillary membrane. In patients with moderate to severe *P. carinii* pneumonia, this deterioration may be sufficient to cause respiratory failure and the need for mechanical ventilation. The routine use of adjuvant corticosteroids in moderate to severe disease has significantly decreased this need for mechanical ventilation. However, the exact mechanism by which corticosteroids protect the lung from this "treatment effect" is unclear. One hypothesis is that corticosteroids may blunt the inflammatory reaction resulting from treatment and thereby protect the lungs from additional injury.

The recognition that impairment of hydrostatic forces across the alveolar-capillary membrane results from active *P. carinii* infection prompted a re-examination of fluid therapy. The parsimonious use of colloids and crystalloids reduces the risk of overhydration and alveolar flooding. In patients who require mechanical ventilation, the judicious use of positive end-expiratory pressure may significantly improve oxygenation. However, the risk of pneumothorax and bronchopleural fistula (BPF) formation versus the potential for improvement in oxygenation and survival must always be balanced.

The prognosis for patients with *P. carinii* pneumonia requiring mechanical ventilation has improved and deteriorated over the course of the epidemic. From 1981 to 1985, only 14% of persons with *P. carinii* pneumonia admitted to an intensive care unit (ICU) at SFGH for ventilatory support survived the hospitalization.[89] From 1986 to 1988, survival improved to nearly 40%.[90] The reason for this improvement is probably multifactorial. Clearly, greater experience with caring for such patients played a role. In addition, more patients received adjunctive corticosteroids compared to the previous era. More careful screening of candidates for ICU admission and mechanical ventilation may have also been a factor. A more recent report suggests that the prognosis for patients with *P. carinii* pneumonia requiring mechanical ventilation has again deteriorated.[91] This report found that overall survival for 37 patients admitted to the ICU at SFGH for mechanical ventilation from 1989 to 1991 was 24%. Predictors of poor outcome were low CD4 lymphocyte count on admission and development of pneumothorax during mechanical ventilation.

Pneumothorax

The emergence of bullous lung disease and spontaneous pneumothorax demonstrated the tissue-destructive potential of *P. carinii*. As inflammation persists and tissue necrosis proceeds, air spaces may enlarge to form frank bullae. These bullae possess an active margin of inflammation that serves as the growth front for further enlargement. As the bullae enlarge, they may impinge upon the subpleural space. As a result, bullae may rupture into the pleural cavity, causing pneumothorax. Small pneumothoraces may not require chest tube thoracostomy and may resolve without active intervention. However, careful observation is always warranted because progressive enlargement is common. Unfortunately, we have seen several life-threatening or fatal tension pneumothoraces caused by failure to vent seemingly clinically insignificant pneumothoraces. Certainly, immediate chest tube thoracostomy is required for all pneumothoraces that impair hemodynamic or respiratory function.[92]

The goal of chest tube placement is full expansion of the lung. However, this may not be attainable depending on the duration that the lung has been collapsed and the degree of lung compliance lost. Frequently, the use of chest tube thoracostomy to expand the lung will entrain a constant flow of air through a BPF. Various interventions have been used to produce closure of a BPF; most have been unqualified failures. At SFGH, we generally have a conservative approach toward management of a BPF. Treatment of the underlying *P. carinii* pneumonia, withdrawal (if possible) of adjuvant corticosteroids or mechanical ventilation, and patience are the hallmarks of BPF management at this institution. If the lungs remain expanded, pleurodesis may be attempted. The instillation of a talc slurry into the pleural space incites pleural inflammation and, ideally, adhesion of the pleural surfaces. If successful, pleurodesis may prevent further pneumothoraces. If only partially successful, the partially adhered pleural surfaces may prevent tension pneumothorax. Thoracoscopy with stapling has been performed with success for rare patients. However, this procedure can only be performed in those patients able to tolerate the procedure who have a single BPF amenable to surgical closure. As a last resort, a patient may be discharged with a chest tube in place connected to a one-way valve (Heimlich valve). Unfortunately, our experience with Heimlich valves has been dismal. Blockage resulting from pleural secretions, tension pneumothorax, and infection are frequent complications seen with one-way valve therapy.[92]

Chronic Airway Disease

Much as we were slow to note the tissue-destructive effects of *P. carinii*, we have been slow to appreciate the chronic airway disease that develops as a consequence of *P. carinii* pneumonia. Patients who have recovered from *P. carinii* pneumonia may display symptoms suggestive of chronic bronchitis, such as a chronic, often debilitating, productive cough. These unfortunate patients frequently become colonized with hospital-acquired bacterial pathogens that are difficult or impossible to eradicate; as a result, pyogenic bacterial infections

are common and result in additional airway destruction. In time, the cycles of infection and airway destruction may produce frank bronchiectasis.[93] The vicious cycle of infection, treatment with broad-spectrum antibiotics, selection of increasingly resistant organisms (particularly *Pseudomonas* and *Staphylococcus* species), and recurrent pneumonia is a common scenario among patients with advanced HIV disease and a history of *P. carinii* pneumonia.

Extrapulmonary Disease

Virtually all cases of *P. carinii* infection involve only the lungs, although the organism's ability to disseminate in rare patients has been recognized for many years. Advances in detection by substrate amplification have affirmed the presence of *P. carinii* organisms in the blood.[36] One review related disseminated *P. carinii* infection to inhaled chemoprophylaxis with aerosolized pentamidine; extrapulmonary disease is generally not seen in patients receiving systemic chemoprophylaxis with trimethoprim-sulfamethoxazole (TMP-SMX), dapsone, or, more recently, atovaquone.[94] Reported sites of dissemination include the lymph nodes, spleen, liver, bone marrow, skin, thyroid, choroid of the eye, adrenal gland, ear, peritoneum, intestine, meninges, and pancreas.[94] Although the relation between aerosolized pentamidine and extrapulmonary pneumocystosis has not been proven, the association is compelling. At SFGH, extrapulmonary *P. carinii* has virtually disappeared with the shift to systemic *P. carinii* prophylaxis. However, clinicians should always consider extrapulmonary *P. carinii* in the differential diagnosis of any febrile HIV-infected patient who is receiving aerosolized pentamidine.

DIAGNOSIS

At SFGH, we have used a diagnostic algorithm for suspected *P. carinii* pneumonia with considerable success (Fig. 20–4). In our algorithm, patients with a clinical presentation suggestive of *P. carinii* pneumonia and a compatible chest radiograph undergo sputum induction for microbiologic identification of *P. carinii*. Patients with a suggestive presentation but a normal or unchanged radiograph undergo pulmonary function testing or chest high-resolution computed tomography (HRCT). On pulmonary function testing, patients with *P. carinii* pneumonia often display a restrictive ventilatory defect with de-

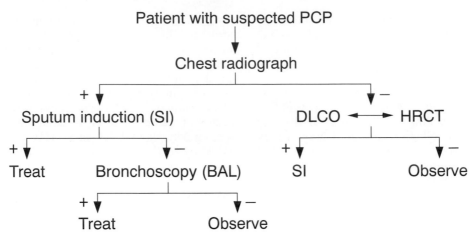

FIGURE 20–4. San Francisco General Hospital diagnostic algorithm for the evaluation of patients with suspected *P. carinii* pneumonia (PCP). BAL, bronchoalveolar lavage; DLCO, single-breath diffusing capacity for carbon monoxide; HRCT, high-resolution computed tomograph of the chest; SI, sputum induction. (From Huang L, Stansell JD: AIDS and the lung. Med Clin North Am 80:775, 1996, with permission.)

creased lung volumes and increased air flows. However, a more sensitive indicator of alveolar-capillary block,[95] and hence *P. carinii* pneumonia, is a decrease in the DL_{CO}.[96,97] The sensitivity of a decreased DL_{CO} (defined as ≤75% of the predicted value, corrected for hemoglobin) for *P. carinii* is 90% in symptomatic patients with normal or unchanged chest radiographs.[98] Moreover, the combination of a normal or unchanged chest radiograph and a DL_{CO} greater than 75% of predicted virtually rules out the possibility of *P. carinii* pneumonia. As a result, we recommend that these patients either be clinically observed without further evaluation or treatment for *P. carinii* or be evaluated/treated for another process. Although a decreased DL_{CO} is a sensitive test for *P. carinii*, it lacks specificity. In the same study reporting a sensitivity of 90% for a DL_{CO} of 75% or less of predicted for *P. carinii*, the specificity was 53%.[98] Therefore, a decreased DL_{CO} is not diagnostic of *P. carinii* pneumonia, and patients with suspected *P. carinii* who have a decreased DL_{CO} still undergo sputum induction in our algorithm.

The low specificity of a decreased DL_{CO} led us to evaluate alternative diagnostic tests. *Pneumocystis carinii* pneumonia has a characteristic appearance on HRCT, that is, patchy areas of ground-glass opacity through which vessels are seen and a background of interlobular septal thickening[99–101] (Fig. 20–5). We studied HRCT in persons with suspected *P. carinii* pneumonia but a normal, unchanged, or equivocal chest radiograph.[102] In this study, no patient with suspected *P. carinii* pneumonia, with a normal, un-

changed, or equivocal chest radiograph, and with an HRCT without ground-glass opacity had a diagnosis of *P. carinii* pneumonia established either on bronchoscopy or after 60 days of clinical follow-up. Unfortunately, similar to a DL_{CO} of 75% or less of predicted, an HRCT with ground-glass opacity lacks specificity for *P. carinii*, and persons with suspected *P. carinii* pneumonia with these findings on HRCT must undergo sputum induction. Whether HRCT will supplant the DL_{CO} in the diagnostic algorithm for suspected pneumonia awaits further analysis.

Gallium scanning is a highly sensitive but nonspecific test for *P. carinii*. In addition, this test suffers from relatively high cost, time delays in obtaining the imaging, and the baseline mild to moderate gallium uptake in the lungs of HIV-infected persons without active pulmonary infection. In our opinion, these factors, combined with the availability and sensitivity of both pulmonary function testing and HRCT scanning, render the test rarely useful in diagnosing *P. carinii* pneumonia.

Although cough productive of clear-white sputum is a frequent presenting complaint in patients with *P. carinii* pneumonia, expectorated sputum is rarely suitable for microscopic evaluation. Similarly, purulent sputum, whether spontaneously produced or induced, is inadequate for *P. carinii* examination. Cells and cellular debris in such specimens make identification of *P. carinii* organisms virtually impossible. Patients in whom there is high suspicion of *P. carinii* pneumonia who have a purulent sputum specimen should be treated with a course of an-

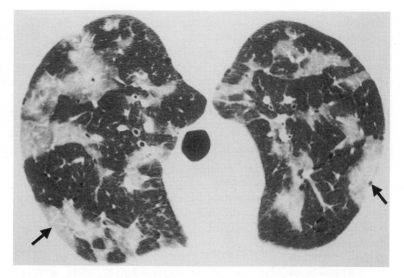

FIGURE 20–5. High-resolution computed tomograph of the chest of an HIV-infected patient with *P. carinii* pneumonia and a normal chest radiograph revealing the characteristic patchy area of ground glass opacities (*arrows*). (From Huang L, Stansell JD: AIDS and the lung. Med Clin North Am 80:775, 1996, with permission.)

tibiotics and possibly *P. carinii* therapy first. If the diagnosis remains in question, then a sputum induction should be obtained after the respiratory secretions have cleared.

Induction of nonpurulent sputum is a simple, inexpensive, and effective means of diagnosing *P. carinii* pneumonia.[103–108] After the patient cleanses the oral cavity with a soft brush and normal saline, a deep sputum specimen is induced by the inhalation of hypertonic (3%) saline. The sample is then digested, centrifuged, plated, and stained.[105] Modified Giemsa, toluidine blue O, or Gomori methenamine silver stain can be used to identify *P. carinii* organisms. Newer direct and indirect fluorescent antibody techniques have improved the sensitivity for induced sputum examination.[105,109] At SFGH, the sensitivity of induced sputum examination for *P. carinii* has been consistently between 74% and 83%.[105,110] However, this range of sensitivities is not high enough to confidently exclude a diagnosis of *P. carinii* pneumonia if a negative result is obtained and, therefore, further diagnostic testing is necessary.

In cases of suspected *P. carinii* pneumonia in which induced sputum examination is negative for *P. carinii* and other pathogens, a fiberoptic bronchoscopy with bronchoalveolar lavage (BAL) should be performed. Bronchoscopy with BAL fluid examination is sensitive for *P. carinii*.[111–114] In contrast to a negative induced sputum examination, a negative BAL fluid examination for *P. carinii* may be sufficient to rule out a diagnosis of *P. carinii* pneumonia. A review at SFGH of 100 HIV-infected patients with suspected *P. carinii* pneumonia who had a negative BAL fluid examination for *P. carinii* and

had no *P. carinii* therapy identified two cases of subsequent *P. carinii* pneumonia within 60 days of the initial negative evaluation (one case after 46 days, the other after 51 days).[110] Thus a negative BAL fluid examination for *P. carinii* may obviate the need for more invasive procedures (i.e., transbronchial biopsy). However, in populations of HIV-infected persons with a high background incidence of *Mycobacterium tuberculosis* infection, the diagnosis of tuberculosis may be enhanced by the use of transbronchial biopsy.

The coordinated effort of a number of services is vital to the optimal use of our diagnostic algorithm. First, clinicians initiate an evaluation and refer those patients with suspected *P. carinii* pneumonia for sputum induction. Next, the Pulmonary Service screens all requests for sputum induction. The Pulmonary Service denies approximately 25% to 30% of all requests (in which case recommendations for further evaluation or treatment are provided). Those patients for whom the request is approved undergo sputum induction the same day as the screening. Third, a pulmonary laboratory technician closely supervises all patients undergoing sputum induction in order to obtain a good specimen. Finally, one of two microbiology technicians processes all specimens for *P. carinii* and reviews each slide with a microbiologist. In our opinion, these factors combine to permit the pursuit of definitive diagnoses of *P. carinii* pneumonia preferable to empiric therapy.

Is empiric *P. carinii* pneumonia therapy a viable option?[115–118] Certainly, there are a host of pressures upon clinicians today that make empiric *P. carinii* pneumonia therapy attractive.

However, empiric therapy should be considered with caution, and appropriate patients should be selected carefully. A number of criteria should be met before empiric therapy is begun (Table 20–1). First, the patient must be at risk for *P. carinii* pneumonia, usually on the basis of a CD4 lymphocyte count of less than 200 cells/μl or a prior history of *P. carinii* pneumonia. Next, the patient should not be on *P. carinii* prophylaxis, especially TMP-SMX. Because the development of *P. carinii* pneumonia while on this combination is infrequent, clinicians who encounter such a patient should make every effort to find an alternate diagnosis before embarking on a course of empiric therapy. Third, the patient should have a clinical and radiographic presentation strongly suggestive of *P. carinii* pneumonia. The presence of atypical features should prompt a consideration of alternate diagnoses. Furthermore, the patient should have mild disease. The potential consequences of a missed or delayed diagnosis in a patient with severe respiratory dysfunction argue strongly for the pursuit of a definitive diagnosis in most, if not all, cases. Next, the patient should be reliable, compliant with medications, able to tolerate the proposed therapy (without nausea/vomiting, diarrhea, or a history of previous adverse drug reactions to that therapy), able to recognize the early progression of symptoms, and willing to return for follow-up visits. In patients fulfilling these criteria, empiric therapy may be a suitable alternative to invasive diagnostic procedures. However, if there is clinical progression or even a slow clinical response to empiric therapy, then diagnostic tests and procedures should be pursued.[119]

TREATMENT

At the time the first cases of AIDS-related *P. carinii* pneumonia were recognized, two drugs, TMP-SMX and pentamidine isethionate, were available for treatment. Indeed, it was the sudden increase in requests for pentamidine that alerted the Centers for Disease Control to a possible new epidemic. Unfortunately, both drugs show a high frequency of adverse reactions and poor tolerability.[120–122] Accordingly, a concerted effort has been made to identify and develop new treatment regimens that are free of serious side effects or at least do not have overlapping toxicity. These efforts have met with mixed success. Currently, several choices are available for treatment of *P. carinii* pneumonia (Tables 20–2 and 20–3).

Trimethoprim-Sulfamethoxazole

TMP-SMX remains the drug of choice for the treatment of *P. carinii* pneumonia. No other drug or drug combination has been shown to be superior to TMP-SMX in efficacy.[123–131] TMP and SMX both act to inhibit key enzymatic steps in folate metabolism. TMP inhibits dihydrofolate reductase (DHFR), preventing the synthesis of tetrahydrofolate from dihydrofolate, while SMX acts upon dihydropteroate synthase (DHPS) to prevent the conversion of *para*-aminobenzoate to dihydrofolic acid. Although TMP alone has no demonstrable anti-*Pneumocystis* activity, when combined with SMX, it produces a synergistic inhibition of *P. carinii*. Significantly, neither of these two agents is the most avid enzyme inhibitor in their class. Pyrimethamine, trimetrexate (TMTX), and methotrexate are orders of magnitude more inhibitory for DHFR than TMP, whereas many sulfones and sulfonamides show greater inhibition of DHPS than SMX. However, TMP-SMX benefits from its availability as a single-combination medication, excellent bioavailability, similar half-lives, and two decades of clinical use. Moreover, utilizing the rat model, Hughes and colleagues have demonstrated the combination

---

TABLE 20–1. Criteria for Empiric *Pneumocystis carinii* Pneumonia Therapy

- Patient is at risk for *P. carinii* pneumonia.
- CD4 lymphocyte count <200 cells/μl
- History of prior *P. carinii* pneumonia
- Patient is not receiving *P. carinii* pneumonia prophylaxis (especially TMP-SMX)
- Patient has a clinical presentation suggestive of *P. carinii* pneumonia
- History of dyspnea on exertion and/or nonproductive cough
- Chest radiograph reveals bilateral interstitial infiltrates
- No evidence of another infectious process
- Patient has mild disease
- Room air PaO_2 >70 mm Hg, alveolar-arterial oxygen difference <35 mm Hg
- Patient is reliable
- Patient is compliant with medications
- Patient can tolerate oral medications
- No complaints of nausea, vomiting, or diarrhea
- No previous adverse reactions to proposed *P. carinii* pneumonia therapy
- Patient is at low risk for tuberculosis, histoplasmosis, coccidioidomycosis, or other infection likely to mimic *P. carinii* pneumonia
- Sputum induction is unavailable or its sensitivity for *P. carinii* is low
- Careful follow-up is available

TABLE 20–2. Treatment Options for Moderate to Severe *P. carinii* Pneumonia

TREATMENT REGIMEN	DOSE(S), ROUTE, FREQUENCY	SIDE EFFECT(S)
Trimethoprim (TMP)– sulfamethoxazole (SMX)	15 mg/kg (TMP), IV, divided every 6– 8 hr*	Rash,[†] fever, N/V, ↑ liver function tests, ↑ K⁺, neutropenia
Pentamidine isethionate	3–4 mg/kg, IV, once daily	Nephrotoxicity, ↑ K⁺, ↓ Ca²⁺/Mg²⁺, ↑ amylase, ↓↑ glucose[‡]
Trimetrexate plus leucovorin ± dapsone[§]	45 mg/m², IV, once daily, plus 20 mg/ m², PO, every 6 hr ± 100 mg, PO, once daily	Neutropenia, thrombocytopenia, rash, fever, ↑ liver function tests, hemolytic anemia (check G6PD level), methemoglobinemia
Clindamycin plus primaquine	1800 mg, IV, divided every 6–8 hr plus 30 mg (base), PO, once daily	Rash, N/V, diarrhea, hemolytic anemia (check G6PD), methemoglobinemia

N/V, nausea and vomiting; G6PD, glucose-6-phosphate dehydrogenase.
*TMP-SMX is dispensed as a fixed combination.
[†]Mild rash that does not cause bullous skin lesions and does not involve mucous membranes can often be treated with antihistamines first and should not necessarily result in discontinuation of drug.
[‡]Avoid other nephrotoxic agents (nonsteroidal anti-inflammatory agents, aminoglycosides, foscarnet, amphotericin B). Risk of hypotension can be minimized if infusion is given over a 2- to 3-hour period.
[§]A study is in progress comparing TMP-SMX to trimetrexate-dapsone (plus leucovorin).

of TMP and SMX to be the most potent inhibitor of *P. carinii* among commonly used medications.[132]

In 1978, Hughes and colleagues documented the efficacy of TMP-SMX in children with cancer and established the dose of the combination at 20 mg/kg/day of the TMP component.[133] Subsequent studies in AIDS patients sought to match this established dose in comparative trials. Wharton and colleagues studied 40 patients with their first episode of *P. carinii* pneumonia in a prospective, randomized trial of TMP-SMX at a dose of 20 mg/kg/day versus pentamidine at a dose of 4 mg/kg/day.[131] Of 20 patients treated with TMP-SMX, 75% survived past the 21-day treatment period but 10% required a switch to pentamidine because of treatment failure and 50% because of adverse drug reactions. Klein and co-workers studied 160 patients with moderate to severe *P. carinii* pneumonia in a prospective, randomized trial of TMP-SMX at a dose of 20 mg/kg/day versus pentamidine at a dose of 4 mg/kg/day.[124] Of 92 patients randomized to TMP-SMX, 67% survived but only 24% were able to successfully complete treatment; in 42% therapy failed because of disease progression and in 34% it failed because of drug toxicity. Similarly, Sattler and colleagues studied 215 patients with moderate to severe disease in a prospective, randomized trial of TMTX at a dose of 45 mg/m²/day (plus leucovorin) versus TMP-SMX at a dose of 20 mg/kg/day.[128] Among those treated with TMP-SMX, 88% survived off respiratory support at day 21 of therapy, while in 20%, TMP-SMX failed because of lack of efficacy and 28% required discontinuation because of drug toxicity. Of note, all of these stud-

ies antedated the routine use of adjunctive corticosteroids.

In 1988, Sattler and colleagues published the results of a prospective, noncrossover trial of TMP-SMX versus pentamidine in 70 patients.[127] Rather than using a fixed dose of TMP-SMX, dosing was adjusted to maintain a TMP serum level of 5 to 8 gm/ml. The average dose received by patients assigned to TMP-SMX was 12 mg/kg/day. Despite this dose reduction, 86% of TMP-SMX–treated patients survived and were without respiratory support at the end of treatment. As a result of this study, TMP-SMX at a dose of 15 mg/kg/day of the TMP component has become the widely accepted dose. Unfortunately, few trials have utilized this dose in comparing therapies for moderate to severe *P. carinii* pneumonia. A randomized trial of TMP-SMX versus clindamycin-primaquine had a mixed population of mild and severe disease, oral and intravenous therapy, and inconsistent steroid use. However, dosing TMP-SMX at 15 to 20 mg/kg/day resulted in successful outcomes in 91% and dose-limiting toxicity in only 20% of patients.[129,130]

The best current insight into the efficacy and tolerability of TMP-SMX comes from trials of oral therapy for mild to moderate *P. carinii* pneumonia. In these studies, 320 mg TMP and 1600 mg SMX (two double-strength tablets) given orally three times daily approximates the 15-mg/kg/day intravenous dosing schedule. In a prospective, randomized trial of 322 patients with mild to moderate *P. carinii* pneumonia who received TMP-SMX at a dose of 320 mg TMP and 1600 mg SMX tid versus atovaquone tablets at a dose of 750 mg tid, 7% of the 146 evaluable

TABLE 20–3. Treatment Options for Mild to Moderate *P. carinii* Pneumonia

TREATMENT REGIMEN	DOSE(S), ROUTE, FREQUENCY	SIDE EFFECT(S)
Trimethoprim (TMP)–sulfamethoxazole (SMX)	15 mg/kg (TMP), PO, divided every 6–8 hr	See Table 20–2
Clindamycin plus primaquine	1800 mg, PO, divided every 6–8 hr plus 30 mg (base), PO, once daily	See Table 20–2
Trimethoprim plus dapsone	15 mg/kg, PO, divided every 6–8 hr plus 100 mg, PO, once daily	Rash, N/V, hemolytic anemia (check G6PD level), methemoglobinemia
Atovaquone	750 mg, PO (suspension), thrice daily	Rash, GI (N/V/diarrhea); well tolerated but poorly absorbed, especially in patients with diarrhea
Pentamidine isethionate	3–4 mg/kg, IV, once daily	See Table 20–2
Trimetrexate plus leucovorin ± dapsone	45 mg/m^2, IV, once daily plus 20 mg/m^2, PO, every 6 hr ± 100 mg, PO, once daily	See Table 20–2

N/V, nausea and vomiting; GI, gastrointestinal; GGPD, glucose-6-phosphate dehydrogenase.

persons assigned to TMP-SMX had therapy fail because of lack of therapeutic efficacy and in 20% it failed because of treatment-limiting adverse reactions.[123] Similar results were obtained in the ACTG 108 study examining the efficacy and safety of three orally available combinations for the treatment of mild to moderate *P. carinii* pneumonia (320 mg TMP and 1600 mg SMX tid versus TMP 300 mg tid plus dapsone 100 mg daily versus clindamycin 600 mg tid with primaquine base 30 mg daily).[126] Overall, 54% of participants completed therapy on the assigned drug, with 50% of those randomized to TMP-SMX completing 3 weeks of assigned treatment. Of patients randomized to TMP-SMX, 9% experienced clinical disease progression on or before day 21, necessitating alternative therapy, and 36% had dose-limiting toxicity. The commonly encountered toxicities associated with TMP-SMX include rash, drug fever, nausea, vomiting, liver function abnormalities, hyperkalemia, and bone marrow suppression, particularly neutropenia (Table 20–2).[120,134] Typically, these toxicities manifest within the first 8 to 12 days of therapy but may develop at any point during treatment.[126] Adverse drug reactions often can be attributed to elevated drug levels of TMP, SMX, or both,[123] suggesting that monitoring drug levels or reducing doses of medications may ameliorate drug toxicity.

Over the course of the HIV epidemic, clinicians have grown increasingly comfortable with managing non–life-threatening drug toxicity caused by TMP-SMX. The routine use of antihistamines to treat rash and antiemetics to treat the gastrointestinal complaints has allowed patients to remain on TMP-SMX treatment. The use of granulocyte colony-stimulating factor and erythropoietin may influence the course of drug-induced cytopenias; however, the role these expensive modalities will play has yet to be determined. Attempts to ameliorate myelosuppression with co-administration of folinic acid have failed to define any beneficial effect. To the contrary, results would indicate a deleterious effect on outcome of *P. carinii* treatment, with an increased risk of therapeutic failure and death among persons receiving such adjunctive therapy.

Pentamidine

Traditionally, pentamidine has been the second-line agent for the treatment of *P. carinii* pneumonia. Typically, clinicians turn to this agent when patients become intolerant of or fail to respond to TMP-SMX. Unfortunately, pentamidine is associated with frequent, severe, and oftentimes permanent toxicities. Today, alternatives to pentamidine are available for the treatment of patients intolerant of or unresponsive to TMP-SMX, and a strategy of using pentamidine as a second-line agent must be reexamined.

Pentamidine isethionate is an aromatic diamine with an uncertain mechanism of action against *P. carinii*. Despite its long use in the treatment of *P. carinii* pneumonia, relatively little is known about the pharmacokinetics and pharmacodynamics of this drug. Studies indicate a large volume of distribution and a long elimination half-life.[135] The drug appears to be preferentially concentrated in certain major organs, particularly the kidneys, and probably requires several days to reach a therapeutic concentration in the lungs.[122] Several clinical trials examined the efficacy and toxicity of pentamidine at a dose of 4 mg/kg/day compared to TMP-SMX.[124,127,131] In 20 patients with a first episode of *P. carinii* pneumonia, 95% of patients treated with pentamidine survived past the 21-day treatment period but only 45% actually completed therapy on pentamidine.[131] In 68 patients with moderate to severe *P. carinii* pneumonia, 74% of patients randomized to receive pentamidine survived, but only 35% were able to successfully complete treatment, with failure in 40% because of disease progression and in 25% because of drug toxicity.[124] Neither of these studies found any significant difference between pentamidine and TMP-SMX in terms of survival, therapeutic failure, or adverse effects.

In a randomized, noncrossover trial involving 70 patients with moderate to severe disease, pentamidine was considerably less effective than TMP-SMX.[127] Only 61% of persons assigned to treatment with pentamidine at a dose of 4 mg/kg/day survived off respiratory support to day 21 of therapy, compared with 86% of persons assigned to TMP-SMX (95% CI for the difference in response, 5% to 45%; $p = .03$). Although the dose of pentamidine was adjusted 30% to 50% for rising serum creatinine, nephrotoxicity occurred in 64%, hypotension in 27%, and hypoglycemia in 21% of pentamidine-treated patients. Finally, a small trial to evaluate an attenuated dose (3.2 ± 0.9 mg/kg/day) of pentamidine in the treatment of mild to moderate *P. carinii* pneumonia found successful outcomes in 81% of patients, with major adverse drug reactions occurring in 14% and minor reactions in 38%.[136]

The major toxicities related to pentamidine administration are renal and pancreatic (Table 20–2). The exact mechanism of nephrotoxicity is incompletely understood. However, special caution must be used to avoid administering pentamidine with other potentially nephrotoxic drugs such as aminoglycosides, nonsteroidal anti-inflammatory agents, foscarnet, or amphotericin B. Hypoglycemia results from direct toxicity to pancreatic islet cells and may presage frank diabetes mellitus. Occurring an average of 8 days into therapy, these toxicities appear to depend upon the cumulative dose. A 5-year retrospective review of the incidence of pentamidine-related adverse drug reactions at SFGH in patients who received at least 5 days of pentamidine therapy found a 72% incidence of treatment-limiting toxicity. Renal toxicity occurred in 49%, hypoglycemia in 24%, and pancreatitis in 9% of pentamidine-treated patients.[137]

Clindamycin-Primaquine

The combination of the lincosamide antibiotic clindamycin (600 to 900 mg every 6 to 8 hours) with the dihydrofolate reductase inhibitor primaquine (15 to 30 mg/day) has gained widespread acceptance and use against all degrees of severity of *P. carinii* pneumonia. Neither drug has activity against *P. carinii* by itself, but animal models confirm the activity of the combination.[138] Unfortunately, rigorous, standardized trials of this combination are largely lacking. Various doses, dosing schedules, and drug formulations have been investigated in a variety of disease severities.[126,130,139–142] The combination was effective in all but 2 of 28 episodes of *P. carinii* pneumonia (25 patients, 17 of whom had been unresponsive to or intolerant of conventional treatment and 8 of whom were being treated for the first time).[142] In a noncomparative, open-label study of 36 patients with mild to moderate *P. carinii* pneumonia and in a similar study of 60 patients, a 92% rate of successful treatment and a 13% incidence of dose-limiting toxicities were found with clindamycin (900 mg every 8 hours intravenously or 450 mg every 6 hours orally) and primaquine (30 mg/day base).[139,140]

A randomized, blinded trial in 65 patients with *P. carinii* pneumonia found virtually identical efficacy using clindamycin plus 15 mg/day of primaquine compared to TMP-SMX.[129] Rash was the most common side effect, occurring in 60% of patients, and gastrointestinal upset was the most common side effect seen with TMP-SMX. An update confirmed the above findings in a cohort of over 100 patients.[130] The ACTG 108 trial offers the best insight into the use of oral clindamycin 600 mg every 8 hours plus primaquine 30 mg/day, versus TMP-SMX or TMP-dapsone.[126] Of the 64 persons with mild to moderate *P. carinii* pneumonia assigned to clindamycin-primaquine, 52% completed 3 weeks of therapy on the study drug combination, 7% experienced clinical disease progression on or before day 21 of therapy, and 33% had dose-limiting toxicity. No statistical differences in efficacy or toxicity were found between any of the three treatment arms. Unfortunately, this study lacked adequate power to find a difference in efficacy but could detect a 25% difference in adverse drug events. Virtually all of the adverse drug events occurred during the first 2 weeks of therapy. Among persons receiving clindamycin-primaquine, rash was the most frequently encountered dose-limiting toxicity, occurring in 21%. Cytopenias occurred in 12%, gastrointestinal intolerance in 3%, and elevations in liver enzymes in 2%. Drug fever accounted for less than 2% of dose-limiting drug reactions in the clindamycin-primaquine group.

Primaquine and clindamycin are strong oxidants and are relatively contraindicated in persons with glucose-6-phosphate dehydrogenase deficiency (Table 20–3). Methemoglobinemia is also a potential dose-limiting toxicity, although modest levels of methemoglobin (<15%) can be found in most primaquine-treated patients and only a few will require treatment with reducing agents or alternative therapy.

Trimetrexate

TMTX is a highly lipophilic folate antagonist structurally related to methotrexate. The drug readily diffuses across cell membranes and inhibits DHFR 1500 times more potently than TMP.[143] TMTX's affinity for DHFR and the potential for interruption of folate metabolism is so great that folinic acid (leucovorin) must be given with TMTX. Herein lies the mechanism of action of TMTX–folinic acid. Folinic acid, a hydrophilic compound, requires active transport across cell membranes. Mammalian cells possess such an active transport system, whereas *P. carinii* apparently lacks such a system. Therefore, human cells are protected from the antifolate effects of TMTX by the administration of folinic acid, whereas *P. carinii* cannot accumulate folinic acid and therefore is fully susceptible to the folate-inhibitory effects of the drug. The long half-life of the drug (8 to 10 hours) permits once-a-day dosing. The drug is principally metabolized by the liver, and the glucuronide or sulfate salt is excreted by the kidney.

An open-label, nonrandomized trial of TMTX (30 mg/m²/day)–folinic acid (20 mg/kg every 6 hours) alone or in combination with sulfadiazine (1 gm every 6 hours) enrolled 49 patients and stratified them by intolerance to or disease progression on TMP/SMX.[143] Eighty-eight percent of the patients with a history of intolerance to sulfonamide treated with TMTX–folinic acid as initial treatment were alive and receiving no respiratory support 2 weeks after completion of therapy. In those treated with TMTX–folinic acid because of disease progression on or intolerance to initial treatment with TMP-SMX, 69% survived. Among those initially treated with TMTX–folinic acid plus sulfadiazine, 77% survived. Initial enthusiasm was somewhat tempered by a 60% relapse rate in the 3 months

following completion of therapy in the group receiving TMTX–folinic acid as initial therapy. The relapse rate was 6% among those receiving TMTX–folinic acid–sulfadiazine and 0% among those receiving TMTX–folinic acid for salvage therapy. However, this study was performed prior to the routine use of secondary *P. carinii* prophylaxis. TMTX was well tolerated, with neutropenia and thrombocytopenia being the most common dose-limiting toxicities. A TMTX dose of 45 mg/m²/day with a folinic acid dose of 80 mg/m²/day was later established as the optimum dose for treatment of *P. carinii* pneumonia.[144]

The clearest insight into monotherapy with TMTX–folinic acid for *P. carinii* pneumonia is provided by the ACTG 029/031 trial.[128] This was a randomized, double-blind multicenter trial comparing TMTX at a dose of 45 mg/m²/day plus folinic acid at a dose of 20 mg/m² every 6 hours to TMP-SMX at a dose of 20 mg/kg/day in patients with moderate to severe *P. carinii* pneumonia. Because the trial began accrual prior to the National Institutes of Health– University of California (NIH-UC) Expert Panel Consensus statement recommendations for steroid use in *P. carinii* pneumonia, use of adjunctive corticosteroids was not permitted. Study endpoints were mortality at day 21 of therapy and clinical response at days 10 and 21. A total of 215 patients were enrolled and maintained in the double-blind portion of the trial until day 10. At that point, patients were assessed as "responders" or "failures." Responders progressed into the open-label phase of the trial comparing oral TMP-SMX to continued intravenous TMTX–folinic acid while "failures" were offered alternative therapy. By day 10 of therapy, the failure rate was 16% in the TMP-SMX group and 27% in the TMTX–folinic acid group (*p* = .064). By day 21, 20% of the TMP-SMX patients and 38% of the TMTX–folinic acid patients were considered clinical failures (*p* = .008). Similarly, there was a trend toward improved survival at day 21 with TMP-SMX compared to TMTX–folinic acid. These differences in mortality were significant by day 49 of therapy (16% versus 31%; *p* = .028). Relapse occurred in 13% of the TMTX treatment group and none of the TMP-SMX treatment group during days 21 through 49. However, dose-limiting toxicity was much more common in the TMP-SMX treatment group, with 29% experiencing toxicity-related discontinuations. Only 10% of the TMTX–folinic acid treatment group had similar dose-limiting toxicity. The most common side effects encountered were hepatitis

(13% with TMP–SMX versus 4% with TMTX), gastrointestinal intolerance (7% with TMP-SMX versus 1% with TMTX), and cytopenias (13% with TMP-SMX versus 4% with TMTX).

These results confirmed that although effective in the treatment of moderate to severe _P. carinii_ pneumonia, TMTX–folinic acid as monotherapy is not as effective as TMP-SMX. Similar results were obtained when single-agent dapsone was evaluated for treatment of _P. carinii_.[145] However, both of these agents have activity against _P. carinii_ and would be an attractive combination because of their efficacy and toxicity profiles. A small Phase I trial of TMTX at a dose of 45 mg/m^2/day, folinic acid at a dose of 80 mg/m^2/day plus dapsone at a dose of 100 mg/day compared to TMP-SMX at a dose of 15 mg/kg/day in moderate to severe _P. carinii_ pneumonia has been completed (J.D. Stansell, unpublished data). All patients received adjunctive corticosteroids at recommended doses. Fifteen patients were randomized to receive TMTX–folinic acid–dapsone and five patients to receive TMP-SMX. Twelve of 15 (80%) TMTX–folinic acid–dapsone patients and 3 of 5 (60%) TMP-SMX patients were responders at day 21. There were two episodes of grade III/IV toxicity among the TMTX–folinic acid–dapsone treatment group and four episodes among the TMP-SMX group. No patient who successfully completed either therapy relapsed during the month following therapy. These data suggest TMTX–folinic acid plus dapsone may be clinically useful against _P. carinii_. Where the combination fits in the armamentarium awaits further large-scale clinical trials.

Trimethoprim-Dapsone

Because oral TMP-SMX is poorly tolerated, alternative oral combinations have been sought for the treatment of mild _P. carinii_ pneumonia. One of the first combinations to receive widespread attention was TMP plus the sulfone antibiotic dapsone. Dapsone is a powerful DHPS inhibitor that has been used successfully to treat murine _P. carinii_.[146] Although dapsone had an unacceptably high rate of treatment failure when used alone,[145] the combination of dapsone plus TMP (dapsone 100 mg/day plus TMP 20 mg/kg/day) was an effective _P. carinii_ pneumonia treatment in an open-label, pilot study of 15 patients at SFGH.[147] Two patients in this small trial experienced dose-limiting toxicity. A subsequent prospective, randomized clinical trial compared the safety and efficacy of TMP at a dose of 20 mg/kg/day plus dapsone at a dose of 100 mg/day with TMP-SMX at a dose of 20 mg/kg/day in 60 patients with mild to moderate _P. carinii_ pneumonia.[125] Disease progression occurred in 2 of 30 patients assigned to TMP-dapsone compared to 3 of 30 assigned to TMP-SMX ($p \geq$ .3). Fifty-seven percent of the TMP-SMX–treated patients encountered dose-limiting toxicity compared to 30% of the TMP-dapsone–treated group ($p <$ .025). The major toxicities with TMP-dapsone were rash and gastrointestinal complaints.

The ACTG 108 trial examined oral TMP-dapsone in a comparative trial with oral TMP-SMX and clindamycin-primaquine. Fifty-nine patients with mild to moderate _P. carinii_ pneumonia were randomized to TMP at a dose of 300 mg tid plus dapsone at a dose of 100 mg/day. Sixty percent of patients on TMP-dapsone completed 21 days of therapy on assigned therapy and 12% experienced disease progression on or before day 21 of therapy, compared to 9% of TMP-SMX– and 7% of clindamycin-primaquine–treated patients ($p =$ .7). There were no differences in death at day 81 between the treatment arms. Twenty-four percent of patients assigned to TMP-dapsone experienced dose-limiting toxicity, compared to 36% of TMP-SMX–treated patients and 33% of clindamycin-primaquine–treated patients. The most frequent dose-limiting adverse drug reactions were rash (10%), nausea and vomiting (8.5%), neutropenia (3%), and diarrhea (3%). Finally, a quality-of-life instrument indicated a trend toward better quality-of-life outcomes with TMP-dapsone compared to the other two study arms at completion of therapy. This study, as did earlier studies, demonstrates TMP-dapsone to be effective and well-tolerated treatment for mild to moderate _P. carinii_ pneumonia.

Atovaquone

Atovaquone, an oral hydroxynapthoquinone, inhibits electron transport in the mitochondrial oxidation-reduction pathway of _P. carinii_. Complicating the use of this medication has been its poor bioavailability, particularly when coupled with chronic diarrhea, although the introduction of a suspension product has somewhat ameliorated concern about achieving adequate serum drug levels. The medication has been evaluated for the treatment of mild to moderate _P. carinii_ pneumonia in both open-label and randomized comparison clinical trials.[123,148,149] In 34 patients with mild to moderate disease (mean room air

PaO$_2$ = 78 mm Hg) treated with several dosages of single-agent atovaquone, treatment was discontinued in four patients for toxicity (rash and drug fever in two patients each) and in five patients for disease progression.[149] Seven (26%) of the 27 successfully treated patients experienced recurrent *P. carinii* pneumonia within 6 months despite secondary *P. carinii* prophylaxis. Outcomes did not appear to be dose related.

A prospective, randomized trial of atovaquone tablets at a dose of 750 mg tid versus TMP-SMX at a dose of 320 mg TMP plus 1600 mg SMX tid in 322 patients with mild to moderate *P. carinii* pneumonia found that treatment failed because of lack of therapeutic efficacy in 20% of 138 evaluable persons assigned to atovaquone, compared with 7% of the TMP-SMX group (*p* = .002); treatment failed in 7% because of treatment-limiting adverse reactions, compared with 20% for the TMP-SMX group (*p* = .001).[123] The most common treatment-limiting adverse effects seen in the atovaquone group were rash (4%) and liver dysfunction (3%). There were 11 deaths in the atovaquone arm compared to a single death in the TMP-SMX arm within 4 weeks of completion of therapy (*p* = .003). These deaths and therapeutic failures on the atovaquone arm were highly correlated with the presence of diarrhea at entry into the study.

A similar randomized, open-label trial has compared atovaquone tablets at a dose of 750 mg every 8 hours to pentamidine at a dose of 4 mg/kg/day in patients with a history of intolerance to TMP-SMX.[148] As in the previous study, atovaquone was less effective (29% disease progression for atovaquone versus 17% for pentamidine; *p* = .18) but better tolerated (4% dose-limiting toxicity compared to 36% for pentamidine; *p* < .001). The mortality rate was similar in both groups (nine deaths) but is generally believed to be unacceptably high compared to other treatment regimens. These studies and continued concerns about the adequacy of drug levels achieved in AIDS patients lend uncertainty to the role of atovaquone (especially as a single agent) in the treatment of HIV-associated *P. carinii* pneumonia. Certainly, at present, this medication cannot be viewed as a first- or second-line agent.

Aerosolized Pentamidine

Two small, open-label trials and a large, double-blind comparative trial with TMP-SMX at a dose of 15 mg/kg/day have shown inhaled pen-

tamidine to be an inferior treatment for *P. carinii* pneumonia.[136,150,151] Significantly higher rates of recrudescence of symptoms and relapse of *P. carinii* pneumonia were found in patients treated with inhaled pentamidine at a dose of 600 mg/day compared to those receiving parenteral pentamidine at a dose of 3 mg/kg/day.[136] Similarly, treatment failure was significantly higher (55%) with inhaled pentamidine compared to parenteral pentamidine at a dose of 4 mg/kg/day (0%).[151] The ACTG 040 trial examined the efficacy of aerosolized pentamidine 600 mg/day versus TMP-SMX at a dose of 15 mg/kg/day in 367 patients with an alveolar-arterial oxygen difference of less than 55 mm Hg.[150] This study documented a significantly higher rate of treatment failure, more protracted recovery, and more frequent relapse among the aerosolized pentamidine–treated group. These studies overwhelmingly affirm the limited, if any, role for aerosolized pentamidine in the treatment of *P. carinii* pneumonia.

Adjuvant Corticosteroid Therapy

Despite the availability of effective anti-*Pneumocystis* drugs, the mortality rate of *P. carinii* pneumonia remains appreciable. The majority of these deaths are caused by progressive lung disease that culminates in intractable hypoxemic respiratory failure. A frequent clinical observation is that worsening often takes place suddenly 3 to 5 days after beginning anti-*Pneumocystis* therapy, even in patients whose disease had been slowly progressive. Several trials have now documented the usefulness of adjunctive corticosteroids in mitigating the sudden deterioration in gas exchange seen several days into standard treatment. Four clinical trials now support the use of corticosteroids in moderate to severe *P. carinii* pneumonia.[152–155] An early deterioration in oxygen saturation occurred in 8 of 19 placebo-treated patients compared to 1 of 18 steroid-treated patients.[154] In the largest study, corticosteroids significantly decreased the early deterioration in gas exchange.[152] These investigators further demonstrated that patients with the most severe disease benefitted the most. In the most severely ill cohort studied, adjunctive corticosteroids significantly ameliorated respiratory failure and death.[153]

Based on these conclusive studies, in 1990 the NIH-UC Expert Panel for Corticosteroids as Adjunctive Therapy for Pneumocystis Pneumonia concluded that such therapy "can clearly reduce the likelihood of death, respiratory failure, or deterioration of oxygenation in patients with moderate-to-severe pneumocystis pneumonia.''[156] The panel further recommended that adjunctive corticosteroids be used in adults or adolescents (children >13 years old) with documented or suspected *P. carinii* pneumonia if they are hypoxic, as defined by an arterial Po_2 of 70 mm Hg or an alveolar-arterial Po_2 difference of 35 mm Hg. Adjunctive corticosteroids, either oral prednisone or intravenous methylprednisolone, should be started when specific anti-*Pneumocystis* treatment is begun; a delay in the administration of corticosteroids may nullify their effectiveness. There is no reason why these drugs cannot be used along with anti-*Pneumocystis* treatment in patients who meet the indications while diagnostic efforts are underway. However, if no diagnosis or some other diagnosis is made, the need for corticosteroids must be carefully re-evaluated.

DIAGNOSTIC APPROACH TO CLINICAL FAILURE OF *PNEUMOCYSTIS CARINII* PNEUMONIA THERAPY

When a patient being treated appropriately for *P. carinii* pneumonia either fails to clinically improve or worsens, a number of factors should be considered (Table 20–4). First, how was the original diagnosis of *P. carinii* established? If the patient was empirically diagnosed, then strong consideration should be given to pursuing a definitive diagnosis. If the patient had a microbiologic diagnosis of *P. carinii*, then a review of the microbiology results may reveal or raise the specter of a coexistent infection such as to warrant further investigation. If the patient had a diagnosis of *P. carinii* pneumonia based on induced sputum examination and is known to have mucocutaneous Kaposi's sarcoma, then bronchoscopy may provide a diagnosis of pulmonary Kaposi's sarcoma. Unless an answer is readily found, diagnostic tests such as the chest radiograph should be repeated to evaluate for a supervening process. Concurrent with these considerations, a review of the patient's *P. carinii* therapy should consider whether the patient is receiving the "best" treatment option, whether adjuvant corticosteroids are warranted, and whether the patient has nausea/vomiting or diarrhea such that a switch to an intravenous route is prudent. As described earlier, patients with *P. carinii* pneumonia may have slow resolution of their disease, and it may be several days to a

TABLE 20–4. Diagnostic Approach to Clinical Failure of *P. carinii* Pneumonia Therapy

Review Diagnosis
How was the initial diagnosis of *P. carinii* pneumonia established?
  Induced sputum? Bronchoscopy? Empiric?
Was there a concurrent process initially?
  Review microbiology results and cultures
Has another process supervened?
  Repeat diagnostic tests (i.e., chest radiograph)

Review Treatment
Is the patient receiving the best *P. carinii* pneumonia treatment?
Is the patient receiving adjuvant corticosteroids?
Is the dose of the medication correct?
Does the patient have nausea/vomiting or diarrhea?
  Switch to intravenous therapy
Allow adequate time for initial therapy to work
  (usually 5–8 days)

Consider Further Evaluation
Consider bronchoscopy
If initial diagnosis of *P. carinii* pneumonia was obtained from induced sputum examination, bronchoscopy may provide higher yield for other infections or may provide a diagnosis of pulmonary Kaposi's sarcoma
If initial diagnosis of *P. carinii* pneumonia was obtained from BAL examination, repeat bronchoscopy may provide evidence for new infection
If initial diagnosis of *P. carinii* pneumonia was empiric, bronchoscopy may confirm diagnosis or provide alternate diagnosis

week or more until their clinical status improves. If a patient fails to improve after this time period or progressively deteriorates, then an evaluation for an alternate process is recommended and a switch in *P. carinii* therapy may be indicated.

PROPHYLAXIS

The definition of when an HIV-infected person is at significant risk for developing *P. carinii* pneumonia and the validation of effective preventive therapies have done more to improve the quantity and quality of life of AIDS patients than any other intervention. Multiple studies convincingly document the benefit of prophylaxis over placebo in preventing *P. carinii* pneumonia and extending life.[157–160] The risk of developing first-episode *P. carinii* pneumonia increases with declining CD4 lymphocyte count or the advent of constitutional symptoms.[59] HIV-infected persons whose CD4 lymphocyte counts decline to fewer than 100 cells/μl have nearly an order of magnitude greater risk of developing *P. carinii* pneumonia compared to persons with CD4 lymphocyte counts between 200 and 400 cells/μl. HIV-infected persons who have experienced an episode of *P. carinii* pneumonia risk a 35% chance of recurrent disease at 6 months and a 60% chance of recurrence at 1 year if prophylaxis is not provided.

TMP-SMX, dapsone with or without pyrimethamine, and aerosolized pentamidine are the three agents most commonly used to prevent *P. carinii* pneumonia (Table 20–5).[161,162] Many studies compared these drugs at different dosages and dosing intervals for primary and secondary prophylaxis. What emerges from these studies is that all of these drugs and combinations have advantages and disadvantages. Nevertheless, none has been shown to be superior to TMP-SMX for prevention of *P. carinii* pneumonia. This fact is best illustrated by two large studies—one of primary prophylaxis and one of secondary prophylaxis.

The ACTG 081 trial was an open-label, randomized trial that evaluated the effectiveness of three treatment strategies in preventing first-episode *P. carinii* pneumonia in HIV-infected persons with CD4 lymphocyte counts less than 200 cells/μl.[161] The study arms were TMP-SMX (one double-strength tablet bid), dapsone (50 mg bid), or aerosolized pentamidine (300 mg once per month). Persons experiencing drug intolerance were assigned to an alternative therapy in a predefined manner. In 842 patients who underwent a median follow-up of 39 months, there were 137 reported cases of *P. carinii* pneumonia. The estimated 36-month risk of *P. carinii* pneumonia was 18%, 17%, and 21% (*p* = NS), respectively, for TMP-SMX, dapsone, and aerosolized pentamidine. However, for persons with a CD4 lymphocyte count less than 100 cells/μl

at study entry, the risk was 33% for aerosolized pentamidine compared to 19% for TMP-SMX and 22% for dapsone (*p* = .04). Moreover, an "as-treated" analysis revealed that only 4 of the 34 patients in the TMP-SMX arm who developed *P. carinii* pneumonia did so while actually receiving the drug, whereas 37 of the 38 treatment failures occurring in the aerosolized pentamidine arm and 21 of the 34 treatment failures in the dapsone arm occurred "on therapy." Thus the oral regimens appear to be superior for *P. carinii* prophylaxis. Unfortunately, only 21% of the TMP-SMX group and 25% of the dapsone group completed the study on their originally assigned drug, compared to 88% of the aerosolized pentamidine group. Twenty-eight percent of the TMP-SMX group and 33% of the dapsone group required dose reduction only during the course of the study. This study clearly demonstrates the advantage of systemic therapy, particularly TMP-SMX, over inhalation therapy, in preventing *P. carinii* pneumonia. Other studies found similar benefits to TMP-SMX prophylaxis strategies at either attenuated doses[163] or different dosing intervals.[164,165]

The bottom line is that TMP-SMX at any dose from 80 to 320 mg TMP per day given at least three times weekly is the first-line choice for primary *P. carinii* pneumonia prophylaxis for the markedly immunocompromised patient. Alternatives include other systemic therapies, usually dapsone with or without pyrimethamine, but also clindamycin-primaquine, clindamycin-pyrimethamine, and combinations with the extended-spectrum macrolides azithromycin and clarithromycin.[166–168] Studies by Hughes and Killmar suggest that most of the prophylactic benefit from TMP-SMX may be achieved by using SMX alone.[168] Aerosolized pentamidine should be considered for possible use in the less

TABLE 20–5. Primary and Secondary Prophylaxis Options for *P. carinii*

PROPHYLAXIS REGIMEN	DOSE(S), ROUTE, FREQUENCY	COMMENTS
Trimethoprim (TMP)–sulfamethoxazole (SMX)*	DS tablet, PO, once daily DS tablet, PO, thrice weekly SS tablet, PO, once daily	Also effective prophylaxis against toxoplasmosis and many bacterial pathogens
Dapsone	100 mg, PO, once daily	
Aerosolized pentamidine	300 mg, via Respirgard II nebulizer, every 4 weeks	Risk of extrapulmonary *P. carinii* infection
Dapsone plus pyrimethamine	100 mg, PO, once daily plus 25 mg, PO, thrice weekly	
Atovaquone†	750 mg, PO, twice daily	

*TMP-SMX is dispensed as a fixed-combination (single strength [SS] tablet = TMP 80 mg/SMX 400 mg, double-strength [DS] tablet = TMP 160 mg/SMX 800 mg).
†Studies are underway comparing atovaquone to dapsone and to aerosolized pentamidine for *P. carinii* prophylaxis.

immunocompromised patient but clearly lacks the efficacy of systemic therapy in persons with a CD4 lymphocyte count less than 100 cells/μl. Trials comparing the efficacy of atovaquone suspension versus dapsone and aerosolized pentamidine in TMP-SMX–intolerant patients are completed. Unpublished analyses of these clinical trails found no difference in efficacy between either atovaquone and dapsone or atovaquone and pentamidine when used as a second-line primary _P. carinii_ prophylaxis. Thus the choice of agent to use when TMP-SMX is unavailable should be guided by the side effect profile and cost of the prophylactic agent.

Similar findings document the superiority of TMP-SMX for secondary _P. carinii_ prophylaxis (maintenance therapy) of AIDS patients after an initial episode of _P. carinii_ pneumonia. In 310 AIDS patients who had recently recovered from _P. carinii_ pneumonia, patients were randomized to receive either TMP-SMX (one double-strength tablet daily) or aerosolized pentamidine (300 mg via nebulizer once per month).[169] All patients received zidovudine, and the median follow-up was 17.4 months. There were 14 (11.4%) _P. carinii_ recurrences among 154 patients assigned to the TMP-SMX arm versus 36 (27.6%) recurrences among the pentamidine-treated group ($p < .001$). By an intent-to-treat analysis, the risk of recurrence was 3.25 times higher for the pentamidine-treatment group. In fact, only four of the participants who received TMP-SMX for more than 3 weeks and tolerated the drug actually developed recurrent disease. In contrast, all of the _P. carinii_ pneumonia recurrences in the aerosolized pentamidine treatment group occurred while the patients were on drug. As expected, aerosolized pentamidine was the better tolerated of the two regimens. Only 4% of the pentamidine treatment group required crossover, compared to 27% of the TMP-SMX group. These data establish the primacy of TMP-SMX for secondary _P. carinii_ prophylaxis in AIDS patients. Unfortunately, there are few data on the role of other systemic antibiotics in secondary _P. carinii_ prophylaxis. What information exists suggests activity of weekly dapsone or dapsone-pyrimethamine comparable to aerosolized pentamidine.[169–172] No study has looked at dapsone with or without pyrimethamine given daily for the prevention of recurrent _P. carinii_ pneumonia. Certainly, the first choice to prevent recurrent _P. carinii_ pneumonia, as with primary _P. carinii_ prophylaxis, should always be systemic antibiotics. Aerosolized pentamidine should be considered only in those patients intolerant of all systemic options.

References

1. Chagas C: Novo trypanomiazaea humana: Ueber eine neve trypanosomiasis de menschen. Mem Inst Oswaldo Cruz 1:159, 1909
2. Gottlieb MS, Schroff R, Schanker HM, et al: _Pneumocystis carinii_ pneumonia and mucosal candidiasis in previously healthy homosexual men: Evidence of a new acquired cellular immunodeficiency. N Engl J Med 305:1425, 1981
3. Masur H, Michelis MA, Greene JB, et al: An outbreak of community-acquired _Pneumocystis carinii_ pneumonia: Initial manifestation of cellular immune dysfunction. N Engl J Med 305:1431, 1981
4. Murray JF, Felton CP, Garay SM, et al: Pulmonary complications of the acquired immunodeficiency syndrome: Report of a National Heart, Lung, and Blood Institute workshop. N Engl J Med 310:1682, 1984
5. Centers for Disease Control: HIV/AIDS Surveillance Report, 6(5):1, 1994
6. Centers for Disease Control: HIV/AIDS Surveillance Report, 6(6):1, 1995
7. Vavra J, Kucera K: _Pneumocystis carinii_: Its ultrastructure and ultrastructural affinities. J Protozool 17:463, 1970
8. Edman JC, Kovacs JA, Masur H, et al: Ribosomal RNA sequence shows _Pneumocystis carinii_ to be a member of the fungi. Nature 334:519, 1988
9. Stringer SL, Stringer JR, Blase MA, et al: _Pneumocystis carinii_: Sequence from ribosomal RNA implies a close relationship with fungi. Exp Parasitol 68:450, 1989
10. Edman JC, Edman U, Cao M, et al: Isolation and expression of the _Pneumocystis carinii_ dihydrofolate reductase gene. Proc Natl Acad Sci USA 86:8625, 1989
11. Edman U, Edman JC, Lundgren B, et al: Isolation and expression of the _Pneumocystis carinii_ thymidylate synthase gene. Proc Natl Acad Sci USA 86:6503, 1989
12. Fletcher LD, McDowell JM, Tidwell RR, et al: Structure, expression and phylogenetic analysis of the gene encoding actin I in _Pneumocystis carinii_. Genetics 137:743, 1994
13. Dyer M, Volpe F, Delves CJ, et al: Cloning and sequence of a beta-tubulin cDNA from _Pneumocystis carinii_: Possible implications for drug therapy. Mol Microbiol 6:991, 1992
14. Meade JC, Stringer JR: Cloning and characterization of an ATPase gene from _Pneumocystis carinii_ which closely resembles fungal H+ ATPases. J Eukaryot Microbiol 42:298, 1995
15. Pixley FJ, Wakefield AE, Banerji S, et al: Mitochondrial gene sequences show fungal homology for _Pneumocystis carinii_. Mol Microbiol 5:1347, 1991
16. Edman JC, Sogin ML: Molecular phylogeny of _Pneumocystis carinii_. In Walzer PD (ed): _Pneumocystis carinii_ Pneumonia (Vol 69/Lung Biology in Health and Disease). New York, Marcel Dekker, 1994, p 91
17. Ruffolo JJ: _Pneumocystis carinii_ cell structure. In Walzer PD (ed): _Pneumocystis carinii_ Pneumonia (Vol 69). New York, Marcel Dekker, 1994, p 25
18. Sinclair K, Wakefield AE, Banerji S, et al: _Pneumocystis carinii_ organisms derived from rat and human hosts are genetically distinct. Mol Biochem Parasitol 45:183, 1991
19. Wakefield AE, Peters SE, Banerji S, et al: _Pneumocystis carinii_ shows DNA homology with the usto-

mycetous red yeast fungi. Mol Microbiol 6:1903, 1992

20. Weinberg GA, Durant PJ: Genetic diversity of *Pneumocystis carinii* derived from infected rats, mice, ferrets, and cell cultures. J Eukaryot Microbiol 41:223, 1994

21. Wakefield GA: Re-examination of epidemiological concepts. In Sattler FR, Walzer PD (eds): *Pneumocystis carinii*, Vol 2. London, Bailliere Tindall, 1995, p 431

22. Hughes WT, Bartley DL, Smith BM: A natural source of infection due to *Pneumocystis carinii*. J Infect Dis 147:595, 1983

23. Hughes WT: Natural mode of acquisition for de novo infection with *Pneumocystis carinii*. J Infect Dis 145:842, 1982

24. Soulez B, Palluault F, Cesbron JY, et al: Introduction of *Pneumocystis carinii* in a colony of SCID mice. J Protozool 38:123S, 1991

25. Wakefield AE, Fritscher CC, Malin AS, et al: Genetic diversity in human-derived *Pneumocystis carinii* isolates from four geographical locations shown by analysis of mitochondrial rRNA gene sequences. J Clin Microbiol 32:2959, 1994

26. Meuwissen J, Tauber I, Leeuwenberg A, et al: Parasitologic and serologic observations of infection with *Pneumocystis* in humans. J Infect Dis 136:43, 1977

27. Peglow SL, Smulian AG, Linke MJ, et al: Serologic responses to *Pneumocystis carinii* in health and disease. J Infect Dis 161:296, 1990

28. Pifer LL, Hughes WT, Stagno S, et al: *Pneumocystis carinii* infection: Evidence for a high prevalence in normal and immunosuppressed children. Pediatrics 61:35, 1978

29. Smulian AG, Sullivan DW, Linke MJ, et al: Geographic variation in the humoral response to *Pneumocystis carinii*. J Infect Dis 167:1243, 1993

30. Peters SE, Wakefield AE, Sinclair K, et al: A search for *Pneumocystis carinii* in post-mortem lungs by DNA amplification. J Pathol 166:195, 1992

31. Millard PR, Heryet AR: Observations favouring *Pneumocystis carinii* pneumonia as a primary infection: A monoclonal antibody study on paraffin sections. J Pathol 154:365, 1988

32. Wakefield AE, Pixley FJ, Banerji S, et al: Detection of *Pneumocystis carinii* with DNA amplification. Lancet 336:451, 1990

33. Eisen D, Ross BC, Fairbairn J, et al: Comparison of *Pneumocystis carinii* detection by toluidine blue O staining, direct immunofluorescence and DNA amplification sputum specimens from HIV positive patients. Pathology 26:198, 1994

34. Evans R, Joss AW, Pennington TH, et al: The use of a nested polymerase chain reaction for detecting *Pneumocystis carinii* from lung and blood in rat and human infection. J Med Microbiol 42:209, 1995

35. Leigh TR, Wakefield AE, Peters SE, et al: Comparison of DNA amplification and immunofluorescence for detecting *Pneumocystis carinii* in patients receiving immunosuppressive therapy. Transplantation 54:468, 1992

36. Lipschik GY, Gill VJ, Lundgren JD, et al: Improved diagnosis of *Pneumocystis carinii* infection by polymerase chain reaction on induced sputum and blood. Lancet 340:203, 1992

37. Tamburrini E, Mencarini P, De Luca A, et al: Diagnosis of *Pneumocystis carinii* pneumonia: Specificity and sensitivity of polymerase chain reaction in comparison with immunofluorescence in bronchoalveolar lavage specimens. J Med Microbiol 38:449, 1993

38. Vargas SL, Hughes WT, Wakefield AE, et al: Limited persistence in and subsequent elimination of *Pneumocystis carinii* from the lungs after *P. carinii* pneumonia. J Infect Dis 172:506, 1995

39. Gajdusek D: *Pneumocystis carinii*—etiologic agent of interstitial plasma cell pneumonia of premature and young infants. Pediatrics 19:543, 1957

40. Perera DR, Western KA, Johnson HD, et al: *Pneumocystis carinii* pneumonia in a hospital for children. JAMA 214:1074, 1970

41. Ruebush TK, Weinstein RA, Baehner RL, et al: An outbreak of *Pneumocystis carinii* pneumonia in children with acute lymphocytic leukemia. Am J Dis Child 132:143, 1978

42. Stiller RA, Paradis IL, Dauber JH: Subclinical pneumonitis due to *Pneumocystis carinii* in a young adult with elevated antibody titers to Epstein-Barr virus. J Infect Dis 166:926, 1992

43. Leigh TR, Millett MJ, Jameson B, et al: Serum titres of *Pneumocystis carinii* antibody in health care workers caring for patients with AIDS. Thorax 48:619, 1993

44. Harmsen AG, Chen W, Gigliotti F: Active immunity to *Pneumocystis carinii* reinfection in T-cell-depleted mice. Infect Immun 63:2391, 1995

45. Gigliotti F, Hughes WT: Passive immunoprophylaxis with specific monoclonal antibody confers partial protection against *Pneumocystis carinii* pneumonitis in animal models. J Clin Invest 81:1666, 1988

46. Harmsen AG, Stankiewicz M: T cells are not sufficient for resistance to *Pneumocystis carinii* pneumonia in mice. J Protozool 38:44S, 1991

47. Roths JB, Sidman CL: Single and combined humoral and cell-mediated immunotherapy of *Pneumocystis carinii* pneumonia in immunodeficient SCID mice. Infect Immun 61:1641, 1993

48. Shellito J, Suzara VV, Blumenfeld W, et al: A new model of *Pneumocystis carinii* infection in mice selectively depleted of helper T lymphocytes. J Clin Invest 85:1686, 1990

49. Harmsen AG, Stankiewicz M: Requirement for CD4+ cells in resistance to *Pneumocystis carinii* pneumonia in mice. J Exp Med 172:937, 1990

50. Roths JB, Sidman CL: Both immunity and hyperresponsiveness to *Pneumocystis carinii* result from transfer of CD4+ but not CD8+ T cells into severe combined immunodeficiency mice. J Clin Invest 90:673, 1992

51. Theus SA, Andrews RP, Steele P, et al: Adoptive transfer of lymphocytes sensitized to the major surface glycoprotein of *Pneumocystis carinii* confers protection in the rat. J Clin Invest 95:2587, 1995

52. Pottratz ST, Martin W: Role of fibronectin in *Pneumocystis carinii* attachment to cultured lung cells. J Clin Invest 85:351, 1990

53. Pottratz ST, Paulsrud J, Smith JS, et al: *Pneumocystis carinii* attachment to cultured lung cells by pneumocystis gp 120, a fibronectin binding protein. J Clin Invest 88:403, 1991

54. Walzer PD: Pathogenic mechanisms. In Walzer PD (ed): *Pneumocystis carinii* Pneumonia (Vol 69/Lung Biology in Health and Disease). New York, Marcel Dekker, 1994, p 251

55. Yoneda K, Walzer PD: Attachment of *Pneumocystis carinii* to type I alveolar cells studied by freeze-fracture electron microscopy. Infect Immun 40:812, 1983

56. Centers for Disease Control and Prevention. HIV/AIDS Surveillance Report, 9(2):18, 1998

57. Centers for Disease Control and Prevention. HIV/ AIDS Surveillance Report, 5(4):16, 1993
58. Centers for Disease Control and Prevention. HIV/ AIDS Surveillance Report, 8(2):18, 1997
59. Phair J, Munoz A, Detels R, et al: The risk of *Pneumocystis carinii* pneumonia among men infected with human immunodeficiency virus type 1: Multicenter AIDS Cohort Study Group. N Engl J Med 322:161, 1990
60. Centers for Disease Control: Recommendations for prophylaxis against *Pneumocystis carinii* pneumonia for adults and adolescents infected with human immunodeficiency virus. MMWR Morb Mortal Wkly Rep 41(RR-4):1, 1992
61. The Pulmonary Complications of HIV Infection Study Group: Design of a prospective study of the pulmonary complications of human immunodeficiency virus infection. J Clin Epidemiol 46:497, 1993
62. Stansell JD, Osmond DH, Charlebois E, et al: Predictors of *Pneumocystis carinii* pneumonia in HIV-infected persons: Pulmonary Complications of HIV Infection Study Group. Am J Respir Crit Care Med 155:60, 1997
63. Kvale PA, Hansen NI, Markowitz N, et al: Routine analysis of induced sputum is not an effective strategy for screening persons infected with human immunodeficiency virus for *Mycobacterium tuberculosis* or *Pneumocystis carinii*: Pulmonary Complications of HIV Infection Study Group. Clin Infect Dis 19:410, 1994
64. Kvale PA, Rosen MJ, Hopewell PC, et al: A decline in the pulmonary diffusing capacity does no indicate opportunistic lung disease in asymptomatic persons infected with the human immunodeficiency virus: Pulmonary Complications of HIV Infection Study Group. Am Rev Respir Dis 148:390, 1993
65. Schneider RF, Hansen NI, Rosen MJ, et al: Lack of usefulness of radiographic screening for pulmonary disease in asymptomatic HIV-infected adults: Pulmonary Complications of HIV Infection Study Group. Arch Intern Med 156:191, 1996
66. Kovacs JA, Hiemenz JW, Macher Am, et al: *Pneumocystis carinii* pneumonia: A comparison between patients with the acquired immunodeficiency syndrome and patients with other immunodeficiencies. Ann Intern Med 100:663, 1984
67. Garay SM, Greene J: Prognostic indicators in the initial presentation of *Pneumocystis carinii* pneumonia. Chest 95:769, 1989
68. Grover SA, Coupal L, Suissa S, et al: The clinical utility of serum lactate dehydrogenase in diagnosing *Pneumocystis carinii* pneumonia among hospitalized AIDS patients. Clin Invest Med 15:309, 1992
69. Kagawa FT, Kirsch CM, Yenokida GG, et al: Serum lactate dehydrogenase activity in patients with AIDS and *Pneumocystis carinii* pneumonia: An adjunct to diagnosis. Chest 94:1031, 1988
70. Kales CP, Murren JR, Torres RA, et al: Early predictors of in-hospital mortality for *Pneumocystis carinii* pneumonia in the acquired immunodeficiency syndrome. Arch Intern Med 147:1413, 1987
71. Katz MH, Baron RB, Grady D: Risk stratification of ambulatory patients suspected of *Pneumocystis pneumonia*. Arch Intern Med 151:105, 1991
72. Lipman ML, Goldstein E: Serum lactic dehydrogenase predicts mortality in patients with AIDS and *Pneumocystis* pneumonia. West J Med 149:486, 1988
73. Quist J, Hill AR: Serum lactate dehydrogenase (LDH) in *Pneumocystis carinii* pneumonia, tuberculosis, and bacterial pneumonia. Chest 108:415, 1995
74. Zaman MK, White DA: Serum lactate dehydrogenase levels and *Pneumocystis carinii* pneumonia: Diagnostic and prognostic significance. Am Rev Respir Dis 137:796, 1988
75. Meeker DP, Matysik GA, Stelmach K, et al: Diagnostic utility of lactate dehydrogenase levels in patients receiving aerosolized pentamidine. Chest 104: 386, 1993
76. Antinori A, Maiuro G, Pallavicini F, et al: Prognostic factors of early fatal outcome and long-term survival in patients with *Pneumocystis carinii* pneumonia and acquired immunodeficiency syndrome. Eur J Epidemiol 9:183, 1993
77. el-Sadr W, Simberkoff MS: Survival and prognostic factors in severe *Pneumocystis carinii* pneumonia requiring mechanical ventilation. Am Rev Respir Dis 137:1264, 1988
78. Cohen BA, Pomeranz S, Robinowitz JG, et al: Pulmonary complications of AIDS: Radiologic features. AJR Am J Roentgenol 143:115, 1984
79. DeLorenzo LJ, Huang CT, Maguire GP, et al: Roentgenographic patterns of *Pneumocystis carinii* pneumonia in 104 patients with AIDS. Chest 91:323, 1987
80. Gamsu G, Hecht ST, Birnberg FA, et al: *Pneumocystis carinii* pneumonia in homosexual men. AJR Am J Roentgenol 139:647, 1982
81. Suster B, Akerman M, Orenstein M, et al: Pulmonary manifestations of AIDS: Review of 106 episodes. Radiology 161:87, 1986
82. Sandhu JS, Goodman PC: Pulmonary cysts associated with *Pneumocystis carinii* pneumonia in patients with AIDS. Radiology 173:33, 1989
83. Goodman PC, Daley C, Minagi H: Spontaneous pneumothorax in AIDS patients with *Pneumocystis carinii* pneumonia. AJR Am J Roentgenol 147:29, 1986
84. Metersky ML, Colt HG, Olson LK, et al: AIDS-related spontaneous pneumothorax: Risk factors and treatment. Chest 108:946, 1995
85. Kennedy CA, Goetz MB: Atypical roentgenographic manifestations of *Pneumocystis carinii* pneumonia. Arch Intern Med 152:1390, 1992
86. Chaffey MH, Klein JS, Gamsu G, et al: Radiographic distribution of *Pneumocystis carinii* pneumonia in patients with AIDS treated with prophylactic inhaled pentamidine. Radiology 175:715, 1990
87. Jules-Elysee KM, Stover DE, Zaman MB, et al: Aerosolized pentamidine: Effect on diagnosis and presentation of *Pneumocystis carinii* pneumonia. Ann Intern Med 112:750, 1990
88. Opravil M, Marincek B, Fuchs WA, et al: Shortcomings of chest radiography in detecting *Pneumocystis carinii* pneumonia. J Acquir Immune Defic Syndr 7: 39, 1994
89. Wachter RM, Luce JM, Turner J, et al: Intensive care of patients with the acquired immunodeficiency syndrome: Outcome and changing patterns of utilization. Am Rev Respir Dis 134:891, 1986
90. Wachter RM, Russi MB, Bloch DA, et al: *Pneumocystis carinii* pneumonia and respiratory failure in AIDS: Improved outcomes and increased use of intensive care units. Am Rev Respir Dis 143:151, 1991
91. Wachter RM, Luce JM, Safrin S, et al: Cost and outcome of intensive care for patients with AIDS, *Pneumocystis carinii* pneumonia, and severe respiratory failure. JAMA 273:130, 1995
92. Stansell JD, Hopewell PC: *Pneumocystis carinii* Pneumonia: Risk factors, clinical presentation, and natural history. In Sattler FR, Walzer PD (eds): *Pneumocystis carinii*, Vol 2. London, Bailliere Tindall, 1995, p 449

93. Holmes AH, Trotman-Dickenson B, Edwards A, et al: Bronchiectasis in HIV disease. Q J Med 85:875, 1992

94. Northfelt DW, Clement MJ, Safrin S: Extrapulmonary pneumocystosis: Clinical features in human immunodeficiency virus infection. Medicine 69:392, 1990

95. Sankary RM, Turner J, Lipavasky A, et al: Alveolar-capillary block in patients with AIDS and *Pneumocystis carinii* pneumonia. Am Rev Respir Dis 137:443, 1988

96. Coleman DL, Dodek PM, Golden JA, et al: Correlation between serial pulmonary function tests and fiberoptic bronchoscopy in patients with *Pneumocystis carinii* pneumonia and the acquired immune deficiency syndrome. Am Rev Respir Dis 129:491, 1984

97. Hopewell PC, Luce JM: Pulmonary involvement in the acquired immunodeficiency syndrome. Chest 87:104, 1985

98. Huang L, Stansell JD, Osmond D, et al: Utility of diffusing capacity (DLco) measurement in subjects with suspected *P. carinii* pneumonia (PCP) and a normal chest radiograph (CXR). Am J Respir Crit Care Med 151:A797, 1995

99. Bergin CJ, Wirth RL, Berry GJ, et al: *Pneumocystis carinii* pneumonia: CT and HRCT observations. J Comput Assist Tomogr 14:756, 1990

100. Moskovic E, Miller R, Pearson M: High resolution computed tomography of *Pneumocystis carinii* pneumonia in AIDS. Clin Radiol 42:239, 1990

101. Rotondo A, Guidi G, Catalano O, et al: High resolution computed tomography (HRCT) of pulmonary infections in AIDS patients. Rays 19:208, 1994

102. Gruden JF, Huang L, Turner J, et al: High-resolution CT in the evaluation of clinically suspected *Pneumocystis carinii* pneumonia in AIDS patients with normal, equivocal, or nonspecific radiographic findings. Am J Roentgenol 169:967, 1997

103. Bigby TD, Margolskee D, Curtis JL, et al: The usefulness of induced sputum in the diagnosis of *Pneumocystis carinii* pneumonia in patients with the acquired immunodeficiency syndrome. Am Rev Respir Dis 133:515, 1986

104. Kovacs JA, Ng VL, Masur H, et al: Diagnosis of *Pneumocystis carinii* pneumonia: Improved detection in sputum with use of monoclonal antibodies. N Engl J Med 318:589, 1988

105. Ng VL, Gartner I, Weymouth LA, et al: The use of mucolysed induced sputum for the identification of pulmonary pathogens associated with human immunodeficiency virus infection. Arch Pathol Lab Med 113:488, 1989

106. O'Brien RF, Quinn JL, Miyahara BT, et al: Diagnosis of *Pneumocystis carinii* pneumonia by induced sputum in a city with moderate incidence of AIDS. Chest 95:136, 1989

107. Pitchenik AE, Ganjei P, Torres A, et al: Sputum examination for the diagnosis of *Pneumocystis carinii* pneumonia in the acquired immunodeficiency syndrome. Am Rev Respir Dis 133:226, 1986

108. Zaman MK, Wooten OJ, Suprahmanya B, et al: Rapid noninvasive diagnosis of *Pneumocystis carinii* from induced liquefied sputum. Ann Intern Med 109:7, 1988

109. Ng VL, Yajko DM, McPhaul LW, et al: Evaluation of an indirect fluorescent-antibody stain for detection of *Pneumocystis carinii* in respiratory specimens. J Clin Microbiol 28:975, 1990

110. Huang L, Hecht FM, Stansell JD, et al: Suspected *Pneumocystis carinii* pneumonia with a negative induced sputum examination: Is early bronchoscopy useful? Am J Respir Crit Care Med 151:1866, 1995

111. Broaddus C, Dake MD, Stulbarg MS, et al: Bronchoalveolar lavage and transbronchial biopsy for the diagnosis of pulmonary infections in the acquired immunodeficiency syndrome. Ann Intern Med 102:747, 1985

112. Golden JA, Hollander H, Stulbarg MS, et al: Bronchoalveolar lavage as the exclusive diagnostic modality for *Pneumocystis carinii* pneumonia: A prospective study among patients with acquired immunodeficiency syndrome. Chest 90:18, 1986

113. Ognibene FP, Shelhamer J, Gill V, et al: The diagnosis of *Pneumocystis carinii* pneumonia in patients with the acquired immunodeficiency syndrome using subsegmental bronchoalveolar lavage. Am Rev Respir Dis 129:929, 1984

114. Orenstein M, Webber CA, Cash M, et al: Value of bronchoalveolar lavage in the diagnosis of pulmonary infection in acquired immune deficiency syndrome. Thorax 41:345, 1986

115. Beck EJ, French PD, Helbert MH, et al: Empirically treated *Pneumocystis carinii* pneumonia in London, 1983–1989. Int J STD AIDS 3:285, 1992

116. Bennett CL, Horner RD, Weinstein RA, et al: Empirically treated *Pneumocystis carinii* pneumonia in Los Angeles, Chicago, and Miami: 1987–1990. J Infect Dis 172:312, 1995

117. Miller RF, Millar AB, Weller IV, et al: Empirical treatment without bronchoscopy for *Pneumocystis carinii* pneumonia in the acquired immunodeficiency syndrome. Thorax 44:559, 1989

118. Tu JV, Biem HJ, Detsky AS: Bronchoscopy versus empirical therapy in HIV-infected patients with presumptive *Pneumocystis carinii* pneumonia: A decision analysis. Am Rev Respir Dis 148:370, 1993

119. Masur H, Shelhamer J: Empiric outpatient management of HIV-related pneumonia: Economical or unwise? Ann Intern Med 111:451, 1996

120. Gordin FM, Simon GL, Wofsy CB, et al: Adverse reactions to trimethoprim-sulfamethoxazole in patients with the acquired immunodeficiency syndrome. Ann Intern Med 100:495, 1984

121. Masur H, Lane HC, Kovacs JA, et al: NIH conference. *Pneumocystis* pneumonia: From bench to clinic. Ann Intern Med 111:813, 1989

122. Stein DS, Stevens RC: Treatment-associated toxicities: Incidence and mechanisms. In Sattler FR, Walzer PD (eds): *Pneumocystis carinii*, Vol. 2. London, Bailliere Tindall, 1995, p 505

123. Hughes W, Leoung G, Kramer F, et al: Comparison of atovaquone (566C80) with trimethoprim-sulfamethoxazole to treat *Pneumocystis carinii* pneumonia in patients with AIDS. N Engl J Med 328;1521, 1993

124. Klein NC, Duncanson FP, Lenox TH, et al: Trimethoprim-sulfamethoxazole versus pentamidine for *Pneumocystis carinii* pneumonia in AIDS patients: Result of a large prospective randomized treatment trial. AIDS 6:301, 1992

125. Medina I, Mills J, Leoung G, et al: Oral therapy for *Pneumocystis carinii* pneumonia in the acquired immunodeficiency syndrome: A controlled trial of trimethoprim-sulfamethoxazole versus trimethoprim-dapsone. N Engl J Med 323:776, 1990

126. Safrin S, Finkelstein DM, Feinberg J, et al: A double-blind, randomized comparison of oral trimethoprim-sulfamethoxazole, dapsone-trimethoprim, and clindamycin-primaquine for treatment of mild-to-moderate *Pneumocystis carinii* pneumonia in patients with AIDS. Ann Intern Med 124:792, 1996

127. Sattler FR, Cowan R, Neilsen DM, et al: Trimethoprim-sulfamethoxazole compared with pentamidine

for treatment of *Pneumocystis carinii* pneumonia in the acquired immunodeficiency syndrome: A prospective, noncrossover study. Ann Intern Med 109:280, 1988

128. Sattler FR, Frame P, Davis R, et al: Trimetrexate with leucovorin versus trimethoprim-sulfamethoxazole for moderate to severe episodes of *Pneumocystis carinii* pneumonia in patients with AIDS: A prospective, controlled multicenter investigation of the AIDS Clinical Trials Group Protocol 029/031. J Infect Dis 170:165, 1994

129. Toma E, Fournier S, Dumont M, et al: Clindamycin/primaquine versus trimethoprim-sulfamethoxazole as primary therapy for *Pneumocystis carinii* pneumonia in AIDS: A randomized, double-blind pilot trial. Clin Infect Dis 17:178, 1993

130. Toma E, Raboud J, Thorne A, et al: Clindamycin-primaquine versus trimethoprim-sulfamethoxazole for PCP in AIDS. In: Abstracts of the 35th Interscience Conference on Antimicrobial Agents and Chemotherapy, San Francisco, 1995, Abstract LM96

131. Wharton JM, Coleman DL, Wofsy CB, et al: Trimethoprim-sulfamethoxazole or pentamidine for *Pneumocystis carinii* pneumonia in the acquired immunodeficiency syndrome: A prospective randomized trial. Ann Intern Med 105:37, 1986

132. Hughes WT, Killmar JT, Oz HS: Relative potency of 10 drugs with anti-*Pneumocystis carinii* activity in an animal model. J Infect Dis 170:906, 1994

133. Hughes WT, Feldman S, Chaudhary SC, et al: Comparison of pentamidine isethionate and trimethoprim-sulfamethoxazole in the treatment of *Pneumocystis carinii* pneumonia. J Pediatr 92:436, 1978

134. Greenberg S, Reiser IW, Chou SY, et al: Trimethoprim-sulfamethoxazole induces reversible hyperkalemia. Ann Intern Med 119:291, 1993

135. Conte J Jr: Pharmacokinetics of intravenous pentamidine in patients with normal renal function or receiving hemodiaylsis. J Infect Dis 163:169, 1991

136. Conte J Jr, Chernoff D, Feigal D Jr, et al: Intravenous or inhaled pentamidine for treating *Pneumocystis carinii* pneumonia in AIDS: A randomized trial. Ann Intern Med 113:203, 1990

137. O'Brien JG, Dong BJ, Coleman RL, et al: Five year retrospective review of the risk factors associated with adverse drug reactions in patients with HIV treated with intravenous pentamidine for *Pneumocystis carinii* pneumonia. In: Abstracts of the 35th Interscience Conference on Antimicrobial Agents and Chemotherapy, San Francisco, 1995, Abstract I-223

138. Queener SF, Bartlett MS, Richardson JD, et al: Activity of clindamycin with primaquine against *Pneumocystis carinii* in vitro and in vivo. Antimicrob Agents Chemother 32:807, 1988

139. Black JR, Feinberg J, Murphy RL, et al: Clindamycin and primaquine as primary treatment for mild and moderately severe *Pneumocystis carinii* pneumonia in patients with AIDS. Eur J Clin Microbiol Infect Dis 10:204, 1991

140. Black JR, Feinberg J, Murphy RL, et al: Clindamycin and primaquine therapy for mild-to-moderate episodes of *Pneumocystis carinii* pneumonia in patients with AIDS: AIDS Clinical Trials Group 044. Clin Infect Dis 18:905, 1994

141. Noskin GA, Murphy RL, Black JR, et al: Salvage therapy with clindamycin/primaquine for *Pneumocystis carinii* pneumonia. Clin Infect Dis 14:183, 1992

142. Toma E, Fournier S, Poisson M, et al: Clindamycin with primaquine for *Pneumocystis carinii* pneumonia. Lancet 1:1046, 1989

143. Allegra CJ, Chabner BA, Tuazon CU, et al: Trimetrexate for the treatment of *Pneumocystis carinii* pneumonia in patients with the acquired immunodeficiency syndrome. N Engl J Med 317:978, 1987

144. Sattler FR, Allegra CJ, Verdegem TD, et al: Trimetrexate-leucovorin dosage evaluation study for treatment of *Pneumocystis carinii* pneumonia. J Infect Dis 161:91, 1990

145. Safrin S, Sattler FR, Lee BL, et al: Dapsone as a single agent is suboptimal therapy for *Pneumocystis carinii* pneumonia. J Acquir Immune Defic Syndr 4:244, 1991

146. Hughes WT, Smith BL: Efficacy of diaminodiphenylsulfone and other drugs in murine *Pneumocystis carinii* pneumonitis. Antimicrob Agents Chemother 26:436, 1984

147. Leoung GS, Mills J, Hopewell PC, et al: Dapsone-trimethoprim for *Pneumocystis carinii* pneumonia in the acquired immunodeficiency syndrome. Ann Intern Med 105:45, 1986

148. Dohn MN, Weinberg WG, Torres RA, et al: Oral atovaquone compared with intravenous pentamidine for *Pneumocystis carinii* pneumonia in patients with AIDS: Atovaquone Study Group. Ann Intern Med 121:174, 1994

149. Falloon J, Kovacs J, Hughes W, et al: A preliminary evaluation of 566C80 for the treatment of *Pneumocystis* pneumonia in patients with the acquired immunodeficiency syndrome. N Engl J Med 325:1534, 1991

150. Montgomery AB, Feigal D Jr, Sattler F, et al: Pentamidine aerosol versus trimethoprim-sulfamethoxazole for *Pneumocystis carinii* in acquired immunodeficiency syndrome. Am J Respir Crit Care Med 151:1068, 1995

151. Soo Hoo GW, Mohsenifar Z, Meyer RD: Inhaled or intravenous pentamidine therapy for *Pneumocystis carinii* pneumonia in AIDS: A randomized trial. Ann Intern Med 113:195, 1990

152. Bozzette SA, Sattler FR, Chiu J, et al: A controlled trial of early adjunctive treatment with corticosteroids for *Pneumocystis carinii* pneumonia in the acquired immunodeficiency syndrome: California Collaborative Treatment Group. N Engl J Med 323:1451, 1990

153. Gagnon S, Boota AM, Fischl MA, et al: Corticosteroids as adjunctive therapy for severe *Pneumocystis carinii* pneumonia in the acquired immunodeficiency syndrome: A double-blind, placebo-controlled trial. N Engl J Med 323:1444, 1990

154. Montaner JS, Lawson LM, Levitt N, et al: Corticosteroids prevent early deterioration in patients with moderately severe *Pneumocystis carinii* pneumonia and the acquired immunodeficiency syndrome (AIDS). Ann Intern Med 113:14, 1990

155. Nielsen TL, Eeftinck Schattenkerk JK, Jensen BN, et al: Adjunctive corticosteroid therapy for *Pneumocystis carinii* pneumonia in AIDS: A randomized European multicenter open label study. J Acquir Immune Defic Syndr 5:726, 1992

156. National Institutes of Health–University of California Expert Panel: Consensus statement on the use of corticosteroids as adjunctive therapy for severe *Pneumocystis carinii* pneumonia in the acquired immunodeficiency syndrome. N Engl J Med 323:1500, 1990

157. Fischl MA, Dickinson GM, La Voie L: Safety and efficacy of sulfamethoxazole and trimethoprim chemoprophylaxis for *Pneumocystis carinii* pneumonia in AIDS. JAMA 259:1185, 1988

158. Girard PM, Landman R, Gaudebout C, et al: Prevention of *Pneumocystis carinii* pneumonia relapse by

pentamidine aerosol in zidovudine-treated AIDS patients. Lancet 1:1348, 1989

159. Hirschel B, Lazzarin A, Chopard P, et al: A controlled study of inhaled pentamidine for primary prevention of *Pneumocystis carinii* pneumonia. N Engl J Med 324:1079, 1991

160. Montaner JS, Lawson LM, Gervais A, et al: Aerosol pentamidine for secondary prophylaxis of AIDS-related *Pneumocystis carinii* pneumonia: A randomized, placebo-controlled study. Ann Intern Med 114: 948, 1991

161. Bozzette SA, Finkelstein DM, Spector SA, et al: A randomized trial of three antipneumocystis agents in patients with advanced human immunodeficiency virus infection: NIAID AIDS Clinical Trials Group. N Engl J Med 332:693, 1995

162. Martin MA, Cox PH, Beck K, et al: A comparison of the effectiveness of three regimens in the prevention of *Pneumocystis carinii* pneumonia in human immunodeficiency virus-infected patients. Arch Intern Med 152:523, 1992

163. Schneider MM, Hoepelman AI, Eeftinck Schattenkerk JK, et al: A controlled trial of aerosolized pentamidine or trimethoprim-sulfamethoxazole as primary prophylaxis against *Pneumocystis carinii* pneumonia in patients with human immunodeficiency virus infection: The Dutch AIDS Treatment Group. N Engl J Med 327:1836, 1992

164. Mallolas J, Zamora L, Gatell JM, et al: Primary prophylaxis for *Pneumocystis carinii* pneumonia: A randomized trial comparing cortimoxazole, aerosolized pentamidine and dapsone plus pyrimethamine. AIDS 7:59, 1993

165. Podzamczer D, Santin M, Jimenez J, et al: Thrice-weekly cotrimoxazole is better than weekly dapsone-pyrimethamine for the primary prevention of *Pneumocystis carinii* pneumonia in HIV-infected patients. AIDS 7:501, 1993

166. Girard PM, Landman R, Gaudebout C, et al: Dapsone-pyrimethamine compared with aerosolized pentamidine as primary prophylaxis against *Pneumocystis carinii* pneumonia and toxoplasmosis in HIV infection: The PRIO Study Group. N Engl J Med 328: 1514, 1993

167. Heald A, Flepp M, Chave JP, et al: Treatment for cerebral toxoplasmosis protects against *Pneumocystis carinii* pneumonia in patients with AIDS: The Swiss HIV Cohort Study. Ann Intern Med 115:760, 1991

168. Hughes WT, Killmar J: Efficacy of sulfonamides alone in prophylaxis for *Pneumocystis carinii* pneumonia. In: Abstracts of the 3rd Conference of Retroviruses and Opportunistic Infections, Washington, DC, 1996, Abstract 572

169. Hardy WD, Feinberg J, Finkelstein DM, et al: A controlled trial of trimethoprim-sulfamethoxazole or aerosolized pentamidine for secondary prophylaxis of *Pneumocystis carinii* pneumonia in patients with the acquired immunodeficiency syndrome: AIDS Clinical Trials Group Protocol 021. N Engl J Med 327:1842, 1992

170. Opravil M, Hirschel B, Lazzarin A, et al: Once-weekly administration of dapsone/pyrimethamine vs. aerosolized pentamidine as combined prophylaxis for *Pneumocystis carinii* pneumonia and toxoplasmic encephalitis in human immunodeficiency virus-infected patients. Clin Infect Dis 20:531, 1995

171. Slavin MA, Hoy JF, Steward K, et al: Oral dapsone versus nebulized pentamidine for *Pneumocystis carinii* pneumonia prophylaxis: An open randomized prospective trial to assess efficacy and haematological toxicity. AIDS 6:1169, 1992

172. Torres RA, Barr M, Thorn M, et al: Randomized trial of dapsone and aerosolized pentamidine for the prophylaxis of *Pneumocystis carinii* pneumonia and toxoplasmic encephalitis. Am J Med 95:573, 1993

21 | Other HIV-Related Pneumonias

JOHN G. BARTLETT

The lower respiratory tract has been, and continues to be, the major site of opportunistic infections in patients with HIV infection. In the period prior to prophylaxis against *Pneumocystis carinii*, this organism accounted for over 70% of initial AIDS-defining diagnoses and was by far the most common identifiable cause of mortality. Despite this historic emphasis on *P. carinii* pneumonia, (PCP), pneumonia caused by other organisms appears to be even more common. There is a substantial spectrum of pathogens, but the majority of cases have no clear etiologic diagnosis. The purpose of this chapter is to review pneumonia, with emphasis on diagnosis and therapy. PCP and mycobacterial infections are not discussed because these are reviewed elsewhere in this book (see Chapters 20, 22 and 23).

FREQUENCY

The most accurate data for incidence of specific respiratory infections are from the multicenter cohort study that prospectively analyzed 1100 HIV-infected patients, including 167 controls, during the 5-year period from 1988 through 1994.[1] This study followed the initial use of PCP prophylaxis and stopped prior to the contemporary period of highly active antiretroviral therapy (HAART). Thus the study reflects the impact of PCP prophylaxis but fails to include the substantial impact of modern antiretroviral therapy. Results are summarized in Table 21–1. This shows that acute bronchitis was the most frequent lower airway infection, with an incidence approximately twofold higher than that in the control group. The frequency data for pneumonia, defined by the presence of typical clinical features accompanied by a demonstrable infiltrate on chest radiograph, indicated that the frequency of bacterial pneumonia was approximately the same as that for PCP. The frequency

of both PCP and non-PCP-associated pneumonia increased with sequential follow-up, presumably reflecting increased rates with progressive decline in CD4 cell count. Among the total of 521 episodes of pneumonia, the frequency of established or suspected pathogens was the following: bacterial infection, 44%; *P. carinii*, 42%; tuberculosis, 5%; and other opportunistic infections, 8%. This rate of non-PCP pulmonary infection is 30- to 100-fold higher than comparable data for the general population.

BACTERIAL PNEUMONIA

The results of three studies of bacterial pneumonia in patients with HIV infection are summarized in Table 21–2.[2–4] These data indicate that the number of pathogens is large, but a relatively small number account for the great majority. *Streptococcus pneumoniae* is consistently the most common identifiable bacterium, and *Haemophilus influenzae* ranks second. In a large number of cases, no etiologic agent is identified, presumably reflecting antecedent antibiotic administration, failure of the patient to produce sputum for diagnostic studies, or microbiologic ineptitude.

Pneumococcal Pneumonia

Streptococcus pneumoniae is by far the most frequent identifiable agent of bacterial pneumonia in patients with HIV infection. The frequency of pneumococcal bacteremia is estimated at approximately 100-fold greater in this group compared to the general population.[3] The increased rate applies to all CD4 strata but increases with a progressive decline, as would be expected.[1,3,4] All patients with HIV infection appear to be at risk, but injection drug use is an independent risk factor for both bacterial pneu-

331

TABLE 21–1. Frequency of Lower Respiratory Tract Infections in Patients with HIV Infection

INFECTION	TOTAL	YEAR 1	YEAR 2	YEAR 5
Bronchitis	586	13*	13	14
Bacterial pneumonia	232	3.9	6.1	7.3
P. carinii pneumonia	220	2.8	5.8	9.5
Tuberculosis	25	0.5	0.5	1.0
Other opportunistic infections[†]	44	0.6	1.1	1.9

*Episodes/100 person-years.
[†]Includes cytomegalovirus (19 cases), aspergillus (12), cryptococcus (7), and herpes simplex (2).
Adapted from Wallace JM, Hansen NI, Lavange L, et al: Respiratory disease trends in the Pulmonary Complications of HIV Infection study cohort. Am J Respir Crit Care Med 155:72, 1997. © American Lung Society, with permission.

monia and *S. pneumoniae* bacteremia. Nevertheless, the rates of pharyngeal carriage of *S. pneumoniae* appear to be similar in persons with and without HIV infection.[5]

The clinical presentation of pneumococcal pneumonia appears to be approximately the same for patients with and without HIV infection except for higher rates of bacteremia in those with HIV.[6] Extrapulmonary involvement, including meningitis, septic arthritis, and endocarditis, is relatively infrequent. Most patients present with symptoms of less than 1 week's duration, which clearly distinguishes this form of pneumonia from PCP, in which the indolent evolution of symptoms is so characteristic. Changes on chest radiograph and other laboratory findings are not unusual except that the absolute leukocyte count is relatively low in patients with more advanced stages of HIV infection. Characteristic changes on chest radiograph include a unilateral infiltrate that may be bronchopneumonia or lobar consolidation. Cavity formation, apical infiltrates, and hilar adenopathy are rare and suggest an alternative or concurrent process. Most patients produce sputum that may be purulent or "rusty." Pleural involvement with pleuritic pain and/or pleural effusion are common. Virtually all patients are febrile.

Recommendations for diagnosis of pneumococcal pneumonia obey the standard recommendations for establishing this diagnosis,[7] which have unfortunately deteriorated substantially in the last decade. Blood cultures and sputum for Gram's stain and culture should be obtained prior to inception of therapy. The probability of recovering *S. pneumoniae* after antibiotics have been given is virtually nil because of the fastidious growth requirements of the organism. The expectorated sputum should be physician procured, expeditiously transported to the laboratory and incubated within 2 hours, and processed by an experienced technician, preferably using a Quellung test to distinguish this organism from other streptococci that are universally present in expectorated sputum samples. Recovery of *S. pneumoniae* from blood, pleural fluid, or another uncontaminated specimen source is regarded as diagnostic; recovery from expectorated sputum requires clinical acumen based

TABLE 21–2. Bacterial Pneumonia in Patients with HIV Infection: Results of Three Series

	HIRSCHTICK ET AL.[2]	MUNDY ET AL.[3]	BOSCHINI ET AL.[4]
Number	237	144	126
Agent			
S. pneumoniae	36 (15%)	38 (21%)	33 (22%)
H. influenzae	12 (5%)	13 (7%)	22 (15%)
S. aureus	13 (5%)	7 (4%)	4 (3%)
Klebsiella	10 (4%)	6 (3%)	—
P. aeruginosa	6 (3%)	11 (6%)	1
GNB (other)*	8 (3%)	9 (5%)	—
Legionella	1	6 (3%)	—
C. pneumoniae	—	7 (4%)	—
M. pneumoniae	—	1	—
Nocardia	1	—	—
No etiologic agent	145 (61%)	46 (26%)	66 (45%)

*GNB, gram-negative bacillus.

on quantitation and clinical correlations. The need for specimen procurement prior to antibiotic therapy is confounded in this patient population by the frequent use of prophylactic sulfamethoxazole-trimethoprim and azithromycin; the prophylactic use of these drugs does substantially reduce the frequency of bacterial pneumonia, including *S. pneumoniae* pneumonia, although most patients will have infections involving strains resistant to these drugs if the disease developed during their administration.[8-10]

The treatment of pneumococcal pneumonia has become complicated in recent years because of escalating rates of antibiotic resistance. The major focus of attention has been on resistance to β-lactams, but this is the source of substantial misunderstanding based on the traditional methods to define susceptibility according to minimum inhibitory concentrations (MIC). The MIC to define "intermediate resistance" to penicillin has been 0.1 to 2 µg/ml, and high-level resistance is defined as a MIC of 2 µg/ml or more. The rate of reduced susceptibility to penicillin for clinical isolates of *S. pneumoniae* in recent years has been 20% to 40%, but most of these are in the "intermediate resistant" category that defines susceptibility based on levels of penicillin achieved in cerebrospinal fluid for patients with pneumococcal meningitis. Thus many authorities now believe that penicillin, amoxicillin,

and selected cephalosporins continue to be the preferred agents for most pneumococcal infections, except for strains showing high-level resistance and cases complicated by meningitis. Of particular interest is the fact that strains with reduced penicillin sensitivity (both intermediate and high-level penicillin resistance) show high rates of resistance to alternative drugs, including macrolides, doxycycline, sulfamethoxazole-trimethoprim, clindamycin, and cephalosporins. Drugs that show good activity against nearly all strains of *S. pneumoniae* regardless of penicillin sensitivity include vancomycin, the fluoroquinolones, and Synercid.[11] Based on these observations, recommendations for the treatment of pneumococcal pneumonia are summarized in Table 21-3.[7] Optimal treatment is obviously facilitated by recovery of the organism, with susceptibility test results to guide antibiotic options, and this is a major justification for quality microbiology studies. Recommendations for empiric antibiotic use, including patients with pending laboratory study, depend on the severity of the illness and regional patterns of susceptibility, which are quite variable. Fluoroquinolones, given orally or parenterally, are attractive options for both inpatients and outpatients based on nearly universal activity in vitro and a substantial clinical experience to verify efficacy. Nevertheless, alternative agents are advocated if supported by in vitro susceptibility tests because

TABLE 21-3. Recommendations for Treatment of Pneumococcal Pneumonia

SETTING	PREFERRED ANTIBIOTIC	ALTERNATIVE
Susceptibility Test Results Known		
Penicillin susceptible (MIC <0.1 µg/ml)	Penicillin G Amoxicillin	Cephalosporins* Macrolides[†] Clindamycin Fluoroquinolones[‡] Doxycycline
Intermediate penicillin resistance (MIC 0.1–1 µg/ml)	Penicillin G IV Amoxicillin Cefotaxime/ceftriaxone	Cephalosporins* Clindamycin Doxycycline
Penicillin resistant (MIC ≥2 µg/ml)	Fluoroquinolones[‡] Vancomycin	Agent selected by susceptibility tests Experimental agents[§]
Empiric Treatment		
Low risk for penicillin resistance and not seriously ill	Penicillin G Amoxicillin Cephalosporins* Macrolides[†]	
High risk for penicillin resistance or seriously ill	Fluoroquinolones[‡] Vancomycin	

*Cephalosporins: cefotaxime, ceftriaxone; oral—cefpodoxime, cefprozil, or cefuroxime.
[†]Macrolides: erythromycin, clarithromycin, and azithromycin.
[‡]Levofloxacin, sparfloxacin, grepafloxacin, trovafloxacin, or other fluoroquinolone with enhanced activity versus *S. pneumoniae*.
[§]Ketolides, oxazolidinones, and streptogramins.

of concern for abuse of fluoroquinolones. It should be noted that none of the antibiotics commonly used for pneumococcal pneumonia show substantial problems with drug interactions with antiretroviral agents, with the exception of clarithromycin. Ritonavir and indinavir increase clarithromycin levels 50% to 77%, while rifabutin and rifampin reduce clarithromycin levels 50% and 120%, respectively.

The mortality rate for bacteremic pneumococcal pneumonia among patients with HIV infection ranges from 5% to 11%.[6,12] This is somewhat lower than the reported experience for bacteremic pneumococcal pneumonia in patients without HIV infection, suggesting a favorable prognosis. One relatively unique feature is a high incidence of recurrent disease, with up to 13% recurrence within 6 months.[6,12]

Prevention of pneumococcal pneumonia is a major goal of current HIV management strategies.[12] Pneumococcal vaccine is recommended for HIV-infected patients at the time of the HIV diagnosis. Response to this vaccine is reduced among those with a CD4 cell count <200/mm^3. The experience with serotypes of strains involved in HIV-infected patients appears to be similar to that with strains causing infection in the general population, which account for approximately 70% to 80% of all pneumococcal infections. The vaccine also includes the predominant strains identified as having reduced susceptibility to penicillin. The duration of protection is not well established, but revaccination is sometimes suggested at 5-year intervals. As noted previously, PCP prophylaxis with sulfamethoxazole-trimethoprim and *Mycobacterium avium* prophylaxis using azithromycin or clarithromycin are associated with reduced rates of pneumococcal pneumonia.[8,9] This is consequently a salutary benefit; current guidelines do not recommend antibiotic prophylaxis to prevent bacterial pneumonia per se.[12]

Haemophilus influenzae

The rate of *H. influenzae* bacteremic pneumonia is increased by at least 100-fold for patients with HIV infection compared to immunocompetent controls.[12,13] Nevertheless, the rate of pneumococcal pneumonia is at least 10- to 100-fold greater than the rate for *H. influenzae*. Again, the clinical features of pneumonia caused by *H. influenzae* are not unique in this population. Chest radiographs usually show bronchopneumonia, symptoms are usually abrupt in onset, and most patients produce expectorated sputum. The diagnosis is best established with blood cultures and sputum Gram's stain plus culture using specimens obtained prior to antibiotic therapy. Most strains are susceptible to sulfamethoxazole-trimethoprim and azithromycin, so that prophylactic use of these drugs should notably reduce frequency and also reduce the diagnostic yield. Approximately two thirds of infections are caused by nontypable strains.[12-14] About 40% of strains produce β-lactamase, conferring resistance to amoxicillin and other penicillins. The preferred drugs are second- or third-generation cephalosporins, doxycycline, β-lactam/β-lactamase inhibitor combinations, fluoroquinolones, azithromycin, and sulfamethoxazole-trimethoprim.[15] The *H. influenzae* vaccine type B is not generally recommended because the rates of this infection are relatively low and because most infections involve nontypable strains.[12]

Staphylococcus aureus

The role of this organism in pneumonia among patients with HIV infection is independent of the retroviral infection per se but reflects the high rate of tricuspid valve endocarditis among injection drug users. The characteristic features of endocarditis, including murmur, embolic lesions, and immune-complex disease, are relatively infrequent. Nevertheless, the clinical constellation of fever, profound constitutional symptoms, and chest radiograph showing diffuse embolic lesions in a susceptible host is strongly suggestive. The CD4 cell count is relatively unimportant in defining susceptibility and response to therapy. Sulfamethoxazole-trimethoprim is active against approximately 95% of strains of *S. aureus*, and this observation emphasizes the potential utility of PCP prophylaxis among injection drug users. Blood cultures are virtually always positive, and most patients have continuous bacteremia. Standard therapy is oxacillin or vancomycin, either with or without gentamicin augmentation. Oral ciprofloxacin is equally effective, but this requires demonstration of in vitro susceptibility because of escalating rates of *S. aureus* resistance to fluoroquinolones.[16] Patients with HIV infection may also develop staphylococcal pneumonia, reflecting the immunosuppressed state, but these infections are relatively infrequent.[2-4] In these cases, the putative agent is relatively easy to recover from expectorated sputum, and these results must be interpreted with caution because of the frequency of sputum contamination, particularly in patients receiving antibiotics.

Pseudomonas aeruginosa

Pneumonia with this organism is infrequent in patients with HIV infection, but is a serious complication of late-stage disease, indicating severe immunosuppression.[17,18] Most patients have a CD4 cell count of less than $50/mm^3$, and some have additional risk factors such as neutropenia or corticosteroid therapy. Many have bacteremia. The morality rate is relatively high, 30% to 40% among those with bacteremic *Pseudomonas* pneumonia. The diagnosis is established with positive blood cultures and should be strongly suspected in those with high concentrations of *P. aeruginosa* in sputum cultures. Standard therapy is appropriate, usually using a combination of an antipseudomonad β-lactam (piperacillin, ticarcillin, ceftazidime, cefepime) or imipenem, usually in combination with tobramycin for prolonged periods. There is a temptation to substitute an oral fluoroquinolone such as ciprofloxacin or trovafloxacin to expedite hospital discharge and reduce the intravenous component of treatment, but my experience indicates high rates of relapse with fluoroquinolone-resistant strains.

Atypical Agents

Established cases of legionella, *Chlamydia pneumoniae* and *Mycoplasma pneumoniae* are relatively uncommon in patients with HIV infection. The agent in this category that is most suspect is *Legionella*, because of its clear association with other conditions that compromise cell-mediated immunity. One study showed a 50-fold increase in the frequency of legionnaires' disease in patients with HIV infection compared to the general population,[19] but this remains an isolated report that has not been substantiated by other authors.[20] Blatt et al.[21] reviewed eight cases of legionnaires' disease encountered in the HIV Natural History Study of the U.S. Air Force. This is an anecdotal collection of cases so the incidence is not known. The median CD4 cell count was $83/mm^3$, five cases were nosocomial, six of the patients had coexistent pulmonary pathogens, and none acquired this infection while receiving sulfamethoxazole-trimethoprim prophylaxis. All patients responded to standard therapy with a macrolide. The diagnosis of legionnaires' disease is best established with the urinary antigen assay and culture on appropriate media, usually by specific request. The urinary antigen detects only *L. pneumophila* serogroup 1, but this accounts for 70% of cases; the culture will detect all species

of *Legionella* but is technically difficult to perform and is fraught with numerous false-negative results.[12] For treatment, the traditional drug of choice has been a macrolide, but more recent studies suggest superior results with a fluoroquinolone such as ciprofloxacin or levofloxacin.[22]

Chlamydia pneumoniae has infrequently been recognized as a pathogen in patients with HIV infection and is not generally associated with immunodeficiency. Comandini et al.[23] described 13 cases verified by the standard serologic microimmunofluorescence assay in a retrospective analysis of 319 cases of pneumonia in patients with HIV infection. Thus this organism accounted for about 2.5% of all pneumonias in this population if one accepts standard serology as an adequate diagnostic test. A similar experience was noted in the report from Johns Hopkins.[2] Most of the patients in Comandini et al.'s review presented with focal pneumonia on chest radiograph, but three had changes suggesting PCP. Patients with mild disease improved spontaneously, but those with more serious illness required changes in treatment to macrolides or doxycycline. *Chlamydia pneumoniae* generally accounts for about 5% to 10% of pneumonia in immunocompetent hosts and should be suspected in patients with HIV infection if routine diagnostic tests are negative, there is failure to respond to β-lactam treatment, and there are accompanying symptoms reflecting upper airway involvement, such as pharyngitis and laryngitis. The CD4 cell count is probably irrelevant to host susceptibility. Unfortunately, few laboratories offer diagnostic tests for detection of this organism. The treatment of choice is a macrolide or doxycycline, although fluoroquinolones are also effective.

Mycoplasma pneumoniae is a common cause of pulmonary infections in young, immunocompetent adults. There is no established association with HIV infection or compromised cell-mediated immunity. As with *C. pneumoniae*, most laboratories do not offer tests that will be clinically useful for establishing the diagnosis in adults. Serology using immunoglobulin M may be useful in children but lacks sensitivity in adults. Clinical clues to this possible diagnosis are the presence of a relatively minor pulmonary infection in a young adult with negative routine diagnostic tests, particularly with extrapulmonary involvement including rash, hemolytic anemia, or aseptic meningitis. The CD4 cell count is probably irrelevant in terms of susceptibility. The preferred treatment is a macrolide or doxycycline, although fluoroquinolones are also effective.

FUNGAL INFECTIONS

Fungi other than *P. carinii* are relatively uncommon in patients with HIV infection, but they represent a diagnostic and therapeutic challenge, and are far more common in patients with HIV infection compared to the general population (Table 21–4). The non–*P. carinii* fungi of greatest importance are *Aspergillus*, *Cryptococcus neoformans*, and the endemic fungi *Histoplasma capsulatum* and *Coccidioides immitis*. Blastomycosis is infrequent in this population, even in the endemic region. *Candida* species may cause an invasive tracheobronchitis in late-stage HIV infection, but this is relatively rare, and *Candida* pneumonia is rare in any patient population; these points are emphasized because *Candida* are relatively common isolates in respiratory secretions as a result of airway contamination, so that interpretation must be cautious.

Pulmonary Aspergillosis

Aspergillus accounts for 1% to 4% of pneumonias in patients with AIDS.[24–26] This occurs late in the course; nearly all patients have CD4 cell counts less than 50/mm[3] and approximately 50% have additional risk factors of neutropenia and/or corticosteroid administration. Additional risk factors include marijuana use, structural disease of the lung, and exposure to broad-spectrum antibiotics.

There are two clinical forms of aspergillosis in this population: invasive parenchymal disease and tracheobronchial disease. Invasive parenchymal aspergillosis is associated with three types of changes on chest radiograph: cavitary disease usually involving the upper lobe, focal infiltrates that are often pleural based, and bilateral infiltrates that may show a nodular or interstitial pattern.[24] The types of tracheobronchial disease include a pseudomembranous form[27] and an ulcerative form,[28] or an obstructive form with mucus plugs.[29] Patients with the invasive parenchymal form usually present with fever, cough, and dyspnea that evolves over a period of weeks or months. There may be pleurisy or hemoptysis.[24] Nearly all patients have the risk factors defined above. The usual clinical features of tracheobronchial disease are dyspnea, cough, and wheezing accompanied by a chest radiograph that is usually normal or shows atelectasis.

The diagnosis requires the recovery of aspergillus or recognition of typical hyphal forms in respiratory secretions.[30,31] Clinical correlations are critical because aspergillus may colonize airways or represent a laboratory contaminant. A biopsy demonstrating fungal invasion is considered diagnostic.

The overall prognosis is poor, with mortality rates up to 90%.[26] This reflects severe immunosuppression complicated by a severe infection. Amphotericin B is considered the drug of choice; itraconazole may be effective but the experience is somewhat limited, and this drug is recommended primarily for long-term follow-up after amphotericin induction.[31] Also important is treatment directed against underlying defects, including neutropenia and corticosteroid use. HAART with immune reconstitution may represent the best option for long-term control of this pathogen.

Pulmonary Cryptococcosis

Cryptococcosis is a common complication of late-stage HIV infection, usually with meningitis that may be accompanied by pulmonary involvement, or, less commonly, there may be pneumonia without extrapulmonary disease. The CD4 cell count is usually less than 100/mm[3].[32]

The usual symptoms associated with pulmonary cryptococcosis are fever, cough, and dyspnea with or without pleurisy that evolves over a period of weeks.[33–35] The chest radiograph usually shows diffuse interstitial infiltrates that often suggest PCP.[34,35] Other features on chest radiograph include focal infiltrates, cavities that may be clinically silent, reticulonodular infiltrates, hilar adenopathy, and/or pleural effusions.

About 90% of patients with cryptococcosis have positive serum antigen assays for *C. neoformans*.[36] A preferred diagnostic test is recovery of the organism in respiratory secretions, including sputum or bronchoalveolar lavage (BAL).[37,38] This organism is a relatively rare contaminant, so recovery is virtually diagnostic. One report indicates that a cryptococcal antigen titer exceeding 1:8 in BAL is highly predictive of pulmonary cryptococcosis.[37] All patients with pulmonary cryptococcosis should have a lumbar puncture to determine the concurrent presence of meningitis that may be clinically silent.

The treatment of cryptococcal meningitis usually consists of amphotericin B followed by lifelong fluconazole as reviewed elsewhere in this

TABLE 21–4. Fungal Agents That Cause Pneumonia in Patients With HIV Infection

AGENT	COURSE	FREQUENCY, SETTING	TYPICAL FINDINGS	DIAGNOSIS
Cryptococcus neoformans	Chronic, subacute, or asymptomatic	Up to 8–10% in AIDS patients; late-stage HIV infection (median CD4 <50); 80% have cryptococcal meningitis	Nodule, cavity, diffuse or nodular infiltrates	Sputum, induced sputum, or FOB stain and culture; serum cryptococcal antigen usually positive; CSF analysis indicated if antigen or organism found at any site
Histoplasma capsulatum	Chronic or subacute	Up to 15% of AIDS patients in endemic area; usually advanced HIV infection with disseminated histoplasmosis (median CD4 <50)	Diffuse nodular infiltrates, nodule, focal infiltrate, cavity, hilar adenopathy	Sputum, induced sputum, or FOB stain and culture; serum and urine polysaccharide antigen assay is best noncultural technique with yield of 85% (blood) and 97% (urine)—available through J. Wheat, Indianapolis (800-HISTO-DG) @ $70/ assay; serology positive in 50–70%; yield with culture of sputum 80%, marrow 80%
Coccidioides immitis	Chronic or subacute	Up to 10% of AIDS patients in endemic area; usually advanced HIV infection (median CD4 <50; disseminated disease in 20–40%	Diffuse nodular infiltrates, focal infiltrate, cavity, hilar adenopathy	Sputum, induced sputum, or FOB stain and culture; KOH of expectorated sputum is rarely positive; PAP stain or silver stain of BAL positive in 40%; culture of BAL usually positive; serology (CF) positive in 70%; skin test positive in <10%; blood cultures positive in 10%
Candida	Chronic or subacute	Common isolate, rare cause of pulmonary disease (median CD4 count <50)	Bronchitis; rare cause of pulmonary infiltrate	Recovery in sputum or FOB specimen is meaningless (up to 30% of all expectorated sputum and FOB cultures in unselected patients yield *Candida* sp.); must have histologic evidence of invasion on biopsy
Aspergillus	Acute or subacute	Up to 4% of AIDS patients; usually advanced HIV infection (median CD4 <30); about 50% have severe neutropenia (ANC <500/mm³) ± chronic steroids; disseminated disease is uncommon	Focal infiltrate; cavity—often pleural based; diffuse infiltrates or reticulonodular infiltrates	Sputum stain and culture; false-positive and false-negative cultures common: most reliable tests are positive stain of respiratory secretions in typical setting or biopsy evidence of tissue invasion; yield with BAL is high; most are *A. fumagitus*

Abbreviations: ANC, absolute neutrophil count; BAL, bronchoalveolar lavage; CF, complement fixation; CSF, cerebrospinal fluid; FOB, fiberoptic bronchoscopy; KOH, potassium hydroxide, PAP, peroxidase–antiperoxidase.
Adapted from Bartlett JG: Medical Management of HIV Infection. Copyright JG Bartlett, Baltimore, 1998, p 244, with permission.

book (see Chapter 24). This should be more than adequate for concurrent pulmonary infection. The main issue concerns cryptococcal pneumonia that is not accompanied by extrapulmonary complications. Experience is limited, but most authorities recommend amphotericin B using the standard formulation or the less toxic, but substantially more expensive, lipid complex or liposomal formulations.[39-41] Patients with less serious disease can probably be treated adequately with fluconazole, although dosage recommendations and duration of treatment are not well defined.[40] The need for long-term prophylaxis in patients with cryptococcosis restricted to the lung is not known. As with virtually all opportunistic infections, effective antiviral therapy for HIV with immune reconstitution probably plays an important role in controlling this disease.

Histoplasmosis

Histoplasma capsulatum is endemic in the Mississippi, Ohio, and St. Lawrence river valleys. Histoplasmosis is found in over 5% of patients with AIDS living in the endemic area.[42] Cases in the endemic area usually represent primary infection with progressive dissemination; patients residing outside the endemic area usually have reactivation of latent infection.[43] Serious and disseminated disease is usually a consequence of severe immunosuppression, and most patients have CD4 cell counts below 100/mm^3.

Most patients with histoplasmosis complicating AIDS have disseminated disease, but pulmonary involvement is seen in up to 70% of these patients.[42,44] Common pulmonary symptoms include cough, fever, and dyspnea that is usually indolent in onset. Other common features that reflect disseminated disease include typical lesions of the skin and mucosal surfaces, wasting, bone marrow suppression, hepatosplenomegaly, lymphadenopathy, and diarrhea.[42-45] The usual changes on chest radiograph are diffuse interstitial or reticulonodular infiltrates; other features found less commonly are focal infiltrates, hilar adenopathy, and pleural effusions.[42,44]

The preferred diagnostic test is detection of *H. capsulatum* polysaccharide antigen in blood and/or urine by radioimmunoassay, a test available from reference laboratories (Table 21–4). The sensitivity of this test is 85% to 97% among patients with disseminated histoplasmosis; the antigen may also be detected in BAL specimens of up to 90% of patients with pulmonary in-

volvement.[46] The organism may also be detected by stain and culture of expectorated sputum in about 30% of patients.[47] Standard serologic tests are relatively insensitive (50% to 70%), and the histoplasmosis skin test is useless.[42]

The standard treatment for disseminated histoplasmosis or the progressive pulmonary form is amphotericin B, and this is recommended for patients with severe disease.[39] Itraconazole may be used for initial treatment in patients with mild or moderately severe infection and for those with more serious disease after amphotericin B induction.[48,49]

Coccidioidomycosis

Coccidioides immitis is endemic in the southwestern United States and represents a significant risk for patients with HIV infection. Up to 10% of AIDS patients in the endemic area develop either primary, progressive coccidioidomycosis or relapse of latent foci.[50,51]

Pulmonary involvement is frequent, and many patients also have extrapulmonary involvement that is most commonly expressed as cutaneous lesions, joint infections, or meningitis. Typical symptoms include cough, fever, and dyspnea, usually with an indolent presentation. The chest radiograph typically shows diffuse or focal infiltrates; less frequent findings are pulmonary nodules, hilar adenopathy, cavity formation, or pleural effusions.[51] The diagnosis is usually established with serology and/or stain and culture of respiratory secretions.[52] The skin test is generally not useful in the HIV-infected population.

Patients with diffuse pulmonary disease or disseminated disease have a poor prognosis and should receive aggressive treatment.[51] The standard treatment is amphotericin B using the standard formulation, the lipid complex, or the liposomal formulations. Azoles are effective in selected cases, but their role as primary agents in treatment is poorly defined.[53,54]

APPROACH TO THE PATIENT WITH SUSPECTED PULMONARY INFECTION

HIV Serology

There is a high rate of HIV infection among patients who are hospitalized with community-acquired pneumonia, especially those between the ages of 17 and 54 years and in urban areas with high rates of HIV infection in general. The experience with hospitalized patients with community-acquired pneumonia at Johns Hopkins Hospital for 1991 showed that 180 (45%) of the 385 patients had HIV infection, and a substantial portion were unaware of this associated condition. This experience emphasizes the importance of HIV serologic testing in young adults who are hospitalized with community-acquired pneumonia.

Decision for Hospitalization

Fine et al. have detailed the clinical observations that would constitute the basis for outpatient versus inpatient management of community-acquired pneumonia.[10] Recommendations are based on probability of mortality as determined by age, comorbid conditions, selected findings on physical exam (altered mental status, pulse >125/min, respiratory rate exceeding 30/min, systolic blood pressure <90 mm Hg, or temperature <35°C or >40°C), and selected laboratory findings (pH < 7.35, blood urea nitrogen >10.7 mmol/l, hematocrit <30%, pO_2 < 60 mm Hg[2], serum sodium <130 mEq/l, and glucose >13.9 mmol/l). Patients are stratified by risk score, and this constitutes the recommendation for hospitalization based on five classes with 19 variables. The rule was validated in a retrospective review of 38,000 patients hospitalized with pneumonia. Although these guidelines regarding admission are not necessarily advocated for HIV-infected patients, there is good reason to consider their application to this population as well.

Diagnostic Evaluation

The differential diagnosis in the HIV-infected patient with a suspected pulmonary infection requires a thoughtful analysis based on history and physical exam. The three variables that constitute the major components to formulate a rational differential diagnosis concern the temporal evolution of disease, the CD4 cell count, and the changes seen on chest radiograph. Exposure to antimicrobial agents for treatment and prophylaxis is also important. The CD4 cell count is critical. Nearly all opportunistic infections are relatively rare in patients with CD4 cell counts exceeding 200/mm[3]; the major exceptions are pneumococcal pneumonia and tuberculosis. Patients with injection drug use have this as an

independent risk factor for pneumococcal pneumonia, tuberculosis, and tricuspid valve endocarditis with septic emboli to the lung. The chest radiograph is critical for establishing pneumonia and for suggesting specific etiologic agents. The differential diagnosis based on chest radiograph changes are summarized in Table 21–5. Nearly all infectious diseases involving the pulmonary parenchyma are associated with demonstrable infiltrates on radiograph. There are relatively few exceptions (Table 21–5); the major exception is PCP, with false-negative radiographs in up to 30% of cases. Computed tomography (CT) scans and high-resolution CT scans are relatively sensitive in terms of detection of subtle lesions and also for defining pathology. Gallium lung scans were once widely advocated for detection of PCP, but this practice was largely abandoned because of the high cost of the scans, the time required for this test, and the availability of alternative diagnostic methods.

Etiologic Diagnosis

Expectorated sputum for stain and culture remains the preferred diagnostic test for recognition of common bacterial pathogens (other than atypical agents), mycobacteria, and occasional fungal infections; these specimens are essentially useless for detection of noninfectious diseases with pulmonary involvement (lymphoma and Kaposi's sarcoma), members of the herpesvirus group, and *P. carinii*. As noted above, this specimen should be procured by the physician, there should be gross evidence of purulence, and it should be transported to the laboratory for processing and incubation within 2 hours of processing; microbiology expertise for Gram's stain, sputum cytology, and culture is regarded as critical. Induced sputum is an alternative method to obtain lower respiratory tract secretions in patients who do not have a productive cough; this technique has established validity for detecting mycobacteria and *P. carinii*. In general, it produces an inferior specimen for routine bacterial cultures because of high concentrations of epithelial cells sloughed from the upper airways during the saline induction. Bronchoscopy is advocated for enigmatic pulmonary infections, especially in the compromised host, including patients with HIV infection. This has become a favored method for detecting *P. carinii*, but it has also proved extremely useful for detecting of mycobacteria in patients who cannot produce expectorated sputum, as well as in patients with selected non-

TABLE 21–5. Differential Diagnosis of Pulmonary Complications Based on Chest Radiograph Changes

CHANGE	COMMON AGENTS	RARE AGENTS
Consolidation	Pyogenic bacteria* Cryptococcosis Kaposi's sarcoma	*Nocardia* *M. tuberculosis* *M. kansasii* *Bordetella bronchiseptica*
Diffuse interstitial or reticulonodular infiltrates	*P. carinii** *P. carinii* + CMV Miliary tuberculosis Histoplasmosis Coccidioidomycosis	Kaposi's sarcoma Lymphocytic interstitial pneumonia *Leishmania donovani* *Toxoplasma gondii*
Nodule	*M. tuberculosis* Cryptococcosis Kaposi's sarcoma	
Cavity	*P. aeruginosa* GNB (other) *M. tuberculosis* *M. kansasii* Cryptococcosis Histoplasmosis Coccidioidomycosis Aspergillosis *Rhodococcus equi* Anaerobic bacteria *S. aureus* (IDU) *Nocardia*	*Legionella* *P. carinii* Lymphoma *M. avium*
Pleural effusion	Pyogenic bacteria* Kaposi's sarcoma *M. tuberculosis* Cryptococcosis *P. carinii* Hypoalbuminemia Septic emboli (IDU) Heart failure Aspergillosis	*Rhodococcus equi* Histoplasmosis Coccidioidomycosis *Leishmania donovani* Lymphoma *M. avium* *Nocardia* *P. carinii*
Hilar adenopathy	*M. tuberculosis* Cryptococcosis *M. avium* Histoplasmosis Coccidioidomycosis Kaposi's sarcoma Lymphoma	
Normal radiograph	*P. carinii** *M. tuberculosis*	*Cryptococcus* *M. avium*

Abbreviations: GNB, gram-negative bacteria; IDU, injection drug user.
*Most common cause.
Adapted from Bartlett JG: Medical Management of HIV Infection. Copyright JG Bartlett, Baltimore, 1998, p 247, with permission.

infectious pulmonary conditions (lymphoma, Kaposi's sarcoma) and some fungal infections. Bronchoscopy is not considered superior to expectorated sputum for detection of acid-fast bacilli (AFB) or for detecting conventional bacteria.

Respiratory secretions, when obtained, should have Gram's stain and sputum cytology, and specimens suggesting *S. pneumoniae* should have laboratory confirmation with a Quellung test. Specialized tests advocated for selective organisms include acid-fast stains for mycobacteria, Gomori methenamine silver stain, potassium hydroxide, and/or calcofluor white stain for fungi; and direct fluorescent antibody staining for influenza virus, respiratory syncytial virus, adenovirus, and parainfluenza. Conventional media are used for detecting the usual bacteria, and specialized media are required for *Legionella* and most fungi other than *Candida*.

Empiric Treatment

It is often necessary to initiate antibiotic therapy before diagnostic studies become available; even when these tests are available, they are often negative. Patients with suspected bacterial pneumonia should be treated according to the guidelines of the Infectious Diseases Society of America[12] or a comparable guideline document.[12] The recommendation for outpatients is a macrolide, fluoroquinolone, or doxycycline. For hospitalized patients on a general medical ward, the recommendation is for a β-lactam (cefotaxime or ceftriaxone) with or without a macrolide; the alternative is a fluoroquinolone. Also acceptable are cefuroxime with or without a macrolide, or monotherapy with azithromycin. For patients hospitalized in the intensive care unit for suspected bacterial pneumonia, the recommendation is for erythromycin, azithromycin or a fluoroquinolone, each given in combination with cefotaxime, ceftriaxone, or a β-lactam/β-lactamase inhibitor. Empiric treatment of suspected fungal infections with amphotericin is rarely given because of the extraordinary toxicity of the drug. The empiric use of an azole in this setting is regarded as ill-advised because selection of agents depends on the putative agent, many of these patients require lifelong therapy, and amphotericin B may be required but is associated with substantial risk as a result of adverse drug reactions. Patients with positive AFB smears from pulmonary secretions should be treated for tuberculosis pending culture. The majority of these isolates are *M. tuberculosis*, and less common species include *M. kansasii* and *M. avium*. Acid-fast organisms that are relatively rare pulmonary pathogens and usually indicate contamination when recovered include *M. gordonae*, *M. flavescens*, *M. simiae*, *M. szulgai*, *M. xenopi*, *M. malmoense*, and *M. terrae*. Mycobacteria that have occasionally been implicated in HIV-infected patients include *M. haemophilum*, *M. gordonae*, and *M. genavense*. It is advised that patients with positive acid-fast bacteria by stain, or with positive culture for these organisms pending identification, be treated for tuberculosis until more definitive information is available. *Nocardia* is an occasional pulmonary pathogen with advanced HIV infection and should be considered in the appropriate setting.

References

1. Wallace JM, Hansen NI, Lavange L, et al: Respiratory disease trends in the Pulmonary Complications of HIV Infection study cohort. Am J Respir Crit Care Med 155: 72, 1997
2. Hirschtick RE, Glassroth J, Jordan MC, et al: Bacterial pneumonia in persons infected with the human immunodeficiency virus. N Engl J Med 333:845, 1995
3. Mundy LM, Auwaerter PC, Oldach D, et al: Community-acquired pneumonia: Impact of immune status. Am J Respir Crit Care Med 152:1309, 1995
4. Boschini A, Smacchia C, DiFine M, et al: Community-acquired pneumonia in a cohort of former injection drug users with and without human immunodeficiency virus infection: Incidence, etiologies, and clinical aspects. Clin Infect Dis 23:107, 1996
5. Redd SC, Rutherford GW III, Sande MA, et al: The role of human immunodeficiency virus infection in pneumococcal bacteremia in San Francisco residents. J Infect Dis 162:1012, 1990
6. Janoff EN, Breiman RF, Daley CL, et al: Pneumococcal disease during HIV infection. Ann Intern Med 117:314, 1992
7. Bartlett JG, Breiman RF, Mandell LA, File TM Jr: Guidelines from the Infectious Diseases Society of America. Community-acquired pneumonia in adults: Guidelines for management. Clin Infect Dis 26:811, 1998
8. Bozzette SA, Finkelstein DM, Spector SA, et al: A randomized trial of three antipneumocystis agents in patients with advanced human immunodeficiency virus infection. N Engl J Med 332:693, 1995
9. Havlir DV, Dubé MP, Sattler FR, et al: Prophylaxis against disseminated *Mycobacterium avium* complex with weekly azithromycin, daily rifabutin, or both. N Engl J Med 335:392, 1996
10. Fine MJ, Auble TE, Yealy DM, et al: A prediction rule to identify low-risk patients with community-acquired pneumonia. N Engl J Med 336:243, 1997
11. Doern GV, Brueggemann A, Holley HP Jr, Rauch AM: Antimicrobial resistance of *Streptococcus pneumoniae* recovered from outpatients in the United States during the winter months of 1994 to 1995: Results of a 30-center national surveillance study. Antimicrob Agents Chemother 40:1208, 1996
12. USPHS/IDSA Prevention of Opportunistic Infections Working Group: 1997 USPHS/IDSA guidelines for the prevention of opportunistic infections in persons infected with human immunodeficiency virus: Disease-specific recommendations. Clin Infect Dis 25(Suppl 3): S313, 1997
13. Munoz P, Miranda ME, Llacaqueo A, et al: *Haemophilus* species bacteremia in adults. Arch Intern Med 157:1869, 1997
14. Steinhart R, Reingold AL, Taylor F, et al: Invasive *Haemophilus influenzae* infections in men with HIV infection. JAMA 268:3350, 1992
15. Thornsberry C, Ogilvie P, Kahn J, et al: Surveillance of antimicrobial resistance in *Streptococcus pneumoniae*, *Haemophilus influenzae*, and *Moraxella catarrhalis* in the United States in 1996–97 respiratory season. Diagn Microbiol Infect Dis 29:249, 1997
16. Heldman AW, Hartert TV, Daoud EG, et al: Oral antibiotic treatment of right-sided staphylococcal endocarditis in intravenous drug-users: prospective randomized comparison with perenteral therapy. Am J Med 101:68, 1996

17. Mendelson MH, Gurtman A, Szabo S, et al: *Pseudomonas aeruginosa* bacteremia in patients with AIDS. Clin Infect Dis 18:886, 1994

18. Shepp DH, Tang IT-L, Ramundo MB, et al: Serious *Pseudomonas aeruginosa* infection in AIDS. J Acquir Immune Defic Syndr Hum Retrovirol 7:823, 1994

19. Marston BJ, Lipman HV, Breiman RF: Surveillance for Legionnaires' disease: Risk factors for morbidity and mortality. Arch Intern Med 154:2417, 1994

20. Stout JE, Yu VL: Legionellosis. N Engl J Med 337:682, 1997

21. Blatt SP, Dolan MJ, Hendrix CW, et al: Legionnaires' disease in human immunodeficiency virus-infected patients: Eight cases and review. Clin Infect Dis 18:227, 1994

22. Edelstein PH: Antimicrobial chemotherapy for Legionnaires' disease: A review. Clin Infect Dis 21:S265, 1995

23. Comandini UV, Maggi P, Santopadre P, et al: *Chlamydia pneumoniae* respiratory infections among patients infected with the human immunodeficiency virus. Eur J Clin Microbiol Infect Dis 16:720, 1997

24. Wallace WT Jr, Sais GJ, Frank I, et al: Pulmonary aspergillosis in patients with AIDS: Clinical and radiographic correlations. Chest 105:37, 1994

25. Denning DW, Follansbee SE, Scolaro M, et al: Pulmonary aspergillosis in the acquired immunodeficiency syndrome. N Engl J Med 324:654, 1991

26. Minamoto GY, Barlam TF, Vander Els NJ: Invasive aspergillosis in patients with AIDS. Clin Infect Dis 14:66, 1992

27. Pervex NK, Kleinerman J, Kattan M, et al: Pseudomembranous necrotizing bronchial aspergillosis: A variant of invasive aspergillosis in patients with hemophilia and acquired immune deficiency syndrome. Am Rev Respir Dis 131:961, 1985

28. Kemper CA, Hostetler JS, Follansbee SE, et al: Ulcerative and plaque-like tracheobronchitis due to infection with *Aspergillus* in patients with AIDS. Clin Infect Dis 17:344, 1993

29. Denning DW: Unusual manifestations of aspergillosis. Thorax 50:812, 1995

30. Lortholary O, Meyoha MC, Dupont B, et al: Invasive aspergillosis in patients with acquired immunodeficiency syndrome: Report of 33 cases. Am J Med 95:171, 1993

31. Denning DW, Tucker RM, Hanson LH, Stevens DA: Treatment of invasive aspergillosis with itraconazole. Am J Med 86:791, 1989

32. Masur H, Ognibene FP, Yarchoan R, et al: CD4 counts as predictors of opportunistic pneumonias in human immunodeficiency virus (HIV) infection. Ann Intern Med 111:223, 1989

33. Chuck SL, Sande MA: Infections with *Cryptococcus neoformans* in the acquired immunodeficiency syndrome. N Engl J Med 321:794, 1989

34. Clark RA, Greer D, Atkinson W, et al: Spectrum of *Cryptococcus neoformans* infection in 68 patients infected with human immunodeficiency virus. Rev Infect Dis 12:768, 1990

35. Chechani V, Kamholz SL: Pulmonary manifestations of disseminated cryptococcosis in patients with AIDS. Chest 98:1060, 1990

36. Eng RH, Bishburg E, Smith SM, et al: Cryptococcal infections in patients with acquired immunodeficiency syndrome. Am J Med 81:19, 1986

37. Baughman RP, Rhodes JC, Dohn MN, et al: Detection of Cryptococcal antigen in bronchoalveolar lavage fluid: A prospective study of diagnostic utility. Am Rev Respir Dis 145:1226, 1992

38. Malabonga VM, Basti J, Kamholz SL: Utility of bronchoscopic sampling techniques for cryptococcal disease in AIDS. Chest 99:370, 1991

39. American Thoracic Society statement: Fungal infections in HIV-infected persons. Am J Respir Crit Care Med 152:816, 1995

40. Nelson MR, Fisher M, Cartledge J, et al: The role of azoles in the treatment and prophylaxis of cryptococcal disease in HIV infection. AIDS 8:651, 1994

41. Coker RJ, Viviani M, Gazzard BG, et al: Treatment of cryptococcosis with liposomal amphotericin B (AmBisome) in 23 patients with AIDS. AIDS 7:829, 1993

42. Wheat LJ, Connolly-Stringfield PA, Baker RL: Disseminated histoplasmosis in the acquired immunodeficiency syndrome: Clinical findings, diagnosis and treatment, and review of the literature. Medicine 69:361, 1990

43. Salzman SH, Smith RL, Aranda CL: Histoplasmosis in patients at risk for the acquired immunodeficiency syndrome in a nonendemic setting. Chest 93:916, 1988

44. Sarosi GA, Johnson PC: Disseminated histoplasmosis in patients infected with human immunodeficiency virus. Clin Infect Dis 14(Suppl 1):S60, 1992

45. Nightingale SD, Parks JM, Pounders SM, et al: Disseminated histoplasmosis in patients with AIDS. South Med J 83:624, 1990

46. Wheat LJ, Connolly-Stringfield P, William B, et al: Diagnosis of histoplasmosis in patients with the acquired immunodeficiency syndrome by detection of Histoplasma capsulatum polysaccharide antigen in bronchoalveolar lavage fluid. Am Rev Respir Dis 145:1421, 1992

47. Prechter GC, Prakash UBS: Bronchoscopy in the diagnosis of pulmonary histoplasmosis. Chest 95:1033, 1989

48. Como JA, Dismukes WE: Oral azole drugs as systemic antifungal therapy. N Engl J Med 330:263, 1994

49. Wheat LJ, Hafner RE, Wulfsohn M, et al: Itraconazole (Itra) is effective treatment for histoplasmosis in AIDS: Prospective multicenter noncomparative trial (abstract). In: Program and Abstracts of the 32nd Interscience Conference on Antimicrobial Agents and Chemotherapy, 1992, p 312

50. Ampel NM, Dols CL, Galgiani JN: Coccidioidomycosis during human immunodeficiency virus infection: Results of a prospective study in coccidioidal endemic area. Am J Med 94:235, 1993

51. Fish DG, Ampel NM, Galgiani JN, et al: Coccidioidomycosis during human immunodeficiency virus infection: A review of 77 patients. Medicine 69:384, 1990

52. DiTomasso JO, Ampel NM, Sobonya RE, Bloom JW: Bronchoscopic diagnosis of pulmonary coccidioidomycosis: Comparison of cytology, culture and transbronchial biopsy. Diagn Microbiol Infect Dis 18:83, 1994

53. Tucker RM, Denning DW, Dupont B, Stevens DA: Itraconazole therapy for chronic coccidioidal meningitis. Ann Intern Med 112:108, 1990

54. Galgiani JN, Cantanzaro A, Cloud GA, et al: Fluconazole therapy for coccidioidal meningitis. Ann Intern Med 119:28, 1993

CHAPTER

22

Disseminated *Mycobacterium avium* Complex and Other Atypical Mycobacterial Infections

MARK A. JACOBSON

DISSEMINATED *MYCOBACTERIUM AVIUM* COMPLEX INFECTION

Epidemiology

Disseminated *Mycobacterium avium* complex (MAC) infection has been one of the most important opportunistic infectious complications associated with AIDS. The association was recognized early in the HIV epidemic[1-8] (disseminated MAC infection had been reported only rarely in patients without HIV disease[3]). Among patients with HIV, disseminated MAC infection historically has occurred almost exclusively in patients with advanced AIDS, those with fewer than 50 CD4 lymphocytes/μl.[4-6] According to Centers for Disease Control and Prevention (CDC) statistics, disseminated MAC was reported as an index AIDS diagnosis in 5.3% of AIDS cases between 1981 and 1987.[7] However, in a large retrospective series from this same time period involving 366 AIDS patients, this opportunistic infection was diagnosed during the course of illness in 18%; the attack rate may have been even higher, because 53% of 79 autopsies in this series showed evidence of disseminated MAC.[8] Subsequent prospective natural history studies conducted prior to the availability of highly active antiretroviral therapy (HAART) or specific antimicrobial prophylaxis for MAC indicated that one third to one half of AIDS patients might develop disseminated MAC infection. Among patients with advanced HIV disease who had serial blood spec-

imens cultured for mycobacteria over a median 1-year period, in the late 1980s, the 2-year actuarial incidence of MAC mycobacteremia was approximately 40%.[6] Also, in a subcohort analysis of 844 men with AIDS in the Multicenter AIDS Cohort Study followed during the same time period, 33.4% of those who received early *Pneumocystis carinii* prophylaxis subsequently developed disseminated MAC infection.[9]

With the advent of MAC prophylaxis in the early 1990s, the incidence of the infection began to decline. Between 1993 and 1994, a marked decrease in the incidence of adult AIDS-defining disseminated MAC or *Mycobacterium kansasii* infection was noted by the CDC, with 4132 cases reported in 1993 compared to 2468 in 1994,[10,11] a 40% decrease that almost certainly resulted from the widespread introduction of rifabutin and macrolide MAC prophylaxis into clinical practice during this time period.

However, between 1994 and 1996, a further significant decrease in the incidence of AIDS-defining MAC infection was noted by the CDC in the United States, a decrease not likely explained by increased utilization of specific antimicrobial prophylaxis. Although the overall number of newly reported adult AIDS cases in 1996 was 14% less than in 1994, the number of AIDS-indicator cases of disseminated MAC or *M. kansasii* infection decreased by 30%.[11,12] Of note, in early 1996, the potent HIV protease inhibitor drugs indinavir and ritonavir became widely available in clinical practice. However, during this same time period, no major changes were reported in the proportion of HIV-infected patients receiving specific MAC prophylaxis. At

Hôpital de la Pitié-Salpêtrière in Paris, the incidence density of disseminated MAC infection decreased from 14/100 patient-years in the second semester of 1995 to 1.8/100 patient-years in the second semester of 1996 among AIDS patients.[13] By the end of 1997, the incidence of new cases of disseminated MAC infection at San Francisco General Hospital had decreased by more than 80% compared to 1994.[14] Data from recent clinical trials provide a more direct link between the use of HAART and decreased incidence of disseminated MAC. For example, in the United States, the AIDS Clinical Trials Group (ACTG) randomized 1156 lamuvidine/protease inhibitor–naive patients with a baseline median CD4 count of 87 cells/μl to zidovudine/lamivudine or zidovudine/lamivudine/indinavir therapy.[15] After a median 38 weeks of follow-up, the incidence density of MAC disease was only 1.8 to 2.1 events per 100 patient-years. It is not known whether this dramatic decrease in new MAC disease will be sustained; for example, MAC incidence could increase again in the future if the new HAART regimens eventually fail in large numbers of patients as a result of virologic resistance.

MAC is a ubiquitous soil and water saprophyte, and epidemiologic data suggest that disseminated MAC infection results from new environmental acquisition of the organism (rather than reactivation of quiescent, endogenous mycobacteria). For example, a common water-source nosocomial outbreak of MAC disease has been reported in an AIDS ward.[16] The route of MAC invasion in AIDS patients may be through the gastrointestinal or respiratory tract. The presence of large clusters of mycobacteria within macrophages of the small bowel lamina propria suggests that the bowel might be the portal of entry. However, respiratory isolation of MAC also frequently precedes disseminated infection, suggesting MAC infection may begin in the lungs as well.[17]

Pathogenesis

In AIDS, the key host defect allowing dissemination of MAC is macrophage dysfunction, specifically the failure of macrophages to kill phagocytized MAC. MAC is able to survive within macrophages unless intracellular killing mechanisms (defective in AIDS) are activated. Cytokines such as interferon-γ, tumor necrosis factor, interleukin-12 and interleukin-2, which play a critical role in this macrophage killing function, are now a major topic of investigation

in understanding MAC pathogenesis and in developing potential new adjunctive treatments for MAC disease.[18–20]

In AIDS, MAC causes high-grade, widely disseminated infection. Nearly all AIDS patients with invasive MAC infection (as opposed to stool, urine, or respiratory secretion colonization) have had positive mycobacterial blood cultures.[8] In the majority of those autopsied, MAC also could be isolated from spleen, lymph nodes (Color Plate I*D*), liver, lung, adrenals, colon, kidney, and bone marrow. The magnitude of mycobacteremia can range from 1^4 to 10^4 colony-forming units per milliliter of blood.[21] At autopsy, bone marrow, spleen, lymph nodes, and liver have yielded even higher microbial loads.[21] Histopathologic studies of involved organs typically have shown absent or poorly formed granulomas and acid-fast bacteria within macrophages.[1] In addition, there have been reports of localized, nondisseminated, MAC infection associated with granuloma formation, tissue destruction, and abscess formation in lymph nodes or skin. These cases have usually occurred soon after antiretroviral therapy was initiated, suggesting some reconstitution of the immune response to MAC.[22–25]

Clinical Manifestations

Because most AIDS patients with disseminated MAC infection have other concomitant infections or neoplasms, and because MAC appears to result in little histopathologic evidence of inflammatory response or tissue destruction, the relationship between constitutional symptoms, organ dysfunction, and MAC infection was initially uncertain. Nevertheless, several large retrospective studies strongly suggest a negative effect of disseminated MAC infection on mortality and morbidity in AIDS. Horsburgh et al. noted a median 4-month survival among 39 patients with untreated disseminated MAC infection compared to 11 months among 39 controls matched for absolute CD4 lymphocyte count, prior AIDS status, history of antiretroviral therapy, history of *Pneumocystis carinii* pneumonia (PCP) prophylaxis, and year of diagnosis ($p < .0001$).[26] At San Francisco General Hospital, we examined the association between disseminated MAC infection and survival after index PCP diagnosis.[17] Among 137 consecutive patients who had a sterile body site cultured for mycobacteria within 3 months of their first AIDS-defining episode of PCP, median survival was significantly shorter in those with disseminated MAC infec-

---

TABLE 22–1. Clinical Syndromes Associated with Disseminated MAC Infection in AIDS

Systemic
Fever, malaise, weight loss, often associated with anemia, neutropenia

Gastrointestinal
Chronic diarrhea and abdominal pain (MAC invasion of colon often observed at autopsy)
Chronic malabsorption (Whipple's-like histopathologic changes in small intestine often observed at autopsy)
Extrabiliary obstructive jaundice secondary to periportal lymphadenopathy

---

Data from Greene JB, Sidhu GS, Lewin S, et al: *Mycobacterium avium-intracellulare*: A cause of disseminated life-threatening infection in homosexuals and drug abusers. Ann Intern Med 97:539, 1982.

tion than in those with negative cultures (107 versus 275 days; $p < .01$), even after controlling for age, absolute lymphocyte count, and hemoglobin concentration.

There are four clinical syndromes, often overlapping, that have been associated anecdotally with disseminated MAC infection. The characteristics of these syndromes are summarized in Table 22–1. In a prospective natural history study of MAC bacteremia underway at San Francisco General Hospital, we interviewed patients regarding symptoms and evaluated laboratory test results at the time of diagnostic evaluation for disseminated MAC infection.[27] We observed that, among patients with fewer than 50 CD4 lymphocytes/μl, a history of fever for more than 30 days, a hemocrit less than 30%, or a serum albumin level less than 3.0 gm/dl were all sensitive predictors of MAC bacteremia. However, neither severe fatigue, diarrhea, weight loss, neutropenia, nor thrombocytopenia discriminated between those who were subsequently found to be blood-culture positive or negative for MAC.

Since 1987, there have been occasional cases reported in which AIDS patients initiating antiretroviral therapy have subsequently developed localized visceral or cutaneous MAC abscesses without mycobacteremia.[22–25] Unlike disseminated infection (see below), these lesions have responded remarkably well to drainage and antimycobacterial therapy. These case series have led to speculation that improved immune function resulting from antiretroviral therapy was responsible for localization of infection. In patients developing such localized abscesses soon after initiating HAART, the clinical course has sometimes been explosive, with large abscess formation and very high fever.

Diagnosis

Special blood culture techniques for isolating mycobacteria, such as the broth-based BACTEC

system or agar-based Dupont Isolator system, appear to be the most sensitive methods for diagnosing disseminated MAC infection.[28] With these techniques, the sensitivity approaches 100%. Specific DNA probes for MAC have recently become available; these probes make it possible to differentiate MAC from other mycobacteria within hours when there is sufficient mycobacterial growth in broth or agar.[29] Time to culture positivity ranges from 5 to 51 days. It is uncommon for blood cultures to be negative when there is a positive histologic diagnosis from lymph node, liver, or bone marrow biopsies. However, one advantage of biopsied specimens is that staining the tissue may demonstrate acid-fast bacteria or granuloma weeks before blood cultures turn positive.

The clinical significance of MAC isolated from sputum or stool remains controversial. In our prospective natural history study, we have found that only two thirds of patients with negative blood cultures but positive stool or sputum cultures for MAC subsequently developed disseminated MAC infection.[30] Therefore, at this time, neither stool nor sputum culture can be recommended as a screening test to identify patients likely to develop MAC bacteremia.

Therapy

MAC is resistant to all standard antituberculous drugs (except ethambutol) at concentrations achievable in plasma. Yet half or more of MAC strains can be inhibited by achievable concentrations of rifabutin, rifampin, clofazimine, cycloserine, amikacin, ethionamide, ethambutol, azithromycin, clarithromycin, ciprofloxacin, or sparfloxacin (Table 22–2).[31–36] Unfortunately, drug levels necessary to kill MAC in vitro (minimum bactericidal concentration) have been 8 to more than 32 times that of inhibitory levels.[35] Whereas combinations of antimycobacterial agents have shown in vitro inhibitory syner-

TABLE 22–2. Drugs Capable of Inhibiting Most MAC Strains at Concentrations Achievable in Plasma

Amikacin
Azithromycin
Ciprofloxacin
Clarithromycin
Clofazimine
Cycloserine
Ethambutol
Ethionamide
Rifabutin
Rifampin
Sparfloxacin

gism, bactericidal synergism has been more difficult to demonstrate.[34,35] In addition, for in vivo killing, drugs must penetrate macrophages as well as the MAC cell wall. Nevertheless, in animal models of disseminated MAC infection, both single and combination antimycobacterial regimens have reduced mycobacterial colony counts by several logs and improved survival.[31]

Results of several sequential trials reported by the California Collaborative Treatment Group (CCTG) highlight the caution needed when interpreting results of treatment trials that have no control arm. In 1990, this group reported striking microbiologic and clinical effects in previously untreated patients with disseminated MAC who were given a combination regimen that included intravenous amikacin and oral rifampin, ethambutol, and ciprofloxacin.[37] Given the modest results that had previously been reported with oral antimycobacterial agents, many drew the conclusion from this uncontrolled trial that the amikacin was primarily responsible for the efficacy of this regimen. Subsequently, the CCTG reported similar microbiologic and clinical results in another similarly designed uncontrolled trial in which intravenous amikacin was replaced by oral clofazimine.[38] More data regarding the clinical utility of intravenous amikacin are now available from a controlled trial conducted by the National Institute of Allergy and Infectious Diseases, which sponsored an ACTG study in which 72 patients with previously untreated disseminated MAC were all given a combination oral regimen of rifampin, ethambutol, ciprofloxacin, and clofazimine and were also randomized to receive or not receive additional intravenous amikacin.[39] In this controlled trial, there were no significant differences in microbiologic or clinical outcomes, demonstrating that the cost, inconvenience, and risk of toxicity of intravenous amikacin is unlikely to

translate into a significant clinical benefit for patients with disseminated MAC.

Data on in vivo microbiologic efficacy against MAC have been most impressive with the new macrolides clarithromycin and azithromycin. A multicenter, randomized, placebo-controlled, dose-ranging trial of clarithromycin monotherapy in patients with previously untreated disseminated MAC reported a median decrease of greater than 2 log in blood MAC colony-forming units—a more potent microbiologic effect than reported in any earlier treatment trials.[40] This microbiologic effect was accompanied by significant clinical improvement according to an analysis of symptoms and quality-of-life indices. However, a globally beneficial dose–response effect was not observed. Unacceptably high gastrointestinal toxicity occurred at the 2000-mg bid dose. Although the 1000-mg bid dose had greater microbiologic efficacy than the 500-gm bid dose, there was actually a trend toward increased mortality in the former group that has subsequently been confirmed in other studies,[41] indicating that a maximum dose for this drug is 500 mg bid. Not surprisingly, drug resistance emerged after 2 to 3 months of monotherapy in this trial, affecting approximately half of patients in all dosing arms. Hence, one or more other antimycobacterial agents must be co-administered with the macrolide in an attempt to prevent or at least delay emergence of resistance, which is almost certain to be associated with clinical deterioration.

Azithromycin is another effective macrolide for MAC treatment. In a similarly designed trial of azithromycin monotherapy, patients with newly diagnosed positive MAC blood cultures were randomized to receive either 600 or 1200 mg/day of azithromycin. At 6 weeks, approximately half of blood cultures were sterile in both groups; the mean reduction in mycobacteremia was 2.0 and 1.55 log, respectively ($p > .05$).[42] Antimycobacterial efficacy was therefore similar to that of clarithromycin monotherapy. Also, as with clarithromycin, there was increased gastrointestinal intolerance with the higher dose.

Preliminary data from a comparative trial of clarithromycin- versus azithromycin-based therapy for newly diagnosed disseminated MAC indicates that clarithromycin may be a more effective agent.[43] Sixty-one patients with MAC-positive blood cultures were treated with ethambutol 15 mg/kg qd and randomized to also receive either clarithromycin 500 mg bid or azithromycin 600 mg qd. The rate of mycobacteremia clearance was significantly different, favoring clarithromycin (92% vs. 33% sterile blood cultures at 16 weeks). However, fewer than half of the patients enrolled were microbiologically evaluable, so the generalizability of these results is uncertain.

Nonmacrolide antimycobacterial agents have been evaluated in several randomized, controlled trials. In order to determine which of the orally bioavailable nonmacrolide antimycobacterial agents might be the most potent in vivo, the CCTG conducted a randomized, controlled trial in which patients with previously untreated disseminated MAC were assigned to receive a 4-week regimen of rifampin, ethambutol, or clofazimine monotherapy.[44] In this trial, only ethambutol resulted in a statistically significant reduction in blood MAC colony-forming units, suggesting that ethambutol might be the most potent of these three antimycobacterial agents. A recent trial has confirmed the clinical benefit of ethambutol when combined with clarithromycin.[45] In this trial, 80 patients with newly diagnosed disseminated MAC infection were all assigned to receive clarithromycin and clofazimine and randomized to receive or not receive ethambutol 800 mg qd. Although 69% of patients initially responded microbiologically, the subsequent mycobacteremia relapse rate at 36 weeks was 50% with ethambutol and 91% without ethambutol ($p = .014$).

Recent data regarding rifabutin treatment for disseminated MAC have also been particularly promising. Interestingly, when rifabutin was evaluated in the 1980s as a treatment for MAC at doses of 100 to 300 mg/day, it was found to be ineffective. In a recent randomized, blind, placebo-controlled trial in which patients with newly diagnosed disseminated MAC were assigned to receive clofazimine/ethambutol or clofazimine/ethambutol/rifabutin (600 mg/day), approximately half of the patients receiving the rifabutin-containing regimen had a greater than 2-log decrease in blood MAC colony-forming units or sterilization of the blood, compared with none of those receiving only clofazimine/ethambutol.[46]

Clofazimine appears to add no clinical efficacy and may actually be harmful when used in macrolide-based combination regimens. A recent trial assigned 106 patients with MAC bacteremia to receive clarithromycin and ethambutol and randomized these patients also to receive or not receive clofazimine 100 mg qd.[47] In this trial, clofazimine was not associated with any benefit in microbiologic response. In fact, patients assigned clofazimine had a significantly higher mortality, indicating that clofazimine should not be used in the initial treatment of disseminated MAC.

The long-term clinical benefit of combination regimens that include both macrolide and nonmacrolide agents for treatment of disseminated MAC has been confirmed recently in a randomized multicenter trial conducted by the Canadian MAC Study Group. In this study, 187 evaluable patients with MAC mycobacteremia were randomized to receive a regimen of clarithromycin 1000 mg bid, rifabutin 600 mg qd, and ethambutol 15 mg/kg/day versus ciprofloxacin 750 mg bid, rifampin 600 mg qd, clofazimine 100 mg qd, and ethambutol 15 mg/kg/day. The in vivo quantitative antimycobacterial effect was significantly better with the macrolide-containing regimen, as was median survival (8.6 versus 5.2 months; $p = .001$).[48]

Table 22–3 summarizes what are currently considered to be the best options for the treatment of disseminated MAC. A macrolide such as clarithromycin or azithromycin should be combined with either rifabutin, ethambutol, or both agents. A multicenter trial is underway to determine which of these options is most effective.

Of note, we have recently reported four patients who had undergone prolonged therapy for disseminated MAC infection, began receiving potent combination antiretroviral regimens after disseminated MAC infection was diagnosed, had absolute CD4 counts rise to more than 100 cells/μl, and had resolution of all MAC-related symptoms. After simultaneous blood and bone marrow cultures were negative, all these individuals discontinued antimycobacterial therapy and have had no relapse after 2 to 12 months of follow-up.[49] In the pre-HAART era, relapse of disseminated MAC would have been predicted

---

TABLE 22–3. Treatment of Disseminated *M. avium* Complex Infection

- Clarithromycin 500 mg PO bid (alternatively azithromycin 500 or 600 mg PO qd)
- PLUS one or both of the following agents:
  1. Ethambutol 15 mg/kg qd
  2. Rifabutin 300 mg PO qd*

*Higher doses may be needed when co-administered with azithromycin rather than clarithromycin. Dose should be reduced to 150 mg qd when co-administered with indinavir or nelfinavir and to 150 mg qod when co-administered with ritonavir.

to occur soon after discontinuing chronic suppressive therapy. Currently, it is not known whether chronic suppressive therapy for MAC disease can be safely discontinued for most or just a few HAART responders. It is also not known how long suppressive therapy can be safely withheld, or, phrased in a different way, when such suppressive therapy must be reinstituted to prevent MAC disease recrudescence.

Finally, in HIV-infected patients, it may be difficult to distinguish tuberculosis from MAC disease. Therefore, an antituberculous regimen should be instituted whenever acid-fast bacteria are demonstrated (and cannot yet be differentiated between MAC and *Mycobacterium tuberculosis*) in a specimen from a patient with HIV infection and clinical evidence of mycobacterial disease.[50]

Prophylaxis

Because 40% of patients with advanced HIV disease (i.e., CD4 counts <50 cells/μl) are likely to develop disseminated MAC, it makes sense to develop a strategy for preventing this disease in patients at risk. There are few specific, clearly defined risk factors for developing disseminated MAC disease, other than a low CD4 lymphocyte count; therefore, any prophylactic strategy has to be applied to the entire population at risk (i.e, those patients with <50 CD4 cells/μl).

Results of combined analysis of two randomized, placebo-controlled trials of rifabutin prophylaxis, conducted in over 1000 patients with advanced HIV disease, demonstrated that prophylactic rifabutin, at a dose of 300 mg/day, reduced the incidence of mycobacteremia by half.[51] Patients who received rifabutin and subsequently developed mycobacteremia had MAC isolates in their blood that retained susceptibility to rifabutin. However, neither trial alone, nor the combined analysis, demonstrated that rifabutin significantly reduced mortality. Nevertheless, a combined analysis of both trials revealed an increased incidence of fever, fatigue, anemia, alkaline phosphatase elevations, and hospitalizations in patients who received placebo compared with those who received rifabutin. Data are also available from a placebo-controlled study in which 667 patients with advanced HIV disease were randomized to receive either clarithromycin 500 mg or placebo bid. During a median 10-month follow-up, only 6% of clarithromycin-assigned patients versus 16% of placebo-assigned patients developed mycobacteremia ($p < .001$).[52] More importantly, median

survival was significantly longer for clarithromycin- than for placebo-assigned patients (32% versus 41% mortality; $p = .026$). However, among the clarithromycin-assigned patients who did develop disseminated MAC infection, 58% had mycobacteremia with MAC isolates that were highly resistant to clarithromycin (minimum inhibitory concentration >512 μg/ml). Clarithromycin at this same dose has also been compared to rifabutin and the combination of clarithromycin and rifabutin in a large randomized trial involving 1216 patients with absolute CD4 counts less than 100 cells/μl. In this trial, clarithromycin was significantly more effective than rifabutin in preventing mycobacteremia (9% vs. 15% of patients; $p < .01$), but addition of rifabutin to clarithromycin provided no significant increase in efficacy compared to clarithromycin alone.[53]

A regimen of weekly azithromycin prophylaxis has been evaluated in a similarly designed trial in which 693 patients with fewer than 100 CD4 cells/μl were randomized to azithromycin 1200 mg once weekly, daily rifabutin, or the combination of both. Azithromycin was more effective than rifabutin in preventing mycobacteremia (7.6% vs. 15.3%; $p = .008$), and the combination of both agents was more effective than either one alone (2.8% incidence of mycobacteremia; $p = .03$).[54]

Based on these data, the U.S. Public Health Service now recommends lifetime prophylaxis with clarithromycin or azithromycin (or rifabutin for macrolide-intolerant patients) for all HIV-infected patients with fewer than 50 CD4 cells/μl.[55] A key remaining question is whether chronic antimycobacterial prophylaxis is needed for patients who at one time had an absolute CD4 count less than 50 cells/μl but now, as a result of potent combination antiretroviral therapy, have absolute CD4 counts that have been sustained well above this threshold level. Because we cannot yet accurately determine which patients can safely discontinue prophylaxis or for how long, prospective trials, randomizing patients to continue or discontinue therapy, are now underway to answer this question.

OTHER ATYPICAL MYCOBACTERIAL INFECTIONS IN AIDS

Disseminated and localized infections caused by *M. kansasii, M. celatum, M. xenopi, M. simiae, M. haemophilum, M. marinum, M. scrofula-*

ceum, M. gordonae, M. genavense, M. fortui- tum, M. chelonei (M. abscessus), and *M. mal- moense* also have been reported in patients with AIDS. Those cases with disseminated disease generally have had clinical presentations similar to that of disseminated MAC infection. In vitro sensitivity of isolates to standard antitubercu- lous drugs has been variable.

Mycobacterium kansasii has been the second most frequently reported of these other atypical mycobacteria, with disseminated infection pres- ent at the time of the index AIDS diagnosis in 0.4% of patients in areas where this organism is endemic (e.g., the southern/midwestern United States).[56] A recent trend toward increased inci- dence of HIV-related *M. kansasii* has been noted in Northern California, with 48 cases reported in 1996 compared to 13 in 1992.[57] This organ- ism, like MAC, is acquired from the environ- ment, and no cases of human–human transmis- sion have been documented.

In three recently published series from New Orleans, Kansas City, and Miami, the clinical features of 119 cases of AIDS-related *M. kan- sasii* infection were reported.[58–60] Ninety-one percent of these cases involved pulmonary dis- ease; 32% had disseminated disease. The me- dian absolute CD4 lymphocyte count at diag- nosis was fewer than 50 cells/μl in all three series. Fever, cough, and weight loss were com- mon in all three series. While cavitation was common in patients with disease limited to the lungs, it was rare in patients with disseminated infection.

Patients with AIDS-related *M. kansasii* infec- tion have been reported to respond to therapy with a combination of agents including isonia- zid, rifampin, ethambutol, clarithromycin, and ciprofloxacin.[58–61] Although the American Tho- racic Society recommends a combination of iso- niazid, rifampin, and ethambutol as therapy for this disease,[62] clinicians must substitute clarith- romycin and/or rifabutin for rifampin in patients receiving protease inhibitors. The recommended duration of therapy is a minimum of 18 months. In vitro, isoniazid resistance and clarithromycin sensitivity are commonly observed.[62–64] Rifam- pin resistance is now an emerging problem.[65] Thus multidrug therapy should be tailored to the results of the in vitro sensitivities of the culture isolate.

Mycobacterium genavense is a newly de- scribed pathogen that causes disseminated in- fection that is clinically similar to disseminated MAC in patients with CD4 counts less than 50 cells/μl.[66–69] This fastidious organism is difficult to detect and does not grow on conventional solid media. Small colonies can be detected in specially supplemented Middlebrook media, and a low growth index can be observed in BAC- TEC broth. Because susceptibilities to drugs cannot be reliably determined, an empiric treat- ment choice must be made. Clinical reports in- dicate that clarithromycin-containing combina- tion regimens may be effective therapy.[66–68]

Mycobacterium haemophilum is an atypical mycobacterium with a particular propensity to cause joint, bone, and ulcerative skin lesions (perhaps related to the lower temperature it re- quires for optimal growth) in addition to dis- seminated infection in patients with AIDS.[70,71] A cluster of cases has been reported in the New York City area. Clarithromycin and rifabutin ap- pear to be the most active therapeutic agents.[72]

Also of note, *M. celatum* is an organism that can be confused microbiologically with *M. xen- opi* and has recently been reported as a cause of disseminated infection in patients with advanced AIDS.[73,74] Susceptibility-directed antimycobac- terial therapy can be beneficial.

References

1. Greene JB, Sidhu GS, Lewin S, et al: *Mycobacterium avium-intracellulare*: A cause of disseminated life- threatening infection in homosexuals and drug abusers. Ann Intern Med 97:539, 1982
2. Macher AM, Kovacs JA, Gill V, et al: Bacteremia due to *Mycobacterium avium-intracellulare* in the acquired immunodeficiency syndrome. Ann Intern Med 99:782, 1983
3. Horsburgh CR, Mason UG, Farhi DC, et al: Dissemi- nated infection with *Mycobacterium avium-intracellu- lare*. Medicine 64:36, 1985
4. Ellner JJ, Goldberger MJ, Parenti DM: *Mycobacterium avium* infection and AIDS: Therapeutic dilemma in rapid evolution. J Infect Dis 163:1326, 1991
5. Havlik JA, Horsburgh CR, Metchock B, et al: Dissem- inated *Mycobacterium avium* complex infection: Clin- ical identification and epidemiologic trends. J Infect Dis 165:577, 1992
6. Nightingale SD, Byrd LT, Southern PM, et al: Inci- dence of *Mycobacterium avium-intracellulare* complex bacteremia in human immunodeficiency virus-positive patients. J Infect Dis 165:1082, 1992
7. Horsburgh CR, Selik MR: The epidemiology of dis- seminated nontuberculosis mycobacterial infection in the acquired immunodeficiency syndrome (AIDS). Am Rev Respir Dis 139:4, 1989
8. Hawkins CC, Gold JWM, Whimbey E, et al: *Myco- bacterium avium* complex infections in patients with the acquired immunodeficiency syndrome. Ann Intern Med 105:184, 1986
9. Hoover DR, Saah A, Bacellar H, et al: Clinical mani- festations of AIDS in the era of *Pneumocystis* prophy- laxis. N Engl J Med 329:1922, 1993
10. Centers for Disease Control and Prevention: AIDS- indicator conditions diagnosed in patients reported in

1993, by age group, United States. HIV/AIDS Surveill Rep 5:16, 1994

11. Centers for Disease Control and Prevention: AIDS-indicator conditions diagnosed in patients reported in 1994, by age group, United States. HIV/AIDS Surveill Rep 6:18, 1995

12. Centers for Disease Control and Prevention: AIDS-indicator conditions diagnosed in patients reported in 1996, by age group, United States. HIV/AIDS Surveill Rep 8:18, 1997

13. Jouan M, Cambau E, Baril L, et al: Decreased incidence of disseminated MAC infection in 689 AIDS patients receiving antiretroviral treatment with protease inhibitors. In Abstracts of the 37th Interscience Conference on Antimicrobial Agents and Chemotherapy, Toronto, 1997, Abstract I-30

14. Holtzer C, Jacobson M, Hadley WK, et al: Decline in specific opportunistic infections at San Francisco General Hospital. In Abstracts of the 5th Conference on Retroviruses and Opportunistic Infections, Chicago, 1998, Abstract 183

15. Hammer SM, Squires KE, Hughes MD, et al: A controlled trial of two nucleoside analogues plus indinavir in persons with human imunodeficiency virus infection and CD4 cell counts of 200 per cubic millimeter or less. N Engl J Med 337:725, 1997

16. Von Reyn CF, Maslow JN, Barber TW, et al: Persistant colonisation of potable water as a source of Mycobacterium avium infection in AIDS. Lancet 343:1137, 1994

17. Jacobson MA, Hopewell PC, Yajko DM, et al: Natural history of disseminated Mycobacterium avium complex infection in AIDS. J Infect Dis 164:994, 1991

18. Appelberg R, Castro AG, Pedrosa J, et al: Role of gamma interferon and tumor necrosis factor alpha during T-cell-independent and dependent phases of Mycobacterium avium infection. Infect Immunol 62:3962, 1994

19. Castro AG, Silva RA, Appelberg R: Endogenously produced IL-12 is required for the induction of protective T cells during Mycobacterium avium infections in mice. J Immunol 155:13, 1995

20. Newman GW, Guarnaccia JR, Vance EA 3rd, et al: Interleukin-12 enhances antigen-specific proliferation of peripheral blood mononuclear cells from HIV-positive and negative donors in response to Mycobacterium avium. AIDS 8:1413, 1994

21. Wong B, Edwards FF, Kiehn TE, et al: Continuous high-grade Mycobacterium avium-intracellulare bacteremia in patients with the acquired immune deficiency syndrome. Am J Med 78:35, 1985

22. Race EM, Adelson-Mitty J, Kriegel GR, et al: Focal mycobacterial lymphadenitis following initiation of protease inhibitor therapy in patients with advanced HIV-1 disease. Lancet 351:252, 1998

23. French MAH, Mallal SA, Dawkins RL: Zidovudine induced restoration of cell-mediated immunity to mycobacteria in immunodeficient HIV-infected patients. AIDS 6:1293, 1992

24. Barbaro DJ, Orcutt VL, Coldiron BM: Mycobacterium avium-Mycobacterium intracellulare infection limited to the skin and lymph nodes in patients with AIDS. Rev Infect Dis 11:625, 1989

25. Packer SJ, Cesario T, Williams JH: Mycobacterium avium complex infection presenting as endobronchial lesions in immunosuppressed patients. Ann Intern Med 109:389, 1988

26. Horsburgh CR, Havlik JA, Ellis DA, et al: Survival of patients with acquired immune deficiency syndrome and disseminated Mycobacterium avium complex infection with and without antimycobacterial chemotherapy. Am Rev Respir Dis 144:557, 1991

27. Chin DP, Reingold AL, Horsburgh CR Jr, et al: Predicting Mycobacterium avium complex bacteremia in patients with the human immunodeficiency virus: A prospectively validated model. Clin Infect Dis 19:668, 1994

28. Young LS: Mycobacterium avium complex infection. J Infect Dis 157:863, 1988

29. Evans KD, Nakasone AS, Sutherland PA, et al: Identification of Mycobacterium tuberculosis and Mycobacterium avium-M. intracellulare directly from primary BACTEC cultures by using acridinium-ester labelled DNA probes. J Clin Microbiol 30:2427, 1992

30. Chin DP, Hopewell PC, Yajko DM, et al: Mycobacterium avium complex in the respiratory or gastrointestinal tract and the risk of M. avium complex bacteremia in patients with the human immunodeficiency virus. J Infect Dis 169:289, 1994

31. Fernandes PB, Hardy DJ, McDaniel D, et al: In vitro and in vivo activities of clarithromycin against Mycobacterium avium. Antimicrob Agents Chemother 33:1531, 1989

32. Gangadharam PRJ, Kesavalu L, Rao PNR, et al: Activity of amikacin against Mycobacterium avium complex under simulated in vivo conditions. Antimicrob Agents Chemother 32:886, 1988

33. Inderlied CB, Kolonoski PT, Wu M, et al: In vitro and in vivo activity of azithromycin (CP 62,993) against the Mycobacterium avium complex. J Infect Dis 159:994, 1989

34. Yajko DM, Kirihara J, Sanders C, et al: Antimicrobial synergism against Mycobacterium avium complex strains isolated from patients with acquired immune deficiency syndrome. Antimicrob Agents Chemother 32:1392, 1988

35. Yajko DM, Nassos PS, Hadley WK: Therapeutic implications of inhibition versus killing of Mycobacterium avium complex by antimicrobial agents. Antimicrob Agents Chemother 31:117, 1987

36. Yajko DM, Sanders CA, Nassos PS, Hadley WK: In vitro susceptibility of Mycobacterium avium complex to the new fluoroquinolone sparfloxacin (CI-978; AT-4140) and comparison with ciprofloxacin. Antimicrob Agents Chemother 34:2442, 1990

37. Chiu J, Nussbaum J, Bozzette S, et al: Treatment of disseminated Mycobacterium avium complex infection in AIDS with amikacin, ethambutol, rifampin, and ciprofloxacin. Ann Intern Med 113:358, 1990

38. Kemper CA, Meng TC, Nussbaum J, et al: Treatment of Mycobacterium avium complex bacteremia in AIDS with a four-drug oral regimen. Ann Intern Med 116:466, 1992

39. Parenti D, Ellner J, Hafner R, et al: A Phase II/III trial of rifampin (RIF), ciprofloxacin (CIPRO), clofazimine (CLOF), ethambutol (ETH), + amikacin (AK) in the treatment (RX) of disseminated Mycobacterium avium (MA) infection in HIV-infected individuals (PTS). In Abstracts of the 2nd National Conference Human Retroviruses and Related Infections, Washington, DC, 1995, Abstract 6

40. Chaisson RE, Benson C, Dube M, et al: Clarithromycin therapy for bacteremic Mycobacterium avium complex disease. Ann Intern Med 121:905, 1994

41. Cohn D, Fisher E, Franchino B, et al: A prospective, randomized trial of four 3-drug regimens for treatment of disseminated MAC disease in AIDS: Excess mor-

tality associated with high-dose clarithromycin. In Abstracts of the 4th Conference on Retroviruses and Opportunistic Infections, Washington, DC, 1997, Abstract 659

42. Berry A, Koletar S, Williams S: Azithromycin therapy for disseminated *Mycobacterium avium-intercellulare* in AIDS patients. In Abstracts of the 1st National Conference on Human Retroviruses, Washington, DC, 1993, Abstract 292

43. Rimland D, Huycke M, Kauffman C: Randomized, open label trial of azithromycin plus ethambutol versus clarithromycin plus ethambutol therapy of MAC bacteremia in AIDS. In Abstracts of the 34th Annual Meeting of the Infectious Diseases Society of America, New Orleans, 1996, Abstract 241

44. Kemper C, Havlir D, Haghighat D, et al: The individual microbiologic effect of three antimycobacterial agents, clofazimine, ethambutol, and rifampin, on *Mycobacterium avium* complex bacteremia in patients with AIDS. J Infect Dis 170:157, 1994

45. Dube MP, Sattler F, Torriani F, et al: A randomized study of clarithromycin plus clofazimine, with or without ethambutol, for treatment and prevention of relapse of disseminated MAC (DMAC) in AIDS. In Abstracts of the 35th Interscience Conference on Antimicrobial Agents and Chemotherapy, San Francisco, CA, 1995, Abstract I-201

46. Sullam P, Gordin F, Wynne B, for the Rifabutin Treatment Group: Efficacy of rifabutin in the treatment of disseminated infection due to *Mycobacterium avium* complex. Clin Infect Dis 19:84, 1994

47. Chaisson RE, Keiser P, Pierce M, et al: Clarithromycin and ethambutol with or without clofazimine for the treatment of bacteremic *Mycobacterium avium* complex disease in patients with HIV infection. AIDS 11:311, 1997

48. Shafran SD, Singer J, Zarowny DP, et al: A comparison of two regimens for the treatment of *Mycobacterium avium* complex bacteremia in AIDS: Rifabutin, ethambutol, and clarithromycin versus rifampin, ethambutol, clofazimine, and ciprofloxacin. N Engl J Med 335:377, 1996

49. Aberg J, Yajko DM, Jacobson MA: Eradication of disseminated *Mycobacterium avium* complex in four patients after twelve months anti-mycobacterial therapy and response to highly active antiretroviral therapy. In Abstracts of the 5th Conference on Retroviruses and Opportunistic Infections, Chicago, 1998, Abstract 729

50. Tuberculosis and human immunodeficiency virus infection: Recommendations of the Advisory Committee for the Elimination of Tuberculosis (ACET). MMWR Morb Mortal Wkly Rep 38:236, 1989

51. Nightingale SD, Cameron DW, Gordin FM, et al: Two controlled trials of rifabutin prophylaxis against *Mycobacterium avium* complex infection in AIDS. N Engl J Med 329:828, 1993

52. Pearce M, Crampton S, Henry D, et al: A randomized trial of clarithromycin as prophylaxis against disseminated *Mycobacterium avium* complex infection in patients with advanced acquired immunodeficiency syndrome. N Engl J Med 335:384, 1995

53. Benson CA, Cohn DL, Williams P, et al: A Phase III prospective, randomized, double-blind study of the safety and efficacy of clarithromycin vs. rifabutin vs. clarithromycin + rifabutin for prevention of *Mycobacterium avium* complex disease in HIV+ patients with CD4 counts ≤100 cell/μL. In Abstracts of the 3rd Conference on Retroviruses and Opportunistic Infections, Washington, DC, 1996, Abstract 205

54. Havlir DV, Dube MP, Sattler FR, et al: Prophylaxis against disseminated *Mycobacterium avium* complex with weekly azithromycin, daily rifabutin or both. N Engl J Med 335:392, 1996

55. Centers for Disease Control and Prevention: 1997 USPHS/IDSA guidelines for prevention of opportunistic infections in persons infected with human immunodeficiency virus. MMWR Morb Mortal Wkly Rep 46(RR-12):1, 1997

56. Horsburgh CR Jr, Selik RM: The epidemiology of disseminated nontuberculous mycobacterial infection in the acquired immunodeficiency syndrome (AIDS). Am Rev Respir Dis 139:4, 1989

57. Bloch K, Pletcher M, Zwerling L, et al: A population-based study of the emergence of *M. kansasii*. In Abstracts of the 4th Conference on Retroviruses and Opportunistic Infections, Washington, DC, 1997, Abstract 66

58. Campo RE, Carlos, CE: *Mycobacterium kansasii* disease in patients infected with human immunodeficiency virus. Clin Infect Dis 24:1233, 1997

59. Bamberger DM, Driks MR, Gupta MR, et al: *Mycobacterium kansasii* among patients infected with human immunodeficiency virus in Kansas City. Clin Infect Dis 18:395, 1994

60. Witzig RS, Fazal BA, Mera RM, et al: Clinical manifestations and implications of coinfection with *Mycobacterium kansasii* and human immunodeficiency virus type 1. Clin Infect Dis 21:77, 1995

61. Levine B, Chaisson RE: *Myocabacterium kansasii*: A cause of treatable pulmonary disease associated with advanced human immunodeficiency virus (HIV) infection. Ann Intern Med 114:861, 1991

62. Wallace RJ Jr., Glassroth J, Griffith DE, et al: Diagnosis and treatment of disease caused by nontuberculous mycobacteria. Am J Respir Crit Care Med 156:S1, 1997

63. Rastogi N, Goh KS: Effect on pH on radiometric MICs of clarithromycin against 18 species of mycobacteria. Antimicrob Agents Chemother 36:2841, 1992

64. Biehle J, Cavalieri S: In vitro susceptibility of *Mycobacterium kansasii* to clarithromycin. Antimicrob Agents Chemother 36:2039, 1992

65. Wallace RJ Jr, Dunbar D, Brown BA, et al: Rifampin-resistant *Mycobacterium kansasii*. Clin Infect Dis 18:736, 1994

66. Pechere M, Opravil M, Wald A, et al: Clinical and epidemiologic features of infection with *Mycobacterium genavense*. Arch Intern Med 155:400, 1995

67. Bessesen MT, Shlay J, Stone-Venohr B, et al: Disseminated *Mycobacterium genavense* infection: Clinical and microbiological features and response to therapy. AIDS 7:1357, 1993

68. Albrecht H, Rusch-Gerdes S, Stellbrink H-J, Greten H: Treatment of disseminated *Mycobacterium genavense* infection. AIDS 9:659, 1995

69. Bottger EC, Teske A, Kirschner P, et al: Disseminated *Mycobacterium genavense* infection in patients with AIDS. Lancet 340:76, 1992

70. Kristjansson M, Bieluch VM, Byeff PD: *Mycobacterium haemophilum* infection in immunocompromised patients: Case report and review of the literature. Rev Infect Dis 13:906, 1991

71. Straus WL, Ostroff SM, Jernigan DB, et al: Clinical and epidemiologic characteristics of *Mycobacterium haemophilum*, an emerging pathogen in immunocompromised patients. Ann Intern Med 120:118, 1994

72. Bernard EM, Edwards FF, Kiehn TE, et al: Activities of antimicrobial agents against clinical isolates of *My-*

cobacterium haemophilum. Antimicrob Agents Chemother 37:2323, 1993

73. Albrecht H, Richter E, Poppinger J, et al: *Mycobacterium celatum* (MC) emerging as an important pathogen in patients with advanced HIV-infection. In Abstracts of the 37th Interscience Conference on Antimicrobial Agents and Chemotherapy, Toronto, 1997, Abstract I-226

74. Piersimoni C, Tortoli E, de Lalla F, et al: Isolation of *Mycobacterium celatum* from patients infected with human immunodeficiency virus. Clin Infect Dis 24:144, 1997

23 | Tuberculosis in the HIV-Infected Patient

HENRY F. CHAMBERS

Introduction of tuberculosis into HIV-infected populations and inadequate funding of tuberculosis control programs were largely responsible for the increase in tuberculosis case rates in the United States in the 1980s. Other factors contributing to the increasing incidence of tuberculosis were reduced sensitivity of the tuberculin skin test as a result of anergy of HIV-infected individuals, a frequently atypical clinical presentation of tuberculosis, presence of a reservoir of drug-resistant strains of *Mycobacterium tuberculosis*, inadequate infection controls, failure to ensure compliance with treatment regimens, and increased toxicity of drugs in HIV-infected individuals. Although tuberculosis is somewhat unique among AIDS-associated infections in that it is transmitted to others, including immunocompetent individuals, once identified and appropriately treated, tuberculosis can be cured and controlled. Successful application of appropriate treatment and control measures has reversed the upward trend of the 1980s, and the tuberculosis case rate is on the decline.[1]

EPIDEMIOLOGY

Reversal of the steady decline in case rates of tuberculosis since the early 20th century began in the mid-1980s.[2–4] Introduction of HIV into populations in which infection with *M. tuberculosis* was prevalent (e.g., the homeless, injection drug users, nonwhite Americans, and recent immigrants and refugees) caused tuberculosis case rates to soar. New York, New Jersey, and, to a somewhat lesser degree, Florida were especially hard hit.[4,5] The incidence of tuberculosis in HIV-infected persons is 100 times that of the general population. Reactivation of latent infection as a result of gradual loss of cell-mediated immunity has accounted for most

cases of tuberculosis associated with HIV infection. In addition, as previously uninfected, highly susceptible individuals with advanced HIV infection have become exposed to active cases, rapidly progressive primary and disseminated infections increasingly are encountered.

The exquisite susceptibility to disease and increasing incidence of tuberculosis in HIV-infected populations has led to nosocomial transmission of tuberculosis to patients and health care workers.[6–10] Tuberculosis has been transmitted by administration of aerosolized pentamidine for prophylaxis of *Pneumocystis carinii* pneumonia (PCP).[8] Failure to establish a diagnosis of tuberculosis and administer appropriate treatment, delayed recognition of the presence of multidrug-resistant (MDR) strains within the community, and inadequate isolation precautions have resulted in several outbreaks of nosocomially acquired tuberculosis caused by MDR strains.[9,10]

Approximately 8% of clinical isolates in the United States are resistant to isoniazid (INH), 6% are resistant to streptomycin, and 2% to 3% are resistant to rifampin, pyrazinamide, or ethambutol.[11] Rifampin resistance is frequently a marker for multidrug resistance, although isolated resistance to rifampin has been reported in association with HIV infections, perhaps as a result of poor absorption of the drug.[12,13] Approximately 2% of U.S. isolates are defined as MDR, that is resistant to both INH and rifampin, but cases tend to be concentrated in certain regions. For example, 38% of cases of tuberculosis caused by MDR strains occur in New York City.[11] The prevalence and incidence of tuberculosis caused by MDR strains has fallen dramatically in recent years as a result of more rapid case identification, improved isolation practices, implementation of early empiric therapy that includes second-line agents active against MDR strains, and use of directly observed therapy. As a result of these measures, the proportion of MDR cases has fallen from 19% to 13% of total cases annually and the MDR case load has been halved.[14]

PATHOGENESIS

Mycobacterium tuberculosis is transmitted by infected aerosol droplets generated by coughing, sneezing, singing, or talking from a person with active pulmonary or laryngeal tuberculosis. Droplets in the range of 1 to 6 μm in size when inhaled can reach the alveoli and initiate infection. *Mycobacterium tuberculosis* then enters alveolar macrophages, in which it readily survives and replicates. The organisms spread by lymphatic drainage to regional lymph nodes and then to the bloodstream, leading to hematogenous dissemination. Cell-mediated immunity develops in the normal host by the second to third month of infection, arresting progression of disease. In approximately 5% of individuals, infection is not contained and primary pulmonary, extrapulmonary, or disseminated tuberculosis occurs. In another 5% of individuals in whom the primary infection is controlled, tuberculosis will reactivate years to decades later. The lifetime risk of developing active tuberculosis in the normal host infected with *M. tuberculosis* is approximately 10%.

HIV infection greatly increases the risk of developing active tuberculosis. As cell-mediated immunity deteriorates (i.e., as the CD4 count falls below 350 cells/mm^3) in the individual latently infected with *M. tuberculosis*, control of replicating organisms is lost and the chance of developing active disease increases. The risk of developing tuberculosis for the HIV-infected patient latently coinfected with *M. tuberculosis* approaches 10% per year instead of 10% in the lifetime of an immunocompetent host.[15] Patients with more advanced HIV infection (e.g., CD4 counts less than 200/mm^3) who are newly infected with *M. tuberculosis* cannot contain the primary infection, which progresses rapidly and is fatal if not appropriately treated.

CLINICAL PRESENTATION AND DIAGNOSIS

The presentation of tuberculosis in patients in early stages of HIV infection (e.g., CD4 counts above 300/mm^3) is similar to that in normal hosts. Pulmonary tuberculosis is the most common presentation. The features are typical for reactivation tuberculosis, including productive cough of several weeks' duration, hemoptysis, fever, and weight loss with presence of focal infiltrates and cavities involving the upper lobes of the lungs on chest radiograph.

Tuberculosis in patients with more advanced stages of HIV infection (CD4 counts less than 200/mm^3) can be atypical, mimicking any of the several AIDS-associated opportunistic infections. Disseminated disease and extrapulmonary involvement of bone, bone marrow, gastrointestinal tract, urinary tract, regional lymph nodes (cervical, perihilar, paratracheal, and mediastinal being particularly suspicious for tuberculosis), liver, soft tissue, and central nervous system are more common.[5,16–21] The chest radiograph may be normal or demonstrate evidence of perihilar or mediastinal lymphadenopathy without parenchymal lung involvement. The clinical and radiographic presentation of pulmonary tuberculosis may be indistinguishable from that of community acquired pneumonia or PCP. Cavitary lung disease is uncommon. More commonly, infiltrates are diffuse or interstitial or involve the lower lung fields. Signs of paratracheal, hilar, or mediastinal lymphadenopathy, which are not features of PCP or other bacterial pneumonias, are highly suggestive of tuberculosis.

Depression of cell-mediated immunity as a result of HIV infection renders the tuberculin skin test insensitive and therefore unreliable. Only 30% to 50% of HIV-infected patients coinfected with *M. tuberculosis* will test positive.[5,17,22] Sputum smears and cultures will be positive in approximately 50% to 70% and 90%, respectively, of HIV-infected patients with pulmonary tuberculosis, frequencies that are similar to those for HIV-negative cases.[20,21,23] The yield depends on the number of specimens examined. A minimum of three samples obtained on consecutive days is recommended. The Amplicor PCR (Roche) and Amplified *Mycobacterium tuberculosis* Direct Test (Gen-Probe) are approved for rapid identification of *M. tuberculosis* in sputum smears that are positive for acid-fast bacilli.[24,25] The sensitivity is approximately 90% to 95% for identifying acid-fast bacilli seen on smear as *M. tuberculosis*. These rapid tests are more sensitive than traditional staining methods (e.g., 75% to 80% vs. 50% to 60%), but they still are not as sensitive as culture. Although useful in confirming or ruling out *M. tuberculosis* in a patient with a sputum smear positive for acid-fast bacilli, these tests should not be relied upon to rule in or rule out tuberculosis in smear-negative cases.

Smears of material from extrapulmonary sites (e.g., bone marrow, lymph node aspirate, cerebrospinal fluid) are often negative for acid-fast bacilli. The sensitivity of culture is 80% to 90%, although this will depend on the number of samples cultured, as well as the site. For example, the sensitivities of culture and smear are less for tuberculous meningitis compared to other sites of infection. Because of the higher frequency of disseminated disease in HIV-infected patients, smear and culture of respiratory samples will occasionally be positive in patients with an apparently normal chest radiograph. Thus multiple samples from several sites—respiratory tract, bone marrow, lymph nodes, brain tissue, cerebrospinal fluid, urine, or blood—may be required to establish a diagnosis of tuberculosis. Empirical therapy should be initiated while awaiting culture results if tuberculosis is strongly suspected. If cultures prove to be negative but the patient has responded to antituberculous therapy, and tuberculosis is strongly suspected on the basis of other evidence (e.g., granulomas on biopsy), continuation of therapy for a full course should be considered.

TREATMENT

HIV-infected patients who have either microbiologic (i.e., a positive smear or culture for acid-fast bacilli) or histopathologic evidence of mycobacterial infection and a clinical course consistent with tuberculosis should be treated for tuberculosis pending final identification of the organism (see Table 23-1 for agents with activity against *M. tuberculosis*). Withholding therapy or initiating therapy directed only against atypical mycobacteria is not advisable because a substantial proportion of patients will prove to have tuberculosis (e.g., acid-fast bacilli isolated from a sputum culture will be identified as *M. tuberculosis* in approximately 50% or more of cases). Regimens that are effective against atypical mycobacteria are not effective against *M. tuberculosis* and could promote selection of resistance. Moreover, untreated or inappropriately treated tuberculosis can be rapidly fatal and poses a public health hazard. Once the clinical isolate is shown to be an atypical mycobacterial organism, the regimen can be modified accordingly.

The response of tuberculosis to combination chemotherapy with first-line agents is generally excellent whether or not the patient is HIV in-

fected. The time to conversion of sputum cultures to negative after initiation of therapy is not affected by HIV infection.[26] The cure rate for the combination of INH, rifampin, pyrazinamide, and ethambutol for 2 months followed by 4 to 7 months of INH plus rifampin for tuberculosis caused by drug-susceptible strains is not substantially different for HIV-infected patients compared to patients not HIV infected.[22] One study[27] comparing relapse in HIV-infected patients with tuberculosis treated with INH and rifampin for 6 months to that with 12 months of treatment reported recurrences in 1.9% of those receiving 12 months of therapy compared to 9% in those receiving 6 months. Survival rates, however, were no different, and it is possible that the higher recurrence rate in the 6-month group was due to reinfection rather than true relapse.[28] Thus recommendations for treatment of tuberculosis until recently have been the same whether a patient is HIV infected or not[29–32] (Table 23-2). The availability of protease inhibitors (saquinavir, ritonavir, indinavir, nelfinavir), which have important drug interactions with rifamycins, rifampin, and rifabutin,[33] has prompted modification of earlier treatment guidelines. As the treatment of HIV infection has become increasingly complex, so has the treatment of tuberculosis in the HIV infected patient. Regimens recommended for treatment of tuberculosis in the HIV-infected patients are summarized below. However, it is strongly advised that these patients be managed by or in consultation with a physician experienced in treatment of both infections.

A Centers for Disease Control advisory panel has revised recommendations for treatment of tuberculosis in the HIV-infected patients.[32,32a] Based on the substantial potential benefit of highly active antiretroviral therapy and availability of numerous drugs active against HIV, withholding antiretroviral therapy until completion of therapy for tuberculosis is no longer recommended. The currently recommended regimens provide three options for treatment of tuberculosis in the HIV-infected patient. The guiding principles of these options are 1) that antiretroviral therapy should be administered when indicated; 2) that a short course regimen (i.e., treatment course of 6 to 9 months, depending on the regimen) administered as directly observed therapy is preferred in treatment of tuberculosis because of improved compliance; and 3) because of its more favorable drug interaction profile, rifabutin is preferred over rifampin. Rifampin is contraindicated for use with protease inhibitors and non-nucleoside reverse

TABLE 23–1. Antituberculous Agents, Typical Dosing for Adults, Cross-Resistances, and Principal Toxicities, Ranked in Order of Preference

DRUG	DOSE, ROUTE	CROSS-RESISTANCES	TOXICITIES
First Line			
Isoniazid	300 mg PO, IV, or IM	Ethionamide (sometimes)	Hepatitis, neuritis
Rifampin	600 mg PO or IV	Rifabutin (usually)	Hepatitis, drug interactions
Ethambutol*	15–25 mg/kg PO	None	Optic neuritis (at higher doses)
Pyrazinamide*	25 mg/kg PO	None	Hyperuricemia, hepatitis
Second Line			
Streptomycin	15 mg/kg IM	None	Ototoxicity and vestibulotoxicity > renal insufficiency
Levofloxacin*	500 mg qd PO or IV	Other quinolones	Gastrointestinal
Ciprofloxacin*	750 mg bid PO	Other quinolones	Gastrointestinal
Amikacin*	15 mg/kg IM	Kanamycin	Same as streptomycin
Capreomycin*	15 mg/kg IM	Possibly amikacin, kanamycin[†]	Same as streptomycin
Kanamycin	15 mg/kg IM	Amikacin	Same as streptomycin, but most toxic
Ethionamide	0.5–1.0 gm PO	INH (sometimes)	Gastrointestinal, hepatitis
Cycloserine	0.5–1.0 gm PO	None	Neuropsychiatric
Clofazimine	200 mg qd	None	Dark skin
Para-aminosalicylic acid	8–12 gm/d	None	Gastrointestinal, rash
Augmentin	1 gm/250 mg tid	None	Diarrhea, rash
Rifabutin	300 mg[‡]	Rifampin	Drug interactions, uveitis, rash

*Core agents around which most treatment regimens are constructed when treating MDR tuberculosis; either capreomycin or amikacin, but not both, should be included.

[†]Although mechanisms of resistance are not the same, resistance to capreomycin frequently is associated with resistance to other aminoglycosides.

[‡]Reduce dose to 150 mg once daily for patients taking protease inhibitors or nevirapine. Rifabutin should not be administered while a patient is receiving ritonavir, hard-gel saquinavir, or delavirdine.

transcriptase inhibitors (e.g., nevirapine and delavirdine) because it is a potent inducer of the cytochrome P-450 enzyme system that metabolizes these drugs and thereby decreases concentrations of these anti-retroviral agents to subtherapeutic levels. Rifabutin is a less potent inducer of cytochrome P-450 enzymes and therefore has less of an effect on protease inhibitor concentrations. Rifabutin is also substrate for cytochrome P-450 enzymes, which protease inhibitors inhibit, leading to accumulation of rifabutin to potentially toxic levels. This interaction, however, permits lowering the dose of rifabutin, which in turn has less of an effect on protease inhibitor levels. Drug interactions between rifabutin and ritonavir, hard-gel saquinavir, or delavirdine are significant, therefore use of any rifamycin with these agents is contraindicated or not recommended. Nucleoside reverse transcriptase inhibitors have no important interactions with rifamycins and may be used. Likewise, antituberculous medications other than the rifamycins have no significant interactions with any nucleoside or non-nucleoside reverse transcriptase inhibitors or protease inhibitors and may be used.

Option one is to use a 6-month INH, rifabutin, pyrazinamide, ethambutol regimen. The dose of rifabutin should be reduced from 300 mg a day to 150 mg a day if the patient is receiving a protease inhibitor or nevirapine. Ritonavir, hard-gel saquinavir, or delavirdine should not be used with rifabutin. After a two-month induction phase, ethambutol and pyrazinamide are discontinued and INH and rifabutin are continued at these same doses administered daily after 4 months. Alternatively, INH at a dose of 900 mg and rifabutin at a dose of 300

TABLE 23–2. Recommended Duration of Antituberculous Therapy for Treatment of Drug-Susceptible Tuberculosis

REGIMEN*	DURATION (MO)
INH + RIF + PZA[†]	6–9
RIF + PZA + EMB + AK (4–6 mo)[‡]	6–9
RIF + PZA + LEVO + AK (4–6 mo)	9–12
RIF + EMB	12
INH + EMB	18–24

*AK, amikacin; EMB, ethambutol; INH, isoniazid; LEVO, levofloxacin; PZA, pyrazinamide; RIF, rifampin.

[†]PZA for the first 2 months only. If PZA is not used, then the INH and RIF combination should be administered for at least 9 months.

[‡]Limited data indicate that amikacin can be omitted provided the other three agents are continued for 6 to 9 months.

mg (no dose adjustment necessary) can be administered twice a week for 4 months. Option two, which avoids the use of either rifampin or rifabutin, is a nine month regimen of INH, streptomycin, pyrazinamide, and ethambutol daily for the first two months at which point the ethambutol is discontinued and the other three agents are continued for an additional seven months. This regimen, which employs agents that are free of drug interactions, may be used with any antiretroviral regimen. Option three is three standard four drug regimen of INH, rifampin, pyrazinamide, and ethambutol. This regimen should not be used for patients who are receiving either protease inhibitors or non-nucleoside reverse transcriptase inhibitors.

Tuberculosis in patients who are infected by a strain that is resistant only to INH, should be treated with a three-drug regimen or rifampin (or rifabutin), pyrazinamide, and ethambutol for the duration of therapy. This regimen may be administered as a daily dosing regimen or a trice weekly regimen for six to nine months, but for at least six months after conversion of cultures to negative. Tuberculosis in patients with disease caused by a mono-rifampin resistant organism should receive the INH, pyrazinamide, ethambutol, and streptomycin regimen (Option 2, Table 23–3).

Approximately 20% of patients will experience side effects in response to antituberculous medications that may require modification of the drug regimen (Table 23–1). The most commonly encountered side effects are rash, neuropathy, gastrointestinal intolerance, hepatitis, thrombocytopenia, and renal failure. Rifampin is often implicated as a cause of side effects. Alternative regimens in addition to those discussed in the previous paragraph for patients intolerant to INH or rifampin are shown in Table 23–2.

Sputum cultures and smears should be monitored monthly to document their conversion to negative. Smears and cultures will have converted to negative by the end of the first month of therapy in 50% of cases and within the second to third month in 95% of cases when an INH-rifampin–based regimen is used. Smears or cultures remaining positive after the third month suggest either noncompliance with medications, drug resistance, or both. Because compliance with medications is critical to prevent emergence of resistance and to assure that cultures become negative as expected, directly observed therapy should be considered for all patients with tuberculosis. Directly observed therapy has been shown to result in improved

TABLE 23–3. Options for Treatment of Tuberculosis in HIV-Infected Patients Who Are Receiving Antiretroviral Therapy

Option 1	1. INH 300 mg + RBT 150 mg* + PZA 25 mg/kg + EMB 15 mg/kg daily for 2 months, then
	2. INH + RBT daily at the same doses for 4 months or INH 900 mg + RBT 300 mg twice weekly for 4 months.
	3. Do not use ritonavir, hard-gel saquinavir, or delavirdine for antiretroviral therapy.
Option 2	1. INH 300 mg + PZA 25 mg/kg + EMB 15 mg/kg + SM 15 mg/kg (1 g) daily for 2 months, then
	2. INH 300 mg + PZA 25 mg/kg + SM 25–30 mg/kg (1.5) two to three times a week for 7 months.
Option 3[†]	1. INH 300 mg + RIF 600 mg + PZA 25 mg/kg + EMB 15 mg/kg daily for 2 months, then
	2. INH 300 mg + RIF 600 mg daily for 4 months or INH 900 mg + RIF 600 mg twice weekly for 4 months.
	3. This regimen should be reserved for patients who either are not receiving antiretroviral therapy or who are receiving antiretroviral therapy consisting only of nucleoside reverse transcriptase inhibitors.

Abbreviations: EMB, ethambutol; INH, isoniazid; PZA, pyrazinamide; RBT, rifabutin; RIF, rifampin; SM, streptomycin.

The dose of indinavir should be increased from 800 mg q8h to 1200 mg q8h. The dose of nelfinavir should be increased from 750 mg tid to 1250 mg tid.

*The dose of rifabutin is 300 mg a day if the patient is not taking a protease inhibitor or a non-nucleoside reverse transcriptase inhibitor.

[†]Alternatively, INH + RIF + PZA + EMB may be administered as a thrice weekly regimen for 6 months.

response rates and lower rates of MDR cases of tuberculosis.[14,34] Sputum should be cultured at 3, 6, and 12 months after therapy to document cure. Patients with negative baseline sputum cultures and tuberculosis at extrapulmonary sites are followed clinically.

HIV infection is a risk factor for tuberculosis caused by MDR strains. Injection drug use and residence in an area when MDR strains are prevalent, New York and New Jersey in particular, also are risk factors.[35] The strongest predictor of whether a patient is likely to have tuberculosis caused by a MDR strain is a history of prior therapy for tuberculosis.[14] Persistence of fever in a patient receiving standard four-drug therapy is an important clinical marker suggesting the possibility of infection caused by an MDR strain.[36] Patients either suspected or documented to have active tuberculosis caused by a MDR strain should have at least two, and preferably several, drugs to which the clinical isolate is likely or known to be susceptible included in the treatment regimen.[37] Exactly which agents to choose if susceptibility tests are pending should be based on relevant exposure history for patients who have been in contact with a MDR case, prior treatment history, and susceptibilities for other MDR strains that are present in the community. For example, for a patient from New York City, where strain W is prevalent, a fluoroquinolone, capreomycin, and cycloserine would be recommended because these drugs are known to be active in vitro against this strain type.[38,39] If a patient has relapsed or failed to respond to a particular drug regimen, every drug that has been used becomes suspect for resistance. One may elect to include previously used agents in a re-treatment regimen, but at least two other new agents lacking cross-resistance to previously used agents should also be included until confirmatory susceptibility data are available. Under no circumstance should a single drug be added to a regimen that is failing or has failed because this runs the risk of resistance emerging to that drug as well. Appropriate early therapy is essential in the treatment of MDR tuberculosis to prevent rapid progression of disease and death and to control an organism that may be transmitted to others.[40] Failure rates and mortality may be high, even with appropriate therapy, although recent data suggest that the inclusion of at least two active drugs in the initial regimen greatly improves outcome compared to the early experience.[36,41] Directly observed therapy has been shown to reduce the prevalence and incidence of MDR tuberculosis and should be used in all MDR cases.[14,35] Given the complexities of managing MDR cases, the likelihood of further emergence of resistance, and the frequent side effects encountered with second-line agents, clinicians are strongly advised to obtain expert consultation in cases of MDR tuberculosis.

Because HIV-infected patients respond no differently to therapy, they do not need to be isolated or excluded from a work setting longer than other tuberculosis patients. The exact period of infectivity once effective chemotherapy has been initiated is not known. Once three consecutive sputum samples are smear-negative for acid-fast bacilli, the patient may safely resume normal social and work activities.

SCREENING AND PREVENTION

All HIV-infected individuals should be screened for tuberculosis by tuberculin skin testing with purified protein derivative (PPD). The test is considered positive if there is 5 mm or more of induration after 48 hours. A 5-mm cutoff is used instead of the standard 10 mm for immunocompetent individuals because impaired cellular immunity blunts the reactivity to the test material. Clinical trials have also demonstrated that the 5-mm cutoff is predictive of latent infection with *M. tuberculosis*.[42] Without preventive therapy, the annual risk for development of active tuberculosis is 7% to 10% in HIV-infected persons with a positive test versus less than 1% in HIV-negative reactors.[15,43] After active tuberculosis has been excluded by appropriate clinical evaluation and chest radiography, INH 300 mg/day should be administered for 12 months.[31,44] INH administered daily for 6 months or in combination with rifampin 600 mg (or rifabutin 300 mg or 150 mg if the patient is receiving protease inhibitors) for 3 months also is effective.[45] Other regimens that may be effective are a 2-month regimen of rifampin (or rifabutin 300 mg) plus pyrazinamide twice weekly, a 6-month regimen of INH twice weekly,[46] or a 6- to 12-month regimen of rifampin (or rifabutin) alone.[47,48] Because of the extremely limited clinical experience, twice-weekly and rifamycin-based regimens should be reserved for patients who, for reasons of poor compliance, documented exposure to an INH-resistant strain of *M. tuberculosis*, necessity for directly observed therapy, or drug toxicity, cannot be treated with daily INH.

Anergy testing has no role in strategies to prevent tuberculosis. More specifically, two randomized controlled trials have shown no benefit in administering INH to anergic individuals.[45, 49] The Centers for Disease Control and Prevention no longer recommends anergy testing for evaluation of skin test reactivity to PPD when evaluating whether chemoprophylaxis for tuberculosis is indicated.[50]

Contacts exposed to HIV-infected patients with a positive sputum smear or culture for *M. tuberculosis* should be screened to determine baseline reactivity. Contacts with a negative test at baseline should be retested at 3 months to determine conversion to a positive test. HIV-negative contacts who convert to a positive skin test or who have a baseline reactivity of 5 mm or more of induration are presumed to have been recently infected and should be treated with 6 months of INH. HIV-positive contacts should be given INH regardless of the skin test result, because anergy may be present. Active tuberculosis must be ruled out prior to initiating prophylaxis. Contacts of patients with tuberculosis caused by a MDR strain should receive prophylaxis with two drugs to which the organism from the index patient is susceptible. A two-drug regimen, such as pyrazinamide and ethambutol or a fluoroquinolone (such as levofloxacin), at standard doses for 12 months has been recommended.[51] Results of noncomparative studies suggest that rifampin 600 mg daily for 6 to 12 months may also be effective if the strain isolated from the index case is rifampin susceptible.[47,48]

All HIV-infected patients being considered for aerosolized pentamidine to prevent *Pneumocystis* pneumonia should be screened for tuberculosis. Administration of aerosolized pentamidine to HIV-infected patients has been associated with transmission of tuberculosis. Patients should be screened with both skin testing and a chest radiograph to exclude active tuberculosis. If tuberculosis is suspected, treatment should be initiated prior to aerosolized pentamidine treatment.

References

1. Centers for Disease Control and Prevention: Tuberculosis morbidity—United States, 1996. MMWR Morb Mortal Wkly Rep 46:695, 1997
2. Centers for Disease Control: Tuberculosis, United States, 1985, and the possible impact of HTLV-III/LAV infections. MMWR Morb Mortal Wkly Rep 35:74, 1986
3. Tuberculosis, final data: United States, 1986. MMWR Morb Mortal Wkly Rep 36:817, 1988
4. Tuberculosis and acquired immunodeficiency syndrome; New York City. MMWR Morb Mortal Wkly Rep 36:785, 1987
5. Pitchenik AE, Cole C, Russell BW, et al: Tuberculosis, atypical mycobacteriosis, and AIDS among Haitian and non-Haitian patients in South Florida. Ann Intern Med 101:641, 1984
6. Di-Perri G, Cruciani M, Danzi MC, et al: Nosocomial epidemic of active tuberculosis among HIV-infected patients. Lancet 2:1502, 1989
7. Daley CL, Small PM, Schecter GF, et al: An outbreak of tuberculosis with accelerated progression among persons infected with the human immunodeficiency virus: An analysis using restriction-fragment-length polymorphisms. N Engl J Med 326:231, 1992
8. *Mycobacterium tuberculosis* transmission in a health clinic; Florida, 1988. MMWR Morb Mortal Wkly Rep 38:256, 1989
9. Centers for Disease Control: Nosocomial transmission of multidrug-resistant tuberculosis to health-care workers and HIV-infected patients in an urban hospital; Florida. MMWR Morb Mortal Wkly Rep 39:718, 1990
10. Beck-Sague C, Dooley SW, Hutton MD, et al: Hospital outbreak of multidrug-resistant *Mycobacterium tuberculosis* infections: Factors in transmission to staff and HIV-infected patients. JAMA 268:1280, 1992
11. Moore M, Onorato IM, McCray E, Castro KG: Trends in drug-resistant tuberculosis in the United States, 1993–1996. JAMA 278:833, 1997
12. Bradford WZ, Martin JN, Reingold AL, et al: The changing epidemiology of acquired drug-resistant tuberculosis in San Francisco, USA. Lancet 348:928, 1996
13. Patel KB, Belmonte R, Crowe HM: Drug malabsorption and resistant tuberculosis in HIV-infected patients. N Engl J Med 332:336, 1995
14. Fujiwara PI, Cook SV, Rutherford CM, et al: A continuing survey of drug-resistant tuberculosis, New York City, April 1994. Arch Intern Med 157:531, 1997
15. Moreno S, Miralles P, Diaz MD, et al: Isoniazid preventive therapy in human immunodeficiency virus-infected persons: Long-term effect on development of tuberculosis and survival. Arch Intern Med 157:1729, 1997
16. Sunderam G, MacDonald RJ, Moniatis T, et al: Tuberculosis as a manifestation of AIDS. JAMA 256:362, 1986
17. Chaisson RE, Schecter GF, Theur CP, et al: Tuberculosis in patients with the acquired immunodeficiency syndrome: Clinical features, response to therapy, and survival. Am Rev Respir Dis 136:570, 1987
18. Moreno S, Pacho E, Lopez-Herce JA, et al: *Mycobacterium tuberculosis* visceral abscesses in the acquired immunodeficiency syndrome (AIDS). Ann Intern Med 109:437, 1988
19. Pitchenik AE, Rubinson HA: The radiographic appearance of tuberculosis in patients with AIDS and pre-AIDS. Am Rev Respir Dis 131:393, 1985
20. Theuer CP, Hopewell PC, Elias D, et al: Human immunodeficiency virus infection in tuberculosis patients. J Infect Dis 162:8, 1990
21. Finch D, Beaty CD: The utility of a single sputum specimen in the diagnosis of tuberculosis: Comparison between HIV-infected and non-HIV-infected patients. Chest 111:1174, 1997
22. Small PM, Schecter GF, Goodman PC, et al: Treatment of tuberculosis in patients with advanced human immunodeficiency virus infection. N Engl J Med 324:289, 1991
23. Alpert PL, Munsiff SS, Gourevitch MN, et al: A prospective study of tuberculosis and human immunodeficiency virus infection: Clinical manifestations and factors associated with survival. Clin Infect Dis 24:661, 1997
24. Dalovisio JR, Montenegro-James S, Kemmerly SA, et al: Comparison of the amplified *Mycobacterium tuberculosis* (MTB) direct test, Amplicor MTB PCR, and IS6110-PCR for detection of MTB in respiratory specimens. Clin Infect Dis 23:1099, 1996
25. Centers for Disease Control and Prevention: Nucleic acid amplification tests for tuberculosis. MMWR Morb Mortal Wkly Rep 45:950, 1996
26. Telzak EE, Fazal BA, Pollard CL, et al: Factors influencing time to sputum conversion among patients with smear-positive pulmonary tuberculosis. Clin Infect Dis 25:666, 1997
27. Perriëns JH, St. Louis ME, Mukadi YB, et al: Pulmonary tuberculosis in HIV-infected patients in Zaire: A controlled trial of treatment for either 6 or 12 months. N Engl J Med 332:779, 1995
28. Godfrey-Faussett P, Githui W, Batchelor B, et al: Recurrence of HIV-related tuberculosis in an endemic area may be due to relapse or reinfection. Tubercle Lung Dis 75:199, 1994
29. Bass JB, Farer LS, Hopewell PC, et al: Treatment of tuberculosis and tuberculous infection in adults and children. Am J Respir Crit Care Med 149:1359, 1994

30. Mycobacterioses and the acquired immunodeficiency syndrome: Joint Position Paper of the American Thoracic Society and the Centers for Disease Control. Am Rev Respir Dis 136:492, 1987

31. Tuberculosis and human immunodeficiency virus infection: Recommendations of the Advisory Committee for the Elimination of Tuberculosis (ACET). MMWR Morb Mortal Wkly Rep 38:236, 1989

32. Centers for Disease Control and Prevention: Clinical update: Impact of HIV protease inhibitors on the treatment of HIV-infected tuberculosis patients with rifampin. MMWR Morb Mortal Wkly Rep 45:921, 1996

32a. Centers for Disease Control. Prevention and treatment of tuberculosis in patients infected with human immunodeficiency virus: principles of therapy and revised recommendations. MMWR Morb Mortal Wkly Rep 47(RR-20):1, 1998

33. Piscitelli SC, Flexner C, Minor JR, et al: Drug interactions in patients infected with human immunodeficiency virus. Clin Infect Dis 23:685, 1996

34. Weis SE, Slocum PC, Blais FX, et al: The effect of directly observed therapy on the rates of drug resistance and relapse in tuberculosis. N Engl J Med 330:1179, 1994

35. Freiden TR, Sterling T, Pablo-Mendez A, et al: The emergence of drug-resistant tuberculosis in New York City. N Engl J Med 328:521, 1993

36. Salomon N, Perlman DC, Friedmann P, et al: Predictors and outcome of multiple-resistant tuberculosis. Clin Infect Dis 21:125, 1995

37. Iseman MD: Treatment of multidrug-resistant tuberculosis. N Engl J Med 329:784, 1993

38. Frieden TR, Sherman LF, Maw KL, et al: A multi-institutional outbreak of highly drug-resistant tuberculosis: Epidemiology and clinical consideration. JAMA 276:1229, 1996

39. Bifani PJ, Plikaytis BB, Kapur V, et al: Origin and interstate spread of a New York City multidrug-resistant Mycobacterium tuberculosis clone family. JAMA 275:452, 1996

40. Pablos-Mendez A, Sterling TR, Freidan TR: The relationship between delayed or incomplete treatment and all-cause mortality in patients with tuberculosis. JAMA 276:1223, 1996

41. Turett GS, Talzak EE, Torian LV, et al: Improved outcomes for patients with multiple-resistant tuberculosis. Clin Infect Dis 21:1238, 1995

42. Markowitz N, Hansen NI, Hopewell PC, et al: Incidence of tuberculosis in the United States among HIV-infected persons: The Pulmonary Complications of HIV Infection Study Group. Ann Intern Med 126:123, 1997

43. Selwyn PA, Hartel D, Lewis VA, et al: A prospective study of the risk of tuberculosis among intravenous drug users with human immunodeficiency virus infection. N Engl J Med 320:545, 1989

44. Centers for Disease Control: Diagnosis and management of mycobacterial infection and disease in persons with HTLV-III/LAV infection. MMWR Morb Mortal Wkly Rep 35:448, 1986

45. Whalen CC, Lohnson JL, Okwera A, et al: A trial of three regimens to prevent tuberculosis in Ugandan adults infected with the human immunodeficiency virus: Uganda-Case Western Reserve University Research Collaboration. N Engl J Med 337:801, 1997

46. Halsey NA, Coberly JS, Desormeaux J, et al: Randomised trial of isoniazid versus rifampicin and pyrazinamide for prevention of tuberculosis in HIV-1 infection. Lancet 351:786, 1998

47. Villarino ME, Ridzon R, Weismuller PC, et al: Rifampin preventive therapy for tuberculosis infection: Experience with 157 adolescents. Am J Resp Crit Care Med 155:1735, 1997

48. Polesky A, Farber HW, Gottlieb DJ, et al: Rifampin preventive therapy for tuberculosis in Boston's homeless. Am J Resp Crit Care Med 154:1473, 1996

49. Gordin FM, Matts JP, Miller C, et al: A controlled trial of isoniazid in persons with anergy and human immunodeficiency virus infection who are at high risk for tuberculosis: Terry Beirn Community Programs for Clinical Research on AIDS. N Engl J Med 337:315, 1997

50. Centers for Disease Control and Prevention: Anergy skin testing and preventive therapy for HIV-infected persons: Revised recommendations. MMWR Morb Mortal Wkly Rep 46:1, 1997

51. Centers for Disease Control: Management of persons exposed to multidrug-resistant tuberculosis. MMWR Morb Mortal Wkly Rep 41:61, 1992

24 | Cryptococcosis and Other Fungal Infections (Histoplasmosis, Coccidioidomycosis)

MICHAEL S. SAAG

Systemic fungal infections generally are late manifestations in HIV disease. Overall, cryptococcal infection is the most common systemic fungal infection in HIV-infected patients. However, in certain endemic regions, histoplasmosis or coccidioidomycosis is the most prevalent mycotic disorder. Although these diseases occur in normal (non–HIV-infected) hosts, among HIV-infected patients they tend to occur when the CD4 count is less than 200/mm[3]. Recent advances in the treatment of systemic fungal infections have substantially reduced both morbidity and mortality of these disorders. Newer diagnostic techniques along with heightened awareness on the part of clinicians have led to more rapid and accurate diagnosis. This chapter reviews the approach to diagnosis and management of cryptococcosis, histoplasmosis, and coccidioidomycosis, the three most commonly occurring systemic mycoses in HIV-infected patients.

CRYPTOCOCCUS

Microbiology

Cryptococcus neoformans is a round or oval yeast (4 to 6 μm in diameter), surrounded by a capsule that can be up to 30 μm thick. The organism grows quite readily on fungal or bacterial culture media and usually is detectable within a week after inoculation, although in some circumstances up to 4 weeks is required for growth. Therefore, clinical cultures should be maintained for a minimum of 2 weeks, and preferably 4 weeks, when *C. neoformans* disease is suspected. The organism is differentiated from other pathogenic yeasts based on its growth characteristics. The organism grows well at 37°C, does not form pseudomycelia on corn-meal or rice-Tween agar, and hydrolyzes urea, a property that allows rapid presumptive identification.[1]

On the basis of antigenic differences in the capsule, biochemical use of nutrients, and distinct DNA base sequences, four serotypes (A, B, C, and D) of *Cryptococcus* have been delineated. Serotypes A and D are classified as *C. neoformans* var. *neoformans*, and serotypes B and C are classified as *C. neoformans* var. *gattii*.[2] *Cryptococcus neoformans* var. *neoformans* is the major cause of cryptococcal disease worldwide. Serotype A is the most common serotype infecting AIDS patients.[3,4] For reasons that are not clearly understood, *C. neoformans* var. *gattii* tends to infect immunocompetent hosts.[5,6] This subtype is found in certain geographic areas, including southern California, Africa, Australia, and Southeast Asia. Interestingly, even within these geographic areas, *C. neoformans* var. *gattii* does not appear to cause disease in HIV-infected patients.[6,7]

Epidemiology

Before the AIDS epidemic, cryptococcal infection occurred in a small number of immunocompetent patients but most often in patients with a compromised immune system. The most frequently affected patients were those with lymphoma, diabetics, transplant recipients, or patients requiring chronic steroid therapy.[8] In the AIDS era, cryptococcal disease is the fourth most common cause of serious opportunistic infection after *Pneumocystis carinii* pneumonia, cytomegalovirus, and myobacterial disease.[9] Disease caused by *C. neoformans* occurs in 6% to 10% of HIV-infected patients. Over the last several years, owing to the more widespread use of azole therapy and improved antiretroviral therapy, the incidence of cryptococcal disease in AIDS has decreased.[10] Among those individuals who develop cryptococcal disease, it is the initial AIDS-defining illness in 40% to 45%.[11-16] At the present time, it is the third most common central nervous system (CNS) disorder in AIDS patients, behind toxoplasmosis and CNS lymphoma.

Cryptococcus neoformans infection is acquired from the environment. The organism, most likely in an unencapsulated form, is inhaled into the lungs and deposited in the small airways. Once there, yeast multiply and compress the surrounding tissue but, remarkably, cause little damage. This pulmonary infection is often asymptomatic. Indeed, in 85% to 95% of patients with cryptococcal meningitis, no evidence of pneumonitis is present.[11,12] As suggested by these data, the organism has a strong propensity for dissemination to the CNS but also may involve skin, bone, and the genitourinary tract.

Clinical Manifestations

The onset of cryptococcal disease usually is insidious. The median time between the onset of symptoms and the diagnosis of cryptococcal disease is 30 days.[11-13] Diagnosis often is delayed by the waxing and waning course of the disease and the absence of specific symptoms. These nonspecific symptoms consist of a prolonged febrile prodrome that is indistinguishable from that of other opportunistic infections. The most common symptoms, in addition to fever, are headache and malaise.[11-13,17] Common symptoms are listed in Table 24–1.

The incidence of extraneural cryptococcal disease in AIDS patients ranges between 20% and 60%.[11,12,14,15] Despite the lung being the portal of entry, evidence of pulmonary disease symptoms is present in only 20% to 30% of cases. Other sites of extraneural involvement include the joints, oral cavity, pericardium, myocardium, skin, mediastinum, and genitourinary tract, which is believed to provide a sanctuary

for *C. neoformans* that may lead to recurring disease.[18]

The physical examination in patients with cryptococcal disease is also nonspecific. In the series reported by Chuck and Sande, 56% of patients were febrile, although less than one third had nuchal rigidity or other focal neurologic deficits.[11] Altered mental status, which is the most important predictor of poor outcome of patients with cryptococcal disease, is present in 20% to 30% of patients. Papilledema is seen in less than 10% of patients. Raised, sometimes umbilicated, skin lesions are reported in 3% to 10% of patients with cryptococcal meningitis. These lesions may resemble those caused by *Molluscum contagiosum* and occasionally have been misdiagnosed as Kaposi's sarcoma.

Diagnosis

The gold standard diagnostic test for cryptococcal meningitis is a positive cerebrospinal fluid (CSF) culture for *C. neoformans*. Therefore, a lumbar puncture is imperative in any individual with suspected cryptococcal meningitis. This procedure is diagnostic but may be therapeutic as well (see "Management of Increased Intracranial Pressure," below). Although controversial, most clinicians will perform an imaging study, such as a computed tomography scan or magnetic resonance imaging, before performing a lumbar puncture in any HIV-infected patient with headache and fever. The rationale supporting this approach is that many space-occupying disease processes, such as CNS toxoplasmosis (Chapter 25) and CNS lymphoma (Chapter 30), may cause similar symptoms. The most common findings noted on brain imaging studies are cerebral atrophy and ventricular enlargement.[11,12,19] On rare occasion, mass lesions caused by *C. neoformans* (cryptococcomas) may be identified.[19] In some patients, especially in those with elevated CSF pressure, the ventricles are normal to small in size, with some evidence of generalized cerebral edema (Fig. 24–1). Assuming these is no evidence of obstructive hydrocephalus, these patients may benefit from serial spinal taps to help relieve the symptoms of elevated intracranial pressure.

After an occult mass lesion has been ruled out, a lumbar puncture should be performed. In patients with non–AIDS-associated cryptococcal meningitis, the most common CSF findings include an elevated opening pressure (>200 mm H_2O), elevated CSF white blood cell count (>20/mm^3), hypoglycorrhachia (<50% of serum

TABLE 24–1. Clinical and Diagnostic Characteristics of Cryptococcal Meningitis in Non-AIDS and AIDS Patients*

	REFERENCE					
	Non-AIDS	AIDS				
	1	*75*	*11*	*12*	*20*	*17*
Clinical Manifestations						
Headache	87	81	73	67	92	89
Fever	60	88	65	62	78	75
Nausea and vomiting	53	†	42	1	8	
Altered mental status	52	19	28		27	21
Stiff neck	50	31	22		37	44
Visual disturbances	33				30	29
Cranial nerve palsies	32				6	
Papilledema	28				6	8
Ataxia	26				10	
Seizures	15	8	4	9		
Aphasia	10					
Malaise		38	76			
Photophobia		19	18		6	
Cough						33
Laboratory Results						
CSF abnormal						
WBC (>20/mm³)	97	31	21	13		
Glucose (<60% of serum level)	75	65	24	17		
Protein (>45 mg/dl)	90	61	55	35		
India ink positive	60	72	74	88	77	83
Opening pressure abnormal (>200 mm H₂O)	65	62	66			
Serology						
CSF antigen positive	>90	92	91	93	99	99
Serum antigen positive	50	95	99	93	99	99
Abnormal Head CT		31	29	19		

*Given as percent of patients.
†Items without entries were not reported by investigators.
Modified from Lapidus W, Saag M: Cryptococcal meningitis. In Johnson S, Johnson FN (series eds), Powderly WG, Van't Wout JW (consultant eds): The Antifungal Agents: Fluconazole. Lancashire, England, Marius Press, 1992, p 137, with permission.

glucose level), elevated CSF protein (>50 mg/dl), and a negative India ink preparation (60% to 70% will be negative) (Table 24–1).[14,43] In contrast, up to 50% of patients with AIDS-associated cryptococcal meningitis have minimal or no abnormalities of their CSF formula.[11,12,16] However, the opening pressure may be elevated (>200 mm H₂O) in over 70% of the patients. Low CSF white blood cell counts (<20/mm³) not only are common but also are associated with a worse prognosis.[17,20] Fortunately, in light of the normal CSF findings in most patients, there are more sensitive and specific tests for cryptococcal disease. The India ink preparation is positive in 74% to 88% of patients with cryptococcal meningitis.[11,12,17,20] When this technique is used, *C. neoformans* is visible as round cells 4 to 6 μm in diameter surrounded by the characteristic thick polysaccharide capsule (Fig 24–2). It is quite important to clearly identify the organism within the capsule because false-positive tests have been reported as a result of an artifact. The frequency of inaccurate readings is minimized through the use of experienced technicians who are familiar with proper interpretation of the microscopic image. Even when a true-positive test is reported, the findings must be confirmed with a CSF cryptococcal antigen (CRAG) test or, ideally, a CSF fungal culture.

CRAG testing of blood and CSF is a reliable and relatively rapid diagnostic technique. Sensitivity of the CRAG test is 93% to 99% in patients with culture-proven cryptococcal meningitis.[11,12] In non–HIV-infected patients, the median CSF titer is between 1:16 and 1:32.[8] In contrast, the median CSF antigen titer in HIV-infected patients is 1:1024. On occasion, CSF titers can exceed 1:1 million. Serum CRAG

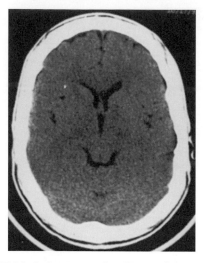

FIGURE 24–1. Representative CT scan from a patient with acute AIDS-associated cryptococcal meningitis, altered mental status, and elevated intracranial pressure (>550 mm H₂O). The paradoxical finding of normal to small-sized ventricles and absence of radiologic hydrocephalus is typical of cryptococcus meningitis. (From Ennis DM, Saag MS: Cryptococcal meningitis in AIDS. Hosp Pract 28:101, 1993, with permission.)

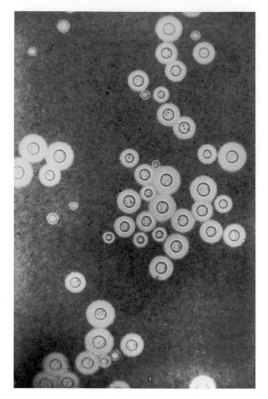

FIGURE 24–2. India ink preparation of CSF demonstrating *C. neoformans* organisms, several of which are budding. The circular organism is encased within a thick polysaccharide capsule. (Courtesy of Dr. Kathleen E. Squires.)

tests are positive in over 99% of patients with *C. neoformans* disease. In patients with AIDS-associated cryptococcal meningitis, the serum antigen tests usually are one tube dilution higher than the CSF antigen test. The serum cryptococcal antigen test is used occasionally as a screening test for an HIV-infected patient with headache and fever. A negative test result reduces the likelihood of cryptococcal disease, whereas a positive test necessitates further evaluation with a CSF work-up. Routine screening of patients with the serum CRAG test is controversial but currently is not recommended. Unfortunately, this test is also not helpful in monitoring patients with proven cryptococcal disease.[21] Specifically, the serum CRAG test is not capable of detecting patients who are about to relapse or to assess the initial response to acute therapy. False-positive CRAG tests have been noted in patients with positive rheumatoid factor, although current techniques have largely eliminated this problem. Patients with *Trichosporon beigelii* infection may also have false-positive CRAG results.[22] *Trichosporon beigelii* infections, however, are quite uncommon. False-positive titers usually do not exceed a 1:8 dilution. Conversely, some patients with cryptococcal infection may have false-negative CRAG tests. Such results may reflect scarce or poorly encapsulated organisms, or, conversely,

the number of organisms may be so large that crosslinking is impaired. This so-called prozone phenomenon may be overcome by ensuring that the tests are performed using an adequate number of dilutions.[23]

A definitive diagnosis of cryptococcal disease requires culturing the organism from body fluids or tissue. CSF fungal cultures require a minimum of 2 ml to obtain maximum sensitivity. By definition, up to 100% of cases of cryptococcal meningitis have positive CSF fungal cultures. In contrast, blood cultures are positive in only one third of patients without AIDS. However, 66% to 80% of patients with AIDS will have positive blood cultures for *C. neoformans*.[8,20]

In patients with extraneural cryptococcal disease, tissue examination can lead to a presumptive diagnosis of cryptococcosis. *Cryptococcus neoformans* organisms are readily identified using methenamine silver, mucicarmine, and periodic acid–Schiff stains. Gram's stain of tissue is generally unreliable in detecting *C. neoformans* organisms.

Prognosis

Left untreated, cryptococcal meningitis is a fatal disorder. Even with aggressive intervention, the mortality among non-AIDS patients with combination amphotericin B and flucytosine therapy is reported to be as high as 30%, depending on underlying disease.[8,13,24] Previously, the reported mortality of acute cryptococcal meningitis in patients with AIDS was between 17% and 20%.[20] However, a recent study has demonstrated a mortality rate of 6% with aggressive therapy (see below).[17] Many studies have evaluated factors associated with treatment failure and mortality in both AIDS and non-AIDS patients. In both populations, the most important baseline prognostic factor is mental status at the time of presentation. Individuals with altered sensorium have a much worse prognosis than those who are awake and alert.[8,20] High fungal burden, as demonstrated by high CRAG titers, positive India ink test, and the presence of extraneural cryptococcal disease, also is associated with poor outcome.[8,20] Elevated intracranial pressure has been shown to be an important factor in morbidity and mortality.[17]

Treatment

Antifungal Agents

Amphotericin B (AMB) is a polyene antimicrobial agent that possesses a broad range of antifungal activity. Its fungicidal activity is due principally to the binding of ergosterol in the fungal membrane, resulting in increased membrane permeability, leakage of cellular components, and resultant cell death. The drug is very poorly absorbed when administered orally (necessitating intravenous administration), has a very high volume of distribution, and is believed to be deposited in fatty tissues throughout the body. However, AMB penetrates into CSF very poorly.

The principal limitation of AMB is its toxicity profile. Virtually all patients who receive this therapy for more than 4 weeks will experience some degree of reversible renal insufficiency. During acute administration, fever, rigors, headache, and thrombophlebitis have been reported. Chronic administration results in electrolyte abnormalities, most notably hypokalemia and hypomagnesemia. Strategies to reduce the toxicity of AMB include slow administration of drug (over 4 to 6 hours), the addition of heparin (1000 U/500 ml) to reduce the incidence of thrombophlebitis, premedication with antipyretics (acetaminophen, diphenhydramine, or both), premedication with meperidine in patients who have experienced severe rigors, and aggressive replacement of electrolytes as needed. Some investigators have attempted to modify the toxicity of AMB by modifying its formulation. Lipid complex formulations (AMB lipid complex) and liposomal preparations of amphotericin have been evaluated in clinical trials, with modest success.[25-29] The advantage of these formulations is that they allow higher doses (up to 3 to 5 mg/kg) of parent drug to be administered. However, preliminary studies reveal success rates that are similar to those with the use of AMB alone, although there seems to be less toxicity.

Flucytosine (5-FC) is a pyrimidine derivative similar in structure to 5-fluorouracil (5-FU). When administered to susceptible fungi, 5-FC is converted to 5-FU and inhibits thymidylate synthetase, a vital enzyme needed for DNA synthesis. 5-FC has a very favorable pharmacokinetic profile, including complete absorption from the gastrointestinal tract when administered orally, a satisfactory half-life of 3 to 4 hours, and very little hepatic metabolism (the drug is excreted virtually unchanged by the kidney). Most importantly, 5-FC reaches high concentrations in the CSF, usually on the order of 70% to 90% of the serum levels. The principal toxicities of 5-FC occur primarily in organ systems that have rapidly dividing cells, namely the bone marrow (leukopenia), gastrointestinal tract (nausea, vomiting, and diarrhea), and skin (rash). Optimally, drug levels should be obtained whenever 5-FC is used to minimize toxicity and maximize effectiveness. The levels should be above 50 μg/ml and below 100 μg/ml.

In the late 1970s and through the 1980s, other oral agents were identified that possessed broad-spectrum antifungal activity (reviewed by Saag and Dismukes[30]). The first of these agents is *ketoconazole*, an imidazole derivative with in vitro activity against *Histoplasma capsulatum*, *Blastomyces dermatitidis*, *Candida* species, and, to a lesser degree, *C. neoformans*. The drug is metabolized predominantly by the liver, requires an acidic environment for absorption, penetrates the CSF poorly, and is highly protein bound. Concomitant administration of ketoconazole with rifampin or rifampin derivatives, dilantin, or carbamazepine results in negligible serum levels because of increased metabolism of drug. Drug absorption is dramatically impaired in an alkaline gastric environment created by histamine$_2$ (H$_2$) blockers or antacids. Nausea and vomiting are the principal dose-related toxicities. Less commonly, hepatic dysfunction or alteration of steroidogenesis has been noted.

Fluconazole, a bistriazole, was the second oral azole agent approved for use in the United States. The pharmacokinetic properties of fluconazole are strikingly different from those of ketoconazole. Fluconazole is well absorbed from the gastrointestinal tract (oral bioavailability 70% to 80%) and is able to achieve adequate serum levels even when exposed to an alkaline gastric environment. The drug is excreted predominantly via the kidney and undergoes minimal metabolism by the liver. Most importantly with regard to cryptococcal disease, fluconazole penetrates well into the CSF, achieving concentrations of 60% to 80%. The most common side effects are gastrointestinal in nature, although skin rash has been reported in up to 3% of patients taking the drug. Rare instances of Stevens-Johnson syndrome have been reported. Fluconazole is active against *C. neoformans*, most *Candida* species, *H. capsulatum*, and *B. dermatitidis* but has little activity against *Aspergillus* species or certain *Candida* species (e.g., *C. krusei*).

Itraconazole is the most recently approved oral antifungal agent in the United States. Although itraconazole is a triazole, its pharmacologic properties are more like those of ketoconazole than those of fluconazole. Like ketoconazole, itraconazole requires an acidic gastric environment for absorption, is metabolized by the liver, and has similar drug interactions with rifampin-like derivatives, dilantin, carbamazepine, H_2 blockers, and antacids. Itraconazole is more potent than ketoconazole on a milligram-per-milligram basis and is better tolerated. The drug demonstrates in vitro activity against *H. capsulatum*, *B. dermatitidis*, *C. neoformans*, *Candida* species, and *Aspergillus* species. Despite its poor penetration into CSF, animal studies demonstrate significant cure rates in murine cryptococcal meningitis models. A new formulation of itraconazole in an oral suspension has been developed that improves absorption in the absence of gastric acidity and results in higher drug levels of itraconazole in the bloodstream.[31] However, this formulation has not been used in clinical studies of cryptococcal disease.

Acute Therapy

The treatment of non–AIDS-associated cryptococcal meningitis consists of AMB (0.5 mg/kg/day) plus 5-FC (150 mg/kg/day in four divided doses) given over 6 weeks. This regimen be-

came firmly established around the same time that the AIDS epidemic was first identified. As a result, the original studies of AIDS-associated cryptococcal meningitis consisted of regimens containing AMB plus 5-FC.[15,16] Although some centers had fairly good success with this regimen, other centers reported much higher toxicity profiles, especially with the 5-FC component of the regimen, than was noted in non-AIDS patients.[11,32]

Several studies have addressed the role of AMB with or without 5-FC as well as the newer triazole agents in the treatment of AIDS-associated cryptococcal meningitis (Table 24–2). In 1985, Kovacs et al. reported success in 10 of 24 patients (42%) treated with either AMB alone (0.4 to 0.6 mg/kg/day) or AMB plus 5-FC (150 mg/kg/day).[15] Nine of the patients in this study died, two patients relapsed after successfully completing initial therapy, and three patients had persistently positive cultures at the end of therapy (quiescent disease). In 1986, Zuger et al. published a report documenting a successful outcome in 75% of patients (18 of 24) treated with AMB with or without 5-FC.[16] In 1989, a retrospective study by Chuck and Sande reported a 79% 6-week survival rate among 89 patients with cryptococcal meningitis.[11] However, the 6-month survival rate was only 38% for those receiving AMB alone compared to 52% for those receiving AMB plus 5-FC. Of note, 53% of the patients receiving 5-FC had their drug discontinued because of toxicities, predominantly cytopenias. Drug levels were not followed routinely in this patient population. In a small study by Larsen et al. in 1990, 6 of 6 patients treated with AMB (0.7 mg/kg/day for the first 2 weeks) plus 5-FC (150 mg/kg/day) converted their cultures to negative with mini-

TABLE 24–2. Outcome of Primary Therapy of Cryptococcal Meningitis in AIDS Patients

	TREATMENT SUCCESS	
REFERENCE	AMB ± 5-FC	Fluconazole
Kovacs et al.[15]	10/24 (42%)	
Zuger et al.[16]	18/24 (75%)	
Dismukes et al.[8]		11/15 (73%)
Stern et al.[34]		4/5 (80%)
Larsen et al.[33]	6/6 (100%)	6/14 (43%)
Saag et al.[20]	25/63 (40%)	44/131 (34%)

Reprinted from Lapidus W, Saag M: Cryptococcal meningitis. In Johnson S, Johnson FN (series eds), Powderly WB, Van't Wout JW (consultant eds): The Antifungal Agents: Fluconazole. Lancashire, England, Marius Press, 1992, p 145, with permission.

mal toxicity.[33] These data, along with historical data reported by Armstrong,[32] suggest that higher doses of AMB (0.7 to 0.8 mg/kg/day) are required for optimal management of AIDS-associated cryptococcal meningitis. Moreover, to minimize toxicity, 5-FC levels should be obtained routinely in patients receiving this drug, especially at higher doses (150 mg/kg/day).

Early pilot studies of oral fluconazole therapy indicated high response rates, although some discrepancies are noted between studies. Stern et al. successfully treated four of five AIDS patients who had cryptococcal meningitis with fluconazole (50 to 200 mg/day), including two patients in whom AMB therapy had previously failed.[34] In contrast to the high success rate in the Stern study, Larsen et al. noted clinical and mycologic success in only 6 of 14 patients (43%) treated with fluconazole (400 mg/day).[33] In that study, among five patients with less severe disease, four experienced CSF culture conversion from positive to negative. Although side effects were much less common in the fluconazole-treated group than the AMB plus 5-FC group, the investigators concluded that the AMB plus 5-FC regimen should be used initially to treat the majority of acute cryptococcal infections in AIDS patients.

In 1992, the National Institute of Allergy and Infectious Diseases Mycoses Study Group (MSG) and AIDS Clinical Trials Group (ACTG), in conjunction with Pfizer Central Research, reported the results of a large study of AIDS-associated cryptococcal meningitis.[20] The Phase II/III study evaluated 194 patients assigned to receive fluconazole (200 mg/day) or AMB (median dose 0.5 mg/kg/day), randomized on a 2:1 (fluconazole/AMB) basis. Only 9 of 63 AMB recipients received concomitant 5-FC. In this study, successful improvement was defined as two negative CSF cultures within a 10-week time period in association with clinical improvement. With this criterion, 25 of 63 AMB patients (40%) and 44 of 131 patients receiving fluconazole (34%) were treated successfully. A remarkable number of patients in each group, 26% receiving fluconazole and 27% receiving AMB, had so-called quiescent disease, defined as clinical improvement but persistently positive CSF cultures at the end of therapy. Although overall survival was similar for the two groups (86% AMB vs. 82% fluconazole), a higher proportion of patients receiving fluconazole died within the first 2 weeks of therapy (19 of 24 compared to 5 of 9 for AMB). In addition, although the overall mycologic success rate was not different between the two groups, patients receiving AMB tended to have their cultures convert to negative more rapidly than those receiving fluconazole (Fig. 24–3).

Based on these results, another large study, ACTG 159/MSG 17, was initiated that evaluated the use of higher dose AMB (0.7 to 0.8 mg/kg) during the first 2 weeks of therapy, followed by fluconazole (400 mg/day) or itraconazole (200 mg twice daily) for the rest of acute therapy (8 to 10 weeks). Before this study, itraconazole had been evaluated in over 50 HIV-infected patients with cryptococcal disease. In a study by Denning et al. among 29 evaluable pa-

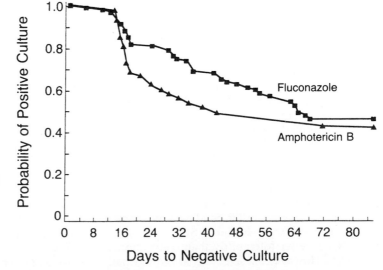

FIGURE 24–3. Kaplan-Meier estimates of the length of time to the first negative CSF culture, according to treatment group. (From Saag MS, Powderly WG, Cloud GA, et al: Comparison of amphotericin B with fluconazole in the treatment of acute AIDS-associated cryptococcal meningitis. N Engl J Med 326:86, 1992, with permission.)

tients with cryptococcal meningitis, 14 patients (48%) had a complete response, 6 patients (21%) had initial responses and then relapsed, and in 9 patients (31%) therapy failed.[35]

ACTG 159/MSG 17 accrued 408 patients over 3 years. No statistical difference was noted between those patients who received AMB plus 5-FC and those who received AMB alone (60% vs. 51% of patients achieved culture-negative status at 2 weeks; $p = .06$). After an additional 8 weeks of treatment, culture-negative status was achieved in 72% of fluconazole recipients compared to 60% of those receiving itraconazole.[17] However, clinical improvement as determined by absence of fever, headache, or meningismus was observed in 70% of itraconazole recipients versus 68% of fluconazole recipients. No difference in survival was noted between any treatment group. Overall mortality at 10 weeks was 6%, substantially lower than that observed in previous studies.

An Italian study utilizing a similar treatment strategy, higher dose AMB followed by oral triazole therapy, demonstrated a high level of success.[36] Among 31 patients treated with this approach, 29 (94%) were characterized as having successful responses. No deaths were reported.

A novel approach using fluconazole in combination with flucytosine has been evaluated by the California Collaborative Treatment Group.[37] The results of this study reveal a mycologic success rate of 75% and a clinical success rate of 63%. Among the 32 patients treated with this regimen, 4 patients (13%) died during the study. Although the results of the study are promising, they are tempered by the high frequency of toxicity noted, principally as a result of the flucytosine component. Over 60% of patients experienced some degree of toxicity that required alteration in dosage, and 28% required discontinuation of study medication. Further evaluation of this approach is warranted before it can be recommended as a treatment option in clinical practice (Table 24–3).

Several studies have evaluated lipid complex and liposomal preparations of AMB. The use of AMB mixed with intralipid resulted in a higher incidence of nephrotoxicity and anemia than did standard AMB in one clinical study.[38] In contrast, a randomized study of AMB lipid complex versus standard AMB resulted in fewer hematologic and nephrologic toxicities among those receiving the lipid complex preparation.[39] Clinical outcomes were similar. Studies of liposomal AMB demonstrated earlier CSF sterilization along with better tolerability than conventional AMB.[28,29] However, these results are from small

---

TABLE 24–3. Recommended Treatment of AIDS-Associated Cryptococcal Meningitis

Acute Therapy
Amphotericin B (0.7–0.8 mg/kg/d) for 2 weeks (minimum) with or without 5-flucytosine (100 mg/kg/d in 4 divided doses)*; followed by
Fluconazole 400 mg by mouth daily for 8–10 weeks (Alternative: Itraconazole[†] 200 mg by mouth twice daily)

Maintenance Therapy
Fluconzaole 200 mg by mouth daily
Alternative: Itraconazole[†] 200 mg by mouth twice daily
             or
             Amphotericin B (1 mg/kg) IV one or two times per week

Primary Prophylaxis
Not recommended (see text)

*Must adjust dose for renal insufficiency; ideally drug levels should be monitored in all patients receiving 5-FC.
[†]Used if patient cannot tolerate fluconazole.

---

studies and should be considered nondefinitive. Larger comparative trials are underway.[39]

Management of Increased Intracranial Pressure

Increased intracranial pressure (ICP), usually in the form of communicating hydrocephalus, is a frequent and potentially life-threatening complication of acute cryptococcal meningitis.[40] Although the cause of increased pressure has not been evaluated systematically, most authorities hypothesize that decreased absorption of CSF via the arachnoid villi is responsible, most likely resulting from impairment of the absorptive mechanism by capsular polysaccharide byproducts or the yeasts themselves.[41] Other proposed mechanisms include cryptococcal-induced vasculitis, microscopic intracerebral abscesses with resultant parenchymal edema, or a combination of all of these effects. A peculiar aspect of the clinical picture of increased ICP is the lack of radiologic evidence of hydrocephalus per se. Indeed, the majority of patients with high CSF pressures have normal to small-sized ventricles (Fig. 24–1). A possible explanation for this phenomenon is equalization of pressures within cranial structures via transependymal flow of CSF from the subarachnoid space into cerebral tissue. An alternative explanation proposes the simultaneous existence of cerebral edema and resistance of outflow, resulting in equalization of CSF pressure with the edematous pressure within the brain tissue itself.

Elevated pressures (>200 mm H_2O) are reported in over two thirds of patients with cryptococcal meningitis. Although the contribution of increased ICP to mortality, especially within the first 2 weeks, is unclear, many investigators believe it plays a critical role in the morbidity and mortality of the disease.[42] In the recently completed MSG/ACTG study, among the 14 patients who died due to cryptococcal disease, 13 had opening pressures of more than 250 mm H_2O at the measurement closest to the time of death.[43] Moreover, the median baseline opening pressures were significantly lower (220 mm H_2O) among those in whom CSF cultures successfully converted to negative compared to those who remained culture positive (median baseline opening pressure of 280 mm H_2O). Anecdotal experience from a number of investigators indicates that mortality is reduced even among high-risk patients when careful attention is paid to management of ICP.

In the absence of obstructive hydrocephalus, serial lumbar punctures provide the best mechanism of relieving the complications of ICP. Ten to 20 ml of spinal fluid can be removed safely at each tap. However, the true therapeutic benefit is most likely due to puncture defects in the dura, with persistent CSF leakage over time. Remarkably, patients with symptomatic elevation of CSF pressure often will experience prompt relief of symptoms (such as headache, nausea, and vomiting) within 30 minutes of the spinal tap and often will request repeat taps when they experience recurrent symptoms. Unfortunately, the effect of aggressive CSF pressure management has not been systematically evaluated. In the large ACTG 159/MSG 17 study, opening pressures were measured in over 60% of patients, and the modes of pressure management were documented. The lower overall mortality (6%) in this study appears to be related to several factors, but the causal relationship of more aggressive pressure management with this outcome remains to be established.

On occasion, serial lumbar punctures are not sufficient to control the symptoms of increased ICP. In those instances, placement of a lumbar drain or ventriculostomy may be of acute benefit. However, placement of a ventricular-peritoneal shunt often is required in this setting to achieve long-term control of symptoms. The use of other measures to control increased ICP, such as acetazolamide or corticosteroids, remains controversial and cannot be recommended for use on a routine basis.

In summary, increased ICP ultimately may prove to be one of the most important predictors of outcome in patients with cryptococcal meningitis. In the setting of AIDS-associated cryp-

toccal disease, where the usual measurements of the spinal fluid formula (such as CSF glucose, protein, and white blood cell count) are within normal limits, ICP often becomes the most important measurement evaluated and should be obtained every time a spinal tap is performed.

Maintenance Therapy

Even after successful treatment of acute cryptococcal meningitis, 50% to 70% of patients will experience recurrent disease within 1 year if no maintenance therapy is administered.[11,12,16] This contrasts with the 12% to 25% relapse rate reported among non–HIV-infected patients.[1] Typically, relapses are associated with the same strain of *C. neoformans* that caused the initial infection.[44,45] Zuger et al. reported no relapses among seven patients treated with weekly amphotericin B after successful initial treatment, compared to a relapse rate of 50% (four of eight patients) among patients receiving maintenance therapy over a 6-month period.[16] Chuck and Sande, in their retrospective review of cases at San Francisco General Hospital, reported a relapse rate of 27% (7 of 26 patients) among those who did not receive maintenance therapy compared to 16% (6 of 37 patients) of those who received either ketoconazole or AMB maintenance therapy.[11] Clark et al. reported a 38% relapse rate (three of eight patients) among those receiving no maintenance therapy versus a 7% rate (2 of 27 patients) among those who received AMB maintenance therapy.[12] Two separate fluconazole maintenance therapy pilot studies each reported 7% relapse rates (1 of 14 patients in a study by Stern et al.[34] and 1 of 15 patients in a study by Sugar and Saunders[46]). A larger placebo-controlled study conducted by the California Collaborative Treatment Group reported a relapse rate of 15% (4 of 27 patients) in the placebo group compared to no relapses among the 24 patients receiving fluconazole therapy (100 to 200 mg/day).[47]

In a large definitive study conducted by the ACTG and the MSG, daily therapy with fluconazole (200 mg/day) was superior to AMB (1 mg/kg/week) as maintenance therapy for AIDS patients who had been treated successfully for acute cryptococcal meningitis.[48] Of 189 evaluable patients, 14 of 78 patients (18%) receiving AMB relapsed compared to 2 of 111 patients (2%) assigned to the fluconazole group. Kaplan-Meier estimates of relapse-free survival demonstrated a 27% difference between the two groups. Therapy-related side effects and bacterial infections were both more common in the

AMB group. The study drug was discontinued because of severe toxicities in 12 patients assigned to AMB versus 6 patients assigned to fluconazole.

Based on this study, along with pilot data from previous studies, fluconazole (200 mg/day) is considered the treatment of choice as maintenance therapy for preventing relapse of cryptococcal meningitis in HIV-infected patients. The use of other triazoles, most notably itraconazole, remains a secondary choice. In a recently published head-to-head study of itraconazole versus fluconazole conducted by the MSG (MSG 25), fluconazole was superior in preventing relapse of cryptococcal disease.[49] The study, which evaluated 107 patients who had been successfully treated for cryptococcal meningitis, was terminated based on a recommendation by an independent Data and Safety Monitoring Board, which noted a disproportionate number of relapses in one of the two study arms. A total of 15 relapses was observed, with 13 of 55 itraconazole recipients experiencing relapse of disease compared to 2 of 52 fluconazole recipients. Of note, in a multivariate analysis of factors predicting the likelihood of relapse, the lack of use of 5-FC during initial acute therapy (the first 2 weeks) was *more* predictive of relapse than any other factor (relative risk 5.88, *p* = .04), including use of itraconazole as maintenance therapy (relative risk 4.32, *p* = .06).

HISTOPLASMOSIS

Epidemiology and Pathogenesis

Histoplasmosis is endemic in the central and south central regions of the United States. The endemic area also extends along the river basins north into the Canadian provinces of Quebec and Ontario and south into Mexico, Central America, and South America. In the southern region of the United States, the endemic area extends to Alabama in the east and southwest Texas in the west, including the San Antonio area. Certain cities, most notably Indianapolis, Indiana, and Kansas City, Missouri, are high-incidence areas of histoplasmosis. In these hyperendemic areas, histoplasmosis has been reported to be the second or third most common opportunistic infection among HIV patients at various times.[50-52]

As with other systemic fungal infections, initial primary infection occurs in the lung after inhalation of arthroconidia, which are rapidly converted into the yeast phase at body temperature. The yeast are phagocytized by reticuloendothelial (RE) cells within the lung, where they continue to multiply. After the infection is well established, the organism disseminates through the body, initially within regional lymph nodes and ultimately within target organs. Two to 3 weeks after the initial infection, specific T-cell–mediated immunity is established, and the infected RE cells are better able to kill the intracellular organisms. In a normal host, the infection is usually brought under control, and the patient does not develop any further clinical manifestations. When the immune system is weakened, however, the initial infection may not be brought under control, and progressive disseminated disease ensues. In the case of an individual with a remote history of histoplasmosis who becomes immunosuppressed, reactivation disease in the form of disseminated histoplasmosis may occur. Patients at highest risk of disseminated histoplasmosis are those with defective T-cell–mediated immunity, such as patients with advanced HIV infection.

Although quite uncommon in an immunologically intact individual, progressive disseminated histoplasmosis (PSH) is the most common form of disease among AIDS patients. In nonendemic areas, PDH most likely represents reactivation disease.[50,53] However, in endemic areas, especially hyperendemic areas, PDH appears to represent disseminated primary infection, although firm epidemiologic data supporting this concept are lacking. Within endemic areas, histoplasmosis represents 5% of the opportunistic infections among AIDS patients. However, in hyperendemic areas, the incidence is as high as 25%.[52] Among these patients who develop histoplasmosis, it is the initial AIDS-defining illness in 50% to 75% of cases.

Clinical Manifestations

Disseminated histoplasmosis is generally a disease of more advanced stages of HIV infection. The median CD4 cell count at the time of diagnosis is $50/mm^3$.[52] Fever, weight loss, and other constitutional signs are present in over 95% of patients with PDH.[51,52] Respiratory complaints are the most common localizing symptoms, occurring in 50% to 60% of patients. Hepatosplenomegaly is noted in 20% to 40% of patients, lymphadenopathy in 20%, and skin or mucosal involvement in 2% to 5% of patients. Importantly, neurologic manifestations are reported in 18% to 20% of histoplasmosis cases.[54,55] This may take the form of meningitis or cerebritis. Approximately 10% of patients have a septicemic picture, characterized by high fever, hypotension, and, on occasion, adult respiratory distress syndrome.[52] On rare occasions, histoplasmosis may occur as retinitis, pericarditis, prostatitis, pancreatitis, pleuritis, or colitis.

Routine laboratory test results are generally nonspecific. Peripheral white blood cell counts are similar to those of other patients with advanced HIV infection. Alkaline phosphatase and γ-glutamyltransferase elevations are seen commonly, especially in those patients with PDH and hepatic involvement. Erythrocyte sedimentation rates are generally elevated. Chest radiographs are abnormal in up to 60% of patients.[52] The most common radiographic abnormality is diffuse infiltration, usually described as an interstitial pattern but possibly also a reticulonodular or alveolar pattern. Interestingly, mediastinal lymphadenopathy is distinctly uncommon in AIDS patients with PDH, occurring on only 3% to 5% of cases described in the literature. Nodular calcification in either the lung or mediastinal lymph nodes is reported in less than 3% of cases.

Diagnosis

Owing to the nonspecific symptoms of disseminated histoplasmosis, the disease may be difficult to diagnose. This is especially true in nonendemic areas, where clinicians may not consider the diagnosis or pathologists may be unaccustomed to identifying *H. capsulatum* in tissue specimens. Fortunately, several techniques have been identified that aid in the diagnosis of histoplasmosis.

The gold standard is a positive culture of the organism from peripheral blood or tissue specimens. The application of lysis-centrifugation blood culture techniques has greatly enhanced the reliability of blood cultures in the diagnosis of disseminated histoplasmosis.[52] Unfortunately, even with lysis-centrifugation systems, the diagnosis can take up to 2 to 3 weeks for confirmation. In experienced hands, this technique is positive in 85% to 95% of patients with disseminated histoplasmosis. Culture of tissues is less sensitive, although still an important means of establishing the diagnosis (Table 24–4).

Histopathologic evaluation of tissues is more rapid than culture and establishes the diagnosis in up to 50% of patients. The most accessible site to biopsy for histopathologic evaluation is the bone marrow. The organism usually can be identified within macrophages, and identification is readily enhanced through the use of special stains, such as methenamine silver (Color Plate II*D*). Other tissues, such as lymph node, liver, and skin, and bronchoalveolar lavage fluid, may yield a diagnosis in individuals with abnormal findings in these organ systems.

Standard serodiagnostic studies, which detect the presence of antibodies against *Histoplasma* antigens, are positive in the majority of patients. The immunodiffusion test usually reveals the presence of an M-band, but the more specific H-band is usually absent. Complement fixation serologic tests are reactive in 75% of patients with disseminated histoplasmosis. Unfortunately, the presence of antibodies does not indicate whether the patient is experiencing an active infection with histoplasmosis or simply has been infected in the past.

During the 1980s, Wheat et al.[56] established a diagnostic histoplasma antigen test (Table 24–4).[5] This test can be applied to both serum and urine, although the urine test is more sensitive and equally specific. In a retrospective study by Wheat et al. the *H. capsulatum* polysaccharide antigen (HPA) was detected in blood, urine, or CSF in 70 of 72 HIV-associated cases (97.3%).[52,57] Negative results in urine occurred in two patients who had asymptomatic pulmonary histoplasmosis.

TABLE 24–4. Sensitivity (%) of Diagnostic Tests for Histoplasmosis

| | TYPE OF *H. Capsulatum* DISEASE | | |
TEST	Disseminated	Chronic Pulmonary	Acute
Histoplasma antigen	92	21	39
Culture	85	85	15
Histopathology	43	17	9
Serology	71	100	98

Data from Joseph Wheat (personal communication).

An important application of the HPA test is its usefulness in following the response to therapy.[52,57,58] In one study, 19 of 19 successfully treated patients demonstrated a two-unit or more fall in serum HPA levels, and 85% of patients had at least a two-unit fall in urine HPA levels.[58] In another study of relapsing disease, 17 of 18 urine samples demonstrated a two-unit increase in HPA levels at the time of relapse. A two-unit increase in HPA serum levels was noted in 12 of 14 relapsing patients. The magnitude of the HPA level may be predictive of long-term outcome. Three of five patients with baseline serum HPA levels of greater than 15 units died within 1 week of initiation of therapy.[52] However, more data are required before this association can be firmly established. Although the HPA test is performed only in Wheat's laboratory, a mechanism is available for practicing clinicians to send specimens to his laboratory for testing on individual patients (for more information, call 1-800-447-8634).

Treatment

AMB has been the gold standard therapy for disseminated histoplasmosis in HIV-infected patients (Table 24–5). Several reports in the literature document 90% success rates in control or resolution of symptoms associated with disseminated histoplasmosis.[50,52,60] In one study, among 56 HIV-infected patients with non–life-threatening manifestations of histoplasmosis, 55 (98%) achieved clinical remission with AMB therapy.[61] Treatment with AMB often results in rapid defervescence within a period of days. Of 29 cases reported by Wheat et al., temperature fell to less than 100°F by day 3 of therapy in 25% and by day 7 of therapy in 73%.[52] Only 7% of patients remained febrile after 2 weeks of AMB therapy. The majority of patients who die of histoplasmosis usually succumb before receiving 500 mg of AMB. Additionally, those patients who are septicemic are at higher risk of death while on therapy.

Ketoconazole, which is effective in the control of histoplasmosis in non-AIDS patients, does not work well in patients with AIDS-associated histoplasmosis.[50,52,60] As induction therapy for control of acute symptoms of disseminated histoplasmosis, ketoconazole is not effective. In one series, only 1 of 11 patients with disseminated histoplasmosis was treated successfully with initial ketoconazole therapy.[52] Even using ketoconazole as maintenance therapy, up to 50% of patients relapsed compared to a relapse rate of 50% to 80% in patients not receiving maintenance therapy. In contrast, AMB at a dose of 1 mg/kg administered one to two times per week is associated with an 80% to 90% relapse-free survival.[52,62]

Unlike ketoconazole, itraconazole has been evaluated in controlled clinical trials as both maintenance therapy (ACTG 084) and acute induction therapy (ACTG 120). The results of the maintenance study demonstrate successful prevention of relapse in 95% of patients (40 of 42 patients) receiving itraconazole (200 mg bid), with a median follow-up time of 109 weeks.[63] Urine HPA levels converted to negative in 43% of patients, whereas serum HPA levels became negative in 75% of the patients in this study. Itraconazole was evaluated as acute primary therapy of disseminated histoplasmosis (ACTG 120). Successful outcome was observed in 50 patients (85%).[64] Among those who were judged to be nonresponders, treatment failed in six (10%) because of progressive disease and in two (4%) because of toxicity, and one (2%) was lost to follow-up by the second week. Although this study was not designed to be a comparative trial, the overall response rate was similar to historical experience with AMB. Based on these data, most investigators favor the use of itraconazole (200 mg three times daily for 3 days, then 200 mg twice daily) as the initial therapy for nonmeningeal, nonsepticemic, AIDS-

TABLE 24–5. Recommendations for Treatment of AIDS-Associated Histoplasmosis

PHASE OF THERAPY	SEVERITY OF DISEASE	PREFERRED DRUG (DOSE)	DURATION OF THERAPY
Induction	Mild	Itraconazole (400 mg/d)	3 months
	Moderate-severe	Amphotericin B (0.7–1.0 mg/kg/d) followed by Itraconazole (400 mg/d)	1–2 weeks 10–12 weeks
Maintenance	Remission/asymptomatic	Itraconazole (200 mg/d)*	Lifelong

*Itraconazole 200 mg twice daily should be continued indefinitely if itraconazole blood levels are less than 4 μg/ml on 400 mg/d.

associated disseminated histoplasmosis. It should be noted that any patient treated with itraconazole should not be receiving contraindicated concomitant medications, such as rifampin, rifabutin, phenytoin, carbamazepine, H_2 blockers, or antacid therapy, in order to assure adequate drug levels. The new liquid formulation of itraconazole is absorbed when H_2 blockers or antacids are co-administered. It is the preferred formulation when these concomitant medications must be used.[31] However, no formal studies of the liquid formulation as treatment of histoplasmosis have been performed.

The use of fluconazole in the treatment of histoplasmosis remains controversial. Anecdotal experience in the literature reveals a response rate of 40% for induction therapy with fluconazole.[65] A study by the ACTG (ACTG 174) demonstrated a lower response rate among those receiving fluconazole for acute histoplasmosis (74% success) than that achieved with itraconazole (historical controls).[66] Based on the lower response rates among the anecdotal reports in the literature, fluconazole should be reserved for patients who are unable to take itraconazole and for whom AMB is not a viable option.

COCCIDIOIDOMYCOSIS

Epidemiology and Pathogenesis

Coccidioidomycosis is caused by *Coccidioides immitis*, an organism that is endemic to the southwestern United States, northern Mexico, and portions of Central and South America. The organism lives in the soil in the mycelial phase, and, when it is disturbed, aerosolized infectious particles are inhaled into the lungs of susceptible hosts. Once in the alveolar space, the organism multiplies, resulting in a giant spherule (Color Plate II*E*). Before development of T-cell immunity, macrophages may ingest the organism but are unable to kill it. Then pathogenesis is similar in many ways to that seen in histoplasmosis, with potential dissemination of the organism before development of an adequate immune system response. Once T-cell immunity develops, the organism can be killed by the cells of the immune system, and the manifestations of disease are arrested. Among patients with impaired cellular immunity, however, progressive coccidioidal disease often develops, manifesting as disseminated disease in the lung, bone, skin, or CNS.

AIDS-associated coccidioidal disease is generally confined to the endemic regions. Reports of cases outside endemic areas probably represent expression of disease after exposure within an endemic area or, potentially, reactivated disease.[67-69] The majority of patients who develop AIDS-associated coccidioidomycosis have CD4 counts of less than $250/mm^3$ and evidence of impaired T-cell function, with negative spherulin skin tests.[68] In Arizona, coccidioidomycosis is the third most frequently reported opportunistic infection after *P. carinii* pneumonia and esophageal candidiasis.[69] The issue of whether disease expression is reactivation of old, arrested disease or acquisition of new infection is not resolved. A recent study by Ampel et al. estimated a 24.6% cumulative incidence of coccidioidal disease among a cohort of HIV-infected patients followed in Arizona.[67] Importantly, the presence of a positive skin test did not predict the development of active coccidioidomycosis in this cohort. Rather, a baseline positive skin test was most associated with the presence of a higher CD4 count at study entry. Nearly 20% of the subjects developed a positive skin test while on study. However, the development of dermal hypersensitivity was not associated with the development of active coccidioidomycosis.

Clinical Manifestations

Coccidioidal infection may occur in a wide variety of forms, ranging from positive serologic tests to life-threatening pneumonitis or meningitis (see review by Fish et al.[68]). Focal pulmonary disease may have focal radiologic abnormalities, which may be multiple and include focal alveolar infiltrates, discrete nodules, hilar adenopathy, or cavitary disease. Rarely, pleural effusions are noted. Diffuse pulmonary disease is more common and may be indistinguishable from other opportunistic infectious processes, such as *P. carinii* pneumonia (Chapters 9 and 20). Occasionally, patients with pulmonary disease may have evidence of cutaneous coccidioidomycosis. Rarely, the skin lesions are noted in the absence of pulmonary manifestations. Unlike cryptococcal meningitis, coccidioidal meningitis is characterized by high CSF cell counts, with white blood cell counts ranging from $2/mm^3$ to more than $1500/mm^3$. CSF glucose is usually suppressed and CSF protein is elevated, but not invariably so. Interestingly, about 50% of patients will have negative CSF cultures at the time of the initial visit. Complement fixation antibody is usually detected in the CSF in the majority of meningitis patients. Localized extrapulmonary disease has been reported in thoracic as well as extrathoracic lymph nodes. Occasionally, hepatic coccidioidal disease is identified.

The majority of patients will have positive serologic titers for *C. immitis* at the time of diagnosis with either the tube precipitin (TP) or complement fixation test.[68] In general, the complement fixation test is more sensitive than the TP test. The likelihood of seropositivity is higher in patients with extrapulmonary disease than in those with focal or diffuse pulmonary manifestations. Complement fixation titers are generally highest in patients with meningitis, with values up to 1:4096. Less than 20% of patients have reactive spherulin skin tests. The CD4 count for patients with coccidioidal disease is generally less than 200/mm³. Among HIV-infected patients, long-term outcome is clearly associated with the type of disease manifestation. Patients with cutaneous or lymph node involvement experience longer median survival times than those with diffuse pulmonary disease or low initial CD4 counts. Survival among meningitis patients is variable but generally better than among those with diffuse pulmonary disease.

Diagnosis

Diagnosis of coccidioidomycosis is made by culturing the organism from clinical specimens or by demonstrating of the organism via histopathologic stains. Spherules are best identified with methenamine silver or Papanicolaou stain (Color Plate II*E*). Blood cultures are positive in less than 30% of patients. Laboratories that attempt culture of *C. immitis* should bear in mind that the organism is extremely infectious and may be easily spread in a laboratory setting. Therefore, laboratory personnel should be notified when *C. immitis* disease is suspected so that appropriate precautions can be taken.

Serologic tests for *C. immitis* are positive in up to 80% of patients with coccidioidomycosis despite evidence of profound immunodeficiency in some patients.

Treatment

AMB remains the principal initial therapy for patients with coccidioidal disease, especially in individuals with diffuse pulmonary disease or meningitis. Several studies evaluating the role of oral azoles, including fluconazole and itraconazole, have demonstrated effectiveness of these agents, especially as maintenance therapy after control of disease has been achieved with AMB.[68,69] As with other systemic mycoses in AIDS patients, chronic suppressive therapy appears warranted. The precise dosage of amphotericin that should be administered before switching to an azole remains unclear. Most investigators suggest a minimum dose of at least 500 to 700 mg of AMB as initial therapy. Newer formulations of AMB, including lipid dispersion (ABLC), colloidal dispersion (ABCD), and liposomal AMB (AmBisome), have been used in small, open-label studies.[70-72] In general, decreased rates of adverse experiences are noted with these preparations (in both human and animal studies), but no reliable efficacy data are available. Itraconazole and fluconazole appear to be effective as maintenance therapy of coccidioidal disease, although the number of patients treated is small.[73,74] Ketoconazole does not work well in AIDS-associated coccidioidomycoses.[75] Some investigators have had success using fluconazole as initial therapy for coccidioidal meningitis, but further data are needed before this therapy can be formally recommended, especially in the acutely ill patient. Intrathecal AMB is reserved for those patients with refractory meningitis.

FUNGAL PROPHYLAXIS

One of the most controversial areas in AIDS therapy is the use of primary prophylaxis for systemic fungal infections.[76] Systemic mycoses occur as late manifestations of HIV disease, usually with CD4 counts of less than 100/mm³.[77] The overall incidence of cryptococcal disease is 8% to 10% of AIDS patients, and the incidence of histoplasmosis and coccidioidomycosis varies with exposure to endemic areas. Many clinicians argue that patients living in endemic areas and patients who have CD4 counts of less than 50/mm³ would benefit from chronic fluconazole prophylaxis, usually at doses of 200 mg/day.[77] Indeed, in surveys of patients with advanced HIV infection who are participating in clinical trials, up to 40% of those with CD4 counts of less than 100/mm³ are on primary antifungal prophylaxis (J. Feinberg, personal communication).

In addition to economic concerns, a major issue in the argument against routine antifungal prophylaxis is that indiscriminate use of these agents may lead to a higher prevalence of resistant organisms in the community.[77-80] Reports of fluconazole-resistant *C. albicans* have increased substantially over the last 3 years. However, the actual incidence of this problem is unknown and is probably quite low. Nonetheless, appropriate concern exists over azole-resistant fungi becoming a more significant problem in the next 5 to 10 years.

Fortunately, an ACTG study (ACTG 981) was initiated in 1988–1989 to evaluate this question.[81] This study enrolled over 400 patients with CD4 counts of less than $100/mm^3$ who were participating in an ongoing study of *P. carinii* pneumonia prophylaxis. Half of the patients were assigned to receive fluconazole (200 mg/day), and the other half received clotrimazole troches five times per day. Median follow-up was more than 35 months. Significantly more serious systemic fungal infections occurred in the clotrimazole group than in the fluconazole group. Most notably, the incidence of cryptococcal meningitis and esophageal candidiasis was substantially higher among the clotrimazole recipients. Interestingly, there were three cases of aspergillosis in the fluconazole-treated patients compared to one in the clotrimazole group. Despite the significant benefit in preventing systemic fungal infections with fluconazole, overall mortality between the two groups was no different; in fact, fewer deaths were noted overall in the clotrimazole-treated patients, although this difference did not reach statistical significance.

These data clearly support several important observations. First, serious systemic mycoses can be prevented with fluconazole when it is used in patients with advanced (CD4 counts <100 cells/mm^3) HIV disease. Second, prevention of systemic mycoses does not necessarily translate into a survival advantage, although morbidity may be reduced. Third, a cost–benefit analysis is needed to assess the overall advantage of preventing systemic fungal infections with no resultant survival advantage versus the monetary costs and potential toxicity costs (including drug interactions and potential development of resistant organisms) in this patient population. These analyses are currently underway. Until then, routine prophylaxis with fluconazole or itraconazole is not recommended.

Acknowledgments

I would like to thank Jane Garrison for her outstanding help in the preparation of this manuscript.

References

1. Sabetta JR, Andriole VT: Cryptococcal infection of the central nervous system. Med Clin North Am 69:333, 1985
2. Wilson DE, Bennett J, Bailey JW: Serologic grouping of *Cryptococcus neoformans*. Proc Soc Exp Biol Med 127:820, 1968
3. Rinaldi MG, Drutz DJ, Howell A, et al: Serotypes of *Cryptococcus neoformans* in patients with AIDS. J Infect Dis 153:642, 1986
4. Shimizu RY, Howard DH, Clancy MN: The variety of *Cryptococcus neoformans* in patients with AIDS. J Infect Dis 154:1042, 1986
5. Saag MS: Clinical and host differences between infections with the two varieties of *Cryptococcus neoformans* [Editorial response]. Clin Infect Dis 21:35, 1995
6. Speed B, Dunt D: Clinical and host differences between infections with the two varieties of *Cryptococcus neoformans*. Clin Infect Dis 21:28, 1995
7. Swinne D, Nkurikiyinfura JB, Muyembe TL: Clinical isolates of *Cryptococcus neoformans* from Zaire. Eur J Clin Microbiol 5:50, 1986
8. Dismukes WE, Cloud G, Gallis H, et al: Treatment of cryptococcal meningitis with combination of amphotericin B and flucytosine for four as compared with six weeks. N Engl J Med 317:334, 1987
9. Centers for Disease Control: HIV/AIDS Surveillance Report. Atlanta, Centers for Disease Control, 1991
10. Hajjeh R, Stephens D, Baughman W, et al: A case-control study of risk factors for cryptococcosis in HIV-infected persons. In: Abstracts of the XIth International Conference on AIDS, Vancouver, 1996, Abstract Tu.B.186
11. Chuck SL, Sande MA: Infections with *Cryptococcus neoformans* in the acquired immunodeficiency syndrome. N Engl J Med 321:794, 1989
12. Clark RA, Greer D, Atkinson W, et al: Spectrum of *Cryptococcus neoformans* infection in 68 patients infected with human immunodeficiency virus. Rev Infect Dis 12:768, 1990
13. Dismukes WE: Cryptococcal meningitis in patients with AIDS. J Infect Dis 157:624, 1988
14. Eng RH, Bishburg E, Smith S, et al: Cryptococcal infections in the acquired immune deficiency syndrome. Am J Med 81:19, 1986
15. Kovacs JA, Kovacs AA, Polis M, et al: Cryptococcosis in the acquired immunodeficiency syndrome. Ann Intern Med 103:533, 1985
16. Zuger A, Louie E, Holzman RS: Cryptococcal disease in patients with the acquired immunodeficiency syndrome: Diagnostic features and outcome of treatment. Ann Intern Med 104:234, 1986
17. Vander Horst C, Saag MS, Cloud G, et al: Treatment of cryptococcal meningitis associated with the acquired immunodeficiency syndrome. N Engl J Med 337:15, 1997
18. Larsen RA, Bozzette S, McCutchan JA, et al: Persistent *Cryptococcus neoformans* of the prostate after successful treatment of meningitis. Ann Intern Med 111:125, 1989
19. Popovich MJ, Arthur R, Helmer E: CT of intracranial cryptococcosis. Am J Radiol 154:603, 1990
20. Saag MS, Powderly WG, Cloud GA, et al: Comparison of amphotericin B with fluconazole in the treatment of acute AIDS-associated cryptococcal meningitis. N Engl J Med 326:83, 1992
21. Powderly WG, Cloud GA, Dismukes WE, et al: Value of serum and cerebrospinal fluid cryptococcal antigen

measurement in the management of AIDS-associated cryptococcal meningitis. Clin Infect Dis 18:789, 1994

22. McManus EJ, Jones JM: Detection of a *Trichosporon beigelii* antigen crossreactive with *Cryptococcus neoformans* capsular polysaccharide in serum from a patient with disseminated *Trichosporon* infection. J Clin Microbiol 21:681, 1985.

23. Hamilton JR, Noble A, Denning DW, et al: Performance of *Cryptococcus* antigen latex agglutination kits on serum and cerebrospinal fluid specimens of AIDS patients before and after pronase treatment. J Clin Microbiol 29:333, 1991

24. Diamond RD, Bennett JE: Prognostic factors in cryptococcal meningitis: A study in 111 cases. Ann Intern Med 80:176, 1974.

25. Coker R, Tomlinson D, Harris J: Successful treatment of cryptococcal meningitis with liposomal amphotericin B after failure of treatment with fluconazole and conventional amphotericin B. AIDS 5:231, 1991

26. Graybill JR, Sharkey PK, Vincent D, et al: Amphotericin B lipid complex (ABLC) in treatment of cryptococcal meningitis in patients with AIDS. In: Abstracts of the 31st Interscience Conference on Antimicrobial Agents and Chemotherapy, Washington, DC, Chicago. American Society for Microbiology, 1991, Abstract 289, p 147

27. Schurmann D, De Matos MB, Grunewald T, et al: Safety and efficacy of liposomal amphotericin B in treating AIDS-associated disseminated cryptococcosis. J Infect Dis 164:620, 1991

28. Coker RJ, Viviani M, Gazzard BG, et al: Treatment of cryptococcosis with liposomal amphotericin B (AmBisome) in 23 patients with AIDS. AIDS 7:829, 1993

29. Leenders ACAP, Reiss P, Portegeis P, et al: A randomized trial of lipsomal amphotericin B (AmBisome) 4 mg/kg vs amphotericin B 0.7 mg/kg for cryptococcal meningitis in HIV-infected patients. In: Abstracts of the 36th Interscience Conference on Antimicrobial Agents and Chemotherapy, New Orleans. Washington, DC, American Society for Microbiology, 1996, Abstract L-035

30. Saag MS, Dismukes WE: Azole antifungal agents: Emphasis on new triazoles. Antimicrob Agents Chemother 32:1, 1988

31. Barone JA, Moskovitz BL, Guarnieri J, et al: Food interaction and steady-state pharmacokinetics of itraconazole oral solution in healthy volunteers. Pharmacotherapy 18:295, 1998

32. Armstrong D: Treatment of opportunistic infections. Clin Infect Dis 16:1, 1993

33. Larsen RA, Leal M, Chan L: Fluconazole compared with amphotericin B plus flucytosine for cryptococcal meningitis in AIDS. Ann Intern Med 113:183, 1990

34. Stern JJ, Hartmen BJ, Sharkey P, et al: Oral fluconazole therapy for patients with acquired immunodeficiency syndrome and crytpococcal meningitis: Experience with 22 patients. Am J Med 85:477, 1988

35. Denning DW, Tucker RM, Hanson LH: Itraconazole therapy for cryptococcal meningitis and cryptococcosis. Arch Intern Med 149:2301, 1989

36. De Lalla F, Pellizzer G, Vaglia A, et al: Amphotericin B as primary therapy for cryptococcosis in AIDS patients: Reliability of relatively high doses administered over a relatively short period. Clin Infect Dis 20:263, 1995

37. Larsen RA, Bozzette SA, Jones BE, et al: Fluconazole combined with flucytosine for treatment of cryptococcal meningitis in patients with AIDS. Clin Infect Dis 19:741, 1994

38. Joly V, Aubry P, Ndayiragide A, et al: Randomized comparison of amphotericin B deoxycholate dissolved in dextrose or Intralipid for the treatment of AIDS-associated cryptococcal meningitis. Clin Infect Dis 23:556, 1996

39. Sharkey PK, Graybill JR, Johnson ES, et al: Amphotericin B lipid complex compared with amphotericin B in the treatment of cryptococcal meningitis in patients with AIDS. Clin Infect Dis 22:315, 1996

40. Johnston SRD, Corbett EL, Foster O, et al: Raised intracranial pressure and visual complication in AIDS patients with cryptococcal meningitis. J Infect 24:185, 1992

41. Denning DW, Armstrong RW, Lewis BH, et al: Elevated cerebrospinal fluid pressure in patients with cryptococcal meningitis and acquired immunodeficiency syndrome. Am J Med 91:267, 1991

42. Ennis DM, Saag MS: Cryptococcal meningitis in AIDS. Hosp Pract 28:99, 1993

43. Graybill JR, Sobel J, Saag M, et al, and the NIAID Mycoses Study Group and AIDS Clinical Trials Group: Cerebrospinal fluid hypertension in patients with AIDS and cryptococcal meningitis. In: Abstracts of the 37th Interscience Conference on Antimicrobial Agents and Chemotherapy, Toronto. Washington, DC, American Society for Microbiology, 1997, Abstract I-153

44. Spitzer ED, Spitzer SG, Freundlich LF, et al: Persistence of initial infection in recurrent *Cryptococcus neoformans* meningitis. Lancet 341:595, 1993

45. Brandt ME, Pfaller MA, Hajjeh R, et al: Molecular subtypes and antifungal susceptibilities of serial Cryptococcus neoformans isolates in human immunodeficiency virus infected patients. J Infect Dis 174:812, 1996

46. Sugar AM, Saunders C: Oral fluconazole as a suppressive therapy of disseminated cryptococcosis in patients with acquired immunodeficiency syndrome. Am J Med 85:481, 1988

47. Bozzette SA, Larsen R, Chiu J, et al: A controlled trial of maintenance therapy with fluconazole after treatment of cryptococcal meningitis in the acquired immunodeficiency syndrome. N Engl J Med 324:580, 1991

48. Powderly WG, Saag MS, Cloud GA, et al: A randomized controlled trial of fluconazole versus amphotericin B as maintenance therapy for prevention of relapse of cryptococcal meningitis in patients with AIDS. N Engl J Med 326:793, 1992

49. Saag MS, Cloud GC, Graybill JR, et al: Comparison of fluconazole versus itraconazole as maintenance therapy in AIDS associated crytpococcal meningitis. Clin Infect Dis 28:291, 1999

50. Graybill JR: Histoplasmosis and AIDS. J Infect Dis 158:623, 1988

51. Sarosi GA, Johnson PC: Disseminated histoplasmosis in patients with human immunodeficiency virus. Clin Infect Dis 14:S60, 1992

52. Wheat LJ, Connolly-Stringfield P, Baker RL, et al: Disseminated histoplasmosis in the acquired immune deficiency syndrome: Clincial findings, diagnosis and treatment, and review of the literature. Medicine (Balt) 69:361, 1990

53. Keath EJ, Kobayashi GS, Medoff G: Typing of *Histoplasma capsulatum* by restriction fragment length polymorphisms in a nuclear gene. J Clin Microbiol 30:2104, 1992

54. Anaissie E, Fainstein V, Samo T, et al: Central nervous system histoplasmosis: An Unappreciated complication of the acquired immune deficiency syndrome. Am J Med 84:215, 1988

55. Wheat LJ, Batteiger BE, Sathapatayavongs B: *Histoplasma capsulatum* infection of the central nervous system. Medicine (Balt) 69:244, 1990

56. Wheat LJ, Kohler RB, Tewari RP: Diagnosis of disseminated histoplasmosis by detection of *Histoplasma capsulatum* antigen in serum and urine specimens. N Engl J Med 314:83, 1986

57. Wheat LJ, Connolly-Stringfield P, Kohler RB, et al: *Histoplasma capsulatum* polysaccharide antigen detection in the diagnosis and management of disseminated histoplasmosis in patients with acquired immunodeficiency syndrome. Am J Med 897:396, 1989

58. Wheat LJ, Connolly-Stringfield P, Blair R, et al: Effect of successful treatment with amphotericin B on *Histoplasma capsulatum* variety *capsulatum* polysaccharide antigen levels in patients with AIDS and histoplasmosis. Am J Med 92:153, 1992

59. Wheat LJ, Connolly-Stringfield P, Blair R, et al: Histoplasmosis relapse in patients with AIDS: Detection using *Histoplasma capsulatum* variety *capsulatum* antigen levels. Ann Intern Med 115:936, 1991

60. Wheat LJ: Histoplasmosis—diagnosis and management. Infect Dis Clin Pract 1:287, 1992

61. Wheat L: Histoplasmosis in the acquired immunodeficiency syndrome. Curr Top Med Mycol 7:7, 1996

62. McKinsey DS, Gupta MR, Riddker SA, et al: Long-term amphotericin B therapy for disseminated histoplasmosis in patients with the acquired immunodeficiency syndrome (AIDS). Ann Intern Med 111:655, 1989

63. Wheat LJ, Hafner RE, Wulfsohn M, et al: Prevention of relapse of histoplasmosis with itraconazole in patients with the acquired immunodeficiency syndrome. Ann Intern Med 118:610, 1993

64. Wheat LJ, Hafner RE, Korzun AM, et al: Itraconazole treatment of disseminated histoplasmosis in patients with AIDS. Am J Med 98:336, 1995

65. Sharkey-Mathis PK, Velez J, Fetchick R, et al: Histoplasmosis in the acquired immunodeficiency syndrome (AIDS): Treatment with itraconazole and fluconazole. J Acquir Immune Defic Syndr 6:809, 1993

66. Wheat J, MaWhinney S, Hafner R, et al: Treatment of histoplasmosis with fluconazole in patients with acquired immunodeficiency syndrome: National Institute of Allergy and Infectious Diseases Acquired Immunodeficiency Syndrome Clinical Trials Group and Mycoses Study Group. Am J Med 103:223, 1997

67. Ampel NM, Dols CS, Galgiani JN: Coccidioidomycosis during human immunodeficiency virus infection: Results of a prospective study in a coccidioidal endemic area. Am J Med 94:235, 1993

68. Fish DG, Ampel NM, Galgiani JN, et al: Coccidioidomycosis during human immunodeficiency virus infection: A review of 77 patients. Medicine (Balt) 69:384, 1990

69. Galgiani JN, Ampel NM: Coccidioidomycosis in human immunodeficiency virus-infected patients. J Infect Dis 162:1165, 1990

70. Sharkey PK, Lipke R, Renteria A, et al: Amphotericin B lipid complex (ABLC) in treatment (Rx) of coccidioidomycosis (C). In: Abstracts of the 31st Interscience Conference on Antimicrobial Agents and Chemotherapy, Chicago. Washington, DC, American Society for Microbiology, 1991, Abstract 742

71. Hotstetler JS, Caldwell JW, Johnson RH, et al: Coccidioidal infections treated with amphotericin B colloid dispersion (Amphocil or ABCD). In: Abstracts of the 32nd Interscience Conference on Antimicrobial Agents and Chemotherapy, Anaheim, CA. Washington, DC, American Society for Microbiology, 1992, Abstract 628

72. Albert MM, Adams K, Luther MJ, et al: Efficacy of AmBisome in murine coccidioidomycosis. J Med Vet Mycol 32:467, 1994

73. Catanzaro A, Fierer J, Friedman PJ: Fluconazole in the treatment of persistent coccidioidomycosis. Chest 97:666, 1990

74. Graybill JR, Stevens DA, Galgiani JN, et al: Itraconazole treatment of coccidioidomycosis. Am J Med 89:282, 1990

75. Zar FA, Fernandez M: Failure of ketoconazole maintenance therapy for disseminated coccidioidomycosis in AIDS [Letter]. J Infect Dis 164:824, 1991

76. Perfect JR: Antifungal prophylaxis: To prevent or not? Am J Med 94:233, 1993

77. Nightingale SD, Cal SX, Peterson DM, et al: Primary prophylaxis with fluconazole against systemic fungal infections in HIV-positive patients. AIDS 6:191, 1991

78. Dupont B, Improvisi L, Eliaszewicz M, et al: Resistance of *Candida albicans* to fluconazole in AIDS patients. Program of the 32nd Interscience Conference on Antimicrobial Agents and Chemotherapy, Anaheim, CA, 1992, p 340, Abstract 1203

79. Troillet N, Durussel C, Billie J, et al: Fluconazole-resistant oral candidiasis in human immunodeficiency virus-infected patients: In vitro—in vivo correlation. Program of the 32nd Interscience Conference on Antimicrobial Agents and Chemotherapy, Anaheim, CA, 1992, Abstract 1202

80. Wingard JR, Merz WG, Rinaldi MG, et al: Increase in *Candida krusei* infection among patients with bone marrow transplantation and neutropenia treated prophylactically with fluconazole. N Engl J Med 325:1274, 1991

81. Powderly WG, Finkelstein D, Feinberg J, et al: A randomized trial comparing fluconazole with clotrimazole troches for the prevention of fungal infections in patients with advanced human immunodeficiency virus infection: NIAID AIDS Clinical Trial Group. N Engl J Med 332:700, 1995

25 AIDS-Associated Toxoplasmosis

CARLOS S. SUBAUSTE • JACK S. REMINGTON

Toxoplasma gondii is among the most prevalent causes of latent infection of the central nervous system (CNS) throughout the world. After an acute infection, cysts of *T. gondii* persist in the CNS and in multiple extraneural tissues. Although normal human hosts maintain infection in a quiescent state, immunocompromised individuals may be at risk for reactivation and dissemination of chronic (latent) infection.[1] Defective cellular immunity in patients with AIDS results in loss of the primary arm of host defense against this parasite. Reactivation of latent infection in patients with AIDS may lead to clinically apparent disease (toxoplasmosis), which most frequently manifests as life-threatening encephalitis. Thus patients with AIDS who have been infected previously with *T. gondii* are at considerable risk for development of CNS toxoplasmosis.

Because AIDS patients in the United States who develop toxoplasmic encephalitis are almost always chronically infected with the protozoan,[2] patients with AIDS (or even individuals without AIDS who have antibody to HIV and who are known also to have antibodies to *T. gondii*) should be considered at significant risk for development of toxoplasmic encephalitis from the outset. Published data have demonstrated that 20% to 47% of AIDS patients who are seropositive for *T. gondii* will ultimately develop toxoplasmic encephalitis.[3-7] Seroprevalence varies between geographic locales and even within subpopulations of the same locale.[8-13] Studies performed in our laboratory have found a prevalence of *T. gondii* antibodies among HIV-positive adults of 8% to 16% in major urban areas of the United States. The prevalence is higher (≥25%) among certain ethnic groups.

CLINICAL PRESENTATION

In the United States, AIDS patients who develop toxoplasmic encephalitis generally do so after the diagnosis of AIDS has been made.[14-17] In areas where seroprevalence of *T. gondii* infection is high, toxoplasmic encephalitis frequently is the initial manifestation of AIDS.[7,18-22]

Ingestion of undercooked or raw meat containing tissue cysts and of vegetables or other food products contaminated with oocysts is a major means of transmission of the parasite, as is more direct contact with cat feces.[23] Independent of category of risk for acquisition of HIV infection, AIDS-associated toxoplasmosis in the United States occurs significantly more often in Hispanic than in white patients.[24] In addition, one study found the frequency of toxoplasmosis to be significantly higher in poor Mexican patients with AIDS than in counterparts with a higher socioeconomic status.[25]

Because multifocal involvement of the CNS is frequent, there may be a wide spectrum of clinical findings, including alteration of mental status, seizures, motor weakness, sensory abnormalities, cerebellar dysfunction, meningismus, movement disorders, and neuropsychiatric manifestations.[15,20,26-30] The characteristic presentation is usually one of subacute onset with focal neurologic abnormalities in 58% to 89% of patients. Altered mental status, manifested by confusion, lethargy, delusional behavior, frank psychosis, global cognitive impairment, anomia, or coma, may be present initially in as many as 60% of patients.[15,20,21,26,27] Seizures are the reason for seeking medical attention in approximately one third of AIDS patients with toxoplasmic encephalitis.[15,20,21,26-28] Focal neurologic deficits are evident on neurologic examination in approximately 60%.[15,20,21,26] Although hemiparesis is the most common focal neurologic finding, patients may have evidence of aphasia, ataxia, visual field loss, cranial nerve palsies, dysmetria, hemichorea-hemiballismus, tremor, parkinsonism, akathisia, or focal dystonia.[15,31–34] In addition, infection of the spinal cord with *T. gondii* has been described in cases of transverse myelitis and conus medullaris syndrome.[35,36] A rapidly fatal panencephalitis form of diffuse cerebral toxoplasmosis also has been described.[37] Unfortunately, computed tomography (CT) of the head was unrevealing in these cases.[9,37,38]

Extracerebral sites with or without concomitant toxoplasmic encephalitis may be involved in HIV-infected individuals.[39–42] Extracerebral toxoplasmosis usually occurs in patients with CD4 counts of less than 100/mm^3.[39,41] In patients with extracerebral toxoplasmosis, ocular and pulmonary sites are most commonly involved (50% and 26% of patients, respectively).[41] However, isolated parasitemia[41] and involvement of the heart,[41,43–47] bone marrow,[41,48] lymph nodes,[41] peritoneum,[49] stomach,[50] liver,[41,51] pancreas,[45] colon,[52] pituitary and adrenal glands,[53,54] bladder,[41] testes,[55,56] skeletal muscle,[57] skin,[41,58] rhinopharynx,[41] and spinal cord[35,36,41] have also been reported.

Pulmonary disease caused by toxoplasmosis has been increasingly reported and recognized.[40,59,60] The most common clinical syndrome is a prolonged febrile illness with cough and dyspnea that is clinically indistinguishable from *Pneumocystis carinii* pneumonia. Associated extrapulmonary disease caused by *T. gondii* has been reported in approximately 50% of the patients at the time of clinical presentation. Toxoplasmic encephalitis may precede or follow pulmonary toxoplasmosis if maintenance therapy is not instituted. A highly lethal syndrome of disseminated toxoplasmosis has been described in AIDS patients that consists of fever and a sepsis-like syndrome with hypotension, disseminated intravascular coagulation, elevated lactate dehydrogenase, and pulmonary infiltrates.[39–41] This syndrome is usually not associated with clinical or radiologic evidence of toxoplasmic encephalitis.[39,40]

Ocular disease caused by toxoplasmosis occurs relatively infrequently in AIDS patients (when compared with the incidence of cytomegalovirus retinitis).[61–64] Ocular pain and loss of visual acuity are common complaints, and funduscopic examination typically reveals findings consistent with necrotizing retinochoroiditis. The lesions are yellow-white areas of retinitis with fluffy borders. In reported series, the lesions were multifocal in 17% to 50%,[61,64] bilateral in 18% to 40%,[61,62,64] and accompanied by optic neuritis in approximately 10%. Vitreal inflammation may vary from mild localized vitreal haze to extensive vitreous inflammation.[61,62] Vasculitis and hemorrhage are uncommon. In most patients, the ocular lesions are located away from areas of pre-existing scars. This suggests that the pathogenesis of these lesions may be secondary to hematogenous seeding rather than local reactivation of infection. The presence of concurrent toxoplasmic encephalitis in AIDS patients with ocular toxoplasmosis has varied from 29% to 63%.[61,62,64] On occasion, ocular toxoplasmosis may precede toxoplasmic encephalitis.[63–66]

In contrast to the immunocompetent host with toxoplasmic retinochoroiditis, in whom gross and histopathologic examination usually will reveal marked inflammation, in patients with AIDS-associated toxoplasmic retinochoroiditis there frequently is only scant retinal inflammation.[64] Thus the features of toxoplasmic retinochoroiditis commonly observed in the immunocompetent host may be absent in patients with AIDS. Toxoplasmic optic neuritis also has been described.[62]

Endocrinopathies secondary to the syndrome of inappropriate antidiuretic hormone secretion or panhypopituitarism may be the primary manifestation or a later complication of CNS toxoplasmosis.[53,54,67]

Abnormalities in routine clinical laboratory tests are too nonspecific to be of diagnostic use. Most AIDS patients with toxoplasmic encephalitis (80% to 95%) have CD4 T-lymphocyte counts of less than 100/mm^3.[6,68–71] Furthermore, the risk of developing toxoplasmic encephalitis appears to be associated with CD4 T-lymphocyte counts.[71,72] The incidence of toxoplasmic encephalitis at 18 months was 12% for patients who had CD4 T-lymphocyte counts above 100/mm^3 at baseline.[72] This increased to 25% and 45% for patients with CD4 T-lymphocyte counts of 50 to 99/mm^3 and less than 50/mm^3, respectively.[72] Approximately 90% of patients who developed this disease had CD4 T-lymphocyte counts of less than 100/mm^3 within 4 months prior to the diagnosis.[72] A case of toxoplasmic encephalitis with laboratory abnormalities of the hypothalamic anterior pituitary–adrenal axis has been described.[54] Cerebrospinal fluid (CSF) may be normal or reveal mild pleocytosis (predominantly lymphocytes and monocytes) and an elevated protein level, whereas the glucose content usually is normal.[15,17,67,73]

CONGENITAL TOXOPLASMOSIS AND THE HIV-INFECTED WOMAN

Women infected with HIV are at risk for transmission of *T. gondii* infection to their fetuses if they are seronegative for *T. gondii* antibodies and acquire *T. gondii* infection during pregnancy or if they are seropositive for *T. gondii* antibodies and suffer reactivation of their latent *T. gondii* infection because of immune deficiency from HIV infection (see Chapter 35). At present, there are insufficient data to quantify the risk of congenital transmission by HIV-infected mothers who have chronic *T. gondii* infection. Preliminary data from Mitchell et al. revealed a congenital transmission rate for women who are dually infected with HIV and *T. gondii* that was more than 400-fold higher when compared to non-HIV-infected, *T. gondii*–seropositive pregnant women. Approximately 4% to 5% of infants born of dually infected mothers had congenital toxoplasmosis.[74,75] However, one of three dually infected mothers with CD4 T-lymphocyte counts less than 100/mm³ transmitted *T. gondii* infection to their babies.[74] When dually infected women developed toxoplasmosis during pregnancy, 75% of their infants were born with congenital toxoplasmosis and HIV infection.[75] All infants with congenital toxoplasmosis born to mothers who were HIV infected also were infected with HIV. The initial clinical presentation of congenital toxoplasmosis in the HIV-infected infant is similar to that in the non-HIV-infected infant but appears to run a more rapid and progressive course. The infants often appear normal at birth. In the ensuing months, they fail to gain weight or develop appropriately. The majority develop multisystem organ involvement, including the CNS, heart, and lungs.[76]

DIAGNOSIS

At present, the definitive diagnosis of toxoplasmosis in AIDS patients can be made only by demonstration of the organism in tissues (Table 25–1). Although the morbidity associated with obtaining a brain biopsy for the diagnosis of toxoplasmic encephalitis is less than that which would accrue from an erroneous diagnosis,[77] neurosurgery is often deferred because many AIDS patients with neurologic syndromes frequently have inaccessible intracerebral lesions. The desire to avoid brain biopsy has resulted in

TABLE 25–1. Methods for Definitive or Presumptive Diagnosis of Toxoplasmosis in Patients with AIDS

- Histologic evaluation, including immunoperoxidase staining of tissue biopsies
- Demonstration of *T. gondii* in body fluids (CSF, BAL) (Wright-Giemsa stain)
- Isolation of *T. gondii* from tissue biopsies or body fluids (CSF, blood, BAL)
- Detection of *T. gondii* DNA by PCR in body fluids (CSF, blood, BAL) or tissue biopsies
- CT scans and/or MR images of the head
- Serology (including titer in agglutination assay, IgG, IgM*)
- Intrathecal production of *T. gondii*–specific antibodies

Abbreviations: BAL, bronchoalveolar lavage; CSF, cerebrospinal fluid; CT, computed tomography, Ig, immunoglobulin; MR, magnetic resonance; PCR, polymerase chain reaction.
*Useful mainly in areas of high seroprevalence.

the almost universal practice of initiating empiric anti–*T. gondii* therapy in AIDS patients who have characteristic findings on neuroradiologic imaging studies. In this setting, alternative causes should be sought when the patient fails to respond clinically or radiographically. Brain biopsy frequently is the only alternative in this situation.

Serology

Because toxoplasmic encephalitis in patients with AIDS in the United States almost always represents reactivation of chronic (latent) infection, the presence of immunoglobulin (Ig)G *T. gondii* antibodies in an AIDS patient must be regarded as a marker for the potential development of toxoplasmosis. If the serologic status of an AIDS patient with suspected toxoplasmic encephalitis is unknown, IgG antibody status should be determined.

Although almost all AIDS patients with toxoplasmic encephalitis have detectable IgG *T. gondii* antibodies in their serum, published series have reported a 0% to 3% seronegativity rate.[21,78,79] Although the prevalence of *T. gondii* infection has not been shown to be higher in HIV-infected individuals than in uninfected individuals,[5] recent data demonstrate that, among *T. gondii*–infected individuals, those with HIV infection have significantly higher titers of *T. gondii* antibodies than do individuals without HIV infection.[78] In some studies, significantly more elevated antibody titers have been observed in AIDS patients with toxoplasmosis compared to those with latent *T. gondii* infection.[4,21,78,80] Although a single determination of IgG antibody titer cannot be used to distinguish latent from active infection, we observed that the magnitude of antibody titer to formalin-fixed *T. gondii* antigen had a high predictive value for the diagnosis of toxoplasmic encephalitis.[79]

When CSF is available, measurement of intrathecal production of antibody to *T. gondii* may serve as a useful ancillary test.[81,82] Whereas a similar investigation demonstrated that determination of antibody load was of little use for the diagnosis of ocular toxoplasmosis in AIDS,[83] a recent study reported that three of five patients with toxoplasmic retinochoroiditis had evidence of intraocular antibody production.[84]

IgM *T. gondii* antibodies, routinely measured to diagnose acute toxoplasmosis in non-AIDS patients, are rarely demonstrable in AIDS patients with toxoplasmic encephalitis and, when present, suggest recently acquired infection.[4,78] The specificity of the IgM immunosorbent agglutination assay (ISAGA) in AIDS patients is unclear.[85,86] IgA *T. gondii* antibodies are rarely elevated in AIDS patients with acute toxoplasmic encephalitis.[87] *Toxoplasma gondii* IgE antibodies measured by enzyme-linked immunosorbent assay and ISAGA have been detected in serum in a limited number of patients with toxoplasmic encephalitis.[88,89]

Isolation Studies

Isolation of *T. gondii* from body fluids or, in the appropriate clinical setting, from tissue obtained from a patient with AIDS should be considered diagnostic of active infection. Because isolation of the organism may not be evident for 6 days to 6 weeks after mice or tissue cultures are inoculated, the results often are not helpful in initial management of the patient. Nevertheless, isolation of the organism may obviate future need for brain biopsy.

Toxoplasma gondii readily forms plaques in tissue cultures of human foreskin fibroblasts and most other cultured cells.[90,91] The plaques, when stained with Wright-Giemsa and examined microscopically, are seen to consist of necrotic and heavily infected cells and numerous extracellular tachyzoites. *Toxoplasma gondii* has been isolated from the blood in 14% to 38% of AIDS patients with toxoplasmosis.[26,92,93] Parasitemia appears to occur more frequently when toxoplasmosis involves extraneural sites.[92] *Toxoplasma gondii* also may be isolated from bronchoalveolar lavage (BAL) fluid in patients with toxoplasmic pneumonitis as early as 48 hours after tissue culture inoculation.[94]

Any diagnostic microbiology or virology laboratory that can inoculate the buffy coat of blood or bronchoalveolar fluid into tissue culture has the capacity to isolate *T. gondii* from patients with active infection.[94,95]

DNA Detection

The use of the polymerase chain reaction (PCR) has enabled detection of *T. gondii* DNA in brain tissue,[51,96–98] CSF (approximately 50% to 70%),[99–102] BAL fluid,[85,103,104] blood (from 16% to 69%),[99,105–107] and aqueous humor[83,98] of AIDS patients with toxoplasmosis. Because *T. gondii* cysts persist in the brain for years after infection, a positive PCR in the brain does not necessarily reflect active infection. Although detection of *T. gondii* DNA by PCR can be useful for the diagnosis of toxoplasmosis, studies indicate that positive PCR can occur in blood samples from patients unlikely to have toxoplasmic encephalitis.[108]

Neuroradiologic Studies

Toxoplasmic encephalitis is the most common cause of focal intracerebral lesions in patients with AIDS.[109–111] Imaging studies of the brain have become indispensable for diagnosis and management of these patients.[112] Typically, multiple, bilateral, hypodense, enhancing mass lesions are found on CT scan.[15,67,113,114] Lesions have a predilection for, but are not limited to, the basal ganglia and hemispheric corticomedullary junction.[67,113–115] A significant degree of enhancement of intracerebral lesions generally is present on CT scan.[15,20,67,110,113–116] *Toxoplasma gondii* abscesses may, however, fail to enhance or be solitary and located anywhere in the brain.[117–120]

Masses demonstrated by magnetic resonance (MR) images may be absent on CT scan,[120,121] whereas the converse apparently is not true. In a review of AIDS patients with focal neurologic symptoms, a CT scan was as good as an MR image in detecting focal brain lesions (70% vs. 74%). However, in AIDS patients with nonfocal neurologic symptoms, only 22% had CT scans that revealed focal lesions, compared to 42% found by MR imaging. As in CT scans, lesions found on MR images of AIDS patients with toxoplasmic encephalitis frequently are bilateral and located in the basal ganglia or cerebral corticomedullary junction.[120,122] Deep lesions, which generally range from 1 to 3 cm in diameter, may show central patterns of both low and high signal intensity, suggestive of necrosis.[119] Unlike CT scans, MR images usually reveal multiple lesions.[117,118,120,122] In fact, a single lesion seen on an MR image should alert the clinician to other possible causes of the focal neuroradiologic findings (e.g., lymphoma, fungal abscesses, tuberculoma, or Kaposi's sarcoma) (see Chapters 23 and 30).[117] When a single lesion is present on an MR image, the probability of CNS lymphoma is at least equal to or higher than the probability of toxoplasmic encephalitis.[117]

As with results of CT scans, MR findings cannot be considered pathognomonic for toxoplasmic encephalitis. Although primary CNS lymphoma cannot be distinguished from toxoplasmosis solely on the basis of neuroradiologic criteria, the most reliable feature distinguishing lymphoma from toxoplasmosis in AIDS patients was the presence of hyperattenuation on nonenhanced CT scans and subependymal location on either CT scans or MR images.[123] The neuroradiologic response of toxoplasmic encephalitis to specific treatment is seen on CT as a reduction in mass effect, number and extent of lesions, and enhancement.[119] Although the time to resolution of lesions may vary from 20 days to 6 months, the vast majority of patients who respond clinically will show radiologic improvement (>50%) by the third week of treatment.[124] The response of abnormalities as seen on MR image to specific therapy also varies with the location and complexity of the mass lesion. Peripheral lesions of uniform signal intensity on MR image frequently resolve after 3 to 5 weeks of therapy, whereas deeper lesions with complex central signal patterns, consistent with necrosis, take longer to resolve and leave residual lesion(s) at the site of necrosis.[119] Persistent enhancement on CT scans or MR images after treatment for toxoplasmic encephalitis has been associated with a higher incidence of subsequent relapse of the encephalitis.[125] Positron emission tomography is reportedly useful in the diagnosis of toxoplasmic encephalitis.[126] Whereas areas of decreased glucose metabolism were seen in brains of all patients with toxoplasmic encephalitis, areas with increased glucose metabolism were observed in all patients with CNS lymphoma.[126] Thallium-201 single-photon emission computer tomography is another radiologic study highly sensitive and specific for the diagnosis of tumors, and thus is helpful in differentiating CNS lymphoma from toxoplasmic encephalitis.[127]

Histopathology

Definitive diagnosis of toxoplasmic encephalitis often requires demonstration of the organism on histopathologic sections of brain tissue obtained at biopsy. Needle brain biopsy or aspiration is limited by lack of sensitivity of the procedure to make a definitive diagnosis, because the size of the specimen may be too small or there may be sampling error.[66] Some evidence suggests the superiority of open excisional biopsy compared to needle biopsy in making the histopathologic diagnosis of toxoplasmic encephalitis.[73] Moreover, the observation of abnormal lymphocytes in areas of involvement demonstrated by needle biopsy or aspiration has led to the erroneous diagnosis of cerebral lymphoma.

The response of the brain to *T. gondii* infection can vary from a granulomatous reaction with gliosis and microglial nodule formation to a severe focal or generalized necrotizing encephalitis.[15,67,111,114,128] Granulomatous lesions with a cellular infiltrate of abnormal lymphocytes, plasma cells, neutrophils, and monocytes may enlarge and develop central regions of necrosis.[15,67,114,128] Perivascular and intimal inflammatory cell infiltrates can lead to fibrosis or necrosis, which can result in hemorrhage[129] or thrombosis, accounting for neurologic signs and symptoms. It has been suggested that the invasion and multiplication of *T. gondii* in the cerebral vascular walls causes focal fibrotic hyperplasia, which leads to an obliterative vasculitis and discrete coagulative necrosis in the CNS.[130,131]

The presence of numerous *T. gondii* tachyzoites or cysts surrounded by an inflammatory reaction is diagnostic.[12] Tachyzoites, when observed, are usually found within the inflammatory reaction surrounding areas of necrosis. Cysts or free organisms not demonstrable on routine histopathologic examination can be identified using the peroxidase-antiperoxidase method.[73,132] This method is significantly more sensitive and no less specific in making the diagnosis of toxoplasmic encephalitis than is direct visualization of the organisms in association with cerebral inflammation and necrosis.[20,132] A rapid, sensitive, and specific method for diagnosis of toxoplasmic encephalitis by electron microscopy has been described.[133] Thus, when routine histopathologic studies fail to provide a definitive diagnosis, appropriately fixed brain tissue should be stained by the immunoperoxidase technique or analyzed by electron microscopy in an attempt to identify *T. gondii* antigens or organisms.

Wright-Giemsa–stained smears or touch preparations should be made as immediately as is feasible from tissue obtained at surgery. If organisms are demonstrated, potentially lifesaving therapy can be initiated promptly. Similarly, Wright-Giemsa stain of a cytocentrifuge preparation of CSF may reveal the presence of tachyzoites.[134] Tachyzoites may be visualized in Giemsa-stained smears of BAL fluid in AIDS patients with pulmonary toxoplasmosis.[135]

Differential Diagnosis

In AIDS patients with focal abnormalities on neurologic examination, multiple enhancing lesions on CT scan and a positive *T. gondii* antibody titer strongly suggest the diagnosis of toxoplasmic encephalitis. Regardless of results of *T. gondii* serology, the differential diagnosis for individuals with nonfocal symptoms and one or two lesions on CT scan includes, in addition to CNS toxoplasmosis, lymphoma, fungal abscess, mycobacterial or cytomegaloviral disease, and Kaposi's sarcoma. Because therapy is available for each of these disorders, brain biopsy for histopathologic diagnosis may be necessary for successful management of the patient. The characteristic appearance of progressive multifocal leukoencephalopathy on neuroimaging studies often permits differentiation of this disorder from other causes of intracerebral mass lesions.

MANAGEMENT

General Principles

Because toxoplasmic encephalitis generally reflects reactivation of a latent infection, all HIV-positive individuals should be tested for *T. gondii*–specific IgG antibody. Patients with positive titers are at risk for development of toxoplasmic encephalitis, and the results of the serologic tests should be clearly available in the chart in case a patient has signs suggestive of toxoplasmosis (Fig. 25–1).

An MR image should be obtained in patients with neurologic abnormalities and a negative CT scan on presentation. Patients with only one lesion on CT scan should undergo MR imaging to attempt to determine if more than a single lesion is present. In patients with nonfocal neurologic abnormalities, MR imaging is the preferred initial evaluation. Because a single lesion on MR imaging is uncharacteristic of *T. gondii* infection and more than 50% of such lesions are lymphomas,[117,118] early biopsy of the involved area should be considered. Expedient and aggressive evaluation of AIDS patients with CNS mass lesions allows earlier use of specific therapies and averts use of erroneous and potentially toxic treatment regimens.

AIDS patients with multiple focal lesions visible on neuroimaging studies should receive therapy for presumptive toxoplasmic encephalitis. Focal intracranial lesions caused by *T. gondii* may occur in association with cerebral lymphoma[136] or *Mycobacterium tuberculosis*.[110] In patients with concurrent focal and diffuse CNS disease, toxoplasmosis also has been found in association with cytomegalovirus encephalitis and cryptococcal meningitis.[110,137]

Diffuse toxoplasmic encephalitis is frequently goes underdiagnosed and should be suspected when a patient with severe CD4 cell depletion and positive *T. gondii* serology experiences unexplained fever and neurologic disease.[38] When diagnostic investigations fail to disclose a specific cause in these cases, a trial of empiric anti–*T. gondii* treatment should be considered.

In regard to what can be expected in relation to clinical and radiologic responses to therapy, a prospective study demonstrated that 71% of the patients had a complete or partial response.[124] The neurologic response was rapid, with 51% of patients showing signs of improvement by day 3 and 91% by day 14.[124] The 29% who were classified as treatment failures all either experienced progression of their baseline neurologic abnormalities or developed new ones within the first 12 days of empiric therapy. Thus brain biopsy with or without change of therapy should be considered in patients whose condition worsens early in the course of therapy or in patients who do not show clinical improvement by 10 to 14 days of therapy.[124] Repeat neuroradiologic study by the same modality as originally selected should be performed 2 to 4 weeks after initiation of therapy in patients who demonstrate a satisfactory clinical response (or earlier if response is poor). Lesions should have diminished in size and possibly in number. Patients with extraneurologic toxoplasmosis should be evaluated for CNS disease, because most will have intracerebral involvement as well.[45,138]

Corticosteroids frequently are required for management of patients with intracranial hyper-

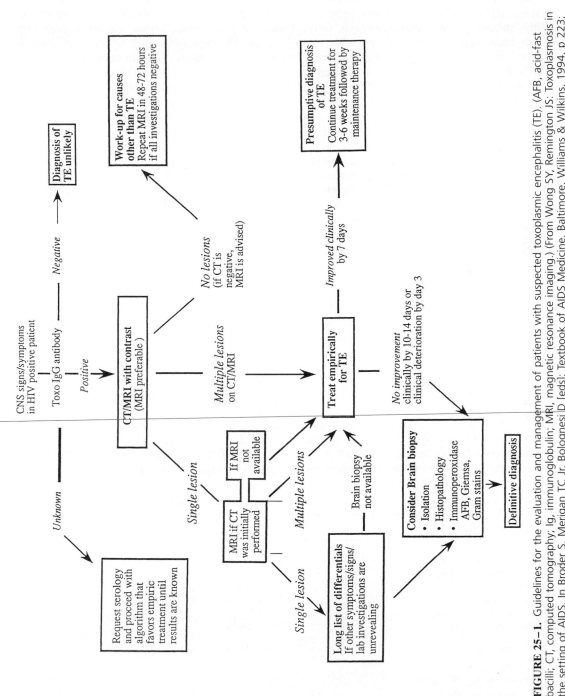

FIGURE 25–1. Guidelines for the evaluation and management of patients with suspected toxoplasmic encephalitis (TE). (AFB, acid-fast bacilli; CT, computed tomography; Ig, immunoglobulin; MRI, magnetic resonance imaging.) (From Wong SY, Remington JS: Toxoplasmosis in the setting of AIDS. In Broder S, Merigan TC Jr, Bolognesi D [eds]: Textbook of AIDS Medicine. Baltimore, Williams & Wilkins, 1994, p 223; reprinted with permission.)

tension caused by the mass effect from *T. gondii* abscesses. A recent study reported that there was no difference in the response rate and the time to response in patients who received corticosteroids when compared to those who did not.[124] At present, AIDS patients with toxoplasmic encephalitis should receive corticosteroids only when it is absolutely necessary. (If possible, no more than 2 weeks of therapy should be given.) Whether administration of anticonvulsant agents is necessary for prevention of seizures has not been determined.

It is important to distinguish between two forms of therapy for toxoplasmic encephalitis in patients with AIDS: primary therapy and maintenance therapy. Primary therapy is administered during the acute disease. Maintenance therapy is administered after an adequate clinical and neuroradiologic response has been observed. Maintenance therapy should be continued for life, because the rate of relapse is prohibitively high when treatment is discontinued.

There is remarkable variability in the susceptibility of different *T. gondii* strains to different antimicrobial agents,[139,140] and the potential for development of drug resistance may complicate the medical management of AIDS-associated toxoplasmosis.

Primary Therapy

Pyrimethamine, a potent dihydrofolate reductase inhibitor, is the cornerstone of current treatment of AIDS-associated toxoplasmic encephalitis. It is standard practice to administer the combination of pyrimethamine plus sulfadiazine or pyrimethamine plus clindamycin (Table 25–2). The half-life of pyrimethamine varies from 20 to 175 hours.[141] Serum concentrations of pyrimethamine in individuals treated with the same dose of drug have great variability.[141–143] This variability may in part reflect erratic absorption of pyrimethamine in patients with AIDS-associated enteropathies. Although serum concentrations cannot be predicted for a given dose[141,143] or even for a given patient on a given day, serum concentrations of pyrimethamine significantly increase with increasing dose.[143] A recent study noted several patients with AIDS-associated CNS toxoplasmosis who were treated daily with 25 or 50 mg of pyrimethamine and who had peak or trough serum concentrations lower than or barely exceeding the concentration of pyrimethamine required in vitro for toxoplasmacidal activity.[143–145] In contrast, all patients who were treated daily with 100 mg of pyrimethamine had peak and trough serum concentrations well above the minimum concentration required in vitro for toxoplasmacidal activity.[143] When CSF penetration of pyrimethamine was studied in small numbers of patients with AIDS[17] and meningeal leukemia,[146,147] the CSF concentration of drug was between 10% and 25% of the serum concentration. Data suggest that pyrimethamine may be concentrated in the brain.[148]

Prospective, randomized studies of treatment of toxoplasmic encephalitis showed that pyrimethamine plus clindamycin and pyrimethamine plus sulfadiazine were equally efficacious during the acute phase of therapy.[26,149,150] When choosing a regimen that includes clindamycin, a panel of experts recommend administration of

TABLE 25–2. Guidelines for Acute or Primary Treatment of AIDS Patients with Toxoplasmic Encephalitis

DRUG	DOSAGE
Recommended Regimens	
Pyrimethamine	PO: 200 mg loading followed by 50–75 mg q24h
Folinic acid	PO, IV, or IM: 10–20 mg q24h
plus	
sulfadiazine	PO: 1 gm q6h
or	
clindamycin	IV or PO: 600 mg q6h
Alternative Regimens	
Trimethoprim-sulfamethoxazole	PO or IV: 5 mg (trimethoprim component)/kg q6h
Pyrimethamine and folinic acid	As in recommended regimen
plus one of the following:	
Clarithromycin	PO: 1 gm q12h
Atovaquone	PO: 750 mg q6h
Azithromycin	PO: 1200–1500 mg q24h
Dapsone	PO: 100 mg q24h

600 mg of clindamycin orally (or intravenously) every 6 hours.

A few studies have revealed that trimethoprim-sulfamethoxazole (TMP-SMX) may be effective for acute therapy of toxoplasmic encephalitis,[151–153] achieving a 75% response rate.[151] However, TMP-SMX cannot, at present, be recommended as a first-line drug for acute therapy of toxoplasmic encephalitis because the activity of this combination against *T. gondii* is significantly inferior to that of the combination of pyrimethamine and sulfadiazine both in vitro and in animal models of toxoplasmosis.[154]

Standard therapy is limited by the high incidence of toxicity associated with both drugs in combination. The most notable toxicity of pyrimethamine is dose-related bone marrow suppression, resulting in thrombocytopenia, granulocytopenia, or megaloblastic anemia.[155–157] At doses of 75 to 100 mg/day, hematologic abnormalities should be anticipated but may be difficult to distinguish from those associated with HIV infection per se. Complete blood counts of patients receiving pyrimethamine should be monitored frequently for the development of drug-associated bone marrow toxicity.

Folinic acid (leucovorin calcium) may prevent marrow toxicity or be used to treat patients with marrow toxicity caused by pyrimethamine[12,155] and is not antagonistic to the activity of pyrimethamine or sulfadiazine against *T. gondii*.[158] The oral dose of folinic acid administered to these patients is usually 10 to 20 mg/day in divided doses[159] (Table 25–2). If hematologic abnormalities develop and malabsorption of the folinic acid is suspected, folinic acid may be administered parenterally. Some investigators increase folinic acid up to 50 mg/day for suspected pyrimethamine-associated hematologic toxicity.[20] Few data suggest that higher doses prevent progression of or reverse the hematologic toxicities. Folic acid must not be used, because it will inhibit the anti–*T. gondii* activity of pyrimethamine.[158] Although 65% to 90% of patients with toxoplasmic encephalitis will have an initial favorable response to pyrimethamine plus sulfadiazine therapy,[15,20,26] untoward reactions to this combination, most frequently rash,[26] may limit duration of therapy. When treating a patient who develops skin rash, it is important to keep in mind that not only sulfadiazine but also pyrimethamine can cause this side effect.[160] Studies reveal that as many as 40% of AIDS patients who receive sulfadiazine and pyrimethamine for toxoplasmic encephalitis manifest signs of toxicity sufficiently severe to

prompt discontinuation of the drug(s) during the primary phase of treatment.[20,27,161]

It is likely that sulfonamide is discontinued prematurely in many cases in which, if it were continued, the rash would lessen or disappear. A number of investigators have stated that the majority of patients with AIDS who experience sulfonamide-associated cutaneous reactions can be successfully desensitized to these agents.[162,163] Crystal-induced nephrotoxicity is another well-recognized adverse reaction to sulfadiazine.[164–166] The most frequent adverse reactions seen in patients treated with pyrimethamine-clindamycin—skin rash and gastrointestinal and hematologic toxicity[26,149]—are similar to those seen with pyrimethamine plus sulfadiazine.[26] The substantial toxicities associated with standard anti–*T. gondii* treatment underscore the urgent need to develop safe and effective alternative drug regimens.

In the search for such regimens, most studies have evaluated the safety and efficacy of a non-sulfonamide agent in combination with pyrimethamine.[149,167–169] Whether toxoplasmic encephalitis can be treated effectively solely with pyrimethamine deserves further investigation.

Almost all the studies on the use of antimicrobial agents that have been described for the treatment of toxoplasmosis in AIDS patients have focused on patients with toxoplasmic encephalitis. Limited data suggest that patients with extracerebral toxoplasmosis also respond to therapy with pyrimethamine-sulfadiazine or pyrimethamine-clindamycin but that the mortality rate in patients with pulmonary or disseminated toxoplasmosis may be much higher than in patients with toxoplasmic encephalitis alone.

Investigational Drugs

A number of other agents have been tried in vitro, in animal models, and in a few case reports[68,168,170–195] (Table 25–3) for the treatment of toxoplasmosis. It is beyond the scope of this chapter to review all of these articles, and interested readers are referred to a review on the topic.[23] Experience with the investigational agents, when they have been used as monotherapy in humans, has been that they are often associated with initial clinical improvement but subsequent relapse even when the agent is continued. *We urge that subsequent trials in humans include at least two agents in combination.*

Spiramycin, used for prevention of transplacental transmission of *T. gondii*, has been reported as ineffective for prevention, treatment,

TABLE 25–3. Newer Antimicrobial/ Investigational Agents and Cytokines Shown to Be Effective Alone or in Combination Against Toxoplasmosis

	REFERENCES
Sulfa Agents	
Dapsone (B, C)*	170, 171
Macrolides/Azalides	
Azithromycin (A, B, C)	172, 173
Clarithromycin (A, B, C)	168, 172, 174
Hydroxynaphthoquinones	
Atovaquone (A, B, C)	175, 176
Folic Acid Reductase Inhibitors	
Trimetrexate (A, C)	177, 178
Piritrexin (B)	68
Others	
Rifabutin (B)	179
Minocycline (B)	180
Doxycycline (B, C)	181, 182
Qinghaosu (A)	183
Arpinocid (B)	184
Pentamidine (A)	185
5-Fluorouracil (A, C)	186, 187
Cytokines	
Interferon-γ (A, B)	188
Interferon-β (B)	189
TNF (B)	190
Interleukin-1 (B)	190
Interleukin-2 (B)	191
Interleukin-7 (B)	192
Interleukin-12 (B)	193, 194
GM-CSF (B)	195

Abbreviations: GM-CSF, granulocyte-macrophage colony-stimulating factor; TNF, tumor necrosis factor.

*A, in vitro; B, in animal models; C, in humans.

or suppression of toxoplasmic encephalitis.[196] The new macrolide-azalide antibiotics azithromycin,[139,197] roxithromycin,[198] and clarithromycin[199] were effective either in vitro or in a murine model of toxoplasmosis. A relatively small, noncomparative clinical trial with clarithromycin plus pyrimethamine demonstrated clinical and radiologic response rates of 80% and 50%, respectively.[168] Similarly, a pilot study of pyrimethamine plus azithromycin reported an overall response rate of 65%.[200] Results of carefully controlled prospective clinical trials are needed before the new macrolide-azalide antibiotics can be recommended routinely for the treatment of acute toxoplasmic encephalitis.

Like pyrimethamine, trimetrexate inhibits *T. gondii* dihydrofolate reductase but more potently.[177] The high incidence of relapse of patients with biopsy-proven toxoplasmic encephalitis who were receiving trimetrexate suggests

that this drug, when used alone, has only transient activity against this disorder.[178]

Atovaquone, a hydroxynaphthoquinone, has remarkable activity against the tachyzoite and cyst (bradyzoite) forms of *T. gondii* both in vitro and in vivo.[140,201] In a small, noncomparative salvage study completed at the National Institutes of Health, atovaquone was found safe and effective.[176] In another study of 24 patients treated presumptively with atovaquone alone for their first episode of toxoplasmic encephalitis, evaluation at 3 weeks of therapy revealed a clinical response in 66%; 13% remained stable and 17% demonstrated clinical or radiologic progression.[175] In this latter study, patients who did not respond to atovaquone therapy responded to pyrimethamine-sulfadiazine. Similarly, a study of patients intolerant to pyrimethamine plus either sulfadiazine or clindamycin, or patients for whom such treatment failed, reported clinical and radiologic improvement in 52% and 37% of cases, respectively, at 6 weeks of atovaquone therapy.[202] Relapse occurred in approximately 50% of patients in whom atovaquone was used for acute therapy and was continued alone as maintenance therapy.[175,176] Whether the combination of pyrimethamine-atovaquone will prove more efficacious is presently being examined by the AIDS Clinical Trials Groups. Atovaquone has not been approved by the Food and Drug Administration for treatment of toxoplasmosis.

Other drugs, including dapsone[171] and doxycycline,[182] have been used to treat toxoplasmic encephalitis. Studies conducted in animal models of toxoplasmosis have demonstrated anti–*T. gondii* activity of rifabutin[179] and remarkable in vivo synergy when the following combinations were used: clarithromycin plus either pyrimethamine, sulfadiazine, or minocycline[174]; azithromycin plus sulfadiazine[172]; atovaquone plus either pyrimethamine or sulfadiazine[203]; and rifabutin plus either pyrimethamine, sulfadiazine, clindamycin, or atovaquone.[179,204] Appropriately designed studies are needed to determine if there is a role for these compounds and combinations in the treatment or prevention of toxoplasmosis in AIDS patients.

Because of the profound defect in cellular immunity in AIDS, there is the possibility that immunologic reconstitution through use of biologic response modifiers might, along with conventional antimicrobial therapy, be useful for treatment of toxoplasmosis in AIDS patients. Of particular interest is interferon (IFN)-γ, which is a known major mediator of host resistance to *T. gondii*.[188] In murine models of toxoplasmosis, significant enhancement of antimicrobial activity was observed when either roxithromycin, azithromycin, pyrimethamine, or clindamycin was combined with recombinant IFN-γ.[198,205,206] Other biologic response modifiers, such as IFN-β,[207] interleukin (IL)-2,[191] IL-7,[192] IL-12,[193,194] tumor necrosis factor-α,[190] and granulocyte-macrophage colony-stimulating factor[195] also had anti–*T. gondii* activity in experimental models but have not been used to treat AIDS-associated toxoplasmosis.

Maintenance Treatment (Secondary Prophylaxis)

Whereas the combination of pyrimethamine plus sulfadiazine is highly active against the proliferative form, neither it nor any of the currently used drugs is effective in eradicating the cyst form of *T. gondii*. It is believed that persistence of the cyst form accounts for relapse of toxoplasmic encephalitis after therapy is discontinued. The relapse rate of toxoplasmic encephalitis in patients who do not receive maintenance therapy is 50% to 80% at 12 months.[21,27] The CT scans or MR images of patients who relapse often demonstrate mass lesions in the same location as at initial presentation.[208] Thus it is essential that AIDS patients who complete a primary course of therapy and who have had a favorable clinical and radiologic response to therapy for toxoplasmic encephalitis receive lifelong anti–*T. gondii* agents.

After successful primary therapy, drug dosages are generally decreased for lifelong maintenance therapy (Table 25–4). There is no single regimen that both is effective and has an acceptable safety profile. Although toxoplasmic encephalitis can recur during maintenance therapy,[21,209] it is important to be aware that some of these failures are due to noncompliance.[208]

The regimen of pyrimethamine plus sulfadiazine appears to have a lower rate of relapse than other regimens and is recommended.[30,209–211] In a prospective, randomized study, patients who received maintenance therapy with pyrimethamine-sulfadiazine (25 mg/day–500 mg four times per day) daily had a lower rate of relapse of toxoplasmic encephalitis (6% at 12 months) than patients receiving pyrimethamine-sulfadiazine twice weekly (30% at 12 months).[211] Patients on maintenance therapy with pyrimethamine-sulfadiazine most likely do not require further prophylaxis for *P. carinii*.[211,212] Although most investigators favor the daily use of pyrimethamine-sulfadiazine, many patients are unable to continue this regimen because of drug toxicity, and alternative regimens will have to be considered (Table 25–4).[209,213,214]

A prospective, randomized study showed no significant differences in clinical outcome of patients who received pyrimethamine plus clindamycin versus pyrimethamine plus sulfadiazine.[26,149] However, another prospective, randomized study reported that, during maintenance therapy, the rate of relapse was double in patients treated with pyrimethamine plus clindamycin (22% vs. 11%).[150] Whether the high

---

TABLE 25–4. Guidelines for Maintenance Treatment of AIDS Patients with Toxoplasmic Encephalitis

	ORAL DOSE	FREQUENCY
Recommended Regimens		
Pyrimethamine* *and*	25–50 mg	q24h
sulfadiazine	0.5–1.0 gm	qid
Pyrimethamine *and*	25–50 mg	q24h
clindamycin	600 mg	q6h
Pyrimethamine/sulfadoxine (Fansidar)	25 mg–500 mg (1 tablet)	tiw
Alternative Regimens		
Pyrimethamine alone	50 mg	q24h
Pyrimethamine	25–50 mg	q24h
plus one of the following:		
Dapsone	100 mg	biw
Atovaquone	750 mg	q6h
Clarithromycin	1000 mg	q12h
Azithromycin	1200–1500 mg	q24h

*Folinic acid (leucovorin calcium) 10–20 mg q24h is recommended for all patients receiving pyrimethamine to help ameliorate the hematologic side effects associated with pyrimethamine. The dose of folinic acid is titrated against the patient's hematologic indices, and up to 50 mg of folinic acid has been used.

relapse rate was due to the low dose of clindamycin (1.2 gm/day) used remains to be determined. In addition, it is important to be aware that pyrimethamine-clindamycin does not prevent *P. carinii* pneumonia.[209,215]

Pyrimethamine-sulfadoxine (Fansidar) administered as one tablet twice weekly has been reported to be effective as maintenance therapy. Side effects were relatively common (40%), with 7% of patients discontinuing therapy because of adverse effects.[216] An uncontrolled, open-label study suggested that atovaquone may be an alternative for secondary prophylaxis in patients who had recovered from toxoplasmic encephalitis and developed intolerance to conventional regimens.[217] In this study, the rate of relapse of toxoplasmic encephalitis was 26% at 1 year. Whether continued maintenance treatment will be necessary in those patients on protease inhibitors whose CD4 T-lymphocyte counts have increased to more than 200/mm³ is being studied.

PREVENTION (PRIMARY PROPHYLAXIS)

Serologic testing for *T. gondii* antibodies will distinguish those HIV-infected individuals who are at risk for reactivation of infection from those at risk for acquisition of infection. All patients who are seronegative for *T. gondii* antibodies and who have evidence of deficient cellular immunity, especially those seronegative for *T. gondii* antibodies, should be educated about appropriate precautions to take to prevent acquisition of *T. gondii* infection (Table 25–5). Seroconversion to *T. gondii* positivity in HIV-infected individuals has been reported to occur in 2% after a mean follow-up of 2 years.[218]

Despite the availability of effective antimicrobial regimens, toxoplasmosis in AIDS patients is associated with a mortality rate of 70% by 12 months after the diagnosis of toxoplasmic encephalitis.[71] Thus the morbidity and mortality associated with toxoplasmosis in AIDS patients strongly support the use of prophylaxis in HIV-infected patients with CD4 T-lymphocyte counts of less than 200/mm³.[219] Given that absolute CD4 T-lymphocyte counts and symptomatic HIV infection (Centers for Disease Control and Prevention stage IV) appear to be independent risk factors for development of toxoplasmic encephalitis, primary prophylaxis is considered appropriate in patients with CD4 T-lymphocyte counts less than 100/mm³ regardless of clinical

TABLE 25–5. Methods for Preventing Toxoplasmosis in Patients with HIV Infection

Individuals Should Take the Following Precautions:
- Cook meat to ~116°C (well done, not pink); smoke it or cure it in brine.
- Avoid touching mucous membranes of mouth and eyes while handling raw meat.
- Wash hands thoroughly after handling raw meat.
- Wash kitchen surfaces that come into contact with raw meat.
- Wash fruits and vegetables before consumption.
- Prevent access of flies, cockroaches, and the like to fruits and vegetables.
- Avoid contact with materials that are potentially contaminated with cat feces (e.g., cat litter boxes) or wear gloves when handling such materials or when gardening.
- Disinfect cat litter box for 5 minutes with nearly boiling water.

status and in patients with CD4 T-lymphocyte counts less than 200/mm³ if they develop AIDS-defining opportunistic infections or malignancies.[72] Numerous studies have reported the efficacy of TMP-SMX,[220–225] pyrimethamine-dapsone,[18,223,226] or pyrimethamine-sulfadoxine,[227] in the prevention of toxoplasmic encephalitis in AIDS patients (Table 25–6). A prospective, randomized study that compared TMP-SMX (160 mg–800 mg orally twice daily on a thrice-weekly regimen) with pyrimethamine-dapsone (50 mg–100 mg orally twice weekly) indicated that both regimens are effective as prophylaxis for toxoplasmosis.[223] However, the TMP-SMX regimen appeared to be more effective for prophylaxis of *P. carinii* pneumonia.[223] It must be emphasized that, among patients receiving primary prophylaxis with TMP-SMX,[224] pyrimethamine-dapsone,[228] or pyrimethamine-sulfadoxine, 40% to 60% will have untoward side effects, and 2% to 12% of the total number of patients will require discontinuation of therapy.

Pyrimethamine alone is currently not considered a first-line regimen for primary prophylaxis against toxoplasmic encephalitis in patients who can tolerate TMP-SMX.[72] Contrary to a previous study that reported a higher death rate among patients receiving pyrimethamine for primary prophylaxis,[229] Leport et al. did not find such an association.[72] Whether the concomitant administration of folinic acid in the study by Leport et al. explains the lack of increased mortality remains to be determined.[72] A trial on the use of clindamycin alone for primary prophylaxis was discontinued because of a high incidence of gastrointestinal side effects.[229] Administration of

TABLE 25–6. Regimens Used for Primary Prophylaxis Against Toxoplasmosis

DRUG	DOSAGE SCHEDULE
TMP-SMX	PO: 1 DS* tab qd
	PO: 2 DS tab biw
	PO: 2 DS tab tiw
Pyrimethamine-dapsone[†]	PO: pyrimethamine 50 mg once a week; dapsone 50 mg qd
	PO: pyrimethamine 50 mg biw; dapsone 100 mg biw
	PO: pyrimethamine 75 mg once a week; dapsone 200 mg once a week
	PO: pyrimethamine 25 mg once a week; dapsone 100 mg once a week
Pyrimethamine-sulfadoxine (Fansidar)[†,‡]	PO: 3 tab every 2 weeks
	PO: 1 tb biw

*DS, double strength.
[†]Folinic acid (Leucovorin) 25 mg qw is recommended for all patients receiving pyrimethamine to help ameliorate the hematologic side effects associated with pyrimethamine. The dose of folinic acid is titrated against the patient's hematologic indices.
[‡]Each tablet contains pyrimethamine 25 mg, sulfadoxine 500 mg.

clarithromycin to AIDS patients as part of regimens for disseminated *Mycobacterium avium* complex infections has not decreased the incidence of toxoplasmic encephalitis,[230] suggesting that clarithromycin may be ineffective for primary prophylaxis for toxoplasmic encephalitis. This failure of clarithromycin may be due to changes in its absorption and/or metabolism caused by co-administration of other drugs (didanosine, rifampin, ethambutol, ciprofloxacin).[230] Spiramycin alone has not been found to be useful in the primary prophylaxis of toxoplasmic encephalitis.

Because even without primary prophylaxis not all HIV-infected individuals who are seropositive for *T. gondii* antibodies develop toxoplasmic encephalitis, it would appear that other factors besides prior infection with *T. gondii* and decreased CD4 T-lymphocyte counts may be involved in determining the risk for this disease. In this regard, an association between the development of toxoplasmic encephalitis and human leukocyte antigen (HLA) molecules has been reported.[231] Compared to controls, HLA-DQ3 was significantly more frequent in white North American AIDS patients with toxoplasmic encephalitis, whereas HLA-DQ1 appeared to be less frequent.[231] Further studies may help to identify populations at greatest risk for toxoplasmic encephalitis and thereby allow for more targeted prophylactic measures.

Although there are no data available on the use of prophylaxis against congenital toxoplasmosis in HIV-infected women who are seropositive for *T. gondii* antibodies, we recommend that these women receive spiramycin 1 gm tid throughout pregnancy if their CD4 lymphocyte counts are less than 100/mm[3]. Whether to use TMP-SMX or pyrimethamine-sulfadiazine after the 17th week of pregnancy should be considered for those who are more severely immunosuppressed.

Acknowledgments

The work discussed in this chapter was supported in part from grants AI04717, AI30230, and AI37936 from the National Institutes of Health, Bethesda, Maryland.

References

1. Frenkel JK, Nelson BM, Arias-Stella J: Immunosuppression and toxoplasmic encephalitis. Hum Pathol 6: 97, 1975
2. Luft BJ, Brooks RG, Conley FK, et al: Toxoplasmic encephalitis in patients with AIDS. JAMA 252:913, 1984
3. Aspöck H, Hassl A: Parasitic infections in HIV patients in Austria: First results of a long-term study. Zentralbl Bakteriol 272:540, 1990
4. Grant IH, Gold JMW, Rosenblum M, et al: *Toxoplasma gondii* serology in HIV-infected patients: The development of central nervous system toxoplasmosis in AIDS. AIDS 4:519, 1990
5. Israelski DM, Chmiel JS, Poggensee L, et al: Prevalence of *Toxoplasma* infection in a cohort of homosexual men at risk of AIDS and toxoplasmic encephalitis. J Acquir Immune Defic Syndr 6:414, 1993
6. Matheron S, Dournon E, Garakhanian S, et al: Prevalence of toxoplasmosis in 365 AIDS and ARC patients before and during zidovudine treatment. In Abstracts of the VIth International Conference on AIDS, San Francisco, 1990, Abstract Th.B.476
7. Zangerle R, Allerberger F, Pohl P, et al: High risk of developing toxoplasmic encephalitis in AIDS patients seropositive to *Toxoplasma gondii*. Med Microbiol Immunol 180:59, 1991
8. Frappier-Davignon L, Walker M, Adrien A, et al: Anti-HIV antibodies and other serological and immunological parameters among normal Haitians in Montreal. J Acquir Immune Defic Syndr 3:166, 1990

9. Greenberg AE, Thomas PA, Landesman SH, et al: The spectrum of HIV-related disease among outpatients in New York City. AIDS 6:849, 1992

10. Liesnard C, Van Vooren JP, Farber CM: Risk of cerebral toxoplasmosis according to toxoplasmosis seroprevalence in African and European HIV seropositive patients and recommendations for cerebral toxoplasmosis primary prevention. In Abstracts of the VIth International Conference on AIDS, San Francisco, 1990, Abstract FB426

11. Luft BJ, Castro KG: An overview of the problem of toxoplasmosis and pneumocystosis in AIDS in the USA: Implications for future therapeutic trials. Eur J Clin Microbiol Infect Dis 10:178, 1991

12. Remington JS, McLeod R, Desmonts G: Toxoplasmosis. In Remington JS, Klein JO (eds): Infectious Diseases of the Fetus and Newborn Infant. Philadelphia, WB Saunders Company, 1995, p 140

13. Zumla A, Savva D, Wheeler RB, et al: *Toxoplasma* serology in Zambian and Ugandan patients infected with the human immunodeficiency virus. Trans R Soc Trop Hyg 85:227, 1991

14. Luft BJ, Conley FK, Remington JS: Outbreak of central nervous system toxoplasmosis in Western Europe and North America. Lancet 1:781, 1983

15. Navia BA, Petito CK, Gold JWM, et al: Cerebral toxoplasmosis complicating AIDS: Clinical and neuropathological findings in 27 patients. Ann Neurol 19:224, 1986

16. Selik RM, Starcher ET, Curran JW: Opportunistic disease reported in AIDS patients: Frequencies, associations, and trends. J Acquir Immune Defic Syndr 1:175, 1987

17. Wong B, Gold JWM, Brown AE, et al: Central nervous system toxoplasmosis in homosexual men and parenteral drug abusers. Ann Intern Med 100:36, 1984

18. Clumeck N: Some aspects of the epidemiology of toxoplasmosis and *Pnemocystis* in AIDS in Europe. Eur J Clin Microbiol Infect Dis 10:177, 1991

19. Clumeck N, Sonnet J, Taelman H, et al: Acquired immunodeficiency syndrome in African patients. N Engl J Med 310:492, 1984

20. Leport C, Raffi F, Katlama C, et al: Treatment of central nervous system toxoplasmosis with pyrimethamine/sulfadiazine combination in 35 patients with acquired immunodeficiency syndrome. Am J Med 84:94, 1988

21. Pedrol E, Gonzalez-Clemente J, Gatell JM, et al: Central nervous system toxoplasmosis in AIDS patients: Efficacy of an intermittent maintenance therapy. AIDS 4:511, 1990

22. Ragnaud JM, Beylot J, Lacut JY, et al: Toxoplasmic encephalitis in 73 AIDS patients (Bordeaux, France 1985–1989). In Abstracts of the VIIth International Conference on AIDS, Florence, 1991, Abstract MB2090

23. Wong SY, Remington JS: Toxoplasmosis in the setting of AIDS. In Broder S, Merigan TC Jr, Bolognesi D (eds): Textbook of AIDS Medicine. Baltimore, Williams & Wilkins, 1994, 223

24. Castro KG, Selik RM, Jaffe HW, et al: Frequency of opportunistic diseases in AIDS patients by race/ethnicity and HIV transmission categories—United States. In Abstracts of the 28th Interscience Conference on Antimicrobial Agents and Chemotherapy, Los Angeles, 1988, Abstract 570

25. Jessurun J, Angeles-Angeles A, Gasman N: Comparative demographic and autopsy findings in AIDS in two Mexican populations. J Acquir Immune Defic Syndr 3:579, 1990

26. Dannemann BR, McCutchan JA, Israelski DM, et al: Treatment of toxoplasmic encephalitis patients with AIDS: A randomized trial comparing pyrimethamine plus clindamycin to pyrimethamine plus sulfonamides. Ann Intern Med 116:33, 1992

27. Haverkos HW: Assessment of therapy for *Toxoplasma* encephalitis. Am J Med 82:907, 1987

28. Levy RM, Bredesen DE: Central nervous system dysfunction in acquired immunodeficiency syndrome. J Acquir Immune Defic Syndr 1:41, 1988

29. Porter SB, Sande MA: Toxoplasmosis of the central nervous system in the acquired immunodeficiency syndrome. N Engl J Med 327:1643, 1992

30. Renold C, Sugar A, Chave J-P, et al: Toxoplasmic encephalitis in patients with the acquired immunodeficiency syndrome. Medicine (Balt) 71:224, 1992

31. Carrazana E, Rossitch E Jr, Martinez J: Unilateral "akathisia" in a patient with AIDS and a toxoplasmosis subthalamic abscess. Neurology 39:349, 1989

32. Carrazana E, Rossitch E Jr, Samuels MA: Parkinsonian symptoms in a patient with AIDS and cerebral toxoplasmosis. J Neurol Neurosurg Psychiatry 52:1445, 1989

33. Koppel B, Daras M: "Rubrual" tremor due to midbrain toxoplasmosis abscess. Mov Disord 5:254, 1990

34. Tolge C, Factor S: Focal dystonia secondary to cerebral toxoplasmosis in a patient with AIDS. Mov Disord 6:69, 1991

35. Herskovitz S, Siegel SE, Schneider AT, et al: Spinal cord toxoplasmosis in AIDS. Neurology 39:1552, 1989

36. Mehren M, Burns PJ, Mamani MD, et al: Toxoplasmic myelitis mimicking intramedullary cord tumor. Neurology 38:1648, 1988

37. Gray F, Gherard R, Wingate E, et al: Diffuse "encephalitic" cerebral toxoplasmosis in AIDS: Report of four cases. J Neurol 236:273, 1989

38. Khuong MA, Matheron S, Marche C, et al: Diffuse toxoplasmic encephalitis without abscess in AIDS patients. In Abstracts of the 30th Interscience Conference on Antimicrobial Agents and Chemotherapy, Atlanta, 1990, Abstract 1157

39. Lucet JC, Bailly MP, Bedos JP, et al: Septic shock due to toxoplasmosis in patients infected with human immunodeficiency virus. Chest 104:1054, 1993

40. Oksenhendler E, Cadranel J, Sarfati C, et al: *Toxoplasma gondii* pneumonia in patients with the acquired immunodeficiency syndrome. Am J Med 88:5N, 1990

41. Rabaud C, May T, Amiel C, et al: Extracerebral toxoplasmosis in patients infected with HIV. Medicine 73:306, 1994

42. Tschirhart D, Klatt EC: Disseminated toxoplasmosis in the acquired immunodeficiency syndrome. Arch Pathol Lab Med 112:1237, 1988

43. Cappell MS, Mikhail N, Ortega A: *Toxoplasma* myocarditis in AIDS. Am Heart J 123:1728, 1992

44. Grange F, Kinney EL, Monsuez JJ, et al: Successful therapy for *Toxoplasma gondii* myocarditis in acquired immunodeficiency syndrome. Am Heart J 120:443, 1990

45. Marche C, Mayorga R, Trophilme D, et al: Pathological study of extraneurological toxoplasmosis (ENT) in AIDS. In: Abstracts of the IVth International Conference on AIDS, Stockholm, 1988, Abstract 7074

46. Moskowitz L, Hensley GT, Chan JC, Adams K: Immediate cause of death in AIDS. Arch Pathol Lab Med 109:735, 1985

47. Roldan EO, Moskowitz L, Hensley GT: Pathology of the heart in AIDS. Arch Pathol Lab Med 111:943, 1987
48. Brouland JP, Audouin J, Hofman P, et al: Bone marrow involvement by disseminated toxoplasmosis in acquired immunodeficiency syndrome: The value of bone marrow trephine biopsy and immunohistochemistry for the diagnosis. Hum Pathol 27.302, 1996
49. Israelski DM, Skowren G, Leventhal JP, et al: *Toxoplasma* peritonitis in a patient with AIDS. Arch Intern Med 148:1655, 1988
50. Smart PE, Weinfeld A, Thompson NE, Defortuna SM: Toxoplasmosis of the stomach: A cause of antral narrowing. Radiology 174:369, 1990
51. Burg JL, Grover CM, Pouletty P, Boothroyd JC: Direct and sensitive detection of a pathogenic protozoan, *Toxoplasma gondii*, by polymerase chain reaction. J Clin Microbiol 27:1787, 1989
52. Pauwels A, Meyohas MC, Eliaszewicz M, et al: Toxoplasmic colitis in the acquired immunodeficiency syndrome. Am J Gastroenterol 87:518, 1992
53. Groll A, Schneider M, et al: Morphology and clinical significance of AIDS-related lesions in the adrenal and pituitary. Deutsche Med Wochenschr 115:483, 1990
54. Milligan SA, Katz MS, Craven PC: Toxoplasmosis presenting as panhypopituitarism in a patient with AIDS. Am J Med 77:760, 1984
55. Crider SR, Horstman WG, Massy GS: Toxoplasma orchitis: Report of a case and a review of the literature. Am J Med 85:421, 1988
56. Nistal M, Santana A, Paniaqua R, Palacios J: Testicular toxoplasmosis in two men with AIDS. Arch Pathol Lab Med 110:746, 1986
57. Gherardi R, Baudrimont M, Lionnet F, et al: Skeletal muscle toxoplasmosis in patients with acquired immunodeficiency syndrome: A clinical and pathological study. Ann Neurol 32:535, 1992
58. Hirschmann JV, Chu AC: Skin lesions with disseminated toxoplasmosis in a patient with the acquired immunodeficiency syndrome [letter]. Arch Dermatol 124:1446, 1988
59. Derouin F, Sarfati C, Beauvais B, et al: Prevalence of pulmonary toxoplasmosis in HIV-infected patients [letter]. AIDS 4:1036, 1990
60. Schanpp L, Geaghan S, Campagna A, et al: *Toxoplasma gondii* pneumonitis in patients infected with the human immunodeficiency virus. Arch Intern Med 152:1073, 1992
61. Cochereau-Massin I, LeHoang P, Lautier-Frau M: Ocular toxoplasmosis in human immunodeficiency virus-infected patients. Am J Ophthalmol 114:130, 1992
62. Friedman D: Neuro-ophthalmic manifestations of human immunodeficiency virus infection. Neurol Clin 9:55, 1991
63. Gagliuso DJ, Teich SA, Friedman AH, Orellana J: Ocular toxoplasmosis in AIDS patients. Trans Am Ophthalmol Soc 88:63, 1990
64. Holland GN, Engstrom RE Jr, Glasgow BJ, et al: Ocular toxoplasmosis in patients with the acquired immunodeficiency syndrome. Am J Ophthalmol 106:653, 1988
65. Parke DW, Font RL: Diffuse toxoplasmic retinochoroiditis in a patient with AIDS. Arch Ophthalmol 104:571, 1986
66. Weiss A, Margo CE, Ledford DK, et al: Toxoplasmic retinochoroiditis as an initial manifestation of AIDS. Am J Opthalmol 101:248, 1986
67. Farkash AE, MacCabbee PJ, Sher JH: Central nervous system toxoplasmosis in AIDS: A clinical-pathological-radiological review of 12 cases. J Neurol Neurosurg Psychiatry 49:744, 1986
68. Araujo FG, Guptil DR, Remington JS: In vivo activity of piritrexin against *Toxoplasma gondii*. J Infect Dis 156:828, 1987
69. Eliaszewicz M, Lecomte I, De Sa M, et al: Relation between decreasing serial CD4 lymphocyte count and outcome of toxoplasmosis in AIDS patients: A basis for primary prophylaxis. In Abstracts of the VIth International Conference on AIDS, San Francisco, 1990, Abstract Th.B.481
70. Miro JM, Buira E, Mallolas J, et al: Relation between CD4 T lymphocyte counts, tuberculosis, other opportunistic infections or Kaposi's sarcoma in Spanish AIDS patients. In Abstracts of the VIIth International Conference on AIDS, Florence, 1991, Abstract MB2347
71. Oksenhendler E, Charreau I, Tournerie C, et al: *Toxoplasma gondii* infection in advanced HIV infection. AIDS 8:483, 1994
72. Leport C, Chene G, Morlat P, et al: Pyrimethamine for primary prophylaxis of toxoplasmic encephalitis in patients with human immunodeficiency virus infection: A double blind placebo-controlled trial. J Infect Dis 173:91, 1996
73. Wanke C, Tuazon CU, Kovacs A, et al: *Toxoplasma* encephalitis in patients with acquired immune deficiency syndrome. Am J Trop Med Hyg 36:509, 1987
74. Minkoff H, Remington JS, Holman S, et al: Vertical transmission of toxoplasma by human immunodeficiency virus-infected women. Am J Obstet Gynecol 176:555, 1997
75. Mitchell CD, Lewis L, McLellan S, et al: Increased risk of congenital toxoplasmosis among infants born to mothers infected with HIV-1 and *Toxoplasma gondii*. In: Abstracts of the 3rd Conference on Retroviruses and Opportunistic Infections, Washington, DC, 1996, Abstract 425
76. Mitchell CD, Erlich SS, Mastrucci MT, et al: Congenital toxoplasmosis occurring in infants perinatally infected with human immunodeficiency virus 1. Pediatr Infect Dis J 9:512, 1990
77. Cimino C, Lipton R, Williams A, et al: The evaluation of patients with human immunodeficiency virus-related disorders and brain mass lesions. Arch Intern Med 151:1381, 1991
78. Derouin F, Thulliez P, Garin YFJ: Value and limitations of toxoplasmosis serology in HIV patients. Pathol Biol (Paris) 39:255, 1991
79. Suzuki Y, Israelski DM, Dannemann BR, et al: Diagnosis of toxoplasmic encephalitis in patients with AIDS by using a new serologic method. J Clin Microbiol 26:2541, 1988
80. Derouin F, Leport C, Pueyo S, et al: Predictive value of *Toxoplasma gondii* antibody titers on the occurrence of toxoplasmic encephalitis in HIV-infected patients. AIDS 10:1521, 1996
81. Orefice G, Carrieri PB, De Marinis T, et al: Use of the intrathecal synthesis of anti-*Toxoplasma* antibodies in the diagnostic assessment and in the follow-up of AIDS patients with cerebral toxoplasmosis. Acta Neurol (Napoli) 12:79, 1990
82. Potasman I, Resnick L, Luft BJ, Remington JS: Intrathecal production of antibodies against *Toxoplasma gondii* in patients with toxoplasmic encephalitis and AIDS. Ann Intern Med 108:49, 1988
83. Chakroun M, Meyohas MC, Pelosse B, et al: Emergence de la toxoplasme oculaire au cours du SIDA. Ann Med Interne (Paris) 141:472, 1990

84. Verbraak FD, Galema M, van den Horn GH, et al: Serological and polymerase chain reaction-based analysis of aqueous humor samples in patients with AIDS and necrotizing retinitis. AIDS 10:1091, 1996

85. Bretagne S, Costa J, Vidaud M, et al: Detection of *Toxoplasma gondii* by competitive DNA amplification of bronchoalveolar lavage samples. J Infect Dis 168: 1585, 1993

86. Holliman RE: Clinical and diagnostic findings in 20 patients with toxoplasmosis and the acquired immune deficiency syndrome. J Med Microbiol 35:1, 1991

87. Stepick BP, Thulliez P, Araujo FG, Remington JS: IgA antibodies for diagnosis of acute congenital and acquired toxoplasmosis. J Infect Dis 162:270, 1990

88. Pinon JM, Toubas D, Marx C, et al: Detection of specific immunoglobulin E in patients with toxoplasmosis. J Clin Microbiol 28:1739, 1990

89. Wong SY, Hadju M-P, Ramirez R, et al: Role of specific immunoglobulin E in diagnosis of acute *Toxoplasma* infection and toxoplasmosis. J Clin Microbiol 29:2952, 1993

90. Derouin F, Mazeron MC, Garin YJF: Comparative study of tissue culture and mouse inoculation methods for demonstration of *Toxoplasma gondii*. J Clin Microbiol 25:1597, 1987

91. Hofflin JM, Remington JS: Tissue culture isolation of *Toxoplasma* from blood of a patient with AIDS. Arch Intern Med 145:925, 1985

92. Derouin F, Garin YJF: Isolement de *Toxoplasma gondii* par culture cellulaire chez les sujets infectes par le VIH. Presse Med 21:10, 1992

93. Tirard V, Niel G, Rosenheim M, et al: Diagnosis of toxoplasmosis in patients with AIDS by isolation of the parasite from the blood [letter]. N Engl J Med 324: 634, 1991

94. Derouin F, Sarfati C, Beauvais B, et al: Laboratory diagnosis of pulmonary toxoplasmosis in patients with acquired immunodeficiency syndrome. J Clin Microbiol 27:1661, 1989

95. Shepp DH, Hackman RC, Conley FK, et al: *Toxoplasma gondii* reactivation identified by detection of parasitemia in tissue culture. Ann Intern Med 103: 218, 1985

96. Holliman RE, Johnson JD, Gillespie SH, et al: New methods in the diagnosis and management of cerebral toxoplasmosis associated with the acquired immune deficiency syndrome. J Infect Dis 22:281, 1991

97. Holliman RE, Johnson JD, Savva D: Diagnosis of cerebral toxoplasmosis in association with AIDS using polymerase chain reaction. Scand J Infect Dis 22:243, 1990

98. Van de Ven E, Melchers W, Galama J, et al: Identification of *Toxoplasma gondii* infections by BI gene amplification. J Clin Microbiol 29:2120, 1991

99. Dupon M, Cazenave J, Pellegrin JL, et al: Detection of *Toxoplasma gondii* by PCR and tissue culture in cerebrospinal fluid and blood of human immunodeficiency virus-seropositive patients. J Clin Microbiol 33:2421, 1995

100. Lebech M: Detection of *Toxoplasma gondii* DNA by polymerase chain reaction in cerebrospinal fluid from AIDS patients with cerebral toxoplasmosis [letter]. J Infect Dis 165:982, 1992

101. Ostergaard L, Nielsen AK, Black FT: DNA amplification on cerebrospinal fluid for diagnosis of cerebral toxoplasmosis among HIV-positive patients with signs or symptoms of neurological disease. Scand J Infect Dis 25:227, 1993

102. Parmley S, Goebel F, Remington JS: Detection of *Toxoplasma gondii* in cerebrospinal fluid from AIDS

103. Bretagne S, Costa JM, Fleury-Feith J, et al: Quantitative competitive PCR with bronchoalveolar lavage fluid for diagnosis of toxoplasmosis in AIDS patients. J Clin Microbiol 33:1662, 1995

104. Lavrard I, Chouaid C, Roux P, et al: Pulmonary toxoplasmosis in HIV-infected patients: Usefulness of polymerase chain reaction and cell culture. Eur Respir J 8:697, 1995

105. Dupouy-Camet J, Lavareda de Souza S, Maslo C, et al: Detection of *Toxoplasma gondii* in venous blood from AIDS patients by polymerase chain reaction. J Clin Microbiol 31:1866, 1993

106. Filice G, Hitt J, Mitchell C, et al: Diagnosis of *Toxoplasma* parasitemia in patients with AIDS by gene detection after amplification with polymerase chain reaction. J Clin Microbiol 31:2327, 1993

107. Lamoril J, Molina JM, de Gouvello A, et al: Detection by PCR of *Toxoplasma gondii* in blood in the diagnosis of cerebral toxoplasmosis in patients with AIDS. J Clin Pathol 49:89, 1996

108. Raffi F, Pelloux H, Dupouy-Camet J, et al: Detection of *Toxoplasma gondii* parasitemia by culture and polymerase chain reaction (PCR) in AIDS patients with suspected toxoplasma encephalitis: A prospective study. In Abstracts of the 2nd National Conference on Human Retroviruses and Related Infections, Washington, DC, 1995, Abstract 303

109. Enzman DR: Imaging of infections and Inflammations of the Central Nervous System: Computed Tomography, Ultrasound and Nuclear Magnetic Resonance. New York, Raven Press, 1984

110. Post MJD, Kursunoglu SJ, Hensley GT, et al: Cranial CT in acquired immunodeficiency syndrome: Spectrum of disease and optimal contrast enhancement technique. AJNR Am J Neuroradiol 6:743, 1985

111. Strittmatter C, Lang W, Wiestler OD, Kleihues P: The changing pattern of human immunodeficiency virus associated cerebral toxoplasmosis: A study of 46 postmortem cases. Acta Neuropathol 83:475, 1992

112. Levy RM, Breit R, Russell R, Dal Canto MC: MRI-guided stereotaxic brain biopsy in neurologically symptomatic AIDS patients. J Acquire Immune Defic Syndr 4:254, 1991

113. Elkin CM, Leon E, Grenell SL, et al: Intracranial lesions in the acquired immunodeficiency syndrome: Radiological (CT) features. JAMA 253:393, 1985

114. Post MJD, Chan JC, Hensley GT, et al: *Toxoplasma* encephalitis in Haitian adults with acquired immunodeficiency syndrome: A clinical-pathologic-CT correlation. AJNR Am J Neuroradiol 4:155, 1983

115. Bursztyn EM, Lee BCP, Bauman J: CT of acquired immunodeficiency syndrome. AJNR Am J Neuroradiol 5:711, 1984

116. Goldstein J, Dickson D, Moser F, et al: Primary central nervous system lymphoma in acquired immunodeficiency syndrome. Cancer 67:2756, 1991

117. Ciricillo SF, Rosenblum ML: Imaging of solitary lesions in AIDS. J Neurosurg 74:1029, 1991

118. Ciricillo S, Rosenblum ML: Use of CT and MR imaging to distinguish intracranial lesions and to define the need for biopsy in AIDS patients. J Neurosurg 73: 720, 1990

119. De La Paz RL, Enzman D: Neuroradiology of acquired immunodeficiency syndrome. In Rosenblum ML, Levy RM, Bredesen DE, et al (eds): AIDS and the Nervous System. New York, Raven Press, 1988, p 121

120. Kupfer M, Zee CS, Colletti PM, et al: MRI evaluation of AIDS-related encephalopathy: Toxoplasmosis vs. lymphoma. MRI 8:51, 1990

121. Levy RM, Mills CM, Posin JP, et al: The efficacy and clinical impact of brain imaging in neurological symptomatic AIDS patients: A prospective CT/MRI study. J Acquir Immune Defic Syndr 3:461, 1990

122. Post MJD, Sheldon JJ, Hensley GT, et al: Central nervous system disease in AIDS: Prospective correlation using CT, MRI and pathologic studies. Radiology 158:141, 1986

123. Dina T: Primary central nervous system lymphoma versus toxoplasmosis in AIDS. Radiology 179:823, 1991

124. Luft BJ, Hafner R, Korzun AH, et al: Toxoplasmic encephalitis in patients with the acquired immunodeficiency syndrome. N Engl J Med 329:995, 1993

125. Laissy JP, Soyer P, Parlier C, et al: Persistent enhancement after treatment for cerebral toxoplasmosis in patients with AIDS: Predictive value for subsequent recurrence. AJNR Am J Neuroradiol 15:1773, 1994

126. Pierce MA, Johnson MD, Maciunas RJ, et al: Evaluating contrast-enhancing brain lesions in patients with AIDS by using positron emission tomography. Ann Intern Med 123:594, 1995

127. Lorberboym M, Estok L, Machac J, et al: Rapid differential diagnosis of cerebral toxoplasmosis and primary central nervous system lymphoma by thallium-201 SPECT. J Nucl Med 37:1150, 1996

128. Luft BJ, Remington JS: Toxoplasmosis of the central nervous system. In Remington JS, Swartz MN (eds): Current Topics in Infectious Disease, Vol 6. New York, McGraw-Hill, 1985, p 315

129. Wijdicks EFM, Borleffs JCC, Hoepelman AIM, Jansen GH: Fatal disseminated hemorrhagic toxoplasmic encephalitis as the initial manifestation of AIDS. Ann Neurol 29:683, 1991

130. De La Torre R, Gorraez M: *Toxoplasma*-induced occlusive hypertrophic arteritis as the cause of discrete coagulative necrosis in the central nervous system. Hum Pathol 20:604, 1989

131. Huang TE, Chou SM: Occlusive hypertrophic arteritis as the cause of discrete necrosis in CNS toxoplasmosis in AIDS. Hum Pathol 19:1210, 1988

132. Conley FK, Jenkins KA, Remington JS: *Toxoplasma gondii* infection of the central nervous system: Use of the peroxidase-antiperoxidase method to demonstrate *Toxoplasma* in formalin-fixed, paraffin-embedded tissue sections. Hum Pathol 12:690, 1981

133. Cerezo L, Alvarez M, Price G: Electron microscopic diagnosis of cerebral toxoplasmosis. J Neurosurg 630:470, 1985

134. Dement SH, Cox MC, Grupta PK: Diagnosis of central nervous system *Toxoplasma gondii* from the cerebrospinal fluid in a patient with AIDS. Diagn Cytopathol 3:148, 1987

135. Bottone EJ: Diagnosis of acute pulmonary toxoplasmosis by visualization of invasive and intracellular tachyzoites in Giemsa-stained smears of bronchoalveolar lavage fluid. J Clin Microbiol 29:2626, 1991

136. Levy RM, Rosenbloom S, Perrett LV: Neuroradiological findings in AIDS: A review of 200 cases. AJNR Am J Neuroradiol 7:833, 1986

137. Catania S, Nobili C, Trinchieri V, et al: Cryptococcal meningitis and *Toxoplasma* encephalitis in an AIDS patient. Acta Neurol (Napoli) 12:82, 1990

138. Leport C, Remington JS: Toxoplasmose au cours du SIDA. Presse Med 21:1165, 1992

139. Araujo FG, Guptil DR, Remington JS: Azithromycin, a macrolide antibiotic with potent activity against *Toxoplasma gondii*. Antimicrob Agents Chemother 32:755, 1988

140. Araujo FG, Huskinson J, Remington JS: Remarkable in vitro and in vivo activities of the hydroxynaphthoquinone 566C80 against tachyzoites and tissue cysts of *Toxoplasma gondii*. Antimicrob Agents Chemother 35:293, 1991

141. Weiss LM, Harris C, Berger M, et al: Pyrimethamine concentrations in serum and cerebrospinal fluid during treatment of acute *Toxoplasma* encephalitis in patients with AIDS. J Infect Dis 157:580, 1988

142. Cavallito JC, Nichol CA, Brenckman WD Jr, et al: Lipid-soluble inhibitors of dihydrofolate reductase. I. Kinetics, tissue distribution and extent of metabolism of pyrimethamine, metroprine, and etoprine in the rat, dog, and man. Drug Metab Dispos 6:329, 1978

143. Leport C, Meulemans A, Robine D, et al: Levels of pyrimethamine in serum and penetration into brain tissue in humans. AIDS 6:1040, 1992

144. Israelski DM, Tom C, Remington JS: Zidovudine antagonizes the action of pyrimethamine in experimental infection with *Toxoplasma gondii*. Antimicrob Agents Chemother 33:30, 1989

145. Mack DG, McLeod R: New micromethod to study the effect of antimicrobial agents on *Toxoplasma gondii*: Comparison of sulfadoxine and sulfadiazine individually and in combination with pyrimethamine and study of clindamycin, metronidazole and cyclosporin A. Antimicrob Agents Chemother 26:26, 1984

146. Geils GF, Scott CW Jr, Baugh CM, Butterworth CE Jr: Treatment of meningeal leukemia with pyrimethamine. Blood 38:131, 1971

147. Stickney DR, Simmons WS, De Angelis RL, et al: Pharmacokinetics of pyrimethamine (PRM) and 2,4-diamino-5(3',4'-dichlorophenyl)-6-methylpyrimide (DMP) relevant to meningeal leukemia. Proc Am Assoc Cancer Res 14:52, 1973

148. Leport C, Meulemans A, Robine D, et al: Penetration of pyrimethamine into human brain tissue after a single dose administration. In Abstracts of the 29th Interscience Conference on Antimicrobial Agents and Chemotherapy, Houston, 1989, Abstract 248

149. Katlama C: Evaluation of the efficacy and safety of clindamycin plus pyrimethamine for induction and maintenance therapy of toxoplasmic encephalitis in AIDS. Eur J Clin Microbiol Infect Dis 10:189, 1991

150. Katlama C, de Witt S, O'Doherty E, et al: Pyrimethamine-clindamycin vs. pyrimethamine-sulfadiazine as acute and long-term therapy for toxoplasmic encephalitis in patients with AIDS. Clin Infect Dis 22:268, 1996

151. Canessa A, Del Bono V, De Leo P, et al: Cotrimoxazole therapy of *Toxoplasma gondii* encephalitis in AIDS patients. Eur J Clin Microbiol Infect Dis 11:125, 1992

152. Herrera G, Villalta O, Visona K, et al: Trimethoprim-sulfamethoxazole treatment of *Toxoplasma* encephalitis in AIDS patients. In Abstracts of the VIIth International Conference on AIDS, Florence, 1991, Abstract WB2321

153. Solbreux P, Sonnet J, Zech F: A retrospective study about the use of cotrimoxazole as diagnostic support and treatment of suspected cerebral toxoplasmosis in AIDS. Acta Clin Belg 45:85, 1990

154. Grossman PL, Remington JS: The effect of trimethoprim and sulfamethoxazole on *Toxoplasma gondii* in vitro and in vivo. Am J Trop Med Hyg 28:445, 1979

155. Kaufman HE, Geisler PH: The hematologic toxicity of pyrimethamine (Daraprim) in man. Arch Ophthalmol 64:140, 1960

156. Myatt AV, Coatney GR, Hernandez T, et al: A further study of the toxicity of pyrimethamine (Daraprim) in man. Am J Trop Med 2:1000, 1953
157. Myatt AV, Hernandez T, Coatney GR: Studies in human malaria. Am J Trop Med 2:788, 1953
158. Frenkel JK, Hitchings GH: Relative reversal by vitamins (*p*-aminobenzoic, folic and folinic acids) of the effects of sulfadiazine and pyrimethamine on *Toxoplasma*, mouse and man. Antibiot Chemother 7:630, 1957
159. Nixon PF, Bertino JR: Effective absorption and utilization of oral formyl-tetrahydrofolate in man. N Engl J Med 186:175, 1972
160. Rousseau F, Pueyo S, Morlat P, et al: Increased risk of toxoplasmic encephalitis in human immunodeficiency virus-infected patients with pyrimethamine-related rash. Clin Infect Dis 24:396, 1997
161. Guichard A, Zamora L, Caumes E, et al: Cutaneous side effects: A major problem in the treatment of toxoplasmosis encephalitis. In Abstracts of the VIIth International Conference on AIDS, Florence, 1991, Abstract MB2188
162. Gluckstein D, Ruskin J: Rapid oral desensitization to trimethoprim-sulfamethoxazole (TMP-SMZ): Use in prophylaxis for *Pneumocystis carinii* pneumonia in patients with AIDS who were previously intolerant to TMP-SMZ. Clin Infect Dis 20:849, 1995
163. Piketty C, Gilquin J, Kazatchkine MD: Efficacy and safety of desensitization to trimethoprim-sulfamethoxazole in human immunodeficiency virus-infected patients. J Infect Dis 172:611, 1995
164. Molina JM, Belenfant X, Doco-LeCompte T, et al: Sulfadiazine-induced crystalluria in AIDS patients with *Toxoplasma* encephalitis. AIDS 5:587, 1991
165. Oster S, Hutchison F, McCabe R: Resolution of acute renal failure in toxoplasmic encephalitis despite continuance of sulfadiazine. Rev Infect Dis 12:618, 1990
166. Simon DI, Brosius FC, Rothstein DM: Sulfadiazine crystalluria revisited. Arch Intern Med 150:2379, 1990
167. Dannemann BR, Israelski DM, Remington JS: Treatment of toxoplasmic encephalitis and intravenous clindamycin. Arch Intern Med 148:2477, 1988
168. Fernandez-Martin J, Leport C, Morlat P, et al: Pyrimethamine-clarithromycin combination for therapy of acute *Toxoplasma* encephalitis in patients with AIDS. Antimicrob Agents Chemother 35:2049, 1991
169. Leport C, Bastuju-Garin S, Perronne C, et al: An open study of the pyrimethamine-clindamycin combination in AIDS patients with brain toxoplasmosis. J Infect Dis 160:577, 1989
170. Derouin F, Piketty C, Chastang C, et al: Anti-toxoplasma effects of dapsone alone and combined with pyrimethamine. Antimicrob Agents Chemother 35:252, 1991
171. Ward DJ: Dapsone/pyrimethamine for treatment of toxoplasmic encephalitis. In Abstracts of the VIII International Conference on AIDS and STD World Congress, Amsterdam, 1992, Abstract Po.B. 3277
172. Araujo FG, Lin T, Remington JS: Synergistic combination of azithromycin and sulfadiazine for treatment of toxoplasmosis in mice. Eur J Clin Microbiol Infect Dis 11:71, 1992
173. Farthing C, Rendel M, Currie B, Seidlin M: Azithromycin for cerebral toxoplasmosis. Lancet 339:437, 1992
174. Araujo FG, Prokocimer P, Lin T, Remington JS: Activity of clarithromycin alone or in combination with other drugs for treatment of murine toxoplasmosis. Antimicrob Agents Chemother 36:2454, 1992
175. Clumeck N, Katlama C, Ferrero T, et al: Atovaquone (14 hydroxynapthoquinone 566C80) in the treatment of acute cerebral toxoplasmosis in AIDS patients. In Abstracts of the VIIIth International Conference on AIDS, Amsterdam, 1992, Abstract 1217
176. Kovacs JA: Efficacy of atovaquone in treatment of toxoplasmosis in patients with AIDS. Lancet 340:637, 1992
177. Kovacs JA, Allergra CJ, Chabner BA, et al: Potent effect of trimetrexate, a lipid-soluble antifolate, on *Toxoplasma gondii*. J Infect Dis 155:1027, 1987
178. Polis MA, Masur H, Tuazon C, et al: Salvage therapy of trimetrexate-leucovorin for treatment of cerebral toxoplasmosis in AIDS patients. Clin Res 37:437A, 1989
179. Araujo FG, Slifer T, Remington JS: Rifabutin is active in the treatment of toxoplasmosis in murine models. Antimicrob Agents Chemother 38:570, 1994
180. Chang HR, Comte R, Piguet PF, et al: Activity of minocycline against *Toxoplasma gondii* infection in mice. J Antimicrob Chemother 27:639, 1991
181. Chang HR, Comte R, Pechere JC: In vitro and in vivo effects of doxycycline on *Toxoplasma gondii*. Antimicrob Agents Chemother 34:775, 1990
182. Pope-Pegram L, Gathe J, Bohn B, et al: Treatment of presumed central nervous system toxoplasmosis with doxycycline. In Abstracts of the VII International Conference on AIDS, Florence, 1991, Abstract MB 2027
183. Ou-Yang K, Krug EC, Marr JJ, Berens RL: Inhibition of growth of *Toxoplasma gondii* by Qinghaosu and derivatives. Antimicrob Agents Chemother 34:1961, 1990
184. Luft BJ: Potent in vivo activity of arpinocid, a purine analogue, against murine toxoplasmosis. J Infect Dis 154:692, 1986
185. Lindsay DS, Balgburn BL, Hall JE, Tidwell RR: Activity of pentamidine and pentamidine analogs against *Toxoplasma gondii* in cell cultures. Antimicrob Agents Chemother 35:1914, 1991
186. Dhiver C, Milandre C, Poizot-Martin I, et al: 5-Fluorouracil-clindamycin for treatment of cerebral toxoplasmosis. AIDS 7:143, 1993
187. Harris C, Miklos P, Tanowitz H, Wittner M: In vitro assessment of antimicrobial agents against *Toxoplasma gondii*. J Infect Dis 157:14, 1988
188. Suzuki Y, Orellana MA, Schreiber RD, et al: Interferon-γ: The major mediator of resistance against *Toxoplasma gondii*. Science 240:516, 1988
189. Orellana MA, Suzuki Y, Araujo FG, Remington JS: Role of beta interferon in resistance to *Toxoplasma gondii* infection. Infect Immun 59:3287, 1991
190. Chang HR, Grau GE, Pechere JC: Role of TNF and IL-1 in infections with *Toxoplasma gondii*. Immunology 69:33, 1990
191. Sharma SD, Hofflin JM, Remington JS: In vivo recombinant interleukin 2 administration enhances survival against a lethal challenge with *Toxoplasma gondii*. J Immunol 135:4160, 1985
192. Kasper LH, Matsuura T, Khan IA: IL-7 stimulates protective immunity in mice against the intracellular pathogen, *Toxoplasma gondii*. J Immunol 155:4798, 1995
193. Araujo FG, Hunter CA, Remington JS: Treatment with a combination of IL-12 and drugs significantly increases survival of mice with acute toxoplasmosis. In Abstracts of the 35th Interscience Conference of Antimicrobial Agents and Chemotherapy, San Francisco, 1995, Abstract G99

194. Hunter CA, Candolfi E, Subauste CS, et al: Studies on the role of interleukin-12 in acute murine toxoplasmosis. Immunology 84:16, 1995

195. Bezares R, Cueva F, Pzenni V, et al: Effects of GM-CSF (granulocyte-macrophage stimulating factor) in mice experimentally infected with *Toxoplasma gondii* [Abstract 2738]. Blood 86:688a, 1990

196. Leport C, Vilde JL, Katlama C, et al: Failure of spiramycin to prevent neurotoxoplasmosis in immunosuppressed patients. JAMA 255:2290, 1987

197. Araujo FG, Shepard RM, Remington JS: In vivo activity of the macrolide antibiotics azithromycin, roxithromycin and spiramycin against *Toxoplasma gondii*. Eur J Clin Microbiol Infect Dis 10:519, 1991

198. Hofflin JM, Remington JS: In vivo synergism of roxithromycin (RU965) and interferon against *Toxoplasma gondii*. Antimicrob Agents Chemother 31:346, 1987

199. Chang HR, Pechere JC: In vitro effects of four macrolides roxithromycin, spiramycin, azithromycin (CP-62, 93) and A-56268 on *Toxoplasma gondii*. Antimicrob Agents Chemother 32:524, 1988

200. Saba J, Morlat P, Raffi F, et al: Pyrimethamine plus azithromycin for treatment of acute toxoplasmic encephalitis in patients with AIDS. Eur J Clin Microbiol Infect Dis 12:853, 1993

201. Araujo FG, Huskinson-Mark J, Gutteridge WE, Remington JS: In vitro and in vivo activities of the hydroxynaphthoquinone 566C80 against the cyst form of *Toxoplasma gondii*. Antimicrob Agents Chemother 36:326, 1992

202. Torres RA, Weinberg W, Stansell J, et al: Atovaquone for salvage treatment and suppression of toxoplasmic encephalitis in patients with AIDS. Clin Infect Dis 24:422, 1997

203. Araujo FG, Lin T, Remington JS: The activity of atovaquone (566C80) in murine toxoplasmosis is markedly augmented when used in combination with pyrimethamine or sulfadiazine. J Infect Dis 167:494, 1993

204. Araujo FG, Suzuki Y, Remington JS: Combinations of rifabutin with atovaquone or clindamycin are effective in treatment of toxoplasmic encephalitis in a murine model. In Abstracts of the 35th Interscience Conference of Antimicrobial Agents and Chemotherapy, San Francisco, 1995, Abstract B55

205. Araujo FG, Remington JS: Synergistic activity of azithromycin and gamma interferon in murine toxoplasmosis. Antimicrob Agents Chemother 35:1672, 1991

206. Israelski DM, Remington JS: Activity of γ interferon in combination with pyrimethamine or clindamycin in treatment of murine toxoplasmosis. Eur J Clin Microbiol Infect Dis 9:358, 1990

207. Schmitz JL, Carlin JM, Borden EC, et al: Beta interferon inhibits *Toxoplasma gondii* growth in human monocyte-derived macrophages. Infect Immun 57:3254, 1989

208. Walckenaer G, Leport C, Longuet P, et al: Relapses of brain toxoplasmosis in 15 AIDS patients. In Abstracts of the 31st Interscience Conference on Antimicrobial Agents and Chemotherapy, Chicago, 1991, Abstract 251

209. Leport C, Tournerie C, Raguin G, et al: Long-term follow-up of patients with AIDS on maintenance therapy for toxoplasmosis. Eur J Clin Microbiol Infect Dis 10:191, 1991

210. Madlener J, Enzensberger W, Herdt P, et al: Neurological outcome and follow-up after successful treatment of CNS toxoplasmosis. In: Abstracts of the VIIIth International Conference on AIDS, Amsterdam, 1992, p B122

211. Podzamczer D, Miro JM, Bolao F, et al: Twice-weekly maintenance therapy with sulfadiazine-pyrimethamine to prevent recurrent toxoplasmic encephalitis in patients with AIDS. Ann Intern Med 123:175, 1995

212. Heald A, Flepp M, Chave J-P, et al: Treatment of cerebral toxoplasmosis protects against *Pneumocystis carinii* pneumonia in patients with AIDS. Ann Intern Med 115:760, 1991

213. de Gans J, Portegies P, Reiss P, et al: Pyrimethamine alone as maintenance therapy for central nervous system toxoplasmosis in 38 patients with AIDS. J Acquir Immune Defic Syndr 5:137, 1992

214. Foppa CU, Bini T, Gregis G, et al: A retrospective study of primary and maintenance therapy of toxoplasmic encephalitis with oral clindamycin and pyrimethamine. Eur J Clin Microbiol Infect Dis 10:187, 1991

215. Girard PM, Lepretre A, Detruchis P, et al: Failure of pyrimethamine-clindamycin combination for prophylaxis of *Pneumocystis carinii* pneumonia. Lancet 1:1459, 1989

216. Ruf B, Schurmann D, Bergmann F, et al: Efficacy of pyrimethamine/sulfadoxine in the prevention of toxoplasmic encephalitis relapses and *Pneumocystis carinii* pneumonia in HIV-infected patients. Eur J Clin Microbiol Infect Dis 12:325, 1993

217. Katlama C, Mouthon B, Gourdon D, et al: Atovaquone as long-term suppressive therapy for toxoplasmic encephalitis in patients with AIDS and multiple drug intolerance. AIDS 10:1107, 1996

218. Wallace MR, Rossetti RJ, Olson PE: Cats and toxoplasmosis risk in HIV-infected adults. JAMA 269:76, 1993

219. Mallolas J, Zamora L, Gatell JM, et al: Primary prophylaxis for *Pneumocystis carinii* pneumonia: A randomized trial comparing cotrimoxazole, aerosolized pentamidine and dapsone, plus pyrimethamine. AIDS 7:59, 1993

220. Carr A, Tindall B, Brew BJ, et al: Low-dose trimethoprim-sulfamethoxazole prophylaxis for toxoplasmic encephalitis in patients with AIDS. Ann Intern Med 117:106, 1992

221. Nicholas P, Pierone G, Lin J, et al: Trimethoprim-sulfamethoxazole in the prevention of cerebral toxoplasmosis. In Abstracts of the VIth International Conference on AIDS, San Francisco, 1990, Abstract Th.B.482

222. O'Farrell N, Bradbeer C, Fitt S, et al: Cerebral toxoplasmosis and cotrimoxazole prophylaxis. Lancet 337:986, 1991

223. Podzamczer D, Salazar A, Jimenez J, et al: Intermittent trimethoprim-sulfamethoxazole compared with dapsone-pyrimethamine for simultaneous primary prophylaxis of Pneumocystis pneumonia and toxoplasmosis in patients infected with HIV. Ann Intern Med 122:755, 1995

224. Podzamczer D, Santin M, Jimenez J, et al: Thrice weekly cotrimoxazole is better than weekly dapsone-pyrimethamine for the primary prevention of *Pneumocystis carinii* pneumonia in HIV-infected patients. AIDS 7:501, 1993

225. Ruskin J, LaRiviere M: Low-dose co-trimoxazole for prevention of *Pneumocystis carinii* pneumonia in human immunodeficiency virus disease. Lancet 337:468, 1991

226. Clotet B, Sirera G, Romeu J, et al: Twice-weekly dapsone-pyrimethamine for preventing PCP and cerebral toxoplasmosis [letter]. AIDS 5:601, 1991
227. Koppen S, Grunewald T, Jautzke G, et al: Prevention of *Pneumocystis carinii* pneumonia and toxoplasmic encephalitis in human immunodeficiency virus-infected patients: A clinical approach comparing aerosolized pentamidine and pyrimethamine/sulfadoxine. Clin Invest 70:508, 1992
228. Girard PM, Landman R, Gaudebout C, et al: Dapsone-pyrimethamine compared with aerosolized pentamidine as primary prophylaxis against *Pneumocystis carinii* pneumonia and toxoplasmosis in HIV infection. N Engl J Med 328:1514, 1993
229. Jacobson MA, Besch CL, Child C, et al: Primary prophylaxis with pyrimethamine for toxoplasmic encephalitis in patients with advanced human immunodeficiency virus disease: Results of a randomized trial. J Infect Dis 169:384, 1994
230. Raffi F, Struillou L, Ninin E, et al: Breakthrough cerebral toxoplasmosis in patients with AIDS who are being treated with clarithromycin. Clin Infect Dis 20:1076, 1995
231. Suzuki Y, Wong SY, Grumet FC, et al: Evidence for genetic regulation of susceptibility to toxoplasmic encephalitis in AIDS patients. J Infect Dis 173:265, 1996

26 | Hepatitis C Infection

MARINA BERENGUER • TERESA L. WRIGHT

An estimated 3.5 million individuals in the United States have chronic hepatitis C virus (HCV) infection. Annually, 8000 to 10,000 chronically infected patients will die of liver-related complications and 1000 will require liver transplantation.[1] Thus HCV is a major public health problem, not only in regard to the number of people infected but also in regard to the number at risk for serious disease.

Because of shared transmission pathways, coinfection with HCV and HIV type 1 is common. However, the efficiency of the transmission of hepatitis viruses and HIV by the parenteral or sexual route appears to differ, thus explaining the wide variability of HCV seropositivity among HIV-infected subjects. Indeed, rates ranging from 4% to 100% have been reported depending on the transmission category, with higher prevalences among intravenous drug users (IDUs) and recipients of blood transfusions than among homosexual men and heterosexual contacts. Furthermore, there is evidence that biologic interaction between these two viruses exists in the same host, which may modify the clinical course or transmissibility of viral infection. These interactive effects are nonetheless complex and subject to ongoing investigation. In particular, there is increasing evidence from the molecular to the clinical level that the effects of HCV infection can be modified by coinfection with HIV. Critical to these interplays are the recent changes in the natural history of HIV infection.[2] As a consequence, certain previously unimportant diseases, such as chronic hepatitis C, are now relevant, and, indeed, chronic hepatitis C is a growing cause of morbidity and mortality in patients coinfected with HIV and HCV. Specific features of HCV infection have been proposed to occur more frequently in coinfected patients than in patients infected with HCV alone. These include (1) lack of sensitivity of serologic assays in diagnosing HCV infection, (2) enhancement of HCV rep-

lication, (3) rapid and more severe course of HCV-related liver disease, and (4) higher risk of heterosexual and perinatal transmission of HCV infection. Data to support these observations are stronger for some than for others. Data regarding the impact of HCV infection on HIV disease progression or HIV transmission are only now emerging, and they are scarce and conflicting.

There is a consensus that HCV infection alone is a progressive disease resulting in liver failure in some, probably the minority, but that progression occurs over decades. As a consequence, the longer patients coinfected with HCV and HIV survive, the more likely it is that they will die of liver failure before they die of HIV-associated complications. Therapeutic strategies are therefore needed to reduce the long-term impact of chronic hepatitis C in coinfected patients. However, no established treatment guidelines for these patients exist.

As the consequences of HCV-related liver disease increasingly become an important problem in the management of HIV-infected patients, the goals of our review are to clarify several issues regarding the interactions between these viruses, including the reciprocal effect of each virus on the natural history of the other, and the resulting prognostic and therapeutic implications of these interactions.

EPIDEMIOLOGY

HCV infection is the major cause of chronic hepatitis among HIV-infected individuals. This high prevalence reflects the shared transmission routes of both viruses, namely the parenteral route, and, to a lesser extent, the sexual/perinatal route. Among HIV-infected subjects, antibodies against HCV are detected in 70% to 92% of hemophiliacs and in 60% to 90% of IDUs but in only 4% to 8% of homosexual men, reflecting the greater likelihood for HCV to be transmitted parenterally than sexually.[3]

The vast majority of persons with hemophilia who were transfused with nontreated clotting factor concentrates before viral inactivation procedures were implemented in 1984 have been infected with HCV,[4] and most have also been infected with HIV.[5] The significant increase in prevalence of anti-HCV and anti-HIV antibodies with age[4] reflects not only an increase in the number of units of clotting factor concentrates received in older patients, but also changes in donor screening and implementation of virus inactivation procedures in the last decade, with anti-HIV screening beginning in 1985 and anti-HCV in 1990.

The introduction of inactivation procedures and blood donor screening for antibodies against HCV has dramatically improved the safety of pooled plasma products.[6] As a consequence, HCV infection has become a rare event among hemophiliac patients in recent years, and IDU currently represents the main risk factor for being coinfected with both viruses.

PATHOGENESIS

There are many parallels between HCV and HIV (Table 26–1). Replication of both viruses is dependent on an error-prone polymerase, which, because of the lack of an efficient proofreading ability, results in considerable viral diversity within individuals known as viral *quasispecies*.[7,8] Quasispecies of both these viruses may influence viral persistence, disease progression, and response to treatment.

Both host immune status and viral factors are likely to be important in the pathogenesis of HCV-related liver injury and in the progression of HCV-related disease.[9] HCV viral factors may be important in the pathogenesis of disease, either directly through cellular injury or indirectly through different immune responses associated with different viral strains. Host cellular and humoral immune response may be important in the initial recognition of virus and persistence of virus with subsequent hepatocellular injury.

Before discussing the possible HIV–HCV interactions, an understanding of the basic mechanisms influencing HIV replication is required.[10-12] HIV infects primarily CD4+ lymphocytes. Viral entry is mediated by the cellular receptor CD4, which binds with high affinity to the external glycoprotein of HIV gp120. Following the viral binding and uptake into the lymphocyte, transcription of viral RNA to double-stranded DNA is catalyzed by a reverse transcriptase/RNA-dependent DNA polymerase. Viral DNA may then become integrated into the genome of the infected cell as a provirus, which either remains in a latent form for years or is activated by both cellular and viral factors to produce replicating virus. HIV replication is known to be affected by a number of cytokines. Tumor necrosis factor has been shown to upregulate HIV expression from chronically infected monocytes.[13] Cell destruction may follow as a consequence of (1) retroviral DNA accumulation within the cytoplasm, and (2) viral packaging and release of viral proteins.

HCV may interact directly with HIV at several stages of the viral life cycle, or it may act indirectly by influencing cytokine production. For a virus to have a direct influence on HIV, it must infect the same cell type. HCV is regarded as predominantly hepatotropic, but the negative strand of HCV or replicative intermediate has also been detected in peripheral blood mononuclear cells (PBMCs),[14] and replication of HCV has been obtained in lymphoid cells in culture.[15] It is therefore a reasonable hypothesis that interactions between these viruses occur in CD4+ cells.

DIAGNOSIS OF HCV INFECTION IN HIV-INFECTED INDIVIDUALS

In HIV-infected individuals, as in immunocompetent ones, HCV infection is generally sus-

TABLE 26–1. Parallels and Differences Between HCV and HIV Infection

	HIV	HCV
Genome (RNA/DNA)	RNA	RNA
U.S. prevalence	750,000	4,000,000
Annual incidence	50,000 (AIDS only)	30,000
Trends in incidence	Increasing since 1980	Decreasing since 1980
Chronicity rate	>99%	>85%
Probable survival	10–15 years	20–40 years
Complications	Immune deficiency	Cirrhosis
Association with cancer	Yes (lymphoma, Kaposi's sarcoma)	Yes (hepatocellular carcinoma)

pected and diagnosed on the basis of elevated liver function test values in an asymptomatic person. Because of the high prevalence of hepatitis markers among HIV-positive patients, a systematic search of HCV infection is increasingly becoming the rule.

Diagnostic assays for HCV can be grouped into serologic and molecular types. A progressive improvement in sensitivity in detecting anti-HCV antibodies has been accomplished with the successive development of second- and third-generation assays that incorporate new antigens. Third-generation supplemental assays are not only more sensitive but also more specific; they have a high correlation with HCV RNA detection in serum. However, in immunosuppressed patients, such as those coinfected with HIV, the rate of indeterminate or false-negative results is higher than in those who are immunocompetent. Diminution or loss of reactivity to HCV antigens has been described in those patients, with a subsequent increase in the number of patients testing indeterminate by recombinant immunoblotting assay (RIBA) (10% to 30%).[16-19] The correlation of such a pattern with HCV viremia appears to be high among HIV-infected individuals, regardless of the transaminase values. In one study[19] of 485 individuals positive for anti-HCV antibody, of whom 167 were seropositive for HIV and 318 were seronegative, 23% of the seropositive group tested indeterminate by second-generation RIBA (RIBA 2), whereas only 15% of the seronegative group were indeterminate. In patients indeterminate by RIBA 2, HCV RNA was more frequently detected in HIV-positive patients (89%) than in those who were HIV-negative (50%). Reactivity to the core antigen c22 appears to be conserved even in HIV-infected individuals.[17] The rate of HCV indeterminate results appears to be related to the degree of immunosuppression. In one study,[18] 62.5% of HIV-infected patients with low CD4 cell counts (<200/mm^3) and AIDS had indeterminate RIBA 2 results, compared to 18% in patients with earlier stages of HIV disease.

In conclusion, an impaired serologic response to HCV occurs frequently in HIV-coinfected individuals, with a high correlation between indeterminate RIBA 2 results and detectable viral RNA. Serologic tests should therefore be interpreted with caution when patients have HIV coinfection. To overcome problems with specificity and sensitivity, the direct detection of viral RNA appears necessary, particularly in patients with indeterminate serologic results or patients without a definitive risk factor for HCV infection.

HIV COINFECTION: IMPACT ON HCV INFECTION

Influence on HCV Replication

Evidence is emerging for the existence of a significant increase in HCV RNA levels in patients coinfected with HIV and HCV compared to those infected with HCV alone.[18,20-25] The role of HIV in the increase of HCV viremia is reinforced by the observation of Eyster et al.,[21] who showed that, in hemophiliacs infected with HCV, HCV viral load significantly increased after HIV seroconversion. However, the mechanisms by which HIV enhances HCV replication are still under investigation. Several hypotheses have been proposed. The first is that immunosuppression secondary to HIV disease progression may facilitate increased HCV replication. A negative correlation between HCV RNA levels and CD4 cell count demonstrated by some,[4,21,25,26] but not all,[18,20,22,23] of the studies supports this hypothesis. Nonetheless, none of the three studies that have looked at the association between HCV and other markers of immunosuppression, such as p24 antigenemia[22,23] or HIV RNA levels,[18,22] have found a positive association between these variables. Moreover, the CD4 count may be an incomplete measure of HIV-induced immunosuppression. Hence the precise contribution of the immune system to controlling viral replication during HCV infection is incompletely understood.

Another hypothesis is that HIV-infected patients are more likely to be coinfected with additional viruses that enhance HCV replication, although there are few findings to support this hypothesis. A third possibility is that of a distinct genotype distribution in HIV-infected versus non-HIV-infected patients, with a subsequent effect on HCV replication. However, findings from three studies comparing the distribution of HCV genotypes in coinfected patients and those infected with HCV alone are conflicting.[18,23,27] There may be increased HCV diversity in coinfected patients, with accumulation of envelope variants of HCV that are ineffectively cleared by the host.[28] Alternatively, there may be differences in the type of patients under investigation (hemophiliacs and IDUs, versus homosexual men). Both hemophiliacs and IDUs coinfected with HIV may have higher viral loads for HCV because of larger numbers of contaminated batches of clotting factors or repeated injections with contaminated needles, but there are no data supporting this hypothesis. Finally, unknown factors induced by HIV may be responsible for increased HCV replication. The possible lymphotropism of HCV[14] would support a possible HIV–HCV interaction of these viruses within the PBMCs.

Increased HCV RNA levels may ultimately lead to (1) enhanced HCV sexual and vertical transmission, which could contribute to high rates of HCV infection in urban populations[1]; (2) more severe liver damage; and (3) nonresponse to treatment with interferon.

Influence on HCV Diversity

RNA viruses, such as HCV and HIV, comprise multiple closely related but nonidentical variants termed *quasispecies*.[7,8,10,11,29] This variability derives from nucleotide substitutions in viral genomes caused by an inherent error-prone replication compounded by an absence of proof-reading repair-enzyme activities. HCV replicates with high mutation rates, in the range of 10^{-3} to 10^{-5} misincorporations per nucleotide and round of copying.[30] Competition between variants exists, the result of which is the transient dominance of one or a few variants highly adapted to the environment (a so-called major variant) over a multitude of "minor variants" that are less capable of replicating efficiently, yet are able to survive the defense mechanisms of the host. Thus the different variants are continuously subjected to a process of mutation, competition, and selection of the ones best fitted to survive and produce infectious progeny. The quasispecies nature of viruses has several implications, such as changes in pathogenicity or in tissue tropism, drug resistance, and evasion of vaccine-induced or natural immunity, with resulting viral persistence.

In order to understand better the role of the immune response in the persistence of HCV infection, pathogenesis of liver damage, and responsiveness to interferon, recent studies have evaluated the effect of HIV coinfection in HCV genomic variability. The variable envelope genes of HCV are believed to be the region most susceptible to immune selection and immune escape.[30] They contain a hypervariable domain (HVR1) that is believed to contain a B-cell epitope[31] that might be the target of neutralizing antibodies. This domain was thus chosen for analysis in all the studies.[28,32,33] Results are conflicting, however, with one study showing a greater HVR1 diversity among coinfected patients[28] and another study[33] showing similar complexity and diversity between coinfected patients and those infected with HCV alone. In

the latter study, however, HCV diversity was shown to decrease in association with decreases in CD4 count, suggesting that a reduction in CD4 count, which is considered to cause a decline in the activity of T-helper lymphocytes, caused changes in the composition of HCV populations.

In conclusion, there are limited data supporting or refuting the notion that the pathogenesis of HCV infection differs in patients with and without HIV infection. Additional studies are needed to assess viral diversity in coinfected patients. However, difficulties in evaluating the importance of viral diversity will not be overcome until new techniques become widely available. Current analyses have been hampered by technical issues because determination of the number of quasispecies by direct sequencing of multiple clones is tedious and determination by indirect methods may be inaccurate.

Influence on the Natural History of HCV-Related Liver Disease

In immunocompetent patients without HIV infection, there is a consensus emerging in which HCV infection is seen as a slowly progressing disease resulting in liver failure in some patients, but probably the minority.

Since the first description by Martin et al.[34] of three patients with HCV–HIV coinfection who developed cirrhosis within 3 years of the onset of hepatitis, a time course that is unusually rapid, several studies have confirmed that, in coinfected individuals, HCV-related liver disease progresses faster than in HIV-seronegative patients.[25,35–40] Eyster et al.[35] found a cumulative incidence of liver failure of 17% 10 years after HIV infection, compared to 0% in non-HIV infected patients. Among HIV-infected individuals, the risk of hepatic decompensation is 3 to 21 times higher than in immunocompetent patients,[36] with a still-higher risk in patients in whom the CD4 cell count drops and p24 antigenemia is detected.[36] Furthermore, the time elapsed between HCV infection and development of severe liver disease is shortened among HIV-coinfected patients.[25,39] In one study,[39] 25% of coinfected patients had cirrhosis 15 years after the estimated date of HCV infection, compared with only 6.5% of those with HCV infection alone. Similar differences in rates were seen during the first 5 and 10 years; most of the HIV-negative group (9/13) developed cirrhosis in a time interval longer than 15 years. In another multicenter cross-sectional study of 547 patients with chronic HCV, 116 of whom were coinfected with HIV,[25] 14.9% of coinfected patients developed cirrhosis in the first 10 years, compared to 6.2% in the HIV-negative group, with similar differences being observed after 5 and 15 years. The mean interval from HCV infection to cirrhosis was longer in HIV-negative patients compared to those coinfected with HIV (23.2 vs. 6.9 years, respectively; $p < .001$).

The reasons why hepatic decompensation develops more rapidly in coinfected patients than in those with HCV infection alone are currently under investigation. Several hypotheses have been raised: (1) HIV does not seem to be cytopathic to hepatocytes, but it can be demonstrated in Kupffer cells in patients with AIDS[41] and could have pathologic effects on the liver by stimulating abnormal production of fibrogenic cytokines; (2) hepatic decompensation could be precipitated by AIDS-related opportunistic infections in patients who have already developed cirrhosis as a result of chronic HCV infection; (3) HIV immunosuppression enhances HCV load, which, in turn, has been shown in some studies to be associated with more severe liver damage; and (4) distribution of HCV genotypes and HCV diversity may be different in coinfected patients compared to those infected with HCV alone. In one study[38] that investigated the influence of HCV genotypes on the histologic severity of chronic hepatitis C in a cohort of 59 IDUs, HIV infection and HCV type 1b were independently associated with histologic severity. Furthermore, a high proportion of genotypically mixed infections were found in this cohort (44%). One can therefore speculate that the simultaneous replication of several HCV subtypes in this population, as well as a wide spectrum of quasispecies populations,[28] might lead to an increased degree of liver damage.

In summary, HIV can modify the natural course of chronic parenterally acquired hepatitis C, leading to an unusually rapid progression to cirrhosis. The factors determining this rapid progression of liver disease remain to be identified.

Influence on the Histologic Picture of Chronic Hepatitis C

Only very recently have studies sought to analyze whether HIV coinfection alters the histopathologic findings of liver disease caused by chronic HCV infection.[42,43] In one study[43] of 68 liver biopsies and 71 livers obtained at autopsy from coinfected and non-coinfected patients, coinfected patients showed less intense portal

lymphoid inflammatory infiltrates than their HIV-seronegative counterparts. Lymphoid portal aggregates, or follicles, frequently found in immunocompetent patients with chronic HCV, were absent in the liver biopsies of patients with coinfection. The difference in portal and periportal infiltrates was not only quantitative but also qualitative, such that HIV-coinfected patients had a predominantly granulocytic portal infiltration in combination with a mild granulocytic cholangiolitis, a pattern of inflammation rarely seen in classic chronic hepatitis C. This reduction of lymphoid infiltrates may be due in part to the advanced disturbance of immune response because the vast majority of coinfected patients in the study had progressed to late stages of AIDS. Additional differences included (1) a significantly more pronounced reticular centrilobular fibrosis in coinfected patients, rarely seen in patients infected with HCV alone and suggesting an independent fibrogenic effect of HIV; and (2) cholestasis in the coinfected patients, a pattern that is very unusual among immunocompetent patients infected with HCV alone but that has recently been described in transplant patients.[44] In either of these immunocompromised groups, marked cholestasis is associated with a poor prognosis.

HCV COINFECTION: IMPACT ON NATURAL HISTORY OF HIV-RELATED IMMUNODEFICIENCY

As survival of HIV-infected patients has progressively improved, clinically significant liver disease caused by HCV infection has become more prevalent. Nonetheless, compared to the number of studies evaluating the effects of HIV infection on the course of HCV disease, there are few studies assessing the overall impact of HCV on the rate of progression to AIDS. The impact of these coinfections on the clinical outcome of HIV-infected patients is, although potentially relevant, unclear. If HCV coinfection were to have a deleterious effect on HIV disease, there would be a rationale for treating HCV infection in coinfected individuals regardless of the stage of liver disease, and a rationale for using antiretroviral therapies for HIV and primary prophylaxis against opportunistic infections at early stages of HIV infection in patients coinfected with HCV.

The results of two early cross-sectional studies[45,46] did not demonstrate a detrimental effect of HCV coinfection on the progression of HIV

TABLE 26–2. Study Findings of HCV Coinfection: Impact on Natural History of HIV-Related Immunodeficiency

STUDY (YEAR)	POPULATION	NUMBER	ASSOCIATION OF HCV WITH AIDS PROGRESSION
Wright et al.[47] (1994)	512 HIV+ male homosexuals (44% AIDS)	HIV+/HCV+ = 74 HIV+/HCV− = 438	No
Dorucci et al.[48] (1997)	416 HIV+; AIDS free	HIV+/HCV+ = 214 HIV+/HCV− = 202	No
Ockenga et al.[3] (1997)	232 HIV+ (47% AIDS)	HIV+/HCV+ = 60 HIV+/HCV− = 172	No/yes*
Sabin et al.[49] (1997)	111 Hemophiliac men: HIV+ and HCV+	HCV type 1: 70%; 2: 13%; 3: 4%; 4: 2%	Yes†

*The incidence of progression to AIDS and actuarial patient survival was not different in the control group versus the HCV-infected group (14% vs. 11% and 590 days vs. 577 days, respectively). However, in patients with AIDS, coinfection with HCV was associated with poorer outcome (actuarial patient survival: 267 days vs. 439 days for non-HCV-infected patients).
†Progression to both AIDS ($p = .009$) and death ($p = .007$) was faster in subjects infected with type 1 than those infected with other types.

disease, although subsequent cohort studies have provided conflicting results[3,47–49] (Table 26–2). The first two studies, which were conducted prior to the availability of effective antiretrovirals, failed to find differences in the natural history of coinfection versus that of HIV infection alone,[47,48] presumably because HIV, but not HCV disease, was determining natural history. In more recent studies, however, HCV coinfection has been associated with shorter survival among patients with AIDS[3] and a more rapid progression to AIDS and death, particularly in patients infected with HCV genotype 1.[49] In the most recent study by Sabin et al.,[49] a cohort of men with hemophilia coinfected with HCV and HIV were evaluated. Of 111 subjects included, genotype was determined in 71%, and genotype 1 was present in 70%. There were no differences in age at HIV seroconversion or CD4 count at time of AIDS diagnosis in patients with genotype 1 infection versus genotype non-1, although progression to both AIDS and death was more rapid in the former than in the latter group ($p = .009$ and $.007$, respectively). After adjustment for differences in patient age at HIV seroconversion and age at hemophilia diagnosis, as well as most recent CD4 count, the relative hazard for progression to AIDS and death was 2.87 and 2.98, respectively, for patients infected with HCV genotype 1 and genotype non-1. Results from this cohort of coinfected hemophiliac men suggest an association between HCV genotype and progression of HIV disease, with genotype 1 being associated with more rapid progression to AIDS and death than genotypes non-1. Caution must be exerted when interpreting these studies because genotype 1 infection has not clearly been shown to alter the pathogenicity of HCV disease.[30] It would appear unlikely, therefore, that genotype 1 infection would clearly accelerate the course of HIV disease unless it is doing so through a mechanism other than HCV-related liver injury.

Reasons for the discrepant results from these studies may include

1. Differences in study design; cross-sectional studies may have masked a possible effect. One problem in the cross-sectional studies, for instance, is that HIV-infected patients did not undergo follow-up from the time of HCV seroconversion, but rather from the time of HCV testing.
2. Differences in the exposure category (hemophiliacs vs. IDUs); different categories may carry different risks for HIV progression.
3. Differences in the time period when the studies were performed, with the availability of new drugs to manage HIV infection and the associated improved survival in later studies. Thus HCV-related liver complications are more prominent in recent studies than in historic studies, and increasingly contribute to mortality.[3,49]

The mechanisms by which HCV interacts with HIV are still unknown, but, theoretically, HCV could interact directly with HIV at several stages of the viral life cycle, or it could act indirectly by influencing cytokine production. Indeed, HCV has been shown to activate HIV replication through cytokines such as tumor necrosis factor.[13]

In conclusion, although early reports in longitudinal cohorts failed to demonstrate a detrimental effect of HCV infection on HIV disease progression, more recent studies that have included HIV-infected individuals treated with new antiretroviral drugs have suggested that HIV-infected patients coinfected with HCV genotype 1 experience more rapid progression to AIDS and death than those infected with other genotypes. Further longitudinal studies are required to confirm the association between HCV infection and/or HCV genotype and HIV disease progression.

HCV VERTICAL AND SEXUAL TRANSMISSION: ASSOCIATION WITH HIV INFECTION

Heterosexual and perinatal transmission of HCV is less efficient than that of HIV, which, in turn, seems to be less efficient than that of hepatitis B virus (HBV). HCV infection is infrequent among sex partners and newborns of coinfected patients, supporting the low rate of vertical or sexual transmission of this virus. Although not confirmed by all studies,[50,51] evidence is accumulating that HIV infection may be a cofactor for heterosexual[52-55] and perinatal transmission of HCV infection.[56] HIV infection is associated with high circulating levels of HCV, and a high titer of HCV viremia is associated with perinatal[57] and sexual[58] transmission of HCV infection, even in the absence of HIV coinfection.

Timing of anti-HCV antibody disappearance in babies has been shown to be affected by the HIV status of the mother, with one study[51] showing 22% of babies of coinfected mothers but only 3% of babies of HIV-seronegative mothers still HCV seropositive at 12 months.

In conclusion, HCV appears to be inefficiently transmitted by sexual or vertical means even in patients who are coinfected with HIV. Whether HIV coinfection facilitates transmission of HCV is controversial.

HIV VERTICAL TRANSMISSION: ASSOCIATION WITH HCV INFECTION

Although several studies have evaluated the influence of HIV coinfection on HCV vertical transmission, few have addressed the converse question, that is, the influence of ongoing HCV infection on HIV vertical transmission.[59,60] In one early study, coinfection was associated with increased perinatal transmission of HIV[59]; HIV was transmitted perinatally by 12 of 25 HIV–HCV coinfected mothers, compared to only 2 of 14 mothers with HIV infection alone. This study was, however, limited by its small number, failure to quantify HCV RNA levels, and inability to control for other factors associated with perinatal transmission of HIV, such as CD4 lymphocyte depletion[61] and IDU during pregnancy.[62]

In a recent study[60] performed as a part of the Women and Infants Transmission Study, a multicenter study that has enrolled a large cohort of HIV-infected pregnant women, 487 mother–infant pairs were evaluated in order to assess the impact of HCV coinfection on HIV perinatal transmission. The study population comprised 161 (33%) coinfected women and 326 (66%) women infected only with HIV. Twenty-six percent of children born to coinfected mothers acquired HIV, as opposed to 16% of children born to non-HCV-infected mothers ($p = .01$). By univariate analysis, several factors were found to be associated with HIV vertical transmission, including coinfection with HCV–HIV, CD4 lymphocyte percent less than 29, HIV culture positive during the entire pregnancy, ruptured membranes for more than 4 hours, and hard drug use (e.g., injection drugs, crack cocaine). However, in a logistic regression model, HCV infection was marginally associated with perinatal transmission ($p = .08$), whereas drug use was not. Women who transmitted HIV perinatally had higher levels of HCV RNA (median 721,254 copies/ml) than those who did not (median 337,561 copies/ml; $p = .01$). Thus these data suggest that maternal HCV infection enhances perinatal HIV transmission. Alternatively, HCV may be a marker for another cofactor, such as maternal drug use, which, in turn, is associated with a high likelihood of transmission. The mechanisms by which HCV affects perinatal HIV transmission are unknown, but may include (1) increased expression of HIV from HCV coinfection through transactivation within the PBMCs, and (2) functional abnormalities in cell-mediated immunity as a consequence of invasion of PBMCs by HCV RNA. Further studies on HIV-infected women with and without HCV coinfection are needed to determine if the association represents a biologic effect of HCV infection or is due to a confounding interaction between HCV and another factor such as drug use.

TREATMENT OF CHRONIC HEPATITIS C IN HIV-INFECTED PATIENTS

Until recently, interferon was the only treatment approved for chronic hepatitis C in immunocompetent patients; long-term virologic and biochemical response rates are approximately 10% to 15% after a standard dosing of 3 million units (MU) thrice weekly for 6 to 12 months. Failure to clear viremia at 1 month appears to be a good predictor of nonresponse. Responsiveness to therapy varies according to genotype, viral load, degree of HCV diversity, different dosing, and the concomitant administration of other drugs. Low pretreatment HCV RNA levels, infection with HCV genotype other than 1, low genomic diversity, longer duration of treatment, and concomitant administration of ribavirin have all been associated with increased initial and/or sustained response to treatment.

The majority of trials with interferon for chronic hepatitis C have excluded patients with HIV coinfection, and, therefore, there are few large studies that have adequately addressed the treatment of HCV disease in this patient population. In theory, administration of interferon-α to patients with HIV infection could accelerate wasting, because endogenous interferon has been shown to contribute to AIDS-associated wasting. However, studies have shown that interferon provides benefits in HIV-infected patients because of the antiviral effects of this drug when adminstered as monotherapy or in association with zidovudine.[63]

There are few trials[64-67] assessing the effectiveness of interferon in dually infected individuals. Most studies published to date lack controls and include a relatively small number of patients. Nonetheless, preliminary results suggest that the rate of response in HIV-infected patients with preserved immune function is similar to that observed in non-HIV-infected individuals with chronic hepatitis C (Table 26–3).

In the largest study published to date,[67] 107 coinfected patients and 27 patients infected with HCV alone were treated with interferon-α 5MU thrice weekly for 3 months. Responders were subsequently treated with 3MU thrice weekly for 9 additional months. Response was assessed both biochemically (normalization of transaminases at the end of treatment and at 12 months of follow-up) and virologically (clearance of HCV RNA from serum at the same time points). Although the rates of response among HIV-infected subjects were always lower than in non-HIV-infected subjects, there were no significant differences between HIV-seropositive and -seronegative individuals regarding early response (at 3 months), complete response (at 12 months), and sustained response (at 12 months of follow-up). These similarities in response rates occurred despite the higher frequency of baseline features typically associated with nonresponse in the HIV-coinfected group. Of the 10 variables (age, sex, route and duration of HCV infection, CD4 cell count, baseline alanine transaminase [ALT] levels, Knodell score, HCV genotype, coinfection with several genotypes, and HCV viral load at baseline), only 2 were found to be independently associated with a positive response to therapy: a CD4 count greater than 500/mm^3 and a baseline HCV viral load less than 10^7 copies/ml. There are two hypotheses that may explain the relationship between these two predictive factors and the response to treatment: (1) HCV RNA levels, which rise with advancing HIV-related immunodeficiency, may explain poor response rates; and (2) response to interferon may depend on an intact immunity. Genotype was not predictive of response, but 43% of the patients were infected with multiple genotypes, complicating the analysis. In a previous study by the same group,[66] low CD4 count at baseline was predictive of nonresponse. Both baseline ALT levels and the Knodell index did not differ between responders and nonresponders.

In all four studies,[64-67] interferon was well tolerated and no significant and serious side effects or opportunistic infections were observed. The only side effect reported in some studies was a dramatic fall in CD4 cell count (reduction of over one half) after beginning interferon; this occurred in 5.2% to 12.5% of the patients treated. In all cases, this happened between the 6th and 14th week of therapy and was transient or partially reversed after stopping the drug in all but a small percentage (~4%). This complication, which has also been described in HIV-infected patients treated with interferon, has been linked to some human leukocyte antigen haplotypes.[68]

In conclusion, interferon therapy results in response rates for HIV-infected patients with CD4 counts greater than 500/mm^3 similar to those for non-HIV-infected patients. Response rates, however are lower among immunosuppressed patients. Because interferon is an expensive drug and sustained response rates are low regardless of HIV status, cost–benefit analyses must be done before general use of interferon can be recommended. Individuals with progressive liver

TABLE 26–3. Study Findings of Chronic Hepatitis C Treatment in Patients Coinfected with HCV and HIV

STUDY YEAR (N)	TYPE OF STUDY*	DOSE[†]	RESPONSE[‡]					SEVERE ADVERSE EFFECTS
			CBR n (%)	CVR n (%)	SBR n (%)	SVR n (%)		
Boyer et al.,[64] 1992 (12)	UC	IFN-α: 1, 3, 5 MU tiw 4–6 mo	4 (30%)	NA	1/9 (11%)	NA		No
Marriott et al.,[65] 1993 (14)	UC	IFN-α: 9 MU/day 3 mo + 9 MU tiw 3 mo + 6 MU tiw 3 mo + 3 MU tiw 3 mo	5/9 (55%)	6/9 (66%)	4/9 (44%)	5/9 (55%)		No
Soriano et al.,[66] 1995 (57)	C, NR; Control: 21 HIV−/ HCV+	IFN: 5 MU tiw 3 mo (in responders: 3 MU tiw 9 mo)	NA	NA	22/57 (38%)[§] vs. 10/21 (47%)	NA		Sharp fall in CD4 in 3 cases (5.8%)
Soriano et al.,[67] 1996 (107)	C, NR; Control: 27 HIV−/ HCV+	IFN: 5 MU tiw 3 mo (in responders: 3 MU tiw 9 mo)	26 (32.5%) vs. 10 (37%)	NA	18 (22.5%) vs. 7 (25.9%)	NA		Sharp fall in CD4 in 10 cases (12.5%)

*C, controlled; UC, uncontrolled; NR, nonrandomized.
[†]IFN, interferon.
[‡]CBR, complete biochemical response (end of treatment); CVR, complete virological response (end of treatment); SBR, sustained biochemical response (end of follow-up); SVR, sustained virological response (end of follow-up).
[§]Response was higher in patients with baseline CD4 count greater than 500 cells/mm³ (58% vs. 24%) and in women (60% vs. 31%).

disease may be candidates for this or other therapies (such as combination interferon and ribavirin) in the setting of randomized controlled trials.

CONCLUSION

Until recent years, the life expectancy of individuals with HIV infection was shortened mainly because of opportunistic infections occurring when the CD4 cell decline reached a critical level ($<200/mm^3$). Because of the overwhelming effect of HIV on the life expectancy of infected individuals, the presence of coexistent viruses such as HBV and HCV, which did not clearly affect the morbidity and mortality of these patients, was largely ignored. However, with longer survival of HIV-infected subjects seen since the introduction of effective antiretroviral drugs in the late 1980s and the wide availability of primary prophylaxis for the most common opportunistic infections, illnesses such as chronic viral hepatitis have assumed greater relevance in this population. Because of similar modes of transmission, coinfection of HCV and HIV is common in patients at risk for either infection. Sexual partners and newborns of coinfected individuals have lower rates of HCV infection than of HIV infection, supporting the inefficient transmission of hepatitis C by these routes. The likely influence of HIV on the clinical course of HCV is beginning to be defined. HCV-related liver disease progresses rapidly in this population. The pathogenesis of this observed progression is as yet unexplained, but potential mechanisms include increased HCV RNA levels and greater HCV diversity in HIV-seropositive patients compared with HIV-seronegative ones. Studies addressing the converse issue, the role of HCV infection on the outcome of HIV, have been few and conflicting, indicating the need for further studies to clarify the complex interactions between these two viruses.

The benefits of using interferon to treat HCV disease in the HIV-infected individual with preserved immune function appear to be similar to those in patients with HCV infection alone. However, in neither population is therapy for HCV infection adequate. Specific inhibitors of HCV replication are awaited.

References

1. Alter MJ: Epidemiology of hepatitis C. Hepatology 26: 62S, 1997
2. Graham NMH, Zeger SL, Park LP, et al: The effects on survival of early treatment of human immunodeficiency virus infection. N Engl J Med 326:1037, 1992
3. Ockenga J, Tillmann HL, Trautwein C, et al: Hepatitis B and C in HIV-infected patients: Prevalence and prognostic value. J Hepatol 27:18, 1997
4. Ghany MG, Leissinger C, Lagier R, et al: Effect of human immunodeficiency virus infection on hepatitis C virus infection in hemophiliacs. Dig Dis Sci 41:1265, 1996
5. Goedert JJ, Kessler CM, Aledort LM, et al: A prospective study of human immunodeficiency virus type 1 infection and the development of AIDS in subjects with hemophilia. N Engl J Med 321:1141, 1989
6. Guo ZP, Yu MW: Hepatitis C virus RNA in factor VIII concentrates. Transfusion 35:112, 1995
7. Domingo E, Menendez-Arias L, Quiñones-Mateu ME, et al: Viral quasispecies and the problem of vaccine-escape and drug-resistant mutants. Prog Food Res 48: 99, 1997
8. Havlir DV, Richman DD: Viral dynamics of HIV: Implications for drug development and therapeutic strategies. Ann Intern Med 124:984, 1996
9. González-Peralta RP, Lau JYN: Pathogenesis of hepatocellular damage in chronic hepatitis C virus infection. Semin Gastrointest Dis 6:28, 1995
10. McNair AN, Main J, Thomas HC: Interactions of the human immunodeficiency virus and the hepatotropic viruses. Semin Liver Dis 12:188, 1992
11. Wei X, Ghosh SK, Taylor ME, et al: Viral dynamics in human immunodeficiency virus type 1 infection. Nature 373:117, 1995
12. Perelson AS, Neumann AU, Markovitz M, et al: HIV-1 dynamics in vivo: Virion clearance rate, infected cell life-span, and viral generation time. Science 271:1582, 1996
13. Horvath J, Raffanti SP: Clinical aspects of the interactions between human immunodeficiency virus and the hepatotropic viruses. Clin Infect Dis 18:339, 1994
14. Zignego AL, Macchia D, Monti M, et al: Infection of peripherial mononuclear blood cells by hepatitis C virus. J Hepatol 15:382, 1992
15. Shimizu YK, Iwamoto A, Hijikata M, et al: Evidence for in vitro replication of hepatitis C virus genome in a human T-cell line. Proc Natl Acad Sci USA 89:5477, 1992
16. Garcia-Smaniego J, Soriano V, Silva E, et al: Significance of HCV RIBA-2 indeterminate results in high-risk individuals: Assessment by a new third generation RIBA (RIBA-3) assay and PCR. Vox Sang 66:48, 1994
17. Cribier B, Rey D, Schmitt C, et al: High hepatitis viremia and impaired antibody response in patients coinfected with HIV. AIDS 9:1131, 1995
18. Picchio GR, Nakatsuno M, Boggiano C, et al: Hepatitis C (HCV) genotype and viral titer distribution among Argentinean hemophilic patients in the presence or absence of human immunodeficiency virus (HIV) coinfection. J Med Virol 52:219, 1997
19. Marcellin P, Martinot-Peignoux M, Elias A, et al: Hepatitis C virus (HCV) viremia in human immunodeficiency virus-seronegative and -seropositive patients with indeterminate HCV recombinant immunoblot assay. J Infect Dis 170:433, 1994
20. Sherman KE, Obrien J, Gutierrez AG, et al: Quantitative evaluation of hepatitis C virus RNA in patients with concurrent human immunodeficiency virus infections. J Clin Microbiol 31:2679, 1993
21. Eyster ME, Fried MW, Di Biscieglie AM, Goedert JJ: Increasing hepatitis C virus RNA levels in hemophili-

acs: Relationship to human immunodeficiency virus infection and liver disease. Multicenter Hemophilia Cohort Study. Blood 84:1020, 1994

22. Telfer P, Brown D, Devereux H, et al: HCV RNA levels and HIV infection: Evidence for a viral interaction in haemophilic patients. Br J Haematol 88:397, 1994

23. Cribier B, Schmidt C, Rey D, et al: HIV increases hepatitis C viremia irrespective of the hepatitis C virus genotype. Res Virol 148:267, 1997

24. Thomas DL, Shih JW, Alter H, et al: Effect of human immunodeficiency virus on hepatitis C virus infection among injecting drug users. J Infect Dis 174:690, 1996

25. Soto B, Sanchez-Quijano A, Rodrigo L, et al: Human immunodeficiency virus infection modifies the natural history of chronic parenterally-acquired hepatitis C with an unusually rapid progression to cirrhosis. J Hepatol 26:1, 1997

26. Soriano V, Bravo R, Mas A, et al: Impact of immunosuppression caused by HIV infection on the replication of hepatitis C virus. Vox Sang 69:259, 1995

27. Chambost B, Gerolami V, Thuret I, et al: Persistent hepatitis C virus RNA replication in haemophilics: Role of co-infection with human immunodeficiency virus. Br J Haematol 91:703, 1995

28. Sherman K, Andreatta C, O'Brien J, et al: Hepatitis C in human immunodeficiency virus-coinfected patients: Increased variability in the hypervariable envelope coding domain. Hepatology 23:688, 1996

29. Martell M, Esteban JI, Quer J, et al: Hepatitis C virus (HCV) circulates as a population of different but closely related genomes: Quasispecies nature of HCV genome distribution. J Virol 66:3225, 1992

30. Bukh J, Miller R, Purcell R: Genetic heterogeneity of hepatitis C virus: Quasispecies and genotypes. Sem Liver Dis 15:41, 1995

31. Weiner AJ, Geysen HM, Christopherson C, et al: Evidence for immune selection of hepatitis C virus (HCV) putative envelope glycoprotein variants: Potential role in chronic HCV infections. Proc Natl Acad Sci USA 89:3468, 1992

32. Mazza C, Puoti M, Ravaggi A, et al: Molecular analysis of mixed infection with hepatitis C virus and human immunodeficiency virus in a patient infected simultaneously. J Med Virol 50:276, 1996

33. Toyoda H, Fukuda Y, Koyama Y, et al: Effect of immunosuppression on composition of quasispecies population of hepatitis C virus in patients with chronic hepatitis C coinfected with human immunodeficiency virus. J Hepatol 26:975, 1997

34. Martin P, Di Biscieglie AM, Kassianides C, et al: Rapidly progressive nonA, nonB hepatitis in patients with human immunodeficiency virus infection. Gastroenterology 97:1559, 1989

35. Eyster ME, Diamondstone LS, Lien JM, et al: Natural history of hepatitis C virus infection in multitransfused hemophiliacs: Effect of coinfection with human immunodeficiency virus. J Acquir Immune Defic Syndr 6:602, 1993

36. Telfer P, Sabin C, Devereux H, et al: The progression of HCV-associated liver disease in a cohort of hemophilia patients. Br J Haematol 87:555, 1994

37. Rockstroh JK, Spengler U, Sudhop T, et al: Immunosuppression may lead to progression of hepatitis C virus-associated liver disease in hemophiliacs coinfected with HIV. Am J Gastroenterol 91:2563, 1996

38. Garcia-Samaniego J, Soriano V, Castilla J, et al: Influence of hepatitis C virus genotypes and HIV infection on histological severity of chronic hepatitis C. Am J Gastroenterol 92:1130, 1997

39. Sanchez-Quijano A, Andreu J, Gavilan F, et al: Influence of human immunodeficiency virus type 1 infection on the natural course of chronic parenterally acquired hepatitis C. Eur J Clin Microbiol Infect Dis 14: 949, 1995

40. Soriano V: High morbidity and mortality of chronic viral liver disease in HIV-infected individuals in Spain. J Infect 28:100, 1994

41. Lafon ME, Kirn A: Human immunodeficiency virus infection of the liver. Semin Liver Dis 12:197, 1992

42. Guido M, Rugge M, Fattovitch G, et al: Human immunodeficiency virus infection and hepatitis C pathology. Liver 14:314, 1994

43. Bierhoff E, Fisher HP, Willsch E, et al: Liver histopathology in patients with concurrent chronic hepatitis C and HIV infection. Virchows Arch 430:271, 1997

44. Schluger L, Sheiner P, Thung S, et al: Severe recurrent cholestatic hepatitis C following orthotopic liver transplantation. Hepatology 23:971, 1996

45. Quan CM, Krajden M, Glynis A, et al: Hepatitis C virus infection in patients infected with the human immunodeficiency virus. Clin Infect Dis 17:117, 1993

46. Llibre JM, Garcia E, Aloy A, Valls J: Hepatitis C virus infection and progression of infection due to human immunodeficiency virus [letter]. Clin Infect Dis 16: 182, 1993

47. Wright TL, Hollander H, Pu X, et al: Hepatitis C in HIV-infected patients with and without AIDS: Prevalence and relationship to patient survival. Hepatology 20:1152, 1994

48. Dorucci M, Pezzotti P, Philips AN, et al: Italian seroconversion study: Coinfection of hepatitis C virus with human immunodeficiency virus and progression to AIDS. J Infect Dis 172:1503, 1995

49. Sabin C, Telfer P, Philips AN, et al: The association between hepatitis C virus genotype and human immunodeficiency virus disease progression in a cohort of hemophilic men. J Infect Dis 175:164, 1997

50. Roudolt-Thoraval F, Pawlotsky JM, Thiers V, et al: Lack of mother-to-infant transmission of hepatitis C virus in human immunodeficiency virus-seronegative women: A prospective study with hepatitis C virus RNA testing. Hepatology 17:772, 1993

51. Manzini P, Saracco G, Cerchier A, et al: Human immunodeficiency virus infection as risk factor for mother-to-child hepatitis C virus transmission: Persistence of anti-hepatitis C virus in children is associated with the mother's anti-hepatitis C virus immunoblottin pattern. Hepatology 21:328, 1995

52. Eyster ME, Alter HJ, Aledort LM, et al: Heterosexual co-transmission of hepatitis C virus (HCV) and human immunodeficiency virus (HIV). Ann Intern Med 115: 764, 1991

53. Novati R, Thiers V, D'Arminio Monforte A, et al: Mother-to-child transmission of hepatitis C virus detected by nested polymerase chain reaction. J Infect Dis 165:720, 1992

54. Soto B, Rodrigo L, Garcia-Bengoechea M, et al: Heterosexual transmission of hepatitis C virus and the possible role of coexistent human immunodeficiency virus infection in the index case: A multicenter study of 423 pairings. J Intern Med 236:515, 1994

55. Thomas DL, Cannon RO, Shapiro C, et al: Hepatitis C, hepatitis B, and human immunodeficiency virus infections among non-intravenous drug-using patients attending clinics for sexually transmitted diseases. J Infect Dis 169:990, 1994

56. Zanetti AR, Tanzi E, Paccagnini S, et al: Mother-to-infant transmission of hepatitis C virus. Lancet 345: 289, 1995

57. Ohto H, Terazawa S, Sasaki N, et al: Transmission of hepatitis C virus from mothers to infants. N Engl J Med 330:744, 1994

58. Thomas DL, Zenilman JM; Alter H, et al: Sexual transmission of hepatitis C virus among patients attending sexually transmitted diseases clinics in Baltimore—an analysis of 309 sex partnerships. J Infect Dis 171:768, 1995

59. Giovanninni M, Tagger A, Ribero ML, et al: Maternal-infant transmission of hepatitis C virus and HIV infections: A possible interaction [letter]. Lancet 335:1166, 1990

60. Hershown RC, Riester K, Lew J, et al: Increased vertical transmission of human immunodeficiency virus from hepatitis C virus-coinfected mothers. J Infect Dis 176:414, 1997

61. Ryder R, Nsa W, Hassig S, et al: Perinatal transmission of the human immunodeficiency virus type 1 to infants of seropositive women in Zaire. N Engl J Med 320: 1637, 1992

62. Rodriguez EM, Mofenson LM, Chang BH, et al: Association of maternal drug use during pregnancy with maternal HIV culture positivity and perinatal HIV transmission. AIDS 10:273, 1996

63. Lane HC: Interferons in HIV and related diseases. AIDS 8:S19, 1994

64. Boyer N, Marcellin P, Degott C, et al: Recombinant interferon-alpha for chronic hepatitis C in patients positive for antibody to human immunodeficiency virus. J Infect Dis 165:723, 1992

65. Marriott E, Navas S, Del Romero J, et al: Treatment with recombinant alpha-interferon of chronic hepatitis C in anti-HIV positive patients. J Med Virol 40:107, 1993

66. Soriano V, Garcia-Samaniego J, Bravo R, et al: Efficacy and safety of alfa-interferon treatment for chronic hepatitis C in HIV-infected patients. J Infect 31:9, 1995

67. Soriano V, Garcia-Samaniego J, Bravo R, et al: Interferon-alfa for the treatment of chronic hepatitis C in patients infected with human immunodeficiency virus. Clin Infect Dis 23:585, 1996

68. Vento S, Di Perri G, Cruciani M, et al: Rapid decline of CD4+ cells after IFN alpha treatment in HIV-1 infection [letter]. Lancet 341:958, 1993

27 Bacillary Angiomatosis and Other Unusual Infections in HIV-Infected Individuals

JANE E. KOEHLER

BARTONELLA INFECTIONS

Historical Perspective

Bacillary angiomatosis (BA) was first described by Stoler and colleagues in 1983,[1] in an HIV-infected patient with multiple subcutaneous nodules. Numerous bacilli were observed by Warthin-Starry staining of the biopsied nodules, and the subcutaneous masses resolved during erythromycin therapy. Subsequently, the BA bacilli visualized using the Warthin-Starry stain were noted to have an appearance similar to that of the cat-scratch disease (CSD) bacillus.[2,3] The BA bacillus remained refractory to isolation attempts for many years, impeding identification efforts. Studies of bacterial DNA extracted from BA lesions subsequently identified the bacillus as closely related to *Rochalimaea quintana*,[4] and, after isolation of the bacillus from the blood of two HIV-infected patients without BA,[5] the organism was further characterized and named *R. henselae* in 1992.[6,7] In 1993, the genus of *Rochalimaea* was merged with the genus *Bartonella*.[8] The genus of *Grahamella* (all of which species have been isolated only from small mammals) also was merged with *Bartonella*,[9] and, most recently, a new species was isolated from pet cats,[10] resulting in a genus that includes nine extant species of *Bartonella*: *B. bacilliformis*, *B. quintana*, *B. vinsonii*, *B. henselae*, *B. elizabethae*, *B. grahamii*, *B. taylorii*, *B. doshiae*, and *B. clarridgeiae*. The BA bacillus was directly cultivated from cutaneous lesions for the first time in 1992, which led to the identification of two species of the genus *Bartonella* as causative agents of BA: *B. henselae* and *B. quintana*.[11] To date, although the species causing BA has been identified in more than 60 cases, only these two species have been found to cause bacillary angiomatosis or peliosis.[11,12]

Clinical Presentation of *Bartonella* Infections

Most patients with BA are immunocompromised, usually as a result of infection with HIV-1.[13] BA occurs as a late manifestation of HIV infection; in a study of 42 patients with BA, the median CD4 lymphocyte count was 21 cells/mm³.[14] In this setting of severe immunosuppression, infection with *B. henselae* and *B. quintana* can produce the unique vascular proliferative lesions known as BA.[15,16] These vascular proliferative lesions can form in many different organs, including skin, bone, brain parenchyma, lymph nodes, bone marrow, and the gastrointestinal and respiratory tracts. A histopathologically different vascular proliferative response is seen in the liver and spleen, known as bacillary peliosis (BP) hepatis.[17] One notable aspect of focal *Bartonella* infection, especially cutaneous BA, is the chronic, indolent nature of the disease: Lesions may be present for as long as 1 year before a diagnosis is made.[11,14]

HIV-infected individuals also can develop manifestations of *Bartonella* infection that lack vascular proliferation. Bacteremia with[18] or without[5,6,19] endocarditis has been reported in HIV-infected individuals, in the absence of focal BA or BP involvement. Patients with higher CD4 cell counts can develop focal necrotizing infections as a result of *B. henselae* in lymph nodes, liver, or spleen that have an appearance similar to that of CSD in immunocompetent in-

411

dividuals. Rarely, HIV-infected individuals with CD4 cell counts below 50/mm[3] have been reported to manifest this necrotizing lymphadenitis without vascular proliferation.[20]

A case–control study comparing clinical findings of 42 patients with BA and BP to 84 control patients found that cases were significantly more likely than controls to have fever, abdominal pain, lymphadenopathy, hepatomegaly, splenomegaly, a low CD4 cell count, anemia, or an elevated serum alkaline phosphatase.[14] With the exception of cutaneous lesions, many of the clinical findings are not specific, and the major obstacle to diagnosis of *Bartonella* infection in the presence of concomitant HIV infection is recognition of the disease by the physician. BP and all forms of BA can be indistinguishable from a number of other infectious or malignant conditions, and the diagnosis can usually be made only after biopsy and careful histopathologic evaluation of tissue, or by direct culture of *Bartonella* species from blood or the affected organ.[21]

The two different species causing focal infection in HIV-infected patients differ in their predilection for forming a specific type of lesion. Only *Bartonella henselae* has been associated with peliosis of the liver, spleen, or both.[12] *Bartonella henselae* also is associated with lymphadenopathy, and *B. quintana* with subcutaneous nodules in late-stage HIV infection.[12]

Cutaneous BA

The most frequently diagnosed BA lesions are those affecting the skin.[21] The cutaneous BA lesions can have myriad presentations, including vascular proliferative lesions with a smooth red or eroded surface (Fig. 27–1) or papules that enlarge to form friable, exophytic lesions (Fig. 27–1). These vascular lesions of cutaneous BA are particularly difficult to distinguish clinically from Kaposi's sarcoma (KS), and thus histopathologic examination of biopsied tissue is essential. BA may appear as a cellulitic plaque, usually overlying an osteolytic lesion (Fig. 27–2A). Less vascular-appearing lesions may be dry and scaly (Fig. 27–3) and some lesions are subcutaneous, with or without overlying erythema (Fig. 27–4). Very deep soft tissue masses (Fig. 27–5) also have been demonstrated to be a manifestation of BA.[11]

Osseous BA

Bartonella infection of the bone results in extremely painful osteolytic lesions. The long bones, including tibia, fibula, and radius, are most commonly involved,[21,22] although osseous BA involvement of a rib[22] and vertebra[23,24] also has been reported. A roentgenogram usually demonstrates well-circumscribed osteolysis (Fig. 27–2B), and these lytic lesions are always detected by technetium-99m methylene diphosphonate bone scans.[22] Osseous BA should be a primary consideration in the differential diagnosis of a lytic bone lesion in HIV-infected patients.

Splenic and Hepatic BP

BP hepatis, a vascular lesion of the liver, was first described in association with bacilli in eight HIV-infected individuals by Perkocha et al.[17] *Bartonella henselae* was cultured from the blood of a patient subsequently found to have BP hepatis.[25] The symptoms of patients with BP hepatitis usually include abdominal pain and fever. All eight patients reported by Perkocha et al.[17] had hepatomegaly, and six also had splenomegaly. Two had a splenectomy, and histopathologic examination revealed BP of the spleen. One fourth of the patients also had cutaneous BA lesions. The alkaline phosphatase level was more highly elevated than were the hepatic transaminase levels in these eight patients with BP. Abdominal computed tomography of the peliotic liver usually reveals numerous hypodense lesions,[21,26] as shown in Figure 27–6, but this appearance is not specific for BP hepatis; therefore, the diagnosis of *Bartonella* infection must be confirmed by histopathologic or microbiologic evaluation. Additionally, some HIV-infected patients with hepatic *Bartonella* infection do not develop peliosis hepatis; three patients described by Slater et al.[27] developed inflammatory nodules in the liver. Patients with splenic BP may have thrombocytopenia or pancytopenia, and abdominal ascites may be present.[25,28,29]

Gastrointestinal and Respiratory Tract BA

Histopathologically proven BA of the gastrointestinal tract has been described by several groups.[30–32] The lesions can involve oral, anal, peritoneal, and gastrointestinal tissue, appearing as raised, nodular, ulcerated intraluminal mucosal abnormalities of the stomach and large and small intestine during endoscopy.[32] Extraluminal, intra-abdominal BA presenting with massive upper gastrointestinal hemorrhage also has been described.[31] Hemorrhage occurred when the highly vascular mass eroded through small intestine; *B. quintana* was cultured from

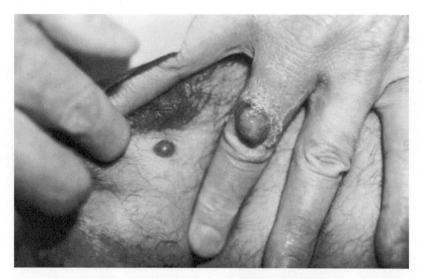

FIGURE 27–1. A friable, exophytic angiomatous BA nodule of the finger and an evolving dome-shaped vascular papule in the same patient. (From Koehler JE, LeBoit PE, Egbert BM, et al: Cutaneous vascular lesions and disseminated cat-scratch disease in patients with the acquired immunodeficiency syndrome [AIDS] and AIDS-related complex. Ann Intern Med 109:449, 1988, with permission.)

tissue obtained by transabdominal needle biopsy of the mass.

BA lesions of the respiratory tract have been observed in the larynx,[30,33] and, in one patient, enlarged to cause an asphyxiative death.[30] Endobronchial BA lesions have been visualized during bronchoscopy, and described as polypoid lesions located in the segmental bronchi in addition to the trachea.[34,35] Several patients with these lesions also had cutaneous BA lesions. *Bartonella* infection also can cause pulmonary nodules in immunocompromised patients; a renal transplant patient with chemotherapy-induced immunocompromise developed high fever (41°C) and bilateral pulmonary nodules.[36] *Bartonella henselae* DNA was demonstrated in the parenchymal lung nodule biopsy specimens obtained at open lung biopsy.

Lymph Node BA

Lymph node involvement has been described frequently in association with cutaneous lesions or peliosis of the liver or spleen.[21] In these cases, the lymph nodes most commonly affected are those draining the BA lesion, and histopathologic examination may reveal angiomatous changes within the lymph node. In other cases, however, BA may involve only a single or several lymph nodes, in the absence of cutaneous or other organ involvement.

Neuropsychiatric Manifestations Associated with **Bartonella** Infection

Bartonella infection has been associated with aseptic meningitis,[20] parenchymal brain masses,[37] chronic central nervous system (CNS) dysfunction,[38] and acute psychiatric decompensation[39] in HIV-infected individuals. A left temporal lobe mass due to BA was reported in an HIV-infected patient with new onset of seizures and facial nerve deficit.[37] The etiology of the mass remained undetermined for 8 months until the patient developed a cutaneous BA lesion. Treatment with erythromycin led to resolution of the cutaneous lesion and neurologic deficit; the parenchymal mass decreased in size during antibiotic treatment. In a study of HIV-infected patients with CNS dysfunction, evaluation for antibodies to *B. henselae* in cerebrospinal fluid (CSF) and serum of 50 HIV-infected patients revealed that 32% of serum samples (16/50) and 26% of the CSF specimens (13/50) had anti–*B. henselae* immunoglobulin G antibodies.[38] Another report details acute psychiatric symptoms that developed in two patients with biopsy-confirmed cutaneous BA, and resolved after the patients were treated with antibiotics appropriate for their BA infection.[39]

Unusual BA Presentations

Several cases of BA involving the bone marrow have been reported.[4,28,40] Hepatosplenomegaly

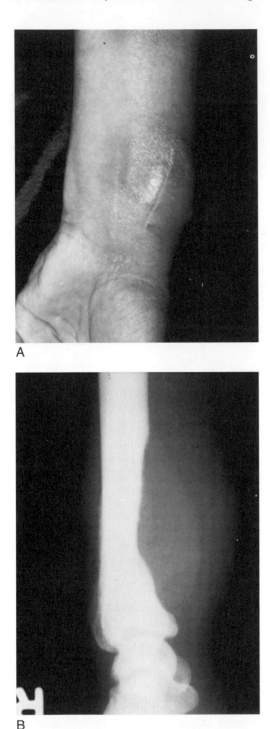

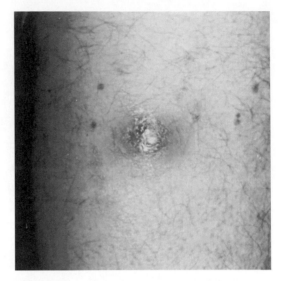

FIGURE 27–3. Unusual-appearing erythematous, dry, scaling plaque of cutaneous BA mimicking staphylococcal pyoderma. *Bartonella quintana* was cultured from this lesion. (From Koehler JE, Tappero JW: AIDS commentary: Bacillary angiomatosis and bacillary peliosis in patients infected with human immunodeficiency virus. Clin Infect Dis 17:612, 1993, with permission.)

FIGURE 27–2. *A*, A tense, firm, erythematous wrist mass due to BA. *B*, A roentgenogram of the wrist of the same patient, demonstrating cortical bone erosion of the radius, with active periostitis, adjacent to the vascular soft tissue mass. (From Koehler JE, LeBoit PE, Egbert BM, et al: Cutaneous vascular lesions and disseminated cat-scratch disease in patients with the human immunodeficiency virus [AIDS] and AIDS-related complex. Ann Intern Med 109:449, 1988, with permission.

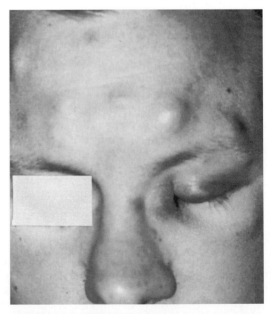

FIGURE 27–4. Multiple subcutaneous BA nodules in a patient with concomitant KS of the medial left eye canthus. (From Koehler JE, Tappero JW: AIDS commentary: Bacillary angiomatosis and bacillary peliosis in patients infected with human immunodeficiency virus. Clin Infect Dis 17:612, 1993, with permission.)

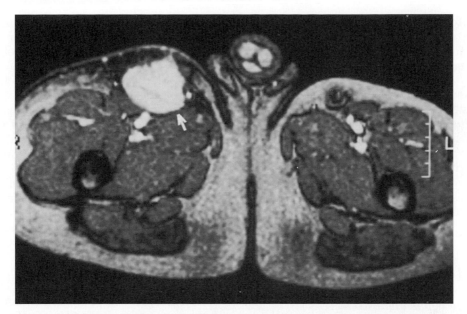

FIGURE 27–5. Magnetic resonance image showing a deep, highly vascular, subcutaneous soft-tissue mass of BA in the anterior right thigh. (From Koehler JE, Tappero JW: AIDS commentary: Bacillary angiomatosis and bacillary peliosis in patients infected with human immunodeficiency virus. Clin Infect Dis 17:612, 1993, with permission.)

and thrombocytopenia were noted in both of these patients, and both resolved after antibiotic treatment. Venous thrombosis of the left upper extremity occurred in an AIDS patient with *B. quintana* bacteremia during relapse.[11] The thrombosis was characterized by multiple non-contiguous, erythematous, tender superficial thromboses in the absence of trauma or intravenous drug use, and all rapidly resolved after institution of antibiotic therapy.

Cutaneous BA complicating pregnancy in an HIV-infected woman has been reported.[41] The cutaneous lesions resolved after antibiotic treatment, and the subsequent pregnancy and delivery were uneventful. BA lesions have been described in pediatric patients: one patient was immunocompromised as a result of chemotherapy,[42] the other had been infected with HIV-1 perinatally.[43]

Bacteremia with Bartonella Species

Some patients with BA and BP also have bacteremia. One half of our patients with culture-

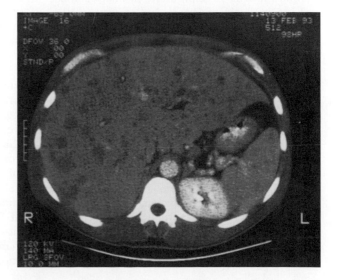

FIGURE 27–6. Computed tomography of the abdomen showing hepatosplenomegaly with numerous low-density hepatic parenchymal lesions. Pelvic ascites and pulmonary effusions were also seen. Percutaneous biopsy of the liver demonstrated peliosis hepatis by histopathology. (From Koehler JE, Tappero JW: AIDS commentary: Bacillary angiomatosis and bacillary peliosis in patients infected with human immunodeficiency virus. Clin Infect Dis 17:612, 1993, with permission.)

positive focal BA or BP also had the corresponding *Bartonella* species simultaneously cultured from the blood.[12] *Bartonella* bacteremia in the absence of focal BA disease has been reported by a number of groups,[5,6,19] and may be more common than focal *Bartonella* disease. Individuals with HIV infection and concomitant *Bartonella* bacteremia usually had systemic symptoms, including fever, chills, and weight loss, that resolved after antibiotic therapy. One patient with HIV infection and culture-proven *B. quintana* bacteremia had endocarditis.[18] A second case of *Bartonella* endocarditis in a patient without apparent immunocompromise was attributed to *B. elizabethae*.[44]

Diagnosis of *Bartonella* Infections

Histopathologic Diagnosis

OBTAINING TISSUE FOR DIAGNOSIS. Biopsy is the principal intervention available for the diagnosis of cutaneous BA. Because KS lesions can be clinically indistinguishable from those of BA, any new vascular lesion should be biopsied. In patients with previously diagnosed KS, any vascular lesion that has a different appearance or rate of growth also should be biopsied, because KS and cutaneous BA can occur simultaneously in the same patient.[45,46] Pedunculated lesions can be biopsied by shave excision, and smaller papular or subcutaneous lesions should be examined by punch biopsy. Biopsy of the cellulitic plaque that frequently overlies osteolytic lesions may be sufficient to yield a diagnosis of BA, but in some patients open excisional bone biopsy is necessary.[11] Fine-needle aspiration of BA lymph nodes has not been useful in diagnosis of BA in our center; open excisional or incisional biopsy remains the optimal technique for diagnosis. For BP of the liver or spleen, the diagnostic procedure with greatest yield appears to be excisional wedge biopsy of the liver or splenectomy; however, peliosis hepatis has been diagnosed by either transvenous liver biopsy[47] or percutaneous liver biopsy.[25] As with cutaneous lesions, several opportunistic infections and malignancies can have a similar appearance on computed tomography of the abdomen; biopsy is therefore extremely important to direct specific treatment. No case of hemorrhage following percutaneous biopsy of a peliotic liver has been reported, but this remains a theoretical concern.

HISTOPATHOLOGIC CHARACTERISTICS. A characteristic vascular proliferation is seen on routine hematoxylin and eosin staining of BA or peliotic tissue (Fig. 27–7A and Color Plate II*H*). Numerous bacilli also can be demonstrated in these lesions by modified silver staining (e.g., Warthin-Starry, Steiner, Dieterle) or electron microscopy (Fig. 27–7B).[16,17,48] Other stains, such as those for tissue Gram's staining, fungi or acid-fast mycobacteria, do not stain *Bartonella* bacilli.

Cutaneous BA lesions may be misdiagnosed histopathologically, most often as KS,[2,3,35,49] angiosarcoma[23,24,30,49] and pyogenic granuloma.[33,50,51] The histopathologic appearance of cutaneous BA lesions may be indistinguishable from pyogenic granuloma (lobular capillary hemangioma) and verruga peruana, the late, chronic phase of infection with *B. bacilliformis*.[3]

A histopathologic diagnosis of pyogenic granuloma, angiosarcoma, or peliosis of the liver or spleen in an HIV-infected patient should prompt further evaluation of the tissue for bacilli, to determine whether the lesion may actually be due to *Bartonella* infection. The presence of bacillary organisms is the diagnostic feature that distinguishes cutaneous BA, extracutaneous BA, and parenchymal BP from these other diagnoses (with the exception of the cutaneous lesions of verruga peruana, which are associated with *B. bacilliformis* bacilli).

Serologic Diagnosis

Bartonella antibodies can be detected by an indirect fluorescence antibody (IFA) test developed at the Centers for Disease Control and Prevention.[52] This test detects *Bartonella* antibodies in the serum of patients with BA.[53] Antibodies to *Bartonella* were detected in seven HIV-infected patients with biopsy-confirmed cutaneous BA, and no antibodies were detected in seven HIV-infected patients without BA. For three of the patients with *Bartonella* antibodies, examination of banked serum revealed the presence of *Bartonella* antibodies as long as 7 years prior to the development of BA disease, suggesting infection with this bacterium occurred years before the diagnosis of BA. Prior to the diagnosis of BA in these three patients, a fourfold rise in titer occurred, raising the possibility of either relapse or reinfection. Culture-proven relapse in another BA patient[11] also was predicted by a rising serum antibody titer.[53] This IFA thus appears to be promising for the diagnosis of BA and other *Bartonella*-associated infections in HIV-infected patients, as well as in monitoring the response to antibiotic treatment.

FIGURE 27–7. *A*, Hematoxylin and eosin staining of a biopsied cutaneous BA lesion demonstrating a dermal vessel. The vessel is lined with protuberant endothelial cells surrounded by myxoid connective tissue containing neutrophils and amphophilic granular material in close proximity to the vascular lumen. *B*, Transmission electron micrograph of cutaneous tissue showing multiple trilaminar cell-walled bacillary organisms. (From Koehler JE, LeBoit PE, Egbert BM, et al: Cutaneous vascular lesions and disseminated cat-scratch disease in patients with the acquired immunodeficiency syndrome [AIDS] and AIDS-related complex. Ann Intern Med 109: 449, 1988, with permission.)

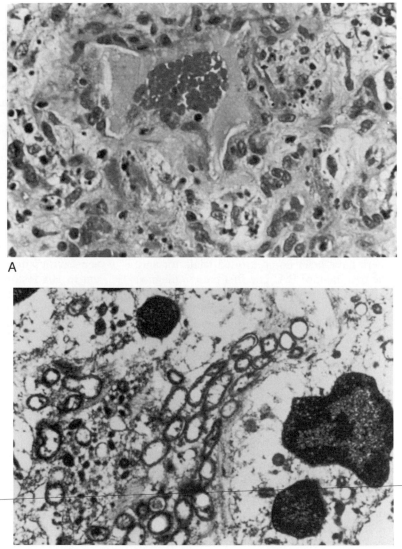

A

B

Culture of Bartonella *Species from Blood and Tissue of Patients with BA*

Slater et al.[5] first reported isolation of *Bartonella* species from blood using lysis–centrifugation tubes (Isostat Tubes; Wampole, Cranbury, NJ) and plating onto fresh chocolate or heart infusion agar with 5% rabbit blood, without antibiotics. Standard blood collection tubes containing EDTA also have been used to isolate *B. henselae* from the blood of an HIV-infected patient.[6] Detection of *B. quintana* bacteremia also has been reported using acridine orange staining of aliquots removed from BACTEC blood culture bottles.[54] The use of quantitative cultures (e.g., lysis–centrifugation tubes) demonstrates

that immunocompromised patients may have a high-grade bacteremia with *Bartonella*, with blood cultures yielding greater than 1000 colony-forming units per milliliter of blood.[11]

Isolation of *Bartonella* species directly from cutaneous BA lesions is difficult because of the fastidious growth characteristics of this genus. Either *B. quintana* or *B. henselae* can be isolated by mincing a sterilely obtained cutaneous,[11] lymph node,[55] splenic,[25] or hepatic biopsy specimen in inoculation media,[11] then spreading onto fresh chocolate or heart infusion agar with 5% rabbit blood and incubating for at least 3 to 4 weeks in 5% CO_2. The highest recovery rate of *Bartonella* species from cutaneous BA lesions has been accomplished using an endothelial cell monolayer co-cultivation system,[11] but this system is not readily available to most microbiology labs.

Because culture of *Bartonella* species from biopsied cutaneous or hepatic tissue remains difficult, culture from blood represents the most accessible method of isolating *Bartonella* species. However, bacteremia is not always present in patients with cutaneous BA or peliosis hepatis.

Treatment of *Bartonella* Infections

Choice of Antibiotics

There have been no controlled trials for antibiotic treatment of BA. The first patient diagnosed with BA was treated empirically with erythromycin, with complete resolution of subcutaneous nodules.[1] From subsequent reports, and our experience at San Francisco General Hospital, it is evident that erythromycin or doxycycline is the drug of first choice for patients with BA and BP (Fig. 27–8). Oral erythromycin therapy of 500 mg four times a day or oral doxycycline therapy with 100 mg twice a day is standard, but intravenous therapy should be given to patients with severe disease or those unable to tolerate oral medication. Resolution of BA caused by *B. henselae* also has been reported in one HIV-infected patient following oral tetracycline treatment[11] and two immunocompetent patients with *B. henselae* bacteremia.[5] Cutaneous BA in an immunocompetent patient also has been successfully treated with minocycline.[56] In several retrospective descriptions of patients with cutaneous BA, resolution of lesions was noted to be temporally related to institution of antimycobacterial therapy[2,3,57–59] presumably as a result of the rifampin component. A summary of the apparent clinical efficacy of antibiotics for *Bartonella* infections in HIV-infected individuals is presented in Table 27–1. It is important to note that some patients develop a Jarisch-Herxheimer reaction after the first several doses of antibiotic, with exacerbation of systemic symptoms and fever.[11] This response may be attenuated by pretreatment with an antipyretic.

The clinical response of patients with BA to treatment with erythromycin, doxycycline, and tetracycline usually corresponds to the in vitro susceptibilities of *B. quintana* and *B. henselae*.[5,44,60,61] However, there is little correlation between the in vivo and in vitro antibiotic susceptibilities for other antibiotics, especially those

that target steps in cell wall synthesis (e.g., penicillins). It is obvious from numerous reports that penicillin, penicillinase-resistant pencillins, aminopenicillins, and first-generation cephalosporins have no activity against the *B. quintana* and *B. henselae* bacilli in BA lesions.[2,3,11,33,45,50,62] Apparent response to some antibiotics (e.g., vancomycin[33] or a first-generation cephalosporin[50] likely represents the treatment of superinfecting skin flora. We pretreated one patient who had superinfected cutaneous BA lesions with cephradine to improve selective recovery of *Bartonella* organisms from the lesions,[11] and *B. quintana* was isolated from the BA lesions of another patient who had received nafcillin and gentamicin for several days prior to biopsy.[12] The differences between in vitro and in vivo sensitivities may result because the bacilli present in BA lesions have different cell wall characteristics from those grown on agar, which changes the susceptibility to cell wall–active antibiotics. Additionally, the fastidious nature of *Bartonella* species makes accurate susceptibility testing difficult to perform.

Rifampin may have clinical efficacy in treating *Bartonella* infections (Table 27–1), but use of this drug alone is not recommended because of the rapid development of resistance. For severely ill patients, we administer rifampin in addition to a first-line drug (erythromycin or doxycycline) during the initial several weeks of therapy. For some other antibiotics with possible clinical efficacy, listed in Table 27–1, single case reports have been associated with improvement in lesions or symptoms, but the response to these antibiotics is not consistent enough to warrant their recommendation at present. It also is difficult to directly attribute improvement of symptoms to treatment with a specific antibiotic when many patients have concomitant infection with other pathogens. The clinical efficacy of ciprofloxacin, trimethoprim-sulfamethoxazole, and third-generation cephalosporins remains inconclusive. One pregnant patient received 2 weeks of ceftizoxime treatment for cutaneous BA and had complete resolution of lesions.[41] In our study of patients with BA, we have observed progression of lesions in patients treated with ciprofloxacin.[48] Although one patient improved when treated with trimethoprim-sulfamethoxazole,[35] most did not or had lesions that progressed,[14,18,41,43,62] and we have isolated *B. henselae* from the tissue of two patients taking prophylactic oral trimethoprim-sulfamethoxazole.[12] In contrast, no *Bartonella* isolate was recovered from any BA patient treated with a tetracycline or erythromycin (even after a single

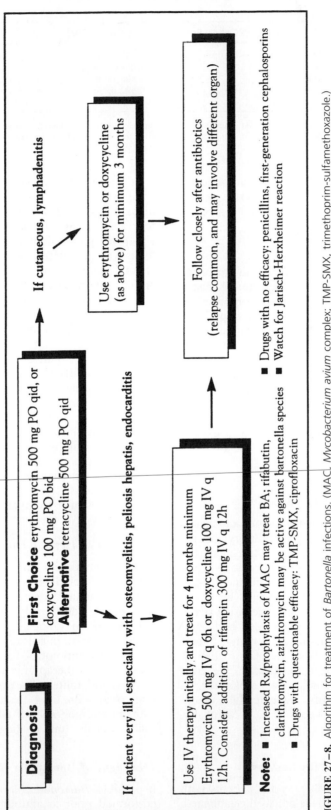

Diagnosis

First Choice erythromycin 500 mg PO qid, or doxycycline 100 mg PO bid
Alternative tetracycline 500 mg PO qid

If cutaneous, lymphadenitis

If patient very ill, especially with osteomyelitis, peliosis hepatis, endocarditis

Use IV therapy initially and treat for 4 months minimum
Erythromycin 500 mg IV q 6h or doxycycline 100 mg IV q 12h. Consider addition of rifampin 300 mg IV q 12h

Use erythromycin or doxycycline (as above) for minimum 3 months

Follow closely after antibiotics (relapse common, and may involve different organ)

Note:
■ Increased Rx/prophylaxis of MAC may treat BA; rifabutin, clarithromycin, azithromycin may be active against bartonella species
■ Drugs with questionable efficacy: TMP-SMX, ciprofloxacin
■ Drugs with no efficacy: penicillins, first-generation cephalosporins
■ Watch for Jarisch-Herxheimer reaction

FIGURE 27–8. Algorithm for treatment of *Bartonella* infections. (MAC, *Mycobacterium avium* complex; TMP-SMX, trimethoprim-sulfamethoxazole.) (From Koehler J: Recurrent bacterial infections: *Bartonella.* Clin Care Options HIV 1:17, 1995, with permission.)

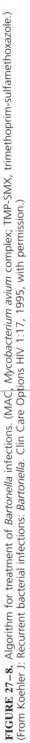

TABLE 27–1. Clinical Efficacy of Antibiotics in the Treatment of BA and BP

DEFINITE	POSSIBLE	INCONCLUSIVE	NONE
Erythromycin	Rifampin	Gentamicin	Penicillin
Doxycycline		Ciprofloxacin	Ceph[1]
Tetracycline		Ceftriaxone	PCN-D
Minocycline		Ceftizoxime	
		TMP/SMX	

Abbreviations: Ceph[1], first-generation cephalosporins; PCN-D, penicillin derivatives (PCNase-resistant penicillins and aminopenicillins); TMP-SMX, trimethoprim-sulfamethoxazole.

dose),[63] and prior treatment with a macrolide has been found to be significantly protective against development of BA.[12]

Relapse

Both *B. qunitana*[64] and *B. henselae*[65] produce relapsing illness in immunocompetent hosts; it is thus not surprising that immunocompromised patients with BA or BP frequently experience relapse despite prolonged antibiotic therapy.[5,6,11,33,45,50,62,66] It should be noted that reinfection remains a possibility in these patients, but the majority of these cases probably represent relapse. The frequency of relapse appears to be increased when patients are treated with antibiotics for a shorter duration; over the past 7 years, as the result of our increased experience, we have increased the duration of treatment for all presentations of BA.

Treatment of Cutaneous BA Lesions

Immunocompromised patients with cutaneous BA should be evaluated for parenchymal and osseous disease before beginning treatment, because the presence of either one requires treatment for a longer duration. For cutaneous disease alone, antibiotic therapy can be given orally. Response of cutaneous lesions is usually rapid, with improvement in 1 week and complete resolution by 1 month,[67] although hyperpigmentation may persist at the site of the lesion. As a result of our experience, we treat patients with cutaneous lesions alone for 12 weeks; if relapse occurs, we extend treatment for an additional 16 weeks and, occasionally, treat indefinitely.

Treatment of Osseous BA Lesions

Duration of antibiotic therapy for patients with *Bartonella* osteomyelitis is not well established. We treated one patient (see Fig. 27–2)

with erythromycin, which the patient self-administered at a dose of 500 mg orally six times a day for 2 months, followed by 500 mg four times a day for an additional two months.[2] The osteolytic lesion resolved completely and there was no relapse of BA during the subsequent 24 months; the patient died of another opportunistic infection. Relapse occurred in another patient with osseous BA[11] despite 4 months of oral treatment with 500 to 1000 mg erythromycin four times a day; the osseous BA healed but the patient relapsed with *B. quintana* bacteremia 1 month after stopping erythromycin. For patients with osseous BA, it may be most appropriate to treat initially with several weeks of intravenous antibiotics (erythromycin or doxycycline), followed by prolonged, and perhaps indefinite, oral antimicrobial therapy. Serial technetium-99m methylene diphosphonate bone scans or roentgenograms can be used to monitor treatment efficacy, although resolution of osseous lesions is delayed, as seen with other causes of osteomyelitis.

Treatment of Hepatic and Splenic BP

Most patients with BP have severe systemic symptoms, including nausea and vomiting, that may substantially decrease absorption or oral antibiotics. Additionally, oral erythromycin or doxycycline may not be tolerated by these patients; therefore, initial treatment should be with intravenous antibiotics for several weeks, followed by oral therapy for at least 4 months, and possibly indefinitely. Treatment progress can be monitored with liver function tests and serial computed tomography if peliotic lesions are visualized at the time of diagnosis (Fig. 27–6).

Treatment of Bartonella *Bacteremia*

If possible, *Bartonella* blood cultures should be performed prior to antibiotic treatment for patients with all forms of BA. Because endocarditis can develop during infection with *B. quintana*,[18,68] *B. henselae*,[69] and *B. elizabethae*,[44] all patients with *Bartonella* bacteremia and a cardiac murmur should be evaluated further with echocardiography. Within 1 week of beginning antibiotic treatment, immunocompromised patients with isolated *Bartonella* bacteremia usually note resolution of fever and most other constitutional symptoms, although one patient did not have permanent remission of fever until he had received 8 weeks of treatment.[5] An initial period of intravenous antibiotic therapy is probably appropriate, followed by at least 3 months of oral antibiotic therapy. If endocarditis is documented, prolonged intravenous antibiotic therapy should be administered.

In summary, the drug of first choice for BA or BP is erythromycin or doxycycline. If neither can be used, alternatives include tetracycline and minocycline. Patients very ill with systemic symptoms, with osteomyelitis, or with endocarditis should initially receive intravenous therapy with erythromycin or doxycycline, probably with rifampin.[70]

Epidemiology and Prevention of *Bartonella* Infections

Arthropods serve as vectors of several *Bartonella* species; for example, *B. quintana* is known to be transmitted from the human reservoir via the body louse to other humans.[64] Ticks also are possible vectors: two patients reported tick bites preceding the diagnosis of *B. henselae* bacteremia.[7,65] However, at present, the vector most strongly implicated in transmission of at least one *Bartonella* species to humans, *B. henselae*, is the domestic cat.

Bartonella henselae has been identified as the principal bacterial agent causing CSD in immunocompetent individuals by serologic studies,[52] by direct culture from lymph nodes with histopathologic characteristics suggestive of CSD,[55] and by demonstrating the presence of *Bartonella* DNA (but not *A. felis* DNA) in the CSD skin test antigen.[71] Similarly, an association between cat exposure and the development of BA has been noted anecdotally in many case reports.[21] The first systematic evaluation of the relationship between cat contact, numerous other environmental exposures, and development of BA was conducted by Tappero et al.[48] This case–control study found a significant epidemiologic association between development of BA and traumatic cat exposure (cat bite or cat scratch). Both CSD and BA caused by *B.*

henselae have been statistically associated with cat exposure,[12,48,72] with the cat as potential vector, reservoir, or both.

The domestic cat is the major reservoir for *B. henselae*. The association between *B. henselae*–infected cats and development of BA in cat owners was demonstrated in 1994, when bacteremia was detected in all seven cat contacts of four patients with BA caused by *B. henselae*.[73] It was further found that about 40% of the domestic cat population sampled in the greater San Francisco Bay Area was bacteremic with *B. henselae*.[73,74]

The cat flea has now been established to be a vector of *B. henselae*.[75] An epidemiologic association between owning a kitten with fleas and development of CSD was found by Zangwill et at.[72] Additionally, a seroprevalence survey of *B. henselae* antibodies in pet cats throughout regions of North America revealed that the regions with the highest average prevalences of antibodies coincided with the geographic areas predicted to have the highest prevalence of the cat flea (e.g., Hawaii, coastal California, the Pacific Northwest, and south central plains).[76] Viable *B. henselae* bacilli were isolated from several fleas combed from a bacteremic cat.[73] Finally, *B. henselae* transmission from cat to cat via the cat flea was demonstrated in 1996.[75]

Despite the high prevalence of infection in the pet cat population (there are 57 million pet cats in the United States), transmission of *B. henselae* to humans is relatively rare, and thus the benefit of these companion animals far outweighs the risk of *B. henselae* infection.[77] We suggest that several practical measures be followed to reduce the risk of *B. henselae* infection in HIV-infected individuals: (1) wash hands after petting and handling pets; (2) wash bites and scratches immediately with soap and water; (3) never allow any pet to lick an open wound; and (4) minimize infestation with fleas.

Although the domestic cat has been identified as the major reservoir and vector for *B. henselae*, it is quite evident that *B. quintana*, which causes nearly half of the BA infections in San Francisco, is not associated with cat contact. In a study of 49 patients and 96 matched controls, patients with BA caused by *B. quintana* infection were significantly more likely than controls to be homeless, have low socioeconomic status, and have had recent infestation with head or body lice.[12] Physicians should consider *B. quintana* infection in homeless patients with fever, whether or not cutaneous lesions are present; strategies to prevent infection with *B. quintana* are currently limited to reducing exposure to body lice.

RHODOCOCCUS EQUI INFECTIONS

Clinical Presentation

Rhodococcus equi has been known to be a veterinary pathogen since the 1920s but was not recognized as a human pathogen until 1967, when the first case report of pulmonary abscess in a human was published.[78] In recent years, increasing numbers of patients with *R. equi* have been described, the majority of whom have concomitant HIV infection. A comprehensive review of 72 cases revealed that 86% of the patients with *R. equi* were immunocompromised, and the majority of these patients developed pulmonary infection.[79] In contrast, the majority of the immunocompetent patients in this series had extrapulmonary disease.

The clinical presentation in HIV-infected patients with *R. equi* includes chest pain, productive cough, dyspnea, hemoptysis, and fever.[79-82] In many patients, symptoms were present for several weeks to months prior to diagnosis, and included anorexia, malaise, and weight loss.[80,81] Roentgenographic findings of *R. equi* infection in HIV-infected patients include pulmonary infiltrates, pleural effusion, empyema, and, most distinctively, cavitary lung disease (more frequently in the upper lobes than the lower lobes in HIV-infected patients) (Fig. 27–9).[79-81,83,84] Because patients with late-stage HIV infection are less likely to develop cavitary disease with *Mycobacterium tuberculosis* infection than early after HIV infection, *R. equi* should be considered to be a potential cause of cavitary pulmonary disease in patients with very low CD4 cell counts.[79] Also included with *Rhodococcus* in the differential diagnosis of cavitary pulmonary disease in late-stage HIV infection are *Nocardia*, *Pseudomonas*, *Mycobacterium kansasii*, and *Aspergillus* infection.[85] In addition to parenchymal and cavitary disease, *R. equi* also has been associated with an endobronchial mass in an HIV-infected patient.[86]

Bacteremia developed in 53% of the immunocompromised patients with *R. equi* infection.[79]

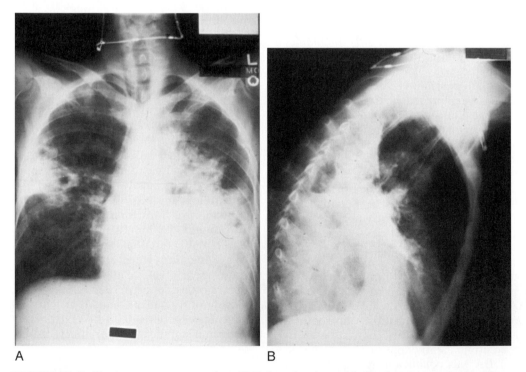

A   B

FIGURE 27–9. Chest roentgenograms of an HIV-infected patient with *Rhodococcus equi* pulmonary infection. Posteroanterior (*A*) and lateral (*B*) views reveal bilateral pulmonary infiltrates with cavitation and air–fluid levels. An undrained empyema also is present in the left chest. (From Verville TD, Huycke MM, Greenfield RA, et al: *Rhodococcus equi* infections of humans: 12 cases and a review of the literature. Medicine 73:119, 1994, with permission.)

Brain abscesses caused by *R. equi* have been documented in several HIV-infected patients, and were presumed to have developed from hematogenous infection in patients with extensive pulmonary disease and bacteremia.[79,82,87] One HIV-infected patient developed a foot mycetoma as a result of *R. equi* that progressed to sequentially involve the ipsilateral inguinal lymph nodes, pulmonary parenchyma, and, probably, brain parenchyma.[87]

Diagnosis of *Rhodococcus* Infections

Rhodococcus equi infection is most readily diagnosed by isolation from sputum or bronchoalveolar lavage fluid and from normally sterile sites, including blood, pleural fluid, and biopsied tissue. The organism is a facultative intracellular, gram-positive, nonmotile, non-spore-forming, aerobic coccobacillus that belongs to the phylogenetic group of nocardioform actinomycetes.[88] The organism grows readily on routine bacteriologic media, including Sabouraud, Lowenstein-Jensen, sheep blood, and chocolate agars and aerobic blood culture media.[82] Distinctive, moist to mucoid, buff to salmon-pink colonies form on agar after 24 to 72 hours of incubation. In broth, bacillary forms predominate, and, on solid agar, cocci are usually seen.[82]

Of note, *R. equi* contains mycolic acids in the cell wall, as do species of the related genera *Mycobacteria* and *Nocardia*; thus *Rhodococcus* may stain weakly positive with acid-fast stains. Two immunocompromised patients received more than 1 month of antituberculous therapy before the acid-fast–staining bacilli from sputum smears were identified correctly as *R. equi*.[84] Additionally, *R. equi* may resemble diphtheroids in respiratory smears and cultures, leading to their erroneous identification as a respiratory contaminant.[81] When *R. equi* is isolated from sterile sites, it should never be considered a contaminating diphtheroid.[82]

Histopathologic findings in resected soft tissue or pulmonary masses include a necrotizing, granulomatous reaction with abundant polymorphonuclear leukocytes and microabscesses.[79,82] Organisms are readily stained in tissue and visualized within histiocytes using tissue Gram's and periodic acid–Schiff stains. Although organisms from young colonies on culture plates may stain acid fast using the Kinyoun stain, tissue acid-fast stains such as Auramine O and modified Fite do not stain *R. equi* in tissue.[82]

Treatment of *Rhodococcus* Infections

Rhodococcus equi isolates are usually susceptible to erythromycin, rifampin, vancomycin, ciprofloxacin, and gentamicin.[79,89] There is usually resistance to pencillins, and, even if an isolate is susceptible initially, resistance to penicillin, ampicillin or first-generation cephalosporins can develop rapidly during treatment with these antibiotics.[88] It is important to perform antimicrobial susceptibility testing on initial patient isolates to direct antimicrobial therapy. Follow-up cultures should be obtained, and, because resistance can develop during therapy with first-line antibiotics, susceptibility testing should be repeated for *R. equi* isolates obtained during antimicrobial therapy. In one case, a patient with *R. equi* foot mycetoma was first treated with trimethoprim-sulfamethoxazole and rifampin, to which the initial isolate was susceptible. However, when pulmonary disease developed, the subsequent isolate from bronchoalveolar lavage fluid was resistant to trimethoprim-sulfamethoxazole.[87] The pulmonary parenchymal lesions resolved completely over the ensuing 5 months during therapy with rifampin and ciprofloxacin. Another patient was treated with rifampin and ciprofloxacin and, although the initial isolate was rifampin sensitive, the *R. equi* isolated after recurrence of pulmonary disease was rifampin resistant.[90] The patient was then treated with the combination of doxycycline and erythromycin and the disease stabilized for the 5 months of subsequent follow-up.

Administration of two or three drugs appears to be important for treatment of patients with concomitant HIV and *R. equi* infection. Efficacy of antibiotics for *R. equi* infection has been studied most extensively in veterinary disease: a combination of rifampin plus erythromycin is apparently superior to combinations of penicillins, aminoglycosides, or trimethoprim-sulfamethoxazole.[80] An immunocompromised transplant patient with vertebral osteomyelitis was treated with erythromycin and imipenem, then erythromycin, but required surgical drainage subsequently. Postoperatively, this patient was then treated successfully with imipenem, vancomycin, and erythromycin, followed by maintenance therapy with clarithromycin and rifabutin.[91] *Rhodococcus equi* is a facultatively intracellular organism that can infect polymorphonuclear leukocytes and macrophages, and can persist in macrophages; it is therefore recommended that the regimen include at least one and preferably two lipid-soluble drugs with good intracellular penetration.[80,81,84] However, vancomycin demonstrated good activity in an animal model and has been used successfully in human regimens despite poor intracellular penetration.[79] A combination of vancomycin and imipenem was used successfully in one patient.[92] Some early case reports suggest that treatment may be facilitated by surgical resection of parenchymal abscesses, but disease recurred in one HIV-infected patient after lobectomy, and the benefit of this approach is unclear at present.[90]

The optimal duration for antimicrobial therapy is not known, but cumulative data from case reports indicate that prolonged, even lifelong therapy may be necessary. Treatment should be initiated with two or three antibiotics and continued for 2 to 6 months; subsequent therapy with one or two antibiotics is probably necessary to prevent relapse in HIV-infected individuals.[80,81,83,84] Even when patients with HIV and *R. equi* co-infection receive appropriate antimicrobial treatment, the infection may be fatal; one review reported that chronic *R. equi* infection occurred in 47% and death occurred in 43% of patients.[79]

Epidemiology and Prevention of *Rhodococcus* Infections

Rhodococcus equi causes chronic suppurative bronchopneumonia in foals less than 6 months of age; pulmonary disease can be complicated by ulcerative colitis and mesenteric adenitis. *Rhodococcus equi* represents a substantial veterinary pathogen, infecting up to 10% of foals in endemic areas and causing death in up to one third of those infected.[79] *Rhodococcus equi* is a common inhabitant of the gut of herbivores, and its presence is widespread: *R. equi* has been demonstrated in the soil of all continents except Antarctica, but it is found especially frequently on horse ranches.[79,81] Both human and equine infection are presumed to result from exposure to soil contaminated with the manure from infected animals, primarily via inhalation. Ingestion has also been implicated as a route of infection, and direct soft tissue inoculation via soil contamination of superficial wounds has been well documented, especially in immunocompetent individuals.[79,82,87]

Approximately one third of patients with *R. equi* infection reported in the literature had potential exposure to contaminated soil,[79] including visiting or working on a horse farm, working as a groom,[80,81,92] or using horse manure

during gardening activities.[93] Some authors have suggested that reactivation of remotely acquired *R. equi* infection may occur, although this has not been clearly demonstrated. Because the majority of HIV-infected patients do not have a defined exposure associated with developing *R. equi* infection, recommendations for prevention of infection with *R. equi* are limited to avoiding exposure to aerosolized soil contaminated with herbivore manure.[94]

PENICILLIUM MARNEFFEI INFECTIONS

Clinical Presentation

Penicillium marneffei is an unusual fungal pathogen in the United States but is the third most common opportunistic infection in HIV-infected patients in some areas of Southeast Asia, after extrapulmonary *M. tuberculosis* infection and cryptococcosis.[95] This infection should be considered in HIV-infected patients who have travelled to or resided in Southeast Asia, where *P. marneffei* is endemic, including Thailand, the Guanxi Province of China, Hong Kong, Vietnam, and Indonesia. Imported cases have been reported in the United States, France, the United Kingdom, the Netherlands, and Australia.[95] The clinical presentation may be very similar to that of disseminated histoplasmosis, and this misdiagnosis has been reported in the literature.[96] In one study of 80 patients with confirmed *P. marneffei* infection, fever was the most common presenting symptom (92%), in addition to other systemic signs and symptoms, including anemia (77%) and weight loss (76%).[95] Distinctive skin lesions were present in 71% of patients at the time of presentation, and the majority of these lesions (87%) had central umbilication, resembling molluscum contagiosum lesions. Larger lesions can form punched-out ulcers.[97] Reactivation after immunosuppression has been reported; disseminated *P. marneffei* infection usually occurs late in HIV infection, and, in two reviews, the CD4 cell counts ranged from 1 to 44/mm³.[95,98]

Diagnosis

Penicillium marneffei is a dimorphic fungus, first isolated from a bamboo rat in Vietnam in 1956. The fungus grows readily on routine fungal culture media in 2 to 5 days, producing an unusual, pinkish-red pigment.[98] *Penicillium marneffei* is most readily isolated from blood, skin lesions, and bone marrow.[95] In endemic regions, where this diagnosis is more frequently encountered, presumptive diagnosis often is made prior to obtaining positive culture results by examination of Wright's-stained samples of bone marrow aspirate or touch smears of skin or lymph node biopsies. In these specimens, *P. marneffei* appears as intrahistiocytic and extracellular basophilic, spherical, oval, and elliptical yeast forms (2 to 6 μ in diameter), some of which contain a clear central septation.[95,99] In contrast, the yeast forms of *Histoplasma capsulatum* usually have narrow-based, unequal budding without septation.[99]

Treatment and Prevention

The majority of patients reported in the literature were treated with amphotericin, and achieved a response. In the largest case series of patients from Thailand, 27 or 39 patients (77%) treated with amphotericin achieved clinical and microbiologic resolution of infection.[95] Seventy-five percent of patients (9/12) responded to treatment with itraconazole, but only 4 of 11 (36%) responded to fluconazole. Like most other systemic fungal infections in HIV-infected patients, there is a propensity for relapse after cessation of antifungal therapy, and lifelong secondary prophylaxis with an antifungal agent (e.g., itraconazole) is recommended. Virtually nothing is known at present about transmission, and therefore prevention, of *P. marneffei* in endemic regions, but is important to note that the high mortality rate attributed to this infection is primarily due to failure to make a timely diagnosis and begin treatment.[95,99]

Acknowledgments

This project was supported by funds from the Universitywide AIDS Research Program and the National Institutes of Health grant AI36075. Dr. Koehler is a Pew Scholar in the Biomedical Sciences.

References

1. Stoler MH, Bonfiglio TA, Steigbigel RT, Pereira M: An atypical subcutaneous infection associated with acquired immune deficiency syndrome. Am J Clin Pathol 80:714, 1983

2. Koehler JE, LeBoit PE, Egbert BM, Berger TG: Cutaneous vascular lesions and disseminated cat-scratch disease in patients with the acquired immunodeficiency syndrome (AIDS) and AIDS-related complex. Ann Intern Med 109:449, 1988

3. LeBoit PE, Berger TG, Egbert BM, et al: Epithelioid haemangioma-like vascular proliferation in AIDS: Manifestation of cat-scratch disease bacillus infection? Lancet 1:960, 1988

4. Relman DA, Loutit JS, Schmidt TM, et al: The agent of bacillary angiomatosis: An approach to the identification of uncultured pathogens. N Engl J Med 323:1573, 1990

5. Slater LN, Welch DF, Hensel D, Coody DW: A newly recognized fastidious gram-negative pathogen as a cause of fever and bacteremia. N Engl J Med 323:1587, 1990

6. Regnery RL, Anderson BE, Clarridge JE, et al: Characterization of a novel *Rochalimaea* species, *R. henselae* sp. nov., isolated from blood of a febrile, human immunodeficiency virus-positive patient. J Clin Microbiol 30:265, 1992

7. Welch DF, Pickett DA, Slater LN, et al: *Rochalimaea henselae* sp. nov., a cause of septicemia, bacillary angiomatosis, and parenchymal bacillary peliosis. J Clin Microbiol 30:275, 1992

8. Brenner DJ, O'Connor SP, Winkler HH, Steigerwalt AG: Proposals to unify the genera *Bartonella* and *Rochalimaea*, with descriptions of *Bartonella quintana* comb. nov., *Bartonella vinsonii* comb. nov., *Bartonella henselae* comb. nov., and *Bartonella elizabethae* comb. nov., and to remove the family *Bartonellaceae* from the order *Rickettsiales*. Int J Syst Bacteriol 43:777, 1993

9. Birtles RJ, Harrison TG, Saunders NA, Molyneux DH: Proposals to unify the genera *Grahamella* and *Bartonella*, with descriptions of *Bartonella talpae* comb. nov., *Bartonella peromysci* comb. nov., and three new species, *Bartonella grahamii* sp. nov., *Bartonella taylorii* sp. nov., and *Bartonella doshiae* sp. nov. Int J Syst Bacteriol 45:1, 1995

10. Lawson PA, Collins MD: Description of *Bartonella clarridgeiae* sp. nov. isolated from the cat of a patient with *Bartonella henselae* septicemia. Med Microbiol Lett 5:64, 1996

11. Koehler JE, Quinn FD, Berger TG, et al: Isolation of *Rochalimaea* species from cutaneous and osseous lesions of bacillary angiomatosis. N Engl J Med 327:1625, 1992

12. Koehler JE, Sanchez MA, Garrido CS, et al: Molecular epidemiology of *Bartonella* infections in patients with bacillary angiomatosis-peliosis. N Engl J Med 337:1876, 1997

13. Adal KA, Cockerell CJ, Petri WA Jr: Cat scratch disease, bacillary angiomatosis, and other infections due to *Rochalimaea*. N Engl J Med 330:1509, 1994

14. Mohle-Boetani JC, Koehler JE, Berger TG, et al: Bacillary angiomatosis and bacillary peliosis in patients infected with human immunodeficiency virus: Clinical characteristics in a case-control study. Clin Infect Dis 22:794, 1996

15. Cockerell CJ, LeBoit PE: Bacillary angiomatosis: A newly characterized, pseudoneoplastic, infectious, cutaneous vascular disorder. J Am Acad Dermatol 22:501, 1990

16. LeBoit PE, Berger TG, Egbert BM, et al: Bacillary angiomatosis: The histopathology and differential diagnosis of a pseudoneoplastic infection in patients with human immunodeficiency virus disease. Am J Surg Pathol 13:909, 1989

17. Perkocha LA, Geaghan SM, Yen TSB, et al: Clinical and pathological features of bacillary peliosis hepatis in association with human immunodeficiency virus infection. N Engl J Med 323:1581, 1990

18. Spach DH, Callis KP, Paauw DS, et al: Endocarditis caused by *Rochalimaea quintana* in a patient infected with human immunodeficiency virus. J Clin Microbiol 31:692, 1993

19. Reed JA, Brigati DJ, Flynn DS, et al: Immunocyto-chemical identification of *Rochalimaea henselae* in bacillary (epithelioid) angiomatosis, parenchymal bacillary peliosis, and persistent fever with bacteremia. Am J Surg Pathol 16:650, 1992

20. Wong MT, Dolan MJ, Lattuada CP Jr, et al: Neuro-retinitis, aseptic meningitis, and lymphadenitis associated with *Bartonella (Rochalimaea) henselae* infection in immunocompetent patients and patients infected with human immunodeficiency virus type 1. Clin Infect Dis 21:352, 1995

21. Koehler JE, Tappero JW: Bacillary angiomatosis and bacillary peliosis in patients infected with human immunodeficiency virus. Clin Infect Dis 17:612, 1993

22. Baron AL, Steinbach LS, LeBoit PE, et al: Osteolytic lesions and bacillary angiomatosis in HIV infection: Radiologic differentiation from AIDS-related Kaposi sarcoma. Radiology 177:77, 1990

23. Herts BR, Rafii M, Spiegel G: Soft-tissue and osseous lesions caused by bacillary angiomatosis: Unusual manifestations of cat-scratch fever in patients with AIDS. Am J Radiol 157:1249, 1991

24. Schinella RA, Greco MA: Bacillary angiomatosis presenting as a soft-tissue tumor without skin involvement. Hum Pathol 21:567, 1990

25. Slater LN, Welch DF, Min KW: *Rochalimaea henselae* causes bacillary angiomatosis and peliosis hepatis. Arch Intern Med 152:602, 1992

26. Wyatt SH, Fishman EK: Hepatic bacillary angiomatosis in a patient with AIDS. Abdom Imaging 18:336, 1993

27. Slater LN, Pitha JV, Herrera L, et al: *Rochalimaea henselae* infection in acquired immunodeficiency syndrome causing inflammatory disease without angiomatosis or peliosis: Demonstration by immunocytochemistry and corroboration by DNA amplification. Arch Pathol Lab Med 118:33 1994

28. Milam M, Balerdi MJ, Toney JF: Epithelioid angiomatosis secondary to disseminated cat scratch disease involving the bone marrow and skin in a patient with acquired immune deficiency syndrome: A case report. Am J Surg 88:180, 1990

29. Schwartzman WA, Marchevsky A, Meyer RD: Epithelioid angiomatosis or cat scratch disease with splenic and hepatic abnormalities in AIDS: Case report and review of the literature. Scand J Infect Dis 22:121, 1990

30. Cockerell CJ, Whitlow MA, Webster GF, Friedman-Kien AE: Epithelioid angiomatosis: A distinct vascular disorder in patients with the acquired immunodeficiency syndrome or AIDS-related complex. Lancet 2:654, 1987

31. Koehler JE, Cederberg L: Intra-abdominal mass associated with gastrointestinal hemorrhage: A new manifestation of bacillary angiomatosis. Gastroenterology 109:2011, 1995

32. Tuur SM, Macher AM, Angritt P, et al: AIDS case for diagnosis series, 1988. Milit Med 153:M57, 1988

33. van der Wouw PA, Hadderingh RJ, Reiss P, et al: Disseminated cat-scratch disease in a patient with AIDS. AIDS 3:751, 1989

34. Foltzer MA, Guiney WB Jr, Wager GC, Alpern HD: Bronchopulmonary bacillary angiomatosis. Chest 104:973, 1993

35. Slater LN, Min KW: Polypoid endobronchial lesions: A manifestation of bacillary angiomatosis. Chest 102:972, 1992

36. Caniza MA, Granger DL, Wilson KH, et al: *Bartonella henselae*: Etiology of pulmonary nodules in a patient with depressed cell-mediated immunity. Clin Infect Dis 20:1505, 1995

37. Spach DH, Panther LA, Thorning DR, et al: Intracerebral bacillary angiomatosis in a patient infected with human immunodeficiency virus. Ann Intern Med 116:740, 1992

38. Schwartzman WA, Patnaik M, Barka NE, Peter JB: *Rochalimaea* antibodies in HIV-associated neurologic disease. Neurology 44:1312, 1994

39. Baker J, Ruiz-Rodriguez R, Whitfeld M, et al: Bacillary angiomatosis: A treatable cause of acute psychiatric symptoms in human immunodeficiency virus infection. J Clin Psychiatry 56:161, 1995

40. Kemper CA, Lombard CM, Deresinski SC, Tompkins LS: Visceral bacillary epithelioid angiomatosis: Possible manifestations of disseminated cat scratch disease in the immunocompromised host: A report of two cases. Am J Med 89:216, 1990

41. Riley LE, Tuomala RE: Bacillary angiomatosis in a pregnant patient with acquired immunodeficiency syndrome. Obstet Gynecol 79:818, 1992

42. Myers SA, Prose NS, Garcia JA, et al: Bacillary angiomatosis in a child undergoing chemotherapy. J Pediatr 121:574, 1992

43. Malane MS, Laude TA, Chen CK, Fikrig S: An HIV-1-positive child with fever and a scalp nodule. Lancet 346:1466, 1995

44. Daly JS, Worthington MG, Brenner DJ, et al: *Rochalimaea elizabethae* sp. nov. isolated from a patient with endocarditis. J Clin Microbiol 31:872, 1993

45. Berger TG, Tappero JW, Kaymen A, LeBoit PE: Bacillary (epithelioid) angiomatosis and concurrent Kaposi's sarcoma in acquired immunodeficiency syndrome. Arch Dermatol 125:1543, 1989

46. Steeper TA, Rosenstein H, Weiser J, et al: Bacillary epithelioid angiomatosis involving the liver, spleen, and skin in an AIDS patient with concurrent Kaposi's sarcoma. Am J Clin Pathol 97:713, 1992

47. Marullo S, Jaccard A, Roulot D, et al: Identification of the *Rochalimaea henselae* 16S rRNA sequence in the liver of a French patient with bacillary peliosis hepatis [letter]. J Infect Dis 166:1462, 1992

48. Tappero JW, Mohle-Boetani J, Koehler JE, et al: The epidemiology of bacillary angiomatosis and bacillary peliosis. JAMA 269:770, 1993

49. Angritt P, Tuur SM, Macher AM, et al: Epithelioid angiomatosis in HIV infection: Neoplasm or cat-scratch disease? [letter] Lancet 1:996, 1988

50. Marasco WA, Lester S, Parsonnet J: Unusual presentation of cat scratch disease in a patient positive for antibody to the human immunodeficiency virus. Rev Infect Dis 11:793, 1989

51. Mui BSK, Mulligan ME, George WL: Response of HIV-associated disseminated cat scratch disease to treatment with doxycycline. Am J Med 89:229, 1990

52. Regnery RL, Olson JG, Perkins BA, Bibb W: Serological response to "*Rochalimaea henselae*" antigen in suspected cat-scratch disease. Lancet 339:1443, 1992

53. Tappero J, Regnery R, Koehler J: Detection of serologic response to Rochalimaea henselae in patients

with bacillary angiomatosis (BA) by immunofluorescent antibody (IFA) testing. In Abstracts of the 32nd Interscience Conference on Antimicrobial Agents and Chemotherapy. Washington, DC, American Society for Microbiology, 1992, Abstract 674

54. Larson AM, Dougherty MJ, Nowowiejski DJ, et al: Detection of *Bartonella* (*Rochalimaea*) *quintana* by routine acridine orange staining of broth blood cultures. J Clin Microbiol 32:1492, 1994

55. Dolan MJ, Wong MT, Regnery RL, et al: Syndrome of *Rochalimaea henselae* adenitis suggesting cat scratch disease. Ann Intern Med 118:331, 1993

56. Tappero JW, Koehler JE, Berger TG, et al: Bacillary angiomatosis and bacillary splenitis in immunocompetent adults. Ann Intern Med 118:363, 1993

57. Hall AV, Roberts CM, Maurice PD, et al: Cat-scratch disease in patient with AIDS: Atypical skin manifestation [letter]. Lancet 2:453, 1988

58. Knobler EH, Silvers DN, Fine KC, et al: Unique vascular skin lesions associated with human immunodeficiency virus. JAMA 260:524, 1988

59. Lopez-Elzaurdia C, Fraga J, Sols M, et al: Bacillary angiomatosis associated with cytomegalovirus infection in a patient with AIDS. Br J Dermatol 125:175, 1991

60. Maurin M, Gasquet S, Ducco C, Raoult D: MICs of 28 antibiotic compounds for 14 *Bartonella* (formerly *Rochalimaea*) isolates. Antimicrob Agents Chemother 39:2387, 1995

61. Myers WF, Grossman DM, Wisseman CLJ: Antibiotic susceptibility patterns in *Rochalimaea quintana*, the agent of trench fever. Antimicrob Agents Chemother 25:690, 1984

62. Szaniawski WK, Don PC, Bitterman SR, Schachner JR: Epithelioid angiomatosis in patients with AIDS. J Am Acad Dermatol 23:41, 1990

63. Whitfeld MJ, Kaveh S, Koehler JE, et al: Bacillary angiomatosis associated with myositis in a patient infected with human immunodeficiency virus. Clin Infect Dis 24:562, 1997

64. Strong RP. Trench Fever: Report of Commission, Medical Research Committee, American Red Cross. Oxford, England, Oxford University Press, 1918

65. Lucey D, Dolan MJ, Moss CW, et al: Relapsing illness due to *Rochalimaea henselae* in immunocompetent hosts: Implication for therapy and new epidemiological associations. Clin Infect Dis 14:638, 1992

66. Krekorian TD, Radner AB, Alcorn JM, et al: Biliary obstruction caused by epithelioid angiomatosis in a patient with AIDS. Am J Med 89:820, 1990

67. Berger TG, Perkocha L: Bacillary angiomatosis. In Volberding P, Jacobson MA (eds): AIDS Clinical Review 1991. New York, Marcel Dekker, 1991, p 83

68. Drancourt M, Mainardi JL, Brouqui P, et al: *Bartonella* (*Rochalimaea*) *quintana* endocarditis in three homeless men. N Engl J Med 332:419, 1995

69. Holmes AH, Greenough TC, Balady GJ, et al: *Bartonella henselae* endocarditis in an immunocompetent adult. Clin Infect Dis 21:1004, 1995

70. Koehler JE: Bartonellosis. In Dolin RH, Masur H, Saag MS (eds): AIDS Therapy. Philadelphia, WB Saunders Company, 1999 (in press)

71. Perkins BA, Swaminathan B, Jackson LA, et al: Case 22-1992—pathogenesis of cat scratch disease [letter]. N Engl J Med 327:1599, 1992

72. Zangwill KM, Hamilton DH, Perkins BA, et al: Cat scratch disease in Connecticut: Epidemiology, risk factors, and evaluation of a new diagnostic test. N Engl J Med 329:8, 1993

73. Koehler JE, Glaser CA, Tappero JW: *Rochalimaea henselae* infection: A new zoonosis with the domestic cat as reservoir. JAMA 271:531, 1994

74. Chomel BB, Abbott RC, Kasten RW, et al: *Bartonella henselae* prevalence in domestic cats in California: Risk factors and association between bacteremia and antibody titers. J Clin Microbiol 33:2445, 1995

75. Chomel BB, Kasten RW, Floyd-Hawkins K, et al: Experimental transmission of *Bartonella henselae* by the cat flea. J Clin Microbiol 34:1952, 1996

76. Jameson P, Greene C, Regnery R, et al: Prevalence of *Bartonella henselae* antibodies in pet cats throughout regions of North America. J Infect Dis 172:1145, 1995

77. Regnery RL, Childs JE, Koehler JE: Infections associated with *Bartonella* species in persons infected with human immunodeficiency virus. Clin Infect Dis 21(Suppl 1):S94, 1995

78. Golub B, Falk G, Spink WW: Lung abscess due to *Corynebacterium equi*: Report of first human infection. Ann Intern Med 66:1174, 1967

79. Verville TD, Huycke MM, Greenfield RA, et al: *Rhodococcus equi* infections of humans: 12 cases and a review of the literature. Medicine 73:119, 1994

80. Gray BM: Case report: *Rhodococcus equi* pneumonia in a patient infected by the human immunodeficiency virus. Am J Med Sci 303:180, 1992

81. Laskey JA, Pulkingham N, Powers MA, Dureack DT: *Rhodococcus equi* causing human pulmonary infection: Review of 29 cases. South Med J 84:1217, 1991

82. Scott MA, Graham BS, Verrall R, et al: *Rhodococcus equi*—an increasingly recognized opportunistic pathogen: Report of 12 cases and review of 65 cases in the literature. Am J Clin Pathol 103:649, 1995

83. Cury JD, Harrington PT, Hosein IK: Successful medical therapy of *Rhodococcus equi* pneumonia in a patient with HIV infection. Chest 102:1619, 1992

84. Takasugi JE, Godwin JD: Lung abscess caused by *Rhodococcus equi*. J Thorac Imaging 6:72, 1991

85. Gallant JE, Ko AH: Cavitary pulmonary lesions in patients infected with human immunodeficiency virus. Clin Infect Dis 22:671, 1996

86. Canfrere I, Germaud P, Roger C: Another cause of endobronchial lesions found in HIV patients [letter]. Chest 108:587, 1995

87. Antinori S, Esposito R, Cernuschi M, et al: Disseminated *Rhodococcus equi* infection initially presenting as foot mycetoma in an HIV-positive patient [letter]. AIDS 6:740, 1992

88. Frame BC, Petkus AF: *Rhodococcus equi* pneumonia: Case report and literature review. Ann Pharmacother 27:1340, 1993

89. Nordmann P, Ronco E: In-vitro antimicrobial susceptibility of *Rhodococcus equi*. J Antimicrobial Chemother 29:383, 1992

90. Nordmann P, Chavanet P, Caillon J, et al: Recurrent pneumonia due to rifampicin-resistant *Rhodococcus equi* in a patient infected with HIV [letter]. J Infect 24:104, 1992

91. Fischer L, Sterneck M, Albrecht H, et al: Vertebral osteomyelitis due to *Rhodococcus equi* in a liver transplant recipient. Clin Infect Dis 26:749, 1998

92. Roquet RM, Clave D, Massip P, et al: Imipenem/vancomycin for *Rhodococcus equi* pulmonary infection in HIV-positive patient [letter]. Lancet 337:375, 1991

93. Adal KA, Shiner PT, Francis JB: Primary subcutaneous abscess caused by *Rhodococcus equi* [letter]. Ann Intern Med 122:317, 1995

94. Glaser CA, Angulo FJ, Rooney JA: Animal-associated opportunistic infections among persons infected with

the human immunodeficiency virus [see comments]. Clin Infect Dis 18:14, 1994

95. Supparatpinyo K, Khamwan C, Baosoung V, et al: Disseminated *Penicillium marneffei* infection in southeast Asia. Lancet 344:110, 1994

96. Borradori L, Schmit JC, Stetzkowski M, et al: Penicilliosis marneffei infection in AIDS. J Am Acad Dermatol 31:843, 1994

97. Liu MT, Wong CK, Fung CP: Disseminated *Penicillium marneffei* infection with cutaneous lesions in

an HIV-positive patient. Br J Dermatol 131:280, 1994

98. Hilmarsdottir I, Meynard JL, Rogeaux O, et al: Disseminated *Penicillium marneffei* infection associated with human immunodeficiency virus: A report of two cases and a review of 35 published cases. J Acquir Immune Defic Syndr 6:466, 1993

99. Wong KF, Tsang DNC, Chan JKC: Bone marrow diagnosis of penicilliosis [letter]. N Engl J Med 330:717, 1994

28 | Management of Herpesvirus Infections (Cytomegalovirus, Herpes Simplex Virus, and Varicella-Zoster Virus)

W. LAWRENCE DREW • MARY JEAN STEMPIEN • MALIKA KHERAJ • KIM S. ERLICH

CYTOMEGALOVIRUS

With the advent of highly active antiretroviral therapy (IIAART), there has been a marked decline in cytomegalovirus (CMV) disease. The syndromes discussed below still occur in the early months of HAART, presumably because the CD4 lymphocytes require weeks to months to become fully functional. CMV disease is also seen in those patients who have eluded medical care and in those who fail or are intolerant of HAART.

Infection with CMV is extremely common in patients with AIDS and can result in several clinical illnesses, including chorioretinitis, esophagitis, colitis, pneumonia, and several neurologic disorders. Not all patients with blood, urine, or tissue cultures positive for CMV will develop clinical illness related to the infection. In patients with advanced AIDS (CD4 lymphocyte counts of less than 50/mm^3) the risk of developing CMV disease and death is directly related to the quantity of CMV nucleic acid in plasma. In a study of over 600 advanced AIDS patients, each $\log_{10}$ increase in baseline CMV DNA load was associated with an approximate threefold increase in CMV disease and twofold increase in mortality at 1 year.[1]

Diagnosis of disease caused by CMV may require tissue biopsy with histologic evidence of viral inclusions and inflammatory response. Detection of CMV antigen or nucleic acid in tissue is an alternative method for establishing that CMV is actually present in tissue. Viral culture is useful only if no other pathogen is identified in tissue. This section reviews the most common clinical manifestations of CMV and their management.

Chorioretinitis

Ocular disease caused by CMV occurs only in patients with severe immunodeficiency and was especially common in patients with AIDS prior to the advent of HIV protease inhibitors. Clinical evidence of CMV retinitis (Color Plate IF) occurred in as many as 40% of AIDS patients, and autopsy series revealed that CMV retinitis was present in up to 30% of patients. With the routine use of prophylaxis against *Pneumocystis*, retinitis became a common presenting manifestation of AIDS, but it more often occurred months to years after the diagnosis of AIDS had been established. The incidence of CMV disease is currently low primarily because of the efficacy of protease inhibitors in controlling primary HIV disease.

Decreased visual acuity, the presence of floaters, or unilateral visual field loss is often the presenting complaint of a patient with retinitis. Ophthalmologic examination typically reveals large creamy to yellowish white granular areas with perivascular exudates and hemorrhages (Fig. 28–1). These lesions initially occur more often at the periphery of the fundus and, if left untreated, progress centrally within 2 to 3 weeks. Retinitis usually begins unilaterally, but progression to bilateral involvement is common because of an associated viremia. Systemic

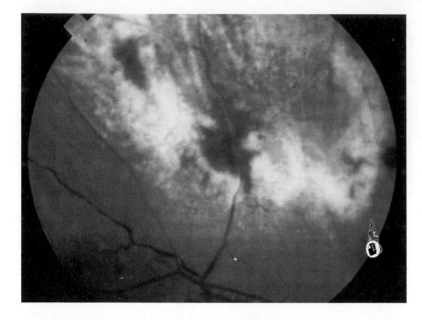

FIGURE 28–1. Funduscopic appearance of CMV retinitis, illustrating "cottage cheese and catsup" appearance resulting from perivascular exudates and hemorrhages. (Courtesy of Dr. L. Schwartz, San Francisco, California.)

CMV infection involving other viscera is frequently present.

CMV accounts for at least 90% of HIV-related infectious retinopathies. Differentiating suspected CMV retinitis lesions from cotton-wool spots is essential. Cotton-wool spots appear as small, fluffy, white lesions with indistinct margins and are not associated with exudates or hemorrhages. They are common in AIDS patients, are usually asymptomatic, and represent areas of focal ischemia. These lesions do not progress and often undergo spontaneous regression. Toxoplasmosis is the second most common opportunistic infection of the eye but is characterized by little if any hemorrhage. It is associated with cerebral toxoplasmosis in the majority of patients. Syphilis, herpes simplex virus (HSV), varicella-zoster virus (VZV), and tuberculosis are other infections that may rarely involve the retina.

Virtually all patients with CMV retinitis have CD4 lymphocyte counts of less than 50/mm^3, and routine ophthalmologic screening of patients with pupillary dilation, as well as indirect ophthalmoscopy, may be valuable when cell counts decline to this level. It is also important to inquire about visual abnormalities, especially increased floaters, and to examine the fundus carefully when there are visual complaints. Patients with confirmed CMV chorioretinitis should be treated with ganciclovir, foscarnet, or cidofovir.[2–4] These agents are equally effective in the initial treatment of CMV chorioretinitis, although disease usually progresses despite continued treatment[5] (see "Treatment of CMV In-

fection," p 433; see also Chapter 11, for additional discussion).

Nervous System

CMV commonly involves the central nervous system (CNS) in AIDS patients. About 20% to 40% of AIDS patients have been identified with CMV CNS involvement in different autopsy series.[6–8] CMV causes a spectrum of neurologic syndromes in AIDS patients, ranging from polyradiculopathy, encephalitis with dementia, and ventriculoencephalitis to mononeuritis multiplex and painful neuropathy.

Polyradiculopathy and Myelitis

The clinical syndrome of CMV polyradiculopathy and myelitis usually has an insidious onset with low back pain radiating to the perianal area and progressive lower extremity weakness, hypo- or areflexia, and variable sensory deficit with usually preserved proprioception and vibratory sensation. In association with bladder and/or anal sphincter dysfunction, most patients develop urinary retention and fecal incontinence. The disease clinically resembles Guillian-Barré syndrome but may be differentiated by lack of sphincter and upper extremity involvement in the latter.

Diagnosis of CMV polyradiculopathy is based on the characteristic neurologic features described above. The cerebrospinal fluid (CSF) abnormalities are very unusual for a viral infection: pleocytosis with predominant polymorphonuclear leukocytosis and hypoglycorrachia. Culture of CSF is usually negative, but antigen or DNA assays are sensitive methods of diagnosis. Magnetic resonance imaging (MRI) may reveal enhancement of leptomeninges and clumping of lumbosacral roots. Characteristic pathologic changes seen in CMV polyradiculopathy are demyelination and destruction of axons.

Acute CMV polyradiculopathy should be differentiated from idiopathic lumbosacral polyradiculopathy, in which CSF pleocytosis is predominantly mononuclear and clinical improvement is seen without CMV treatment. Lymphoma, tuberculosis, syphilis, and toxoplasmosis also cause similar clinical syndromes.

Encephalitis with Dementia and Ventriculoencephalitis

Cytomegalovirus encephalitis (CMVE) with a distinct clinical syndrome of dementia and CMV ventriculoencephalitis are the two syndromes of CMVE described in AIDS patients. CMVE with dementia, the more common of the two syndromes, is well described neuropathologically[9] as a multifocal, scattered micronodular encephalitis that resembles HIV encephalitis, which causes HIV-associated dementia (HIVD). CMV ventriculoencephalitis is a late and terminal event with acute onset of encephalitis often associated with cranial nerve involvement and nystagmus. CMVE-associated dementia has been described and compared with HIVD.[10] The significance of differentiating CMVE and HIVD lies in the different drugs available for treatment.

CMVE is seen more commonly among homosexual men, which may reflect the increased CMV seroprevalence in homosexual men.[11] CMVE always occurs in patients with CD4 counts of less than 100/mm[3] and should be suspected in homosexual men presenting with a subacute encephalopathy who have had AIDS for more than 1 year. Clinicians should suspect a diagnosis of CMVE in patients who have a history of systemic CMV infection, especially those with CMV retinitis who develop encephalopathic features and change in mental status.

Patients with dementia caused by CMVE usually have a more acute onset and rapid progression than patients with HIVD. The encephalopathic symptoms include delirium and confusion, lethargy and somnolence, apathy and withdrawal, personality changes, and focal neurologic signs with cranial nerve involvement. During the course of illness, recurrent fever episodes may occur that may be attributed to other opportunistic infections (e.g., *Mycobacterium avium-intracellulare*). Psychomotor slowing, primitive reflexes, and peripheral neuropathy may also be seen in CMVE. Distal sensory polyneuropathy usually antedates the onset of CMVE.[12]

The course of encephalopathic illness in both CMVE and HIVD includes progressive worsening in mental status until death. The median survival of CMVE patients is significantly shorter (weeks) compared to that of HIVD patients (months). Autopsies reveal a range of neuropathology including ependymal and subependymal necrosis, areas of demyelination, and microglial nodules that are more frequently encountered than typical nuclear and cytoplasmic CMV inclusions.[13] Neuropathologic evaluations of CMVE and HIV coinfection of single cells suggests that CMV and HIV mutually help each other's replication in the brain.[14]

It is difficult to make a definitive diagnosis of CMVE, and laboratory investigations are not very helpful in distinguishing CMV from HIVD. Electrolyte abnormality, especially hyponatremia, is more commonly present in CMVE patients.[10] There are insufficient data to determine whether CMV antigen or DNA is regularly detected in CSF. Imaging study with MRI brain scans showing meningeal enhancement consistent with ventriculitis and periventricular enhancement are helpful in differentiating CMVE from HIVD. However, periventricular enhancement may also be seen in lymphoma, toxoplasmosis, and pyogenic brain abscesses. Progressive ventriculomegaly, if seen in serial computed tomography scans, is highly suspicious of CMVE.[15,16]

Combination therapy with ganciclovir and foscarnet is recommended, especially when disease progression is noted with single-agent therapy.

Mononeuritis Multiplex

This is the least common of all the neurologic syndromes attributed to CMV. Clinical characteristics of CMV mononeuritis are more varied than the polyradiculopathy/myelitis. Patients may present with multifocal, patchy and/or asymmetrical sensory and motor deficits. Cranial nerve palsies caused by CMV, especially in the recurrent laryngeal nerve in the setting of severe immunosuppression, have been reported.[17] This symptom may occur with other neurologic manifestations of CMV (e.g., polyradiculopathy, encephalitis, or retinitis). Pathologic findings in peripheral nerve biopsies have shown endoneurial necrosis with cellular infiltrates and Schwann cells showing CMV inclusions.

Painful Distal Neuropathy

This syndrome of painful distal symmetrical neuropathy of subacute onset limited to the feet and associated with some numbness and weakness has been reported with CMV infection.[18]

Gastrointestinal System

CMV colitis previously occurred in at least 5% to 10% of AIDS patients but is now uncommon (see Chapter 13). Diarrhea, weight loss, anorexia, and fever frequently are present. The differential diagnosis includes infection by other gastrointestinal pathogens, including *Cryptosporidium*, *Giardia*, *Entamoeba*, *Mycobacterium*, *Shigella*, *Campylobacter*, and *Strongyloides stercoralis*, and involvement by lymphoma or Kaposi's sarcoma. Endoscopy usually reveals diffuse submucosal hemorrhages and mucosal ulcerations, although a grossly normal-appearing mucosa may be encountered in up to 10% of those with histologic evidence of CMV colitis (Fig. 28–2). Biopsy reveals vasculitis, neutrophilic infiltration, and nonspecific inflammation, but the diagnosis is confirmed by the presence of characteristic CMV inclusions, antigen, or nucleic acid and the absence of other pathogens.

Clinically evident esophagitis in AIDS patients most commonly is due to either *Candida albicans* or HSV, but may also be caused by CMV (see Chapter 13). Patients with CMV eso-phagitis are apt to have pain on swallowing and distal ulceration on endoscopy. As in colitis, diagnosis should be established through endoscopic examination and biopsy.

Patients with symptomatic esophagitis or enterocolitis who have CMV (and not other pathogens) detected by endoscopy, histology, or culture should benefit from anti-CMV treatment for 3 to 6 weeks and should be considered for continued maintenance treatment in part as a means of preventing retinitis.[19]

The efficacy of anti-CMV treatment in patients with enterocolitis is not dramatic.[20] When compared to placebo, a significant antiviral effect was observed but a clinical benefit was less apparent. Diarrhea and abdominal discomfort were not relieved, but in general patients seemed to improve with this therapy.[20]

Pulmonary System

Pulmonary Manifestations

Isolation of CMV from pulmonary secretions or lung tissue in AIDS patients with pneumonia who undergo bronchoscopy is common, but a true pathogenic role of the virus in the disease process is not readily established. Many patients with pulmonary disease and CMV isolation from the lung have concomitant infection with other pathogens, especially *Pneumocystis carinii*. Many of the patients respond to therapy directed at *P. carinii* pneumonia alone, raising the question of whether CMV is a true pulmonary pathogen in AIDS patients. However, patients with positive CMV cultures and histologic find-

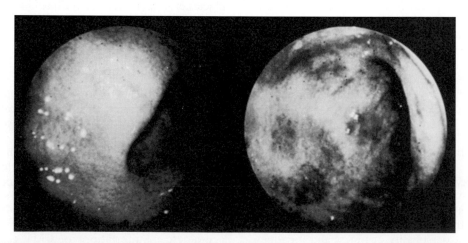

FIGURE 28–2. Sigmoidoscopic appearance of CMV colitis (two views), demonstrating diffuse submucosal hemorrhages and mucosal ulcerations. (Courtesy of Dr. D. Dieterich, New York, New York.)

ings from lung tissue and no other pathogens identified on diagnostic bronchoscopy may truly have invasive CMV pneumonia.

When CMV causes pulmonary disease in AIDS patients, the syndrome is that of an interstitial pneumonitis. Patients often complain of gradually worsening shortness of breath, dyspnea on exertion, and a dry, nonproductive cough. The heart and respiratory rates are elevated, but auscultation of the lungs often reveals minimal findings with no evidence of consolidation. Chest radiographs show diffuse interstitial infiltrates similar to those in patients with *P. carinii* pneumonia. Hypoxemia is invariably present.

Anti-CMV therapy should be considered when a patient has documented CMV pulmonary infection as the only pathogen identified and a progressive, deteriorating clinical course.[21-23]

Treatment of CMV Infection

Ganciclovir

STRUCTURE AND MECHANISM OF ACTION. Ganciclovir (DHPG, Cytovene) is a nucleoside analog that differs from acyclovir (Zovirax) by a single carboxyl side chain. This structural change confers on the drug approximately 50 times greater activity than acyclovir against CMV. Acyclovir has low activity against CMV because it is not well phosphorylated in CMV-infected cells. This is due to the absence of the gene for thymidine kinase (TK) in CMV. Ganciclovir, however, is active against CMV because it does not require TK for phosphorylation. Instead another viral-encoded phosphorylating enzyme (UL 97) is present in CMV-infected cells.[24] It is capable of phosphorylating ganciclovir and converting it to the monophosphate. Cellular enzymes then convert the monophosphate to the active compound, ganciclovir triphosphate. Ganciclovir triphosphate acts to inhibit the viral DNA polymerase.

PHARMACOLOGY AND DOSAGE. Ganciclovir is available for clinical use in intravenous and oral formulations, as well as a sustained-release intraocular implant. Intravenous ganciclovir is used for initial induction therapy, followed by either intravenous or oral ganciclovir for maintenance therapy. A more recently studied highly effective treatment alternative is the combination of oral ganciclovir and the intraocular ganciclovir implant.[25] Oral ganciclovir is also used for prevention (see "Prevention of CMV Infection," p 437).

Initial intravenous induction treatment for CMV disease consists of 5 mg/kg twice daily for 14 to 21 days or until there is an adequate clinical response. The standard intravenous dosage for maintenance therapy is approximately one half the induction dose (i.e., 5 mg/kg/day 7 days/week) or, if given orally, 1000 mg three times daily with food.

When administered by intravenous infusion over 1 hour in the usual dosage of 5 mg/kg, peak ganciclovir blood levels are approximately 8 to 9 µg/ml, and the serum half-life is 3.5 hours. The absolute bioavailability of oral ganciclovir capsules is 6% to 9%. When administered orally as 1000 mg three times daily with food, peak serum levels are approximately 1 µg/ml, and the serum half-life is approximately 5 hours. Because ganciclovir is excreted unchanged through the kidneys, dosage for intravenous ganciclovir must be reduced in patients with renal impairment. Dosage adjustments should also be considered for oral ganciclovir. The appropriate dose reductions are presented in Table 28–1. Initial response in retinitis (improvement or stabilization in vision or ophthalmoscopic appearance) occurs in approximately 75% of treated patients.[4] By comparison, the disease is relentlessly progressive in 90% of patients if left untreated. Visual-field defects present at the onset of therapy do not reverse, but a decrease in visual acuity caused by edema of the macula may improve with treatment. Retinal detachment may occur in later stages as the necrotic retina scars and thins.

Prior to the availability of HAART, maintenance therapy throughout the life of the patient was critical for CMV retinitis because the virus is only suppressed by ganciclovir and is not eliminated. Even with continued maintenance therapy, CMV retinitis eventually progressed. Why this occurred is not clearly understood, but it is likely related to suboptimal drug delivery to the retina. This hypothesis is supported by the longer times to progression achieved with the ganciclovir intraocular implant, which delivers greater concentrations of ganciclovir to the vitreous.[26] Viral resistance does not appear to be involved in most progressions of CMV retinitis (see "Resistance," p 434).

With successful HAART, it may be possible for selected patients with CMV retinitis to discontinue maintenance therapy. This is not recommended at present because the influence of HAART on the course of CMV disease is not understood.[19] Studies are currently underway to determine which patients can safely omit or dis-

TABLE 28–1. Ganciclovir Dosage Adjustment in Patients with Impaired Renal Function

CREATININE CLEARANCE (ml/min)*	IV INDUCTION DOSE (mg/kg)	INDUCTION DOSING INTERVAL (hr)	MAINTENANCE DOSE (mg/kg)	MAINTENANCE DOSING INTERVAL (hr)	ORAL DOSE
>70	5.0	12	5.0	24	1000 mg tid
50–69	2.5	12	2.5	24	1500 mg qd
25–49	2.5	24	1.25	24	1000 mg qd
10–24	1.25	24	0.625	24	500 mg qd
<10	1.25	3 times/wk, following hemodialysis	0.625	3 times/wk, following hemodialysis	500 mg 3 times/wk, following hemodialysis

*Creatinine clearance can be related to serum creatinine by the following formulas:

$$\text{For males: } \frac{(140 - \text{age [yr]})(\text{body weight [kg]})}{72 \ (\text{serum creatinine [mg/dl]})}$$

For females: $0.85 \times$ male value

continue maintenance treatment and how they should be monitored.

Oral ganciclovir maintenance therapy is associated with a risk of more rapid rate of retinitis progression compared to intravenous therapy (mean of 5 to 12 days' earlier progression in three studies), but can be used where this risk is balanced by the benefit of avoiding daily intravenous infusions.[27,28] Patients with stable, non-sight-threatening retinitis appear to be appropriate candidates for oral maintenance therapy.

Intravitreal injection of ganciclovir has been used in certain special situations, such as in patients in whom neutropenia limited the systemic use of the drug, and in one series[29] appeared effective and relatively safe. Sustained intravitreal release of ganciclovir has been accomplished using a surgically implantable device.[30–32] This implant, which is designed to deliver ganciclovir into the vitreous over several months, has been shown to be highly efficacious for local control of retinitis. In addition, in a large controlled study that evaluated combined oral ganciclovir (4500 mg/day) and the implant for treatment of CMV retinitis, the combination not only delayed progression of retinitis but reduced the risk of developing contralateral retinitis or extraocular CMV disease. The incidence of Kaposi's sarcoma was also reduced.[25]

CLINICAL USE. Administration of ganciclovir is indicated for the treatment of acute CMV infection, but other herpesviruses, including HSV-1, HSV-2, VZV, human herpesvirus (HHV)-6, and HHV-8, the virus responsible for Kaposi's sarcoma, are also susceptible to the drug in vitro. Because AIDS patients with severe CMV infection frequently have illnesses caused by other herpesviruses, a bonus of ganciclovir ther-

apy may be an associated prevention or improvement of these infections. Ganciclovir is probably also active against Epstein-Barr virus.

VIROLOGIC RESPONSE TO GANCICLOVIR. CMV cultures of blood and urine rapidly become negative in patients treated with ganciclovir[33] (Fig. 28–3). Most of these patients had CMV retinitis, although AIDS patients with CMV infections of other organ systems are included. Of these patients, 87% had a complete virologic response (conversions of culture from positive to negative or a more than 100-fold reduction in CMV titer) in urine, and 83% had a complete response in blood culture. The median time until response was 8 days for both blood and urine cultures.

RESISTANCE. Erice et al.[34] reported three patients whose clinical course suggested the emergence of resistance and whose CMV isolates exhibited increases in the concentration of ganciclovir required to inhibit the virus in tissue culture over baseline determinations. In a separate report, after 3 months of continuous intravenous ganciclovir therapy, approximately 10% of patients were excreting resistant strains of CMV (arbitrarily defined as strains that are only inhibited by four times or more the median concentration of ganciclovir required to inhibit a group of pretherapy isolates).[35] In virtually all isolates, there was a mutation in the phosphorylating gene. These strains remain sensitive to foscarnet, which may be used as an alternative therapy.[36]

In another investigation of CMV resistance in 38 retinitis patients treated with intravenous or oral ganciclovir, the in vitro 50% inhibitory concentration (IC_{50}) increased with duration of ganciclovir exposure (W. L. Drew et al., submitted for publication, J Infect Dis, 1999). Resistant

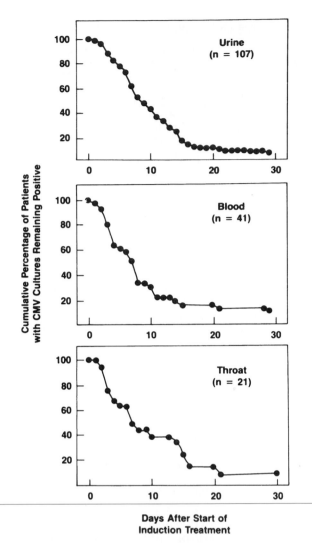

Days After Start of Induction Treatment

FIGURE 28–3. Time course of conversion of CMV cultures of specimens of urine, blood, or throat washings from positive (before treatment) to negative (after treatment with ganciclovir). Cultures from individual patients were performed at various times after start of treatment. Numbers in parentheses are the number of patients in whom the particular body fluid or site was sequentially cultured. (Reprinted from Buhles WC Jr, Mastre BJ, Tinker AJ, et al: Ganciclovir treatment of life- or sight-threatening cytomegalovirus infection: Experience in 314 immunocompromised patients. Rev Infect Dis 10[suppl 3]:S495, 1988, with permission.)

strains (defined as having an $IC_{50} > 6$ µM) were first identified after 50 days of treatment, but resistance was infrequent, occurring in about 6% of patients treated with oral ganciclovir and about 3% of patients treated with intravenous ganciclovir. Most patients did not shed CMV at the time of retinitis progression, but a patient with "breakthrough" shedding of virus during treatment was more likely to demonstrate resistance.

In another report of 76 retinitis patients initially treated with ganciclovir, 11.4% had a resistant strain of CMV ($IC_{50} > 6$ µM) by 6 months.[37]

TOXICITY. Toxicity may limit therapy with ganciclovir. The following adverse effects may occur.

Effects on Hematopoiesis. Leukopenia and anemia may affect up to 40% and 25%, respectively, of patients receiving intravenous ganciclovir for treatment of CMV disease. The incidence of both is lower during administration of oral ganciclovir (3000 mg daily) for either maintenance treatment of retinitis or primary prevention of CMV disease (Table 28–2). Many AIDS patients have low white blood cell counts before therapy, so the contribution of ganciclovir to leukopenia is not always clear. Neutropenia may develop at any time and is usually reversible, although at least five patients are known to have had irreversible suppression. Cytokines, such as granulocyte colony-stimulating factor (G-CSF; filgrastim), are effective in reversing ganciclovir-induced neutropenia. Severe neutropenia (absolute neutrophil count <500/mm³) requires a ganciclovir dose interruption until evidence of marrow recovery is observed and neutrophil counts have risen, preferably to greater than 1000/mm³. Thrombocytopenia occurs in up to 6% of ganciclovir-treated patients.

Toxicities in Other Organ Systems. Gastrointestinal adverse events, most commonly diarrhea, nausea, anorexia, and vomiting, affect a substantial number of patients treated with intravenous or oral ganciclovir. Data from a large double-blind safety comparison of oral ganciclovir (3000 mg daily) to placebo, however, suggest that the rates of these events are only modestly higher among ganciclovir-treated patients; 48% developed diarrhea (vs. 42% of placebo-treated patients, 19% developed anorexia (placebo, 16%), and 14% developed vomiting (placebo, 11%).[43] Neuropathy and paresthesia are the most frequent adverse events involving the nervous system, affecting up to 21% and 10% of patients, respectively, but only neuropathy occurred more often in ganciclovir-versus placebo-treated patients (21% vs. 15%, respectively). A minority of ganciclovir-treated patients will experience modest elevations in serum creatinine (maximum levels of at least 1.5 mg/dl, or greater than 25% increases over pretreatment levels).

Therapeutic Drug Interactions

Ganciclovir Plus Zidovudine. Because both zidovudine and ganciclovir can cause neutropenia and anemia, some patients may not tolerate this combination at full dosage. The use of

TABLE 28–2. Selected Laboratory Abnormalities in Patients Receiving Ganciclovir for Treatment of CMV Retinitis and Prevention of CMV Disease

| | CMV RETINITIS TREATMENT | | CMV DISEASE PREVENTION | |
	Oral (3000 mg/d)	IV (5 mg/kg/d)	Oral (3000 mg/d)	Placebo
Number of patients	320	175	478	234
Neutropenia (ANC/L)*				
<500	18%	25%	10%	6%
500 to <749	17%	14%	16%	7%
750 to <1000	19%	26%	22%	16%
Anemia (Hgb, gm/dl)*				
<6.5	2%	5%	1%	<1%
6.5 to <8.0	10%	16%	5%	3%
8.0 to <9.5	25%	26%	15%	16%

*Data are percentages of patients. ANC, absolute neutrophil count; Hgb, hemoglobin.

filgrastim (G-CSF) may counter the neutropenia caused by these drugs. Antiretroviral agents with less hematologic toxicity provide another means of maintaining antiretroviral activity during ganciclovir therapy.

Ganciclovir Plus Didanosine (ddI). Blood levels of ddI are significantly increased during concomitant ganciclovir use.[38] The clinical significance of these increased levels is not yet known, but patients should be monitored for possible increased ddI-associated toxicity.

Gonadal Toxicity. In preclinical animal studies, ganciclovir is a potent inhibitor of spermatogenesis and may also suppress female fertility. Sperm counts in humans before and during ganciclovir therapy, however, have been performed too infrequently to provide meaningful information on spermatogenesis. Patients wishing to have children should use ganciclovir only for the strongest indications.

Teratogenesis. Because ganciclovir is a mutagen and teratogen in animals, effective contraception should be practiced by men and women with childbearing potential during treatment. Ganciclovir should be used during pregnancy only if the potential benefit justifies the potential risk to the fetus.

Foscarnet

Foscarnet, also known as phosphonoformate or phosphonoformic acid, is a pyrophosphate that inhibits the DNA polymerase of CMV. Specifically, the drug blocks the pyrophosphate-binding site of the viral DNA polymerase, preventing cleavage of pyrophosphate from deoxyadenosine triphosphate.[39] This action is relatively selective in that CMV DNA polymerase is inhibited at concentrations less than 1%

of that required to inhibit cellular DNA polymerase. Unlike such nucleosides as acyclovir and ganciclovir, foscarnet does not require phosphorylation intracellularly to be an active inhibitor of viral DNA polymerases. This biochemical fact becomes especially important in regard to viral resistance, because the principal mode of viral resistance to nucleoside analogs is a mutation that eliminates phosphorylation of the drug in virus-infected cells. Foscarnet can be used to treat patients with ganciclovir-resistant CMV, unless the virus is one of the 10% that are resistant because of a polymerase mutation and is cross-resistant to foscarnet.

PHARMACOLOGY. The recommended initial therapy is foscarnet administered intravenously as 60 mg/kg every 8 hours or as 90 mg/kg every 12 hours. A dose of 120 mg/kg/day may be superior in efficacy to 90 mg/kg/day,[40] but this dose may also be more toxic.

CSF concentrations of foscarnet are approximately 40% of serum levels. Excretion is entirely renal, without a hepatic component. Oral bioavailability is estimated at 12% to 22%, but it is poorly tolerated.

Adverse effects include renal impairment, anemia, hypocalcemia (especially ionized calcium), hypomagnesemia, and hypophosphatemia. It is important to measure renal function frequently and adjust dosage accordingly to minimize toxicity. Daily preinfusion of 1 liter of saline may reduce nephrotoxicity during maintenance therapy.

Palestine et al.[3] reported a randomized control trial of foscarnet in the treatment of CMV retinitis in AIDS patients. Patients were assigned to receive either no therapy or immediate treatment with intravenous foscarnet. The justification for the design was that the lesions were peripheral and not threatening visual acuity. The mean time to progression of retinitis was 3 weeks in the control group versus 13 weeks in the treatment group, thereby proving that foscarnet is effective therapy. Also, an excellent antiviral effect was achieved in the treatment group (i.e., 9 of 13 patients had positive blood cultures for CMV at entry, and all 9 had CMV cleared from their blood by the end of the 3-week induction period). Adverse effects were seizures, hypomagnesemia, hypocalcemia, and elevated serum creatinine levels.

A study comparing foscarnet with ganciclovir in the treatment of sight-threatening CMV retinitis was reported.[5] The two drugs were equivalently effective in treating retinitis. The mean time to progression of retinitis was approximately 56 days in both groups. The notable difference in the study was that patients treated with foscarnet had a 4-month longer survival time than those receiving ganciclovir. The explanation for the difference in survival time is not clear and does not seem entirely attributable to differences in the ability to take concurrent antiretroviral medications. However, this analysis was based on tabulating whether a patient had ever received any antiretroviral therapy (e.g., zidovudine, dideoxycytidine [ddC], or ddI) and did not assess the quantitative ability of patients to take these medications. Presumably, it was more difficult for the patient to be on concurrent zidovudine therapy while taking ganciclovir because of additive myelosuppression. Thus whether the survival benefit of foscarnet was due to these other medications or was an inherent effect of foscarnet therapy itself remains unclear. Now that cytokines (e.g., granulocyte-macrophage colony-stimulating factor and G-CSF) and other antiretrovirals (ddI, ddC) without extreme myelosuppressive toxicity are available, it should be possible for patients to continue receiving antiretroviral medications while taking ganciclovir.

Ganciclovir and Foscarnet

The results of a Studies of Ocular Complications of AIDS trial of combination therapy versus monotherapy for relapsed CMV retinitis were published in early 1996.[41] Combination therapy (5 mg/kg/day ganciclovir and 90 mg/kg/day foscarnet) was significantly superior in delaying progression than either ganciclovir alone (10 mg/day) or foscarnet alone (120 mg/kg/day). This study also showed no advantage in switching monotherapy. That is, patients in whom monotherapy failed with ganciclovir and

then switched to high-dose foscarnet did not do better than patients who continued ganciclovir at the higher dose. The median times to progression were: foscarnet group, 1.3 months; ganciclovir group, 2.0 months; and combination group, 4.3 months ($p < 0.001$). Side effects were not statistically significantly different in any group, but the quality of life was poorest in the combination group as a result of the prolonged daily infusion time of 3.1 hours.

Cidofovir

Cidofovir, or HPMPC, represents a departure from previous nucleoside analogs because it appears to the cell as a nucleotide. It has a phosphonate moiety attached to a cytosine analog and does not require phosphorylation by viral-encoded enzyme. It is therefore active against the majority of ganciclovir-resistant CMV strains that have resistance mutations in the UL97 or phosphorylating gene. The drug also has an extremely long half-life, permitting intravenous administration as infrequently as every 2 weeks during maintenance treatment.[42]

Cidofovir is nephrotoxic, especially to the proximal renal tubule, but this can apparently be diminished by prehydration and concomitant probenecid therapy. Renal function and toxicity must be monitored carefully, and proteinuria or a rising creatinine level are reasons for dosage reduction, interruption, or discontinuation. Concurrent administration of other nephrotoxic drugs must be avoided and there must be at least a 7-day period of "washout" of these drugs if their use precedes administration of cidofovir. Despite its potential for toxicity, the drug is effective and convenient and it may find an important niche in anti-CMV therapy.

Prevention of CMV Infection

Ganciclovir

The oral form of ganciclovir is currently the only agent approved by the Food and Drug Administration (FDA) for prevention of CMV disease in patients with advanced HIV infection. The approval was based on a placebo-controlled study of 725 patients known to be CMV sero- or culture positive, the majority of whom had CD4 lymphocyte cell counts under 50/mm³. Ganciclovir taken prophylactically as 1000 mg orally three times daily decreased the cumulative risk of developing CMV disease over 12 months from 26% to 14% (an overall risk reduction of nearly 50%).[43] Ganciclovir also effectively decreased and suppressed CMV excretion throughout the treatment period as measured by prevalence of CMV-positive urine cultures.

HERPES SIMPLEX VIRUS

Herpes simplex virus types 1 and 2 (HSV-1, HSV-2) cause disease in both normal and immunocompromised hosts and are responsible for substantial morbidity in patients with AIDS. Most adult patients with AIDS have been infected with one or both HSV types before the development of AIDS, and are not susceptible to primary HSV infection following new exposure. During initial HSV infection, viral latency develops in the nerve root ganglia corresponding to the site of mucocutaneous inoculation. Latent virus can then reactivate at any time throughout the life of the host, and all infected persons are at risk for virus shedding and recurrent symptomatic disease. Recurrent HSV mucocutaneous eruptions are common in patients with HIV infection and can be severe, with extensive tissue destruction and prolonged viral shedding.[44-46]

Recent studies confirm the high prevalence of both HSV-1 and HSV-2 in the general population.[47-49] Type-specific serologic studies conclude that up to 70% of the population are infected with HSV-1, and up to 21.9% are infected with HSV-2. HSV-2 infection rates are higher in women than in men and higher in African-Americans and Mexican-Americans than in Caucasians.[47-49] The prevalence of HSV infection in homosexual AIDS patients exceeds that of the general population and likely reflects the common risk factor for transmission of both HSV and HIV (sexual contact). Serologic studies have revealed that up to 77% of HIV-infected patients have been previously infected with HSV. AIDS subgroups who did not acquire HIV infection through sexual contact, such as hemophiliacs and transfusion recipients, have rates of HSV infection that are lower than the incidence in AIDS as a whole, and are likely comparable to those in the general population. The presence of latent HSV infection in this high percentage of patients with HIV infection explains the frequency of clinical disease in this population. Clinical observations suggest that the frequency and severity of HSV recurrences may increase with advancing immunosuppressions.[49-53]

Clinical Presentation

Because most HIV-infected patients have been infected with HSV before acquiring HIV, recurrent HSV is much more common than primary HSV infection in this population. HSV infection in AIDS patients may appear similar to the typical HSV lesions observed in the normal host or, alternatively, lesions may appear quite atypical and unusual because of the immunosuppressed state associated with HIV infection. The severity of clinical illness depends on several factors, including the anatomic site of initial infection, the degree of immunosuppression, and whether the clinical episode represents initial primary infection (no previous exposure to either HSV type), initial nonprimary infection (previous exposure to the heterologous HSV type), or recurrent infection.[44-46]

Localized mucocutaneous ulcerative lesions, without visceral or cutaneous dissemination, is the most frequent presentation of HSV infection in HIV-infected patients. Because the lesions may appear atypical, a high index of suspicion is required by the clinician in evaluating any mucocutaneous lesion in a patient with HIV infection. Chronic or persistent HSV infection may lead to an initial diagnosis of AIDS; an individual with confirmed HIV infection and no other cause of immunodeficiency who has ulcerative HSV infection present for longer than 1 month has sufficient criteria for a diagnosis of AIDS.

Orolabial Infection

Orolabial infection in adults with AIDS is usually due to recurrent disease from previously latent infection. Primary infection of the mouth or nose may occur, however, in a seronegative individual who acquires infection at this site for the first time. Primary infection is more likely to occur in children with AIDS than in adults, because HIV infection in children (especially those infected prenatally) is more likely to precede initial exposure to HSV.

The incubation period of primary HSV infection ranges between 2 and 12 days. In the normal host, primary orolabial infection may be asymptomatic or result in clinically apparent gingivostomatitis.[46,49,54] Immunocompromised patients are at greater risk than normal hosts of developing a severe clinical illness during primary HSV-1 infection, with a painful vesicular eruption occurring along the lips, tongue, pharynx, or buccal mucosa. The vesicles rapidly coalesce and rupture to form large ulcers covered by a whitish yellow necrotic film.[54,55] Fever, pharyngitis, and cervical lymphadenopathy are often present in adults, whereas infants may display poor feeding and persistent drooling.

Following initial or primary infection, all infected patients remain at risk for virus reactivation and recurrent disease. Recurrent HSV gingivostomatitis ("fever blisters") may occur spontaneously or as a result of external stimuli, such as a febrile illness, excessive wind or ultraviolet light exposure to the lips, surgical manipulation of the trigeminal nerve, or stress. Prodromal symptoms, consisting of tingling or numbness at the site of the impending recurrence, may be present from 12 to 24 hours before the onset of an HSV recurrence. Instituting antiviral chemotherapy during the prodrome may have a beneficial effect on the illness and may abort the development of visible cutaneous lesions (see "Treatment of HSV Infection," below). Recurrences may increase in frequency and severity as immunosuppression worsens, although many AIDS patients will have only infrequent, mild, self-limiting recurrences throughout their disease.[50,54]

In the normal host, orolabial herpes lesions usually heal in 7 to 10 days. By comparison, AIDS patients often have a prolonged illness with markedly delayed healing of mucocutaneous lesions. If left untreated, chronic ulcerative lesions with persistent viral shedding may last for several weeks.[55]

Genital Infection

After a 2- to 12-day incubation period, many individuals with primary genital herpes develop local symptoms.[44–46] Symptoms will be most apparent in patients with primary genital infection (no prior infection with the heterologous HSV type) as compared to patients with nonprimary initial infection (prior infection with the heterologous HSV type). When present, signs and symptoms include small papules that rapidly evolve into fluid-filled vesicles. These lesions are usually painful and tender to palpation. The vesicles ulcerate rapidly and, in the normal host, heal over 3 to 4 weeks by crusting and reepithelialization. Tender inguinal adenopathy is common, and dysuria may be present even if the urethra is not infected. Systemic symptoms, such as fever, headache, myalgias, malaise, and meningismus, may be present during primary infection.[44–46]

In the normal host, recurrent genital herpes is less severe than primary infection. Compared with primary infection, recurrent herpes typi-cally results in fewer external lesions, a shorter duration of illness, and the absence of systemic symptoms.[44–46] As with primary infection, recurrent genital herpes in patients with AIDS may be more severe and prolonged as compared to that seen in the normal host. Prolonged new lesion formation, continued tissue destruction, persistent virus shedding, and severe local pain are not uncommon findings in this setting. As with orolabial herpes, the frequency and severity of genital recurrences may increase with advancing immunosuppression, and symptoms may last for several weeks if left untreated.[50,56]

Asymptomatic genital HSV shedding in nonimmunocompromised patients occurs on between 1% and 6% of the days on which cultures are obtained.[57,58] HIV-infected patients infected with HSV shed HSV at even higher rates, and asymptomatic shedding may increase with advancing immunosuppression.[59] All HSV-infected individuals (whether HIV infected or not) should be counseled about asymptomatic HSV shedding and the risk of transmission to sexual partners despite the absence of symptoms or visible lesions.[60]

Anorectal Infection

Chronic perianal herpes was among the first reported opportunistic infections associated with AIDS. HSV is the most frequent cause of nongonococcal proctitis in sexually active homosexual men.[61,62] HSV proctitis usually results from primary HSV-2 infection but may also occur as a result of HSV-1 infection or recurrent disease caused by either viral type. Severe anorectal pain, perianal ulcerations, constipation, tenesmus, and neurologic symptoms in the distribution of the sacral plexus (sacral radiculopathy, impotence, and neurogenic bladder) are common findings of HSV proctitis. These signs and symptoms help differentiate HSV proctitis from proctitis from other causes[61] (Fig. 28–4). Anorectal or sigmoidoscopic examination in patients with HSV proctitis typically reveals a friable mucosa, diffuse ulcerations, and occasional intact vesicular or pustular lesions.[61]

Recurrent perianal lesions caused by HSV in the absence of true proctitis is a common finding in patients with AIDS. Local pain, tenderness, itching, and pain on defecation are prominent symptoms of these lesions. Shallow ulcers in the perianal region are often visible on external examination, and ulcerative lesions frequently coalesce and extend along the gluteal crease to involve the area overlying the sacrum. These lesions are often atypical in appearance and may

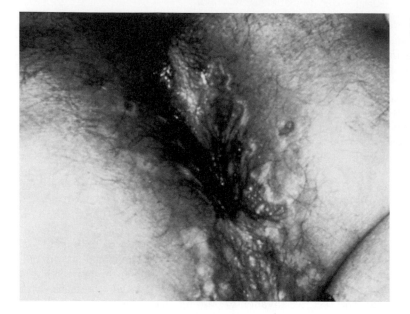

FIGURE 28–4. Perianal ulcerations typical of herpes simplex.

be confused with pressure decubiti (Color Plate II*F*). To prevent misdiagnosis, all perianal ulcerations and anal fissures in patients with AIDS should be examined for the presence of HSV by culture or direct antigen detection.

Esophagitis

Symptoms of HSV esophagitis typically include retrosternal pain and odynophagia (see Chapter 13). Patients may present with acute onset of dysphagia or with chronic swallowing complaints, and symptoms may be severe enough to interfere with eating and adequate nutrition. Visible herpetic lesions in the oropharynx may not be present, and the clinical picture may be confused with *Candida* or CMV esophagitis. Radiographic contrast studies typically reveal a cobblestone appearance of the esophageal mucosa, but this finding is nonspecific and is also present with esophagitis from other causes (Fig. 28–5). Definitive diagnosis of HSV esophagitis should be made by direct endoscopic visualization of the esophageal mucosa with positive viral studies and histopathologic evidence of invasive viral infection.[63]

Encephalitis

HSV encephalitis occurs rarely in AIDS but is the most life-threatening complication of HSV infection (see Chapter 14). Both HSV-1 and HSV-2 have been identified in brain tissue of AIDS patients, and simultaneous brain infections with HSV and CMV have been reported.[64–66] In adults with AIDS, HSV encephalitis usually occurs as a complication of primary or reactivated orolabial HSV infection. In neonates, the disease may occur as a result of primary HSV infection at the time of birth.[46]

The presentation of HSV encephalitis in adults with AIDS is often highly atypical. A subacute illness with subtle neurologic abnormalities is common in AIDS patients with HSV encephalitis, suggesting that host immune responses contribute to the clinical manifestations of the disease.[64–66] Headache, meningismus, and personality changes may develop gradually as the illness progresses. Alternatively, however, some AIDS patients with HSV encephalitis present with acute onset of symptoms. Abrupt onset of fever, headache, nausea, lethargy, and confusion may occur with temporal lobe abnormalities, cranial nerve defects, and focal seizures. Grand mal seizures, obtundation, coma, and death may eventually ensue.

The clinical diagnosis of HSV encephalitis may be extremely difficult, because other central nervous system infections (including HIV encephalopathy, *Cryptococcus neoformans*, and *Toxoplasma gondii*) may present with similar features. CSF usually reveals nonspecific findings, including elevated protein and a lymphocytic pleocytosis. Viral CSF cultures are usually negative.[67] Noninvasive diagnostic studies (such as computed tomography scan, radionuclide brain scan, or electroencephalography) are rarely diagnostic but may reveal localized abnormalities (often in the temporal lobes) to guide diagnostic brain biopsy. Definitive diag-

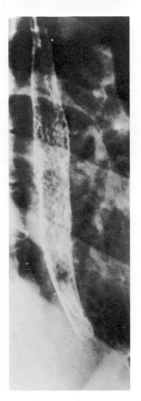

FIGURE 28–5. Barium esophagram revealing a cobblestone appearance of the esophageal mucosa. These findings are typical in both HSV esophagitis and *Candida* esophagitis. (Reprinted from Farthing CF, Brown SE, Staughton RCD: A Colour Atlas of AIDS and HIV Disease Slide Set, 2nd ed. London, Mosby-Year Book/Wolfe, 1989, with permission.)

mised hosts has been estimated as 4% to 5%,[71] but the exact incidence of this problem in the AIDS population has not been determined. The most common mechanism of acyclovir resistance in patients with AIDS is the selection and overgrowth of HSV strains deficient in the enzyme thymidine kinase. These mutated TK-deficient strains do not phosphorylate acyclovir or famciclovir to the active antiviral compounds, and these viruses are resistant to standard dosages of acyclovir, valacyclovir and famciclovir. Although these strains have reduced virulence in animal models[72] and only rarely cause clinical disease in nonimmunocompromised hosts,[74] they are capable of causing severe clinical illness in patients with AIDS.[72] Other mechanisms of drug resistance, including alteration of TK and DNA polymerase specificity, have been described but occur much less frequently. Most reports of drug-resistant HSV have cited localized chronic mucocutaneous infection, but cases of disseminated mucocutaneous disease,[73] meningoencephalitis,[75] and esophagitis[71] caused by these strains have been described.

Treatment of HSV Infection

Mucocutaneous HSV infections in patients with AIDS are often symptomatic and can be a source of great discomfort. Visceral involvement or disseminated HSV disease can be life threatening, and all symptomatic HSV infections should be treated aggressively even if they are reactivations. The prompt administration of antiviral chemotherapy in patients with acute HSV infection reduces morbidity and the risk of serious complications. Currently, several effective antiviral drugs are available, and the clinician must choose the appropriate medication and the optimal route of administration (topical, oral, or intravenous).

Acyclovir

Acyclovir, a synthetic purine nucleoside analog, was the first antiviral agent approved by the FDA for treatment of mucocutaneous HSV infection. Acyclovir has been available and widely used since the early 1980s and, until recently, has been the undisputed antiviral agent of choice for HSV infections in patients with AIDS and for other immunocompromised and nonimmunocompromised hosts.[76] The drug has significant activity against HSV-1, HSV-2, and VZV. Despite excellent in vitro activity against these viruses, the bioavailability of oral acyclo-

nosis may require brain biopsy and the recovery of virus or demonstration of viral antigens from tissue specimens.[67] The histopathologic abnormalities typically observed in normal hosts (hemorrhagic cortical necrosis and lymphocytic infiltration) may be absent in AIDS patients.[64,66,68] Recent studies have demonstrated the utility of detecting HSV DNA in CSF by the polymerase chain reaction technique as a method of noninvasive diagnosis of HSV encephalitis, although false-positive and false-negative results do occur.[69,70] AIDS patients with suspected HSV encephalitis should be treated with high-dose intravenous acyclovir pending results of diagnostic studies.

Drug-Resistant HSV Infection

Since the initial description of acyclovir-resistant HSV infection in patients with AIDS, numerous additional reports have appeared in the literature.[71–73] The incidence of acyclovir-resistant HSV infections in immunocompro-

vir is only about 20%, resulting in relatively low serum drug levels following oral administration as compared to levels achieved with intravenous therapy. Despite these findings, the serum levels of acyclovir achieved with standard acyclovir dosing (200 mg five times daily or 400 mg tid) exceed the levels required to inhibit the growth of HSV-1 and HSV-2, although higher oral doses (800 mg five times daily) are needed to achieve inhibitory serum drug levels to treat the more resistant VZV (see below).[76] Acyclovir has a high therapeutic-to-toxic ratio because it undergoes selective activation and phosphorylation by virus-induced TK only in HSV- and VZV-infected cells. Acyclovir triphosphate selectively inhibits HSV DNA polymerase and results in early termination of DNA chain synthesis. The drug has slightly higher activity against HSV-1 than HSV-2.

Acyclovir distributes into all tissues, including the brain and CSF, and is cleared by renal mechanisms. The serum half-life in patients with normal renal function is 2.5 to 3.3 hours. The dose of intravenous acyclovir is 15 mg/kg/day in three divided doses for treatment of mucocutaneous infection and 30 mg/kg/day for HSV encephalitis. Although oral dosage adjustment is not required because of poor bioavailability, the intravenous dose should be reduced in patients with impaired renal function (Table 28–3). High-dose intravenous therapy can be associated with crystalluria, and adequate hydration should be maintained in patients on intravenous acyclovir to prevent this complication.[76]

Numerous studies have shown acyclovir to be effective for treatment of primary as well as recurrent HSV infection, and as suppressive therapy for patients with frequently recurring HSV. In the immunocompromised patient treatment of recurrence is only marginally beneficial, but in AIDS patients with more severe recurrence treatment is more likely to impact the disease. The drug has an excellent safety record and is usually well tolerated, although some patients may complain of headache or nausea. Acyclovir can be administered orally,[77–83] intravenously,[84,85] or topically,[56,80] and the optimal route of administration, dosage, and duration of therapy depend on the site and severity of the HSV infection. Oral acyclovir is usually appropriate for outpatients with localized, non-life-threatening mucocutaneous HSV infection. Intravenous therapy should be prescribed for patients with disseminated disease, HSV encephalitis, or visceral organ involvement. Additionally, intravenous therapy is indicated for those patients who do not respond adequately to oral treatment, raising concern over issues such as poor drug absorption, poor compliance with oral therapy, or the development of drug-resistant infection. Topical acyclovir ointment is only minimally effective and should not be prescribed in the place of systemic antiviral therapy.

Valacyclovir

Valacyclovir hydrochloride is the L-valyl ester of acyclovir, and is available and effective in the treatment of HSV[86] and VZV[87] infections. Following oral administration, valacyclovir is rapidly absorbed from the gastrointestinal tract. The drug is rapidly and extensively converted to acyclovir in vivo, and the resulting acyclovir serum levels are much higher than those achieved with oral acyclovir. Pharmacokinetic studies reveal that a therapeutic drug level equivalent to acyclovir 800 mg five times daily can be achieved with 1000 mg valacyclovir given every 8 hours.[86–88]

Because of the improved bioavailability of valacyclovir as compared to acyclovir, studies have evaluated less frequent dosing for patients with HSV infection. Valacyclovir is effective in the treatment of first-episode HSV infection at a dose of 500 mg to 1 gm twice daily, and in the treatment of recurrent HSV infection at a dose of 500 mg twice daily if initiated within the first 24 hours of signs or symptoms. Therapy should be continued until all lesions are dry and crusted. Additionally, valacyclovir is effective as suppressive therapy at a dose of 250 mg twice daily, 500 mg once daily (for patients with fewer than 10 recurrences per year), and 1 gm once daily (for patients with 10 or more recurrences per year).[88] Dosage reduction is recommended in patients with a creatinine clearance less than 50 ml/min (Table 28–4).

TABLE 28–3. Dosage Adjustment of Intravenous Acyclovir in Patients with Renal Dysfunction

CREATININE CLEARANCE (ml/min/1.73 m²)	PERCENT OF STANDARD DOSE*	DOSING INTERVAL (hr)
>50	100	8
25–50	100	12
10–25	100	12
0–10	50	24

*Usually 5 mg/kg; 10 mg/kg is used for HSV CNS infections and in some instances for VZV infection.

TABLE 28–4. Dosage Adjustment of Valacyclovir in Patients with Renal Dysfunction

CREATININE CLEARANCE (mL/min)	DOSAGE FOR HERPES ZOSTER	DOSAGE FOR GENITAL HERPES	
		Initial Treatment	Recurrent Episodes
≥50	1 g every 8 hours	1 g every 12 hours	500 mg every 12 hours
30–49	1 g every 12 hours	1 g every 12 hours	500 mg every 12 hours
10–29	1 g every 24 hours	1 g every 24 hours	500 mg every 24 hours
<10	500 mg every 24 hours	500 mg every 24 hours	500 mg every 24 hours

A study evaluating very high valacyclovir dosing (8 gm/day) for suppression of CMV in patients with advanced HIV disease suggested a possible association between valacyclovir and the syndromes of thrombotic thrombocytopenic purpura and hemolytic–uremic syndrome (TTP/HUS). A cause-and-effect relationship has not been firmly established, however, and these findings have not been observed in patients receiving standard dosages of valacyclovir. In view of these observations, however, caution should be used when prescribing valacyclovir in HIV-infected patients, and the standard recommended dosages should not be exceeded.[88]

Famciclovir

Famciclovir is the diacetyl 6-deoxy analog of the active antiviral compound penciclovir. When taken orally, famciclovir is readily absorbed from the upper gastrointestinal tract, and is rapidly converted into penciclovir. In a manner similar to acyclovir, penciclovir undergoes phosphorylation to the triphosphate compound by viral-induced TK and cellular enzymes. Penciclovir triphosphate acts as a competitive inhibitor of the natural substrate required for viral DNA replication, but does not irreversibly terminate DNA replication. The drug has a very long half-life (10 to 20 hours) in HSV-infected cells, ensuring prolonged antiviral activity.[89–93]

Clinical studies have shown that oral famciclovir is effective in the treatment of first-episode HSV infections at a dose of 250 mg three times daily (but as of June 1998 is not approved by FDA for this purpose) and is effective in the treatment of recurrent HSV infection at a dose of 125 mg twice daily if given within the first 6 hours of symptoms or signs. Therapy should be continued until all lesions are dry and crusted. Additionally, famciclovir is effective as suppressive therapy at a dose of 250 mg twice daily.[88,90,91,93] Dosage reduction is rec-

ommended in patients with creatinine clearance less than 60 ml/min (Table 28–5).

Topical penciclovir has been approved by the FDA for the treatment of recurrent HSV gingivostomatitis. Unlike topical acyclovir, penciclovir appears to have a beneficial effect on recurrent mucocutaneous HSV infection when compared to placebo.[94] Topical penciclovir has not been extensively evaluated in patients with HIV infection, however, and may not be as effective as systemic therapy in this immunocompromised population.

Foscarnet

Foscarnet (phosphonoformic acid) is an inorganic pyrophosphate with a broad range of antiviral activities against herpesviruses as well as HIV.[39] Studies have demonstrated foscarnet to be effective in the treatment of CMV disease and in the treatment of drug-resistant HSV and VZV infections. Unlike acyclovir and famciclovir, foscarnet does not require viral enzyme-mediated phosphorylation for activity. Hence,

TABLE 28–5. Dosage Adjustment of Famciclovir in Patients with Zoster and Renal Dysfunction

CREATININE CLEARANCE (mL/min)	DOSAGE REGIMEN
≥60	500 mg every 8 hours
40–59	500 mg every 12 hours
20–39	500 mg every 24 hours

There are insufficient data to recommend a dosage for patients with creatinine clearance <20 mL/min.

Famvir is supplied as 50 mg white, oval, film-coated tablets debossed with FAMVIR on one side and 500 on the other, in bottles of 30 and in Single Unit Packages (blister packs) of 50 (intended for institutional use only). 500 mg 30's: NDC 0007-4117-13; 500 mg SUP 50's: NDC 0007-4117-19. Store at controlled room temperature (15° to 30°C; 59° to 86°F).

foscarnet remains an effective antiviral agent for treatment of TK-deficient, drug-resistant HSV.[95–97] Foscarnet is superior to vidarabine in the treatment of acyclovir-resistant HSV infections in patients with AIDS, and remains a treatment of choice for this illness at a dose of 40 mg/kg three times daily.[97]

Foscarnet must be given intravenously, and side effects (including nausea, fever, headache, anemia, and renal failure) are common. Because of the potential for nephrotoxic effects and electrolyte imbalances, close monitoring of renal function and serum levels of potassium, calcium, phosphate, and magnesium is required. Variable penetration into the CSF has been reported. Dosage adjustments are required in patients with renal dysfunction.

Other Antiviral Drugs

Cidofovir is a long-acting antiviral drug approved by the FDA for the treatment of CMV retinitis, and also appears to be effective in the treatment of drug-resistant HSV.[98,99] Cidofovir has a prolonged serum half-life, allowing for once-weekly intravenous administration. Nephrotoxicity can occur with therapy, however, and pretreatment with intravenous fluids and probenecid is recommended. A gel form of cidofovir for topical use is effective for mucocutaneous drug-resistant HSV infections.[100]

Management of Patients with HSV Infection (Table 28–6)

Most AIDS patients with primary or recurrent mucocutaneous HSV infections are not ill enough to require hospitalization and are suitable candidates for outpatient treatment. The treatment of choice for most HSV infections in AIDS is either oral acyclovir, oral valacyclovir, or oral famciclovir. Because therapy with valacyclovir or famciclovir results in serum antiviral levels comparable to those with intravenous acyclovir, many AIDS patients with severe HSV infections who can tolerate oral therapy can be treated as outpatients.

Although the bioavailability and resultant serum drug levels with oral acyclovir are not as favorable as those with valacyclovir or famciclovir, acyclovir remains a safe, effective, and well-tolerated treatment regimen in HIV-infected patients with HSV infection. Most HIV-infected patients respond well to oral acyclovir, although many clinicians use higher doses of acyclovir in HIV-infected patients than those recommended in nonimmunocompromised patients.

Patients with symptomatic HSV disease should be treated as early as possible with acyclovir 400 mg three to five times daily, valacyclovir 500 to 1000 mg twice daily, or famciclovir 125 to 250 mg two to three times daily until all lesions are healed.

Patients requiring suppressive therapy because of frequent or exceptionally severe recurrences can be treated with acyclovir 400 mg two to three times daily, valacyclovir 250 mg twice daily, valacyclovir 500 to 1000 mg once daily, or famciclovir 250 mg twice daily. As mentioned above, FDA-approved doses of valacyclovir should not be exceeded in patients with HIV infection because of the observation of TTP/HUS with high-dose (8 gm/day) therapy.

Intravenous acyclovir should be reserved for patients with severe or extensive mucocutaneous HSV infection and for patients with viral dissemination, visceral organ infection (e.g., brain, esophagus, eye), or neurologic complications (atonic bladder, transverse myelitis). Intravenous therapy may also be indicated for AIDS patients who require antiviral chemotherapy but are unable to tolerate or absorb oral antiviral therapy because of nausea, dysphagia, or protracted diarrhea. The dose of intravenous acyclovir for patients with mucocutaneous HSV infection and normal renal function is 15 mg/kg/day in three divided doses.[84] Patients with life-threatening HSV infection (encephalitis, neonatal infection, disseminated infection) or visceral organ involvement (esophagitis, proctitis)

TABLE 28–6. Management of HSV Infections in AIDS

CLINICAL PRESENTATION	TREATMENT
Mucocutaneous infection, mild	Acyclovir, 200 mg PO 5 times daily or famciclovir 500–750 mg PO tid × 7 days
Mucocutaneous infection, severe	Acyclovir, 15 mg/kg/d IV
Visceral organ infection	Acyclovir, 30 mg/kg/d IV
Recurrent mucocutaneous infection	Acyclovir, 200–400 mg tid or qid
Severe infection caused by acyclovir-resistant HSV	Foscarnet, 40 mg/kg IV tid

Modified from Drew WL: The medical management of AIDS. Infect Dis Clin North AM 2:505,1988, with permission.

should receive intravenous acyclovir 30 mg/kg/day in three divided doses.[85] Treatment should last for a minimum of 10 days, but longer therapy may be necessary if response to therapy is slow. As noted above, the dose of intravenous acyclovir should be adjusted in patients with impaired renal function (Table 28–3). Oral treatment with acyclovir, valacyclovir, or famciclovir can be substituted for IV acyclovir once the patient is ready for hospital discharge.

Because of their limited absorption, topical acyclovir and topical penciclovir are probably much less effective than either oral or intravenous therapy in the treatment of HSV infections in AIDS. Although topical therapy slightly decreases the duration of viral shedding in immunocompromised hosts with mucocutaneous HSV infection, these nonsystemic therapies do not reduce new lesion formation or the risk of dissemination. There is no added benefit to combining topical therapy with either oral or intravenous antiviral therapy. Topical therapy has little, if any, usefulness in the clinical setting.[80]

Systemic antiviral therapy should be continued until all mucocutaneous lesions have crusted or re-epithelialized. This may require longer treatment than the usual duration of therapy prescribed in the nonimmunocompromised host, because HSV lesions may heal slowly in AIDS patients even with optimal antiviral chemotherapy. If lesions do not heal while the patient is receiving antiviral therapy, repeat viral cultures should be obtained, high-dose oral therapy (e.g., acyclovir 800 mg 5 times daily, famciclovir 500 mg tid, valacyclovir 1 gm tid, or intravenous acyclovir 30 mg/kg/day) may be given, and the possibility of drug-resistant HSV infection should be considered. If available, antiviral susceptibility testing should be performed in this setting to determine whether drug-resistant HSV infection is present. If antiviral testing is not available, patients who continue to have positive cultures for HSV and no evidence of clinical response despite high-dose intravenous acyclovir should be treated presumptively for drug-resistant infection with intravenous foscarnet.

Suppressive Acyclovir Therapy for HSV Infection

Many AIDS patients suffer from frequently recurring HSV infection or develop new HSV recurrences shortly after antiherpes chemotherapy is discontinued. These patients can often be managed with suppressive antiviral therapy.[77–79,82,83,88,90,93,101] AIDS patients requiring suppressive therapy should initially be treated with a regimen of oral acyclovir 400 mg two to three times daily, valacyclovir 250 mg twice daily, valacyclovir 500 to 1000 mg once daily, or famciclovir 250 mg twice daily. Increase of the daily dosage may be necessary to control recurrences, but gastrointestinal intolerance may limit the amount of drug that can be taken. Breakthrough recurrences that develop while the patient is receiving suppressive therapy may be controlled by increasing the daily suppressive dose. Breakthrough recurrences may or may not represent the emergence of drug-resistant strains.[102] Patients who demonstrate a good response to suppressive therapy at high doses may attempt a reduction in the daily suppressive dose. Although suppressive therapy is approved for no longer than 12 months, patients have received daily acyclovir for up to 11 years with no evidence of adverse reactions or cumulative toxicity.[79,101] Studies have shown that the incidence of asymptomatic virus shedding is decreased while a patient is on acyclovir suppression.[103] Individuals maintained on long-term suppressive therapy should be cautioned, however, that recurrences will likely develop after discontinuation of therapy and that the first recurrence may be more severe than those previously experienced.[77,78,82,83] Many HIV-positive patients receiving acyclovir may also be taking zidovudine or other antiretroviral agents. There is no evidence that the combination of these drugs and acyclovir results in synergistic activity against HIV.

Management of Drug-Resistant HSV Infection

With the increased incidence of drug-resistant HSV infections observed in patients with AIDS, several studies have examined the utility of alternate antiviral agents and treatment regimens. Standard doses of intravenous or oral acyclovir have no clinical benefit if the HSV isolate is resistant to acyclovir (ID_{50} >3.0 μg/ml) in vitro. Most acyclovir-resistant strains isolated from patients with AIDS have been TK deficient and are therefore also resistant to valacyclovir and famciclovir. These strains remain susceptible in vitro to vidarabine, which is phosphorylated without TK, and to foscarnet, which does not require phosphorylation for activity. Studies have confirmed that foscarnet is superior to vidarabine in the treatment of these TK-deficient, drug-resistant HSV infections, and foscarnet remains the treatment of choice in this setting.[39,95–97] The dosage of foscarnet used for the treatment of acyclovir-resistant HSV infections in AIDS patients is 40 mg/kg every 8 hours (with reduction in dose for renal dysfunction).

Continuous-infusion acyclovir therapy has been effective in a few AIDS patients with severe acyclovir-resistant HSV infection. Acyclovir has been administered at a dosage of 1.5 to 2.0 mg/kg/hr for 6 weeks, and complete resolution of acyclovir-resistant HSV proctitis has been reported.[104] Other investigational agents for possible treatment of drug-resistant HSV infections include topical trifluridine,[105] topical cidofovir gel,[100] and intravenous cidofovir.[98]

As with many opportunistic infections in AIDS patients, there is a high incidence of recurrent HSV disease after successful treatment for drug-resistant HSV. Some (but not all) relapses in this setting have been due to drug-resistant strains, suggesting that these mutant viruses are capable of causing latency in the immunocompromised host. Chronic prophylaxis with daily acyclovir, valacyclovir, famciclovir, or foscarnet can be considered in patients who are treated successfully for drug-resistant HSV, although there are no data to confirm efficacy in this setting. Foscarnet-resistant strains of HSV have been reported, raising concerns over the possible selection for multi-drug-resistant HSV with suppressive therapy.[99,106]

VARICELLA-ZOSTER VIRUS

Primary VZV infection is usually a childhood illness, with attack rates exceeding 90% in susceptible household contacts.[107] Most adults with AIDS have been previously infected with VZV and (as with HSV) are not susceptible to primary infection.

AIDS patients develop recurrent VZV infection (zoster) more frequently than do age-matched immunocompetent hosts. A retrospective review of 300 AIDS patients with Kaposi's sarcoma revealed that 8% of patients had at least one prior attack of zoster, an incidence seven times greater than expected by the age of the study group. Zoster also occurs with a higher-than-expected frequency in HIV-infected individuals who appear otherwise healthy. Additionally, some HIV-infected patients develop more than one episode of zoster in a relatively short period of time, an uncommon occurrence in immunocompetent hosts.[108–112]

Primary Infection—Varicella

Varicella in immunocompetent children is usually a benign illness. Adults, however, are more likely to develop complications during primary VZV infection. Viral dissemination to visceral organs occurs in up to one third of immunocompetent adults with primary infection.[107] Although most adults with AIDS have been previously infected with VZV and are not susceptible to primary infection,[113] for those who are, a protracted and potentially life-threatening illness could follow.[108]

Recurrent Infection—Zoster

Unlike primary VZV infection, recurrent VZV infection (zoster) is common in patients with AIDS. The illness usually begins with radicular pain and is followed by a localized or segmental erythematous rash covering one to three dermatomes. Maculopapules develop in the dermatomal area, and the patient experiences increasing pain. The maculopapules progress to fluid-filled vesicles, and contiguous vesicles may become confluent, with true bullae formation. In most HIV-infected patients, the lesions remain confined to a dermatomal distribution and heal by crusting and re-epithelialization. Occasionally, however, widespread cutaneous or visceral dissemination may occur. Extensive cutaneous dissemination may appear identical to primary varicella. Visceral dissemination to lung, liver, or the CNS may produce a life-threatening illness.[108–111,114]

Reactivated infection involving the ophthalmic division of the trigeminal nerve often results in infection of the cornea (zoster ophthalmicus). The presence of vesicles on the tip of the nose is often associated with involvement of the eye. Although healing without sequelae may occur, untreated patients are at increased risk to develop anterior uveitis, corneal scarring, and permanent visual loss.[109] Acyclovir-resistant zoster is a rare complication, and has a peculiar dermatomal wart-like, nonhealing appearance.[115]

Complications

Complications of VZV infection are common in immunocompromised patients and may cause prolonged morbidity and death. Dissemination of virus to the lung, liver, and CNS has been associated with a mortality rate of 6% to 17%. Varicella pneumonia may occur during primary VZV infection or during reactivated infection with visceral dissemination in immunocompromised patients. Symptoms are variable. Many patients develop only mild respiratory symptoms, whereas others suffer from severe hypoxemia and succumb to respiratory failure. Radiographic abnormalities are usually out of proportion to the clinical findings, with diffuse nodular densities on chest radiograph and occasional pleural effusions.[107,116]

Encephalitis is a rare complication of VZV infection in AIDS patients but may occur with or without visceral dissemination. The illness begins 3 to 8 days after the onset of varicella or 1 to 2 weeks after the development of zoster, although occasional AIDS patients have developed progressive neurologic disease caused by VZV up to 3 months after the onset of localized zoster.[114] Headache, vomiting, lethargy, and cerebellar symptoms (ataxia, tremors, dizziness) are prominent findings. Diagnosis based on clinical criteria alone can be difficult, because other CNS infections can present in a similar fashion. The diagnosis of VZV encephalitis is documented by finding VZ DNA by polymerase chain reaction or VZV antibody in CSF. Postherpetic neuralgia, defined as prolonged pain following resolution of the cutaneous lesions from zoster, can be severe and disabling.[107,117,118] Although postherpetic neuralgia is a more common occurrence in elderly individuals with zoster, AIDS patients also may be at risk for this complication. Polyradiculopathy similar to that caused by CMV may rarely be due to VZV. In these cases VZV may be isolated from CSF.

Management of VZV Infection
(Table 28–7)

HIV-infected patients who develop primary or recurrent VZV infection should be treated promptly with an effective antiviral regimen. Acyclovir, valacyclovir, and famciclovir are safe and effective in the treatment of patients with primary or recurrent VZV infection. Treatment should be started as soon as the diagnosis is made (preferably within 72 hours of rash onset), and should be continued until all the external lesions are dry and crusted (usually 7 to 10 days).

Because VZV is less susceptible than is HSV to acyclovir, valacyclovir, and famciclovir, the dosages of antiviral therapy used for treatment of VZV infections must be higher than those recommended for HSV. Oral acyclovir in the dosage used to treat HSV does not produce serum drug levels high enough to inhibit VZV in tissue culture, and is unlikely to be effective in patients with active VZV infection. To treat VZV with oral acyclovir, a dose of 800 mg five times daily should be prescribed.[116,119–121] This higher dose does produce serum drug levels high enough to inhibit the growth of VZV in vitro, and this regimen has been shown to modestly decrease the incidence and severity of postherpetic neuralgia in nonimmunocompromised patients.[118,122]

Valacyclovir and famciclovir (discussed in detail above) are also effective agents against VZV and are suitable for oral treatment of acute VZV infections. Because of their improved bioavailability, these drugs have the advantage of producing higher seum drug levels than that achieved with oral acyclovir. Treatment with valacyclovir 1 gm tid[87] or famciclovir 500 mg tid[92,123] reduces the severity of acute VZV infection and appears to reduce the severity and duration of postherpetic neuralgia.[89,117] Although the favorable pharmacokinetics and higher serum drug levels achieved with these agents could be expected to offer a therapeutic advantage as compared to oral acyclovir, no comparative trials evaluating clinical outcome in HIV-infected patients have been reported.

As mentioned in the section on treatment of HSV, the possible association between valacyclovir and TTP/HUS in patients with advanced HIV disease must be kept in mind when prescribing valacyclovir. Although a cause-and-effect relationship has not been firmly established, caution should be used when prescribing valacyclovir in HIV-infected patients, and the standard, FDA-recommended dosages should not be exceeded.[88]

Most AIDS patients with localized zoster are not ill enough to require hospitalization, and are suitable for outpatient therapy with oral acyclovir, oral valacyclovir, or oral famciclovir. Intravenous acyclovir remains an available option, however, and has been shown to be effective in the treatment of patients with VZV infection. Treatment with intravenous acyclovir reduces the duration of viral shedding, new lesion formation, the incidence of dissemination, and mortality rates in immunocompromised hosts with VZV infection.[119,124] Intravenous acyclovir should be prescribed for those patients with disseminated disease or visceral organ involvement, and for those patients who are unable to tolerate oral therapy. The dosage of intravenous acyclovir for patients with VZV infection is 30 mg/kg/day in three divided doses (with dosage adjustments for renal dysfunction; see Table 28–3). Treatment should be continued for at least 7 days or until all external lesions are crusted. The decision whether to hospitalize an individual patient for intravenous acyclovir must be based on several factors, including the severity of the in-

TABLE 28–7. Management of VZV Infections in AIDS

CLINICAL PRESENTATION	TREATMENT
Primary infection (varicella)	Acyclovir, 30 mg/kg/d IV, *or* acyclovir, 600–800 mg PO 5 times daily
Recurrent infection (localized zoster)	Acyclovir, 30 mg/kg/d IV, *or* acyclovir, 600–800 mg PO 5 times daily
Recurrent infection, disseminated	Acyclovir, 30 mg/kg/d IV
Severe infection caused by acyclovir-resistant VZV	Foscarnet, 40 mg/kg tid IV (not FDA approved)

Modified from Drew WL: The medical management of AIDS. Infect Dis Clin North Am 2:507, 1988, with permission.

fection, the immune status of the host, and whether visceral or cutaneous dissemination has occurred.

Treatment with steroids to prevent postherpetic neuralgia remains a controversial topic in regard to the nonimmunocompromised population, but recent studies have failed to document the efficacy of this practice,[125,126] although the general quality of life may be improved. Because of the potential for further immunosuppression and increasing the risk of VZV dissemination in patients with AIDS, however, steroids should not be prescribed for this indication in this population.

Treatment of Drug-Resistant VZV Infection

Drug-resistant VZV has been identified in patients with AIDS. These patients may present with atypical-appearing cutaneous lesions that shed VZV intermittently despite ongoing high-dose antiviral therapy. All strains have been isolated from patients previously treated with acyclovir for recurrent VZV or HSV infection, and these strains may be resistant to acyclovir, valacyclovir, and famciclovir by deficiency of the enzyme thymidine kinase.[127] Foscarnet has been shown to be effective in small studies, but remains investigational for this purpose.[115]

Prevention of VZV Infection

Varicella-zoster immune globulin (VZIG) is effective in preventing severe primary VZV infection in susceptible (i.e., seronegative) immunocompromised hosts if administered within 96 hours from the time of a significant exposure. Care should be taken to ensure that an exposed individual is truly susceptible to infection (by serologic testing if there is no history of chickenpox) prior to administration of VZIG. VZIG is contraindicated in individuals with a history of prior chickenpox and in those who have serologic evidence of previous VZV infection. VZIG is not effective as treatment in individuals who present with acute VZV infection.

The attenuated, live VZV vaccine is licensed in the United States for prevention of varicella in history- and VZ antibody–negative nonimmunocompromised hosts.[128,129] The efficacy and safety of the vaccine in HIV-infected patients has not been well studied, and caution should be used because the vaccine is a live virus and is transmissible. Patients receiving the VZV vaccine can develop a varicella-like rash after administration.[130] Because the vaccine strain produces latency after administration, vaccinated individuals remain at low risk to develop zoster later in life.[128,129,131]

SUMMARY

Herpesvirus (CMV, HSV, VZV) infections are common in AIDS patients and often exist in a chronic or progressive form. Oral ganciclovir prophylaxis can reduce the risk of developing CMV disease. CMV retinitis occurs in up to 40% of AIDS patients and can be treated effectively with ganciclovir or foscarnet. Perianal ulcers, proctitis, and other clinical syndromes caused by HSV can be treated effectively with acyclovir, valacyclovir, or famciclovir. These drugs can be administered daily to prevent HSV recurrences. Herpes zoster in a young adult may be the first indication of immune deficiency resulting from HIV. Because VZV is less susceptible to antiviral drugs than is HSV, higher doses of acyclovir, valacyclovir, or famciclovir are required to achieve inhibitory blood levels. HSV and VZV resistant to acyclovir and related drugs are usually susceptible to foscarnet.

References

1. Spector SA, Wong R, Hsia K, et al: Plasma cytomegalovirus (CMV) DNA load predicts CMV disease and survival in AIDS patients. J Clin Invest 101:497, 1998

2. Felsenstein D, D'Amico DJ, Hirsch MS, et al: Treatment of cytomegalovirus retinitis with 9-[2-hydroxy-1-(hydroxymethyl)ethoxymethyl]guanine. Ann Intern Med 103:377, 1985

3. Palestine AG, Polis MA, De Smet MD, et al: A randomized, controlled trial of foscarnet in the treatment of cytomegalovirus retinitis in patients with AIDS. Ann Intern Med 115:665, 1991

4. Spector SA, Weingeist T, Pollard RB, et al: A randomized, controlled study of intravenous ganciclovir therapy for cytomegalovirus peripheral retinitis in patients with AIDS. J Infect Dis 168:557, 1993

5. Jabs D, and the Studies of Ocular Complications of AIDS Research Group, in collaboration with the AIDS Clinical Trials Group: Mortality in patients with the acquired immunodeficiency syndrome treated with either foscarnet or ganciclovir for cytomegalovirus retinitis. N Engl J Med 326:213, 1992

6. Budka H, Costanzi G, Cristina S, et al: Brain pathology induced by infection with the human immunodeficiency virus (HIV): A histological, immunocytochemical and electron microscopical study of 100 autopsy cases. Acta Neuropathol (Berl) 75:185, 1987

7. Petito CK, Cho E-S, Lehman W, et al: Neuropathology of acquired immunodeficiency syndrome (AIDS): An autopsy review. J Neuropathol Exp Neurol 45:635, 1986

8. Snider WD, Simpson DM, Nielsen S, et al: Neurological complications of acquired immune deficiency syndrome: Analysis of 50 patients. Ann Neurol 14:403, 1983

9. Morgello S, Cho E, Nielsen S, et al: Cytomegalovirus encephalitis in patients with acquired immunodeficiency syndrome: An autopsy study of 30 cases and review of literature. Hum Pathol 18:289, 1987

10. Holland NR, Power C, Mathews VP, et al: Cytomegalovirus encephalitis in AIDS. Neurology 44:507, 1994

11. Drew WL, Mintz L, Miner RC, et al: Prevalence of cytomegalovirus infection in homosexual men. J Infect Dis 143:188, 1981

12. Fiala M, Singer EJ, Graves MC et al: AIDS dementia complex complicated by cytomegalovirus encephalopathy. J Neurol 240:223, 1993

13. Vinters HV, Kwok MK, HO HW, et al: Cytomegalovirus in the nervous system of patients with the acquired immune deficiency syndrome. Brain 112:245, 1989

14. Casareale D, Fiala M, Chang CM, et al: Cytomegalovirus enhances lysis of HIV infected T lymphoblasts. Int J Cancer 44:124, 1989

15. Walot I, Miller BL, Chang L, Mehringer CM: Neuroimaging findings in patients with AIDS. Clin Infect Dis 22:906, 1996

16. Clough LA, Clough JA, Maciunsas RJ, Haas DW: Diagnosing CNS mass lesions in patients with AIDS. AIDS Reader 7:83, 1997

17. Small PM, McPhaul LW, Sooy CD, et al: Cytomegalovirus infection of the laryngeal nerve presenting as hoarseness in patients with acquired immunodeficiency syndrome. Am J Med 86:108, 1989

18. Fuller GN, Jacobs JM, Guiloff RJ: Axonal atrophy in the painful peripheral neuropathy in AIDS. Acta Neuropathol 81:198, 1990

19. Whitley RJ, Jacobson MA, Friedberg DN, et al: Guidelines for the treatment of cytomegalovirus diseases in patients with AIDS in the era of potent antiretroviral therapy. Arch Intern Med 158:957, 1998

20. Dieterich DT, Kotler DP, Busch DF: Ganciclovir treatment of cytomegalovirus colitis in AIDS: A randomized, double-blind, placebo-controlled multicenter study. J Infect Dis 167:278, 1993

21. Emanuel D, Cunningham I, Jules-Elysee K, et al: Cytomegalovirus pneumonia after bone-marrow transplantation successfully treated with the combination of ganciclovir and high-dose intravenous immune globulin. Ann Intern Med 109:777, 1988

22. Reed EC, Bowden RA, Dandliker PS, et al: Treatment of cytomegalovirus pneumonia with ganciclovir and intravenous cytomegalovirus immunoglobulin in patients with bone marrow transplants. Ann Intern Med 109:783, 1988

23. Shepp DH, Dandliker PS, de Miranda P, et al: Activity of 9-[2-hydroxy-1-(hydroxymethyl)ethoxymethyl]guanine in the treatment of cytomegalovirus pneumonia. Ann Intern Med 103:368, 1985

24. Sullivan V, Taliarico CL, Stanat SC, et al: A protein kinase homologue controls phosphorylation of ganciclovir in human cytomegalovirus-infected cells. Nature 358:162, 1992

25. Martin D, Kuppermann B, Wolitz R, et al: Combined oral ganciclovir and intravitreal ganciclovir implant for treatment of patients with cytomegalovirus retinitis: A randomized, controlled study. Program and Abstracts of the 37th Interscience Conference on Antimicrobial Agents and Chemotherapy, Toronto, 1997, Abstract LB-9

26. Musch DC, Martin DF, Gordon JF, et al: Treatment of cytomegalovirus retinitis with a sustained-release ganciclovir implant. N Engl J Med 337:83, 1997

27. Drew WL, Ives D, Lalezari JP, et al: Oral ganciclovir as maintenance treatment for cytomegalovirus retinitis in patients with AIDS. N Engl J Med 333:615, 1995

28. The Oral Ganciclovir European and Australian Cooperative Study Group: Intravenous versus oral ganciclovir: European/Australian comparative study of efficacy and safety in the prevention of cytomegalovirus retinitis recurrence in patients with AIDS. AIDS 9:471, 1995

29. Cantrill HL, Henry K, Melroe H, et al: Treatment of cytomegalovirus retinitis with intravitreal ganciclovir: Long-term results. Ophthalmology 96:367, 1989

30. Anand R, Nightingale D, Fish RH, et al: Control of cytomegalovirus retinitis using sustained release of intraocular ganciclovir. Arch Ophthalmol 111:223, 1993

31. Martin DF, Parks DJ, Mellow D, et al: Treatment of cytomegalovirus retinitis with an intraocular sustained-release ganciclovir implant. Arch Ophthalmol 112:1531, 1994

32. Sanborn GE, Anand R, Torti RE, et al: Sustained-release ganciclovir therapy for treatment of cytomegalovirus retinitis. Arch Ophthalmol 110:188, 1992

33. Buhles WC Jr, Mastre BJ, Tinker AJ, et al: Ganciclovir treatment of life- or sight-threatening cytomegalovirus infection: Experience in 314 immunocompromised patients. Rev Infect Dis 10(Suppl 3):S495, 1988

34. Erice A, Chou S, Biron K, et al: Progressive disease due to ganciclovir-resistant cytomegalovirus in immunocompromised patients. N Engl J Med 320:289, 1989

35. Drew WL, Miner RC, Busch DF, et al: Prevalence of resistance in patients receiving ganciclovir for serious cytomegalovirus infection. J Infect Dis 163:716, 1991

36. Jacobson MA, Drew WL, Feinberg J, et al: Foscarnet therapy for ganciclovir-resistant cytomegalovirus retinitis in patients with AIDS. J Infect Dis 163:1348, 1991

37. Jabs DA, Enger C, Dunn JP, et al: Cytomegalovirus retinitis and viral resistance: Ganciclovir resistance. J Infect Dis 177:770, 1998

38. Cimoch PJ, Lavelle J, Pollard R, et al: Pharmacokinetics of oral ganciclovir alone and in combination with zidovudine, didanosine, and probenecid in HIV-infected subjects. J AIDS Acquir Immune Defic Syndr Hum Retrovirol 17:227, 1998

39. Chrisp P, Clissold SP: Foscarnet: A review of its antiviral activity, pharmacokinetic properties and therapeutic use in immunocompromised patients with cytomegalovirus retinitis. Drugs 41:104, 1991

40. Jacobson MA, Causey D, Polsky B: A dose-ranging study of daily maintenance intravenous foscarnet therapy for cytomegalovirus retinitis in AIDS. J Infect Dis 168:444, 1993

41. Studies of Ocular Complications of AIDS Research Group in Collaboration with the AIDS Clinical Trials Group: Combination foscarnet and ganciclovir therapy vs monotherapy for the treatment of relapsed cytomegalovirus retinitis in patients with AIDS: The cytomegalovirus Retreatment Trial. Arch Ophthalmol 114:23, 1996

42. Lalezari, JP, Drew WL, Glutzer E, et al: (S)-1-[3-hydroxy-2-(phosphonylmethoxy)propyl]cytosine (cidofovir): Results of a Phase I/II study of a novel antiviral nucleotide analogue. J Infect Dis 171:788, 1995

43. Spector SA, McKinley GF, Lalezari JP, et al: Oral ganciclovir for the prevention of cytomegalovirus disease in persons with AIDS. N Engl J Med 334:1491, 1996

44. Corey L, Adams HG, Brown ZA, et al: Genital herpes simplex virus infections: Clinical manifestations, course, and complications. Ann Intern Med 98:958, 1983

45. Corey L, Homes KK: Genital herpes simplex virus infections: Current concepts in diagnosis, therapy, and prevention. Ann Intern Med 98:973, 1983

46. Corey L, Spear PG: Infections with herpes simplex viruses (parts 1 and 2). N Engl J Med 314:686, 749, 1986

47. Fleming DT, McQuillan GM, Johnson RE, et al: Herpes simplex virus type 2 in the United States, 1976 to 1995. N Engl J Med 337:1105, 1997

48. Johnson RE, Nahmias AJ, Magder LS, et al: A seroepidemiologic survey of the prevalence of herpes simplex virus type 2 infection in the United States. N Engl J Med 321:7, 1989

49. Nahmias AJ, Keyserling H, Lee FK: Herpes simplex viruses 1 and 2. In Evans A (ed): Viral Infections of Humans: Epidemiology and Control, 3rd ed. New York, Plenum Press, 1989, p 393

50. Quinnan GV, Masur H, Rook AH, et al: Herpes simplex infections in the acquired immune deficiency syndrome. JAMA 252:72, 1984

51. Safrin S, Arvin A, Mills J, Ashley R: Comparison of the Western immunoblot assay and a glycoprotein G enzyme immunosassay for detection of serum antibodies to herpes simplex virus type 2 in patients with AIDS. J Clin Microbiol 30:1312, 1992

52. Siegel D, Golden E, Washington E, et al: Prevalence and correlates of herpes simplex infections: The population-based AIDS in Multiethnic Neighborhoods study. JAMA 268:1702, 1992

53. Stewart JA, Reef SE, Pellett PE, et al: Herpesvirus infections in persons infected with human immunodeficiency virus. Clin Infect Dis 21 (Suppl 1):S114, 1995

54. Spruance SI, Overall JC, Kern ER, et al: The natural history of recurrent herpes simplex labialis: Implications for antiviral therapy. N Engl J Med 297:68, 1977

55. Straus SE, Smith HA, Brickman C, et al: Acyclovir for chronic mucocutaneous herpes simplex virus infection in immunosuppressed patients. Ann Intern Med 96:270, 1982

56. Whitley RJ, Levin M, Barton N, et al: Infections caused by herpes simplex virus in the immunocompromised host: Natural history and topical acyclovir therapy. J Infect Dis 150:323, 1984

57. Brock BV, Selke S, Benedetti J, et al: Frequency of asymptomatic shedding of herpes simplex virus in women with genital herpes. JAMA 263:418, 1990

58. Koelle DM, Benedetti J, Langenberg A, Corey L: Asymptomatic reactivation of herpes simplex virus in women after the first episode of genital herpes. Ann Intern Med 116:433, 1992

59. Augenbraun M, Feldman J, Chirgwin K, et al: Increased genital shedding of herpes simplex virus type 2 in HIV-seropositive women. Ann Intern Med 123:845, 1995

60. Wald A, Zeh J, Selke S, et al: Virologic characteristics of subclinical and symptomatic genital herpes infections. N Engl J Med 333:770, 1995

61. Goodell SE, Quinn TC, Mkrtichian F, et al: Herpes simplex proctitis in homosexual men: Clinical, sigmoidoscopic, and histopathologic features. N Engl J Med 308:868, 1983

62. Siegel FP, Lopez C, Hammer BS, et al: Severe acquired immunodeficiency in male homosexuals, manifested by chronic perianal ulcerative herpes simplex lesions. N Engl J Med 305:1439, 1981

63. Genereau T, Lortholary O, Bouchaud O, et al: Herpes simplex esophagitis in patients with AIDS: Report of 34 cases. Clin Infect Dis 22:926, 1996

64. Dix RD, Bredesen DE, Davis RL, Mills J: Herpesvirus neurological diseases associated with AIDS: Recovery of viruses from central nervous system (CNS) tissues, peripheral nerve, and cerebrospinal fluid (CSF). In: Program and Abstracts of the International Conference on AIDS, Atlanta, 1985, Abstract 43

65. Dix RD, Bredesen DE, Erlich KS, et al: Recovery of herpes-viruses from cerebrospinal fluid of immunodeficient homosexual men. Ann Neurol 18:611, 1985

66. Dix RD, Waitzman DM, Follansbee S, et al: Herpes simplex virus type 2 encephalitis in two homosexual men with persistent adenopathy. Ann Neurol 17:203, 1985

67. Nahmias AJ, Whitley RD, Visintine AN, et al: Herpes simplex virus type 2 encephalitis: Laboratory evaluations and their diagnostic significance. J Infect Dis 146:829, 1982

68. Kahlon J, Chatterjee S, Lakeman FD, et al: Detection of antibodies to herpes simplex virus in the cerebrospinal fluid of patients with herpes simplex encephalitis. J Infect Dis 155:38, 1987

69. Lakeman FD, Whitley RJ, and the National Institute of Allergy and Infectious Diseases Collaborative Antiviral Study Group: Diagnosis of herpes simplex encephalitis: Application of polymerase chain reaction to cerebrospinal fluid from brain-biopsied patients and correlation with disease. J Infect Dis 171:857, 1995

70. Landry ML: False-positive polymerase chain reaction results in the diagnosis of herpes simplex encephalitis. J Infect Dis 172:1641, 1995

71. Englund JA, Zimmerman ME, Swierkosz EM, et al: Herpes simplex virus resistant to acyclovir: A study in a tertiary care center. Ann Intern Med 112:416, 1990

72. Erlich KS, Mills J, Chatis P, et al: Acyclovir-resistant herpes simplex virus infections in patients with the acquired immunodeficiency syndrome. N Engl J Med 320:293, 1989
73. Marks GL, Nolan PE, Erlich KS, Ellis MN: Mucocutaneous dissemination of acyclovir-resistant herpes simplex virus in a patient with AIDS. Rev Infect Dis 11:474, 1989
74. Kost RG, Hill EL, Tigges M, et al: Recurrent acyclovir-resistant genital herpes in an immunocompetent patient. N Engl J Med 329:1777, 1993
75. Gateley A, Gander RM, Johnson PC, et al: Herpes simplex type 2 meningoencephalitis resistant to acyclovir in a patient with AIDS. J Infect Dis 161:711, 1990
76. Whitley RJ, Gnann JW. Acyclovir: A decade later. N Engl J Med 327:782, 1993
77. Douglas JM, Critchlow C, Benedetti J, et al: Double blind study of oral acyclovir for suppression of recurrences of genital herpes simplex virus infection. N Engl J Med 310:1551, 1984
78. Fife KH, Crumpacker CS, Mertz CJ, et al: Recurrence and resistance patterns of herpes simplex virus following cessation of >6 years of chronic suppression with acyclovir. J Infect Dis 169:1338, 1994
79. Kaplowitz LG, Baker D, Gelb L, et al: Prolonged continuous acyclovir treatment of normal adults with frequently recurring genital herpes simplex virus infection. JAMA 265:747, 1991
80. Kinghorn GR, Abeywickreme I, Jeavons M, et al: Efficacy of combined treatment with oral and topical acyclovir in first episode genital herpes. Genitourin Med 62:186, 1986
81. Shepp DH, Newton BA, Dandliker PS, et al: Oral acyclovir therapy for mucocutaneous herpes simplex virus infections in immunocompromised marrow transplant recipients. Ann Intern Med 102:783, 1985
82. Straus SE, Seidlin M, Takiff H, et al: Oral acyclovir to suppress recurring herpes simplex virus infections in immunodeficient patients. Ann Intern Med 100:522, 1984
83. Wade JC, Newton B, Flournoy N, et al: Oral acyclovir for prevention of herpes simplex virus reactivation after marrow transplantation. Ann Intern Med 100:823, 1984
84. Wade JC, Newton B, McLaren C, et al: Intravenous acyclovir to treat mucocutaneous herpes simplex virus infection after marrow transplantation. Ann Intern Med 96:265, 1982
85. Whitley RJ, Alford CA, Hirsch MS, et al: Vidarabine versus acyclovir therapy in herpes simplex encephalitis. N Engl J Med 314:144, 1986
86. Spruance SL, Tyring SK, DeGregorio B, et al: A large-scale, placebo-controlled, dose-ranging trial of peroral valaciclovir for episodic treatment of recurrent herpes genitalis. Arch Intern Med 156:1729, 1996
87. Beutner KR, Friedman DJ, Forszpaniak C, et al: Valaciclovir compared with acyclovir for improved therapy for herpes zoster in immunocompetent adults. Antimicrob Agents Chemother 39:1546, 1995
88. Centers for Disease Control and Prevention. 1998 guidelines for treatment of sexually transmitted diseases. MMWR Morb Mortal Wkly Rep 47(RR-1):20, 1998
89. Gnann JW: New antivirals with activity against varicella-zoster virus. Ann Neurol 34:S69, 1994
90. Mertz GJ, Loveless MO, Levin MJ, et al: Oral famciclovir for suppression of recurrent genital herpes simplex virus infection in women: A multicenter, dou-

91. Sacks SL, Aoki FY, Diaz-Mitoma F, et al. Patient-initiated, twice-daily oral famciclovir for early recurrent genital herpes: A randomized, double-blind multicenter trial. JAMA 276:44, 1996
92. Saltzman R, Jurewicz R, Boon R: Safety of famciclovir in patients with herpes zoster and genital herpes. Antimicrob Agents Chemother 38:2454, 1994
93. Schacker T, Hu H, Koelle DM, et al: Famciclovir for the suppression of symptomatic and asymptomatic herpes simplex virus reactivation in HIV-infected persons: A double-blind, placebo-controlled trial. Ann Intern Med 128:21, 1998
94. Spruance SL, Rea TL, Thoming C, et al: Penciclovir cream for the treatment of herpes simplex labialis: A randomized, multicenter, double-blind, placebo-controlled trial. JAMA 277:1374, 1997
95. Chatis PA, Miller CH, Schrager LE, Crumpacker CS: Successful treatment with foscarnet of an acyclovir-resistant mucocutaneous infection with herpes simplex virus in a patient with acquired immunodeficiency syndrome. N Engl J Med 320:297, 1989
96. Erlich KS, Jacobson MA, Koehler JE, et al: Foscarnet therapy for severe acyclovir-resistant herpes simplex virus type-2 infections in patients with the acquired immunodeficiency syndrome (AIDS): An uncontrolled trial. Ann Intern Med 110:710, 1989
97. Safrin S, Crumpacker C, Chatis P, et al: A controlled trial comparing foscarnet with vidarabine for acyclovir-resistant mucocutaneous herpes simplex in the acquired immunodeficiency syndrome. N Engl J Med 325:551, 1991
98. Lalezari JP, Drew WL, Glutzer E, et al: Treatment with intravenous (s)-1[3-hydroxy-2-(phosphonylmethoxy)propyl]-cytosine of acyclovir-resistant mucocutaneous infection with herpes simplex virus in a patient with AIDS. J Infect Dis 170:570, 1994
99. Snoeck R, Andrei G, Gerard M, et al. Successful treatment of progressive mucocutaneous infection due to acyclovir- and foscarnet-resistant herpes simplex virus with (S)-1-(3-hydroxy-2-phosphonylmethoxypropyl)-cytosine (HPMPC). J Infect Dis 18:570, 1994
100. Lalezari J, Schacker T, Feinberg J, et al: A randomized, double-blind placebo-controlled trial of cidofovir gel for the treatment of acyclovir-unresponsive mucocutaneous herpes simplex virus infection in patients with AIDS. J Infect Dis 176:892, 1997
101. Goldberg LH, Kaufman R, Kurtz TO, et al: Long-term suppression of recurrent genital herpes with acyclovir: A 5-year benchmark study. Arch Dermatol 129:582, 1993
102. Nusinoff-Lehrman S, Douglas JM, Corey L, et al: Recurrent genital herpes and suppressive oral acyclovir therapy: Relation between clinical outcome and in-vitro sensitivity. Ann Intern Med 104:786, 1986
103. Wald A, Zeh J, Barnum G, et al: Suppression of subclinical shedding of herpes simplex virus type 2 with acyclovir. Ann Intern Med 124:8, 1996
104. Engel JP, Englund JA, Fletcher CV, Hill EL: Treatment of resistant herpes simplex virus with continuous-infusion acyclovir. JAMA 263:1662, 1990
105. Kessler HA, Hurwitz, S, Farthing C, et al: Pilot study of topical trifluridine for the treatment of acyclovir-resistant mucocutaneous herpes simplex disease in patients with AIDS (ACTG 172). J Acquir Immune Defic Syndr Hum Retrovirol 12:147, 1996
106. Safrin S, Kemmerly S, Plotkin B, et al: Foscarnet-resistant herpes simplex virus infection in patients with AIDS. J Infect Dis 169:193, 1994

107. Weller TH: Varicella and herpes zoster: Changing concepts of the natural history, control, and importance of a not-so-benign virus (parts 1 and 2). N Engl J Med 309:1362, 1434, 1983

108. Buchbinder SP, Katz MH, Hessol NA, et al: Herpes zoster and human immunodeficiency virus infection. J Infect Dis 166:1153, 1992

109. Cole EL, Meisler DM, Calabrese LH, et al: Herpes zoster ophthalmicus and acquired immune deficiency syndrome. Arch Ophthalmol 102:1027, 1984

110. Cone LA, Schiffman HA: Herpes zoster and the acquired immunodeficiency syndrome [letter]. Ann Intern Med 100:462, 1984

111. Friedman-Kien AE, Lafleur FL, Gendler E, et al: Herpes zoster: A possible early clinical sign for development of acquired immunodeficiency syndrome in high-risk individuals. J Am Acad Dermatol 14:1023, 1986

112. Gershon AA, Mervish N, LaRussa P, et al. Varicella-zoster virus infection in children with underlying human immunodeficiency virus infection. J Infect Dis 176:1496, 1997

113. Rogers MF, Morens DM, Stewart JA, et al: National case-control study of Kaposi's sarcoma and Pneumocystis carinii pneumonia in homosexual men: Part 2, Laboratory results. Ann Intern Med 99:151, 1983

114. Ryder JW, Croen K, Kleinschmidt-DeMasters BK, et al: Progressive encephalitis three months after resolution of cutaneous zoster in a patient with AIDS. Ann Neurol 19:182, 1986

115. Safrin S, Berger TG, Gilson I, et al: Foscarnet therapy in five patients with AIDS and acyclovir-resistant varicella-zoster virus infection. Ann Intern Med 115:19, 1991

116. Wallace MR, Katz MH, Hessol NA, et al: Treatment of adult varicella with oral acyclovir: A randomized, placebo-controlled trial. Ann Intern Med 117:358, 1992

117. Gilden DH: Herpes zoster with postherpetic neuralgia—persisting pain and frustration. N Engl J Med 330:932, 1994

118. Huff JC, Drucker JL, Clemmer A, et al: Effect of oral acyclovir on pain resolution in herpes zoster: A reanalysis. J Med Virol 1(Suppl):93, 1993

119. Balfour HH, Bean B, Laskin OL, et al: Acyclovir halts progression of herpes zoster in immunocompromised patients. N Engl J Med 308:1448, 1983

120. Laskin O: Acyclovir: Pharmacology and clinical experience. Arch Intern Med 144:1241, 1984

121. Haake DA, Zakowski PC, Haake DL, Bryson YJ: Early treatment with acyclovir for varicella pneumonia in otherwise healthy adults: Retrospective controlled study and review. Rev Infect Dis 12:788, 1990

122. Huff JC, Bean B, Balfour HH, et al: Therapy of herpes zoster with oral acyclovir. Am J Med 85 (Suppl 2A): 84, 1988

123. Tyring S, Barbarash RA, Nahlik JE, et al: Famciclovir for the treatment of acute herpes zoster: Effects on acute disease and postherpetic neuralgia. A randomized, double blind, placebo controlled trial. Ann Intern Med 123:89, 1995

124. Shepp DH, Dandliker PS, Meyers JD: Treatment of varicella zoster virus infection in severely immunocompromised patients. N Engl J Med 314:208, 1986

125. Whitley RJ, Weiss H, Gnann JW, et al. Acyclovir with and without prednisone for the treatment of herpes zoster: A randomized, placebo controlled trial. Ann Intern Med 125:376, 1996

126. Wood MJ, Johnson RW, McKendrick MW, et al: A randomized trial of acyclovir for 7 days or 21 days with and without prednisolone for treatment of acute herpes zoster. N Engl J Med 330:896, 1994

127. Jacobson MA, Berger TG, Fikrig S, et al: Acyclovir (ACV)-resistant varicella zoster virus (VZV) infection following chronic oral ACV therapy in patients with AIDS. Ann Intern Med 112:187, 1990

128. Gershon AA, Steinberg SP, LaRussa P, et al: Immunization of healthy adults with live attenuated varicella vaccine. J Infect Dis 158:132, 1988

129. White CJ, Kuter BJ, Hidebrand CS, et al: Varicella vaccine (VARIVAX) in healthy children and adolescents: Results from clinical trials, 1987 to 1989. Pediatrics 87:604, 1991

130. LaRussa P, Steinberg S, Meurice F, Gershon A: Transmission of vaccine strain varicella-zoster virus from a healthy adult with vaccine-associated rash to susceptible household contacts. J Infect Dis 176:1072, 1997

131. Hardy I, Gershon AA, Steinberg SP, et al: The incidence of zoster after immunization with live attenuated varicella vaccine. N Engl J Med 325:1545, 1991

29 | Management of Syphilis in HIV-Infected Persons

GAIL BOLAN

The management of syphilis in persons with co-existing HIV infection is a complex problem.[1-8] Epidemiologic studies have demonstrated that a history of sexually transmitted diseases (STDs), including syphilis, is associated with an increased risk for HIV infection and AIDS and that STDs causing genital ulceration may be cofactors for acquiring HIV infection.[9-11] More recently, isolated case reports have suggested that coexistent HIV infection may alter the natural history of syphilis or the dosage or duration of treatment required to cure syphilis.[12-16] Also, reports of false-negative and false-positive serologic test results for syphilis in HIV-infected persons raise questions about the sensitivity and specificity of serologic diagnostic tests in such patients.[17-21] Questions about the significance of cerebrospinal fluid (CSF) abnormalities in patients with early syphilis may assume greater importance in the presence of HIV infection.[1,2,4,5,22,23]

Because data from prospective controlled studies are not available to answer many of these questions, definitive recommendations for managing HIV-infected patients with syphilis are limited. Management options are presented here for clinicians to consider until more definitive recommendations can be made. Options to consider in treating HIV infected patients include

1. Evaluating CSF for evidence of neurosyphilis earlier in the course of infection
2. Treating patients with penicillin regimens of longer duration, higher dose, and better CSF penetration
3. Obtaining biopsy specimens from suspicious lesions and using special stains for spirochetes in patients with serologic test results negative for syphilis

4. Testing syphilitic patients for antibodies to HIV and testing HIV-infected patients for syphilis

EPIDEMIOLOGY

Epidemiologic studies demonstrate that a history of an STD, including syphilis, is associated with an increased risk for HIV infection and AIDS among both homosexuals[9,11] and heterosexuals,[24] presumably because sexual behaviors that increase the risk for acquiring other STDs also increase the risk for acquiring HIV (see Chapter 1). Furthermore, STDs that cause genital ulcerations have been implicated as cofactors for acquiring HIV infection.[10] Therefore, increases in the incidence of STDs in any population may presage future HIV-related disease.

Since 1982, the significant decreases seen in syphilis morbidity in the United States have occurred primarily among homosexual and bisexual men.[25] In areas reporting high rates of syphilis infection, the percentage of early syphilis cases occurring among homosexual and bisexual men decreased from 50% to 70% in the late 1970s to 5% to 15% in 1990.[25] These data presumably reflect changes in sexual practices that reduce the risk of HIV infection among homosexual and bisexual men. They suggest that education efforts encouraging safer sex practices have been effective among homosexual men. However, safer sex practices, such as oral sex without ejaculation, may reduce the risk of HIV infection but may not reduce the risk of syphilis unless a condom is used. In addition, because many patients with syphilis are not routinely tested for neurosyphilis or HIV infection, and because these conditions (if diagnosed) are not reportable in many areas, the incidence of syphilis—especially neurosyphilis—in HIV-infected patients is unknown. Thus it is not known whether patients with HIV infection are at higher risk for acquired syphilis or neurosyphilis than persons without HIV infection.

PATHOGENESIS

It is plausible that impairment of both cell-mediated and humoral immunity by HIV[26] could limit the host's defenses against *Treponema pallidum*, thereby altering the clinical manifestations or natural course of syphilis infection, or both. Host immunity, especially cell-mediated immunity, plays an important role in protecting the host against syphilis.[27] In animal models, selective impairment of cell-mediated immunity alters the host response to syphilis infection. Incubation time is shorter, lesions are more numerous and widespread, and healing time is slower.[28] Furthermore, HIV-induced meningeal inflammation may facilitate penetration of spirochetes into the central nervous system (CNS) and thus contribute to the development of symptomatic neurosyphilis.

CLINICAL MANIFESTATIONS AND COURSE

Case reports have suggested that the clinical manifestations of syphilis may be unusual and the course more rapid in patients with HIV infection.[5,15] These anecdotal reports have led to the hypothesis that, in patients co-infected with HIV and *T. pallidum*, symptomatic neurosyphilis may be more likely to develop, the latency period before development of meningovascular syphilis may be shorter, and the efficacy of standard therapy for syphilis may be reduced.

Neurosyphilis

Several cases of neurosyphilis have been reported in patients with HIV infection[15,29–31] (see Chapter 14). One patient had a diffuse maculopapular rash, hepatomegaly, and unilateral facial palsy. Laboratory data were remarkable for transient elevation of serum transaminases, a rapid plasma reagin (RPR) titer of 1:512, and a positive fluorescent treponemal antibody-absorbed (FTA-abs) test result. CSF examina-

tion revealed mononuclear pleocytosis (66 cells/mm³), an elevated protein level (182 mg/dl), and a CSF–Venereal Disease Research Laboratories (VDRL) titer of 1:4. This case is consistent with secondary syphilis accompanied by acute syphilitic meningitis and cranial nerve involvement.

Another patient presented with a pure motor hemiplegia that appeared after a 2-month prodrome of fatigue, malaise, and headache. No previous history of syphilis or chancre was reported. Laboratory data were remarkable for transient elevation of serum transaminases, an RPR titer of 1:256, and a positive FTA-abs test result. CSF examination revealed lymphocytic pleocytosis (234 cells/mm³), an elevated protein level (94 mg/dl), hypoglycorrhachia (glucose 33 mm/dl), and a CSF-VDRL titer of 1:1. This case is consistent with meningovascular syphilis. A third patient had posterior uveitis, neurosensory hearing loss, and meningovascular syphilis (pure motor hemiparesis) 4 months after the diagnosis of primary syphilis. Another patient presented with an unsteady gait, sensory deficits, generalized areflexia, and a positive Romberg sign. The RPR titer was 1:8 and the FTA-abs test result was positive. CSF examination revealed lymphocytic pleocytosis (54 cells/mm³) and a CSF-VDRL titer of 1:2.

These case reports of neurosyphilis in HIV-infected persons are similar to cases reported before the AIDS epidemic.[32–34] Neurosyphilis may occur at any stage of syphilis. The clinical spectrum and time between primary infection and neurologic symptoms are well described.[34] Approximately 35% to 40% of persons with secondary syphilis have asymptomatic CNS involvement, with an abnormal cell count, protein level, glucose level, or reactive CSF-VDRL found on CSF examination. Acute syphilitic meningitis usually occurs within the first 2 years of infection; 10% of cases are diagnosed at the time of the secondary rash. Patients experience headache, meningeal irritation, and cranial nerve abnormalities. Typically, cranial nerves at the base of the brain (especially cranial nerves II, III, VI, VII, and VIII) are involved. Meningovascular syphilis can occur a few months to 10 years after the primary infection (average, 7 years).

Unlike the sudden onset of thrombotic or embolic stroke syndromes, meningovascular syphilis is associated with prodromal symptoms for weeks to months before focal defects of a vascular syndrome are identified. Prodromal symptoms include headache, vertigo, insomnia, and psychiatric abnormalities, such as personality changes. The focal defects initially are intermittent or progress slowly over a few days. In contrast, general paresis and tabes dorsalis are the parenchymatous forms of neurosyphilis that occur, in general, 10 to 30 years later. General paresis causes symptoms similar to those of any dementia, and syndromes similar to many psychiatric illnesses also have been described. Tabes dorsalis is associated with a triad of symptoms (lightning pains, dysuria, and ataxia) and a triad of signs (Argyll Robertson pupils, areflexia, and loss of proprioceptive sense).

Most symptomatic neurosyphilis cases reported among HIV-infected persons have been the early forms of neurosyphilis, namely, acute syphilitic meningitis and meningovascular neurosyphilis. Tabes dorsalis was reported in one HIV-infected man who had been treated for primary syphilis 7 years earlier[35] and in another man exposed 7 years earlier.[30] In addition, cases of syphilitic meningomyelitis with spastic paraparesis[36] and syphilitic polyradiculopathy with progressive leg pain and weakness[37] have been published.

Although it is clear that the neurosyphilis cases involving persons with concurrent HIV infection published to date do not represent unusual clinical manifestations, neurologic complications may occur more frequently and earlier in HIV-infected patients. Until better data from controlled studies are available, most experts believe that HIV-infected patients with syphilis are at increased risk of neurologic complications, but the magnitude of the risk is probably very small.[38] However, the importance of a careful neurologic evaluation in any patient with syphilis or in any patient with HIV is obvious. Of note, Lukehart et al.[22] found viable *T. pallidum* in the CSF of 12 of 40 patients with primary or secondary syphilis and no neurologic symptoms. In this study, isolation of *T. pallidum* was associated with two or more abnormal CSF findings, including pleocytosis, elevated protein concentration, or a reactive CSF-VDRL test, but was not associated with coexisting HIV infection. These data suggest that asymptomatic CNS involvement at the time of early syphilis infection is common, but not more common, in HIV-infected individuals.

Ocular and Otologic Syphilis

A number of case reports of ocular and otologic manifestations of syphilis in HIV-infected persons have been published.[39–45] The most common ocular findings in patients with concurrent HIV infection are uveitis, chorioretinitis, and re-trobulbar neuritis. Retinitis or neuroretinitis, papillitis, vitreitis, and optic perineuritis also have been described. The most common presenting symptoms are decreased vision, eye pain, or both. In addition to the abnormalities of the optic cranial nerve and ocular motor nerves III and VI that can occur with acute syphilitic meningitis, these other ocular manifestations of syphilis commonly have been associated with the secondary state of infection and CNS involvement. One case report of a gumma of the optic nerve has been published.[46]

Otologic syphilis is one of the few forms of sensorineural hearing loss that can be reversed if diagnosed and treated appropriately. Although the incidence of otologic symptoms in patients with HIV infection apparently is low, five cases of otosyphilis in persons with coexisting HIV infection have been reported.[44] Otologic findings in these patients included progressive hearing loss, tinnitus, imbalance, and a sensation of ear fullness. Three patients had been treated for primary syphilis 2 to 5 years before the onset of symptoms. Only one patient with acute syphilis meningitis had evidence of CNS involvement coincident with the diagnosis of otosyphilis. One case report of otosyphilis from an internal auditory canal gumma has been published.[41]

These clinical manifestations of ocular and otologic syphilis among persons with concurrent HIV infection have been described among persons without HIV infection. However, as is the case for neurologic complications, it is possible that ocular and otologic findings may occur more frequently in HIV-infected persons, albeit very infrequently. Performing careful opthalmologic and otologic examinations of symptomatic HIV-infected persons and any symptomatic persons with syphilis is essential.

Mucocutaneous Syphilis

Most HIV-infected patients with *T. pallidum* have typical dermatologic clinical features of primary and secondary disease, such as chancres and diffuse maculopapular rashes.[1,47–49] In one study among patients seen in an STD clinic, however, patients with HIV infection were more likely to present with signs and symptoms of secondary syphilis and were more likely to have overlap between the primary and secondary stages of syphilis (i.e., chancres were still present at the time of the secondary syphilis diagnosis). In addition, atypical chancres have been reported,[50] and two patients in our clinic presented with lesions that looked like a fissure and an abrasion; serous fluid from both were positive for *T. pallidum* by darkfield examination. Gummatous penile ulcerations have also been reported.[51,52]

Case reports of unusual rashes include papular or nodular eruptions,[18,53] nodular or ulcerative lesions with necrotic centers (i.e., lues maligna),[18,54,55] and keratoderma.[56] These skin lesions have been characterized as more aggressive forms of secondary syphilis in HIV-infected persons, yet the same dermatologic presentations have been described in non–HIV-infected persons. The frequency of these uncommon cutaneous findings cannot be determined by these case reports, and additional studies are needed to define the clinical spectrum of syphilis in both HIV-infected and non–HIV-infected populations.

Other Forms of Syphilis

It is important to remember that syphilis is a systemic infection that disseminates early in the course of infection and can ultimately involve any organ system. Symptomatic involvement of organs other than skin, mucous membranes, and CNS is very rare but has been described prior to the AIDS era. Case reports of one HIV-infected patient with pneumonitis and hepatitis[57] and another with osteitis[58] have been published. Gummatous syphilis, a tertiary form of syphilis, also has been described in persons with HIV infection.[59–61]

DIAGNOSIS

Diagnosing syphilis may be more complicated in HIV-infected patients because of false-negative and false-positive serologic test results and atypical clinical presentations in the presence of HIV infection. The diagnosis should be based on a number of factors, including the patient's history, the clinical findings, direct examination of lesion material for spirochetes, and the results of serologic tests for syphilis. The importance of a careful clinical examination of HIV-infected patients with syphilis cannot be overstated. CNS disease may occur during any stage of syphilis. Clinical evidence of neurologic involvement warrants examination of the CSF.

Darkfield examination or direct fluorescent antibody (DFA) staining of exudate from lesions suspected of being primary syphilis always should be done if feasible because, in patients with suspicious lesions but negative serologies, a positive darkfield examination or DFA stain is diagnostic. Darkfield examination or DFA staining of selected secondary lesions should be used in establishing the diagnosis of secondary syphilis. It is important to confirm by DFA that the treponema seen in darkfield-positive oral lesions are *T. pallidum*, since nonpathogenic spirochetes are found in the mouth.

Serologic tests for syphilis remain the cornerstone of diagnosing untreated syphilis infection—even in HIV-infected patients. Serum samples should be obtained from any patient in whom the diagnosis of syphilis is suspected. All patients with known HIV infection should be screened for possible untreated syphilis infection. Nontreponemal antibody test results should be reported quantitatively and titered to a final endpoint.

A negative RPR or VDRL test result may not rule out syphilis in patients with HIV infection. Although the sensitivity of these serologic tests in diagnosing secondary syphilis generally is very high, case reports of seronegative secondary syphilis in patients with HIV infection have raised concerns that some patients may fail to develop a normal antibody response to *T. pallidum*.[18,19,21] Even though these patients eventually seroconverted before treatment, more data are needed on the serologic response to *T. pallidum* in HIV-infected patients. However, until better data are available, most experts believe that syphilis serologic tests appear to be accurate and reliable for diagnosis of syphilis and evaluation of treatment response in the vast majority of HIV-infected patients.[38]

When clinical syndromes compatible with primary or secondary syphilis occur and darkfield examinations and serologic test results are negative, the prozone phenomenon (i.e., falsely reading a nontreponemal serologic test as negative because the specimen was not tested after sufficient dilution so that the high concentration of antigen did not allow detectable antigen–antibody complex formation) should be ruled out.[62] A biopsy should be performed on suspicious lesions, and such biopsy specimens should be evaluated for spirochetes using special stains or isolation techniques or both. A silver stain, such as the Steiner stain,[63] has been used successfully. Specific DFA stains for *T. pallidum* also can be used. Because *T. pallidum* cannot be grown on artificial media, inoculation of laboratory animals (usually rabbit testicles) is the only method available to isolate the organism. This method is available only in a few research laboratories.

Clinicians should consult with infectious disease specialists or pathologists about special tests available in their areas. If spirochetes are not demonstrated on biopsy material or if special techniques are not available to identify spirochetes but clinical suspicion of syphilis remains high, the clinician may wish to treat HIV-infected patients presumptively for syphilis. Such patients should be followed closely with serial serologic testing at 1, 2, 3, and 6 months to detect any delayed antibody response.

The specificity of the nontreponemal serologic tests for syphilis can be compromised in HIV-infected persons.[17,20,64] Very high VDRL/RPR titers of greater than 1:64 have been reported in HIV-infected patients without syphilis (SA Larsen, personal communication). However, the majority of biologically false-positive results among HIV-infected persons are titers of less than 1:8.[16,20] The nontreponemal tests detect antibodies directed against a cardiolipin-lecithin antigen. In patients with immunoglobulin abnormalities, the RPR or VDRL test result may falsely be positive. Many persons with HIV infection have both anti−cardiolipin-lecithin antibodies and polyclonal gammopathy. Thus a positive RPR or VDRL test result may not represent active syphilis infection. However, in a patient with a history of adequately treated syphilis, it is best to assume a reactive nontreponemal test indicates active disease unless a serofast state has been well documented, because reinfection is difficult to rule out and reactivation or relapse of a previously treated infection is possible in a person with HIV infection.

Treponemal tests in HIV-infected patients previously treated for syphilis may not remain reactive after treatment. Haas et al.[65] demonstrated that seroreversion rates of treponemal tests were significantly associated with falling T-cell counts. Rates of seroreversion were 7% for patients with asymptomatic HIV infection and 38% for patients with AIDS. More recently, Romanowski et al.[66] reported that seroreversion of treponemal tests also occurs in non−HIV-infected persons treated early in the course of their syphilis infection. In this study, 13% of microhemagglutination−*T. pallidum* (MHA-TP) test results and 25% of FTA-abs test results were negative at 36 months following therapy for primary syphilis. Seroreversion was not found in patients treated for secondary or early latent syphilis. With progression of HIV disease, anti−treponemal antibody reactivity may be lost in patients previously treated for syphilis. However, no data about the serologic response of treponemal tests in HIV-infected persons with very low T-cell counts and active syphilis infection

exist. Until additional data are available, the sensitivity of treponemal tests in HIV-infected individuals should be considered high in patients with syphilis beyond the primary stage of infection. If asymptomatic patients have a positive nontreponemal test and a negative confirmatory treponemal test result, it is unlikely that they have active syphilis.

Diagnosis of Neurosyphilis

The diagnosis of neurosyphilis is based on the CSF findings of cells, elevated protein concentration, and a positive CSF-VDRL test result. Even if the CSF-VDRL test result is negative, the finding of increased CSF leukocytes (5/mm^3) and protein (0.4 mg/ml) requires consideration of a diagnosis of neurosyphilis.[67] If the CSF-VDRL test result is negative, the diagnosis of neurosyphilis is complicated by the lack of another reliable diagnostic test and the difficulty of distinguishing between neurologic disease caused by *T. pallidum* and that caused by HIV or other CNS pathogens found in patients with AIDS.

The majority of symptomatic neurosyphilis cases among persons with coexisting HIV infection have a positive CSF-VDRL test result.[68] However, case reports of symptomatic neurosyphilis in HIV-infected patients whose initial CSF-VDRL test results were negative suggest that cases of neurosyphilis will go untreated if the CSF-VDRL is the only finding used to guide therapeutic decisions.[67] In these patients, the CSF-VDRL test result became positive after penicillin therapy. These reports underscore the need for clinical judgment in establishing the diagnosis of active neurosyphilis in HIV-infected individuals. Better diagnostic tests for neurosyphilis are needed. The CSF FTA-abs test may help rule out neurosyphilis if it is negative, but a positive result is nonspecific. Measurement of immunoglobulins or treponemal antigens and isolation of treponemes have been suggested,[69] but these techniques have not yet been adequately studied.[70] Detection of treponemal DNA using the polymerase chain reaction is under development, and it may be a potentially useful test for diagnosing neurosyphilis.[71,72] Until better diagnostic tests are available, clinicians may wish to treat for neurosyphilis in patients whose CSF leukocytes and protein concentration are elevated but in whom the CSF-VDRL is negative and all other possible causes have been excluded. If this empiric approach is undertaken, then it is essential that such patients be followed closely with repeat lumbar punctures at 3, 6, and 12 months to determine if the CSF returns to normal after aqueous penicillin G therapy.

Indications for CSF Examination

It is unclear when to examine the CSF in patients with syphilis and concurrent HIV infection,[1,4,6,22] but recommendations regarding indications for CSF examination in HIV-infected patients with untreated syphilis have changed based on a growing body of anecdotal evidence. The Centers for Disease Control and Prevention (CDC) now recommends CSF examination in all HIV-infected patients diagnosed with latent syphilis regardless of the apparent duration of infection.[38] Previous guidelines recommended CSF examination only for HIV-infected patients who had latent syphilis for longer than 1 year. Examination of CSF for evidence of neurosyphilis also should be performed in all HIV-infected patients (or patients at risk for HIV infection) who have any unexplained behavioral abnormalities; psychological dysfunction; or ocular, auditory, or other neurologic symptoms or signs, especially those consistent with neurosyphilis. In addition, the CSF of HIV-infected patients should be examined for evidence of neurosyphilis if treatment for primary or secondary syphilis fails (i.e., if the titer does not decrease appropriately—fourfold [two dilutions] decrease by 3 months) or if a fourfold or greater increase occurs.

Because of case reports of neurosyphilis or isolation of *T. pallidum* from the CSF of HIV-infected patients who had completed standard therapy for early syphilis, some experts believe that routine CSF examination in all HIV-infected patients with syphilis is indicated and that therapy for neurosyphilis should be offered to those patients with a positive CSF-VDRL test result or with an abnormal cell count and protein concentration.[4,7,22,73] Other clinicians believe that all HIV-infected patients should be treated empirically with neurosyphilis regimens, even if the CSF examination is entirely normal. Many experts, however, believe that these isolated case reports do not justify the need for routine CSF examinations in patients with primary and secondary syphilis and that additional studies are needed to determine the significance of these reports. CSF abnormalities are common in HIV-infected patients with primary and secondary syphilis and are of unknown diagnostic significance. The vast majority of HIV-infected patients with primary or secondary syphilis respond appropriately to clinically recommended benzathine penicillin therapy. The CDC does not recommend routine CSF examination in patients with primary and secondary syphilis.[38] Until data are available to address the need for evaluating the CSF in patients with primary and secondary syphilis, the patients should be informed about the current dilemma, and their available treatment options should be discussed with them.

Indications for Screening for HIV Infection

Many of the diagnostic options discussed previously (e.g., lumbar punctures in patients with latent syphilis) and the therapeutic options to be discussed are recommended only for patients with coexisting HIV infection. Therefore, it is important to know the HIV antibody status of patients with syphilis when choosing diagnostic and therapeutic options. All patients with syphilis should be tested for HIV antibodies and counseled. If HIV antibody testing is not possible, the clinician provides treatment, keeping in mind that HIV co-infection may be present.

TREATMENT

The isolated case reports discussed previously have raised questions about the efficacy of current treatment recommendations for syphilis in the HIV-infected patient. Until further studies determine the optimum therapeutic regimen for syphilis and neurosyphilis in HIV-infected patients and the significance of abnormal CSF findings in primary and secondary syphilis, treatment in such patients will remain controversial.[1,3,4,6,22,74,75] The CDC currently recommends that penicillin regimens be used whenever possible for all stages of syphilis in HIV-infected patients (Table 29–1). Erythromycin is not recommended. Doxycycline and cephalosporins are also not recommended by the CDC because no studies establishing an effective dose and duration have been done. In addition, no proven alternative therapies to penicillin are available for treating patients with neurosyphilis, congenital syphilis, or syphilis in pregnancy. Therefore, confirmation of penicillin allergy and desensitization is recommended for these patients. The following treatment recommendations are based on available data and the

TABLE 29–1. Treatment of Syphilis in HIV-Infected Patients

Primary and Secondary Syphilis*
Treatment Recommended[†]
Benzathine penicillin G, 2.4 million units IM
Unstudied Treatment Considerations
Benzathine penicillin G, 4.8 million units IM
  (administered as two doses of 2.4 million units IM
  weekly for 2 successive weeks)
Regimens for neurosyphilis as outlined below

Latent Syphilis with Normal CSF Examination
Treatment Recommended[†]
Benzathine penicillin G, 7.2 million units IM
  (administered as three doses of 2.4 million units IM
  weekly for 3 successive weeks)
Unstudied Treatment Considerations
Regimens for neurosyphilis as outlined below

Neurosyphilis
Treatment Recommended[†]
Aqueous crystalline penicillin G, 12–24 million units
  IV per day for 14 days (administered as 2–4 million
  units every 4 hr each day)
  or
Aqueous procaine penicillin G, 2.4 million units IM
  daily for 14 days, plus probenecid, 500 mg PO four
  times a day for 14 days
  plus
Benzathine penicillin G, 2.4 million units IM, after
  completion of the above aqueous penicillin G 14-day
  regimen

---

*Without clinical evidence of neurosyphilis.
[†]Penicillin-allergic patients should be densensitized if skin testing confirms penicillin allergy or is unavailable.

consensus recommendations published by the CDC.[38,75] These recommendations have been changed to include 7.2 million units of benzathine penicillin G total (administered in three doses of 2.4 million units IM weekly for 3 weeks) for treatment of non-neurologic latent syphilis regardless of the apparent duration of infection. Previous guidelines recommended 7.2 million units of benzathine penicillin G only for patients with non-neurologic latent syphilis of greater than 1 year's duration.

Treatment of Non-neurologic Primary and Secondary Syphilis

A careful clinical examination to rule out clinical evidence of neurologic involvement (e.g., optic and auditory symptoms and cranial nerve palsies) must be done before treatment of HIV-infected patients with primary and secondary syphilis. For HIV-infected patients with incubating, primary, or secondary syphilis and no clinical evidence of neurologic involvement, the same treatment regimen as for patients without

HIV infection is recommended: 2.4 million units of benzathine penicillin G administered IM at a single session. In penicillin-sensitive patients, allergy should be confirmed. If compliance and close follow-up are ensured, use of doxycycline (100 mg orally two times a day for 2 weeks) may be considered if the patient refuses desensitization. However, no data are available on the efficacy of tetracyclines in treating syphilis in HIV-infected patients, and, if compliance and close follow-up cannot be ensured in patients taking tetracyclines, desensitization to penicillin and management in consultation with an infectious disease expert are recommended.

Treatment of Non-neurologic Latent Syphilis

A careful clinical and CSF examination should precede and guide treatment of HIV-infected patients with latent syphilis. If CSF examination is not possible, patients should be treated for presumed neurosyphilis. If the CSF examination yields no evidence of neurosyphilis, administration of 7.2 million units of benzathine penicillin G total (administered as three doses of 2.4 million units by IM injection weekly for 3 successive weeks) is recommended. In penicillin-sensitive patients, allergy should be confirmed, after which desensitization to penicillin and management in consultation with an infectious disease expert are recommended. Doxycycline is not recommended.

All patients should be warned about the possibility of a Jarisch-Herxheimer reaction before any treatment is given. In addition, HIV-infected patients should be informed that currently recommended regimens may be less effective for them than for patients without HIV infection and that follow-up care is essential.

Treatment of Neurosyphilis

For HIV-infected patients with any type of symptomatic neurosyphilis (including ocular or otologic syphilis), aqueous crystalline penicillin G is the treatment of choice (12 to 24 million units IV per day [i.e., 2 to 4 million units every 4 hours for 14 days]). Penicillin-sensitive patients should be desensitized to penicillin.

If hospitalization is impossible, administration of aqueous procaine penicillin G (2.4 million units IM daily) plus probenecid (500 mg by mouth four times daily) for 14 days is another option. However, these injections are painful, and patient compliance may be difficult to ensure. Most experts also recommend the addition of benzathine penicillin G 2.4 million units IM after completion of aqueous crystalline or aqueous procaine penicillin G therapy to provide comparable duration of therapy for latent syphilis.

Treatment Alternatives

Other outpatient regimens have been used in the treatment of neurosyphilis patients with normal immune function. These regimens include amoxicillin (2 gm) with probenecid (500 mg) by mouth three times daily for 14 days,[76–78] although the minimum inhibitory concentrations of the drug for *T. pallidum* are 10 to 20 times higher than that of penicillin, doxycycline (200 mg by mouth twice a day for 21 days),[79] and ceftriaxone (1 gm IM daily for 14 days).[80] However, tetracyclines and cephalosporins are less active than penicillin for syphilis therapy. The efficacy of these regimens for treating syphilis in HIV-infected patients is unknown.

Because of concerns about neurologic relapse and persistence of treponemes in the CSF in HIV-infected patients treated with benzathine penicillin G for primary and secondary syphilis, some experts believe that, until better data are available, HIV-infected patients with primary and secondary syphilis and abnormal CSF (i.e., with asymptomatic neurosyphilis) should be offered treatment regimens of longer duration, higher dosage, and better CSF penetration (e.g., the antibiotic regimens for neurosyphilis outlined previously).[22] Other experts emphasize that HIV-infected patients treated for syphilis who fail to respond (as defined below) to standard benzathine penicillin G therapy should also be offered antibiotic regimens of higher dose, longer duration, and better CSF penetration. Some clinicians believe that all HIV-infected patients with syphilis should be treated with penicillin regimens effective for neurosyphilis, an approach considered by others as of unproven benefit, impractical, and costly.[1] Still other experts suggest that HIV-infected patients with primary and secondary syphilis should receive a longer course of benzathine penicillin G therapy, such as 2.4 million units IM weekly for 2 or 3 weeks.[4,74] Others have considered adding oral amoxicillin to the benzathine penicillin G regimen to supplement levels of penicillin in the blood.[7] The justification for using any of these alternative regimens is only theoretical. No studies comparing the efficacy of 2.4 million units of benzathine penicillin G with other treatment options for the treatment of syphilis in HIV-infected patients have been completed. Eradication of *T. pallidum* from patients with HIV infection may be impossible, and such patients may require chronic penicillin therapy to control their infection.

FOLLOW-UP

Until the efficacy of treatment regimens is better defined, the importance of close follow-up of HIV-infected patients with syphilis cannot be overstated. All patients should be watched carefully for persistent or recurrent symptoms, for any signs of neurologic involvement, and for increasing serologic titers.[81]

All patients treated for syphilis should be examined and retested with a quantitative nontreponemal test at 1 to 2 weeks and at 1, 2, 3, 6, 9, and 12 months after treatment. The reasons for the follow-up intervals include

- Verifying that the level of the nontreponemal test result falls and does not increase
- Documenting a Jarisch-Herxheimer reaction
- Monitoring resolution, persistence, or recurrence of clinical signs and symptoms and development of any new signs or symptoms, especially those involving the CNS
- Ensuring compliance with treatment, effective partner notification, and safer sex practices

Although of unproven benefit, some experts recommend performing a CSF examination 6 months after therapy. Patients should be followed longer if any questions about the adequacy of their clinical or serologic response exist. Patients must be followed using the same nontreponemal test because titers from the VDRL and RPR tests are not interchangeable. In the absence of HIV infection and no previous history of *T. pallidum* infection, treatment usually produces seronegativity within 1 year in patients with primary syphilis and within 2 years in patients with secondary syphilis. The serologic response in HIV-infected patients and patients with a history of syphilis infection needs further study. One retrospective case–control study found no difference in serologic response in HIV-infected patients treated for early syphilis when compared with non–HIV-infected patients treated for a comparable stage of syphilis.[82]

Determining what constitutes a therapeutic cure for syphilis in patients with coexisting HIV infection is problematic because no simple test is available. Moreover, symptoms and signs of early syphilis may resolve even without treatment. Criteria defining treatment failure are currently based on curves of serologic response to treatment established in patients with normal immune function.[83–85] Treatment failure criteria include the following findings

1. Persistence or recurrence of signs or symptoms of syphilis
2. A sustained, fourfold (two dilutions) increase in the titer of nontreponemal tests of greater than 2 weeks' duration
3. Failure of the nontreponemal test titer in patients with primary and secondary syphilis to decrease fourfold (two dilutions) by 3 months

Until additional follow-up data on HIV-infected patients treated for syphilis are available, it is recommended that all patients with a documented clinical or serologic relapse as evidenced by persisting or recurring signs or symptoms of syphilis or by a sustained fourfold increase in nontreponemal test titer undergo a CSF examination. If there is no evidence of neurosyphilis, retreatment with three weekly injections of benzathine penicillin G 2.4 million units IM (7.2 million units, total) is recommended.

For HIV-infected patients treated for primary and secondary syphilis whose serologic titers have not decreased fourfold at 3 months after therapy, a CSF examination is indicated. If there is no evidence of neurosyphilis, most clinicians would treat the patient with 7.2 million units of benzathine penicillin G IM (i.e., 2.4 million units IM weekly for 3 weeks) and follow the patient with repeat serologic testing every 6 months. Unless the patient has recurrent or new clinical signs or symptoms or a sustained fourfold increase in the serologic titer, no further therapy is offered.

For patients with neurosyphilis, repeat serologic testing as described previously and CSF examination at 6-month intervals are recommended until the findings have stabilized. Abnormal CSF white blood cell (WBC) counts and protein levels should decrease by 6 months if no coexisting CNS infections are present, but CSF-VDRL tests may not return to nonreactivity. If the CSF WBC count is not normal by 2 years, retreatment using an antibiotic regimen for neurosyphilis is recommended.

For HIV-infected patients treated for latent syphilis, follow-up guidelines are less clear because limited data are available to guide the evaluation of the serologic response. Current guidelines suggest that, in patients treated for latent disease in whom an initially high titer (1 : 32) fails to decline at least fourfold (two dilutions) within 12 months, another evaluation for neurosyphilis should be done. If the CSF examination is normal, some experts re-treat with 7.2 million units of benzathine penicillin G IM (i.e., 2.4 million units IM weekly for 3 weeks), and other clinicians do not re-treat but simply follow such patients for evidence of clinical or serologic relapse. Recommendations regarding management of patients treated for latent syphilis in whom the initial nontreponemal titer is low are less clear. Although of unproven benefit, some experts recommend performing a CSF examination if a low titer fails to decrease after 12 months and re-treatment with 7.2 million units of benzathine penicillin G if the CSF examination is normal. Other experts follow these patients for evidence of clinical or serologic relapse.

TREATMENT FAILURES

Neurosyphilis

Several cases of neurologic relapse after benzathine penicillin G and ceftriaxone therapy for syphilis have been reported in patients with HIV infection.[12,14,15,37,73,81] One patient was seen initially with eye pain, double vision, dizziness, and headache. Two weeks later, he was found in a stuporous state with hemiparesis, homonymous hemianopsia, and expressive aphasia. CSF evaluation revealed mononuclear pleocytosis (32 cells/mm^3), an elevated protein level (92 mg/dl), and a CSF-VDRL titer of 1 : 4. This presentation is consistent with meningovascular syphilis. The patient had been treated with benzathine penicillin G for secondary syphilis 5 months before this neurologic event, and his serum VDRL titer had decreased from 1 : 256 to 1 : 16. Although a serum VDRL titer around the time of the stroke was 1 : 256, careful contact tracing and close follow-up after the initial treatment suggested that reinfection did not occur.[12] Meningovascular neurosyphilis was diagnosed also in a patient within 6 months after treatment with 2 gm of ceftriaxone IV daily for 14 days for latent syphilis.[81] Another patient developed syphilitic ophthalmitis with irreversible blindness 96 hours after starting the high-dose IV penicillin treatment for syphilitic meningitis.

Twenty-four weeks after completing the 10-day course of 24 million units of crystalline penicillin G daily, she developed meningovascular neurosyphilis. Prior to her treatment for syphilitic meningitis, she had recently received 7.2 million units of benzathine penicillin for early syphilis.[14]

Neurologic relapse following penicillin therapy is not unique to HIV-infected patients[13,34,86] but is uncommon in non–HIV-infected patients. Additional studies are needed to determine the response of HIV-infected patients to currently recommended therapy.

Persistence of Treponemes

Lukehart et al.[22] found viable treponemes in the CSF of two of three HIV-infected patients with secondary syphilis 3 to 6 months after treatment with a single dose of 2.4 million units of benzathine penicillin G. In these two patients, no signs or symptoms of neurologic relapse were reported, CSF-VDRL titers seroreverted, and the CSF WBC count decreased; in one patient, the serum VDRL titer decreased. In another HIV-infected patient with early syphilis who was treated with a single dose of benzathine penicillin G, serum and CSF-VDRL titers were unchanged but no treponemes were isolated 8 months after therapy. This patient also had no signs or symptoms of neurologic relapse. Long-term studies on larger numbers of patients are needed to determine whether persistence of treponemes is common and reflects inadequate therapy or whether the usual course after therapy is eventually to clear the CSF of organisms, albeit slowly.

Other Treatment Failure Issues

Clinicians have reported slow resolution of skin lesions in patients with HIV infection after penicillin therapy, although the time period from treatment to resolution of the signs and symptoms of primary or secondary syphilis has never been well defined, even in patients without HIV infection. In addition, relapse of mucocutaneous signs and symptoms of secondary syphilis has been reported[16] and was documented in a sexually inactive AIDS patient treated with penicillin for infectious syphilis 3 years earlier in our clinic. It is plausible that, in addition to neurologic relapse, other signs and symptoms of syphilis recur in HIV-infected individuals after treatment. Furthermore, the question of treat-

ment failure has been raised about HIV-infected patients whose nontreponemal serologic titers fail to decrease following therapy for early syphilis.[64] As discussed previously, a positive RPR or VDRL test result may not represent active syphilis infection but rather a high serofast state. Additional studies are needed to determine the clinical and serologic response to currently recommended therapy among HIV-infected patients. Of note, well-documented treatment failures following erythromycin therapy for primary or secondary syphilis have been reported in patients with concurrent HIV infection. In these cases, chancres and mucocutaneous signs and symptoms failed to resolve or relapsed within a few days after 2 weeks of erythromycin therapy.[87]

SEXUAL CONTACTS

An effort must be made to identify and treat any possible contacts of patients with early syphilis. In patients with primary syphilis, all contacts for 3 months before the appearance of the chancre should be evaluated clinically and serologically. In patients with secondary syphilis, contacts for the prior 6 months should be evaluated clinically and serologically. In patients with early latent syphilis and no history of symptoms or signs suggestive of primary or secondary syphilis, contacts for the prior 12 months should be evaluated clinically and serologically. Efforts should be made to establish a diagnosis of syphilis by history, clinical findings, and serologic testing before treating such contacts. However, persons exposed to a patient with early syphilis within the previous 3 months may be infected and seronegative and, therefore, should be treated presumptively for early syphilis, even without an established diagnosis.

Follow-up serologic tests should also be done at 1 week and 3 months to establish the diagnosis of syphilis in these contacts if they are HIV infected or at risk of HIV infection. All cases of infectious syphilis (primary, secondary, and early latent) must be reported to the local health department. In addition, some state and local health departments (e.g., in San Francisco) require that health care providers notify the director of STD control about HIV-infected patients who have

1. Neurosyphilis confirmed by CSF examination (i.e., positive CSF-VDRL) or histopathology (DFA or special stains of biopsy material)

2. Negative serologic test results for syphilis (nontreponemal [VDRL, RPR] or treponemal [FTA-abs, MHA-TP] tests) during secondary syphilis diagnosed by darkfield microscopy or histopathology of lesion material
3. Failed treatment for syphilis as defined previously

EDUCATION

All patients with syphilis and their contacts must be given education and counseling to reduce their risk of future STDs. Safer sex messages should include reducing the number of sexual partners, knowing the health status of partners (if possible), avoiding unsafe sexual practices, and using condoms.

Acknowledgments

Our studies on the clinical management and therapy of syphilis in HIV-infected patients are supported by Public Health Service grant no. H25/CCH 904371-02.

References

1. Hook EW III: Syphilis and HIV infection. J Infect Dis 160:530, 1989
2. Hook EW III: Treatment of syphilis: Current recommendations, alternatives and continuing problems. Rev Infect Dis 11:S1511, 1989
3. Hook EW III: Management of syphilis in human immunodeficiency virus-infected patients. Am J Med 93:477, 1992
4. Musher DM: Syphilis, neurosyphilis, penicillin and AIDS. J Infect Dis 163:1201, 1991
5. Musher DM, Hamill RJ, Baughn RE: Effect of human immunodeficiency virus (HIV) infection on the course of syphilis and on the response to treatment. Ann Intern Med 113:872, 1990
6. Centers for Disease Control: Recommendations for diagnosing and treating syphilis in HIV-infected patients. MMWR Morbid Mortal Wkly Rep 37:600, 607, 1988
7. Tramont EC: Syphilis in the AIDS era. N Engl J Med 316:1600, 1987
8. Tramont EC: Syphilis in adults: From Christopher Columbus to Sir Alexander Fleming to AIDS. Clin Infect Dis 21:1361, 1995
9. Darrow WW, Echenberg DF, Jaffe HW, et al: Risk factors for human immunodeficiency virus (HIV) infections in homosexual men. Am J Public Health 77:479, 1987
10. Greenblatt RM, Lukehart SA, Plummer FA, et al: Genital ulcerations as a risk factor for human immunodeficiency virus infection. AIDS 2:47, 1988
11. Jaffe HW, Choi K, Thomas PA, et al: National case-control study of Kaposi's sarcoma and *Pneumocystis carinii* pneumonia in homosexual men. Part 1. Epidemiologic results. Ann Intern Med 99:145, 1983
12. Berry CD, Hooton TM, Collier AC, Lukehart SA: Neurologic relapse after benzathine penicillin therapy for secondary syphilis in a patient with HVI infection. N Engl J Med 316:1587, 1987
13. DiNubile MJ, Copare FJ, Gekowski KM: Neurosyphilis developing during treatment of secondary syphilis with benzathine penicillin in a patient without serologic evidence of human immunodeficiency virus infection. Am J Med 88:45N, 1990
14. Gordon SM, Eaton ME, George R, et al: The response of symptomatic neurosyphilis to high-dose intravenous penicillin G in patients with human immunodeficiency virus infection. N Engl J Med 331:1469, 1994
15. Johns DR, Tierney M, Felsenstein D: Alteration in the natural history of neurosyphilis by concurrent infection with the human immunodeficiency virus. N Engl J Med 316:1569, 1987
16. Malone JR, Wallace MR, Hendrick BB, et al: Syphilis and neurosyphilis in a human immunodeficiency virus type-1 seropositive population: Evidence for frequent serologic relapse after therapy. Am J Med 99:55, 1995
17. Augenbraun MH, Dehovitz JA, Feldman J, et al: Biological false-positive syphilis test results for women infected with human immunodeficiency virus. Clin Infect Dis 19:1040, 1994
18. Gregory N, Sanchez M, Buchness MR: The spectrum of syphilis in patients with human immunodeficiency virus infection. J Am Acad Dermatol 22:1061, 1990
19. Hicks CB, Benson PM, Lupton GP, Tramont EC: Seronegative secondary syphilis in a patient infected with the human immunodeficiency virus (HIV) with Kaposi's sarcoma: A diagnostic dilemma. Ann Intern Med 107:492, 1987
20. Rompalo AM, Cannon RO, Quinn TC, Hook EW III: Association of biologic false-positive reactions for syphilis with human immunodeficiency virus infection. J Infect Dis 165:1124, 1992
21. Tikjob G, Russel M, Petersen CS, et al: Seronegative secondary syphilis in a patient with AIDS: Identification of *Treponema pallidum* in biopsy specimen. J Am Acad Dermatol 24:506, 1991
22. Lukehart SA, Hook EW III, Baker-Zander SA, et al: Invasion of the central nervous system by *Treponema pallidum*: Implications for diagnosis and treatment. Ann Intern Med 109:855, 1988
23. Musher DM: How much penicillin cures early syphilis? Ann Intern Med 109:849, 1988
24. Collaborative Study Group of AIDS in Haitian-Americans: Risk factors for AIDS among Haitians in the United States: Evidence of heterosexual transmission. JAMA 257:635, 1987
25. Rolfs RT, Nakashima AK: Epidemiology of primary and secondary syphilis in the United States: 1981–1989. JAMA 264:1432, 1990
26. Bowen DL, Lane HC, Fauci AS: Immunopathogenesis of the acquired immunodeficiency syndrome. Ann Intern Med 103:704, 1985
27. Pavia CS, Folds JD, Baseman JB: Cell-mediated immunity during syphilis: A review. Br J Venereal Dis 54:144, 1978
28. Pacha N, Metzger M, Smogor W, et al: Effects of immunosuppressive agents on the course of experimental syphilis in rabbits. Arch Immunol Ther 27:45, 1979
29. Berger JR: Neurosyphilis in human immunodeficiency virus type 1-seropositive individuals. Arch Neurol 48:700, 1991

30. Gue JW, Wang SJ, Lin YY, et al: Neurosyphilis presenting as tabes dorsalis in a HIV-carrier. China Med J 51:389, 1993

31. Katz DA, Berger JR: Neurosyphilis in acquired immunodeficiency syndrome. Arch Neurol 46:895, 1989

32. Jordan KG: Modern Neurosyphilis—a critical analysis. West J Med 149:47, 1988

33. Merritt HH, Adams RD, Soloman HC: Neurosyphilis. New York, Oxford University Press, 1946

34. Simon RP: Neurosyphilis. Arch Neurol 42:606, 1985

35. Calderon W, Danville H, Nigro M, et al: Concomitant syphilitic and HIV infection: A case report. Acta Neurol 45:132, 1990

36. Strom T, Schneck SA: Syphilis meningomyelitis. Neurology 41:325, 1991

37. Lanska MJ, Lanska DJ, Schmidley JW: Syphilitic polyradiculopathy in an HIV-positive man. Neurology 38:1297, 1988

38. Centers for Disease Control: 1993 Sexually transmitted diseases treatment guideline. MMWR Morbid Mortal Wkly Rep 42:RR-14, 1993

39. Becerra LI, Ksiazek SM, Savino PJ, et al: Syphilitic uveitis in human immunodeficiency virus infected and noninfected patients. Ophthalmology 96:1727, 1989

40. Gass JD, Braunstein RA, Chenoweth RG: Acute syphilitic posterior placoid chorioretinitis. Ophthalmology 97:1288, 1990

41. Little JP, Gardner G, Acker JD, Land MA: Otosyphilis in a patient with human immunodeficiency virus: Internal auditory canal gumma. Otolaryngol Head Neck Surg 112:488, 1995

42. Levy JH, Liss RA, Maguire AM: Neurosyphilis and ocular syphilis in patients with concurrent human immunodeficiency virus infection. Retina 9:175, 1989

43. McLeish WM, Pulido JS, Holland S, et al: The ocular manifestations of syphilis in the human immunodeficiency virus type-1 infected host. Ophthalmology 97:196, 1990

44. Smith ME, Canalis RF: Otologic manifestations of AIDS: The otosyphilis connection. Laryngoscope 99:365, 1989

45. Tamesis RR, Foster CS: Ocular syphilis. Ophthalmology 97:1281, 1990

46. Smith JL, Byrne SF, Cambron GR: Syphilmoa/gumma of the optic nerve and human immunodeficiency virus seropositivity. J Clin Neurol Ophthalmol 10:175, 1990

47. Gourevitch MN, Selwyn PA, Davenny K, et al: Ann Intern Med 118:350, 1993

48. Hook EW III, Marra CM: Acquired syphilis in adults. N Engl J Med 326:1060, 1992

49. Hutchinson CM, Hood EW III, Shepherd M, et al: Altered clinical presentation of early syphilis in patients with human immunodeficiency virus infection. Ann Intern Med 121:94, 1994

50. Garcia-Silva J, Velasco-Benito JA, Pena-Penabad C: Primary syphilis with multiple chancres and porphyria cutanea tarda in an HIV-infected patient. Dermatology 188:163, 1994

51. Hay PE, Tam FWK, Kitchen VS, et al: Gummatous lesions in men infected with human immunodeficiency virus and syphilis. Genitourin Med 66:374, 1990

52. Kitchen VS, Cook T, Doble A, Harris JR: Gummatous penile ulceration and generalized lymphadenopathy in homosexual man: Case report. Genitourin Med 64:276, 1988

53. Cusini M, Zerboni R, Muratori S, et al: Atypical early syphilis in a HIV-infected homosexual male. Dermatologica 177:300, 1988

54. Sands M, Markus A: Lues maligna, or ulceronodular syphilis, in a man infected with human immunodeficiency virus: Case report and review. Clin Infect Dis 20:387, 1995

55. Schlossbert D, Morley J, Montero M, Krouse T: Rupia syphilitica. Arch Dermatol 129:514, 1993

56. Radolph JD, Kaplan RP: Unusual manifestations of secondary syphilis and abnormal humoral immune response to *Treponema pallidum* antigens in a homosexual man with asymptomatic human immunodeficiency virus infection. J Am Acad Dermatol 18:423, 1988

57. Dooley DP, Tomski S: Syphilitic pneumonitis in an HIV-infected patient. Chest 105:629, 1994

58. Kastner RJ, Malone JL, Decker CF: Syphilitic osteitis in a patient with secondary syphilis and concurrent human immunodeficiency virus infection. Clin Infect Dis 18:250, 1994

59. Dawson S, Evans BA, Lawrence AG: Benign tertiary syphilis and HIV infection. AIDS 2:315, 1988

60. Horowitz HW, Valsamis MP, Wicher V, et al: Cerebral syphilitic gumma confirmed by the polymerase chain reaction in a man with human immunodeficiency virus infection. N Engl J Med 331:1488, 1994

61. Kerns G, Pogrel MA, Honda G: Intraoral tertiary syphilis (gumma) in a human immunodeficiency virus-positive man. J Oral Maxillofac Surg 51:85, 1993

62. Jurado RL, Campbell J, Martin PD: Prozone phenomenon in secondary syphilis. Arch Intern Med 153:2496, 1993

63. Swisher BL: Modified Steiner procedure for microwave staining of spirochetes and non-filamentous bacteria. J Histotechnol 10:241, 1987

64. Drabick JJ, Tramont EC: Utility of the VDRL test in HIV-seropositive patients. N Engl J Med 322:271, 1990

65. Haas JS, Bolan G, Larsen SA, et al: Sensitivity of treponemal tests for detecting prior treated syphilis during human immunodeficiency virus infection. J Infect Dis 162:862, 1990

66. Romanowski B, Sutherland R, Fick GH, et al: Serologic response to treatment of infectious syphilis. Ann Intern Med 144:1005, 1991

67. Feraru ER, Aronow HA, Lipton RB: Neurosyphilis in AIDS patients: Initial CSF VDRL may be negative. Neurology 40:541, 1990

68. Matlow AG, Rachlis AR: Syphilis serology in human immunodeficiency virus-infected patients with symptomatic neurosyphilis: Case report and review. Rev Infect Dis 12:703, 1990

69. Tomberlin MG, Holtom PD, Owens JL, Larsen RA: Evaluation of neurosyphilis in human immunodeficiency virus-infected individuals. Clin Infect Dis 18:288, 1994

70. Hart G: Syphilis tests in diagnostic and therapeutic decision making. Ann Intern Med 104:368, 1986

71. Burstain JM, Frimprel E, Lukehart SA, et al: Sensitive detection of *Treponema pallidum* by using the polymerase chain reaction. J Clin Microbiol 29:62, 1991

72. Hay PE, Clark JR, Taylor-Robinson D, Goldmeier D: Detection of treponema DNA in the CSF of patients with syphilis and HIV infection using the polymerase chain reaction. Genitourin Med 66:428, 1990

73. Tramont EC: Persistence of *Treponema pallidum* following penicillin G therapy: Report of 2 cases. JAMA 236:2206, 1976

74. Fiumara N: Human immunodeficiency virus infection and syphilis. J Am Acad Dermatol 21:141, 1989

75. Zenker PN, Rolfs RT: Treatment of syphilis, 1989. Rev Infect Dis 12:S590, 1990

76. Faber WR, Bos JD, Reitra PJ, et al: Treponemicidal levels of amoxicillin in cerebrospinal fluid after oral administration. Sex Transm Dis 10:148, 1983

77. Hay PE, Taylor-Robinson D, Waldron S, Goldmeier D: Amoxicillin, syphilis, and HIV infection. Lancet 335: 474, 1990

78. Morrison RE, Harrison SM, Tramont EC: Oral amoxicillin: An alternative treatment for neurosyphilis. Genitourin Med 61:359, 1985

79. Yim CW, Flynn NM, Fitzgerald FT: Penetration of oral doxycycline into the cerebrospinal fluid of patients with latent or neurosyphilis. Antimicrob Agents Chemother 28:347, 1985

80. Hook EW III, Baker-Zander SA, Moskovitz BL, et al: Ceftriaxone therapy for asymptomatic neurosyphilis: Case report and Western blot analysis of serum and cerebrospinal fluid IgG response to therapy. Sex Transm Dis Suppl 3: 185S, 1986

81. Dowell ME, Ross PG, Musher DM, et al: Response of latent syphilis or neurosyphilis to ceftriaxone therapy in persons infected with human immunodeficiency virus. Am J Med 93:481, 1992

82. Telzak EE, Greenberg MSZ, Harrison J, et al: Syphilis treatment response in HIV-infected individuals. AIDS 5:591, 1991

83. Brown ST, Zaidi A, Larsen SA, Reynolds GH: Serologic response to syphilis treatment: A new analysis of old data. JAMA 253:1296, 1985

84. Guinan ME: Treatment of primary and secondary syphilis: Defining failure at three- and six-month follow-up. JAMA 257:359, 1987

85. Schroeter AL, Lucas JB, Price EV, Falcon VH: Treatment for early syphilis and reactivity of serologic tests. JAMA 221:471, 1972

86. Bayne LL, Schmidley JW, Goodin DS: Acute syphilitic meningitis: Its occurrence after clinical and serologic cure of secondary syphilis with penicillin G. Arch Neurol 43:137, 1986

87. Duncan WC: Failure of erythromycin to cure secondary syphilis in a patient infected with the human immunodeficiency virus. Arch Dermatol 125:82, 1989

30 Malignancies Associated with AIDS

LAWRENCE D. KAPLAN • DONALD W. NORTHFELT

Malignancies as a complication of immunodeficiency have been well described in the literature, being recognized long before the advent of the HIV epidemic.[1-3] The incidences of both Kaposi's sarcoma (KS) and non-Hodgkin's lymphoma (NHL) are markedly increased in immunosuppressed allograft recipients. It is therefore not surprising that patients with HIV infection, who also have profound defects in cell-mediated immunity, develop these two malignancies. The marked rise in the incidence of both KS and B-cell lymphoma in populations at risk for HIV infection in the years since 1982 strongly suggests a causal relationship between immunodeficiency and the development of these malignancies.[4] Neoplasms are considered to be "AIDS associated" if their incidence is significantly increased in the seropositive population relative to the general population. For example, although rare in the United States, squamous carcinoma of the conjunctiva is observed with high frequency in HIV-seropositive individuals in Central Africa.[5] Table 30–1 lists the three neoplasms for which epidemiologic data clearly document an increased incidence.

Recent epidemiologic data from several large prospective cohort studies[6-9] have suggested that several other neoplasms may be increased in incidence in the setting of HIV disease. This second category of neoplasms is referred to as "probably AIDS associated" in Table 30–1. Because the relative risk of these other neoplasms is significantly less than that of KS and NHL, follow-up of large numbers of patients over a long period of time was required to identify the increased risk of the neoplasms associated with the presence of HIV infection.

The third group listed in Table 30–1 comprises those neoplasms considered "AIDS defining" by the Centers for Disease Control and Prevention (CDC).[10] Although invasive cervical carcinoma is included in the CDC case definition of AIDS,[10] epidemiologic data to date do not indicate an increased incidence of this neoplasm among HIV-seropositive women in the United States, with the exception of one study indicating a relative risk of 2.8 (range 2.2 to 3.4) in HIV-seropositive women in New York City compared to the general population.[11] However, despite the smaller number of cases of invasive disease seen in this patient population, several investigators have now documented a significantly increased risk of preinvasive disease of the cervix among HIV-seropositive women relative to those who are HIV seronegative.[12-14] The characteristics and management of individuals with preinvasive squamous lesions of the cervix are discussed later in this chapter.

Other studies have suggested small increases in the relative risk of nonmelanoma carcinomas of the skin, lung cancer, and melanoma. However, these observations have not been consistent among different cohort studies and at this time are not considered to be significant.

Regardless of the causal relationship between various malignancies and the underlying immunodeficiency state, reports in the literature suggest that the natural history of cancer may be altered in the setting of HIV infection.[15-17] Patients tend to present with more advanced disease that is more rapidly progressive and responds less well to therapy than in the non-HIV-infected population. Lung cancer, which is particularly difficult to treat in the general population, is associated with a very poor clinical outcome in HIV-infected patients.[18] However, for neoplastic disease that is normally highly responsive to therapeutic intervention, such as testicular germ cell tumors, treatment when these neoplasms occur in the setting of HIV infection can be highly successful.[19,20]

TABLE 30–1. Neoplasms in HIV Disease

Definitely AIDS Associated
Kaposi's sarcoma
Non-Hodgkin's lymphoma
Squamous carcinoma conjunctiva

Probably AIDS Associated
Hodgkin's disease
Plasmacytoma
Leiomyosarcoma (pediatric)
Seminoma

AIDS Defining*
Kaposi's sarcoma
Non-Hodgkin's lymphoma
Invasive cervical cancer

*From the Centers for Disease Control Prevention: Revision of the case definition of acquired immunodeficiency syndrome for national reporting—United States. MMWR Morb Mortal Wkly Rep 34:373, 1985.

Management of the HIV-infected patient with a malignancy imposes obstacles rarely encountered in the non-HIV-infected population. Poor bone marrow reserve and the risk of intercurrent opportunistic infections, problems frequently observed in this patient population, can compromise the delivery of adequate dose intensity. In addition, administration of chemotherapy may lead to further immunosuppression, resulting in a greater likelihood of opportunistic infection. Finally, the toxicity of chemotherapeutic agents, antibiotics, and radiation therapy is excessive and often severe, further impairing the physician's ability to administer adequate therapy.

This chapter focuses on the most common AIDS-associated neoplasms from primarily a clinical perspective. KS, NHL, and the human papillomavirus (HPV)–associated anogenital neoplasms are discussed. The natural history of these malignancies is presented along with various therapeutic options.

The advent of highly active antiretroviral therapy (HAART) is having a significant effect on both the incidence and management of neoplastic disease in this population. Use of these antiretroviral agents as part of the management of HIV patients with neoplasias is discussed.

KAPOSI'S SARCOMA

Epidemiology

KS, once a rarely reported malignancy, is the most common neoplasm affecting HIV-infected individuals. It is seen primarily in homosexual men and is less commonly reported in IV drug users or other risk groups.[21,22] The proportion of AIDS patients with KS as the initial AIDS diagnosis has changed since the first cases were reported in 1981.[23] In New York City, KS was the initial AIDS diagnosis in 50% of non-IV-drug-using homosexual men diagnosed between 1981 and 1983. Between 1984 and 1987, however, this proportion had fallen to 30%. Similar trends have been reported from San Francisco.[24] In a study of infectious diseases and cancers among persons dying of HIV infection, national multiple-cause mortality data showed no significant trend in the prevalence of KS between 1987 (10.4%) and 1992 (12.1%).[25] However, more recent data from the Multicenter AIDS Cohort Study (MACS) indicate a steady decline in the incidence of Kaposi's sarcoma through January of 1995, followed by a more precipitous fall through January of 1997 corresponding with the more widespread use of HAART.[26] The number of new KS cases in the cohort fell from 25.6/1000 person-years in the early 1990s to an average incidence of 7.5 cases/100 person-years in 1996–1997.[26] Additional evidence suggesting a decline in the occurrence of KS in conjunction with widespread use of HAART has been reported from the San Francisco City Clinic Cohort Study[27] and the Adult Spectrum of HIV-Disease Project.[28] Tumor registry data from San Francisco General Hospital demonstrate a decline in the number of newly diagnosed cases of KS from 103 in 1995 to 62 in 1996 to 36 in 1997.

Pathogenesis

The pathogenesis of KS in HIV-infected patients is complex and involves both viral processes and dysregulation of cytokine pathways. The decline in the incidence of KS in the homosexual male population during a period of time when sexual practices were changing, as well as the nearly exclusive confinement of this neoplasm to the homosexual male population, have always supported the concept of the involvement of another sexually transmitted agent in the pathogenesis of KS.[29] When KS occurs in women, it is seen almost exclusively in women whose sexual partners are bisexual males.[30] Chang et al.[31] used the molecular technique of representational difference analysis to identify the presence of novel herpesvirus sequences that were present in KS tissue but not present in other tissues in a given individual. This virus was termed human herpesvirus-8 (HHV8), or Kaposi's sarcoma herpesvirus, and has since

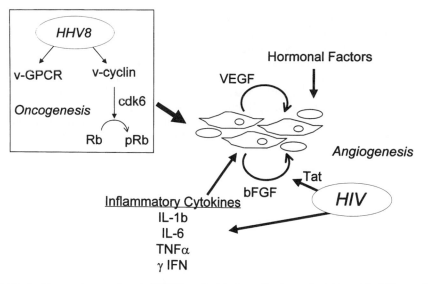

FIGURE 30–1. Human herpesvirus-8 (HHV8) cyclin binds cyclin-dependent kinase (cdk6), resulting in phosphorylation (pRb) or Rb and activation of cell cycle. G-protein–coupled receptor (GPCR) may be primary HHV8 oncogene. Inflammatory cytokines enhance basic fibroblast growth factor (bFGF) release by KS spindle cells. Tat enhances angiogenic response to bFGF. (IFN, interferon; IL, interleukin; TNF, tumor necrosis factor; VEGF, vascular epidermal growth factor.)

been identified in association with all of the various epidemiologic forms of KS in addition to that associated with HIV.[32,33] The virus is predominantly present in a latent form within the spindle cells of the lesions.[34] HHV8 has recently been cultured from a body cavity–based lymphoma cell line and intact virions have been visualized. The viral genome has been sequenced and several viral genes have been identified that have homology to genes encoding a variety of human cytokines and cell cycle–regulatory proteins, raising the possibility that this virus may be capable of influencing the cell division cycle.[35–37] A viral G-protein–coupled receptor has been identified that appears to function as a viral oncogene.[38]

KS can be best characterized as a hyperplastic proliferative disease mediated by the cooperation of inflammatory cytokines, which may be induced by HHV8, and angiogenic factors (Fig. 30–1). The Tat protein of HIV-1 plays a direct role in KS pathogenesis by synergizing with basic fibroblast growth factor (bFGF), an angiogenic factor highly expressed in KS lesions, in inducing angiogenesis and KS lesion formation.[39] Tat provides the KS cells with an adhesion signal required for cell growth in response to angiogenic stimuli.[40,41] Inflammatory cytokines, which are required to induce the production and release of bFGF and the expression of integrin receptors,[40,42] are highly expressed in KS lesions. Similarly, these integrins are ex-

pressed by endothelial and spindle cells of the lesions and co-stain with extracellular Tat,[39] indicating that these mechanisms are operating in vivo. Thus there are a number of potential sites for intervention with pathogenesis-based approaches to therapy for Kaposi's sarcoma. Such approaches might include the use of agents to block production of or activity of inflammatory cytokines such as interleukin-6 (IL-6), inhibitors of vascular endothelial growth factor, anti-Tat agents, or agents that might block the interaction between bFGF and integrins.

The reason for the male predominance in Kaposi's sarcoma is not clear. IL-6 production in cultured KS-derived spindle cells was enhanced by glucocorticoids and testosterone,[43] whereas marked inhibition of IL-6 production was noted with the addition of 17-β-estradiol.[43,44] Other in vitro studies have suggested inhibitory activity of β-human chorionic gonadotropin against cultured spindle cells.[45] Some of these observations have been used in the design of newer therapeutic approaches.

Clinical Presentation and Diagnosis

Unlike the more indolent, endemic form of KS, KS in the HIV-infected individual usually is an aggressive and unpredictable disease.[21,22] The skin is most commonly the first site of presentation. Palpable, firm, cutaneous nodules ranging from 0.5 to 2 cm in diameter frequently are observed. However, in early stages, smaller, nonpalpable lesions may be seen. Some early lesions can appear like small ecchymoses. In more advanced disease, cutaneous lesions can become confluent and form large tumor masses involving extensive cutaneous surfaces. In light-skinned individuals, the lesions are typically violaeous in appearance (Color Plate I*G*), whereas in dark-skinned individuals, the lesions acquire a more hyperpigmented appearance, appearing brown or even black. KS lesions may follow Langer's lines, may be symmetrical, and have a particular predilection for the tip of the nose and the penis. Rather than being limited to a single cutaneous site as in classic KS, KS in individuals with HIV infection can involve any cutaneous surface. Involvement of the head and neck is frequent, and the appearance of oral KS lesions is often the first sign of disease (Color Plate I*H*).

The natural history of KS associated with HIV infection more closely resembles that observed in immunosuppressed allograft recipients. The disease tends to progress with time and is associated with the appearance of larger and more numerous cutaneous lesions. However, the course of the disease is unpredictable. A patient may have relatively few lesions that remain stable over time. New cutaneous lesions may not appear for many months but may be followed by a sudden and rapid increase in disease activity. Visceral involvement with KS is extremely common and can involve almost any visceral site. Careful endoscopic examination will reveal gastrointestinal (GI) sites of disease in 40% of patients with asymptomatic cutaneous KS at the time of diagnosis.[46]

Although KS is usually not a direct cause of death in HIV-infected patients, the morbidity associated with more advanced disease can be significant. Bulky cutaneous lesions may become painful and, if large cutaneous surfaces are involved, can restrict movement. Lymphatic obstruction is common and can result in severe edema, most commonly involving the extremities (Color Plate I*E*) or the face. Visceral spread of KS is rarely symptomatic, particularly when it involves the GI tract. However, rare cases of obstruction, perforation, or GI bleeding have been reported.[47] Often, pulmonary KS results in cough, bronchospasm, and dyspnea, and death caused by respiratory failure is not uncommon.[48,49] Finally, the social problems associated with this disfiguring neoplasm in the setting of an already socially stigmatizing disease cannot be overemphasized.

Pulmonary involvement with KS deserves special attention because this is becoming an increasingly common complication of KS. In contrast to other visceral sites of involvement, pulmonary KS is generally symptomatic. This complication tends to occur in the setting of poor immune function, and most individuals will have a CD4 lymphocyte count of less than 100/mm^3.[50] Pulmonary involvement also tends to occur more frequently in individuals who have more than 50 cutaneous lesions, although the disease has been seen in individuals with minimal or even absent cutaneous KS.[51] The disease may be rapidly progressive when it involves the lungs, and clinically may be difficult to distinguish from a rapidly progressive pneumonitis. Survival is relatively short in these patients, with median survival times of between 2 and 6 months reported.[48,50] The typical chest radiographic appearance is variable, with the characteristic reticular-nodular pattern being seen in approximately one third of patients[48] (Chapter 9). More commonly, diffuse interstitial infiltrates are observed that may be difficult to distinguish from *Pneumocystis carinii* pneumonitis.[48,50,52,53] Pleural effusions are seen frequently,[48,50,52,53] and hilar adenopathy is observed in approximately 50% of cases.[50] Death caused by respiratory failure is not uncommon in the patient with pulmonary KS.

Careful examination of the skin and oral cavity at each clinic visit is the key to early diagnosis. Once lesions are identified, histologic confirmation should be obtained. This is particularly important because other cutaneous diseases, some of which can mimic KS, are common in the HIV-infected patient (Chapter 12). For cutaneous lesions, a small punch biopsy specimen generally is obtained. Conventional biopsy techniques can be used at other sites. In patients with suspected pulmonary KS, violaceous endobronchial lesions are typically observed on bronchoscopic examination. Unfortunately, attempts at endobronchial biopsy frequently are unsuccessful because of the submucosal nature of the lesions. However, bronchoscopic visualization of typical lesions is generally accepted for the purpose of diagnosis of pulmonary disease in patients who have had KS at other sites.[48] In the patient for whom treatment with chemotherapy is anticipated for KS at other sites and who has respiratory symptoms or an abnormal chest radiograph, gallium scanning can be sufficient to rule out a pulmonary opportunistic infection, making chemotherapy administration more acceptable. KS is not gallium avid.[48]

Although historically the most common cause of death in individuals with HIV and KS is opportunistic infection, there is evidence that, as survival is prolonged in individuals with HIV infection as a result of improvements in medical care, pulmonary involvement with KS is becoming an increasingly common cause of death.

Staging

Currently used staging systems are based primarily on tumor bulk. A modification of this staging system to include the presence or absence of constitutional symptoms is shown in Table 30–2. Unfortunately, these systems have not proved useful because a majority of patients fall into the most advanced stages. In addition, tumor bulk may not be the most important predictor of survival in this group of patients.

Analysis of data from 190 individuals with HIV-associated KS at the University of California at Los Angeles Medical Center demonstrated that the most important predictor of survival is the absolute CD4+ lymphocyte count[54] (Fig. 30–2). Only 30% of patients with fewer than 100 CD4 lymphocytes survived for 1 year. Other features associated with a negative impact on survival in various studies have included prior history of opportunistic infection,[55] bulky tumor,[55,56] the presence of constitutional symptoms,[55,56] and initial presentation that involves a mucosal surface or cutaneous site other than the lower extremities or the lymph nodes.[56]

Based on these known predictors of survival in patients with AIDS-associated KS, the Oncology Subcommittee of the National Institutes of Health–sponsored AIDS Clinical Trials Group (ACTG) has been using a newer staging

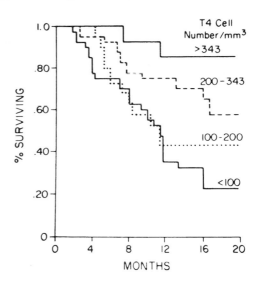

FIGURE 30–2. Relationship of various levels of (CD4) cell numbers to survival in AIDS KS patients (Kaplan-Meier graph). (From Taylor J, Afrasiabi R, Fahey JL, et al: Prognostically significant classification of immune changes in AIDS with Kaposi's sarcoma. Blood 67:666, 1986, with permission.)

classification, illustrated in Table 30–3.[57] This system takes into account tumor bulk, immune function, and the presence of other systemic illness, including history of opportunistic infection by the presence of constitutional symptoms. This staging system has recently been validated by comparing survival times among patients staged using this classification who participated in ACTG KS clinical trials between 1986 and 1994.[57a]

Treatment

Because most patients do not die as a direct result of KS, it would seem unlikely that therapy directed toward this neoplasm would have a significant impact on survival. Although the data are retrospective, a review of 194 cases of KS by Volberding et al.[59] suggests that this is, in fact, the case. There was no significant difference in survival time between the group of patients treated with chemotherapy (or α-interferon) and those who received no treatment.

Most patients with KS require treatment of some type. Treatment may range from antiviral therapy to systemic chemotherapy. It is important to recognize that KS is a *systemic* disease, and that most often systemic treatment is the most appropriate choice of treatment modalities. The primary goals of therapy for patients with KS are palliation of symptoms and cosmesis.

TABLE 30–2. Staging of Kaposi's Sarcoma

STAGE	CHARACTERISTICS
I	Limited cutaneous lesions (<10 or in one anatomic area)
II	Disseminated cutaneous lesions (>10 or in more than one anatomic area)
III	Visceral lesions only (gastrointestinal, lymph node)
IV	Cutaneous and visceral lesions
Subtypes	
A	No systemic signs or symptoms
B	Fevers >37.8°C, unrelated to identifiable infection for >2 weeks or weight loss >10% of body weight

From Mitsuyasu RT, Groopman JE: Biology and therapy of Kaposi's sarcoma. Semin Oncol 11:53, 1984, with permission.

TABLE 30–3. ACTG Staging Classification for Kaposi's Sarcoma

GOOD RISK (0): ALL OF THE FOLLOWING	POOR RISK (1): ANY OF THE FOLLOWING
Tumor (I)	
Confined to skin and/or lymph nodes and/or minimum oral disease*	Tumor associated edema or ulceration
	Extensive oral Kaposi's sarcoma (KS) lesions
	Gastrointestinal KS lesions
	KS lesions in other nonnodal viscera
Immune System (I)	
CD4 cells ≥200/μl	
Systemic Illness (S)	
No history of opportunistic infection (OI) or thrush	History of OI or thrush or both
No "B" symptoms†	B symptoms present
Karnofsky performance status ≥70	Karnofsky performance status <70
	Other HIV-related illness (e.g., neurologic disease, lymphoma)

Modified from Krown SE, Metroka C, Wernz J: Kaposi's sarcoma in the acquired immune deficiency syndrome: A proposal for uniform evaluation, response, and staging criteria. J Clin Oncol 7:1201, 1989, with permission.

*Minimum oral disease in nonnodular KS confined to the palate.

†B symptoms are unexplained fever, night sweats, >10% involuntary weight loss, or diarrhea persisting for more than 2 weeks.

Achievement of good cosmetic results may not only improve appearance but also significantly improve the patient's overall outlook.

Palliative therapy may be indicated in the following situations:

1. Painful or uncomfortable intraoral or pharyngeal lesions can interfere with eating or swallowing. Bulky KS can even result in airway compromise.
2. Lymphedema is a common complication of advanced KS. Because of its propensity for infiltrating lymphatic tissue, obstruction and edema formation can occur relatively early. The face and the lower extremities are the sites most commonly affected. Lower extremity edema can form as a result of bulky lymphadenopathy in the femoral, inguinal, or iliac regions, in the setting of confluent bulky cutaneous lesions, or even in the absence of bulky visible KS.
3. Painful or bulky lesions can occur at any site. Lesions involving the plantar surfaces of the feet may be particularly uncomfortable during ambulation.
4. Pulmonary KS is frequently symptomatic and can result in a variety of respiratory symptoms. This is becoming a more frequent complication of KS as patients survive for longer periods of time with the disease. Disease progression can be rapid, resulting in severe respiratory compromise and death.[48,50]

Another indication for therapy is rapidly progressive disease. Although it is impossible to prove benefit without a randomized trial, it is likely that, without treatment, such patients will rapidly develop either symptomatic disease requiring palliative therapy or cosmetically problematic disease.

Treatment options include a variety of local therapies, such as radiation, cryotherapy, and intralesional chemotherapy, as well as systemic therapy (e.g., chemotherapy, α-interferon). Systemic chemotherapy can result in subjective toxicities, myelosuppression, and immunosuppression, leaving the patient more susceptible to a variety of opportunistic infections. Therefore, the use of systemic chemotherapy should be approached cautiously. Local forms of therapy should be selected whenever possible.

Local Therapy

Local forms of therapy are most useful for the management of nonbulky local disease.

RADIATION THERAPY. Radiation therapy has been the most frequently used local therapeutic modality. A single dose of 800 cGy or the equivalent fractionated dose can be highly effective in achieving local palliation in selected patients.[60,61]

Radiation therapy is not appropriate for the patient with widespread symptomatic disease but is best suited for the patient with a single or a few locally symptomatic areas. It is highly effective in relieving facial edema and can be applied to a field encompassing the whole face. Generally, electron-beam therapy is used in treating the face. Radiation therapy has been frequently used, although less effectively, in the treatment of lower extremity edema,[61] and is not recommended as first-line therapy for the treatment of this complication because of the frequent occurrence of lymphedema and loss of skin compliance as complications. In addition, larger facial lesions, painful lesions, or other unsightly cutaneous lesions can be treated with this modality, as can intraoral and pharyngeal lesions. However, a high frequency of severe mucositis has been observed in the latter two groups of patients.[61] In addition, late complications of radiotherapy fibrosis, loss of skin compliance, and chronic lymphedema are common and may result in significant discomfort after 6 to 12 months.

INTRALESIONAL CHEMOTHERAPY. Small cutaneous lesions can be treated with intralesional chemotherapy for cosmetic purposes.[62] This is generally accomplished by intralesional injection of 0.01 mg of vinblastine in 0.1 ml sterile water using a tuberculin syringe. Repeated treatments may be necessary. A hyperpigmented area frequently remains after treatment.

CRYOTHERAPY. Cryotherapy using liquid nitrogen has been used successfully for the treatment of isolated small KS lesions.[63] This modality is particularly useful for the treatment of cosmetically unsightly lesions.

PHOTODYNAMIC THERAPY. Phase I results of the use of photodynamic therapy using intravenously administered Photofrin 48 hours prior to exposure to 100 to 300 J/cm^2 of 630-nm light demonstrated that up to 68% of lesions exposed to 300 J/cm^2 showed evidence of partial response.[58] This therapeutic approach remains investigational at the present time but may be useful for small, cosmetically unsightly lesions.

Systemic Therapy

Its pathogenesis would indicate that KS is a systemic disease, and therefore systemic therapy will be appropriate for a majority of patients. Systemic therapy may include antiretroviral therapy alone (described below) or the KS-directed therapies that follow.

ANTINEOPLASTIC AGENTS. Several antineoplastic agents used alone or in combination are active against KS (Table 30–4).[6,50,65–73]

Liposomal Anthracyclenes. These agents should now be considered the first-line treatment of choice for relatively advanced KS as a result of their efficacy and low incidence of toxicity. Phase I and II studies have shown the liposome-encapsulated anthracyclines doxorubicin and daunorubicin to be a promising new approach to the administration of chemotherapy to individuals with KS. In one trial, intralesional concentrations of doxorubicin after administration of the liposome-encapsulated agent were shown to be 5 to 11 times the levels achieved after administration of the non-liposome-encapsulated agent.[53] Subsequent Phase II trials with both liposome-encapsulated daunorubicin and doxorubicin have demonstrated response rates of 30% to 100% in patients treated with the single agents.[69,73] Most of the treated individuals had advanced KS with visceral involvement and their disease was refractory to previous chemotherapy. Significant responses have also been observed in patients previously unresponsive to doxorubicin-containing combination chemotherapy regimens.[68,69] The results of a Phase III clinical trial in which liposomal

TABLE 30–4. Chemotherapy in AIDS—Kaposi's Sarcoma

AGENTS	DOSE	REPORTED RESPONSE (%)	REFERENCES
Vincristine	2 mg/wk	20–59	64
Vinblastine	0.05–0.1 mg/kg/wk	25–30	65
Etoposide	150 mg/m^2 IV qd for 3 days every 3–4 wk, or 50 mg PO qd	75	66
Doxorubicin (Adriamycin)	20 mg/m^2 every other week	53	67
Bleomycin	10–15 U/m^2 every 2 wk		
Liposomal doxorubicin	20 mg/m^2 every 2–3 wk	30–95	6, 68
Liposomal daunorubicin	40 mg/m^2 every 2–3 wk	30–95	69, 70
Paclitaxel	135 mg/m^2 every 2–3 wk	53	71
Vinorelbine	100 mg/m^2 every 2 wk	44	72
Combination Chemotherapy			
Vincristine	2 mg	100	50
plus bleomycin	10 mg/m^2 (every 14 days)		
Doxorubicin	10–20 mg/m^2	87	67
plus bleomycin	10 mg/m^2		
plus vincristine	2 mg (every 14 days)		

doxorubicin was compared to the standard Adriamycin-bleomycin-vincristine (ABV) regimen have been reported.[74] This trial demonstrated that liposome-encapsulated doxorubicin is associated with a lower incidence of toxicities such as nausea, fatigue, and alopecia. Mild mucositis appears to occur more commonly with liposomal doxorubicin than with the non-liposome-encapsulated product, and neutropenia occurs as frequently with the liposomal drugs as with the standard combination regimen. In this study, liposomal doxorubicin was associated with a significantly higher response rate than ABV when used as initial therapy.[74] The addition of vincristine and bleomycin to liposomal doxorubicin does not improve the response rate over the liposomal agent alone.[75] Both liposomal agents have received recent Food and Drug Administration (FDA) approval and are currently available for use in patients with KS.

A similar trial in which liposomal daunorubicin was compared with ABV[76] also revealed a lower incidence of toxicities (alopecia, nausea, neuropathy) with the liposomal agent. Response rates in the two treatment arms were similar.

Paclitaxel. Clinical trials of the drug paclitaxel (Taxol) have demonstrated significant antitumor activity in patients with both previously untreated[71] and refractory[71,77] KS. Response rates are over 50% regardless of prior therapy. Outstanding clinical responses have been seen in patients with advanced refractory symptomatic disease. The drug has been well tolerated, with generally only mild toxicities reported. Paclitaxel is significantly myelosuppressive, and most patients in these trials have required adjunctive therapy with a myeloid colony-stimulating factor (CSF). This agent should be considered the treatment of choice for refractory KS and was recently FDA-approved for this indication.

Etoposide (VP16). Etoposide also is an active agent in treating KS.[66] The frequent occurrence of alopecia in patients treated with etoposide makes it a poor choice for patients being treated primarily for cosmetic purposes. However, the more recent availability of an oral formulation of etoposide makes this an attractive agent for systemic therapy in other situations. When administered orally, etoposide is 50% bioavailable. Therefore, an appropriate oral dose is generally twice the standard IV dose. The use of daily administration of low-dose oral etoposide is under study.

Doxorubicin (Adriamycin).[67] Doxorubicin may be useful in the management of patients with more advanced disease or in those in whom prior therapy has failed to produce a response. A randomized trial has suggested that the ABV combination regimen is more efficacious against KS than doxorubicin used as a single agent.[67] This regimen has been used successfully in patients with widespread, advanced KS, including those with peripheral edema and pulmonary involvement.[67] It is not unusual to see rapid improvement in peripheral edema or in respiratory symptoms after administration of this combination. In one study, the overall response rate to ABV in pulmonary KS was 60%.[67] The major short-term toxicity associated with doxorubicin is myelosuppression, which may require periodic dose reductions or the use of a myeloid growth factor.

The combination of vincristine and bleomycin has significant antitumor activity and may be especially useful for those patients with granulocytopenia, who are likely to be intolerant of more myelosuppressive regimens.[50,78-80]

The recent availability of the myeloid growth factors granulocyte colony-stimulating factor (G-CSF) and granulocyte-macrophage colony-stimulating factor (GM-CSF) make it possible to administer myelosuppressive chemotherapy to individuals in whom this may not have been possible in the past. Because many individuals with advanced KS have poor myeloid reserve, these agents can be valuable adjuncts to chemotherapy. For most individuals with KS, the use of a CSF is unnecessary. The use of a relatively nonmyelosuppressive regimen, such as vincristine with bleomycin, will be adequate therapy for many patients. At San Francisco General Hospital, we usually reserve the use of myeloid growth factors for those patients who require the use of an anthracycline or paclitaxel as a part of their chemotherapeutic regimen and who have a neutrophil count of less than 1500/mm^3 before initiating therapy in any chemotherapy cycle. Although no specific guidelines exist for administering CSFs in this setting, we generally begin administration 1 to 4 days after chemotherapy. In our experience, a dose of 300 μg (5 μg/kg) administered on alternate days for a total of five doses often is adequate. However, therapy must be individualized, and frequent neutrophil counts should be made during the first cycle of therapy to establish the optimal dosage regimen.

INTERFERON. α-Interferon is an active agent for use in the treatment of AIDS-associated KS because it possesses both antiproliferative[81] and apparent anti-HIV[82,83] activity. α-Interferon used as a single agent in the treatment of HIV-associated KS has significant antitumor activity,

TABLE 30–5. α-Interferon in AIDS-Related Kaposi's Sarcoma: Efficacy of Low-Dose Versus High-Dose Therapy

RESPONSE	LOW DOSE ($<$20 million U/m^2), $n = 65$	HIGH DOSE ($\geq$20 million U/m^2), $n = 105$
Complete	1 (2%)	18 (17%)
Partial	3 (5%)	27 (26%)
Minor or stable	13 (20%)	17 (16%)
Progression	48 (74%)	43 (41%)

Data compiled from published studies at San Francisco General Hospital, the University of California at Los Angeles, Memorial Sloan-Kettering Cancer Center, the M.D. Anderson Hospital and Tumor Institute, and the National Cancer Institute.

as demonstrated in a large number of clinical trials.[81,84–89] The importance of dose intensity in the administration of α-interferon is demonstrated in Table 30–5. These data, compiled from several institutions,[85–87,89] demonstrate that high doses ($>$20 million units/m^2) of α-interferon are more effective in inducing antitumor responses than are lower doses. Several studies have demonstrated that patients with better immune function (higher CD4 cell counts), without a prior history of opportunistic infection and without B symptoms, are more likely to respond to α-interferon than those whose cellular immune function is more compromised and who have had a prior opportunistic infection and are symptomatic.[81,89]

Despite the frequency of objective responses and reports of long disease-free remissions, the use of α-interferon in high doses as a single agent has been limited by its toxicity. With chronic administration, many patients experience a flu-like syndrome, with low-grade fever, anorexia, malaise, myalgias, and weight loss. Although many patients develop tachyphylaxis to these symptoms during the first several weeks of treatment, these symptoms may persist and become sufficiently disabling to warrant either dosage reduction or discontinuation of the agent.

Most patients who go on to have significant antitumor response usually show evidence of tumor regression after 4 to 8 weeks of high-dose treatment. Often 6 or more months of therapy are required to achieve maximum tumor regression. Because tumor recurrence is usual after discontinuation of treatment, it is suggested that alpha-interferon therapy be maintained for as long as the antitumor response persists.

α-Interferon and Nucleoside Analogs. The use of combinations of interferon and nucleoside analogs is currently being investigated in several Phase I and II trials and in large clinical trials. From the standpoint of antiretroviral therapy the combination of α-interferon with a nucleoside analog is an attractive one, because each of these agents appears to inhibit HIV-1 replication at a different stage of the viral life cycle, and the combination has shown synergistic in vitro inhibition of HIV-1 replication.[91] Although the nucleoside analogs have failed to show any significant antitumor activity in patients with KS when used as single agents,[92] the use of these agents is associated with improvement in immune function, a factor clearly associated with responsiveness of KS to interferon. Furthermore, the use of α-interferon is not associated with the decline in immune function normally associated with the use of standard cytotoxic chemotherapeutic agents.

The results of three clinical trials investigating the use of combination α-interferon with zidovudine are shown in Table 30–6.[93–95] It appears that daily 600-mg doses of zidovudine can be combined safely with α-interferon doses of

TABLE 30–6. Trials of α-Interferon with Zidovudine for Kaposi's Sarcoma

α-INTERFERON	α-INTERFERON DOSES OR RANGE (million units)	ZIDOVUDINE DOSES (mg q4h)	COMPLETE OR PARTIAL RESPONSE TOTAL (%)	REFERENCES
α-2A or α-nl	4, 5, 9, 18	100 or 200	17/37 (46)	93
α-2 or α-nl	9, 18, 27	100 or 200	20/43 (47)	94
α-nl	$<$5 to $>$25	50, 100, or 250	11/26 (42)	95
TOTAL			48/108 (45)	

4 to 18 million units daily. The most common dose-limiting toxicity has been neutropenia. Response rates of over 40% have been observed in all these trials and apparently are better at all levels of immune function when the results of treatment with these two agents are compared with historical data for the use of single-agent α-interferon. These response rates are particularly striking in view of the fact that α-interferon doses used in these trials were significantly lower than those known to have single-agent antitumor activity. The ability to use these lower doses of α-interferon may significantly reduce the incidence of subjective toxicities that frequently are dose limiting in patients treated with high-dose single-agent α-interferon.

Because the most common dose-limiting toxicity of the combination of α-interferon and zidovudine is neutropenia, two clinical trials have explored the addition of GM-CSF to this regimen.[96,97] Scadden et al.[97] found that GM-CSF administered at a dosage of 125 $\mu g/m^2$ reversed neutropenia in patients whose neutrophil counts fell to less than $1000/mm^3$ while on the drug combination. Krown et al.[96] titrated the dose of GM-CSF to maintain neutrophil counts between 1000 and $5000/mm^3$ in patients receiving 1200 mg zidovudine and 5, 10, or 20 million units of α-interferon daily. On average, a dose of only 1.25 $\mu g/kg/day$ was sufficient to maintain the neutrophil count within this range.

Because the addition of a CSF to the combination of α-interferon and zidovudine adds the additional expense of a potentially toxic agent, it seems more appropriate to combine α-interferon with other relatively nonmyelosuppressive antiretroviral agents. An ongoing ACTG clinical trial (ACTG 206) is investigating combinations of α-interferon with didanosine without a CSF. Therapy appears to be well tolerated, and antitumor responses have been seen in both arms of the study, including those patients receiving α-interferon doses as low as 1 million units/day. Other investigators have also documented responses with combinations of antiretroviral therapy and a 1-million-unit dose of α-interferon.[98] It is unclear whether response rates with this very low dose are comparable to those seen with somewhat higher interferon dosages.

Appropriate candidates for therapy with α-interferon and antiretrovirals include those patients with relatively intact immune function (CD4 count not below $100/mm^3$) whose KS is not significantly symptomatic, given that tumor regression may not be observed for up to 8 weeks after initiation of therapy. At San Francisco General Hospital, we generally begin patients on an α-interferon dose of 5 million units/day administered by subcutaneous injection 5 days/week. Patients are instructed in self-administration of their medication. Any combination of agents is acceptable to use concurrently with interferon; however, nonmyelosuppressive agents are preferable (excluding zidovudine) so as to avoid overlapping myelosuppression with α-interferon. Clinical trials of α-interferon with HAART are currently in progress.

ANTIRETROVIRAL THERAPY. The advent of HAART has had a significant impact on the management of individuals with Kaposi's sarcoma. In addition to being the likely cause of the recent decline in the incidence of KS, these agents have also altered the natural history of the disease itself. There have been several anecdotal reports[99-103] of anti-KS responses to antiretrovirals alone, and most clinicians who care for large numbers of patients with HIV disease have recognized that, in some patients, KS will respond to the introduction of HAART in the absence of any specific KS-directed therapy (L. Kaplan, unpublished observations). This phenomenon is generally associated with an effective antiviral response.[100] There is, indeed, precedent for this in the allograft population. In these iatrogenically immunosuppressed individuals, discontinuation of immunosuppressive therapy often leads to regression of KS. The use of these agents is of particular importance in the management of individuals with asymptomatic KS, in whom a trial of antiviral therapy alone may prove effective enough to eliminate the need for KS-specific therapy.

Others have presented data in patients receiving HAART indicating that, following discontinuation of chemotherapy in patients whose KS has responded to therapy, no progression of KS was observed at a median follow-up of 10 weeks.[104] These observations differ significantly from past experience, in which progression of KS following discontinuation of chemotherapy was the rule. Thus it is now possible to discontinue chemotherapy in individuals who have had good virologic response to HAART. Many of these patients will remain stable for prolonged periods of time. This may eliminate the need in some patients for a prolonged administration of chemotherapy.

Therapeutic Recommendations

Table 30–7 summarizes the recommendations for treatment of patients with AIDS-associated

TABLE 30–7. Kaposi's Sarcoma: Recommendations for Treatment

Minimal Disease	
Stable or slowly progressive	1. HAART
	2. HAART + α-interferon
	3. Chemotherapy if unresponsive to above
Rapidly progressive	1. HAART
	2. Consider liposomal anthracycline (Doxil, Daunoxome)
Widespread Disease	
Symptomatic	1. Liposomal anthracycline
	2. Other chemotherapy: doxorubicin/bleomycin/vincristine (ABV)
Refractory to liposomal agent	3. Paclitaxel
Locally Symptomatic	1. Radiotherapy
	2. Chemotherapy
Local Cosmesis	1. Intralesional chemotherapy
	2. Radiotherapy
	3. Cryotherapy
	4. Photodynamic therapy
Cytopenic Patients	1. Vincristine and/or
	2. Bleomycin
	3. G-/GM-CSF with liposomal anthracycline

KS. One should not lose sight of the fact that KS is a systemic illness and that, in most cases, systemic therapy is the most appropriate choice. In some cases systemic therapy can be defined as combination antiretroviral therapy rather than chemotherapy. Local therapeutic modalities such as intralesional vinblastine and radiotherapy should be reserved for the most minimal or locally symptomatic disease in patients who are concurrently receiving some form of systemic therapy (including antiviral therapy). Patients with asymptomatic KS should be started on combination antiretroviral therapy if they are not already receiving it. This alone may be effective therapy for KS in some individuals.

α-Interferon is a good choice for the relatively asymptomatic individual whose KS is not responding to antiretroviral therapy alone and in whom the KS is presenting predominantly a cosmetic problem.

Chemotherapy is most useful in those individuals who have symptomatic disease, in whom a more rapid response to therapy is required. Because responses to both α-interferon and antiretroviral therapy may be quite slow, chemotherapy is the treatment of choice for these more symptomatic patients. Chemotherapy may be discontinued at the time of maximal response to therapy in patients whose viral load is well controlled on HAART. The liposomal antracyclenes (liposomal doxorubicin, liposomal daunorubicin) are the agents of choice for initial chemotherapy, while paclitaxel is the agent of choice for individuals who have refractory disease.

NON-HODGKIN'S LYMPHOMA

The NHLs are a heterogeneous group of malignancies. Their biologic behavior ranges from indolent, requiring no therapy, to aggressive with few long-term survivors. Approximately 70% of NHLs originate in B cells, and another 20% derive from T cells.

In the most commonly used classification system for the NHLs,[105] these malignancies are divided into three major categories—low grade, intermediate grade, and high grade—according to pathologic characteristics of involved lymph nodes and morphologic criteria of the lymphoma cells.

The first cases of NHL in homosexual men were reported in 1982,[106] and increasing numbers of cases have been reported since that time. The finding of an intermediate- or high-grade B-cell NHL in an HIV-infected individual constitutes an AIDS diagnosis as defined by the CDC.[10] Advanced extranodal disease is commonly found at presentation, and median survival times have been short.

Epidemiology

The incidence of NHL is increased markedly in individuals with impaired cell-mediated immunity.[1,3] The best described group is immunosuppressed allograft recipients, in whom the incidence of NHL is 30 to 50 times that of the general population.[3,107,108] Similarly, Harnly et al.[4] have demonstrated a statistically significant increase in the incidence of NHL among never-married men ages 25 to 44 years in San Francisco in the years 1980 to 1985. The increase in census tracts with a high incidence of AIDS was greater than the increase in other San Francisco census tracts. In 1985, the incidence of NHL was five times greater than the rate in 1980. However, increases in incidence rates were not observed for other malignancies. Similar trends have been observed for New York City.[64]

Recently reported data from both prospective cohort studies and single institutions indicate a significant fall in the incidence of KS since the advent of HAART.[26-28] During this same period the Multicenter AIDS Cohort Study (MACS) continued to exhibit the same 21% per year increase in cases of NHL observed since 1985.[26] From 1994 through 1997, the Adult Spectrum of HIV Disease project, which includes more than 40,000 persons followed at 100 clinics and hospitals, documented a significant fall in the incidence of primary central nervous system (CNS) lymphoma but no significant change in the incidence of systemic lymphoma.[28]

Tumor registry data from San Francisco General Hospital indicate a dramatic decline in new diagnosis of primary CNS lymphoma, with 17 cases in 1995 and only 4 diagnosed in 1997. During this period there was no change in the number of diagnoses of systemic lymphoma.

Pathogenesis/Etiology

The etiology of NHL in patients with HIV infection appears to be multifactorial. In immunosuppressed allograft recipients, molecular data have implicated Epstein-Barr virus (EBV) as a potential causative agent in the development of NHL. Several studies have documented the presence of EBV DNA sequences in the vast majority of B-cell lymphomas from transplant recipients.[51,107,109] The majority of lymphomas described in this population have been classified as immunoblastic lymphomas. However, in this patient population, aggressive lymphoproliferative processes also have been described that apparently are polyclonal by both immunologic and morphologic criteria.[51,110,111] In some of these cases, a typical monoclonal lymphoma has subsequently developed.[112]

Although the finding of chromosome 8;14 translocations, like those seen with Burkitt's lymphoma, and the finding of EBV nuclear antigen in some tumors[113-116] suggested that EBV might also be implicated in the etiology of HIV-associated lymphomas, more recent observations indicate that EBV DNA sequences are present in only approximately 40% of systemic HIV-associated lymphomas.[117-120] However, there is also information suggesting that EBV DNA sequences are present in a majority of primary CNS lymphomas in patients with HIV infection.[118,121] Other viruses have been implicated in the pathogenesis of specific subcategories of HIV-associated NHL. The observation of a clonally integrated HIV genome in either the malignant cells themselves or tumor-associated macrophages within certain HIV-associated T-cell lymphomas has raised the possibility of a more direct role for HIV in lymphomagenesis in a small number of cases.[6,122] HIV, by infecting macrophages, may act in a nonspecific way to enhance cytokine expression. Cytokine overexpression may then drive polyclonal B-cell proliferation. In addition, recent laboratory studies have identified HHV8 sequences associated with HIV-associated primary effusion lymphomas.[123]

Evaluation of immunoglobulin gene rearrangements using Southern blot hybridization techniques demonstrates that, although many of the B-cell tumors observed in this patient population have clonal immunoglobulin gene rearrangements, clonal rearrangements are not observed in other lymphomas.[118,119,124,125] These tumors may represent polyclonal processes not unlike those observed in allograft recipients.[111]

Emilie et al.[126] recently demonstrated high levels of the cytokine IL-6 associated with immunoblastic lymphoma. Others have identified overexpression of both IL-6 and interleukin-10 in some HIV-associated NHLs,[127] and higher IL-6 levels have been observed in individuals with HIV-associated NHL than in those with HIV disease only,[128] suggesting that a cytokine-driven process may be involved in pathogenesis.

This heterogeneity of molecular characteristics, including clonality and the presence or absence of EBV, suggests that lymphomagenesis may occur through several different mechanisms. Although EBV may be involved in the pathogenesis of some HIV-associated lymphomas, other viruses, spontaneous genetic changes, cytokines, or even the underlying immune disregulation itself may give rise to NHL.

Clinical Characteristics

Like the molecular features of the lymphomas themselves, the individuals with HIV-associated NHL are also a heterogeneous group. Individuals with HIV-associated NHL are not all severely immunocompromised. Patients seen at San Francisco General Hospital with peripheral (as opposed to primary CNS) NHL have exhibited a wide range of CD4 lymphocyte counts, with a mean value of 200/mm^3 (n = 95). Over one third of these individuals had CD4 lymphocyte counts above 200/mm^3. NHL was the initial AIDS-defining diagnosis in 70. In a recent multicenter study of 192 patients with HIV-associated NHL, the median pretreatment CD4 count was 100/mm^3.[129] Patients with primary CNS lymphoma represent a very different patient population. These individuals are almost universally severely immunocompromised, with CD4 lymphocyte counts below 50/mm^3.[130]

The vast majority of the NHLs observed in patients with HIV infection are classified as B-cell malignancies.[131,132] A small number of NHLs of other histologic and immunologic subtypes have been observed, including T-cell lymphoma[117,133,134] and others of uncertain lineage.[135] Of 327 cases reported in the literature from five centers, 73% of the lymphomas were classified as high grade, 24% as intermediate grade, and 3% as low grade.[117,132,136–139] Most B-cell lymphomas in these individuals are classified as diffuse large-cell tumors of either intermediate-grade type or the high-grade immunoblastic type (Color Plate IIG). In addition, approximately one third of patients have tumors of the high-grade, small, noncleaved cell variety.

Widespread disease involving extranodal sites is the hallmark of AIDS-associated lymphoma at the time of diagnosis. Ziegler et al.[132] reported that 95% of patients had evidence of extranodal disease, 42% of patients had CNS disease, and 33% had bone marrow involvement. In a series of 89 patients diagnosed at New York University, 87% had extranodal disease at presentation.[138] The most common sites of disease included the GI tract, CNS, bone marrow, and liver. At San Francisco General Hospital, two thirds of the patients had stage W disease, and 31% had extranodal disease alone, with no identifiable site of nodal disease.

As observed in other immunosuppressed patients with NHL, unusual extralymphatic presentations are common. Sites of disease have included the rectum,[140] heart and pericardium,[141,142] and common bile ducts.[143] GI involvement has been reported in up to 27% of individuals with lymphoma,[144] and virtually any site in the GI tract or hepatobiliary tree can be involved. In the San Francisco General Hospital series, other unusual sites of disease included subcutaneous and soft tissue, epidural space, appendix, gingiva, parotid gland, and paranasal sinus.[117]

NHL confined to the CNS frequently has been reported in association with HIV infection.[145–148] The most common presenting symptoms have been confusion, lethargy, and memory loss. Other symptoms have included hemiparesis, aphasia, seizures, cranial nerve palsies, and headache. Single or multiple discrete, contrast-enhancing lesions are the most common findings on computed tomographic (CT) scans or magnetic resonance (MR) images of the brain. The radiographic appearance of primary CNS lymphoma is generally not easily distinguished from that of toxoplasmosis. Solitary lesions are observed in approximately 21% of MR images from individuals with toxoplasmosis, and therefore solitary lesions are somewhat more likely to be associated with lymphoma. However, 50% of CNS lymphomas present as multiple lesions, creating an even more difficult diagnostic dilemma.[149]

Patients with neurologic symptoms should be evaluated promptly with CT scans or MR images of the brain. Lumbar puncture should be performed if not contraindicated by the findings. A serum specimen from patients with focal lesions should be sent for cryptococcal antigen and toxoplasma titers. Because toxoplasmosis is infrequent in individuals with negative *Toxoplasma* serologies,[150,151] brain biopsy should be performed in a timely fashion in this group of patients. Individuals with focal intracerebral lesions and positive serologic studies for *Toxoplasma* typically are started on antitoxoplasma therapy and observed closely for signs of improvement or deterioration.

Recently, thallium-201 single-photon emission CT (SPECT) scanning has been utilized as a means for distinguishing between these two entities. In one series, all 24 individuals with toxoplasmosis had negative scans whereas all 12 with CNS lymphoma had positive scans.[152] In a second study, nine cases of CNS lymphoma were all positive on thallium SPECT scanning.[153] Of concern, however, was the fact that 3 of 10 cases of toxoplasmosis also had positive scans. Although these series are small and data from larger numbers of patients are needed, these observations do suggest a potential utility for this nuclear medicine study in the diagnosis of CNS lymphoma.

Of even greater interest are observations made using polymerase chain reaction (PCR) for detecting EBV DNA sequences in cerebral spinal fluid. De Luca et al. showed that 7 of 8 individuals with documented CNS lymphoma had positive PCR for EBV in cerebral spinal fluid.[154] All 11 cases with brain lesions and no lymphoma were negative, and 21 individuals with AIDS but no CNS lesions were also negative. In a second series, all 17 individuals with CNS lymphoma were positive for EBV by PCR, and 67 of 68 individuals with HIV and no lymphoma were negative.[155] Data from a much larger series of patients confirm these results and have been reported elsewhere in this volume. These data strongly suggest PCR is a useful means of noninvasive diagnosis of primary CNS lymphoma in patients with HIV disease. This may be particularly powerful when used in conjunction with thallium SPECT scanning and the results of toxoplasma serologic studies.

At the present time, the standard of care for diagnosis of CNS lymphoma is brain biopsy. Because treatment outcome is strongly dependent upon early diagnosis and institution of therapy, it is strongly recommended that individuals who are *Toxoplasma* seronegative, and therefore unlikely to have a diagnosis of toxoplasmosis, be referred for early brain biopsy if cerebral spinal fluid cytology is negative. Once the diagnosis of CNS lymphoma has been established, all patients should undergo a slit-lamp examination to rule out the presence of ocular lymphoma prior to initiation of therapy.

Treatment and Prognosis in Systemic Lymphoma

The use of multiagent chemotherapeutic regimens for the treatment of intermediate- and high-grade NHL in the non-HIV-infected individual has resulted in a dramatic improvement in prognosis for this group.[156] A complete response rate as high as 86% and long-term survival rates as high as 65% have been reported in patients treated for aggressive, large-cell lymphomas.[157]

In HIV-infected individuals, however, the use of similar chemotherapeutic regimens has not resulted in as favorable an outcome (Table 30–8).[48,130,137,161,162] Complete response rates are lower than the corresponding rates in the non-HIV-infected population, and these responses are usually of short duration. In a retrospective review by Ziegler et al.[132] of patients treated at multiple institutions, 53% of 66 patients who could be evaluated achieved complete response to combination chemotherapy. However, 54% of the complete responders subsequently relapsed. In a series of patients from San Francisco General Hospital, 54% of 59 patients who could be evaluated and who were treated with a variety of combinations of chemotherapeutic regimens

had complete responses.[117] Twenty-three percent of these complete responders subsequently relapsed (Fig. 30–3).

Morphologic subtype appeared to predict response to chemotherapy in one series of patients reported from New York University.[138] The best complete response rate was reported for those patients classified as having a large, noncleaved cell lymphoma (52%), whereas those having a small, noncleaved cell lymphoma and immunoblastic lymphoma had response rates of 26% and 21%, respectively.

Survival times from a number of large series of patients reported in the literature are shown in Table 30–8. Median survival times in these groups range from 4 to 7 months. In the series of 23 patients who received chemotherapy at the Pacific Medical Center, the median survival time was 20 months in those patients who had complete response to therapy.[136]

Although overall survival times in patients with AIDS-associated NHL are disappointing, subgroups of patients can be identified in which the therapeutic outcome is significantly worse than for other groups of patients (Table 30–9). Morphologic subtypes predictive of response to therapy in patients treated at New York University were also predictive of survival in this same series.[138] Patients with intermediate-grade large-cell lymphoma had the longest median survival time (7.5 months); those with small, noncleaved cell lymphoma had a median survival time of 5.5 months; and those with immunoblastic lymphoma had a median survival time of only 2 months.

In the San Francisco General Hospital series, median survival time for all patients receiving chemotherapy ($n = 65$) was only 5.5 months. However, life-table analysis for subgroups within this population illustrates the importance of prognostic features. Those features identified as being predictive of significantly shorter survival time included an absolute CD4+ lymphocyte count less than 100/mm³, a prior AIDS diagnosis, a Karnofsky performance score of less than 70%, and the presence of an extranodal site of disease.

Data from more recent studies, such as the prospective data in 192 patients enrolled in the ACTG 142 study,[129] a study of low-dose versus standard-dose chemotherapy, more closely resemble those factors identified in the International Prognostic Index[163] (Table 30–9) for non-immunodeficiency-associated aggressive NHLs. In this study,[129] factors associated with poor prognosis included age greater than 35 years, CD4 count of less than 100/mm³, history of IV

TABLE 30–8. HIV-Associated NHL: Treatment Outcome

REGIMEN*	NO. OF PATIENTS	MEDIAN CD/mm³	COMPLETE RESPONSE (%)	MEDIAN SURVIVAL TIME (mo)	REFERENCES
HDAraC/HD MTX	9	173	33	6.0	137
COMP, ProMACE-MOPP	83		33	5.0	138
COMET-A	38	164	58	5.2	117
COMLA, m-BACOD, CHOP	27	169	46	11.3	117
L-17, CHOP, NHL-7, m-BACOD, MACOP-B	30		56	6.0	139
LNH-84	141	227	63	9.0	161
Low-dose m-BACOD	35	150	46	6.5	168
ProMACE-MOPP/CytaBOM	72		35	4.0	162

*HDAraC/HD MTX, high-dose cytarabine/high-dose methotrexate; COMP, cyclophosphamide, vincristine, methotrexate, and prednisone; ProMACE-MOPP, prednisone, methotrexate, doxorubicin, cyclophosphamide, and etoposide; COMET-A, cyclophosphamide, vincristine, methotrexate, etoposide, and cytarabine; COMLA, cyclophosphamide, vincristine, methotrexate, leukovorin, and cytarabine; m-BACOD, methotrexate, bleomycin, doxorubicin, cyclophosphamide, vincristine, and dexamethasone; CHOP, cyclophosphamide, doxorubicin, vincristine, and prednisone; L-17, cyclophosphamide, vincristine, intrathecal methotrexate, doxorubicin, and prednisone; NHL-7, cyclophosphamide, NGBG, bleomycin, prednisone, doxorubicin, and vincristine; MACOP-B, methotrexate, doxorubicin, cyclophosphamide, vincristine, prednisone, and bleomycin; LNH-84, *induction*: doxorubicin, cyclophosphamide, vindesine, bleomycin, prednisone, intrathecal methotrexate, *consolidation*: methotrexate, hyfosphamide, etoposide, L-asparaginase, and cytarabine; ProMACE-CytaBOM, cyclophosphamide, doxorubicin, etoposide, cytarabine, bleomycin, vincristine, methotrexate, and prednisone.

TABLE 30–9. Predictors of Poor Clinical Outcome in Chemotherapy-Treated Patients with HIV-Associated NHL

KAPLAN ET AL.[117]	ACTG 142[129]	VACCHER ET AL.[163a]
CD4 count <100/mm³	CD4 count <100/mm³	CD4 count <100/mm³
Prior AIDS	Age >35	Age >40
Karnofsky performance score <70%	Stage III/IV	Stage III/IV
Extranodal disease	IV drug use	Abnormal lactate dehydrogenase

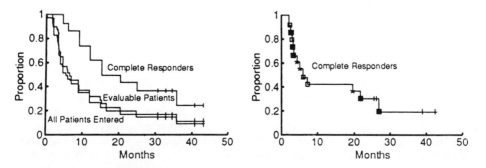

FIGURE 30–3. *Left,* Overall survival in patients with AIDS-related lymphoma. Tick marks indicate patients who are alive at the given time interval. *Right,* Event-free survival in 16 complete responders. Tick marks indicate patients who are still alive in continuous complete remission; solid boxes, development of intercurrent HIV-related illness; open boxes, development of relapse of lymphoma; asterisks, death from unknown cause. Event-free survival is taken from the time of achievement of complete remission to the time of relapse, HIV-related illness, or death. (From Levine AM, Wernz JC, Kaplan L, et al: Low-dose chemotherapy with central nervous system prophylaxis and zidovudine maintenance in AIDS-related lymphoma. JAMA 266:84, 1991, with permission. Copyright 1991, American Medical Association.)

drug use, and, for the first time, tumor bulk as measured by stage of disease. Advanced stage III and stage IV disease were associated with a poor outcome. Similarly, a recent retrospective review of 96 patients treated for aggressive HIV-associated lymphomas indicated that bulky tumor as measured by elevation of serum lactate dehydrogenase was again associated with a poor clinical outcome.[90]

Evaluation of newly diagnosed patients for these prognostic features may help determine how to approach therapy in individuals with this disease. The patient without a prior AIDS diagnosis whose immune function is relatively good will tolerate therapy better and have a more favorable outcome than a patient whose diagnosis of lymphoma comes after a history of multiple opportunistic infections. Because many patients will fall between these extremes, these prognostic characteristics can serve only as rough guidelines in determining which patients to treat.

The most appropriate therapeutic regimen for a given patient also must be individualized, because there is no known best regimen. Poor bone marrow reserve and the occurrence of opportunistic infections often result in dose reductions and delays in therapy. In addition, the risk of further immunosuppression when treating HIV-infected patients with aggressive combination chemotherapy must be considered. The impact of HAART on therapeutic outcome and on tolerance of chemotherapy is unclear because published reports have yet to evaluate this recent change in managing HIV disease.

Contrary to the belief that more intensive chemotherapy is associated with improved clinical outcome in non-HIV-associated lymphoma, retrospective data from two centers have suggested that, in HIV-infected individuals with NHL, survival may be improved in those treated with less aggressive regimens. Survival data from the San Francisco General Hospital cohort of chemotherapy-treated patients with NHL revealed that patients receiving chemotherapy regimens containing 1 gm/m^2 or more of cyclophosphamide had a median survival time of only 4.6 months compared to those treated with regimens containing less than 1 gm/m^2 of cyclophosphamide, who had a median survival time of 12.2 months ($p = .02$).[117] Similarly, in a study of nine patients treated with a novel, more aggressive chemotherapeutic regimen consisting of high-dose cytosine arabinoside, L-asparaginase, vincristine, prednisone, cyclophosphamide (high dose), methotrexate, and leucovorin, only three patients had complete re-

mission.[137] This intensive regimen was associated with a high risk of mortality caused by opportunistic infection.

Two different approaches to therapy have been studied and reported. In the first of these clinical trials, 35 patients with HIV-associated NHL and a mean CD4 lymphocyte count of 150/mm^3 were treated with a modification of the standard methotrexate, bleomycin, doxorubicin, cyclophosphamide, vincristine, and dexamethasone (m-BACOD) regimen.[168] Instead of administering cyclophosphamide at 600 mg/m^2 and doxorubicin at 45 mg/m^2, these two agents were administered at 300 mg/m^2 and 25 mg/m^2, respectively. All patients received CNS prophylaxis and zidovudine maintenance after the completion of chemotherapy. Complete remission was observed in 16 of 35 individuals (46%), and the median survival time for the 35 patients who could be evaluated was 6.5 months. These results are not significantly different from those reported previously using a variety of more standard chemotherapeutic regimens. However, these results were achieved with significantly less hematologic toxicity; only 10% of chemotherapeutic cycles were complicated by an absolute neutrophil count of less than 500/mm^3. Fifteen cycles (12%) were delayed because of neutropenia. The survival curves shown in Figure 30–3 demonstrate that durable, complete remissions were achieved in some individuals, with a median survival time of 15 months in the 16 complete responders. It is noteworthy, however, that, when a similar regimen was used in a group of individuals with a mean CD4 count of 35/mm^3,[164] only 19% had complete remission and the median survival was only 3 months. These observations again point out the strong relationship between immune function and clinical outcome.

In a second approach to therapy, more standard doses of cyclophosphamide, doxorubicin, vincristine, and prednisone (CHOP) chemotherapy were used in a trial in which patients receiving chemotherapy were randomized to receive either concurrent therapy with GM-CSF or no further adjunctive treatment.[165] Table 30–10 demonstrates that individuals receiving GM-CSF had a significantly higher mean nadir of absolute neutrophil counts and a significantly shorter duration of life-threatening neutropenia compared with those in the control group. As a result, those patients who received GM-CSF spent a mean time of 5.9 days in the hospital for febrile neutropenic episodes through the course of their treatment, compared with a mean of 18.6 days in the control group. This small

TABLE 30–10. Low-Dose Versus Standard-Dose Chemotherapy for HIV-Associated NHL

PARAMETER	STANDARD DOSE	LOW DOSE	P VALUE
Complete response	42/81 (52%)	39/94 (41%)	NS
Time to progression	30 wk	39 wk	NS
Median survival	31 wk	35 wk	NS
Time to grade 3/4 toxicity	7 wk	17 wk	.001
Toxicity ≥grade 3	70% patients	51% patients	.008
Grade 4 neuropenia	39% cycles	24% cycles	.001
NHL at time of death	60%	70%	NS

Data from ACTG 142 trial. Kaplan L, Straus D, Testa M, et al: Low-dose compared with standard-dose m-BACOD chemotherapy for non-Hodgkin's lymphoma associated with human immunodeficiency virus infection. N Engl J Med 336:1641, 1997.

clinical trial was not designed to evaluate response or survival, but it clearly demonstrated that one of the most significant morbidities associated with chemotherapy in this patient population can be reduced with the adjunctive use of a myeloid growth factor.

Result from a French-Italian trial indicate that an aggressive, multiagent chemotherapy regimen can be tolerated by patients with good immune function (CD4 count >200/mm^3).[161] In this study, 140 patients received the aggressive LNH84 regimen. Treatment was associated with a complete remission rate of 63% and a median survival time of 9 months. It is more likely, however, that these results simply reflect the favorable outcome associated with good immune function rather than an advance in chemotherapy.

The ACTG 142 study was a large, multicenter, randomized clinical trial designed to directly address the question of the importance of chemotherapy dose intensity in determining clinical outcome of treatment for HIV-associated NHL. In this study, 198 patients were randomized to receive either standard-dose m-BACOD chemotherapy with adjunctive administration of GM-CSF or the same low-dose m-BACOD regimen described earlier with GM-CSF administered only as required for management of neutropenia.[129] The results of this trial (Table 30–10) demonstrated no significant difference in response rate or survival time. However, toxicity was more severe in those patients randomized to standard-dose therapy, particularly with respect to the occurrence of grade IV neutropenia. Survival differences were not even observed for those patients with CD4 counts above 100/mm^3, suggesting that most individuals with HIV-associated NHL should be treated with a low-dose chemotherapeutic regimen. However, in this trial only 40 individuals with CD4 greater than 200/mm^3 were enrolled. Of these patients,

those randomized to low-dose therapy survived for a median of 66 months, while those assigned to standard-dose survived for a median of 73 months. This difference was not statistically significant, and the number of patients was too small to determine whether some might have benefited from the use of standard-dose therapy. Because patients with higher CD4 counts are more tolerant of chemotherapy, consideration might therefore still be given to the use of a standard-dose regimen in those with CD4 counts greater than 200/mm^3.

Another more recent approach to therapy is the use of continuous infusion chemotherapy. In a pilot study, Sparano et al.[166] treated 25 patients with a 96-hour continuous infusion of cyclophosphamide, doxorubicin, and etoposide. All patients received antiviral therapy with didanosine. Complete response occurred in 58% and median survival was 18.4 months, longer than reported in previous trials. Whether this longer survival time is the result of a more effective chemotherapy regimen or is due to more effective management of HIV disease in recent years is unclear. This regimen is currently being studied in a large Phase II trial in the Eastern Cooperative Oncology Group.

It is clear that, ultimately, variations in standard cytotoxic regimens will probably not have a major impact on survival. In the presence of the underlying immunodeficiency state, novel approaches using nonmyelosuppressive and nonimmunosuppressive treatment modalities, either alone or as an adjunct to cytotoxic therapy, are needed. Clinical trials are currently evaluating the use of monoclonal antibodies and immunotoxins directed toward cell surface determinants that are unique to HIV-associated NHLs. Other studies are evaluating the use of cytokines such as interleukins 2 and 12 to enhance α-interferon production and the cellular immune response. Adoptive immunotherapy and approaches directed at inhibition of clonal macrophages are also in clinical trials. It is hoped that, as we continue to learn more about the biology of the HIV-associated lymphomas, we can develop more rational and effective treatment modalities that take advantage of the unique molecular characteristics of these tumors.

Treatment of Primary CNS Lymphoma

Primary CNS lymphoma has been particularly difficult to treat. Many cases have been diagnosed at autopsy,[132] and those occurring antemortem often have been in patients who had advanced immunodeficiency and had suffered multiple previous bouts of opportunistic infections.[145]

In the largest published series of treated patients, Baumgartner et al.[145] observed that 76% of 29 patients treated with 4000 cGy of whole-brain radiation therapy showed evidence of significant clinical improvement, and 69% demonstrated complete or partial radiographic response. Similar results have been reported in smaller series from other institutions. In a series reported by Formenti et al.,[144] complete responses to cranial irradiation occurred in 6 of the 10 patients. Despite this good response rate, survival times remain short, with median survival time for treated patients reported as between 2 and 5 months.[145,146] In patients with CNS lymphoma, opportunistic infection has been the most common cause of death.[145,146] In Formenti et al.'s series,[146] 50% of the patients died of opportunistic infection, and only two died of recurrent lymphoma. In Baumgartner et al.'s series,[145] of those patients who had postmortem examinations, the only patient who died as a result of uncontrolled lymphoma had developed a site of disease outside of the radiation portal in the cervical spinal cord. However, in a University of California at San Francisco series of 56 patients with HIV-associated primary CNS lymphoma, 29 of whom received radiation therapy, CNS lymphoma was the most commonly documented cause of death (63%), with only 21% dying of opportunistic infection.[170]

The results of treatment of primary CNS lymphoma from both retrospective and prospective clinical series are shown in Table 30–11.[130,145,167,169–173] These data confirm that most patients with CNS lymphoma treated with radiotherapy alone do have improvement in their neurologic symptoms. However, survival is short, with most individuals dying from complications of HIV disease. Of note is the observation that, in a small pilot study of chemoradiotherapy for CNS lymphoma, survival was not improved by the addition of chemotherapy despite a very high complete response rate.[172]

Because most CNS lymphoma patients have severe immunodeficiency, they are highly susceptible to a variety of opportunistic infections. In addition, at least 20% do not respond to therapeutic intervention directed at the CNS lymphoma. Progress in the management of this disease will therefore depend on advances in the management of both the neoplastic disease and the underlying HIV infection.

Treatment Recommendations

In selecting therapy for patients with HIV-associated NHL, emphasis should be placed on individualized therapy. Although standard-dose chemotherapy may be appropriate for the patient with good immune function (CD4 >200/mm^3) and no prior opportunistic infection, a lower dose treatment regimen might be selected for

TABLE 30–11. Treatment of HIV-Related Primary CNS Lymphoma

STUDY	N	CD4	Rx	CLINICALLY IMPROVED	OVERALL RESPONSE	SURVIVAL (mo)	DEATH WITH NHL
Rubio et al.[167]	81	32	RT	—	70%	2.0	55
Baumgartner et al.[145]	29	—	RT	76%	69%	3.9	13
Levine et al.[130]	11	30	RT	—	—	2.5	33
Nisce et al.[169]	24	—	RT	79%	87%	4.8	—
Lee et al.[170]	24	20	RT	62%	52%	4.0	63
Ling et al.[171]	41	—	RT	—	—	3.0	—
Forsyth et al.[172]	10	40	CT/RT	—	86% (CR)	3.5	0%
Chamberlain[173]	11	—	CT/RT	—	69%	4.0	—

Abbreviations: CT, chemotherapy; RT, radiotherapy.

the patient with more severe immunologic compromise, marginal performance score, and a history of opportunistic infection. For some patients who are severely ill, a decision may be made to withhold therapy altogether. These decisions must take into account not only the patient's history and present condition but also the patient's own desires for a given therapeutic approach. Regardless of the chemotherapeutic approach used, it is strongly recommended that all patients treated with chemotherapy receive adjunctive antibiotic prophylaxis against *P. carinii* pneumonia.

HODGKINS' DISEASE

As discussed previously, Hodgkin's disease is not an AIDS-defining illness. The precise relationship of this malignancy to the underlying immunodeficiency state is unclear. The observation that the frequency of Hodgkin's disease in the single male population ages 20 to 49 years in San Francisco had not increased between 1979 and 1987, when HIV seroprevalence markedly increased,[64,174] argued against a direct causal relationship between HIV-related immunodeficiency and the occurrence of Hodgkin's disease in this population. This is in striking contrast to the earlier sharp rise in the frequency of NHL observed in the same population during the same time period.[4,64] However, data from several recently reported epidemiologic studies, including the San Francisco Clinic Cohort study[175] and the Multicenter AIDS Cohort Study (MACS),[176] suggest a significant increased risk of Hodgkin's disease in HIV-seropositive individuals. The reported relative risks fall between two- and fivefold, significantly lower than that observed for NHL, possibly explaining why a greater period of observation of larger populations was required to identify these differences.

Clinical observations suggest that Hodgkin's disease in a patient with HIV infection has a different natural history and therapeutic outcome than do cases of Hodgkin's disease in the general population. The clinical features and therapeutic outcome in 14 homosexual men with Hodgkin's disease diagnosed at San Francisco General Hospital have been compared with those in a group of 35 single men 20 to 49 years of age diagnosed with Hodgkin's disease between the years 1973 and 1979.[174] Mixed cellularity was the most common histologic pattern among the 14 risk-group patients, whereas nodular sclerosis was significantly more common in

the control population. All but one of the risk-group patients had advanced (stage III or IV) disease. Bone marrow and liver were the most common sites of extranodal disease. Similar observations were made in a series of 22 patients reported from a cooperative study of six hospitals[177] in which 68% of patients presented with either mixed cellularity or lymphocyte-depleted histology and 91% presented with stage III or IV disease.

The outcome of therapy in these patients has been disappointing. Of 12 patients treated at San Francisco General Hospital who could be evaluated, 7 had complete responses to either nitrogen mustard, vincristine, procarbazine, and prednisone (MOPP) or MOPP with doxorubicin, bleomycin, vinblastine, and dacarbazine (ABVD).[174] Six of these patients had subsequent relapses. Eight patients (62%) developed *P. carinii* pneumonia during treatment. None of these patients is alive; half died with advanced Hodgkin's disease, and the others died as a result of opportunistic infections. Median survival time was less than 1 year in this group, compared with 12 years in the control population. There were no differences in either response or survival time between those patients treated with MOPP alone and those treated with MOPP-ABVD.

The mean dose intensity of chemotherapy delivered to our patients was only 41% of the planned therapeutic dose. This was a result of the need for frequent dose reductions and delays in chemotherapy because of poor bone marrow reserve and intercurrent opportunistic infections. The very low dose intensity of chemotherapy may account for the high relapse rate observed in complete responders.

The Italian cooperative group for AIDS-related tumors reported on 35 cases of Hodgkin's disease occurring in HIV-infected individuals.[162] Eighty-nine percent of these patients were IV drug abusers, 3% were homosexual males, and 9% were IV-drug-using homosexual males. Fifty-three percent of the patients had mixed-cellularity histologic type, 31% had nodular sclerosis, and 16% had lymphocyte depletion. Seventy-eight percent of patients had either stage III or stage IV disease. Seventeen patients were treated with either MOPP, ABVD, ABV, or MOPP alternating with ABVD. Only 8 patients (30%) had complete remission. Of 13 patients who died, 7 (54%) died of opportunistic infections, 3 of progression of Hodgkin's disease, and 2 of disseminated intravascular coagulation. In one patient, the cause of death could not be determined. The median survival time of these patients was 15 months.

In a series of 22 patients in Spain treated with a variety of standard combination chemotherapeutic regimens,[177] the median survival for all patients was 18 months. No significant differences were found between survival and stages of Hodgkin's disease, histologic subgroup, or CD4 count; however, the sample size was quite small. Nonetheless, patients with a prior AIDS-defining diagnosis had a median survival time of 13 months, which was significantly shorter than that in other patients.

As is the case for NHLs in HIV-seropositive patients, experience does not suggest that survival with Hodgkin's disease will be improved with more aggressive chemotherapeutic regimens. Poor bone marrow reserve and the occurrence of opportunistic infections have made it difficult to administer full doses of standard Hodgkin's disease chemotherapy to these patients. Preliminary results of a clinical trial using a relatively nonmyelosuppressive combination chemotherapeutic regimen for Hodgkin's disease in patients with HIV infection were encouraging.[178] This treatment regimen used a combination of bleomycin, vincristine, streptozocin, and etoposide. Of the first five patients treated with this regimen, four had complete responses to chemotherapy alone, and the fifth had a complete response when chemotherapy and radiation therapy were completed. Myelosuppression was not observed, and all patients remain alive and well.

More recently, Levine et al. studied the use of standard ABVD chemotherapy combined with G-CSF in an effort to reduce the myelosuppression associated with standard chemotherapy.[179] In this trial, 60% of 21 treated individuals achieved complete remission with a median survival of 78 weeks (19 months). Overall this regimen was tolerated well, although considerable hematologic toxicity did occur.

At this time there are not sufficient data available to allow us to determine which chemotherapeutic regimen may be more efficacious. It is recommended that standard treatment regimens (this will usually be ABVD) be utilized for the majority of patients with myeloid CSF support. However, for those individuals with severe immunocompromise (CD4 count $<100/mm^3$) and for those with poor hematologic reserve, consideration may be given to dose-modified standard regimens or the use of less myelosuppressive chemotherapeutic combinations such as those described above.

HUMAN PAPILLOMAVIRUS INFECTION AND ANOGENITAL NEOPLASIA

Published reports suggest that HIV-induced immunodeficiency may promote the development of neoplasia in the cervical and anal mucosa. Cervical and anal cancers probably will become increasingly common manifestations of HIV disease as patients with profound immunodeficiency who would have succumbed to opportunistic infections earlier in the epidemic survive for extended periods of time because they receive more effective antiretroviral, prophylactic, and antimicrobial therapies. The resulting state of prolonged, severe immunodeficiency provides the necessary milieu for the emergence of diseases that develop after longer latency, such as anogenital carcinomas.

HPV Infection, Immunosuppression, and Anogenital Neoplasia

Anogenital neoplasia has a recognized association with chronic immunodeficiency. Studies of cohorts of immunosuppressed organ transplant recipients, for example, have demonstrated a 100-fold increase in incidence of vulvar and anal carcinomas and a 14-fold increase in the incidence of cervical carcinoma as compared with controls.[180,181]

Considerable evidence links the development of anogenital carcinoma to HPV infection. The so-called oncogenic HPV genotypes (HPV-16, HPV-18, and HPV-31) have been detected in 80% to 90% of cervical intraepithelial neoplasia grade 3 lesions and invasive cervical cancers.[182] HPV infection has been presumed to play a similar causative role in the development of anal carcinoma, as suggested by the presence of HPV DNA and mRNA in tumor tissues from that site.[183] The high incidence of anogenital cancer in immunosuppressed transplant recipients is probably a consequence of the high prevalence of detectable anogenital HPV infection in that population. The prevalence of HPV infection is 5 to 17 times greater in immunosuppressed transplant recipients than in the general population.[14]

HIV Infection, HPV Infection, and Cervical Neoplasia

Over the past 10 years, numerous studies have identified HIV infection as an important risk factor for HPV infection and the development of HPV-associated neoplasia of the female anogenital tract. These findings suggest that HIV-associated immunodeficiency increases a woman's susceptibility to HPV infection, and that HIV infection alters the natural history of IIPV infection in a way that makes development of anogenital neoplasia more likely. Table 30–12 details the general conclusions reached from reviewing numerous such studies.

A more detailed review of some representative recent studies illustrates these points. For example, a recent report described a large prospective cohort study in which the natural history of HPV infection was compared in HIV-infected and non-HIV-infected women.[184] Two hundred twenty HIV-infected and 231 non-HIV-infected women in the New York City area were evaluated at two or more semiannual gynecologic examinations that included a test of cervicovaginal lavage specimens for HPV DNA. Among women without neoplastic lesions identified at their first visit, the investigators found that HPV infection was more common and more persistent in the HIV-infected women. Specimens from the HIV-infected women were also more likely to contain the HPV genotypes known to be most strongly associated with high-grade squamous intraepithelial lesions and invasive cancer.

Results of another recent study were also described in which anal and cervical HPV infection and cytologic abnormalities were evaluated in HIV-infected and non-HIV-infected women.[185] Anal and cervical Pap smears, dot-blot and PCR tests for HPV, and peripheral blood CD4+ T-lymphocyte counts were performed in this cross-sectional study of 114 women enrolled in a community-based study of HIV infection. Anal HPV infection was twice as common as cervical HPV infection, and was also strongly statistically associated with HIV infection. Cervical and anal cytologic abnormalities were also strongly statistically associated with HIV infection, as well as with more advanced immunodeficiency as indicated by lower mean CD4+ T-lymphocyte counts. The authors concluded that HPV-associated epithelial abnormalities were associated with immunodeficiency among HIV-infected women, and that anal HPV infection was at least as common as cervical infection and disease among HIV-infected women.

An important report by Maiman et al. described a cohort of HIV-infected women in New York with invasive and preinvasive cervical neoplasia.[186] In comparison to a group of non-HIV-infected women from the same institution, cervical neoplasia in HIV-infected women was more advanced at presentation, was more likely to recur, was associated more commonly with perianal involvement, and was associated more often with cytologic or histologic evidence of HPV infection. The authors concluded that HPV-related neoplasia was having a significant impact on their female patients. In a study expanding on their initial observations, these authors confirmed that HIV-infected women appear to have more advanced disease at initial presentation with cervical cancer.[187] They also showed that standard treatment approaches for advanced cervical cancer in HIV-infected women resulted in significantly shorter mean time intervals until disease recurrence and death than were experienced in uninfected women. The same authors recently obtained additional evidence from New York City cancer and AIDS registries from 1987 through 1995 confirming that the cervical cancer recurrence rate was high in HIV-infected women, and that cervical cancer led to death in 95% of HIV-infected women who contracted the disease.[188] Cervical cancer was the most common AIDS-related malignancy in the cohort that they studied.

Despite the apparent high prevalence of cervical neoplasia in HIV-infected women, only a few cases of invasive cervical cancer have been reported.[186,187,189–191] However, the experience with immunosuppressed transplant recipients suggests that a prolonged period of immunosuppression (mean of 88 months) may be necessary to permit development of anogenital cancer.[180] Until recently, most patients died of other complications of their HIV infection after a much shorter period of immunodeficiency and, therefore, may not have survived long enough to de-

---

TABLE 30–12. Summary of Findings from Studies of Anogenital Intraepithelial Neoplasia in Persons with HIV Infection

1. HIV-infected subjects are more likely to have cervical or anal intraepithelial neoplasia than non-HIV-infected controls.
2. HIV-infected subjects are more likely to have detectable cervical or anal HPV infection than non-HIV-infected controls.
3. Cervical or anal intraepithelial neoplasia is more common among HIV-infected subjects with lower CD4+ T-lymphocyte counts or more advanced clinical stage of HIV disease.
4. Detectable cervical or anal HPV infection is more common among HIV-infected subjects with lower CD4+ T-lymphocyte counts.

velop cervical cancer. With the improvements in survival now being achieved through the use of effective antiretroviral, prophylactic, and antimicrobial therapies, the duration of severe immunodeficiency may become long enough for women co-infected with HPV and HIV to develop cervical cancer with increasing frequency.

HIV Infection, HPV Infection, and Anal Neoplasia

The relationship of HIV infection, HPV infection, and anal neoplasia also has been described. Although an association of anal neoplasia and HPV infection in homosexual men has been recognized for some time,[192,193] it is now apparent that HIV-infected, immunosuppressed men are particularly at risk for the development of HPV-related anal neoplasia.

Several early investigations provided preliminary evidence of the relationship of HIV infection, HPV infection, and anal neoplasia. Two small studies demonstrated HPV in neoplastic anal lesions of homosexual men by histopathologic and immunohistochemical techniques.[159,194] One individual in each study had a diagnosis of AIDS at the time that anal neoplasia was found. Frazer et al.[195] examined a larger cohort of homosexual men using anorectal cytologic smears, HIV antibody testing, and T-lymphocyte phenotyping. They found that HIV seropositivity, lower CD4+ T-lymphocyte counts, and lower CD4+: CD8+ ratios were significantly associated with more pronounced cytologic atypia.

More recently, Palefsky et al.[196] assessed the prevalence of anal HPV infection and precancerous abnormalities of the anal epithelium in 97 severely immunodeficient, HIV-infected homosexual men. Thirty-nine percent of the men had abnormal anal cytology, and 54% had HPV DNA in their anal cytologic specimens. Abnormalities on anal cytologic smear were significantly associated with the presence of HPV DNA (risk ratio, 4.6), and median CD4+ T-lymphocyte counts of men with abnormal cytologic findings were significantly lower than those of men with normal findings ($p = .05$).

Another cohort of 105 homosexual men, including men with and without HIV infection, took part in a similar study conducted by Caussy et al.[197] HPV DNA was found in anal cytologic specimens from 53% of HIV-infected men, compared to 29% of non-HIV-infected men ($p = .012$). Anal neoplasia was present more frequently in HIV-infected men (24% vs. 7%; $p = .03$). Multivariate logistic regression

analysis of data from the HIV-infected men showed that low CD4+ T-lymphocyte count was an independent risk factor for detection of HPV DNA ($p = .04$). Similar findings have been reported from a study of 120 Danish homosexual men[198] and from a study of 101 homosexual men attending a sexually transmitted diseases clinic in Seattle.[158] The results of a variety of studies of this nature are summarized in Table 32–12.

Lorenz et al.[160] reviewed the surgical experience with anal carcinoma in HIV-infected men at the University of California at San Francisco. They noted poor treatment outcomes and short survival in their patients, similar to the experience described above with HIV-associated cervical cancer.

Holland and Swift[199] reported on a retrospective review of the anal cancer treatment outcomes of seven HIV-seropositive patients and 55 patients whose HIV serostatus was negative or unknown. The patients were treated with standard radiotherapy with or without adjunctive chemotherapy. It was found that HIV-infected patients required more treatment delays and hospitalizations because of treatment-related toxicities. Relapses were more common and the mean time to treatment failure was shorter in HIV-infected patients. Other reports of single cases[200,201] and small case series[202,203] have described varying treatment outcomes with standard therapeutic approaches, with a suggestion that HIV-infected patients can benefit from standard therapies for anal cancer when HIV-related immunodeficiency is not advanced.

Clinical Implications of HIV-Related Anogenital Neoplasia

The studies cited previously demonstrate that anogenital HPV infection and neoplasia are common in persons with HIV infection. Information on the natural history of these conditions is limited, but it should be presumed that these lesions are precancerous and likely to evolve into invasive cancer over time. Early detection of preinvasive or minimally invasive cancers of the anogenital region can provide the opportunity to cure these diseases, as has been demonstrated by the successful use of Pap smears in screening programs in the general population. It therefore seems reasonable that some patients with HIV infection, particularly those with relatively better prognosis (higher CD4+ T-lymphocyte count, no prior opportunistic infections or malignancies), would benefit from early detection and treatment of anogenital neoplasia. Palefsky, of the University of California at San Francisco, has proposed guidelines (Table 30–13) for the management of cervical and anal neoplasia in HIV-infected persons.[204]

A study is underway in which a large population of HIV-infected men will be examined with anal Pap smears and biopsies to validate the use of the Pap smear as a screening tool in this setting (J. Palefsky, personal communication). Recommendations about the widespread use of the anal Pap smear for population screening must await the results of this or similar studies.

Cervical cancer and anal cancer are likely to become more common problems in patients with HIV-induced immunodeficiency as the epidemic progresses. Observations about the development of malignancies in other states of immunosuppression suggest that these cancers will become more frequent as therapeutic interventions prolong survival. Strategies for prevention, detection, and treatment of HIV-associated anogenital malignancies will be needed.

TABLE 30–13. Proposed Guidelines for Management of HIV-Associated Anogenital Neoplasia

---

Screening for Cervical Neoplasia
All HIV-infected women:
   Annual Pap smear of cervix
   Consider baseline colposcopy
HIV-infected women at high risk for HPV infection*:
   Pap smear every 6 months
   Careful inspection of vulvar, vaginal, and anal
     epithelium

Treatment for Cervical Neoplasia
Refer to a gynecologist for standard treatment

Screening for Anal Neoplasia
HIV-infected men with history of anal intercourse:
   Anal Pap smear[†]
   Anoscopy on a routine basis
   Biopsy of any abnormality identified on anoscopy
   Frequent anoscopic follow-up if abnormalities were
     identified previously

Treatment for Anal Neoplasia
Anal intraepithelial neoplasia: electrocautery or
   cryotherapy

Invasive Cancer
Surgical excision or radiation therapy or both

---

*Those with a history of multiple sexual partners or sexual partners with HIV infection.
[†]Studies evaluating the use of anal Pap smears are currently underway.

SUMMARY

Patients with HIV infection, like immunosuppressed transplant recipients, are at high risk for the development of both KS and B-cell NHL. Although other malignancies may occur in the HIV-infected patient, epidemiologic evidence does not suggest a causal relationship between the underlying immunodeficiency state and the subsequent development of malignancy. Whether causally related or not, however, any malignancy occurring in a patient with HIV infection is likely to have a more aggressive course and to be associated with short survival time.

KS is the most common malignancy seen in HIV-infected patients. The etiology of KS is uncertain, as are the reasons for its nearly exclusive confinement to the homosexual male population with HIV infection. Prognosis is related to the extent of the disease, immune function, and the presence of systemic and local symptoms. A variety of local and systemic therapeutic modalities are available, including radiation therapy, cryotherapy, chemotherapy, and α-interferon. Which treatment approach is most appropriate for an individual depends on the extent of disease; the presence of local symptoms, including pain or edema; and the presence of cosmetically unsightly disease. HAART is an important component of KS therapy which may induce antitumor response and prolong chemotherapy-induced responses.

Patients with B-cell lymphoma tend to present with advanced extranodal disease, and primary lymphoma of the CNS frequently has been reported as well. Not unlike B-cell lymphoma seen in allograft recipients, lymphoma in the presence of HIV infection appears to arise out of a background of polyclonal B-cell activation. Although a viral cause has been suspected, the cause of lymphoma in these patients remains unknown. Response to therapy in these patients has been disappointing. Response rates to chemotherapy have been lower than those observed in other lymphoma patients, and treatment has been complicated by lack of adequate bone marrow reserve and by the occurrence of frequent opportunistic infections. Although overall survival times have been short, factors predictive of improved survival time include better immune function, absence of a prior AIDS diagnosis, good performance score, and absence of an extranodal site of disease. Experience suggests that, in some patients, more aggressive chemotherapy may be associated with shortened survival time. Recent clinical trials have demonstrated that reduced-dosage chemotherapy may be associated with clinical outcome that is comparable to that associated with the use of standard-dose therapy in a majority of individuals. Determining which of these treatment approaches will be of the greatest benefit with respect to response and survival time must await the results of ongoing clinical trials.

Cervical and anal neoplasia related to HPV infection also can occur as a consequence of HIV-induced immunodeficiency. Longstanding, profound immunodeficiency increases the risk of developing HPV-related anogenital neoplasia, as has been described in transplant recipients requiring prolonged immunosuppression. As the survival time of patients with HIV infection is extended through the use of more effective antiretroviral, prophylactic, and antimicrobial therapies, the resulting state of profound, prolonged immunodeficiency will provide the necessary milieu for the emergence of anogenital neoplasia.

Treatment of the patient with an HIV-associated malignancy imposes obstacles and challenges that are unique in medicine. For this reason, it is especially important that treatment be individualized carefully, with the patient playing an important role in determining which therapeutic alternative is most appropriate.

References

1. Frizzera G, Rosai J, Dehner LP, et al: Lymphoreticular disorders in primary immunodeficiencies: New findings based on an up-to-date histologic classification of 35 cases. Cancer 46:692, 1980
2. Harwood AR, Osoba D, Hofstader SL, et al: Kaposi's sarcoma in recipients of renal transplants. Am J Med 67:759, 1979
3. Hoover R, Fraumeni JF: Risk of cancer in renal transplant recipients. Lancet 2:55, 1973
4. Harnly ME, Swan SH, Holly EA, et al: Temporal trends in the incidence of non-Hodgkin's lymphoma and selected malignancies in a population with a high incidence of acquired immunodeficiency syndrome (AIDS). Am J Epidemiol 128:261, 1988
5. Ateenyi-Agaba C: Conjunctival squamous-cell carcinoma associated with HIV infection in Kampala, Uganda. Lancet 341:695, 1995
6. Herndier BG, Shiramizu BT, Jewett NE, et al: Acquired immunodeficiency syndrome-associated T-cell lymphoma: Evidence for human immunodeficiency virus type 1-associated T-cell transformation. Blood 79:1768, 1992
7. Biggar RJ, Rabkin CS: The epidemiology of AIDS-related neoplasms. Hematol Oncol Clin North Am 10:997, 1996
8. Lyter DW, Bryant J, Thackeray R, et al: Incidence of human immunodeficiency virus-related and non-related malignancies in a large cohort of homosexual men. J Clin Oncol 13:2540, 1995
9. Biggar RJ: Epidemiologic clues to the etiology of cancer in AIDS. In Abstracts of the 2nd National AIDS Malignancy Conference, Bethesda, MD, 1998, Abstract S2
10. Centers for Disease Control: Revision of the case definition of acquired immunodeficiency syndrome for national reporting—United States. MMWR Morb Mortal Wkly Rep 34:373, 1985
11. Chiasson MA, Kelley K, Vazquez F, et al: Increased incidence of invasive cervical cancer (ICC) in HIV+ women in New York City. In Abstracts of the 2nd National AIDS Malignancy Conference, Bethesda, MD, 1998, Abstract 4
12. Vadhan-Raj S, Wong G, Gnecco C, et al: Immunological variables as predictors of prognosis in patients with Kaposi's sarcoma and the acquired immunodeficiency syndrome. Cancer 46:417, 1986
13. Mandelblatt JS, Fahs M, Garibaldi K, et al: Association between HIV infection and cervical neoplasia: Implications for clinical care of women at risk for both conditions. AIDS 6:173, 1992
14. Sillman FH, Sedlis A: Anogenital papillomavirus infection and neoplasia in immunodeficient women. Obstet Gynecol Clin North Am 14:537, 1987
15. Frager DH, Wolf EL, Competiello LS, et al: Squamous cell carcinoma of the esophagus in patients with acquired immunodeficiency syndrome. Gastrointest Radiol 13:358, 1988
16. Ravalli S, Chabon AB, Khan AA: Gastrointestinal neoplasia in young HIV-positive patients. Am J Clin Pathol 91:458, 1989
17. Tirelli U, Vaccher E, Sinicco A, et al: Forty-nine unusual HIV-related malignant tumors. In Abstracts of the Vth International Conference on AIDS, Montreal, 1989, Abstract W.C.P.50
18. Karp J, Profeta G, Marantz PR, Karpel JP: Lung cancer in patients with immunodeficiency syndrome. Chest 103:401, 1993
19. Bernardi D, Salvioni R, Vaccher E, et al: Testicular germ cell tumors and HIV infection: A report of 26 cases. J Clin Oncol 13:2705, 1995
20. Timmerman JM, Northfelt DW, Small EJ: Malignant germ cell tumors in men infected with the human immunodeficiency virus: Natural history and results of therapy. J Clin Oncol 13:1391, 1995
21. Mitsuyasu RT, Groopman JE: Biology and therapy of Kaposi's sarcoma. Semin Oncol 11:53, 1984
22. Safai B: Pathophysiology and epidemiology of epidemic Kaposi's sarcoma. Semin Oncol 2(Suppl 3):7, 1987
23. Des Jarlais DC, Stoneburner R, Thomas P: Declines in proportion of Kaposi's sarcoma among cases of AIDS in multiple risk groups in New York City. Lancet 2:1024, 1987
24. Rutherford GW, Schwarcz SK, Lemp GF, et al: The epidemiology of AIDS-related Kaposi's sarcoma in San Francisco. J Infect Dis 159:569, 1989
25. Selik RM, Chu SY, Ward JW: Trends in infectious disease and cancers among persons dying of HIV infection in the United States from 1987 to 1992. Ann Intern Med 123:933, 1995
26. Jacobson LP: Impact of highly effective antiretroviral therapy on the incidence of malignancies among HIV-infected individuals. In Abstracts of the 2nd National AIDS Malignancy Conference, Bethesda, MD, Abstract S5
27. Buchbinder SP, Vittinghoff E, Colfax G, Holmberg S: Declines in AIDS incidence associated with highly active antiretroviral therapy (HAART) are not

reflected in KS and lymphoma incidence. In Abstracts of the 2nd National AIDS Malignancy Conference, Bethesda, MD, 1998, Abstract S7

28. Jones JL, Hanson DL, Ward JW: Effect of antiretroviral therapy on recent trends in cancer among HIV-infected persons. In Abstracts of the 2nd National AIDS Malignancy Conference, Bethesda, MD, 1998, Abstract S3

29. Drew WL, Mills J, Hauer LB, et al: Declining prevalence of Kaposi's sarcoma in homosexual AIDS patients paralleled by fall in cytomegalovirus transmission. Lancet 1:66, 1988

30. Beral V, Peterman TA, Berkelman RL, et al: Kaposi's sarcoma among persons with AIDS: A sexually transmitted infection? Lancet 1:123, 1990

31. Chang Y, Cesarman E, Pessin MS, et al: Identification of herpesvirus-like DNA sequences in AIDS-associated Kaposi's sarcoma. Science 266:1865, 1995

32. Moore PS, Chang Y: Detection of herpesvirus-like DNA sequences in Kaposi's sarcoma in patients with and without HIV infection. N Engl J Med 332:1181, 1995

33. Huang YQ, Li JJ, Kaplan MH, et al: Human herpesvirus-like nucleic acid in various forms of Kaposi's sarcoma [see comments]. Lancet 345:759, 1995

34. Zhong W, Wang H, Herndier B, Ganem D: Restricted expression of Kaposi's sarcoma-associated herpesvirus (human herpesvirus 8) genes in Kaposi's sarcoma. Proc Natl Acad Sci USA 93:6641, 1996

35. Nicholas J, Ruvolo V, Zong J, et al: A single 13-kilobase divergent locus in the Kaposi's sarcoma-associated herpesvirus (human herpesvirus 80 genome contains nine open reading frames that are homologous to or related to cellular proteins. J Virol 71:1963, 1997

36. Cesarman E, Nador RG, Bai F, et al: Kaposi's sarcoma-associated herpesvirus contains G protein-coupled receptor and cyclin D homologs which are expressed in Kaposi's sarcoma and malignant lymphoma. J Virol 70:8218, 1996

37. Godden-Kent D, Talbot SJ, Boshoff C, et al: The cyclin encoded by Kaposi's sarcoma-associated herpesvirus stimulates cdk6 to phosphorylate the retinoblastoma protein and histone H1. J Virol 71:4193, 1997

38. Bais C, Santomasso B, Coso O, et al: G-protein-coupled receptor of Kaposi's sarcoma-associated herpesvirus is a vital oncogene and angiogenesis activator. Nature 391:86, 1998

39. Ensoli B, Gendelman R, Markham P, et al: Synergy between basic fibroblast growth factor and HIV-1 Tat protein in induction of Kaposi's sarcoma. Nature 371:674, 1994

40. Barillari G, Gendelman R, Gallo RC, Ensoli B: The Tat protein of human immunodeficiency virus type 1, a growth factor for AIDS Kaposi's sarcoma and cytokine-activated vascular cells, induces adhesion of the same cell types by using integrin receptors recognizing the RGD amino acid sequence. Proc Natl Acad Sci U S A 90:7941, 1993

41. Albini A, Barillari G, Benelli R, et al: Angiogenic properties of human immunodeficiency virus type 1 Tat protein. Proc Natl Acad Sci U S A 92:4838, 1995

42. Samaniego F, Markham PD, Gallo RC, Ensoli B: Inflammatory cytokines induce AIDS-Kaposi's sarcoma-derived spindle cells to produce and release basic fibroblast growth factor and enhance Kaposi's sarcoma-like lesion formation in nude mice. J Immunol 154:3582, 1995

43. Gill PS, Naidu Y, Nakamura S, et al: IL-6 regulation by steroid hormones and autocrine activity in Kaposi's sarcoma. AIDS Res Hum Retroviruses 7:220, 1991

44. Ziegler J, Katongole-Mbidde E, Wabinga H, Dollbaum CM: Absence of sex-hormone receptors in Kaposi's sarcoma. N Engl J Med 345:925, 1995

45. Lunardi-Iskandar Y, Bryant JL, Zeman RA, et al: Tumorigenesis and metastasis of neoplastic Kaposi's sarcoma cell line in immunodeficient mice blocked by a human pregnancy hormone. Nature 375:64, 1995

46. Friedman SL, Wright TL, Altman DF: Gastrointestinal Kaposi's sarcoma in patients with acquired immunodeficiency syndrome: Endoscopic and autopsy findings. Gastroenterology 89:102, 1985

47. Friedman SL: Gastrointestinal and hepatobiliary neoplasms in AIDS. Gastroenterol Clin North Am 17: 465, 1988

48. Kaplan LD, Hopewell PC, Jaffe H, et al: Kaposi's sarcoma involving the lung in patients with the acquired immunodeficiency syndrome. J Acquir Immune Defic Syndr 1:23, 1988

49. Ognibene FP, Steis RG, Macher AM, et al: Kaposi's sarcoma causing pulmonary infiltrates and respiratory failure in the acquired immunodeficiency syndrome. Ann Intern Med 102:471, 1985

50. Gill PS, Akil B, Colletti P, et al: Pulmonary Kaposi's sarcoma: Clinical findings and results of therapy. Am J Med 87:57, 1989

51. Hanto DW, Frizzera G, Purtilo, et al: Clinical spectrum of lymphoproliferative disorders in renal transplant recipients and evidence for the role of Epstein-Barr virus. Cancer Res 41:4253, 1981

52. Davis SD, Henschke CI, Chamides BK, Westcott JL: Intrathoracic Kaposi sarcoma in AIDS patients: Radiographic-pathologic correlation. Radiology 163: 495, 1987

53. Northfelt DW, Martin FJ, Kaplan LD, et al: Pharmacokinetics (PK), tumor localization (TL), and safety of doxil (liposomal doxorubicin) in AIDS patients with Kaposi's sarcoma (AIDS-KS) [abstract 8]. Proc Am Soc Clin Oncol 12:51, 1993

54. Taylor J, Afrasiabi R, Fahey JL, et al: Prognostically significant classification of immune changes in AIDS with Kaposi's sarcoma. Blood 67:666, 1986

55. Mitsuyasu R, Taylor J, Glaspy A, et al: Heterogeneity of epidemic Kaposi's sarcoma: Implications for therapy. Cancer 57:1657, 1986

56. Myskowski PL, Niedzweicki D, Shurgot BA, et al: AIDS-associated Kaposi's sarcoma: Variable associated with increased survival. J Am Acad Dermatol 18:1299, 1988

57. Krown SE, Metroka C, Wernz JC: Kaposi's sarcoma in the acquired immunodeficiency syndrome: A proposal for uniform evaluation, response, and staging criteria. J Clin Oncol 7:1201, 1989

57a. Krown SE, Testa M, Huang J: Validation of the AIDS clinical trials group (ACTG) staging classification for AIDS-associated Kaposi's sarcoma (AIDS/KS) [abstract 844]. Proc Am Soc Clin Oncol 15:303, 1996

58. Bernstein ZP, Wilson D, Summers K, et al: Pilot/Phase I study—photodynamic therapy (PDT) for treatment of AIDS-associated Kaposi's sarcoma (AIDS/KS). Proc Am Soc Clin Oncol 14:289, 1995

59. Volberding PA, Kusick P, Feigal D: Effects of chemotherapy for HIV-associated Kaposi's sarcoma on long-term survival [abstract 11]. Proc Am Soc Clin Oncol 8:3, 1989

60. Chak LY, Gill PS, Levine AM, et al: Radiation therapy for AIDS-related Kaposi's sarcoma. J Clin Oncol 6:863, 1988

61. Hill DR: The role of radiotherapy for epidemic Kaposi's sarcoma. Semin Oncol 14(Suppl 3):1207, 1987

62. Newman SB: Treatment of epidemic Kaposi's sarcoma (KS) with intralesional vinblastine injection (IL-VLB) [abstract 19]. Proc Am Soc Clin Oncol 7: 5, 1988

63. Tappero JW, Berger TG, Kaplan LD, et al: Cryotherapy for cutaneous Kaposi's sarcoma (KS) associated with acquired immune deficiency syndrome (AIDS): A phase II trial. J Acquir Immune Defic Syndr 4:839, 1991

64. Kristal AR, Nasca PC, Burnett WS, Mikl J: Changes in the epidemiology of non-Hodgkin's lymphoma associated with epidemic human immunodeficiency virus (HIV) infection. Am J Epidemiol 128:711, 1988

65. Volberding PA, Abrams DI, Conant M, et al: Vinblastine therapy for Kaposi's sarcoma in the acquired immunodeficiency syndrome. Ann Intern Med 103: 335, 1985

66. Laubenstein LJ, Krigel RL, Odajnyk CM, et al: Treatment of epidemic Kaposi's sarcoma with etoposide or a combination of doxorubicin, bleomycin and vinblastine. J Clin Oncol 2:1115, 1984

67. Gill PS, Krailo M, Slater L, et al: Randomized trial of ABV (Adriamycin, bleomycin and vinblastine) vs A (Adriamycin) in advanced Kaposi's sarcoma (KS) [abstract 11]. Proc Am Soc Clin Oncol 7:3, 1988

68. Harrison M, Tomlinson D, Stewart S: Liposomal-entrapped doxorubicin: An active agent in AIDS-related Kaposi's sarcoma. J Clin Oncol 13:914, 1995

69. Presant CA, Scolaro M, Kennedy P, et al: Liposomal daunorubicin treatment of HIV-associated Kaposi's sarcoma. Lancet 341:1242, 1993

70. Sharma D, Muggia F, Lucci L, et al: Liposomal daunorubicin (VS103): Tolerance and clinical effects in AIDS-related Kaposi's sarcoma (KS) during a phase I study [abstract 9]. Proc Am Soc Clin Oncol 9:4, 1990

71. Gill PS, Hadienberg J, Espina BM, et al: Low dose paclitaxel (taxol) every two weeks over 3 hours is safe and effective in the treatment of advanced AIDS-related Kaposi's sarcoma. In Abstracts of the 39th Annual Meeting of the American Society of Hematology, Seattle, 1995, Abstract 1516

72. Errante D, Spina M, Tavio M, et al: Evidence of activity of vinorelbine (VNR) in patients (pts) with previously treated endemic Kaposi's sarcoma (KS). Proc Am Soc Clin Oncol 16:1997, Abstract 146

73. Goebel FD, Bogner JR, Spathling S, et al: Efficacy and toxicity of liposomal doxorubicin in advanced AIDS-related Kaposi's sarcoma (KS): An open study [abstract WSB15-6]. In Abstracts of the IXth International Conference on AIDS, Berlin, 1993, p 120

74. Northfelt DW, Dezube BJ, Thommes JA, et al: Pegylated-liposomal doxorubicin versus doxorubicin, bleomycin, and vincristine in the treatment of AIDS-related Kaposi's sarcoma: Results of a randomized phase III clinical trial. J Clin Oncol 16: 2445, 1998

75. Mitsuyasu R, von Roenn J, Krown S, et al: Comparison study of liposomal doxorubicin (DOX) alone or with bleomycin and vincristine (DVB) for treatment of advanced AIDS-associated Kaposi's sarcoma (AIDS-KS): AIDS Clinical Trial Group (ACTG) protocol 286 [abstract 191]. Proc Am Soc Clin Oncol 16:55a, 1997

76. Gill PS, Wernz J, Scadden DT, et al: Randomized Phase III trial of liposomal daunorubicin versus doxorubicin, bleomycin, and vincristine in AIDS-related Kaposi's sarcoma. J Clin Oncol 14:2353, 1996

77. Saville MW, Lietzau J, Pluda JM, et al: Activity of paclitaxel (taxol) as therapy for HIV-associated Kaposi's sarcoma. Lancet 346:26, 1995

78. Gill PS, Rarick MU, Espina B, et al: Advanced acquired immune deficiency syndrome-related Kaposi's sarcoma: Results of pilot studies using combination chemotherapy. Cancer 65:1074, 1990

79. Glaspy J, Miles S, McCarthy S: Treatment of advanced stage Kaposi's sarcoma with vincristine and bleomycin [abstract 10]. Proc Am Soc Clin Oncol 5: 3, 1986

80. Mintzer DM, Real FX, Jovino L, Krown SE: Treatment of Kaposi's sarcoma and thrombocytopenia with vincristine in patients with the acquired immunodeficiency syndrome. Ann Intern Med 102:200, 1985

81. Krown SE: The role of interferon in the therapy of epidemic Kaposi's sarcoma. Semin Oncol 14(Suppl 3):27, 1987

82. Kovacs JA, Lance HC, Masur H, et al: A Phase III, placebo-controlled trial of recombinant alpha interferon in asymptomatic individuals seropositive for the acquired immunodeficiency syndrome. Clin Res 35:479A, 1987

83. Lane HC, Feinberg J, Davery V, et al: Anti-retroviral effects of interferon-alpha in AIDS-associated Kaposi's sarcoma. Lancet 2:1218, 1988

84. deWit R, Schatenkerk JKME, Boucher CAB, et al: Clinical and virological effects of high-dose recombinant interferon-α in disseminated AIDS-related Kaposi's sarcoma. Lancet 2:1214, 1988

85. Groopman JE, Gottlieb MS, Goodman J, et al: Recombinant alpha-2 interferon therapy for Kaposi's sarcoma associated with the acquired immunodeficiency syndrome. Ann Intern Med 100:671, 1984

86. Real FX, Oettgen HF, Krown SE: Kaposi's sarcoma and the acquired immunodeficiency syndrome: Treatment with high and low doses of leukocyte A interferon. J Clin Oncol 4:544, 1986

87. Rios A, Mansell PWA, Newell GR, et al: Treatment of acquired immunodeficiency syndrome-related Kaposi's sarcoma with lymphoblastoid interferon. J Clin Oncol 3:506, 1985

88. Volberding PA, Mitsuyasu R: Recombinant interferon alpha in the treatment of acquired immune deficiency syndrome-related Kaposi's sarcoma. Semin Oncol 2(Suppl 5):2, 1985

89. Volberding PA, Mitsuyasu RT, Golando JP, et al: Treatment of Kaposi's sarcoma with interferon alfa-2 (Intron A). Cancer 59:620, 1987

90. Vaccher E, Tirelli U, Spina M, et al: Age and serum lactate dehydrogenase level are independent prognostic factors in human immunodeficiency virus-related non-Hodgkin's lymphomas: A single-institute study of 96 patients. J Clin Oncol 14:2217, 1996

91. Hartshorn KL, Vogt MW, Chou TC, et al: Synergistic inhibition of human immunodeficiency virus in vitro by azidothymidine and recombinant interferon alpha-A. Antimicrob Agents Chemother 31:168, 1987

92. Lane HC, Falloon J, Walker RE, et al: Zidovudine in patients with human immunodeficiency virus (HIV) infection and Kaposi's sarcoma. Ann Intern Med 111:41, 1989

93. Krown SE, Gold JWM, Niedzwiecki D, et al: Interferon-α with zidovudine: Safety, tolerance, and clin-

ical and virologic effects in patients with Kaposi sarcoma associated with the acquired immunodeficiency syndrome (AIDS). Ann Intern Med 112:812, 1990

94. Fischl MA, Uttamchandani R, Resnick L, et al: A Phase I study of recombinant human interferon alfa-2 or human lymphoblastoid interferon alfa-n1 and concomitant zidovudine in patients with AIDS-related Kaposi's sarcoma. J Acquir Immune Defic Syndr 4:4, 1991

95. Kovacs JA, Deyton L, Davey R, et al: Combined zidovudine and interferon-α therapy in patients with Kaposi's sarcoma and the acquired immunodeficiency syndrome (AIDS). Ann Intern Med 111:280, 1989

96. Krown SE, Paredes J, Bundow D, et al: Interferon-α, zidovudine, and granulocyte-macrophage colony-stimulating factor: A Phase I AIDS clinical trials group study in patients with Kaposi's sarcoma associated with AIDS. J Clin Oncol 10:1344, 1992

97. Scadden DT, Bering HA, Levine JD, et al: Granulocyte-macrophage colony-stimulating factor mitigates the neutropenia of combined interferon alpha and zidovudine treatment of acquired immune deficiency syndrome-associated Kaposi's sarcoma. J Clin Oncol 9:802, 1991

98. Shepherd F, Beaulieu R, Murphy K, et al: A randomized trial of 2 doses of alpha interferon (IFN) added to AZT for the treatment of epidemic Kaposi's sarcoma (KS). Proc Am Soc Clin Oncol 13:50, 1994

99. Workman C, Lewis C, Smith DO: Resolution of Kaposi's sarcoma associated with saquinavir therapy—case report. In Abstracts of the International Conference on AIDS, 1996, Abstract Tu.B.2217

100. Henry K, Worley J, Sullivan C, et al: Documented improvement in late stage manifestations of AIDS after starting ritonavir in combination with two reverse transcriptase inhibitors. In Abstracts of the 4th Conference of Retroviruses and Opportunistic Infections, Washington, DC, 1997, Abstract 356

101. Aboulafa DM: Regression of acquired immunodeficiency syndrome-related pulmonary Kaposi's sarcoma after highly active antiretroviral therapy. Mayo Clinic Proc 73:439, 1998

102. Wit FW, Sol CJ, Renwick N, et al: Regression of AIDS-related Kaposi's sarcoma associated with clearance of human herpesvirus-8 from peripheral blood mononuclear cells following initiation of antiretroviral therapy [letter]. AIDS 12:218, 1998

103. Parra R, Leal M, Delgado J, et al: Regression of invasive AIDS-related Kaposi's sarcoma following antiretroviral therapy. Clin Infect Dis 26:218, 1998

104. Volm MD, Wernz J: Patients with advanced AIDS-related Kaposi's sarcoma (EKS) no longer require systemic therapy after introduction of effective antiretroviral therapy [abstract 162]. Proc Am Soc Clin Oncol 16:46a, 1997

105. National Cancer Institute: NCI-sponsored study of classifications of non-Hodgkin's lymphoma: Summary and description of a working formulation for clinical usage. The Non-Hodgkin's Lymphoma Pathologic Classification Project. Cancer 49:2112, 1982

106. Ziegler JL, Drew WL, Miner RC, et al: Outbreak of Burkitt's-like lymphoma in homosexual men. Lancet 2:631, 1982

107. Penn I: Lymphomas complicating organ transplantation. Transplant Proc 15(Suppl 1):2790, 1983

108. Penn I: The incidence of malignancies in transplant recipients. Transplant Proc 7:323, 1975

109. Shearer WT, Ritz J, Finego MJ, et al: Epstein-Barr virus-associated B-cell proliferations of diverse clonal origins after bone marrow transplantation in a 12-year-old patient with severe combined immunodeficiency. N Engl J Med 312:1151, 1985

110. Frizzera G, Hanto DW, Gajl Peczalkska K, et al: Polymorphic diffuse B-cell hyperplasias and lymphomas in renal transplant recipients. Cancer Res 41:4262, 1981

111. Hanto DW, Gajl-Peczalkska KJ, Frizzera G, et al: Epstein-Barr virus-induced polyclonal and monoclonal B-cell lymphoproliferative disease occurring after renal transplantation. Ann Surg 198:356, 1983

112. Hanto DW, Frizzera G, Gajl-Peczalkska K, et al: Epstein-Barr virus induced B-cell lymphoma after renal transplantation. N Engl J Med 306:913, 1982

113. Bernheim A, Berger R: Cytogenetic studies of Burkitt lymphoma-leukemia in patients with acquired immunodeficiency syndrome. Cancer Genet Cytogenet 32:67, 1988

114. Chaganti R, Jhanwar S, Koziner B, et al: Specific translocations characterize Burkitt's-like lymphoma of homosexual men with the acquired immunodeficiency syndrome. Blood 61:1269, 1983

115. Groopman J, Sullivan J, Mulder C, et al: Pathogenesis of B-cell lymphoma in a patient with AIDS. Blood 67:612, 1986

116. Petersen JM, Tubbs RR, Savage RA, et al: Small non-cleaved B-cell Burkitt-like lymphoma with chromosome t(8;14) translocation and Epstein-Barr virus nuclear-associated antigen in a homosexual man with acquired immune deficiency syndrome. Am J Med 78:141, 1985

117. Kaplan LD, Abrams DI, Feigal E, et al: AIDS-associated non-Hodgkin's lymphoma in San Francisco. JAMA 261:719, 1989

118. Meeker TC, Shiramizu B, Kaplan L, et al: Evidence for molecular subtypes of HIV-associated lymphoma: Division into peripheral monoclonal, polyclonal and central nervous system lymphoma. AIDS 5:669, 1991

119. Shiramizu B, Herndier B, Meeker T, et al: Molecular and immunophenotypic characterization of AIDS-associated EBV-negative polyclonal lymphoma. J Clin Oncol 10:383, 1992

120. Subar M, Neri A, Inghirami G, et al: Frequent c-myc oncogene activation and infrequent presence of Epstein-Barr virus genome in AIDS-associated lymphoma. Blood 72:667, 1988

121. MacMahon EME, Glass JD, Hayward SD, et al: Epstein-Barr virus in AIDS-related primary central nervous system lymphoma. Lancet 338:969, 1991

122. Shiramizu B, Herndier BG, McGrath MS: Identification of a common clonal human immunodeficiency virus integration site in human immunodeficiency virus-associated lymphomas. Cancer Res 54:2069, 1994

123. Nador RG, Cesarman E, Knowles DM, Said JW: Herpes-like DNA sequences in a body-cavity-based lymphoma in an HIV-negative patient. N Engl J Med 333:943, 1995

124. Delecluse HJ, Raphael M, Magaud JP, Felman P: Variable morphology of human immunodeficiency virus-associated lymphomas with c-myc rearrangements. Blood 82:552, 1993

125. Strigle SM, Martin SE, Levine AM, Rarick MU: The use of fine needle aspiration cytology in the management of human immunodeficiency virus-related non-Hodgkin's lymphoma and Hodgkin's disease. J Acquir Immune Defic Syndr 6:1329, 1993

126. Emilie D, Coumbaras J, Raphael M, et al: Interleukin 6 production in high-grade B lymphomas: Correlation with the presence of malignant immunoblasts in acquired immunodeficiency syndrome and in human immunodeficiency virus-seronegative patients. Blood 80:498, 1992

127. Herndier BG, Kaplan LD, McGrath MS: Pathogenesis of AIDS lymphoma. AIDS 8:1025, 1994

128. Pluda JM, Venzon DJ, Tosato G, et al: Parameters affecting the development of non-Hodgkin's lymphoma in patients with severe human immunodeficiency virus infection receiving antiretroviral therapy. J Clin Oncol 11:1099, 1993

129. Kaplan L, Straus D, Testa M, et al: Low-dose compared with standard-dose mBACOD chemotherapy for non-Hodgkin's lymphoma associated with human immunodeficiency virus infection. N Engl J Med 336:1641, 1997

130. Levine AM, Sullivan-Halley J, Pike MC, et al: Human immunodeficiency virus-related lymphoma: Prognostic factors predictive of survival. Cancer 68:2466, 1991

131. Levine A, Meyer P, Begandy M, et al: Development of B-cell lymphoma in homosexual men. Ann Intern Med 100:7, 1984

132. Ziegler J, Beckstead J, Volberding P, et al: Non-Hodgkin's lymphoma in 90 homosexual men: Relation to generalized lymphadenopathy and the acquired immunodeficiency syndrome. N Engl J Med 311:565, 1984

133. Nasr S, Brynes R, Garrison C, Chan W: Peripheral T-cell lymphoma in a patient with acquired immunodeficiency syndrome. Cancer 61:947, 1988

134. Presant CA, Gala K, Wiseman C, et al: Human immunodeficiency virus-associated T-cell lymphoblastic lymphoma in AIDS. Cancer 60:1459, 1987

135. Knowles DM, Inghirami G, Ubraico A, Dalla-Favera R: Molecular genetic analysis of three AIDS-associated neoplasms of uncertain lineage demonstrates their B-cell derivation and the possible pathogenic role of Epstein-Barr virus. Blood 73:792, 1989

136. Bermudez M, Grant K, Rodvien R, Mendes F: Non-Hodgkin's lymphoma in a population with or at risk for acquired immunodeficiency syndrome: Indications for intensive chemotherapy. Am J Med 86:71, 1989

137. Gill P, Levine A, Krailo M, et al: AIDS-related malignant lymphoma: Results of prospective treatment trials. J Clin Oncol 5:1322, 1987

138. Knowles DM, Chamulak G, Subar M, et al: Lymphoid neoplasia associated with the acquired immunodeficiency syndrome (AIDS). Ann Intern Med 108:744, 1988

139. Lowenthal D, Straus D, Campbell S, et al: AIDS-related lymphoid neoplasia: The Memorial Hospital Experience. Cancer 61:2325, 1988

140. Burkes RL, Meyer PR, Gill PS, et al: Rectal lymphoma in homosexual men. Arch Intern Med 146:913, 1986

141. Balasubramanyam A, Waxman M, Kazal HL, Lee MH: Malignant lymphoma of the heart in acquired immunodeficiency syndrome. Chest 90:243, 1986

142. Guarner J, Brynes RK, Chan WC, et al: Primary non-Hodgkin's lymphoma of the heart in two patients with the acquired immunodeficiency syndrome. Arch Pathol Lab Med 111:254, 1987

143. Kaplan L, Kahn J, Jacobson M, et al: Primary bile duct lymphoma in the acquired immunodeficiency syndrome (AIDS). Ann Intern Med 110:162, 1989

144. Daling JR, Weiss NS, Klopfenstein LL, et al: Correlates of homosexual behavior and the incidence of anal cancer. JAMA 247:1988, 1982

145. Baumgartner J, Rachlin J, Beckstead J, et al: Primary central nervous system lymphomas: Natural history and response to radiation therapy in 55 patients with acquired immunodeficiency syndrome. J Neurosurg 73:206, 1990

146. Formenti SC, Gill PS, Rarick M, et al: Primary central nervous system lymphoma in AIDS: Results of radiation therapy. Cancer 63:1101, 1989

147. Gill PS, Levine A, Meyer P, et al: Primary central nervous system lymphoma in homosexual men. Am J Med 78:742, 1985

148. So YT, Beckstead J, Davis R: Primary central nervous system lymphoma in acquired immunodeficiency syndrome: A clinical and pathological study. Ann Neurol 20:566, 1986

149. Ciricillo S, Rosenblum M: Use of CT and MR imaging to distinguish intracranial lesions and to define the need for biopsy in AIDS patients. J Neurosurg 73:720, 1990

150. Grant I, Gold J, Armstrong D: Risk of CNS toxoplasmosis in patients with acquired immunodeficiency syndrome [abstract 441]. In Abstracts of the Interscience Conference on Antimicrobial Agents and Chemotherapy New Orleans, 1986, p 177

151. Porter SB, Sande MA: Toxoplasmosis of the central nervous system in the acquired immunodeficiency syndrome. N Engl J Med 327:1643, 1992

152. Ruiz A, Ganz WI, Post MJ, et al: Use of thallium-201 brain SPECT to differentiate cerebral lymphoma from toxoplasma encephalitis in AIDS patients. Am J Neuroradiol 15:1885, 1994

153. Barker DE, Trepashko D, DeMarais P, et al: Utility of thallium brain SPECT in the exclusion of CNS lymphoma in AIDS [abstract 708]. In Abstracts of the 4th Conference on Retroviruses and Opportunistic Infections, Washington, DC, 1997, p 195

154. De Luca A, Antinori A, Cingolani A, et al: Evaluation of cerebrospinal fluid EBV-DNA and IL-10 as markers for *in vivo* diagnosis of AIDS-related primary central nervous system lymphoma. Br J Haematol 90:844, 1995

155. Cinque P, Brytting M, Vago L, et al: Epstein-Barr virus DNA in cerebrospinal fluid from patients with AIDS-related primary lymphoma of the central nervous system. Lancet 342:398, 1993

156. DeVita VT, Hubbard SM, Young RC, Longo DL: The role of chemotherapy in diffuse aggressive lymphoma. Semin Hematol 25(Suppl 2):2, 1988

157. Connors JM, Klimo P: MACOP-B chemotherapy for malignant lymphomas and related conditions: 1987 update and additional observations. Semin Hematol 25(Suppl 2):41, 1988

158. Kiviat N, Rompalo A, Bowden R, et al: Anal human papillomavirus infection among human immunodeficiency virus-seropositive and seronegative men. J Infect Dis 162:358, 1990

159. Gal AA, Meyer PR, Taylor CR: Papillomavirus antigens in anorectal condyloma and carcinoma in homosexual men. JAMA 257:337, 1987

160. Lorenz HP, Wilson W, Leigh B, et al: Squamous cell carcinoma of the anus and HIV infection. Dis Colon Rectum 34:336, 1991

161. Gisselbrecht C, Oksenhendler E, Tirelli U, et al: High-dose chemotherapy (LNH84) for HIV-associated non-Hodgkin's lymphoma. Am J Med 95:188, 1993

162. Italian Cooperative Group for AIDS-Related Tumors: Malignant lymphomas in patients with or at risk for AIDS in Italy: Reports. J Natl Cancer Inst 80:855, 1988

163. The International Non-Hodgkin's Lymphoma Prognostic Factors Project: A predictive model for aggressive non-Hodgkin's lymphoma. N Engl J Med 329:987, 1993

163a. Vaccher E, Tirelli V, Spina M, et al: Age and serum lactate dehydrogenase level are independent prognostic factors in human immunodeficiency virus-related non-Hodgkin's lymphoma: single institute study of 96 patients. J Clin Oncol 14:2217, 1996

164. Tirelli U, Errante D, Oksenhendler E, et al, for the French-Italian Cooperative Study Group: Prospective study with combined low-dose chemotherapy and zidovudine in 37 patients with poor-prognosis AIDS-related non-Hodgkin's lymphoma. Ann Oncol 3:843, 1992

165. Kaplan LD, Kahn JO, Crowe S, et al: Clinical and virologic effects of recombinant human granulocyte-macrophage colony-stimulating factor in patients receiving chemotherapy for human immunodeficiency virus-associated non-Hodgkin's lymphoma: Results of a randomized trial. J Clin Oncol 9:929, 1991

166. Sparano JA, Wiernik PH, Xiaoping H, et al: Pilot trial of infusional cyclophosphamide, doxorubicin, and etoposide plus didanosine and filgrastim in patients with human immunodeficiency virus-associated non-Hodgkin's lymphoma. J Clin Oncol 14:3026, 1996

167. Rubio R, Rubio M, Grauss F, et al: Primary central nervous system lymphoma (PCNSL) in AIDS: A multicentric clinical study. In Abstracts of the XIth International Conference on AIDS, Vancouver, 1996, p 291

168. Levine AM, Wernz JC, Kaplan L, et al: Low-dose chemotherapy with central nervous system prophylaxis and zidovudine maintenance in AIDS-related lymphoma. JAMA 266:84, 1991

169. Nisce L, Kaufmann T, Metroka C: Radiation therapy in patients with AIDS-related central nervous system lymphomas. JAMA 267:1921, 1992

170. Lee J, Kaplan LD, Conant M, Northfelt DW: Natural history, treatment outcome and causes of death in AIDS-related primary central nervous system lymphoma (PCNSL) [abstract 18]. Proc Am Soc Clin Oncol 13:54, 1994

171. Ling SM, Roach IM, Larson DA, Wara WM: Radiotherapy of primary central nervous system lymphoma in patients with and without human immunodeficiency virus: Ten years of treatment experience at the University of California, San Francisco. Cancer 73:2570, 1994

172. Forsyth PA, Yahalom J, DeAngelis LM: Combined-modality therapy in the treatment of primary central nervous system lymphoma in AIDS. Neurology 44:1473, 1994

173. Chamberlain MC: Long survival in patients with acquired immunodeficiency syndrome-related primary central nervous system lymphoma. Cancer 73:1728, 1994

174. Kaplan LD, Abrams DA, Volberding PA: Clinical course and epidemiology of Hodgkin's disease in homosexual men in San Francisco. In Abstracts of the IIIrd International Conference of AIDS, Washington, DC, 1987, Abstract M.11.3

175. Hessol NA, Katz MH, Lui JY, et al: Increased incidence of Hodgkin's disease in homosexual men with HIV infection. Ann Intern Med 117:309, 1992

176. Lyter DW, Kingsley LA, Rinaldo CR, Bryant J: Malignancies in the multicenter AIDS cohort study (MACS), 1984–1994 [abstract 852]. Proc Am Soc Clin Oncol 15:305, 1996

177. Serrano M, Bellas C, Campo E, et al: Hodgkin's disease in patients with antibodies to human immunodeficiency virus: A study of 22 patients. Cancer 65:2248, 1990

178. Kaplan L, Kahn J, Northfelt D, et al: Novel combination chemotherapy for Hodgkin's disease (HD) in HIV-infected individuals [abstract 7]. Proc Am Soc Clin Oncol 10:33, 1991

179. Levine AM, Cheung T, Tulpule A, et al: Preliminary results of AIDS Clinical Trials Group (ACTG) study #149: Phase II trial of ABVD chemotherapy with G-CSF in HIV infected patients with Hodgkin's disease (HD). In Abstracts of the National AIDS Malignancy Conference, Bethesda, MD, 1997, Abstract S7

180. Penn I: Cancers of the anogenital region in renal transplant recipients: Analysis of 65 cases. Cancer 58:611, 1986

181. Penn I: Tumors of the immunocompromised patient. Annu Rev Med 39:63, 1988

182. Pfister H: Relationship of papillomaviruses to anogenital cancer. Obstet Gynecol Clin North Am 14:349, 1987

183. Gal AA, Saul SH, Stoler MH: In situ hybridization analysis of human papillomavirus in anal squamous cell carcinoma. Mod Pathol 2:439, 1989

184. Sun X-W, Kuhn L, Ellerbrock TV, et al: Human papillomavirus infection in women infected with the human immunodeficiency virus. N Engl J Med 337:1343, 1997

185. Wright AB, Darragh TM, Vranizan K, et al: Anal and cervical papillomavirus infection and risk of anal and cervical epithelial abnormalities in human immunodeficiency virus-infected women. Obstet Gynecol 89:76, 1997

186. Maiman M, Fruchter RG, Serur E, et al: Human immunodeficiency virus infection and cervical neoplasia. Gynecol Oncol 38:377, 1990.

187. Maiman M, Fructer RG, Guy L, et al: Human immunodeficiency virus infection and invasive cervical carcinoma. Cancer 71:402, 1993

188. Maiman M, Fructer RG, Clark M, et al: Cervical cancer as an AIDS-defining illness. Obstet Gynecol 89:76, 1997

189. Monfardini S, Vaccher E, Pizzocaro G, et al: Unusual malignant tumors in 49 patients with HIV infection. AIDS 3:449, 1989

190. Rellihan MA, Dooley DP, Burke TW, et al: Rapidly progressing cervical cancer in a patient with human immunodeficiency virus infection. Gynecol Oncol 36:435, 1990

191. Saccucci P, Mastrone M, Are P, et al: Rapidly progressive squamous cell carcinoma of the cervix in a patient with acquired immunodeficiency syndrome: Case report. Eur J Gynaecol Oncol 17:306, 1996

192. Daling JR, Weiss NS, Hislop TG, et al: Sexual practices, sexually transmitted disease, and the incidence of anal cancer. N Engl J Med 317:973, 1987

193. Holly EA, Whittemore AS, Aston DA, et al: Anal cancer incidence: Genital warts, anal fissure or fistula, hemorrhoids, and smoking. J Natl Cancer Inst 81:1726, 1989

194. Croxson T, Chabon AB, Rorat E, Barash IM: Intraepithelial carcinoma of the anus in homosexual men. Dis Colon Rectum 27:325, 1984

195. Frazer IH, Crapper RM, Medley G, et al: Association between anorectal dysplasia, human papillomavirus, and human immunodeficiency virus infection in homosexual men. Lancet 2:657, 1986

196. Palefsky JM, Gonzales J, Greenblatt RM, et al: Anal intraepithelial neoplasia and anal papillomavirus infection among homosexual males with group IV HIV disease, JAMA 263:2911, 1990

197. Caussy D, Goedert JJ, Palefsky J, et al: Interaction of human immunodeficiency and papilloma viruses: Association with anal intraepithelial abnormality in homosexual men. Int J Cancer 46:214, 1990

198. Melbye M, Palefsky J, Gonzales J, et al: Immune status as a determinant of human papillomavirus detection and its association with anal epithelial abnormalities. Int J Cancer 46:203, 1990

199. Holland JM, Swift PS: Tolerance of patients with human immunodeficiency virus and carcinoma to treatment with combined chemotherapy and radiation therapy. Radiology 193:251, 1994

200. Nasti G, Santarossa S, Vaccher E, et al: Anal cancer in patients with HIV infection: A report of two cases without evidence of immunological dysfunction. AIDS 8:1507, 1994

201. Svensson C, Kaigas M, Lidbrink E, et al: Carcinoma of the anal canal in a patient with AIDS. Acta Oncol 30:8986, 1991

202. Bottomley DM, Agel N, Selvaratnam G, Phillips RH: Epidermoid anal cancer in HIV-infected patients. Clin Oncol (R Coll Radiol) 8:319, 1996

203. Peddada AV, Smith DE, Rao AR, et al: Chemotherapy and low-dose radiotherapy in the treatment of HIV-infected patients with carcinoma of the anal canal. Int J Radiat Oncol Biol Phys 37:1101 1997

204. Palefsky J: Human papillomavirus infection among HIV-infected individuals. Hematol Oncol Clin North Am 5:357, 1991

Special Aspects of HIV and Population-Specific Management

31 | The Global Prevention of HIV

MYRON S. COHEN • GINA DALLABETTA •
WILLARD CATES, JR. • KING K. HOLMES

HIV is now endemic throughout the world, with epidemic epicenters in sub-Saharan Africa and Asia.[1] Unlike many other infectious diseases, HIV infection has no geographic or socioeconomic boundaries, and it ties together the entire human species. Accordingly, HIV prevention must represent a coordinated global effort, with varying regional emphasis depending on the most important modes of transmission, the medical and public health infrastructure available, governmental and nongovernmental resources, and, perhaps most importantly, political will. This chapter briefly reviews interventions designed to prevent transmission of HIV.

DETERMINANTS OF HIV TRANSMISSION

The spread of HIV can be ascribed to bloodborne transmission (contaminated blood supply, IV drug use, needlestick injuries), vertical transmission (mother to her offspring), and sexual transmission.[2] Sexual transmission accounts for most HIV infections in the world.[3]

At the individual level, transmission of HIV depends upon infectiousness of the index case[4] and susceptibility of the exposed host.[5,5a] Infectiousness of a biologic secretion can be defined by the concentration of the virus in the secretion and the virologic factors expected to facilitate transmission. Increased concentration of HIV in blood can be correlated with enhanced transmission by all three routes.[6,7]

The concentration of HIV in genital tract secretions from males and females is increased at times when sexual transmission is thought to be enhanced.[4,8–11] Antiretroviral therapy that reduces the concentration of the free virus in plasma reduces perinatal transmission[12] and may reduce sexual transmission,[13] and, although conclusive data on this point are still lacking, appears to reduce infectiousness of the index case.[12,13]

Virologic factors required for HIV transmission are only poorly understood, but some viral quasispecies in a swarm appear to be favored,[14] and inconclusive evidence suggests that different viral clades (subtypes) found in different parts of the world may be transmitted with different levels of efficiency.[15] In general, the viral envelope probably plays a critical role in determining transmissibility of simian immunodeficiency virus (SIV) and HIV.[16]

Susceptibility to HIV infection depends on the lack of immunity in the exposed host[17] and lack of hereditary resistance.[18] Cells receptive to HIV infection can be found in the bloodstream and in all mucosal surfaces.[19] These cells express a variety of different surface receptors able to recognize and accept the viral envelope.[19] People with cell receptor mutations that lead to resistance to HIV infection of cells in vitro have been described.[18,19]

A variety of cofactors appear to amplify HIV transmission by increasing either the infectiousness of the index case or the susceptibility of the exposed host.[2,20] The most important cofactors for HIV transmission cause inflammation of the genital mucosa. In some countries, sexual practices allow trauma to the mucosa.[21,22] Sexually transmitted diseases (STDs) are common in the same geographic locations and populations as HIV, and untreated STDs appear to increase both infectiousness and susceptibility to HIV.[20,23] Lack of circumcision appears to be an important cofactor facilitating transmission of disease to men, perhaps by increasing the number of receptive cells.[24]

At the population level, transmission of sexually acquired HIV has been described in a mathematical model as $R_o = \beta \times D \times c$, where R_o represents the number of secondary infections arising from a given infection early in the epidemic, β the mean efficiency of transmission, D the mean duration of infectiousness, and c the mean partner change rate (a surrogate for the rate of exposure of susceptibles to infecteds in the population).[25] When R_o exceeds 1, the epidemic spreads. Successful prevention strategies must be designed to reduce R_o to less than 1; these include (1) lowering the rate of partner change, (2) reducing the efficiency of transmission, and (3) shortening the duration of infectiousness.

The efficiency of transmission per exposure of a susceptible to an infected person can be reduced by promoting condom use and safe sex practices (e.g., masturbation is the most safe and receptive anal intercourse is the most unsafe with respect to acquiring HIV). The efficiency of transmitting HIV can also be reduced by controlling other STDs. Promoting circumcision might be warranted to reduce the acquisition of chancroid and HIV infection in countries where these diseases are highly endemic.

The average number of new partners acquired by an infected individual could be lowered if everyone in the population chose to have fewer sex partners. Alternatively, reducing exposures to or by those with high-risk behaviors, who are likely to be infected, would more specifically target this behavioral approach. In the case of HIV infection, identifying those who are infected and encouraging them to have fewer partners, and to employ measures to reduce the efficiency of STD transmission, are essential.

The duration of infectiousness for HIV is a subject of continuing research. Individuals who spontaneously develop a low plasma viral load (i.e., "viral set point") early in the natural history of acute infection have prolonged survival. By identifying individuals early in the course of infection, and administering combination antiviral therapies, the viral set point can be lowered; by inference, the individual's prognosis for survival may be improved. It is plausible that this lower plasma viral load also will translate to a decreased infectiousness, either on a per-sexual-act basis or as a decreased lifetime cumulative risk of transmission, but this remains to be determined. In any case, the primary HIV infection interval (i.e., viremia until antibodies against HIV can be detected) remains a key target for both clinical and prevention outcomes.[26]

Depending upon whether HIV prevention strategies are viewed from the individual or population perspective, a different emphasis emerges. From the perspective of the interaction of an individual patient with the clinician, the main objectives are to prevent acquisition of HIV infection, to prevent HIV disease progression, to prevent HIV-related opportunistic infections, and to protect the patient's own sex partners. However, from a population perspective, the objective is to lower the overall rate of spread of HIV, and to intervene with those most likely to spread HIV within a community. Therefore, the individual-level intervention generally emphasizes safer practices in uninfected persons and/or notifying exposed partners; however, the population perspective would approach the HIV-infected "source partner" to counsel and treat as a way of reducing further HIV transmission. Interestingly, this was an important aspect of early HIV prevention intervention in Sweden, which recognized the epidemic while the prevalence of infection in high-risk groups was still very low; whereas in the United States, which already had a relatively high prevalence of infection in high-risk groups by the time specific testing first became possible, emphasis has been on changing behaviors of high-risk individuals who are still uninfected.

SPECIFIC INTERVENTION STRATEGIES

To accomplish reduction of HIV transmission, prevention strategies must include overlapping behavioral and biologic approaches. Comprehensive HIV prevention strategies are now multisectoral (involving the activities of many sectors or agencies) and are aimed not only at individuals but at families, groups, communities, institutions, and the contextual or structural barriers to behavior change.[27–29] Approaches have been broadened to address the social, political, infrastructural, and environmental factors that influence risk behaviors.[28]

Behavior Change Interventions

Behavior change interventions, unlike older health communication efforts, draw upon contemporary marketing principles, including (1) audience segmentation based on variables such as age, sex, attitudes, and values; (2) audience research; (3) concept development and pretesting; (4) multiple message development to target various segments of the audience; (5) design of messages that offer benefits meaningful to the audience; and (6) ensuring accessibility to needed services or products.[30] A variety of HIV prevention messages are needed to reduce risk for and vulnerability to HIV infection (e.g., abstinence, delayed sexual debut, sexual monogamy and choice of safer partners, correct and consistent condom use, safer injecting drug habits, and appropriate early treatment-seeking behavior for sexually transmitted infections.)

Behavior change as a result of risk reduction counseling has now been well documented in people at risk for HIV.[31–33] For example, Project Respect is a recent behavior change clinical trial conducted in the United States. A total of 5872 persons attending STD clinics were randomized to receive individualized standard brief HIV health education messages, client-centered counseling in two 20-minute clinic sessions, or a more intensive theory-based risk reduction intervention. At 6-month follow-up, significant increase in condom usage and reduction in incident STDs were demonstrated with both the client-centered and the more intensive interventions.[33] Clinicians and managed care organizations therefore can and should become much more active in routinely assessing the risk for STD/HIV exposure in patients undergoing initial examination, annual follow-up exams, or contraceptive care, as well as those with symptoms suggesting STD, especially in adolescents.[34] For those with positive risk factors, the standard of care should include client-centered risk reduction counseling or other interventions of proven efficacy.

Challenges in behavior change programs include (1) the most effective way to measure intermediate stages of change and actual reduction in disease occurrence to assess a program's effectiveness and (2) how to sustain behavior change. A behavior change intervention strategy must be comprehensive and designed to address specific target groups in which HIV is spreading,[35–37] should consider the stage and the progress of the epidemic, and should combine an array of media and interpersonal methods. Adolescent African-Americans have a particularly high risk of HIV acquisition. A very recent randomized controlled trial of interventions in adolescents has demonstrated the feasibility and effectiveness of a harm-reduction-model promotion of condoms to reduce risk-taking behavior, and found that promotion of abstinence was less effective.[38] In addition, promotion of norms that foster behavior changes at the societal level are essential.[39]

From the perspective of the clinician, much greater attention must be given to interventions that prevent the transmission of infection from HIV-positive individuals. As noted above, HIV prevention interventions have generally focused on acquisition of infection. In the past, many clinicians, as advocates for their patients with HIV infections, have felt reluctant to consider partner notification or risk reduction counseling. However, 25 states in the United States now require name-based reporting of HIV infection, and increasingly they participate in HIV partner notification. Most HIV-infected patients do want to prevent transmission of infection to current or new partners for altruistic reasons. Prevention services for HIV-affected individuals are also essential.[40,41] Advances in health care for people with HIV infection can greatly reduce morbidity and mortality,[41] and also can be expected to reduce infectiousness (discussed below). Perhaps the availability of better therapy will actually help reduce the discrimination suffered by HIV-infected individuals.

Improving the Availability and Use of Condoms

Male latex condoms, when used consistently and properly, prevent transmission of HIV[42,43] (Fig. 31–1), but ensuring their availability and proper usage are continuing challenges.[43–46] The accumulated data on condom use and HIV infection provide convincing evidence. In 10 cohort studies of high-risk populations in seven countries where both the level of condom use

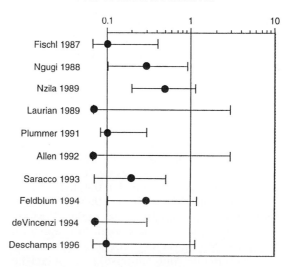

FIGURE 31–1. Risk of HIV infection among heterosexual couples using condoms, selected cohort studies. (From Cates W: Contraception, contraceptive technology and STD. In Holmes KK, et al. (eds): Sexually Transmitted Diseases, 3rd ed. New York, McGraw-Hill, 1998, with permission.)

(exposure) and HIV incidence (outcome) were prospectively measured, all showed that consistent use of male condoms protected against HIV acquisition, with a level of protection ranging from 50% to 100%. Two studies involving HIV-discordant couples are the most persuasive. In Europe, none of the 123 seronegative partners prospectively reporting consistent condom use became infected.[42] In Haiti, only 1 of 42 seronegative partners consistently using condoms became infected.[43] In both studies, among HIV-discordant couples who either used condoms inconsistently or did not use them at all, between 7% and 14% became infected. Thus, when used regularly and correctly, condoms worked.

At the population level, targeting condom use to key environments where HIV is spreading can have a marked impact on reducing HIV transmission. The Thailand "100 Percent Condom Program" is a remarkable success story.[47] In 1991, the Thai government implemented a national strategy to require widespread condom use in commercial sex facilities. The proportion of commercial sex acts in Thailand in which condoms were used increased from 25% in 1989 to 94% in 1995. During the same interval, the incidence of curable STDs reported to government clinics decreased dramatically, as has HIV prevalence among Thai military recruits.[32] Likewise, in the United States, Nevada brothels which have instituted similar "100 percent condom policies" have not had a reported case of HIV transmission during the duration of epidemic in this country.[48]

The male latex condom is available in many countries through private pharmacies, maternal/child health and family planning clinics, STD services, community-based distribution systems linked with peer education programs, and condom social marketing. Condom social marketing programs have been extremely successful in expanding condom accessibility by making condoms available to consumers at an affordable price (usually subsidized) and in convenient places by using nontraditional outlets such as bars, taxis, and hotels. For example, in Ethiopia, condom sales went from 300,000 in 1990 to 19.8 million in 1995 with over 90% of the condoms sold from nontraditional outlets.[49] Moreover, the aggressive promotion of condoms through social marketing programs makes them more acceptable and diminishes the social taboos surrounding them. Social marketing approaches are also being used to increase STD treatment and prevention services.[50]

Although the male latex condom remains a key element in HIV prevention programs, this method is used only at the discretion of the male partner. Female condoms are now available in some countries. Their efficacy against HIV transmission has not been proven. The female condom is currently expensive (several times the cost of a male latex condom) and can only be used once. High cost as well as issues of acceptability have limited its use.[51] However, there is evidence that when female condoms are made available as an alternative to the male condom in high-risk settings, total condom use can increase. In Zambia the majority of high-risk couples use the female condom as part of an array of barrier method options (including spermicides and male condoms) in about one quarter of their coital acts. This intervention includes counseling and free distribution of barrier methods.[52]

Biomedical HIV Prevention Strategies

Biomedical interventions include vaccines, elimination of cofactors that facilitate the transmission of HIV, and the use of antiretroviral drugs.

Vaccines

Vaccines that offer sustained immunity rank with improved hygiene and sanitation as the most cost-effective ways to prevent transmission of infectious diseases. Development of vaccines is particularly important for STDs because change in sexual behavior is so difficult. Unfortunately, vaccine development is time consuming and expensive, and, even when a vaccine is available (as with hepatitis B vaccine), vaccine deployment for an STD remains a formidable challenge. An ideal vaccine for HIV would work by increasing immunity of the susceptible host to prevent both mucosal and systemic infection.[53,54] Alternatively, an HIV vaccine might provide enough immunity to reduce the initial viral burden, thereby making the spread of the disease to the next sexual partner less likely.

Work on development of a vaccine to prevent HIV began almost 15 years ago with the recognition of the pathogen, but this has proven a daunting task because of the variability of the virus and our lack of understanding of the immunity required to prevent infection. In addition, HIV-1 vaccine efforts to date have focused primarily on the subtype B virus in the United States and Western Europe, whereas perhaps 90% of HIV infections occurring globally involve other subtypes, especially subtypes E and C in the epidemic epicenters.

Some progress has been made in Phase I (safety) studies of a subtype B vaccine.[55] Available candidate vaccines generally include critical viral immunogens packaged in a viral vector and/or an adjuvant, and several novel approaches are also being evaluated.[53-55] Trials are now planned for vaccine evaluations in a variety of developing countries, with the hope that a subtype B vaccine might prevent infection caused by other subtypes. Development of subtype C and E vaccines is also in progress.

Cytotoxic T-lymphocyte responses to vaccines have been of increasing interest as potential surrogates of immunity, because some people exposed to HIV who remain uninfected have demonstrated a strong cytotoxic T-lymphocyte response to HIV antigens.[53,56]

Concern remains that a vaccine that is less than 100% effective could increase transmission of HIV by adversely affecting safer sex behavior.[57] Such a vaccine might also increase the incidence of the other classic STDs, which could be synergistic with relapsing high-risk exposures in promoting HIV transmission.

Antiretroviral Therapy

Antiretroviral drugs, especially azidothymidine (AZT; zidovudine) have been used as HIV postexposure prophylaxis (PEP)[58] and to prevent vertical transmission of HIV.[59] AZT and other antiretroviral drugs can reduce the shedding of cell-free HIV in genital secretions.[60-64] Reducing the concentration of HIV in genital secretions is likely to reduce sexual transmission.[13,60] However, the effects of antiretroviral drugs are not so predictive as to provide any reassurance to an individual patient about his/her infectiousness.[60] Indeed, recent studies suggest that HIV-positive people taking antiretroviral therapy realize they remain contagious. On the other hand, knowledge of the availability of more effective therapy could lead to increased risk-taking behavior by those still uninfected. In addition, poor adherence to therapy or use of therapy that fails to penetrate the urogenital tract could facilitate resistance,[65] and resistant isolates have been sexually transmitted.[65a] We anticipate development of antiretroviral drugs designed to concentrate in genital secretions, which would have unique public health benefit.

Antiretroviral agents can also be used as PEP after high-risk sex.[58,66,67] Experimental antiretroviral agents such as (R)-9-(2-phosphonylmethoxypropyl) adenine (PMPA) provide some protection to macaques from a vaginal inoculation of HIV. Indeed, PEP is recommended after sexual assault.[66] However, it is not known if available drugs can prevent HIV transmission after sexual exposure.[68] In addition, PEP after consensual sex with a partner whose HIV status is unknown represents an untenable strategy given the costs and side effects of antiretroviral drugs.[67]

Some mathematical models indicate that most HIV transmission occurs through the sexual activity of people with primary HIV infection,[26] who generally have a very high blood viral burden. These people do not know their infection status, and antibody testing would not be useful because they have not had time to seroconvert. If this hypothesis proves correct, a strategy to detect and treat people with primary infection will provide both public health and long-term benefit to patients receiving early therapy.[26]

Elimination of Cofactors That Amplify Transmission of HIV

Increased concentrations of HIV in blood can be correlated with enhanced transmission by all routes.[68] In developing countries systemic infections such as malaria[69] and tuberculosis[70] increase the blood burden of HIV, and treatment of these infections reduces the concentration of free virus in plasma.

The concentration of HIV in the genital tract probably correlates even more directly with vertical and sexual transmission of HIV, although this has not yet been proven. The concentration of HIV in the genital tract increases in association with vitamin A deficiency,[11,20] with use of Depo-Provera, and the high-dose oral contraceptives still available in some developing countries,[11] and with classic STDs.[10,71-74] STDs and hormonal contraception may also increase susceptibility to HIV.[75-77] Recent studies suggest that the changes in the vaginal flora that characterize bacterial vaginosis also increase susceptibility of women to acquisition of HIV.[78,79] Accordingly, interventions to reduce the blood and/or genital tract concentration of both free and cell-associated HIV could become key elements in an HIV prevention strategy.

SPECIFIC APPROACHES TO HIV PREVENTION

Blood-borne Transmission

Blood-borne transmission of HIV can occur when the blood supply is not adequately protected, or from IV drug use or needlestick injury. The protection of the blood supply can generally be accomplished by appropriate screening. With recognition of the value of ensuring a safe blood supply, it has been possible to improve the recruitment of donors, blood screening procedures, and policies for transfusion practices (e.g., by eliminating administration of injection of small volumes of blood). Enzyme-linked immunosorbent assay (ELISA) testing is the standard approach; it has reduced the risk of HIV to 1 in every 450,000 to 660,000 donations of screened blood in the United States.[80] In order to further secure the blood supply in the United States, blood is also screened for p24 antigen or RNA.[81] This test is designed to try to detect patients who have recently acquired HIV but remain antibody negative. Such an approach is generally untenable for developing countries, and may not be warranted even in more developed countries because detecting even a single patient with negative ELISA and positive p24 may require screening hundreds of thousands or millions of donors. Furthermore, neither the p24 antigen test nor the newer HIV RNA detection procedures can guarantee the sensitivity required to find all possible infected donors.

A comprehensive approach for protection of the blood supply includes (1) recruitment of donors who are healthy and unlikely to be HIV infected, (2) excluding donors who have been exposed to blood-transmissible diseases, (3) following and testing manufacturer protocols, (4) emphasizing public health support of governmental policies to protect the blood supply, and (5) reducing demand for blood supply so that only essential components are employed.[81] In Lusaka, Zambia, a change in the blood collection policy that emphasized collection from voluntary donors (usually family members) reduced the prevalence of HIV infection in units collected from 20.3% to 7% between 1990 and 1994.[82]

Although sexual transmission of HIV remains the most important transmission route at the global level, injection drug use has played a major role in the epidemics in the United States,[83] and in some countries in Asia, Eastern Europe, and the former Soviet Union. Injection drug users (IDUs) who share injection equipment and also have many sex partners represent a "bridge population" that is extremely important in fueling the growing heterosexual epidemic of HIV infection in the United States.[84,85] Interventions directed at IDUs include behavior change strategies to reduce sharing of injecting equipment, to reduce sharing partners, and to increase access to clean injection equipment (needle

exchange programs, needle sterilization or cleaning); behavioral and medical interventions to detoxify IDUs and stop injection drug use; and interventions to reduce sexual transmission to nonusing partners.[86] Implementation of successful interventions, however, has often been limited or obstructed because of the political, legal, and regulatory barriers to dealing with this population.

Whereas transfusion of HIV-infected blood products and injection drug use have a high probability of transmitting HIV, needlestick injuries appear less efficient,[2,58] probably because the volume of blood inoculated is lower. Blood-drawing, large-bore needles present a 1:250 risk for transmission of HIV during needlesticks. Protection of health care workers from HIV disease after needlestick injury is discussed elsewhere in this book.[58]

Vertical Transmission of HIV: Childbirth and Breast-feeding

Babies born to infected mothers appear to have approximately a 30% to 50% risk of acquiring HIV. The concentration of HIV in the mother's blood is a risk factor.[87,88] In addition, it seems likely that untreated STDs facilitate the vertical transmission of HIV, because they increase genital shedding of HIV during pregnancy.[20] Vitamin A deficiency also is associated with increased genital shedding of HIV.[89]

HIV may be transmitted prepartum, intrapartum, or postpartum.[90] Intrapartum transmission probably accounts for the largest proportion of mother-to-child transmission, but the precise contribution of each, and the factors associated with transmission, are subjects of ongoing studies. Potential interventions being studied include prepartum vaginal chlorhexidine or benzalkonium vaginal disinfection, cesarean section, vitamin A or micronutrient replacement therapy, breast milk alternatives, and hyperimmune globulin administration.[91–97]

Treatment of the mother and neonate with AZT has had a dramatic effect. In ACTG Study 076, mothers were treated with AZT during the third trimester and at delivery, and neonates received 6 weeks of additional therapy.[59] Transmission was reduced from 25.5% in the placebo group to 8.3% in those who received therapy. Unfortunately, this trial did not define the effects of AZT per se on the mother or the infant, or the least amount of AZT effective. Recent work in Thailand has shown that a short course of AZT offered to the mother late in pregnancy also reduced transmission of HIV, by about one half. AZT is not the most potent antiretroviral drug available, and vertical transmission of AZT-resistant isolates has been reported.[98] Accordingly, several trials have been launched to determine the effects of other antiretroviral drugs and drug combinations on mother-to-child transmission.[97]

HIV transmission also occurs during breast-feeding.[99] One analysis suggested a 14% risk of postnatal transmission attributable to breast-feeding.[92] High viral burden and low levels of antibodies directed against HIV may facilitate HIV transmission. The timing of breast-feeding may also be important. Some investigators report that HIV is detected most readily in colostrum, although this finding has not been consistent in all studies. Transmission of HIV by breast-feeding later in infancy has also been well defined.[100,101] Transmission of HIV through breast-feeding is especially likely by a mother who develops primary infection shortly after pregnancy, probably because of the high viral burden and lack of immunity associated with primary infection. The risk of transmission from mother to infant by women who have become HIV positive after pregnancy was 29% in one study.[92]

In the United States, HIV-positive women are instructed to use infant formula as an alternative to breast-feeding. However, in many developing countries breast-feeding is essential to avoid infant diarrhea and dehydration.[102] The results of a randomized controlled trial of breast feeding versus formula feeding by HIV-positive mothers to prevent postnatal vertical HIV transmission in Nairobi, Kenya, will soon become available. Meanwhile, the balance between the risks of breast-feeding by HIV-positive women and the benefits of breast-feeding for all infants is confounding current global strategies to limit vertical transmission. The issue is particularly important as short-course AZT comes into use, because the risk of transmission of HIV through breast-feeding remains following a short-course antiretroviral regimen.

Sexual Transmission of HIV

Worldwide, HIV is primarily a sexually transmitted disease, affecting both men and women.[3] Accordingly, the greatest efforts (and progress) in prevention of transmission of HIV have focused on sexual transmission. Indeed, it can be argued that all the tools needed for HIV prevention have already been developed, but not prop-

erly deployed.[39] Transmission of HIV from men to their partners is more efficient than from women to men.[3] Transmission of HIV through anal intercourse is more efficient than by other routes. Oral sexual behavior between women (cunnilingus) appears to confer almost no risk, and performing fellatio appears to have much lower risk than sexual intercourse.[3] Patients with primary and late-stage HIV are probably more infectious that those at other stages of disease[26,103]; to the extent this is true, it has profound implications for HIV prevention.

The main HIV prevention strategies employed to date concomitantly emphasize fewer and less risky partners; safer sex practices, including use of condoms especially in casual or commercial sex; and early detection and therapy of classic STDs.[104] These strategies were developed at a time before the biology of HIV transmission was well understood, and were based solely on epidemiologic considerations. Adoption of safer sex practices had a dramatic effect on the incidence of HIV in men having sex with men, and in several other groups.[39,105] A key debate involves targeting of messages. Recent National Academy of Sciences and World Bank reports suggest a focused approach to prevention behavior,[36,37] whereas others have argued such targeting is stigmatizing and ignores the risk of HIV to the entire species.[106] It is important to consider the need to develop messages specific to HIV-infected individuals, because they represent a target audience of great importance. Focusing on HIV-infected individuals can have a dramatic effect on the epidemic, provided appropriate, effective, ethical interventions are available. Cuba appears to have avoided an HIV epidemic (at least thus far) through mass screening and quarantine with re-education of HIV-infected individuals,[107] an approach used by other totalitarian countries to control STDs.[108] It should be noted that even Sweden, a country with a generally nondiscriminatory approach to HIV infection, has at least temporarily quarantined for further counseling those few HIV-infected individuals who initially continued to practice high-risk behaviors after having been informed and counseled about being infected. As better therapy for HIV infection becomes available (see below), dealing with HIV-infected individuals will become of even greater importance.

Treatment of STDs has proven a successful HIV intervention. Several biologic studies have demonstrated that STDs increase the shedding of HIV in both male and female genital secretions,[10,11,20,72,73] and that treatment of STDs reduces shedding of HIV. In addition, STDs probably reduce mucosal resistance to HIV and recruit cells receptive to the virus.[77] In Tanzania, strengthened syndromic treatment of symptomatic STDs reduced the incidence of new HIV infections in the population as a whole by 42%[109]; this was an extremely cost-effective approach to HIV prevention.[110]

The role of alternative approaches, such as broad population-level screening programs to detect asymptomatic infections or periodic selective mass treatment of high-risk "core" transmitters such as sex workers, is not well studied. In Welcom, South Africa, a four-pronged approach to an STD intervention targeting sex workers serving a mining community included (1) monthly use of azithromycin, (2) serologic testing and treatment of syphilis, (3) syndromic treatment of vaginal discharge and genital ulcer disease, and (4) condom promotion. This targeted intervention led to lower levels of gonorrhea and chlamydia in the sex workers themselves and also their male clients (R. Steen et al., unpublished data). The impact on HIV transmission has not yet been defined. In rural Uganda, a community randomization trial of mass therapy with azithromycin plus cefixime or ciprofloxacin administered every 9 months to all adults of reproductive ages,[111] reduced the incidence of trichomoniasis and syphilis, with very modest or no reduction in other STDs.[112] There was no impact on HIV transmission.[112]

The different results from the Mwanza and Rakai community trials suggested that syndromic treatment of symptomatic STDs had a greater effect on HIV transmission than did mass administration of antibiotics to the entire population (in an effort mainly to cure asymptomatic STDs). Those STDs that cause inflammatory symptoms sufficient to have persons seek health care may have a disproportionate effect on either the transmission or acquisition of HIV. Such biologic factors as higher viral load, more exposed inflamed area to provide a portal of entry or egress, or more CD4 target cells for viral attack may provide the basis for the greater impact of the symptomatic STDs.

Topical microbicides continue to hold hope for the prevention of HIV in women. However, the only microbicide tested extensively in field trials to date is the detergent spermicide nonoxynol-9 (N-9). Although this compound has in vitro activity against many STD pathogens (including HIV), its results in human trials have been disappointing. Three randomized controlled trials have compared three different N-9 products—a gel,[113-115] the sponge, and the film.[116] Taken together, these studies have shown that N-9 reduces the risks of both gonorrhea and chlamydial infections, albeit at relatively low levels of protection (Fig. 31-2). Of the two studies looking at HIV, the trial of the N-9 sponge showed a nonsignificant trend toward increased HIV acquisition (despite reduced gonorrhea acquisition) among sponge users,[115] whereas the study of the N-9 film found no effect of N-9 on HIV, gonorrhea, of *Chlamydia trachomatis* acquisition. Clearly, studying other preparations of N-9, as well as developing alternative microbicides that may be more active against HIV, are important. In macaques vaginally inoculated with SIV, the compound PMPA

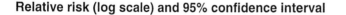

Relative risk (log scale) and 95% confidence interval

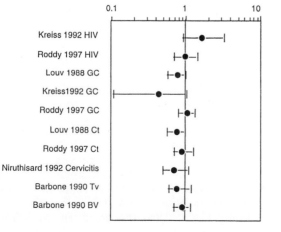

FIGURE 31-2. Risk of STD among women using nonoxynol-9–containing spermicides, by organism, among highest quality randomized controlled trials.

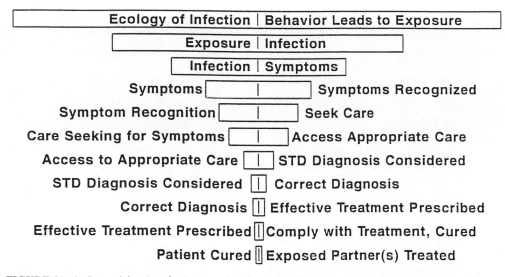

FIGURE 31–3. Potential points for intervention through STD care management and other public health intervention, to reduce acquisition of STD and detected and treat asymptomatic and symptomatic infections that occur. (From Ryan CA, Holmes KK: STD care management. In Holmes KK, et al. (eds): Sexually Transmitted Diseases, 3rd ed. New York, McGraw-Hill, 1998, with permission.)

has reduced the rates of infection.[117] Multiple Phase I and Phase II studies are underway to contribute different microbicidal products to the pipeline. Additional Phase III studies should be initiated immediately.

Controlling STDs, including HIV, within any sexually active community can be viewed as a cascading series of phased interventions addressing different components of STD prevention[118] (Fig. 31–3). Four stages of STD control are involved: (1) promote behavior change, (2) assure availability of effective STD care for those seeking care, (3) promote early health care seeking for symptoms of STD, and (4) detect and treat asymptomatic infections. At Stage 1, prevention is concerned with the entire socio-sexual network. Efforts to prevent populations from becoming infected include overall promotion of safer behaviors, which means avoiding risky sexual behaviors, reducing the number of sex partners and choosing them more carefully, and using condoms during all sexual acts. Stage 2 requires clinicians providing treatment for persons with an STD to have an adequate knowledge of the principles of STD management and guidelines for treatment, as well as an available supply of effective drugs with which to cure diagnosed STDs. Stage 3 involves helping both individuals and populations to recognize the possible symptoms of STDs and providing them with access to convenient diagnostic and treatment services. Stage 4, a

more advanced stage in STD control, involves active screening for asymptomatic infection and treating those with asymptomatic infections. This involves widespread community screening programs for those unsuspecting individuals who might be infected. Depending on such factors as community resources, prevalence of infection within a community, and availability of trained clinicians, different combinations of these four stages will be necessary to provide effective STD control within specific communities, in general, increasing resources allow progression from stage 1 to stage 4.[119]

CONCLUSION

The recognition of the etiology of HIV disease led to a serologic test and a misplaced belief that a preventive vaccine would soon follow. Behavioral interventions for prevention were developed in the absence of supportive biologic data, focused almost exclusively on promotion of condoms and safe sex practices (rather than, for example, on patterns of partnership formation). Now, more than 20 years after HIV began to spread, the true nature and ferocity of this epidemic is apparent, but its emotional, financial, social, and biologic implications have not been fully realized. In addition, biomedical and behavioral approaches have yet to be properly integrated, or even appreciated by different segments of the research community. Some social and behavioral scientists and many policy makers remain poorly informed about the biology of HIV transmission, or the ramifications of discoveries related to immunity or therapy of STDs and of HIV infection. Conversely, some biologists and clinicians have been dismissive of behavior change and prevention science, as have many funding agencies accustomed to supporting more traditional biologic research. From this discussion, it should be clear that biomedical and behavioral approaches to HIV prevention are complementary, and must evolve together. The biomedical interventions cannot be implemented without the behavioral change components to support and amplify them. Conversely comprehensive HIV prevention programs must utilize the full array of prevention strategies and be constantly re-evaluated to incorporate the ever-changing biomedical and behavioral advances.

References

1. Stanecki KA: The dynamic HIV/AIDS pandemic. In Mann J, Tarantola D (eds): AIDS in the World II. New York, Oxford University Press, 1996, p 41
2. Royce RA, Seny Y, Cates W, et al: Sexual transmission of HIV: Host factors that shape the epidemic and implications for prevention. N Engl J Med 269:2853, 1997
3. UNAIDS/WHO Working Group on Global HIV/AIDS and STD Surveillance: Report on the Global HIV/AIDS Epidemic. Geneva, World Health Organization, 1997
4. Vernazza PL, Gilliam BL, Dyer J, et al: Quantification of HIV in semen: Correlation with antiviral treatment and immune status. AIDS 11:987, 1997
5. Buchacz KA, Wilkinson DA, Krowka JF, et al: Genetic and immunological host factors associated with susceptibility to HIV-1 infection. AIDS 12 (Suppl A): 587, 1998
5a. Padian NS, Shiboski SC, Jewell NP: The effect of number of exposures on the risk of heterosexual HIV transmission. J Infect Dis 161:883, 1990
6. Busch MP, Operskalski EA, Mosley JW, et al: Factors influencing human immunodeficiency virus type 1 transmission by blood transfusion. J Infect Dis 174: 26, 1996
7. Lee TH, Sakahara N, Fiebig E, et al: Correlation of HIV-1 RNA levels in plasma and heterosexual transmission of HIV-1 from infected transfusion recipients [letter]. J Acquir Immune Defic Syndr Hum Retrovirol 12:427, 1996
8. Coombs RW, Speck CE, Hughes JP, et al: Association between culturable human immunodeficiency virus type 1 (HIV-1) in semen and HIV-1 RNA levels in semen and blood: Evidence for compartmentalization of HIV-1 between semen and blood. J Infect Dis 177: 320, 1998
9. Dyer JR, Gilliam BL, Eron JJ, et al: Shedding of HIV-1 in semen during primary infection. AIDS 11: 543, 1997

10. Ghys PD, Fransen K, Diallo MO, et al: The associations between cervicovaginal HIV shedding, sexually transmitted diseases and immunosuppression in female sex workers in Abidjan, Cote d'Ivoire. AIDS 11: F85, 1997
11. Mostad SB, Overbaugh J, DeVange DM, et al: Hormonal contraception, vitamin A deficiency, and other risk factors for shedding of HIV-1 infected cells from the cervix. Lancet 350:922, 1997
12. Anonymous: Administration of zidovudine during late pregnancy and delivery to prevent perinatal HIV transmission—Thailand, 1996–1998. MMWR Morb Mortal Wkly Rep 47:151, 1998
13. Musicco M, Lazzarin A, Nicolosi A, et al: Antiretroviral treatment of men infected with human immunodeficiency virus type 1 reduces the incidence of heterosexual transmission. Arch Intern Med 154:1971, 1994
14. Zhu T, Wang N, Carr A, et al: Genetic characterization of human immunodeficiency virus type 1 in blood and genital secretions: Evidence for viral compartmentalization and selection during sexual transmission. J Virol 70:3098, 1996
15. Kunanusont C, Foy HM, Kreiss JK, et al: HIV-1 subtypes and male-to-female transmission in Thailand. Lancet 345:1078, 1995
16. Lu Y, Brosio P, Lafaile M, et al: Vaginal transmission of chimeric simian/human immunodeficiency viruses in Rhesus macaques. J Virol 70:3045, 1996
17. Clerici M, Giorgi JV, Chou CC, et al: Cell-mediated immune response to human immunodeficiency virus (HIV) type 1 in seronegative homosexual men with recent sexual exposure to HIV-1. J Infect Dis 165: 1012, 1992
18. Dragic T, Litwin V, Allaway JP, et al: HIV-1 entry into CD4+ cells is mediated by the chemokine receptor CC-CKR-5. Nature 381:667, 1996
19. Graziosi C, Pantaleo G: The multi-faceted personality of HIV. Nature 3:1318, 1997
20. John GC, Nduati RW, Mbori-Ngacha D, et al: Genital shedding of human immunodeficiency virus type 1 DNA during pregnancy: Association with immunosuppression, abnormal cervical or vaginal discharge, and severe vitamin A deficiency. J Infect Dis 175:57, 1997
21. Hellman NS, Desmond-Hellman S, Nsubuga PSJ, et al: Genital trauma during sex is a risk factor for HIV in Uganda. In: Abstracts of the VIIth International Conference on AIDS, Florence, 1991, Abstract MC3079
22. Dallabetta GA, Miotti PG, Chiphangwi JD, et al: Traditional vaginal agents: Use and association with HIV infection in Malawian women. AIDS 9:293, 1995
23. Wasserheit JN: Epidemiological synergy: Interrelationships between human immunodeficiency virus infection and other sexually transmitted diseases. Sex Transm Dis 19:61, 1992
24. Moses S, Plummer FA, Bradley JE, et al: Association between lack of male circumcision and risk for HIV infection: Review of epidemiologic evidence. In: Abstracts of the XIth International Conference on AIDS. Vancouver, 1996, Abstract We.C.452
25. Anderson RM, May RM: Epidemiologic parameters of HIV transmission. Nature 333:415, 1988
26. Cates W, Chesney M, Cohen MS: Primary HIV disease: A publich health emergency. Am J Public Health 87:1928, 1997
27. Sweat MD, Denison JA: Reducing HIV incidence in developing countries with structural and environmental interventions. AIDS 9(Suppl A):S251, 1995

28. O'Reilly KR, Piot P: International perspectives on individual and community approaches to the prevention of sexually transmitted disease and human immunodeficiency virus infection. J Infect Dis 174(Suppl 2): S214, 1996

29. Lamptey PR, Kamenga MC, Weir SS: Prevention of sexual transmission of HIV in sub-Saharan Africa: Lessons learned. AIDS 11(Suppl B):S63, 1997

30. Kotler P: Social Marketing: Changing Public Behavior by Persuasion. New York, Free Press, 1989

31. Family Health International: AIDS Control and Prevention Project, August 27, 1991–December 31, 1997, Final Report. Arlington, VA, Family Health International, 1998

32. Nelson KE, Celentano DD, Eiumtrakol S, et al: Changes in sexual behavior and a decline in HIV infection among young men in Thailand. N Engl J Med 335:297, 1996

33. Kamb ML, Dougles JM, Rhodes F, et al: A multicenter randomized controlled trial evaluating HIV prevention counseling (Project Respect): Preliminary results. In: Abstracts of the XIth International Conference on AIDS, Vancouver, 1996, Abstract Th.C.4380

34. Curtis R, Holmes KK: Individual-level risk assessment for STD/HIV infection. In Homes KK, et al. (eds): Sexually Transmitted Diseases, 3rd ed. New York, McGraw-Hill, 1998

35. Kahn JG: The cost-effectiveness of HIV prevention targeting: How much more bang for the buck? Am J Public Health 86:1, 1996

36. National Academy of Sciences: Assessing the Social and Behavioral Science Base for HIV/AIDS Prevention and Intervention: Workshop Summary. Washington, DC, National Academy Press, 1995

37. The World Bank: Confronting AIDS: Public Priorities in a Global Epidemic. New York, Oxford University Press, 1997

38. Jemmott JB III, Jemmott LS, Fong GT: Abstinence and safer sex HIV risk-reduction interventions for African American adolescents: A randomized controlled trial. JAMA 279:1529, 1998

39. Coates TJ, Collins C: Preventing HIV infection. Sci Am 279:96, 1998

40. Des Jarlais DC, Padian NS, Winkelstein W Jr: Targeted HIV-prevention programs. N Engl J Med 331: 1451, 1994

41. MacNeil JM, Anderson S: Beyond the dichotomy: Linking HIV prevention with care. AIDS 1998 (in press)

42. De Vincenzi I: A longitudinal study of human immunodeficiency virus transmission by heterosexual partners. N Engl J Med 331:341, 1994

43. Deschamps MM, Pape JW, Hafner A, et al: Heterosexual transmission of HIV in Haiti. Ann Intern Med 125:324, 1996

44. Rietmeijer CA, Wolitski RJ, Fishbein M, et al: Sex hustling, injection drug use, and non-gay identification by men who have sex with men: Associations with high-risk sexual behaviors and condom use. Sex Transm Dis 25:353, 1998

45. Warner L, Clay-Warner J, Boles J, Williamson J: Assessing condom use practices: Implications for evaluating method and user effectiveness. Sex Transm Dis 25:273, 1998

46. Sangi-Haghpeykar H, Poindexter AN 3rd: Planned condom use among women undergoing tubal sterilization. Sex Transm Dis 25:335, 1998

47. Hanenberg RS, Rojanapithayakorn W, Kunasol P, et al: Impact of Thailand's HIV-control programme as indicated by the decline of sexually transmitted diseases. Lancet 344:243, 1994

48. Albert AE, Warner DL, Hatcher RA: Facilitating condom use with clients during commercial sex in Nevada's legal brothels. Am J Public Health 88:643, 1998

49. Ethiopia Condom Social Marketing Project: Project Sales Figures. Washington, DC, Population Services International, 1996

50. Crabbé F, Tchupo JP, Manchester T, et al: Prepackaged therapy for urethritis: The "MSTOP" experience in Cameroon. Sex Transm Infect 1998 (in press)

51. UNDP/UNFPA/WHO/World Bank Special Programme of Research, Development and Research Training in Human Reproduction: The Female Condom: A Review. Geneva, World Health Organization, 1997

52. Musuba E, Morrison DS, Sunkutu MR, et al: Longterm use of the female condom among couples at high risk of human immunodeficiency virus infection in Zambia. Sex Transm Dis 25:260, 1998

53. Burton DR, Moore JP: why do we not have an HIV vaccine and how can we make one? Nature Med 4: 495, 1998

54. Heilman CA, Baltimore D: HIV vaccines—where are we going? Nature Med 4:532, 1998

55. AIDS Vaccine Evaluation Group: The AVEG Information Handbook. Data Coordinating Analysis Center, Potomac, MD, 1998

56. Moore A, McGuirk P, Adams S, et al: Immunization with a soluble recombinant HIV protein entrapped in biodegradable microparticles induces HIV-specific CD8+ cytotoxic T lymphocytes and CD4+ Th1 cells. Vaccine 13:1741, 1995

57. Blower SM, McLean AR: Prophylactic vaccines, risk behavior change, and the probability of eradicating HIV in San Francisco. Science 265:1451, 1994

58. Gerberding JL: Prophylaxis for occupational exposure to HIV. Ann Intern Med 125:497, 1996

59. Connor EM, Sperling RS, Gelber R, et al: Reduction of maternal-infant transmission of human immunodeficiency virus type 1 with zidovudine treatment. N Engl J Med 331:1173, 1994

60. Vernazza PL, Gilliam BL, Flepp M, et al: Effect of antiviral treatment on the shedding of HIV-1 in semen. AIDS 11:1249, 1997

61. Gilliam BL, Dyer JR, Fiscus SA, et al: Effects of reverse transcriptase inhibitor therapy on the HIV-1 viral burden in semen. J Acquir Immune Defic Syndr Hum Retrovirol 15:54, 1997

62. Gupta P, Mellors J, Kingsley L, et al: High viral load in semen of HIV-1 infected men at all stages of disease and its reduction by therapy with protease and nonnucleoside RT inhibitors. J Virol 71:6271, 1997

63. Cu-Uvin S, Caliendo A, Flanigan TP, et al: Cervicovaginal HIV-1 secretion and plasma viral load in HIV seropositive women. In: Abstracts of the 1997 National Conference on Women and HIV, 1997, p 113

64. Cu-Uvin S, Caliendo A, Russo R, et al: HIV-1 RNA levels in the genital tract of women on antiretroviral therapy. In: Abstracts of the 5th Conference on Retroviruses and Opportunistic Infections, Chicago, 1998, p 212, Abstract 713

65. Eron JJ, Vernazza PL, Johnston DM, et al: Resistance of HIV-1 to antiretroviral agents in blood and seminal plasma: Implications for transmission. AIDS 1998 (in press)

65a. Hecht FM, Grant RM, Petropoulos CJ, et al. Sexual transmission of an HIV-1 variant resistant to multiple reverse-transcriptase and protease inhibitors. N Engl J Med 339:307, 1998

66. Katz M, Gerberding J: Postexposure treatment of people exposed to the human immunodeficiency virus through sexual contact or injection-drug use. N Engl J Med 336:1097, 1997

67. Evans B, Derbyshire J, Cartledge J: Should preventive antiretroviral treatment be offered following sexual exposure to HIV? Not yet! Sex Transm Infect 74:146, 1998

68. Vernazza PL, Eron JJ, Fiscus SA, et al: Sexual transmission of HIV: Infectiousness and prevention. AIDS 13:155, 1998

69. Hoffman IF, Jere CS, Taylor TE, et al: The effect of P. falciparum malaria on HIV-1 blood plasma concentration: Implications for HIV-1 progressions and transmission. J Infect Dis (in press)

70. Goletti D, Weissman D, Jackson RW, et al: Effect of Mycobacterium tuberculosis on HIV replication: Role of immune activation. J Immunol 157:1271, 1996

71. Plummer FA, Simonsen JN, Cameron DW, et al: Cofactors in male-female sexual transmission of human immunodeficiency virus type 1. J Infect Dis 163:233, 1991

72. Cohen M, Hoffman I, Royce R, et al: Reduction of concentration of HIV-1 in semen after treatment of urethritis: Implications for prevention of sexual transmission of HIV-1. Lancet 349:1868, 1997

73. Kreiss J, Willerford DM, Hensel M, et al: Association between cervical inflammation and cervical shedding of human immunodeficiency virus DNA. J Infect Dis 170:1597, 1994

74. Moss GB, Overbaugh J, Welch M, et al: Human immunodeficiency virus DNA in urethral secretions in men: Association with gonococcal urethritis and CD4 cell depletion. J Infect Dis 172:1469, 1995

75. Cameron DW, Simonsen JN, D'costa LJ, et al: Female to male transmission of human immunodeficiency virus type 1: Risk factors for seroconversion in men. Lancet 2:403, 1989

76. Laga M, Alary M, Nzila N, et al: Condom promotion, sexually transmitted disease treatment, and declining incidence of HIV-1 infection in female Zairian sex workers. Lancet 244:243, 1994

77. Levine WC, Pope V, Bhoomkar A, et al: Increase in endocervical CD4 lymphocytes among women with nonulcerative sexually transmitted diseases. J Infect Dis 177:164, 1998

78. Sewankambo N, Gray RH, Wawer MJ, et al: HIV-1 infection associated with abnormal vaginal flora morphology and bacterial vaginosis. Lancet 350:546, 1997

79. Taha TE, Dallabetta GA, Hoover DR, et al: Trends of HIV-1 and sexually transmitted diseases among pregnant and postpartum women in urban Malawi. AIDS 12:197, 1998

80. Lacritz EM, Satten GA, Aberle-Grasse J, et al: Estimated risk of transmission of the human immunodeficiency virus by screened blood in the United States. N Engl J Med 333:1721, 1995

81. Gilmore N: Blood and blood product safety. In Mann J, Tarantola D (eds): AIDS In The World II. New York, Oxford University Press, 1996, p 287

82. Watts C, Goodman H, Muyinda G: Estimation of the number of HIV infections averted by screening of blood. Lancet 345:783, 1995

83. Holmberg SD: The estimated prevalence and incidence of HIV in 96 large US metropolitan areas. Am J Public Health 86:642, 1996

84. Anderson RM: The spread of HIV and sexual mixing patterns. In Mann J, Tarantola D (eds): AIDS In The World II. New York, Oxford University Press, 1996, p 71

85. Anderson RM, May RM, Boily MC, et al: The spread of HIV-1 in Africa: Sexual contact patterns and the predicted demographic impact of AIDS. Nature 352: 581, 1991

86. National AIDS Programme Management: Prevention of HIV Transmission Through Injection Drug Use. Geneva, Global Programme on AIDS, World Health Organization, 1993

87. Sperling RS, Shapiro DE, Coombs RW, et al: Maternal viral load, zidovudine treatment, and the risk of transmission of human immunodeficiency virus type 1 from mother to infant. N Engl J Med 335:1621, 1996

88. Gabiano C, Rovo PA, de Martino M, et al: Mother-to-child transmission of human immunodeficiency virus type 1: Risk of infection and correlates with transmission. Pediatrics 90:369, 1992

89. Kreiss J: Breastfeeding and vertical transmission of HIV-1. Acta Paediatr Suppl 421:113, 1997

90. Newell ML: Mechanisms and timing of mother-to-child transmission of HIV-1. AIDS 12:831, 1998

91. Bigger JR, Miotti PG, Taha TE, et al: Perinatal intervention trial in Africa: Effect of a birth canal cleansing intervention to prevent HIV transmission. Lancet 347:1647, 1996

92. Dunn DT, Newell ML, Ades AE, et al: Risk of human immunodeficiency virus type 1 transmission through breastfeeding. Lancet 340:585, 1992

93. Dunn DT, Newell ML, Mayaux MJ, et al: Mode of delivery and vertical transmission of HIV-1: a review of prospective studies. J Acquir Immune Defic Syndr 7:1064, 1994

94. Kuhn L, Bobat R, Coutsoudis A, et al: Cesarean deliveries and maternal-infant HIV transmission: Results from a prospective study in South Africa. J Acquir Immune Defic Syndr Hum Retrovirol 11:478, 1996

95. European Collaborative Study: Risk factors for mother-to-child transmission of HIV-1. Lancet 339: 1007, 1992

96. Mayaux MN, Blanche S, Rouzioux C, et al: Maternal factors associated with perinatal HIV-1 transmission: The French cohort study: 7 years of follow-up observation. J Acquir Immune Defic Syndr 8:188, 1995

97. Wiktor SZ, Edpini E, Nduati RW: Prevention of mother-to-child transmission of HIV-1 in Africa. AIDS 11(Suppl B):S79, 1997

98. Calgrove R, Pitt J, Chung PH, et al: Selective vertical transmission of HIV-1 zidovudine resistance mutations. In: Abstracts of the 5th Conference on Retroviruses and Opportunistic Infections, 1998, Abstract 265

99. John GC, Kreiss J: Mother-to-child transmission of human immunodeficiency virus type 1. Epidemiol Rev 18:149, 1996

100. Bertolli J, St. Louis ME, Simonds RJ, et al: Estimating the timing of mother-to-child transmission of human immunodeficiency virus in a breast-feeding population, Kinshasa, Zaire. J Infect Dis 174:722, 1996

101. Ekpini ER, Wikton SZ, Satten GA, et al: Late postnatal mother-to-child transmission of HIV-1 in Abidjan, Cote d'Ivoire. Lancet 349:253, 1997

102. Brown KH, Black RE, Dreed de Kanashiro H, et al: Infant feeding practices and their relationship with diarrheal and other diseases in Huascar (Lima), Peru. Pediatrics 83:31, 1989

103. Jacquez JA, Koopman JS, Simon CP, et al: Role of the primary infection in epidemics of HIV infection in gay cohorts. J Acquir Immune Defic Syndr 7:1169, 1994

104. Cohen MS, Dallabetta G, Holmes KK: A new deal in HIV prevention: Lessions from the global approach. Ann Intern Med 120:340, 1994

105. Stryker J, Coates TJ, DeCarlo P, et al: Looking back, looking ahead. JAMA 273:1143, 1995

106. Osborn JE: AIDS prevention: Issues and strategies. AIDS 2(Suppl 1):S229, 1998

107. Scheper-Hughes N: AIDS, public health, and human rights in Cuba. Lancet 342:965, 1993

108. Cohen MS, Henderson GE, Hamilton H, et al: Eradication of syphilis in China—lessons for the 20th century? J Infect Dis 174(Suppl 2):S223, 1996

109. Grosskurth H, Mosha F, Todd J, et al: Impact of improved treatment of sexually transmitted disease on HIV infection in rural Tanzania: Randomized control trial. Lancet 346:530, 1995

110. Gilson L, Mkanje R, Grosskurth H, et al: Cost-effectiveness of improved STD treatment services as a preventive intervention against HIV in Mwanza region, Tanzania. Lancet 350:1805, 1997

111. Wawer MJ, Sewankambo NK, Gray RH, et al: Community-based trial of mass STD treatment for HIV control, Rakai, Uganda: Preliminary data on STD declines. In: Abstracts of the XIth International Conference on AIDS, Vancouver, 1996, Abstract C.443

112. Wawer MJ, Sewankambo NK, Serwadda D, et al: Control of sexually transmitted diseases for AIDS prevention in Uganda: A randomised community trial. Lancet 353:525, 1999

113. Louv WC, Austin H, Alesander WJ, et al: A clinical trial of nonoxynol-9 for preventing gonococcal and chlamydial infections. J Infect Dis 158:518, 1988

114. Barbone F, Austin H, Louv WC, et al: A follow-up study of methods of contraception, sexual activity and rates of trichomoniasis, candidiasis, and bacterial vaginosis. Am J Obstet Gynecol 163:510, 1990

115. Kreiss J, Ngugi E, Holmes K, et al: Efficacy of nonoxynol 9 contraceptive sponge use in preventing heterosexual acquisition of HIV in Nairobi prostitutes. JAMA 268:477, 1992

116. Roddy RE, Zekeng L, Ryan KA, et al: A controlled trial of nonoxynol-9 film to reduce male-to-female transmission of sexually transmitted diseases. N Engl J Med 339:504, 1998

117. Tsai CC, Emau P, Follis KE, et al: Effectiveness of postinoculation (R)-9-(2-phosphonylmethoxypropyl) adenine treatment for prevention of persistent simian immunodeficiency virus SIVmne infection depends critically on timing of initiation and duration of treatment. J Virol 72:4265, 1998

118. Hayes R, Wawer M, Gray R, et al: Randomized trials of STD treatment for HIV prevention: Report of an international workshop. Genitourinary Med 73:432, 1997

119. St. Louis M, Holmes KK: A critical assessment of STD prevention. In Holmes KK, et al. (eds): Sexually Transmitted Diseases, 3rd ed. New York, McGraw-Hill, 1998

32 HIV Exposure Risk Assessment and Prophylactic Treatment

JULIE LOUISE GERBERDING

Health care workers exposed to blood and other body fluids risk infection with HIV. Although rare, nosocomial transmission of HIV to patients is also an important issue. Defining the risks of HIV transmission in health care settings and developing policies for protecting health care workers and their patients are important aspects of care delivery in the AIDS era. In the past 2 years, advances in both primary prevention (exposure prevention) and secondary prevention (postexposure prophylaxis) have contributed to occupational safety. Not surprisingly, interest in postexposure treatment has moved beyond the realm of occupational exposure in health care settings to the community, where persons at risk through recent sexual and injection drug use behaviors could benefit from prophylactic antiviral treatment. In this chapter, the current status of occupational exposure prevention, exposure risk assessment, and postexposure treatment are reviewed. In addition, the rationale for extending the principles of occupational exposure management to nonoccupational exposures in the community are reviewed.

PATIENT-TO-PROVIDER TRANSMISSION

The risk of occupational HIV transmission has been evaluated in prospective studies of exposed health care workers at several medical centers around the world.[1-12] In these studies, both the numerator (number of infections) and the denominator (number of HIV exposures) are known and so the probability of transmission through various exposure routes can be estimated. Pooled data indicate that the average risk of HIV transmission associated with needle punctures or similar percutaneous injuries is 0.32% (21 infections following 6498 exposures; 95% confidence interval = 0.18% to 0.46%).[1] The current estimate of mucocutaneous transmission risk is 0.09% (one infection following 2885 exposures through mucous membranes or nonintact skin).[3] This mucocutaneous risk estimate may be biased, however, because the single-transmission event was actually reported before prospective data were collected from the involved institution.

These risk estimates are useful in evaluating populations of exposed persons but do not necessarily pertain to the probability of infection in individual cases. The factors influencing infectivity have not been completely defined, but the amount of virus transmitted during the exposure (inoculum) may be very important. The exposure inoculum is dependent on the titer of virus in the source fluid and the volume of that fluid. Virus titer is the sum of cell-free virus (viral load) plus cell-associated virus, but only viral load measurements are readily available in most clinical settings.

To some extent, the titer of circulating HIV can be approximated (albeit imperfectly) by ascertaining the clinical stage of HIV infection in the source patient. In general, circulating titers of infectious HIV are highest at the time of seroconversion and during advanced stages of AIDS.[13-15] Recent data from the Centers for Disease Control and Prevention (CDC) suggest that the odds of acquiring infection after percutaneous exposure are almost six times higher when the source patient has preterminal AIDS (defined by death within 2 months) than when the source has earlier stages of infection (Table 32-1).[16] This may be a consequence of high

TABLE 32–1. Factors Independently Associated with Percutaneous Injury Transmission Risk ($p < .05$) by Logistic Regression Analysis in a Case–Control Study[16]

RISK FACTOR	ODDS RATIO
Deep injury	15.0
Visible blood on sharp device	6.2
Device used to enter blood vessel	4.3
Source patient with terminal AIDS	5.6
Postexposure zidovudine treatment	0.19

Data from Centers for Disease Control and Prevention.

virus titers in these patients, or could also reflect differences in HIV phenotype or genetic subtypes present in late-stage disease. Viral load per se is not a reliable predictor of risk. To date, at least three cases of HIV transmission from source patients with "undetectable" viral loads have been documented.[17,18]

Deep (intramuscular) penetrations, large-bore hollow needles, and injections of blood are factors associated with most of the reported needlestick accidents causing occupational infections. In a laboratory model of needle injuries, these same factors predicted the amount of blood transferred to the skin (exposure volume).[19] Deep punctures (defined as injuries penetrating the skin and resulting in spontaneous bleeding), injuries caused by devices visibly contaminated with blood before the accident, and injuries caused by devices that had entered an artery or vein prior to the accident were independently associated with infection risk in the CDC's retrospective study. (Table 32–1).[16] Large volumes of blood, prolonged duration of contact, and a portal of entry are common features in the reported cases of infection through mucosal surfaces or skin, but the number of cases is too small to identify and quantify risk factors for infections through these routes.[1]

The efficiency of occupational transmission could be influenced by other factors. The presence of intracellular (as opposed to cell-free) virus in the inoculum or the genotype or phenotype of the virus strain may be relevant to transcutaneous infectivity. The immunologic response of the recipient health care provider could affect the probability of successful infection. Recent in vitro studies demonstrate that circulating T lymphocytes from uninfected health care workers who were exposed to HIV proliferate in vitro in response to HIV antigens.[20–22] This observation suggests that the cellular immune system may be an important host response, capable of "aborting" transcutaneous HIV infection.

Blood or bloody fluid has been implicated as the source of the exposure in all infections occurring in clinical health care workers. Other body fluids, including saliva, tears, and urine, may contain HIV, but the titer of HIV in these fluids is usually much lower than the titer found in blood and semen. While HIV transmission is very unlikely following exposure to most non-bloody body fluids, these fluids could contain other viruses or pathogens and should be considered potentially infectious when planning infection control interventions.

Cutaneous exposure involving intact skin has not been linked to HIV infection in any setting. Although Langerhans' cells and other subcutaneous cells possess CD4 receptors, these cells are protected from primary infection by an intact integument. However, transcutaneous inoculation during parenteral needlestick injury, or contamination of skin wounds or lesions, is hypothesized to promote primary infection of subcutaneous target cells. No HIV transmission risk from close personal contact with patients, exposure to airborne droplets, or contact with contaminated environmental surfaces or fomites has been observed, nor have aerosols been associated with HIV infection in any setting to date.

As of June 1997, 52 cases of documented occupational HIV transmission among health care workers in the United States were reported to the CDC.[23] Occupational transmission was proven by demonstrating HIV antibody seroconversion temporally related to a discreet accidental HIV exposure event. Needlestick exposure or laceration was the cause of infection in the majority. Exposure to HIV through breaks in the skin or mucous membrane inoculation was the route of transmission in only five cases. In addition, 114 health care workers with possible occupational infection were reported to the CDC.[23] These health care workers provided no history of nonoccupational exposure risks and all recalled contact with blood or body fluids. However, the relationship between exposure and infection could not be proven because a baseline HIV test at the time of exposure was not performed.

The infections reported to the CDC almost certainly do not include all cases of occupational infection. In many states, HIV is not a reportable condition until AIDS develops, and some occupational infections may not yet be recognized or reported. Most experts agree that the CDC data do include a large majority of the occupational infections. Efforts to improve surveillance and reporting of cases are in progress. In the future, a more complete assessment of the frequency of such events may be possible. Success will depend, at least in part, on the willingness of exposed health care workers to undergo HIV testing and disclose their serostatus to public health agencies. Concerns about employment, loss of insurance, and stigmatization are strong disincentives for participating in a voluntary HIV reporting system, and must be addressed before reliable surveillance can be accomplished.

PROVIDER-TO-PATIENT TRANSMISSION

Transmission of HIV to patients could occur by direct inoculation of blood or other infected body fluids or through use of contaminated materials or equipment. Direct inoculation is possible when an infected health care provider is injured and then bleeds into the patient, when the contaminated instrument or object causing injury recontacts the patient's tissue, or when the provider is injured by bone, hardware, or other sharps fixed in the patient.[24-36] The frequency of injuries severe enough to cause bleeding into the wounds or tissues of patients undergoing invasive procedures is unknown but likely to be low. Recontact exposures, when an instrument that injured a provider then passes through the tissue of the patient, are more common. "Shear injuries" (trauma to the hand while manually tightening sutures) have been proposed as a related mechanism of exposure.[27,28]

The HIV transmission risk associated with recontact exposures is unknown. To date, a single case of HIV infection has been attributed to transmission during a surgical procedure, but the exact mode of transmission has not been determined[29]. The only other reported case of probable provider-to-patient HIV transmission occurred in a single cluster involving a Florida dentist with AIDS.[30] Six patients in this practice were infected with virus strains that were genetically similar to the dentist's isolates. The exact mechanism by which the patients were infected has not been established. Speculations about the routes of infection include direct inoculation of blood or recontact with a contaminated instrument following sharps injuries to the provider (though no injuries were recalled), cross-contamination via handpieces or instruments that were used on the provider and then

subsequently reused without proper disinfection, and intentional exposure. Insufficient evidence is available to identify which, if any, of these potential exposure routes played a role in the transmission events in this practice.

It is probable that additional cases of provider-to-patient HIV transmission will eventually emerge. Even so, these events must be extremely rare.[31] From the public health perspective, nosocomial transmission does not contribute to the AIDS epidemic, and special policies to restrict the practice of infected health care workers will have little if any measurable impact on the spread of the infection. However, implementing safer surgical techniques that prevent provider injuries and recontacts could be very effective in preventing the growing list of blood-borne pathogens that pose a risk to providers and (albeit rarely) their patients.[32]

PATIENT-TO-PATIENT TRANSMISSION

Instruments contaminated with blood from infected patients could transmit HIV to other patients when proper disinfection procedures are not followed.[33] Even though HIV is a relatively fragile virus, survival in clots of blood or tissue (especially in a warm or moist environment) for several hours is possible. If disinfection protocols are not rigorously followed, then nosocomial transmission from one patient to another is potentially a more likely event than is transmission from an infected provider to a patient. The practice of obtaining medication from a vial contaminated by a needle used on a previous patient is contraindicated, but does occasionally occur.[34,35] Although HIV transmission through this route has not been proven, hepatitis B virus transmission has been associated with multiple-use medication vials. Needle reuse has also been associated with nosocomial infections, including a number of cases of HIV transmission to children.[36]

Accidental infusion of radiolabeled blood products from HIV-infected products for nuclear medicine studies into the wrong patient has resulted in patient infections.[37] A cluster of outpatient surgical patients who received care on the same day as an infected patient has also been reported, but the route of cross-contamination has not been determined.[38] Although rare, these anecdotes clearly illustrate the potential for patient infection when safety protocols and disinfection techniques are not followed.

RISK REDUCTION: INFECTION CONTROL

Avoiding contact with potentially infected body fluids and tissues is an essential component of risk reduction for health care workers. Preventing needlestick injuries and other parenteral exposures is likely to have the biggest impact on reducing HIV transmission in most health care settings. Although nearly all cases of occupational HIV transmission involved exposure to blood, common sense and concern for preventing transmission of other nosocomial pathogens dictate that other body fluids also should be considered potentially infectious.

Universal precautions were recommended by the CDC for all patients, regardless of diagnosis, for preventing transmission of blood-borne pathogens.[39-41] These precautions include the use of gloves for procedures where contact with blood, bloody body fluids, and certain other fluids (amniotic fluid, semen, vaginal fluid, cerebrospinal fluid, serial transudates/exudates, and inflammatory exudates) might occur, the use of masks and protective eyewear when splatter of such body fluids is anticipated, and the use of gowns or other protective garments when clothing is likely to be soiled. Body substance isolation (BSI) is an alternative system of infection control practiced by many institutions.[42-44] A single standard of precautions, based on the anticipated degree of exposure to all body fluids and tissues regardless of the infectious disease diagnosed or suspected, is implemented at the moment of initial contact with the patient. The main difference between these two infection control systems is that the CDC isolation system considers the type of infection suspected, whereas BSI is based on the degree of contact anticipated. The CDC has recently developed a new isolation system for hospitalized patients.[45] In this new system, components of universal precautions and BSI are merged into "standard precautions." Standard precautions apply to all patients and require the use of gloves, protective clothing, and other barriers as needed to prevent direct contact with all body fluids (except sweat).

All three of these isolation protocols emphasize prevention of needlestick injury and use of barrier protection for avoiding exposure to potentially infectious materials, and do not require labeling of patients or specimens in order to be implemented. Safer needle devices, which are engineered to retract, cover, or blunt the needle after use, are gaining acceptance. These new devices may contribute to a reduction in the frequency of postuse injuries, providing that training is adequate to ensure their proper use, but they are less likely to have an impact on during-use injury rates.[46,47]

Needles and other sharps used during invasive procedures are undergoing scrutiny to prevent injuries that could expose the provider (and then the patient). Blunt suture needles are gaining acceptance and are associated with a reduction in needle injury risk without adverse patient outcomes.[48] Using the index finger of the nondominant hand to retract tissue or to palpate the needle tip during suturing accounts for a large proportion of intraoperative injuries. Substituting instruments for manual manipulations or use of special protective coverings is advocated to ameliorate this problem. Gloves constructed of monofilament polymers resistant to tears have become available for use when manipulation of bone fragments or suture wires is needed, but use is not widespread because of the associated decrease in tactile sensation. The benefit of double gloving, glove reinforcement, and new glove materials in preventing tissue trauma during suture manipulations has not been evaluated. Efforts are underway to identify other changes that may impact favorably on injury risks during invasive procedures.

MANAGING OCCUPATIONAL EXPOSURES TO HIV

Determining whether or not exposure has actually occurred is not always simple. Health care workers may not report exposures for a variety of reasons, and may under- or overestimate the severity of the exposure. A careful history will usually permit assignment of the exposure into one of the following broad categories: (1) needle puncture, (2) injury by non-needle sharps (or similar injury resulting in direct transcutaneous exposure), (3) mucous membrane inoculation, (4) contamination of open skin wound or lesion, (5) contamination of nonintact skin, or (6) a bite.

Needlesticks and other percutaneous accidents should be further characterized to help assess the exposure severity. The presence of factors known or suspected to affect the virus titer (viral load, clinical stage of HIV illness in the source patient, antiviral treatment history) and exposure volume (deep punctures, visible bloody device, device used in an artery or vein, actual injection of blood) should be recorded

(Table 32–1).[23,49] In addition, the size and type of needle or instrument involved (suture needle, hollow-bore needle, scalpel, etc.), volume of blood actually injected (if any), location of the injury, wound appearance, amount of bleeding (spontaneous or induced), method and timing of decontamination, and duration of time that the contaminating fluid was ex vivo before the exposure occurred all should be established. Similarly, the type, volume, and duration of contact should be estimated for fluids implicated in mucous membrane and skin wound contacts.

Establishing the presence of HIV infection in the source patient can be difficult. HIV exposure can be assumed when patients are diagnosed with AIDS or are known to be HIV infected. Institutions vary in guidelines for testing source patients whose HIV status is unclear. In most, the probability of HIV infection is assessed by clinical and epidemiologic criteria. Patients perceived to be at risk are then counseled and asked to consent to testing. Routine testing of all source patients is gaining acceptance, especially where legislation has guaranteed access to this information. Rapid tests can help exclude infection when negative, but only when conducted and interpreted in reliable laboratories. Positive rapid tests must be confirmed before disclosure to patients.

In the past 5 years, more than 95% of all source patients with HIV infection at San Francisco General Hospital, an institution with an aggressive source patient testing program, were already known to have HIV at the time the exposure occurred. The only previously undiagnosed infected source patients had obvious behavioral risks for infection (men who had sex with men and/or used injection drugs). In other words, the pretest probability of HIV infection among source patients who were not injection drug users or men who had sex with men was zero at this institution. This experience argues against the presumption of HIV infection in untested source patients until proven otherwise (i.e., until a negative HIV test is obtained) unless the source is at high risk for HIV.

The exposed health care worker should be encouraged to have a HIV test or have serum banked as soon as possible after exposure has occurred (baseline).[1,23,49] Without a negative baseline HIV test, proving that infection was temporally related to the exposure event is extremely difficult. In rare cases, demonstrating close genetic similarity in virus sequences obtained from the source patient and the infected health care provider can confirm the source of exposure, but these studies are expensive, difficult to obtain, and sometimes difficult to interpret. Subsequent HIV testing, usually performed 6 weeks, 3 months, and 6 months after exposure, is recommended when HIV is present or potentially present in the exposure source. Sequential testing is extremely useful in allaying fears, documenting seronegativity, and, rarely, diagnosing HIV infection. HIV seroconversion occurs within 3 months of exposure in more than half of occupational infections, and is expected within 6 months in virtually all. For this reason, testing beyond 6 months is not routinely advised.[23,50,51]

Most cases of occupational infection documented more than 6 months after exposure did not have a 6-month test, so the time of seroconversion could not be ascertained. However, seroconversion beyond 6 months has been reported; in two cases, the health care worker was co-infected with hepatitis C virus (HCV) and developed early and severe hepatitis.[23] Although anecdotal, these cases suggest that health care workers who are exposed to both HIV and HCV, and who acquire HCV (seroconvert), should be tested for HIV for up to 12 to 18 months after exposure, especially if clinical hepatitis C is apparent.

Because symptoms of acute retroviral infection (fever, lymphadenopathy, rash, headache, profound fatigue) are associated with approximately 80% of reported occupational infections, persons sustaining exposures should be advised to return for evaluation if a compatible illness occurs. Enzyme-linked immunosorbent assay HIV antibody tests may be negative or indeterminate during the early phases of seroconversion illness. Viral load tests (HIV RNA polymerase chain reaction [PCR]) immunoblot, virus cultures, or HIV p24 antigen tests may be more sensitive methods for detecting early infection. In the absence of a compatible illness, viral load testing or other gene amplification studies should *not* be used to follow exposed health care workers. False-positive results (which occur in 2% to 3% of tests) result in enormous anxiety for the health care worker and further complicate treatment. Moreover, latent infections detected by HIV RNA or DNA PCR rarely, if ever, are detected in seronegative health care workers.[2]) In at least one case of seroconversion, HIV antibody was detected before a DNA PCR test was positive.[5]

Postexposure counseling by experienced care providers familiar with the special medical and psychological needs of exposed health care workers is essential.[52] Counseling should provide information about the degree of risk present, options for follow-up, a description of the confidentiality procedures in place, and infection control procedures to prevent similar occurrences in the future. Counselors should be alert to the concerns of the sexual partners, co-workers, family, and friends of the exposed worker. Referral for ongoing supportive therapy during the follow-up interval is helpful for the minority of exposed persons who experience difficulty in adjusting to the stress inherent in waiting the 6 months for testing to be complete.

The CDC recommends "safer" sexual practices and other behavior changes to minimize the potential for transmission until infection has been ruled out by a negative antibody test 6 months after the exposure.[23] Unfortunately, this advice frequently produces confusion and anxiety in the exposed person. Counselors are faced with the difficult task of communicating a "mixed message" about the risk of infection: reassurance that occupational transmission is statistically unlikely, and conversely, advocacy of behaviors to prevent exchange of body fluids, to avoid pregnancy, and to defer blood donation until infection has been ruled out.

In some centers, advice is individualized to the specific situation. For example, persons sustaining trivial punctures with small-bore non-hollow needles minimally contaminated by blood from a low-risk untested source patient may decide to return for follow-up HIV testing for 6 months, but to comply with safer sex guidelines for a shorter interval of time. Likewise, recipients of deep intramuscular injections of infected blood may be cautioned to compulsively follow all guidelines for preventing transmission.

Patients exposed to provider's blood should be managed with the same standard of care applied to occupational exposures. A system for confidential reporting of such exposures should be developed and communicated to hospital staff. It is the ethical and professional responsibility of the involved provider to undergo testing for blood-borne pathogens and to communicate test results to the clinician responsible for the patient's postexposure care.

POSTEXPOSURE PROPHYLAXIS FOR OCCUPATIONAL EXPOSURES

Interest in postexposure chemoprophylaxis for occupationally exposed health care workers has increased since zidovudine was licensed for pal-

liating HIV infection in persons with advanced disease.[1,23,49,53,54] Zidovudine or other antiretroviral drugs may prevent or help abort HIV infection when administered soon after exposure (during the putative "window of opportunity") by preventing HIV replication in the initial target cells and allowing the antigen-independent or antigen-dependent host defenses to clear the exposure inoculum. This hypothesis is supported by animal studies of HIV pathogenesis. For example, in rhesus macaques exposed to intravaginal simian immunodeficiency virus, virus appears to remain associated with the mucosal dendritic cells without proprogation for the first 24 hours after infection, but after 24 to 48 hours, active replication in the regional lymph nodes is evident.[55] Virus is disseminated to the peripheral blood by 5 days after exposure in this model.

The relevance of animal models of retrovirus infection to human infection with HIV is not established. Experiments using murine, feline, and human retroviruses in animal inoculated with high titers of virus indicate that zidovudine can prevent viremia and illness under some conditions. Protection is most apparent when treatment is started within 24 hours of exposure. Recent primate studies indicate that at least four factors affect the efficacy of prophylactic treatment: virus inoculum, duration of treatment, antiviral treatment regimen, and delay until onset of treatment.[56,57] From this perspective, current standards for chemoprophylaxis are designed to maximize the potential treatment benefit: occupational exposure almost always involves a relatively small inoculum, treatment with two or more drugs is started within hours of the exposure, and treatment is continued for 4 weeks.

The outcome of two studies prompted renewed enthusiasm for postexposure antiretroviral treatment. First, data from ACTG protocol 076 demonstrated that zidovudine treatment could reduce the risk of perinatal HIV transmission by 80%.[58,59] This study included only women who had never received zidovudine before, and involved treatment of the infected mothers during the last two trimesters and of the newborns for 6 weeks. Although this experience cannot be generalized to transcutaneous exposures experienced by health care workers, it does demonstrate the prophylactic efficacy of antiretroviral treatment under some clinical circumstances.

The second study, the CDC's retrospective case–control study of occupational HIV transmission, is directly relevant to health care workers.[16] In this study, those who received zidovudine treatment after exposure were 81% less likely (odds ratio = .19) to acquire infection than those who did not receive treatment (Table 33–1), independent of the other variables affecting the probability of transmission. Cases and controls had equal access to treatment. The study's retrospective design precluded determination of the dosing regimen or treatment duration most likely to be effective. Based on this study, the U.S. Public Health Service (USPHS) changed its postexposure treatment guidelines and is now recommending prophylactic antiviral treatment for percutaneous exposures, especially when other risks for infection are present.[23]

The frequency of zidovudine resistance among source patients undergoing treatment increases with the duration of therapy. In addition, transmission of zidovudine-resistant virus has been documented. Zidovudine prophylaxis is unlikely to be effective when the exposure involves resistant virus. New postexposure treatment guidelines recommend combination therapy with zidovudine *and* lamivudine for most occupational exposures (basic regimen)[23] (Table 32–2). A protease inhibitor, usually indinavir or nelfinavir, is recommend in addition to the nucleoside analogs when the exposure is especially high risk and/or the source patient has recently taken both zidovudine and lamivudine (expanded regimen).

Failure of zidovudine prophylaxis has been documented in at least 11 health care workers who were treated after occupational exposures.[60] These cases indicate that zidovudine treatment is not always successful, but, in the absence of a controlled trial, the efficacy of postexposure treatment cannot be established. Conduct of such a study is difficult given the relatively low rate of seroconversion, which necessitates evaluation of an extremely large sample of exposed persons to measure efficacy.

Most parenteral exposures to HIV (99.7%) do not transmit HIV infection. Antiretroviral chemoprophylaxis is a promising but unproved prevention strategy that appears to be protective in select cases. While it is hoped that the incidence of serious adverse events associated with combination treatment will be low, experience with the new agents alone or in combination with zidovudine is limited.[61,62] In my view, prophylactic treatment is still experimental therapy, despite the USPHS endorsement. Health care workers electing treatment should carefully consider the potential risks as well as benefits associated with treatment and provide written consent (or perhaps declension) to document their decision about treatment.

Prophylactic treatment should be started as soon as possible (within hours) after the exposure to maximize the chance of efficacy.[23,49] The optimal dose and duration of treatment have not been established. Treatment is usually recommended for 4 weeks. Treatment of pregnant or breast-feeding women or persons not practicing effective contraception is not contraindicated when the exposure imposes a risk of HIV infection, but the decision must be made with full disclosure of potential risks, ideally in conjunction with an expert in perinatal HIV treatment. Close monitoring for hematologic, hepatic, pancreatic, renal, and neurologic dysfunction is essential for all who elect treatment.[23,29] Adverse reactions should be reported to the Food and Drug Administration and to the drug manufacturer(s).

At San Francisco General Hospital, alternatives to the basic regimen have been developed to help manage exposures when the source patient is taking antiretroviral drugs and drug resistance is suspected[63] (Table 32–3). This approach is based on a "worst-case scenario" and assumes that circulating infectious virions are apt to be resistant to antivirals taken by the source patient in the past 30 days. Hopefully, when tests for HIV drug resistance are more readily available, and/or reliable predictors of drug resistance are identified, choosing drugs for prophylaxis will involve less guesswork.

Several guides to exposure risk assessment have been prepared to assist persons making treatment decisions,[23,49,63] but none has been validated in clinical studies. They are intended to provide general guidance but not an absolute measure of exposure risk. Treating clinicians who lack expertise in managing antiviral treatments are encouraged to seek consultation with local experts, or to call the National Clinicians' Post-exposure Prophylaxis Hotline (PEPLine; 1-888-HIV-4911). This service, supported by the CDC and Health Resources and Services Administration is designed to assist clinicians who need immediate advice about managing an occupationally exposed health care worker, and is available 24 hours a day 7 days a week.

POSTEXPOSURE PROPHYLAXIS FOR SEXUAL AND INJECTION DRUG USE EXPOSURES TO HIV

The USPHS guidelines for managing occupational exposures advise that prophylaxis should be offered after mucosal as well as percutaneous

TABLE 32–2. Basic and Expanded Postexposure Prophylaxis Regimens

REGIMEN CATEGORY	APPLICATION	DRUG REGIMEN
Basic	Occupational HIV exposures for which there is a recognized transmission risk	4 weeks of both zidovudine 600 mg every day (in 2 or 3 divided doses) and lamivudine 150 mg twice a day
Expanded	Occupational HIV exposures that pose an increased risk for transmission (e.g., larger volume of blood and/or higher viral load)	Basic regimen plus either indinavir (800 mg every 8 hr) or nelfinavir (750 mg three times a day) for 4 wk

Adapted from Centers for Disease Control and Prevention. Public Health Service guidelines for the management of health-care worker exposures to HIV and recommendations for post-exposure prophylaxis. MMWR Morb Mortal Wkly Rep 47:1, 1998.

exposures to HIV.[23] These recommendations led to advocacy for access to treatment after sexual (mucosal) and injection drug use (percutaneous) exposures to HIV.[64–66] In fact, prophylactic antiretroviral treatment for community exposures to HIV is analogous to treatment after occupational exposures in several ways (Table 32–4). Although imperfect, available data suggest that, for anal and vaginal sex and injection drug use, the per-episode transmission risk is similar to (within an order of magnitude of) the risk associated with a typical needle puncture.[65–67] Moreover, the animal data that support the concept of a "window of opportunity" to intervene before infection is established (biologic plausibility) are based on a vaginal model of simian retrovirus infection (sexual), not a transcutaneous route (occupational).[56] The safety of antiviral treatment is a concern in both cases, and there is no reason to assume there are major differences in type, frequency, or severity of side effects when treating health care workers compared to persons in the community.[65,66]

Despite these similarities, providing treatment for community exposures presents unique challenges. One major question must be addressed before such programs become standard: What impact will access to postexposure prophylaxis for sexual and injection drug use exposures have on the overall rate of HIV transmission in the community? The optimistic view is that "marketing" access to preventive treatment will result in a net decrease in HIV transmission incidence. Persons at highest risk for acquiring or transmitting HIV, an otherwise very "hard-to-reach" group, will seek medical care, get an HIV test, and participate in risk-reduction counseling programs.[65,66] Those who are already infected will be diagnosed and referred for antiviral treatment, an intervention that not only will improve their prognosis but also will reduce their risk of infecting others. Those in the "window of opportunity" whose exposures do pose a risk of infection may benefit from prophylactic treatment. Finally, all who seek care could benefit from risk reduction counseling, and might be especially motivated to adopt safer behaviors in the context of realizing their personal risk.

The more pessimistic position is that providing postexposure treatments in the community will create a false sense of security and actually encourage risky behaviors.[65–67] As a result,

TABLE 33–3. Post-exposure Treatment Regimens at San Francisco General Hospital

CATEGORY	USE	REGIMEN
Basic	Exposures where treatment is indicated and the source patient/partner has not taken either drug in the past 30 days	4 wk of both zidovudine 600 mg every day (in 2 or 3 divided doses) and lamivudine (3TC) (150 mg twice a day)
Alternate I	Used when the source patient/partner has taken zidovudine in the past 30 days or is known to have AZT-resistant virus	4 wk of both 3TC (150 mg twice a day) and stavudine (d4T) (40 mg twice a day or 30 mg twice a day if <60 kg)
Alternate II	Used when the source patient/partner has taken both zidovudine and lamivudine in the past 30 days or is known to have resistant virus	4 wk of both d4T (40 mg twice a day or 30 mg twice a day if <60 kg) and didanosine (200 mg twice a day or 125 mg twice a day if <60 kg)
Protease inhibitor regimen	Used when the exposure is very high risk (large volume and high titer) or when drug resistance is suspected in the source patient/partner	4 wk of standard or alternate regimen plus either indinavir (800 mg every 8 hr) or nelfinavir (750 mg three times a day) the past 30 days

TABLE 32–4. Comparison of Occupational and Community HIV Exposures

	OCCUPATIONAL EXPOSURE	COMMUNITY EXPOSURE
Per episode transmission risk	0.03% (needle puncture)	0.03–0.6%[65,66]
Biologic plausibility of prophylactic efficacy	Yes (animal studies, efficacy in preventing perinatal HIV transmission)	Yes (animal studies, efficacy in preventing perinatal HIV transmission)
Safety	Serious objective toxicity unusual; subjective intolerance common	Likely to be similar
Feasibility of starting treatment soon after exposure	Feasible wihtin 4 hr, especially with "hotlines"	Feasibility not established; delays expected
Access to treatment	Available in most medical centers	Not easily available; emergency rooms, sexual assault crisis centers, and sexually transmitted disease clinics have some capacity in some locales
Cost-effective?	Yes	Probably, at least for high-risk exposures
Efficacious?	Not proven, but likely	No data
Overall public health impact	Very small impact on HIV incidence; indirect impact on access to care for infected persons	Potentially very large, but could be positive (decreased HIV incidence) or negative (increased HIV incidence)

overall HIV incidence will increase. Uncertainties about the net impact of a postexposure treatment program for community exposures of HIV on transmission rates and the relatively high cost of antiviral prophylaxis influenced the CDC to withhold support for widespread implementation of community treatment programs until more data are available.[67] However, the CDC does recommend HIV prophylaxis after exposures resulting from sexual assault.[68]

The San Francisco Department of Public Health, in conjunction with the University of California at San Francisco, has launched a demonstration project to evaluate thc feasibility and impact of postexposure treatment for sexual and injection drug use exposures in the community. In this program, chemoprophylaxis is just one component of a comprehensive prevention program that stresses safer behavior and avoidance of future risks, and is used only as a backup when other prevention efforts fail.[65,66] Carefully constructed public health messages that place prophylaxis in the overall context of health promotion are disseminated in the communities at risk.

Eligible exposures include parenteral blood contact, rectal and vaginal sexual exposure, and oral receptive sex with ejaculation.[65,66] For activities less likely to transmit HIV, the risks of treatment may outweigh the benefits, and treatment is not routinely offered. However, the presence of factors facilitating transmission (e.g., traumatic intercourse, presence of genital mucosal lesions) could increase the infection risk and the potential benefit of treatment. The

decisions about treatment also reflect the patient's willingness to adhere to a drug regimen and avoid unsafe practices in the future. The best option for persons who are repeatedly exposed to HIV is usually enhanced prevention counseling and case management, not repeated courses of antiviral treatment. Treatment requires written informed consent.

The drug regimen used in San Francisco is the same as that used for occupational exposures (Table 32–3). Treatment with both zidovudine and lamivudine for 4 weeks is appropriate in most cases, but alternatives are available in special cases, depending on exposure risk and probability of drug resistance. The importance of initiating treatment as soon as possible is emphasized in the community awareness campaign, but this may not prove feasible.

For now, there is no mandate for clinicians to provide antiretroviral treatment to individuals exposed to HIV in the community. However, when the potential benefits appear to outweigh the risks, treatment should be offered. Until further clinical guidance is published, the guidelines for managing occupational exposures provide an excellent resource to aid in selecting and monitoring drug regimens, evaluating and testing source partners, and counseling exposed persons.

References

1. Gerberding JL: Management of occupational exposures to blood-borne viruses. N Engl J Med 332:444, 1995

2. Gerberding JL: Incidence and prevalence of human immunodeficiency virus, hepatitis B virus, hepatitis C virus, and cytomegalovirus among health care personnel at risk for blood exposure: Final report from a longitudinal study. J Infect Dis 170:1410, 1994

3. Ippolito G, Puro V, DeCarlt G, and the Italian Study Group on Occupational Risk of HIV Infection: The risk of occupational human immunodeficiency virus infection in health care workers. Arch Intern Med 153:1431, 1993

4. Tokars JI, Marcus R, Culver DH, et al: Surveillance of human immunodeficiency virus infection and zidovudine use among health care workers after occupational exposure to HIV-infected blood: The CDC Cooperative Needlestick Group. Ann Intern Med 118:913, 1993

5. Henderson DK, Fahey BJ, Willy M, et al: Risk for occupational transmission of human immunodeficiency virus type-1 (HIV-1) associated with clinical exposures. A prospective evaluation. Ann Intern Med 113:47, 1990

6. Cavalcante NJF, Abreu ES, Fernandes ME, et al: Risk of health care professionals acquiring HIV infection in Latin America. AIDS Care 3:311, 1991

7. Centers for Disease Control: Surveillance for occupationally acquired HIV infection—United States, 1981–1992. MMWR Morb Mortal Wkly Rep 41:823, 1992

8. Kuhls TL, Viker S, Parris NB, et al: Occupational risk of HIV, HBV and HSV-2 in health care personnel caring for AIDS patients. Am J Public Health 77:1306, 1987

9. Josephson A, Bottone M, Gerber M, Oppermann N: Blood and body fluid exposure followup in the AIDS era: A two year experience. Am J Infect Control 18:136, 1990

10. Wormser GP, Joline C, Sivak S, Arlin ZA: Human immunodeficiency virus infection: Considerations for health care workers. Bull N Y Acad Med 64:203, 1988

11. Pereira LIA, Souza LCS, Souza MA, et al: Acidentes profissionais com material biologico de paclantes com sindrome da immunodeficiencia adquirida-accompanhamento clinico-serologico. Rev Soc Bras Med Trop 24:169, 1991

12. Heptonstall J, Porter K, Gill ON: Occupational HIV: Summary of Published Reports. London, Public Health Laboratory Services Communicable Disease Surveillance Centre, 1995

13. Daar ES, Moudgil T, Meyer RD, Ho DD: Transient high levels of viremia in patients with primary human immunodeficiency virus type 1 infection. N Engl J Med 325:733, 1991

14. Saag MS, Crain MJ, Decker WD, et al: High-level viremia in adults and children infected with human immunodeficiency virus in relation to disease stage and CD4+ lymphocyte levels. J Infect Dis 164:72, 1991

15. Ho DD, Moudgil T, Alam M: Quantitation of human immunodeficiency virus type 1 in the blood of infected persons. N Engl J Med 321:1622, 1989

16. Cardo DM, Culver DH, Ciesielski CA, et al: A case-control study of HIV seroconversion in health care workers after percutaneous exposures. N Engl J Med 337:1485, 1997

17. Cao Y, Krogstad P, Korber BT, et al: Maternal HIV-1 viral load, zidovudine treatment, and the risk of transmission of human immunodeficiency virus type 1 from mother to infant. N Engl J Med 3:549, 1997

18. Sperling RS, Shapiro DE, Coombs RW, et al: Maternal viral load, zidovudine treatment, and the risk of transmission of human immunodeficiency virus type 1 from mother to infant. N Engl J Med 335:1621, 1996

19. Mast S, Woolwine J, Gerberding JL: Efficacy of gloves in reducing blood volumes transferred during simulated needlestick injury. J Infect Dis 168:1589, 1993

20. Clerici M, Levin JM, Kessler HA, et al: HIV-specific T-helper activity in seronegative health care workers exposed to contaminated blood. JAMA 271:42, 1994

21. Clerici M, Berzofsky JA, Shearer GM, Tacket CO: Exposure to HIV-1 indicated by HIV-specific T helper cell responses before detection of infection by polymerase chain reaction and serum antibodies. J Infect Dis 165:1012, 1992

22. Pioto LA, Landay AL, Berzofsky JA, et al: Immune response to human immunodeficiency virus (HIV) in health care workers occupationally exposed to HIV-contaminated blood. Am J Med 102:21, 1997

23. Centers for Disease Control and Prevention: Public Health Service guidelines for the management of health-care worker exposures to HIV and recommendations for post-exposure prophylaxis. MMWR Morb Mortal Wkly Rep 47:1, 1998

24. Tokars JI, Bell DM, Culver D, et al: Percutaneous injuries during surgical procedures. JAMA 267:2899, 1992

25. Rose DA, Ramiro N, Perlman J, et al: Usage rates and perforation patterns of 6306 gloves from intraoperative procedures at San Francisco General Hospital. Infect Control Hosp Epidemiol 15:349, 1994

26. Centers for Disease Control: Recommendations for preventing transmission of human immunodeficiency virus and hepatitis B virus to patients during exposure-prone invasive procedures. MMWR Morb Mortal Wkly Rep 40:1, 1991

27. Harpaz R, Von Seidlein L, Averhoff FM, et al: Transmission of hepatitis B virus to multiple patients from a surgeon without evidence of inadequate infection control. N Engl J Med 334:549, 1996

28. Gerberding JL: The infected health care provider. N Engl J Med 334:594, 1996

29. Blanchard, Ferris S, Charmaret S, et al: Molecular evidence for nosocomial HIV transmission from a surgeon to one of his patients. J Virol 72:4537, 1998

30. Ciesielski C, Marianos D, Ou CY, et al: Transmission of human immunodeficiency virus in a dental practice. Ann Intern Med 116:798, 1992

31. Centers for Disease Control: Update: Investigations of persons treated by HIV-infected health-care workers—United States. MMWR Morb Mortal Wkly Rep 42:329, 1993

32. Gerberding JL: Procedure-specific infection control for preventing intraoperative blood exposures. Am J Infect Control 21:364, 1993

33. Centers for Disease Control: Improper infection-control procedures during employee vaccination programs—District of Columbia and Pennsylvania. MMWR Morb Mortal Wkly Rep 42:969, 1993

34. Alter MJ, Ahtone J, Maynard JE: Hepatitis B transmission associated with a multiple-dose vial in a hemodialysis unit. Ann Intern Med 99:330, 1983

35. Oren I, Hershow RC, Ben-Porath E, et al: A common-source outbreak of fulminant hepatitis B in a hospital. Ann Inten Med 110:691, 1989

36. Hersh BS, Popovici F, Apertrei RC, et al: Acquired immunodeficiency syndrome in Rumania. Lancet 338:645, 1991

37. Centers for Disease Control: Patient exposures to HIV during nuclear medicine procedures. MMWR Morb Mortal Wkly Rep 41:575, 1992

38. Medically acquired HIV. Lancet 43:42, 1994

39. Centers for Disease Control: Recommendations for prevention of HIV transmission in health-care settings.

MMWR Morb Mortal Wkly Rep 36(Suppl 2S):1S, 1987

40. Centers for Disease Control: Update: Universal precautions for prevention of transmission of human immunodeficiency virus, hepatitis B virus, and other bloodborne pathogens in health care settings. MMWR Morb Mortal Wkly Rep 37:377, 1988

41. U.S. Department of Labor, Occupational Safety and Health Administration: Occupational exposure to bloodborne pathogens: Final rule. Federal Register 56: 64004, 1991

42. Gerberding JL, and the University of California, San Francisco Task Force on AIDS: Recommended infection-control policies for patients with human immunodeficiency virus infection: An update. N Engl J Med 315:1562, 1986

43. Lynch P, Jackson MM, Cummings MJ, Stamm WE: Rethinking the role of isolation practices in the prevention of nosocomial infections. Ann Intern Med 107: 243, 1987

44. Gerberding JL, Henderson DK: Design of rational infection control guidelines for human immunodeficiency virus infection. J Infect Dis 156:861, 1987

45. Garner JL: Guidelines for isolation precautions in hospitals. Infect Control Hosp Epidemiol 17:54, 1996

46. Jagger J, Hunt EH, Bland-Elnaggar J, Pearson RD: Rates of needlestick injury caused by various devices in a university hospital. N Engl J Med 319:284, 1988

47. Evaluation of safety devices for preventing percutaneous injuries among health-care workers during phlebotomy procedures—Minneapolis–St. Paul, New York City, and San Francisco. MMWR Morb Mortal Wkly Rep 46:21, 1997

48. Evaluation of blunt suture needles in preventing percutaneous injuries among health-care workers during gynecologic surgical procedures—New York City, March 1993–June 1994. MMWR Morb Mortal Wkly Rep 46:25, 119

49. Gerberding JL: Prophylaxis for occupational exposures to HIV. Ann Intern Med 125:497, 1996

50. Busch MP, Statten GA: Time course of viremia and antibody seroconversion following human immunodeficiency virus exposure. Am J Med 102:117, 1997

51. Ciesielski CA, Metler RP: Duration of time between exposure and seroconversion in healthcare workers with occupationally acquired infection with human immunodeficiency virus. Am J Med 102:115, 1997

52. Dilley JW: Counseling health care workers after accidental exposures. Focus 5:3, 1990

53. LaFon SW, Lehrman SN, Barry DW: Prophylactically administered Retrovir in health care workers potentially exposed to the human immunodeficiency virus. J Infec Dis 158:503, 1988

54. LaFon SW, Mooney BD, McMullen JP, et al: A double-blind, placebo-controlled study of the safety and effi-cacy of Retrovir (zidovudine, ZDV) as a chemoprophylactic agent in health care workers. In: Program and Abstracts of the 30th Interscience Conference on Antimicrobial Agents and Chemotherapy. Washington, DC, American Society for Microbiology, 1990, Abstract 489

55. Spira AI, Marx PA, Patterson BK, et al: Cellular targets of infection and route of vital dissemination after an intravaginal inoculation of simian immunodeficiency virus into rhesus macaques. J Exp Med 183:215, 1996

56. Black RJ: Animal studies of prophylaxis. Am J Med 102:39, 1997

57. Van Rompay KKA, Marthas ML, Ramos RA, et al: Simian immunodeficiency virus (SIV) infection of infant rhesus macaques as a model to test antiretroviral drug prophylaxis and therapy: Oral 3'-azido-3'- deoxy-thymidine prevents SIV infection. Antimicrob Agents Chemother 36:2381, 1992

58. Centers for Disease Control: Zidovudine for the prevention of HIV transmission from mother to infant. MMWR Morb Mortal Wkly Rep 43:285, 1994

59. Centers for Disease Control: Recommendations of the U.S. Public Health Service task force on the use of zidovudine to reduce perinatal transmission of HIV. MMWR Morb Mortal Wkly Rep 43(RR-11):1, 1994

60. Jochimsen EM: Failures of zidovudine postexposure prophylaxis. Am J Med 102:52, 1997

61. Puro V, Ippolito G, Guzzanti E, et al: Zidovudine prophylaxis after accidental exposure to HIV: The Italian experience. The Italian Study Group on Occupational Risk of HIV Infection. AIDS 6:963, 1992

62. Beekmann SE, Fahrner R, Henderson DK, Gerberding JL: Zidovudine safety and tolerance among uninfected health care workers: A brief update. Am J Med 102: 63, 1997

63. Gerberding JL: Post-exposure prophylaxis for human immunodeficiency virus at San Francisco General Hospital. Am J Med 102:85, 1997

64. Carpenter CCJ, Fischl MA, Hammer SM, et al: Antiretroviral therapy for HIV infection in 1996: Recommendations of an international panel. JAMA 276:146, 1996

65. Katz MH, Gerberding JL: Postexposure treatment of people exposed to the human immunodeficiency virus through sexual contact or injection-drug use. N Engl J Med 336:1097, 1997

66. Katz MH, Gerberding JL: Managing recent sexual exposures to HIV. Ann Intern Med 128:306, 1998

67. Centers for Disease Control and Prevention. Management of sexual, injection-drug-use, and other non-occupational exposures to HIV, including considerations regarding antiretroviral therapy. MMWR Morb Mortal Wkly Rep 47:1, 1998

68. Centers for Disease Control and Prevention: Guidelines for treatment of sexually transmitted diseases. MMWR Morb Mortal Wkly Rep 47(RR-1):109, 1998

33 Pediatric AIDS

ANDREW T. PAVIA • JOHN C. CHRISTENSON

EPIDEMIOLOGY

The epidemiology of HIV disease in children reflects the epidemiology of HIV in women, although this relationship has been profoundly altered by the ability of antiretroviral therapy during pregnancy to prevent transmission from mother to child. In spite of the 11% decline in the total number of new AIDS cases in the United States in 1997, the number of new cases among women has remained relatively constant (13,105 in 1997). Women continue to make up an increasing proportion of AIDS cases and new HIV infections (for more discussion of this topic, see Chapter 34).

An estimated 6000 to 7000 infants are born to HIV-infected women each year in the United States. In the last 4 years, there has been a dramatic 47% decline in the number of new AIDS cases among children under 13.[1] In 1997, 473 new cases were reported, compared to a peak of 959 cases in 1993. This decline represents the combined effects of several factors: the use of zidovudine to prevent perinatal HIV transmission based on the findings of Pediatric AIDS Clinical Trial Group (PACTG) 076,[2] increased use of antiretroviral drugs to treat HIV infection in pregnant women, and delayed disease progression in infected children as a result of improved antiretroviral therapy and prophylaxis. In developed countries, this decline in new AIDS cases among children should continue, and vertical transmission of HIV can potentially be all but eliminated. However, worldwide, the picture is far bleaker: An estimated 1600 children with HIV infection are born every day.[3] More than 90% live in developing countries where the benefits of new combination therapies are not available. A less appreciated but devastating impact of HIV on children is the loss of their mothers; there are an estimated 8 million children worldwide who have been orphaned by HIV.[3]

In the United States, about 50% of children with HIV are concentrated in four regions: New York, Florida, California, and Puerto Rico. HIV disproportionately affects minority children; 58% are African-American, 23% are Hispanic, and 18% are white, non-Hispanic.

RISK FACTORS FOR PERINATAL TRANSMISSION

Perinatal transmission of HIV is complex and multifactorial, as recently reviewed by Mofenson[4] and in Chapter 35 of this book. Transmission rates vary widely in different parts of the world, ranging from 14% to 40% without treatment.[4-8] Transmission can occur during gestation, intrapartum, and postpartum through breast feeding. Intrapartum transmission is estimated to account for 50% to 70% of infections. A working definition of in utero transmission is based on the presence of viremia within 48 hours of birth, demonstrated by culture or polymerase chain reaction (PCR).[9] Children who have no detectable virus within 48 hours but become viremic within 1 to 2 weeks of birth are thought to have been infected around the time of delivery.

Risk factors for vertical transmission can be divided into maternal and obstetric factors. Maternal factors most consistently associated with increased risk of transmission are those that reflect advanced disease in the mother (AIDS, low CD4 count, high plasma HIV RNA, high titer of infectious virus). Other factors identified in some studies but not others include maternal hard drug use, sexually transmitted disease, multiple sexual partners, primary HIV infection during pregnancy, viral phenotype, and lack of neutralizing antibody against the maternal viral isolate.[4,10-15] Higher plasma viral loads have been consistently associated with the risk of transmission, but there is no threshold value for transmission. Transmission may occur in women with very low viral loads, and some women with high levels of RNA do not transmit.[16]

Obstetric risk factors include duration of ruptured membranes, abruptio placenta, birth order, and chorioamnionitis.[4,17–19] The role of cesarian section remains controversial.[20,21] Avoiding prolonged rupture of membranes may be the major benefit,[19] and more aggressive antiviral treatment in pregnancy may reduce transmission to as low as 1% to 3%. At least one study has suggested that elective cesarian section, performed before the onset of labor, provides additive protection when used with azidothymidine (AZT; zidovudine).[20] Cost and maternal morbidity remain barriers to the widespread use of elective cesarian, in the absence of definitive trials (see Chapter 35 for detailed discussion of this issue).

NATURAL HISTORY

Timing of Infection

HIV progresses more rapidly in children with perinatal infection than among children infected at an older age or among adults. The median survival time of HIV-infected children in recent studies is 5 to 8 years.[22–25] It has long been recognized that there was a bimodal distribution of clinical progression.[22,26] One subset of children has early onset of symptoms, usually in the first year of life. These children have a rapid downhill course with rapid decline in CD4 count and development of clinical symptoms, often including *Pneumocystis carinii* pneumonia (PCP), and have high mortality.[23,25]

There appear to be a number of predictors of rapid progression, including evidence of in utero transmission (positive PCR, culture, or p24 antigen assay at birth),[27,28] hepatosplenomegaly at birth,[27] and higher viral loads after 1 month of life.[28–30] CD4 and CD8 counts below the fifth percentile in infancy are associated with rapid progression among babies infected in utero, perhaps reflecting early destruction of the thymus.[31]

Declining CD4 count and CD4 percent are the hallmarks of HIV disease progression in children. CD4 count normally declines with age, making interpretation somewhat problematic. CD4 percent is less age dependent and is very useful in disease staging (Table 33–1). The revised Centers for Disease Control and Prevention (CDC) classification uses both immunologic status and clinical status and is useful for staging.[32]

Plasma Viral Load

Quantitative measurement of plasma viral RNA levels revolutionized the management of HIV in adults. Studies to define the natural history and prognostic value of plasma viral RNA levels and the interpretation of specific levels in children have lagged behind. Several studies have convincingly demonstrated the prognostic value of baseline plasma RNA levels and the independent value of CD4 count.[11,29,30,33–36] However, the kinetics of plasma HIV RNA in children differ from those in adults in several ways. First, children tend to have higher viral loads, with median peak values between 100,000 and 1,000,000 copies. In one study, the median peak value was 318,000 copies.[30] Second, after primary infection, the viral load slowly declines during the first year of life, in contrast to the rapid 2- to 3-log drop in adults over the first 2 to 4 months.[30] Finally, although viral load is consistently associated with prognosis, it has been difficult to establish specific levels that are sensitive and specific for high risk.[33,34] These differences may reflect greater numbers of target cells and a limited ability to mount an immune response by the immature immune system. Chil-

TABLE 33–1. 1994 Revised HIV Pediatric Classification System: Immune Categories Based on Age-Specific CD4+ T-Lymphocyte Count and Percent

IMMUNE CATEGORY	CD4+ T-LYMPHOCYTE COUNT/ml (%)		
	<12 mo	1–5 yr	6–12 yrs
1—no suppression	>1500 (>25)	>1000 (>25)	>500 (>25)
2—moderate suppression	750–1499 (15–24)	500–999 (15–24)	200–499 (15–24)
3—severe suppression	<750 (<15)	<500 (<15)	<200 (<15)

From Centers for Disease Control and Prevention: 1994 revised classification system for human immunodeficiency virus infection in children less than 13 years of age. MMWR Morb Mortal Wkly Rep 43(RR-12):1, 1994.

dren infected in utero tend to have modest viral loads at birth, but their peak values at 1 to 2 months are higher than in children with presumed intrapartum infection.[30,34]

Growth failure and neurodevelopmental decline are sensitive indicators of disease activity. Improvements in these areas are markers of successful antiviral therapy.[37]

EARLY DIAGNOSIS AND MANAGEMENT OF INFANTS EXPOSED TO HIV

Diagnosis of HIV Infection

Early diagnosis of HIV infection in children born to HIV-infected mothers has been challenging. Currently however, the diagnosis can be made in most infants by 1 month of age using methods that directly detect virus. Detection of virus by peripheral blood mononuclear cell (PBMC) co-culture, DNA PCR of the infant's PBMCs, or HIV RNA in plasma is presumptive evidence of infection but *must* be confirmed by repeat testing.

Viral culture is considered the gold standard[38] but is slow, cumbersome, and expensive. Currently, DNA PCR is the method of choice for diagnosis of HIV in infants.[39,40] In a meta-analysis of data from 271 infected children,[41] HIV DNA PCR was only moderately sensitive in the first 48 hours of life (38%; 90% confidence interval [CI], 29% to 46%). Sensitivity rose rapidly during the second week; 93% of infected children (90% CI, 76% to 97%) were PCR positive by 14 days of age. Preliminary data suggest that quantitative RNA PCR is at least as sensitive and specific as DNA PCR, and offers the advantage of providing important prognostic data.[42,43] Additional studies are needed before quantitative plasma RNA testing can replace DNA PCR for initial diagnosis. Measurement of p24 antigen, either conventionally or with immune dissociation, is not recommended for the diagnosis of neonatal HIV infection because it is less sensitive than PCR or culture, and false positives may occasionally occur.[44]

Most experts recommend obtaining a first sample for DNA PCR or culture during the first 48 hours of an infant's life.[45,46] Cord blood should not be used because of the possibility of contamination with maternal blood. A positive viral test in the first 48 hours of life presumptively identifies children who were infected in utero,[9] who may have a more rapid disease course.[27,28] However, in one study, plasma RNA measurement after the first month of life appeared to be more prognostic than time of first positive test.[30]

For infants with an initial negative test, testing should be repeated at 14 to 28 days of life. Testing at 14 days offers the potential to stop AZT monotherapy for patients with presumed infection and begin combination therapy during the period of acute infection. For infants with initial negative tests, testing should be repeated again at 3 to 6 months of age. Any positive test should be confirmed immediately by testing of a separate blood sample, and two positive tests should be considered diagnostic of infection. We recommend obtaining quantitative plasma RNA (viral load) concentrations as well as DNA PCR for confirmatory testing. This provides independent confirmation and important prognostic information. Two negative blood samples for DNA PCR or culture, one after at least 1 month of age and another after 3 months of age, reasonably exclude HIV infection. In these children, HIV antibodies should be monitored until they become undetectable.

Use of PCP Prophylaxis

PCP occurs most often between 3 and 6 months of age in perinatally infected children. Disease may develop before HIV infection is confirmed or before a drop in CD4 counts has been documented. Because of continuing mortality with CD4-based guidelines for prophylaxis, the CDC published revised guidelines[47] recommending that PCP prophylaxis be initiated at 4 to 6 weeks of life for all HIV-exposed infants. Prophylaxis should be continued until HIV-infection can be excluded (see above). In all infected infants, prophylaxis should be continued until 12 months of age. After that age, prophylaxis is recommended for all children who have evidence of severe immunosuppression (CDC category 3). Trimethoprim-sulfamethoxazole is the preferred drug. The recommended dose is 150 mg/m^2/day in divided doses on 3 consecutive days each week, but there are several acceptable alternatives.[47]

Monitoring the HIV-Exposed or HIV-Infected Infant

Infants born to HIV-infected women should receive oral AZT (2 mg/kg every 6 h) during the

TABLE 33–2. Suggested Schedule for Routine Monitoring of HIV-Exposed and -Infected Infants

INTERVENTION	BIRTH	4 wk	6 wk	2 mo	3 mo	4 mo	6 mo
AZT per ACTG-076	X	X	X				
PCP prophylaxis			X	X	X	X	X*
CBC with differential	X	X	X	X	X	X	X
HIV DNA PCR	X	X			X		
CD4 absolute and %					X		X†
HIV plasma RNA‡							
Quantitative immunoglobulins					X		

*PCP prophylaxis is continued until HIV is excluded or for the first 12 months of life in children who are infected or whose infection status is unknown.

†CD4 counts should be repeated every 2 to 3 months in children who are infected or whose infection status is unknown.

‡HIV plasma RNA should be measured immediately if infection is suspected based on a positive HIV DNA PCR. If no treatment is initiated, plasma RNA should be monitored every 3 months. If treatment is initiated or changed, plasma RNA should be monitored 4 weeks and 8 weeks after changing therapy and every 3 months thereafter.

first 6 weeks of life based on the PACTG 076 protocol, followed by trimethoprim-sulfame-thoxazole for PCP prophylaxis. Both agents can cause myelosuppression, and the complete blood count should be monitored in all infants.[45] Plasma viral RNA and CD4 count and percent should be monitored once the diagnosis of HIV is established. These are measured at baseline, 1 and 2 months after starting antiretroviral therapy, and at least every 3 months thereafter. Screening for hypogammaglobulinemia can be performed at 6 months in infected children. A suggested monitoring scheme is shown in Table 33–2.

Vaccination

Timely vaccination is important in HIV-infected children. Recent guidelines are available.[48] Inactivated vaccines (hepatitis B, *Haemophilus influenzae* type B, diptheria-tetanus-pertussis) are given according to the schedule recommended for all children. Inactivated polio should be substituted for oral polio vaccine. The measles, mumps, and rubella vaccine is a live vaccine, which poses a theoretical risk to severely immunocompromised children. HIV-infected children without immunosuppression should receive their first dose as soon as possible after their first birthday. The second dose need not be delayed until school entry; it can be given as soon as 1 month after the first dose. Annual immunization against influenza is recommended for all HIV-infected children. Initially, two doses of split-virus vaccine are given, separated by at least 1 month. Because infections with encapsulated organisms are prominent among HIV-infected children, the potential benefit of pneumococcal vaccine is large. Unfortunately, children younger than 2 years old respond poorly to polysaccharide vaccines; the response to some serotypes is poor until after 6 years of age. Vaccination with the 23-valent pneumococcal vaccine should be given at 24 months. Revaccination should be offered after 3 to 5 years.

ANTIRETROVIRAL THERAPY

Principles of Therapy

Based on available evidence, antiretroviral therapy of HIV in children is guided by principles similar to those for therapy in adults. Ongoing viral replication is the driving force behind immunologic destruction. Plasma viral RNA load is a useful measure of viral replication and is therefore important in determining prognosis and assessing the effects of therapy. The goal of antiretroviral therapy in children should be to suppress viral replication to extremely low levels; if replication continues, ongoing mutation will lead to drug resistance. Combination therapy with three or more agents offers the greatest opportunity to achieve maximal suppression. However, the ability to adhere to a regimen is a key determinant of continued viral suppression. The complexity of HIV therapy in children and adolescents and the rapid rate of change suggest that children with HIV should receive care from physicians with substantial expertise in HIV and in conjunction with multidisciplinary teams. Whenever possible, children should be offered the opportunity to participate in clinical trials.

It is important, however, to appreciate ways in which children differ from adults. The majority of HIV-infected children are infected around the time of delivery, and therapy can potentially be started during primary infection. Theoretically, this offers children an advantage that is rare in adults.[49] Intact thymic architecture offers the potential for greater immune reconstitution, and, in one study, thymic volume on computed tomography scan correlated with completeness of immune reconstitution.[50]

However, many of the differences lead to challenges. In general, clinical trial data in children are limited, and pharmacokinetic studies may be inadequate. The disposition of drugs changes during growth and development, changing from infancy into childhood, and again during adolescence. In general, volume of distribution is larger and clearance is faster, which may require more frequent dosing. The developing central nervous system (CNS) of children appears to be more vulnerable to damage by HIV. Regimens therefore should be highly active in the CNS. Young children usually require liquid formulations, which may be unpalatable or simply not available. Young children are dependent on the caregiver's ability to give medications consistently, on schedule, and in spite of protests. Older children may be concerned about taking antiretroviral therapy in public or at school. The social problems that are common in families with HIV-infected children (poverty, homelessness, parents who may be ill or absent, substance abuse, mental illness, isolation, fear of disclosure) compound the problems of complex regimens, frequent dosing, and sometimes resistance from the child or adolescent. Thus problems with adherence can be daunting.

When to Start Therapy

In agreement with the 1998 report from the Working Group on Pediatric HIV Disease,[46] we strongly recommend initiating therapy for all children with symptoms of HIV disease (CDC category A, B, or C) or with evidence of immunologic deterioration (CDC category 2 or 3). Children who are diagnosed with HIV infection in the first year of life should be considered for antiretroviral therapy regardless of clinical or immunologic status. The high viral loads and poor host control of HIV replication argue for aggressive therapy. Treatment during primary infection in adults may alter the immune response and the clinical course of HIV disease.[49,51,52] Moreover, despite the prognostic value of HIV RNA level and CD4 count, these markers cannot completely predict who will

progress slowly enough to safely delay therapy. The likely benefits of early therapy, however, have not yet been demonstrated in clinical trials, and must be weighed against the need for life-long treatment, the risk of selecting for viral resistance, and the potential long-term risks of protease inhibitor therapy. Therefore, the clinicians should have extensive discussions with the family or caregivers. Continuing efforts to support adherence are vital.

Treatment for children older than 1 year who are asymptomatic is more problematic. The majority of children will have symptoms or decreases in CD4 percent.[22] One approach would be to treat all children who have preserved immune function. This approach can be considered when the family or caregivers are committed to aggressive therapy, there is adequate medical and social support, and there is a high likelihood of good adherence.

A second approach is to defer therapy in older children who have no symptoms and no evidence of immune dysfunction and are at low risk of rapid progression based on plasma HIV RNA levels. Unlike adults, in children the levels of viral load that define low risk of progression are unclear.[29,30,33,34] In one study, fewer than 10,000 copies of viral RNA and relatively normal CD4 counts for age identified a group with a 2-year progression rate of less than 5%.[34] In other studies, however, RNA levels greater than 100,000 copies were associated with a high risk of death[33] or clinical progression.[53] In light of this uncertainty, patients in whom therapy might be deferred are older children with low viral loads and stable CD4 counts and percents. Perhaps the most important consideration, and one that requires thoughtful clinical judgment, is whether to defer therapy in low-risk patients because the risk of poor adherence and development of resistance outweighs the benefit of immediate therapy. If antiretroviral therapy is deferred, it is wise to consider starting therapy if new symptoms develop, if the CD4 percent is falling rapidly or falls below 25, or if the viral load increases by more than 0.7 log (confirmed by repeated measures). Although our knowledge is rapidly evolving based on ongoing studies, at present it is reasonable to encourage therapy for any child with a viral load greater than 50,000 to 100,000 copies regardless of other factors.[53]

Initial Therapy

The choice of initial therapy must balance efficacy at reducing viral load and maintaining immune function, complexity, long-term tolerability, with the ability to preserve future options. Compared to monotherapy, combination therapy has demonstrated better clinical outcome, longer survival time, greater reductions in viral load, greater increases in CD4 count, and decreased emergence of resistance.[54-57] Monotherapy with didanosine (ddI) performed as well as the combination of AZT and ddI in PACTG trial 152,[55] but triple combination therapy is superior to two-drug therapy in adults[58] and in children.[59]

Combination therapy using two nucleoside reverse transcriptase inhibitors (NRTIs) and a potent protease inhibitor is the initial therapy of choice for children, as for adults (Table 33–3). The greatest amount of data in children for NRTI combinations is for AZT and ddI[55] or AZT and lamivudine (3TC)[54]; however, small studies suggest that stavudine (d4T) and ddI[60] or d4T and 3TC are also safe and effective. The combination of AZT plus 3TC can be used in sequence with d4T plus ddI, with either combination used initially. Alternatively, AZT plus ddI can be followed by d4T plus 3TC. Unfortunately, no studies have directly compared the safety and efficacy of the protease inhibitors.

Only nelfinavir and ritonavir are available in pediatric formulation. Nelfinavir is available as a powder that is fairly palatable when mixed in breast milk, milk, formula, water, pudding, or ice cream. It tastes bitter if mixed with acidic juices. Some data suggest that patients for whom nelfinavir fails may be more likely to respond to salvage therapy with a regimen containing two protease inhibitors, although this is unproven. In the largest controlled trial to date, regimens containing ritonavir have been able to reduce viral loads below the limit of quantification in more than 50% of patients.[59,61] Dramatic clinical improvements can occur in children with advanced disease.[62] The liquid formulation of ritonavir tastes very unpleasant, however. Coating the mouth with peanut butter or chocolate syrup before the dose, and ice cream or pudding as a "chaser," can help. Indinavir has been used successfully in children who can swallow capsules.[63,64] In general, the response rate of children to protease-containing regimens is not as good as for adults. There are more limited data on the use of two nucleosides with nevirapine as initial therapy. In one study, seven of eight infants had initial responses of greater than 1.5 log to treatment with AZT, ddI, and nevirapine.[65] Two of the eight maintained undetectable viral loads; the remainder had significant rebound. Nevirapine-containing regimens should be considered for children with more modest initial viral loads, and those who

---

TABLE 33–3. Options for Initial Antiretroviral Therapy in Children with HIV Infection

A: Preferred (Greatest Clinical and Antiviral Efficacy Expected)

2 nucleoside reverse transcriptase inhibitors* plus Potent protease inhibitor

AZT and 3TC	Nelfinavir
d4T and ddI	Ritonavir
AZT and ddI	Indinavir[†]
d4T and 3TC	Saquinavir soft gel[†]
	Ritonavir and saquinavir[†,‡]
	Efavirenz or efavirenz plus nelfinavir[†]

B. Alternative (Less Likely to Have Long-Term Efficacy)

2 nucleoside reverse transcriptase inhibitors plus nevirapine

C. Secondary Alternative (Clinical Efficacy but Less Than Other Options)

2 nucleodise reverse transcriptase inhibitors[§]

D. Not Recommended

All monotherapy
ddI and ddC
AZT and d4T
3TC and ddC
d4T and ddC

*AZT, azidothymidine (zidovudine); ddC, zalcitabine; ddI, didanosine; d4T, stavudine; 3TC, lamivudine.
[†]For children who can take capsules.
[‡]Very limited data in children.
[§]3TC should not be used in dual therapy because of rapid emergence of resistance and the importance of 3TC in protease-containing regimens.
Adapted from Centers for Disease Control and Prevention: Guidelines for the use of antiretroviral agents in the treatment of pediatric HIV infection. MMWR Morb Mortal Wkly Rep 47(RR-4):1, 1998.

may be able to take nelfinavir three times daily. Preliminary data from ACTG 382 suggest that efavirenz plus nelfinavir plus two NRTIs is superior to 3-drug regimens; 78% had fewer than 400 copies at week 12.[65a]

At present, there are insufficient data to suggest that the mother's treatment history should influence the choice of initial therapy. In PACTG 076, AZT resistance among mothers was rare and did not result in transmission of resistant virus.[66] However, cases of transmission of resistant virus have been reported,[67,68] and it is reasonable to expect that, as women with extensive antiretroviral experience become pregnant, transmission of resistant virus will increase. At present, routine use of baseline resistance testing cannot be recommended; this may change based on ongoing studies.

When to Change Therapy

In children, even more than in adults, the decision to change therapy must balance the need to better control viral replication and the higher likelihood of control with earlier switching against the limited number of active drugs and the problems of cross-resistance. In children, there is a real need not to exhaust too quickly the limited options. When there is major toxicity or if new data suggest that the current therapy is inadequate, the regimen must be changed. For minor clinical or laboratory toxicities, it is worth trying to manage the symptoms.

When therapy appears to be failing, the issues are more complex. When the initial regimen is failing, there may be several acceptable options. Unfortunately, many children have been treated with sequential monotherapy or dual nucleosides, and the choice of new drugs is limited. Before changing therapy, it is essential to carefully assess adherence and to try to solve adherence problems. Otherwise, the new regimen is doomed to fail. There are three broad indicators of drug failure, as suggested by the Working Group on Antiretroviral Therapy in Children: virologic, immunologic, and clinical.[46] Virologic indicators have the advantage of being easily quantifiable and often correlate with the emergence of drug-resistant virus. If a change is observed, RNA measurements should be repeated before deciding to change therapy. Failure to achieve a minimally acceptable response (1 log for protease inhibitor-containing regimens) after 8 to 12 weeks should prompt a change. The repeated detection of viral RNA after a period when it fell below limits of quan-

tification, or an increase of 0.7 to 1 log from the nadir, indicate virologic failure. However, virologic failure may not be an indicator of immediate clinical or immunologic failure, and a decision to change therapy should weigh the available options and the CD4 response. Failure to achieve a viral load less than 400 to 500 copies/ml 4 to 6 months after beginning an aggressive initial regimen is an inadequate response. However, because of high baseline viral loads, it appears that only 50% to 65% of children will achieve this goal.[59,63,64,69,70]

Immunologic progression is an indicator of increased risk of death. Therefore, therapy should be changed in the face of immunologic progression and detectable virus as indicated by CD4 percent, which is less affected by age and mild illness than is absolute CD4 count and is often a better indicator. A change to a new immunologic category, or, for those with CD4 percent less than 15, a decrease of 5 percentiles, is a clear indicator of immunologic progression. However, rate of change should also be considered. Several measurements should be used to determine rate of change. A 30% change in absolute CD4 count or CD4 percent in 6 months is worrisome. For example, a decline from a CD4 percent of 40 to 30% over 2 years may be acceptable. A similar decline over 6 months indicates the need to consider new treatment.

Certain types of clinical progression are ominous and should prompt changes in therapy. Growth failure (e.g., failure to maintain the expected growth velocity) or progressive neurodevelopmental decline is a clear indicator of disease progression. Although definitive data are lacking on clinical efficacy, agents that produce good antiretroviral activity in the cerebrospinal fluid should be used. These include AZT, d4T, 3TC, and nevirapine. Among protease inhibitors, indinavir currently has more data to support activity in the CNS.

The choice of agents for "salvage" therapy is difficult to make, and there are few clear guidelines. Strategies recommended in adults[71] also make sense for children. Whenever possible, three to four new agents that the child has not already taken and that are not predicted to be cross-resistant should be used. Four-drug regimens using dual protease inhibitors or combining a non-nucleotide reverse transcriptase inhibitor with protease inhibitors have had moderate success in adults and should be considered. There are no data yet on the use of hydroxyurea in children, but in adults it enhances the activity of ddI and nucleotide analogs and partially reverses ddI resistance. Experience in children with sickle cell disease suggests hydroxyurea is safe, but bone marrow toxicity can occur.

PROPHYLAXIS OF OTHER OPPORTUNISTIC INFECTIONS

Primary prevention of specific opportunistic infections is extremely important for children with advanced immunosuppression. Guidelines have been formulated by the Infectious Diseases Society of America with the CDC that categorize the advisability of prophylaxis, the CD4 levels at which to begin prophylaxis, and the agents of choice.[48] Secondary prevention to prevent recurrence is continued lifelong for most opportunistic infections in children, including PCP, disseminated *Mycobacterium avium* complex, toxoplasmosis, cryptococcosis, and the endemic mycoses.

With the progressive immune restoration achievable with multidrug antiretroviral therapy, important questions have emerged about primary and secondary prophylaxis. Can primary prophylaxis be stopped if the CD4 count remains elevated? Can secondary prophylaxis be stopped for some or all opportunistic infections, and, if so, after how long? At present, there are insufficient data to recommend stopping prophylaxis in children under most circumstances, but this is an area of active research and recommendations may change.

MANAGEMENT

Comprehensive management of the HIV-infected child is beyond the scope of this chapter. Optimal care requires a multidisciplinary approach and, if possible, a dedicated team. Careful attention must be given to nutrition, developmental assessment, psychosocial issues, and education. Teaching about HIV and multiple strategies to support adherence are critical. Medical care of the mother is important to the child's health as well as the mother's (see also Chapters 34 and 35). It is not uncommon for mothers to ignore their own health care while providing excellent care to an infected child. If possible, HIV services for mother and child should be available at the same site and should be coordinated. Periodic case management meetings to coordinate issues among providers and agencies are extremely useful.

ADOLESCENTS

Adolescents infected with HIV pose unique challenges. The needs of children who were infected perinatally who have survived into adolescence are different than those who are infected during adolescence. Survivors of perinatal infection have demonstrated slow disease progression, but often have advanced disease and may have been extensively pretreated. They have often outlived their parents. Most adolescents who are recently infected were infected through sexual activity. HIV infection through sexual abuse occurs, and can only be diagnosed if there is awareness and careful investigation.[72] Adolescent behavior problems, including drug use or being a runaway, are relatively common.[73] The clinical course of disease for adolescents infected sexually or through drug use is more similar to that in adults; adult treatment guidelines are appropriate.[71, 74]

Some issues are common among adolescents. Rapid growth, change in metabolism, and increases in muscle mass in males and in fat for women affect drug metabolism. Adolescents in early puberty (Tanner stages I and II) should be dosed as children. Those in late puberty (Tanner stage V) should be dosed as adults. There are no clear guidelines for those at intermediate stages.

Adherence to medical care and antiretroviral therapy is particularly difficult for adolescents. The need for autonomy, a distrust of authority, embarrassment, lack of support, and low self-esteem may be issues. Adolescents are often unable to grasp long-term risks and consequences. Some have chaotic lives. Medical care and medications may make the adolescent feel different and vulnerable. Multidisciplinary teams, including mental health, social work, educators, and perhaps peer counseling may be helpful. In adolescents at low or moderate risk of progression, it may often be wise to delay antiretroviral therapy until adherence is more likely.

UNANSWERED QUESTIONS

Despite the important gains in antiviral therapy and the promise of further improvement, there remain frustrating gaps in our knowledge and our ability to deliver antiviral therapy to children. Early diagnosis of HIV-infected children and early treatment with fully suppressive regimens hold enormous promise. However, we need to learn much more about the pharmacology of antiretroviral drugs in all stages of growth and the long-term safety of these drugs in growing children. All agents must be studied in infants and children during the early phase of development. As with adults, we do not yet know the optimal combinations and sequences of drugs, or the best way to ensure adherence to difficult and complex regimens. The potential for immune reconstitution and preservation in children is much greater given the intact thymic network and bone marrow reserve, and successfully treated children may provide important insights into immune reconstitution in adults.

The prevention of perinatal transmission is the ultimate answer to controlling pediatric AIDS. In developed countries, it should be possible to virtually eliminate perinatal transmission of HIV through universal screening of pregnant women, use of effective antiviral regimens during pregnancy and delivery, and optimal obstetric management.

References

1. Centers for Disease Control and Prevention: Update: Perinatally acquired HIV/AIDS—United States 1997. MMWR Morbid Mortal Wkly Rep 46:1086, 1997
2. Connor EM, Sperling RS, Gelber R, et al: Reduction of maternal-infant transmission of human immunodeficiency virus type 1 with zidovudine treatment: Pediatric AIDS Clinical Trials Group Protocol 076 Study Group. N Engl J Med 331:1173, 1994
3. Joint United Nations Programme on HIV/AIDS: Report on the Global HIV/AIDS Epidemic, June 1998. Geneva, Joint United Nations Programme on HIV/AIDS, 1998
4. Mofenson LM: Mother-child HIV-1 transmission: Timing and determinants. Obstet Gynecol Clin North Am 24:759, 1997
5. Hira SK, Kamanga J, Bhat GJ, et al: Perinatal transmission of HIV-I in Zambia. BMJ 299:1250, 1989
6. Ryder RW, Nsa W, Hassig SE, et al: Perinatal transmission of the human immunodeficiency virus type 1 to infants of seropositive women in Zaire. N Engl J Med 320:1637, 1989
7. Matheson PB, Abrams EJ, Thomas PA, et al: Efficacy of antenatal zidovudine in reducing perinatal transmission of human immunodeficiency virus type 1: The New York City Perinatal HIV Transmission Collaborative Study Group. J Infect Dis 172:353, 1995
8. European Collaborative Study: Risk factors for mother-to-child transmission of HIV-1. Lancet 339:1007, 1992
9. Bryson Y, Luzuriaga K, Sullivan J, Wara D: Proposed definitions for in utero versus intrapartum transmission of HIV-1. N Engl J Med 327:1246, 1993
10. Cao Y, Krogstad P, Korber BT, et al: Maternal HIV-1 viral load and vertical transmission of infection: The Ariel Project for the prevention of HIV transmission from mother to infant. Nature Med 3:549, 1997
11. Dickover RE, Garratty EM, Herman SA, et al: Identification of levels of maternal HIV-1 RNA associated with risk of perinatal transmission: Effect of maternal zidovudine treatment on viral load. JAMA 275:599, 1996
12. Mayaux MJ, Dussaix E, Isopet J, et al: Maternal virus load during pregnancy and mother-to-child transmission of human immunodeficiency virus type 1: The French perinatal cohort studies, SEROGEST Cohort Group. J Infect Dis 175:172, 1997
13. Sperling R, Shapiro D, Coombs R, et al: Maternal plasma HIV-1 RNA and the success of zidovudine (ZDV) in the prevention of mother-child transmission. In: Abstracts of the 3rd Conference on Retroviruses and Opportunistic Infections, Washington, DC, 1996, Abstract LB-1
14. St. Louis ME, Kamenga M, Brown C, et al: Risk for perinatal HIV-1 transmission according to maternal immunologic, virologic, and placental factors. JAMA 269:2853, 1993
15. Shaffer N, Bhiraleus P, Chinayon P, et al: High viral load predicts perinatal HIV-1 subtype E transmission, Bangkok, Thailand. In: Abstracts of the XIth International Conference on AIDS, Vancouver, 1996, Abstract Tu.C.343
16. Contopoulos-Ioannidis DG, Ioannidis JP: Maternal cell-free viremia in the natural history of perinatal HIV-1 transmission: A meta-analysis. J Acquir Immune Defic Syndr Hum Retrovirol 18:126, 1998
17. Burns DN, Landesman S, Wright DJ, et al: Influence of other maternal variables on the relationship between maternal virus load and mother-to-infant transmission of human immunodeficiency virus type 1. J Infect Dis 175:1206, 1997
18. Goedert J, Duliege A, Amos C, et al: High risk of HIV-1 infection for first-born twins. Lancet 338:1471, 1991
19. Landesman SH, Kalish LA, Burns DN, et al: Obstetrical factors and the transmission of human immunodeficiency virus type 1 from mother to child: The Women and Infants Transmission Study. N Engl J Med 334:1617, 1996
20. Mandelbrot L, Le Chenadec J, Berrebi A, et al: Perinatal HIV-1 transmission: Interaction between zidovudine prophylaxis and mode of delivery in the French Perinatal Cohort. JAMA 280:55, 1998
21. Dunn DT, Newell ML, Mayaux MJ, et al: Mode of delivery and vertical transmission of HIV-1: A review of prospective studies. Perinatal AIDS Collaborative Transmission Studies. J Acquir Immune Defic Syndr 7:1064, 1994
22. Blanche S, Newell ML, Mayaux MJ, et al: Morbidity and mortality in European children vertically infected by HIV-1: The French Pediatric HIV Infection Study Group and European Collaborative Study. J Acquir Immune Defic Syndr Hum Retrovirol 14:442, 1997
23. European Collaborative Study: Natural history of vertically acquired human immunodeficiency virus-1 infection. Pediatrics 94:815, 1994
24. Wei X, Ghosh SK, Taylor ME, et al: Viral dynamics in human immunodeficiency virus type 1 infection. Nature 373:117, 1995
25. Pizzo PA, Wilfert C, Wilfert CM, et al: Markers and determinants of disease progression in children with HIV infection. The Pediatric AIDS Siena Workshop II. J Acquir Immune Defic Syndr Hum Retrovirol 8:30, 1995
26. Scott GB, Hutto C, Makuch RW, et al: Survival in children with perinatally acquired human immunodeficiency virus type 1 infection. N Engl J Med 321:1791, 1989

27. Mayaux MJ, Burgard M, Teglas JP, et al: Neonatal characteristics in rapidly progressive perinatally acquired HIV-1 disease: The French Pediatric HIV Infection Study Group. JAMA 275:606, 1996
28. Dickover RE, Dillon M, Leung KM, et al: Early prognostic indicators in primary perinatal human immunodeficiency virus type 1 infection: Importance of viral RNA and the timing of transmission on long-term outcome [in process citation]. J Infect Dis 178:375, 1998
29. Abrams EJ, Weedon JC, Lambert G, Steketee R: HIV viral load early in life as a predictor of disease progression in HIV-infected infants. In: Abstracts of the XIth International Conference on AIDS, Vancouver, 1996, Abstract We.B.311
30. Shearer WT, Quinn TC, LaRussa P, et al: Viral load and disease progression in infants infected with human immunodeficiency virus type 1: Women and Infants Transmission Study Group. N Engl J Med 336: 1337, 1997
31. Nahmias AJ, Clark WS, Kourtis AP, et al: Thymic dysfunction and time of infection predict mortality in human immunodeficiency virus-infected infants. J Infect Dis 178:680, 1998
32. Centers for Disease Control and Prevention: 1994 revised classification system for human immunodeficiency virus infection in children less than 13 years of age. MMWR Morbid Mortal Wkly Rep 43 (RR-12):1, 1994
33. Mofenson LM, Korelitz J, Meyer WAR, et al: The relationship between serum human immunodeficiency virus type 1 (HIV-1) RNA level, CD4 lymphocyte percent, and long-term mortality risk in HIV-1-infected children: National Institute of Child Health and Human Development Intravenous Immunoglobulin Clinical Trial Study Group. J Infect Dis 175:1029, 1997
34. Palumbo PE, Raskino C, Fiscus S, et al: Predictive value of quantitative plasma HIV RNA and CD4+ lymphocyte count in HIV-infected infants and children. JAMA 279:756, 1998
35. Tetali S, Than S, Pahwa S, et al: Plasma virus load evaluation in relation to disease progression in HIV-infected children. In: Abstracts of the 4th Conference on Retroviruses and Opportunistic Infections, Washington, DC, 1997, Abstract 484
36. Ramos JT, Rodriguez-Cerrato V, Ruiz-Contreras J, et al: Plasma viral load and disease progression in HIV-infected children. In: Abstracts fo the 4th Conference of Retroviruses and Opportunistic Infections, Washington, DC, 1997, Abstract 483
37. McKinney RE Jr, Wilfert C: Growth as a prognostic indicator in children with human immunodeficiency virus infection treated with zidovudine: AIDS Clinical Trials Group Protocol 043 Study Group. J Pediatr 125: 728, 1994
38. McIntosh K, Pitt J, Brambilla D, et al: Blood culture in the first 6 months of life for diagnosis of vertically transmitted human immunodeficiency virus infection. J Infect Dis 170:996, 1994
39. Luzuriaga K, Sullivan JL, Owens DK, et al: DNA polymerase chain reaction for the diagnosis of vertical HIV infection. JAMA 275:1360, 1996
40. Paul MO, Tetali S, Lesser ML, et al: Laboratory diagnosis of infection status in infants perinatally exposed to human immunodeficiency virus type 1. J Infect Dis 173:68, 1996
41. Dunn DT, Brandt CD, Krivine A, et al: The sensitivity of HIV-1 DNA polymerase chain reaction in the neonatal period and the relative contributions of intra-

uterine and intra-partum transmission. AIDS 9:F7, 1995
42. Steketee R, Abrams E, Thea D, et al: Early detection of perinatal human immunodeficiency virus (HIV) type 1 infection using HIV RNA amplification and detection. J Infect Dis 175:707, 1997
43. Young NL, Shaffer N, Chaowanachan T, et al: RNA and DNA PCR for early diagnosis of infants born to HIV-infected mothers, Thailand. In: Abstracts of the XIIth International Conference on AIDS, Geneva, 1998, Abstract 166
44. Nesheim S, Lee F, Kalish ML, et al: Diagnosis of perinatal human immunodeficiency virus infection by polymerase chain reaction and p24 antigen detection after immune complex dissociation in an urban community hospital. J Infect Dis 175:1333, 1997
45. American Academy of Pediatrics Committee on Pediatric AIDS: Evaluation and medical treatment of the HIV-exposed infant. Pediatrics 99:909, 1997
46. Centers for Disease Control and Prevention: Guidelines for the use of antiretroviral agents in the treatment of pediatric HIV infection. MMWR Morbid Mortal Wkly Rep 47(RR-4):1, 1998
47. Centers for Disease Control and Prevention: 1995 revised guidelines for prophylaxis against Pneumocystis carinii pneumonia for children infected with or perinatally exposed to human immunodeficiency virus. MMWR Morbid Mortal Wkly Rep 44(RR-4):1, 1995
48. Centers for Disease Control and Prevention: 1997 USPHS/IDSA guidelines for the prevention of opportunistic infections in persons infected with human immunodeficiency virus. MMWR Morbid Mortal Wkly Rep 46(RR-12):1, 1997
49. Kahn JO, Walker BD: Acute human immunodeficiency virus type 1 infection. N Engl J Med 339:33, 1998
50. Vigano A, Clerici M, Bricalli D, et al: Immune reconstitution and role of thymus during potent antiretroviral therapy in vertically HIV-infected children. In: Abstracts of the XIIth International Conference on AIDS, Geneva, 1998, Abstract 114
51. Rosenberg ES, Billingsley JM, Caliendo AM, et al: Vigorous HIV-1-specific CD4+ T cell responses associated with control of viremia. Science 278:1447, 1997
52. Kinloch-de Loes S, Perneger TV: Primary HIV infection: Follow-up of patients initially randomized to zidovudine or placebo. J Infect 35:111, 1997
53. Valentine ME, Jackson CR, Vavro C, et al: Evaluation of surrogate markers and clinical outcomes in two-year follow-up of eighty-six human immunodeficiency virus-infected pediatric patients. Pediatr Infect Dis J 17:18, 1998
54. McKinney RE, for the PACTG Protocol 300 Team: Pediatric ACTG Trial 300: Clinical efficacy of ZDV/3TC vs ddI vs ZDV/ddI in symptomatic, HIV-infected children. In: Program and Abstracts of the 35th Annual Meeting of the Infectious Diseases Society of America, San Francisco, 1997, Abstract 768
55. Englund JA, Baker CJ, Raskino C, et al: Zidovudine, didanosine, or both as the initial treatment for symptomatic HIV-infected children: AIDS Clinical Trials Group (ACTG) Study 152 Team. N Engl J Med 336: 1704, 1997
56. Hammer SM, Katzenstein DA, Hughes MD, et al: A trial comparing nucleoside monotherapy with combination therapy in HIV-infected adults with CD4 cell counts from 200 to 500 per cubic millimeter: AIDS Clinical Trials Group Study 175 Study Team. N Engl J Med 335:1081, 1996

57. Katzenstein DA, Hammer SM, Hughes MD, et al: The relation of virologic and immunologic markers to clinical outcomes after nucleoside therapy in HIV-infected adults with 200 to 500 CD4 cells per cubic millimeter. N Engl J Med 335:1091, 1996

58. Hammer SM, Squires KE, Hughes MD, et al: A controlled trial of two nucleoside analogues plus indinavir in persons with human immunodeficiency virus infection and CD4 cell counts of 200 per cubic millimeter or less: AIDS Clinical Trials Group 320 Study Team [see comments]. N Engl J Med 337:725, 1997

59. Yogev R, Stanley K, Nachman S, et al: Virologic efficacy of ZDV+3TC vs d4T+ritonavir (RTV) vs ZDV+3TC+RTV in stable antiretroviral experienced HIV-infected children (Pediatric ACTG Trial 338). In: Abstracts and Proceedings of the 37th Interscience Conference on Antimicrobial Agents and Chemotherapy, Toronto, 1997, Abstract LB-6

60. Kline MW, Fletcher CV, Federici ME, et al: Combination therapy with stavudine and didanosine in children with advanced human immunodeficiency virus infection: Pharmacokinetic properties, safety, and immunologic and virologic effects. Pediatrics 97:886, 1996

61. Mueller BU, Nelson RP Jr, Sleasman J, et al: A Phase I/II study of the protease inhibitor ritonavir in children with human immunodeficiency virus infection. Pediatrics 101:335, 1998

62. Tepper VJ, Farley JJ, Rothman MI, et al: Neurodevelopmental/neuroradiologic recovery of a child infected with HIV after treatment with combination antiretroviral therapy using the HIV-specific protease inhibitor ritonavir. Pediatrics 101:7, 1998

63. Kline MW, Fletcher CV, Harris AT, et al: A pilot study of combination therapy with indinavir, stavudine (d4T), and didanosine (ddI) in children infected with the human immunodeficiency virus. J Pediatr 132:543, 1998

64. Wintergerst U, Hoffmann F, Solder B, et al: Comparison of two antiretroviral triple combinations including the protease inhibitor indinavir in children infected with human immunodeficiency virus. Pediatr Infect Dis J 17:495, 1998

65. Luzuriaga K, Bryson Y, Krogstad P, et al: Combination treatment with zidovudine, didanosine, and nevirapine in infants with human immunodeficiency virus type 1 infection. N Engl J Med 336:1343, 1997

65a. Starr SE, Fletcher CV, Spector SA, et al: Efavirenz in combination with nelfinavir and nucleoside reverse transcriptase inhibitors (NRTIs) is safe and virologically effective in HIV-infected children. In: Abstracts and Proceedings of the 38th Interscience Conference on Antimicrobial Agents and Chemotherapy, San Diego, 1998, Abstract LB-6

66. Eastman PS, Shapiro DE, Coombs RW, et al: Maternal viral genotypic zidovudine resistance and infrequent failure of zidovudine therapy to prevent perinatal transmission of human immunodeficiency virus type 1 in pediatric AIDS Clinical Trials Group Protocol 076. J Infect Dis 177:557, 1998

67. Payan C, Fialaire P, Vitour D, et al: Mother-to-child transmission of Pol mutant T215Y HIV-1 isolates related to a high viral load under AZT treatment. In: Abstracts of the XIIth International Conference on AIDS, Geneva, 1998, Abstract 23308

68. Siegrist CA, Yerly S, Kaiser L, et al: Mother to child transmission of zidovudine-resistant HIV-1. Lancet 344:1771, 1994

69. Martel L, Valentine M, Ferguson M, et al: Virologic and CD4 response to treatment with nelfinavir in therapy experienced but protease inhibitor naïve HIV-infected children. In: Abstracts of the 5th Conference on Retroviruses and Opportunistic Infections, Chicago, 1998, Abstract 233

70. Pelton SI, Yogev R, Johnson D: Changes in viral load and immunologic markers in children treated with triple therapy including ritonavir. In: Abstracts of the 5th Conference on Retroviruses and Opportunistic Infections, Chicago, 1998, Abstract 234

71. Carpenter CC, Fischl MA, Hammer SM, et al: Antiretroviral therapy for HIV infection in 1998: Updated recommendations of the International AIDS Society—USA Panel. JAMA 280:78, 1998

72. Gutman LT, Herman-Giddens ME, McKinney RE: Pediatric acquired immunodeficiency syndrome: Barriers to recognizing the role of child sexual abuse. Am J Dis Child 147:775, 1993

73. Grubman S: Older children and adolescents living with perinatally acquired human immunodeficiency virus. Pediatrics 95:657, 1995

74. Department of Health and Human Services and Henry J. Kaiser Family Foundation: Guidelines for the use of antiretroviral agents in HIV-infected adults and adolescents. MMWR Morbid Mortal Wkly Rep 47:43, 1998

34 | Women and HIV Disease

MEG D. NEWMAN • CONSTANCE B. WOFSY*

EPIDEMIOLOGY

In December of 1997, almost 30.6 million adults worldwide were living with HIV/AIDS. Women constituted 42% or 12.8 million, of those infected.[1] It is estimated by the U.S. Agency for International Development that 40 million children in developing nations will lose one or both parents to AIDS by 2010. In the United States, women comprise the fastest growing population of persons with AIDS. Each year the proportion of cases among women continues to increase. Women comprised 22% of all the new cases recognized from January 1997 until December 31, 1997.[2,3] Women now account for 15% of the total cumulative cases, up from 8% of the cases in 1981–1987.[2-6]

Cumulative national data through December 1997 reveal that 44% of women have contracted AIDS from their own personal intravenous (IV) drug use and 39% from heterosexual contact (44% of the latter from sex with an IV drug user, 46% from sex with an HIV-infected person whose source of infection is unknown, and 7.5% from sex with a bisexual man). Another 4% of women developed AIDS from transfusion or other blood products; in 13% of the cases, the transmission route remains unidentified or not fully evaluated.[2,3]

In younger women ages 13 to 25, heterosexual contact dominates as a means of transmission, whereas it is a relatively uncommon mode of transmission in young men (54% compared to 4%).[2,3] In this same age group, injection drug use (IDU) accounts for 28% of infections in women and an injecting heterosexual partner is the source in 42.5% of heterosexually acquired cases. Thus IV drug use directly or indirectly accounts for over 60% of HIV in all women in the United States.[2,3,7]

In the United States as of December 1997 there were 98,468 women with AIDS. Of these women, 56% were African-American and 20% were Hispanic.[2,3] In 1996, among women ages 25 to 44, HIV infection was the third leading cause of death overall (11% of deaths), the fifth leading cause for Caucasian women (6% of deaths), and the leading cause for African-American women (22% of deaths). AIDS, especially heterosexually acquired AIDS, is found disproportionately among women of color.[8] It is estimated that the increasing death rate for women will leave 125,000 to 150,000 orphaned children when a projected 80,000 HIV-infected women die this decade in the United States.[1,9,10]

Increased Rates of Heterosexual Transmission

Heterosexuals represent the fastest growing risk group nationally, increasing from 3% of all AIDS cases among women in 1983 and 1984 to 38% as of December 31, 1997.[2-6] In 1995, heterosexual contact was the dominant mode of transmission for the majority of women in most regions of the United States, including 58% of AIDS cases in women reported in the south. Regions with the highest rates in women correspond to those where seroprevalence is highest in male IDUs.[11]

The true incidence of heterosexually transmitted cases is probably even higher, but cases are sometimes unrecognized because of the Centers for Disease Control and Prevention (CDC) reporting hierarchy. For example, if a woman had heterosexual contact multiple times and injected IV drugs once, she is categorized as having IDU as the source of her infection. Of the 90,837 cases ever classified as "risk not reported or identified" through December 1997, 41,391 have been reclassified. Of these, 10,201 are women, and 6835 (67%) of them have been

*Deceased.

reclassified as "transmission through heterosexual contact."[4,5] Reports suggest that, within the heterosexual transmission group, up to 50% of women did not know that they had been exposed to HIV.[2-4,12,13]

The AIDS Epidemic in Young Women

Not surprisingly, the IDU epidemic in men is reflected in the heterosexual epidemic in women, which is in turn reflected in the epidemic among children. The most alarming trends of heterosexual transmission are now occurring in young women.[2-4] In 1995 the largest increases in AIDS incidence rates were observed in women who were 14 to 18 years old in 1988, presumably a time period when they were likely to be infected.[14] A number of factors, both social and physiologic, are influential. In New York City, where one third of all women diagnosed with AIDS reside, infections in women under 30 outnumber those in men under 30 except for those in men having sex with men. Most of these young women have not reported IV drug use and are likely to have partners that are an average of 5 years older than themselves. It is well documented that women frequently have trouble negotiating with their male sexual partners for condom use, and one could speculate that the age gap between younger women and their sexual partners is likely to worsen this trend.[15-17] Finally, normal physiology in young women includes cervical ectopy, wherein the columnar cells of the endocervix are more exposed and allow more efficient transmission of HIV. Younger populations of women, particularly women of color, constitute a focus group that requires urgent outreach and intervention measures.[18-20]

Older Women and Heterosexual Transmission of HIV

An increasing number of transmissions have been noted in women over 60. In 1986, 102 cases were reported and by 1996, 305 cases had been reported to the CDC. The majority of the 102 cases reported in 1986 were linked to contaminated blood transfusions, whereas 69% of infections evaluated in 1996 were transmitted through heterosexual sex.[21] Most women who do not inject drugs, who do not have multiple sexual partners, who are over 45, or who have not received a blood transfusion do not perceive themselves as at risk for HIV. Too often providers also perceive women with these characteristics as having no HIV risk factors. Older women are often misdiagnosed and forfeit the benefits of highly active antiretroviral medication.

TRANSMISSION OF HIV

Heterosexual Transmission

Among HIV-discordant couples (those with only a single HIV-positive partner), heterosexual transmission is approximately eight times more efficient from male to female. Most infections have occurred by the vaginal route, although participation in rectal sex enhances the risk.[22-24] The cumulative incidence of transmission between discordant couples suggests an approximate 20% risk of transmission from male to female after unprotected sex over a sustained period in a fixed partnership. Female-to-male transmission is less efficient, at least in prospectively followed research subjects.[25,26] A study from Northern California that began prospectively following patients in 1985 found that only 2 (2.4%) of the 82 male partners of HIV-infected females became infected, but 68 (19%) of the 360 female partners became infected.[22,23]

Risk Factors Associated with Heterosexual Transmission

Factors associated with increased transmission include other sexually transmitted diseases (STDs), lack of condom use, advanced disease state (measured by CD4 count, viral load, or AIDS diagnosis), anal intercourse, number of sexual contacts, genital ulcerative disease, and intrauterine contraceptive device use[13,22,27,28] (Table 34–1). Cervical ectopy is emerging as a risk for acquisition by women from HIV-infected men. It is possible that the increased levels of heterosexual transmission in adolescent women may be partially explained by the natural occurrence of cervical ectopy in this age group.[29-31]

Recent research suggests that specific HIV subtypes (E and C) replicate more efficiently than subtype B in the Langerhans cells, the cells hypothesized to be the antigen-presenting cells responsible for vaginal transmission. In regions such as Thailand and India, where subtypes E and C, respectively, are common, heterosexual transmission is increased. In North America, however, subtype B predominates and hetero-

TABLE 34–1. Factors Associated with Heterosexual Transmission of HIV

FACTOR	MALE TO FEMALE	FEMALE TO MALE
Lack of condom	Yes	Yes
Anal intercourse	Yes	No
Sex during menses	No	Yes
Number of sexual contacts	Yes	Yes
Advanced disease state*	Yes	Yes
Zidovudine decreases risk	Possibly	Unknown
Genital sores, infections, or inflammation	Yes	Yes
Oral contraceptives[†]	Yes	Unknown
Intrauterine contraceptive device use	Possibly	Unknown
Cervical ectopy	Yes	Unknown

*As measured by CD4, p24 antigen, or AIDS diagnosis.
[†]Whether oral contraceptives are protective or increase the likelihood of transmission is controversial.
Modified from Padian N: Epidemiology of AIDS and heterosexually transmitted HIV in women. AIDS File 5:12, 1991, with permission.

sexual transmission is less common. It is speculated that the introduction of subtypes E or C into North America could augment heterosexual transmission.[32,33]

In men, HIV could be cultured from 30% of semen specimens from HIV-infected men with early disease. Sperm morphology and seminal characteristics were not affected even in men on zidovudine, but direct fertility studies are not available.[34] Lack of circumcision had been associated with increased risk of transmission in Africa, and Kreiss and Hopkins found that uncircumcised homosexual men in the United States had a twofold increased risk of HIV infection.[35] In men, zidovudine may decrease the prevalence or titer of HIV in seminal fluid but should not be considered an effective means of preventing transmission in either direction.[36–39]

Contraception and HIV Transmission

World health leaders have universally proclaimed the need for female-controlled contraceptive anti-infectives and microbicides. Women throughout the world identified fear of nonconsensual sex, domestic violence, or economic abandonment as limiting their ability to use the male condom. The ideal female-controlled method would be easy to use, would prevent other STDs, and could be used without a partner's consent or knowledge. The female condom, first marketed in 1993, is a polyurethane sheath that partially covers the external genitalia and may offer more protection against all STDs. The polyurethane membrane is 40% stronger than latex and inhibits HIV, cytomegalovirus (CMV), and hepatitis B. As a contraceptive, it is comparable to other barrier methods, including the male condom, diaphragm, cervical cap, and contraceptive sponge. The female condom has yet to attain full acceptability but has the potential to emerge as an important female-controlled contraceptive.

Nonoxynol 9 is another promising agent because of its potent viricidal effect in vitro and its effectiveness at killing other STD-causing agents.[41–45] However, it may produce vaginal irritation when used frequently.[41–45] At the Research Clinic for Prostitutes in Nairobi, Kenya, 138 seronegative prostitutes were evaluated, half routinely using a nonoxynol-9–treated sponge and half using a placebo. There were more genital ulcers and vulvitis in the nonoxynol 9 group, and the rate of HIV acquisition was similar; thus nonoxynol 9 was not protective.[41] The role of nonoxynol 9 in women with less frequent sexual contact remains to be determined. Because of the inherent value of nonoxynol 9, it is now being evaluated in a Phase III trial in South Africa and Thailand, formulated in a potentially less irritating bioadhesive compound named Col-1492.

Other microbicides under evaluation include C31G, an amphoteric surfactant that may have greater antichlamydial efficacy than nonoxynol 9. A vaginal suppository containing *Lactobacillus crispatus* is being tested, and sulfated polymer gels in Phase 1 trials appear well tolerated. Inhibitors of viral replication are also being considered. A small study in simian immunodeficiency virus (SIN)-positive macaques using a vaginal gel of PMPA was encouraging, as was a trial using loviride and chlorhexidine in a suppository.[46,47] The lack of in vitro systems and small animal models for testing, as well as deficient commercial interest, has slowed development of all of these products.[46] More knowledge about Langerhans cells and other sites for HIV and STD acquisition in the female genital tract is urgently needed so that effective and affordable methods can be developed.

The role of oral contraceptives in facilitating transmission to HIV-uninfected women or in transmitting HIV from HIV-infected women to their male partners has not been clearly delineated. Progesterone is known to thin vaginal epithelium, which may increase viral access to Langerhans and other cells. Studies have been indeterminate and inconsistent because of many factors, including that some women who use oral contraceptives may not also use a barrier method. In the rhesus macaque model, it has been documented that progesterone causes thinning of vaginal epithelium with increased SIV infection after intravaginal SIV exposure.[31] Although this study is not generalizable necessarily to humans, it does identify an important issue. In a study of HIV-infected women in Kenya, cervical proviral shedding was significantly associated with low T-cells count, vitamin A deficiency, medroxyprogesterone acetate, and both low- and high-dose oral contraceptives. Even when the analysis was adjusted for low T-cell count, it identified medroxyprogesterone acetate and oral contraceptives as risk factors for increased viral shedding.[48] Large, well-controlled studies need to address the issue further before final recommendations can be made.

Transmission of HIV in Lesbians

Transmission of HIV between women was documented as early as 1984.[49] A number of small studies have been conducted but are plagued by small numbers of women having sex with women (WSW) who have no other HIV risk factors, especially IDU. Through September 1989, 79 women with AIDS had reported sex with a female only, but 95% were IDUs.[50] Sporadic cases of direct transmission have been reported, but analysis is hampered by lack of data regarding baseline serology or blood exposure during sex.[51]

When the CDC surveillance hierarchy of risk factors is used, an infected WSW who has injected drugs or had heterosexual contact will be classified into the highest category: IDU and heterosexual transmission. Currently, WSW who are HIV infected but have no other risk factors are classified as "no identified risk"; that is, they have not reported behaviors known to efficiently transmit HIV. These regulations can shroud the true risk of HIV among WSW. Although HIV is present in the cervical and vaginal secretions of HIV-infected women, there is still a paucity of data on women's genital fluids and the risks of transmission from myriad WSW sexual practices.[52] Of note, a recent study of 21 lesbian monogamous partners suggests strongly that bacterial vaginosis can be sexually transmitted between women.[53]

There has been no evidence of female-to-female transmission in a study of 960,000 female blood donors in the United States. Of the total, there were 96 seropositive women, of whom 3 reported sex with men and women and none with women only.[54] Raiteri and colleagues looked at a group of 10 HIV-infected lesbians and their seronegative partners from 1992 through 1995. In the final analysis, 26 discordant lesbian couples were examined and no seroconversions occurred.[55] Lesbians have thus been considered at low risk. However, if providers assume that lesbians are not engaging in sex with men, especially gay men and IDU men, they may be overlooking risk behaviors that may be (or are) more common than most providers suspect. In 1993, the San Francisco Department of Health studied 498 women recruited at public social events aimed at lesbian and bisexual women in San Francisco and Berkeley, California. In the cohort, of whom 68% self-identified as lesbians and 22% as bisexuals, 81% reported having sex with men, including unprotected oral (56.3%), vaginal (39%), and anal (10.9%) sex. High rates of unprotected oral, vaginal, or anal sex with gay/bisexual men (14.6%, 9.6%, and 3.2%, respectively) were also noted.[56] Multiple other studies conducted in New York City, Milwaukee, and Seattle corroborate these results; however, they are not ideal for deriving precise prevalence data about WSW and probably involve only segments of the WSW community. These studies re-emphasize the important point that sexual identity is a poor marker for sexual behaviors. Because they have been considered "safe," lesbians have not been targeted for AIDS education and may be engaging in multiple unsafe sexual practices.[57]

WSW may engage in sexual activity with men for pleasure, during commercial sex work, or through sexual assault. Some women IDUs who engage in sex with other women are associated with riskier IDU and sexual behaviors and therefore are at a higher risk of acquiring HIV than other women IDUs.[52] WSW who also use injection drugs were more likely to share needles, to exchange sex for drugs or money, to be homeless, and to seroconvert. This more marginalized group and their sexual partners would likely benefit from specially targeted pre-

TABLE 34–2. Prevention Strategies for Women Who Have Sex with Women

1. Remember to focus on behavior, not labels. Remember to ask if your patient is sexually active with women, men, or both even if she defines herself as a lesbian.
2. Don't be alarmist but be informative about female-to-female transmission.
3. Focus on WSW who have high-risk behaviors such as drug use or sex with men at risk for HIV.
4. Focus on female partners of women who also have sex with men at risk for HIV.
5. Behaviors that are higher risk are likely to include acts that result in vaginal trauma.

vention programs. Although the reservoir of HIV is low in WSW at this juncture, there is no doubt about the transmissibility of the disease between WSW. Women partners of women infected with HIV need to observe the same principles of safer sexual activity and avoid mucous membrane contact of all potentially infectious secretions[58,59] (Table 34–2). Lesbian women who are attempting artificial insemination from unknown donors should chose facilities that carefully test donors for HIV at the time of donation and then again at six months before using their stored product.

PROGRESSION OF DISEASE

Results of initial early studies analyzing progression and survival suggested there was a difference based on gender. Many early studies indicated that the prognosis for women was worse than that for men regardless of the risk group or race. A study done in New York City early in the epidemic looked at 544 women compared to 2526 men with first-episode *Pneumocystis carinii* pneumonia. Fewer women were white, more women were admitted through emergency rooms, more women received care at hospitals with less experience in caring for PCP, and fewer women underwent bronchoscopy. In addition, more women were admitted to the intensive care unit. This study reflected late access to decreased care—a common scenario for women early in the AIDS epidemic.[60] All of the more recent work disputes the notion that women have increased levels of morbidity and mortality as a result of gender and supports the contention that earlier results that suggest so were just markers for poor access to care.[61,62]

Studies of disease progression in women are limited and, when available, are derived from three principal sources: large national data bases, which usually include the diagnosis of AIDS and the date of death with little additional interval information; small to moderate-sized cohort studies of 50 to 200 women, often followed for less than 3 years; and large cohort studies conducted in other regions (e.g., Africa) from which conclusions may not be applicable to the United States or western Europe because of great differences in economic, sociologic, medical, and public health conditions.[63] In the Bronx, New York, access to or adherence to follow-up care strongly influenced survival time, with survival substantially shortened in women who had no prior care before a severe HIV-related infection. A recently published trial of 1372 patients followed by Chaisson and colleagues in Baltimore found that gender had no relationship to disease progression.[64]

Among New York Medicaid recipients (of whom 60% of the men and women were IDUs), treatment with zidovudine and PCP prophylaxis was equal in IDUs, but non-IDU women were less likely to get on zidovudine or PCP prophylaxis. Among drug users, women survived slightly longer than men, and among non–drug users, survival was similar for both sexes.[65]

A Community Programs for Clinical Research on AIDS study looked at 3779 men and at 768 women with median T-cell counts higher than the men (median 240 in women versus 137 in men) and found that women were at increased risk of death (with a relative risk of 1.3) during a 15-month period. It is important to note that there was no increased risk of HIV disease progression in women. Equally important, the increased risk of death was found primarily among IDUs, and the deaths were secondary to bacterial pneumonia and endocarditis, both of which are probably related to IDU. The study authors concluded that these findings may represent differential access to care, treatments, or social support.[61] The most important predictors of survival or progression appear to be CD4 count, viral load, and the specific AIDS-defining diagnosis, not gender.[16,63,66–70]

In a review of AIDS in women reported to the CDC by December 1990, 73% of women with AIDS were residents of large metropolitan areas of over 1 million population. Most of these areas are on the Atlantic seaboard, and suggested a target for interventions. The other 26% were from smaller cities, making it harder to target a specific population. Because women frequently use emergency rooms, family planning clinics, STD clinics, youth guidance centers, jail clinic facilities, and drug treatment units, these are the sites for targeting efforts at

TABLE 34–3. Proposed Recommendations for Referral for HIV Counseling and Testing (Clinical Conditions Warranting HIV Counseling and Testing)

Possible immunosuppression must be considered with the following gynecologic conditions:
1. Recurrent genital herpes simplex (more than 2 episodes within 6 months or 4 per year, or the frequency of episodes doubled over a year)
2. Severe or coalescing lesions of genital herpes simplex or candidiasis
3. Other genital ulcer disease (chancroid, syphilis, apthous genital ulcers, or lymphogranuloma venereum)
4. Condyloma acuminata that is recalcitrant to conventional therapy or involves multiple sites
5. Pap test with abnormalities*
6. Any PID or any STD
7. Persistent or recurrent vaginal candidiasis (persistence after 2 treatment courses, or more than 2 episodes within 6 months, or 4 per year, or the frequency of episodes doubled over a year)

*The vast majority of abnormal Pap smears are in women without HIV.

early diagnosis and use of early intervention with antiviral and prophylactic therapies.[71]

Lack of access to care, minimal self-motivation, attention to the health care of their children over that of themselves, and disenfranchisement among a large proportion of women all contribute to decreased rates of early detection and intervention.[60] Medical providers need to maintain a low threshold to counsel and test for HIV, remembering that women in the United States who have HIV through heterosexual transmission may be unaware of their partners' HIV status and therefore do not perceive themselves as at risk for HIV (Table 34–3). HIV and AIDs for women is an issue of access to health care, and the care system is not always well suited to their needs.[3,4,72,73]

RESOURCES FOR WOMEN

One valuable resource for women with AIDS is Women Organized to Respond to Life Threatening Diseases (WORLD), a diverse community of women living with HIV/AIDS and their supporters. They provide support, information, education, and inspiration as well as promote public awareness about AIDS (contact by phone: 510-658-6930 or fax: 510-601-9746).

CLINICAL MANIFESTATIONS

Several factors may influence the presentation of HIV or response to therapy in women. These include altered pharmacokinetics of drugs resulting from either gender or interactions between commonly associated drugs (such as methadone or oral contraceptive pills). Presentation and response to therapy are possibly also related to differences in the immune system; medical literature suggests autoimmune diseases are more frequent in women than in men. Symptoms of middle-stage HIV in women, as in men, may be nonspecific, including night sweats, diarrhea, fatigue, cough, and weight loss.[74–76] There are no glaring differences between the sexes in the presentation or natural history of common AIDS-defining diseases such as PCP, disseminated *Mycobacterium avium* complex, cryptococcus, and toxoplasmosis.[77,78]

Opportunistic Infections and HIV-Associated Infections

AIDS-defining diagnoses seen with frequency in data combined from a number of small female cohorts include PCP, esophageal candidiasis, disseminated *Mycobacterium avium*, and mucocutaneous herpes simplex virus (HSV).[73] Women are not protected from any of the other AIDS-defining opportunistic infections.[79] Bacterial infections, especially respiratory infections with such encapsulated organisms as *Streptococcus pneumoniae* and *Haemophilus influenzae*, occur more frequently in IV drug users than in homosexual men and occur with equal frequency in heterosexual men and women.[27,80] One of the earliest and largest prospectively followed cohorts of women with HIV, initiated in the early 1980s, comes from Rhode Island, where 200 HIV-infected women have been followed at regular intervals. The initial clinical manifestations of HIV infection in 117 symptomatic women were *Candida* vaginitis (*n* = 43), lymphadenopathy (*n* = 17), bacterial pneumonia (*n* = 15), acute retroviral syndrome (*n* = 8), and constitutional symptoms, such as unexplained weight loss of 10 pounds or more or diarrhea for 4 weeks or more (*n* = 8). The rest had syndromes that would suggest to most clinicians a consideration of HIV infection (i.e., thrush, tuberculosis, hairy leukoplakia, herpes zoster, PCP, AIDS encephalopathy, and CMV retinitis).[74] Nonspecific conditions of vaginitis, pneumonia, and constitutional symptoms associated with HIV infection were more frequent. In this cohort, PCP was the AIDS-defining manifestation in only 20%, and 34% presented with esophageal candidiasis as their AIDS-defining diagnosis. This cohort differs from others, particularly in having a smaller percentage of non-white subjects, which is in accord with the demographics of Rhode Island. Another study from France found that esophageal candidiasis was also more common in a cohort of women than was PCP. These studies are in sharp contrast to national data and other cohorts in which, prior to 1993, PCP was the leading AIDS diagnosis.[68,81–83]

Opportunistic Infection Prophylaxis and CMV Antibody Screening

Appropriate opportunistic infection prophylaxis is necessary for both women and men, and no gender-specific recommendations can be made. Immunoglobulin G antibodies to CMV are almost always positive in homosexual men, but the rates in women are more like the rates in the general population, in which approximately 50% of adults are seropositive. The CMV-negative patient in need of a transfusion should always receive CMV-negative blood to avoid future risk of CMV end-organ disease.[84,85]

Malignancies

Kaposi's Sarcoma

Kaposi's sarcoma (KS), seen frequently in homosexual men, is found in less than 2% of HIV-infected women as an initial AIDS diagnosis. When KS has been seen in women, it most frequently has been associated with sex with a bisexual man, but it has been seen in women whose risk was IDU or transfusion.[86] There is strong evidence that KS in persons with or without HIV infection is associated with newly identified human herpesvirus 8 (HHV8) and can be transmitted sexually.[87,88] HHV8 has been identified in tissues from people with all kinds of KS, including KS associated with AIDS, endemic cases in Africa, classic KS in elderly men of Mediterranean descent, and in KS arising from organ transplant. HHV8 has been detected in semen and sperm, peripheral blood lymphocytes, nasal secretions, and saliva as well as endothelial cells. The presence or absence of HHV8 in myriad women's fluids (breast milk, vaginal and cervical secretions) has not been determined.

HHV8 appears to be present in 3% of normal blood donors from the United States and United Kingdom and in substantially higher numbers in Greece (20%) and Africa (35% to 65%). Approximately 4% of women with AIDS in the United States have antibody to HHV8.[89] HHV8 appears to be a cofactor for the development of KS, but the other factors that contribute to expression of KS have not been elucidated.[90]

In one cohort of 1239 patients, 123 had KS diagnoses between 1988 and 1995; 12 were women. All of the women had heterosexual contact with men at risk for HIV, 5 of the 12 had contact with bisexual men, and 3 of the women were commercial sex workers. Both the men and the women in the cohort were matched for stage of HIV disease at the time of initial presentation. KS in these women was more aggressive and advanced, with more noncutaneous disease, more lymphedema, and more lymph node and visceral involvement.[91] Several reports suggest the course of KS in women can be aggressive, even when KS is the initial manifestation of AIDS.[86,92]

The case of a 22-year-old woman whose KS and HIV were diagnosed when she went to her dentist because of a violaceous lesion on her hard palate emphasizes that all health practitioners must be alert for signs of HIV in both high-risk and seemingly low-risk populations.[93] This is particularly germane to women who may contract HIV or HHV8 disease through heterosexual transmission because they often are unaware of their risk factors and do not perceive themselves to be at any risk.[92,94] A recent report describes an HIV-infected woman who presented with vulvar pain, vaginal discharge, and a vulvar mass that proved to be KS.[95] This case emphasizes the point that unusual presentations of KS are likely to occur.[42,96]

Other Malignancies

Non-Hodgkin's lymphoma, an AIDS-defining diagnosis, is encountered too infrequently in women to compare gender-specific incidence rates.[97,98] However, it does constitute an AIDS-defining diagnosis in both sexes. To date, it appears that the occurrence of lung cancer is greater in HIV-positive individuals. One initial report suggests the natural history is distinct in the HIV-infected person, with the diagnosis occurring at a younger age, almost entirely in males, presenting at a later stage, with a decreased survival.[99] Kaplan provides observational data from 797 HIV-infected women suggesting that these women are experiencing a wide array of cancers, including lung cancers, especially when their T cell counts are less than 200 cells/mm^3.[100] Other sporadic case reports have observed a few cases of aggressive breast cancer.

Because both women and men are surviving longer, it will be important to document the frequency and natural history of these malignancies over the next decade. A discussion of cervical dysplasia is included in the next section on gynecologic manifestations.

Gynecologic Manifestations

Much attention has been given to four disorders that may be more frequent, more severe, and less responsive to therapy in HIV-infected women than in HIV-uninfected women: human papillomavirus (HPV), associated cervical disorders such as cervical intraepithelial neoplasia (CIN), *Candida* vaginitis, and pelvic inflammatory disease (PID).[8,101–105] These disorders are recognized as HIV-associated conditions in the expanded CDC case definition.[106,107]

Cervical Disorders

HPV AND CERVICAL NEOPLASIA. As of 1993, cervical cancer constitutes an AIDS diagnosis.[81,106,108] Limited evidence suggests an increased occurrence and aggressiveness of cervical cancer in women with HIV infection. In data from 1994–1995, Weber et al. appreciated a rate of invasive cervical cancer of 10.4 per 1000 in HIV-infected women versus 6.2 per 1000 in HIV-negative controls.[109] Higher rates of invasive cervical cancer were noted in HIV-infected African-American and Hispanic women ages 20 to 34 when compared to their HIV-uninfected controls. In the general population, invasive cervical cancer is more common among black women living in the south and is typical of women diagnosed with AIDS as a result of their invasive cervical cancer.[110–114]

HPV is believed to be an etiologic factor in human cervical cancer and has been investigated since the 1970s. Approximately 95% of cervical condyloma, all grades of CIN, and invasive cervical cancer contain HPV DNA. HPV types 16 and 18 have been found most commonly in cervical cancer, and types 6 and 11 are most frequently associated with benign condylomas or low-grade squamous intraepithelial lesions (SILs).[115,116]

Immune suppression appears to make one particularly susceptible to infection by HPV. Reports indicate that autograft transplant recipients receiving immunosuppressive treatments have a nine times increased incidence of HPV anogenital infection and 16 times increased incidence of CIN compared with the general population.

HPV prevalence, acquisition, and retention are higher in HIV-positive women than in matched controls. By DNA analysis, types 16, 18, and 33 are associated most frequently with CIN in HIV-positive women and controls,[95,103,117] especially in women with CD4 counts of less than 200 cells/mm^3.[22,107,118–128] An increased frequency of abnormal Papanicolaou (Pap) smear results was first noted in women attending clinics for HIV, methadone maintenance, and cervical dysplasia.[8,102] In an early study, 40% of 35 HIV-positive women had SILs on cervical cytologic examinations, compared with 9% of 32 HIV-negative women.[102]

In another early study of 32 HIV-infected women, 78% had a normal Pap smear result, and only 3% had cytologic Pap smear findings suggesting CIN. However, colposcopy associated with biopsy disclosed that 41% had cervical abnormalities.[104] This had profound implications, since colposcopy is more costly and more time consuming and requires specially trained personnel for proper interpretation.

Subsequent studies have not confirmed these findings and, in fact, suggest that a correctly obtained and expertly read Pap smear (at least under research conditions) has sufficient sensitivity and specificity to detect cervical abnormalities.[129] A large, prospective, multicenter study conducted by the CDC in conjunction with investigators in Miami and New York compared HIV-positive and negative women, all of whom had Pap smears, colposcopy, and evaluation for HPV by polymerase chain reaction. This controlled trial confirmed numerous prior uncontrolled studies of HIV-positive cohorts in finding that CIN is more frequent in HIV-positive women (20% in HIV-positive compared with 4% in HIV-negative women) and that more advanced CIN is more likely with more advanced stage of immunosuppression. By multivariate analysis, HPV (odds ratio [OR] 9.8), HIV infection (OR 3.5), and CD4 count (OR 2.7) were independently associated with CIN.[114,125] A large cohort from the Women's Interagency HIV Study (WIHS) reported on 2015 HIV-infected women and 577 HIV-seronegative controls. Those women who were HIV infected had the highest rates of HPV infection (58%) compared with seronegative controls (26%). HIV-infected women also demonstrated a 42% prevalence of infection with multiple types of HPV versus a 16% prevalence in uninfected women. Risk factors for CIN/SIL were CD4 lymphocytes <200 cell/mm^3, higher risk HPV types and multiple types of HPV.[130] In a meta-analysis examining 19 studies incorporating 728 HIV infected women, Korn and Landers found dysplasia occurring in 64% of those with AIDS and in 36% of HIV-positive women.[131]

ARE PAP SMEARS AS SENSITIVE IN HIV-INFECTED WOMEN? Because CIN is more frequent and more aggressive in women with severe immunosuppression, some practitioners routinely recommend a Pap smear every 6 months, particularly for women with more advanced immunodeficiency.[132] The WIHS study also suggested that Pap smears were highly sensitive in HIV-positive women. Subsequent studies confirm that Pap smears also were equally sensitive for detecting cervical disorders in HIV-positive and HIV-negative women.[131,133] One study also demonstrated that 15% of the dysplasia in HIV-positive women seen in a large dysplasia referral clinic was limited to vulvar, vaginal, or perianal lesions detected only by colposcopy. These lesions would have been missed if only a cervical Pap smear had been performed.[131] Although colposcopy would be the most sensitive and specific diagnostic tool, the general lack of availability and standardization require assiduous attention to appropriate Pap smear tests and follow-up.

The Women's Interagency HIV Study (WIHS), a large natural history study of HIV-infected women, is currently being conducted, and the results will define the optimum interval for Pap screening. At this time, performing a Pap screening every 6 months along with careful vulvar, vaginal, and anal inspection appears prudent, especially with more immunosuppressed patients with T-cell counts less than 200/mm^3. Colposcopic evaluation of women should be performed with any atypical squamous cells of unknown significance, atypical glandular cells of unknown significance, low-grade and high-grade SIL on any Pap smear, or any persistent inflammation that is unresolved after treatment for gonococcus, *Trichomonas*, or chlamydia. Initial colposcopy could be considered for women with poor likelihood of follow-up or suspicion of extracervical disease[131,134] (Table 34–4). Pregnancy did not affect the incidence of abnormal smears in women enrolled in the Women and Infants Transmission Study.[135]

TREATMENT OF CIN. CIN I that is documented on biopsy (not just Pap smear) does not appear to progress to invasive cervical cancer, although it requires follow-up to detect progression to a higher grade of CIN. CIN II and CIN III require definitive therapy to avoid invasive cervical cancer. Modalities such as loop electrosurgical excision procedure, cryotherapy, and laser vaporization are effective when the endo-

TABLE 34–4. Proposed Recommendations for Routine Gynecologic Care of HIV-Infected Women

1. Perform baseline colposcopy at HIV diagnosis if available.
2. Perform a pelvic exam and Pap smear every 6 months with careful vulvar, vaginal, and anal inspection.
3. Refer for colposcopic evaluation women with any atypia, ASCUS, AGCUS, low-grade and high-grade SIL, or persistent inflammation (that is unresolved after treatment for GC or chlamydia) on any Pap smear.*
4. Treat genital warts.
5. Assess for syphilis.
6. Perform a wet mount to rule out bacterial vaginosis, trichomonas, and *Candida*.
7. Counsel on STDs, cervical cancer, HPV, contraception, pregnancy, and safer sex.

*AGCUS, atypical glandular cells of undetermined significance; ASCUS, atypical squamous cells of undetermined significance; SIL, squamous intraepithelial lesion; GC, gonococcus.

cervical region can be well visualized and there is no endocervical involvement.

Cervical conization is indicated for women who do not meet those criteria. In seronegative women there is a small risk of 5% to 10% of CIN II or III recurring after therapy. All of the treatments for CIN appear less effective in HIV-infected women, especially those with more advanced immunosuppression. In HIV-positive women, the risk of recurrence is much higher and requires careful surveillance.[136] The treating clinician should be prepared to treat recurrences with the knowledge that doing so is preventing the development of invasive cervical cancer.

Genital Warts

Genital warts in HIV-infected women may be large, multifocal, and more prone to recurrence than in non-HIV-infected women. Traditional treatments with trichloroacetic acid, cryotherapy with liquid nitrogen, or cryoprobe usually work. Laser or surgical excision may be required in difficult cases.

Anal Squamous Intraepithelial Lesions

Anal squamous intraepithelial lesions (ASIL) are also more prevalent and increasingly recognized in HIV-infected individuals.[137] As noted earlier, immunosuppression allows HPV to be more persistent and aggressive, resulting in ASIL and invasive anal cancer. Receptive anal intercourse undoubtedly plays a role in the transmission of anal HPV in women and men.[123,138,139] It is uncertain if fingers or sexual tools with HPV contamination are capable of establishing infection in either men or women. In one study of 102 HIV-infected women and 96 HIV-uninfected women, anal cytologic abnormalities were significantly more common in HIV-infected women (26%) than in HIV-uninfected women (7%). In the HIV-infected group, 95% of the abnormalities were mild squamous cytologic atypia and only 5% were low-grade anal intraepithelial neoplasia. Notably, the likelihood of cytologic abnormalities was greater in women with lower CD4 lymphocyte counts.[120] In a group of women IDUs in San Francisco, ASIL was as prevalent as CIN.[117,123,139,140,141]

At this time it is difficult to make specific recommendations for screening or for treatment for ASIL in women, because the natural history of ASIL and the likelihood of progression to anal carcinoma in women is unknown. Studies are ongoing in the United States to determine optimum screening and treatment regimens for both men and women.

If women have other sites of HPV anogenital disease and lower CD4 lymphocyte counts, they are more likely to have ASIL. If a decrease in morbidity and mortality can be demonstrated from screening and treatment, it would be justified for women with low CD4 lymphocytes, and it would even be justified in women without known HPV but with clinical prognosticators suggesting long survival. In all cases morbidity and mortality considerations for the individual patient should weigh heavily into a decision of whether to screen or treat for ASIL.

Vaginal Candidiasis

Vaginal candidiasis, a frequent disorder in women in the general population, may be a source of morbidity for HIV-infected women.[74,83,142–144] In the revised CDC case definition of 1993, severe vaginal candidiasis became a designated HIV-associated symptomatic disorder.[106] Early studies such as that of the Rhode Island cohort demonstrated vulvovaginitis in 44 of 200 prospectively followed women, and vulvovaginitis was the most common initial HIV-associated clinical condition. Other uncontrolled studies have shown a moderate prevalence of disease, but no comparison to non-HIV-infected patients could be made. Although it is clear that vulvovaginitis and HIV occur together, it is unclear that vulvovaginitis is significantly worse or more common in HIV-infected women. Recent work by Sobel et al. evaluated 833 HIV-infected women and 427 non-HIV-infected women and found that, although HIV-infected women were vaginally colonized more often with Candida, their incidence of vulvovaginitis was the same.[145,146] Many women with HIV disease experience vulvovaginitis (it can occur at any time in HIV disease) and many women, even with severe immunosuppression, do not experience vulvovaginitis. We think it is important to have a low threshold for testing and counseling for HIV disease, especially in women who acquire this disease through heterosexual transmission. Contrary to prior thinking, recurrent vulvovaginitis alone may not be sensitive or specific of an HIV diagnosis. As with many other topics in women and AIDS, this domain warrants further study.

Candida can be cultured readily from the vagina in the absence of symptoms, so a diagnosis must include clinical symptoms and a potassium hydroxide preparation. Cultures are not indicated initially. Cultures should be considered in patients with recurrent or recalcitrant cases of fungal vulvovaginitis. Torulopsis glabrata can be difficult to diagnose without a culture because it does not form hyphae or pseudohyphae, may not demonstrate a cheesy discharge, is often associated with recurrent vulvovaginitis, and can be resistant to imidazoles.[147,148]

Response of vulvovaginitis to such topical agents as clotrimazole or miconazole is usually quite good in HIV-infected women. Vaginal secretions maintain increased concentrations of fluconazole for 72 hours or more, and 150 mg for 1 to 3 days can be extremely effective. Sometimes a higher dose or longer duration is necessary for more refractory cases. Fluconazole is notable for some resistance to non-albicans species (Torulopsis, lambica, and krusei).

Genital Ulcerative Disease

Genital ulcerative disease is a well-described risk factor for transmission of HIV, particularly in studies in Africa, where STDs are more prevalent.[149] A wide array of agents may be causative, including HSV, CMV, syphilis, chancroid, gonorrhea, acid-fast bacteria, other bacterial or fungal pathogens, and malignancies. Genital ulcers are painful, disabling, and difficult to treat. Such ulcers should be evaluated with a full work-up.

HERPES SIMPLEX VIRUS. Severe ulcerative genital herpes was the AIDS-defining diagnosis in 18% of 44 HIV-infected women prospectively followed who developed AIDS.[74] Genital HSV infections are very prevalent in the population at large and may be particularly refractory in HIV-infected men and women. HSV may present atypically and recur frequently. Common sites of presentation include the labia majora, labia minora, sacrum, and buttocks.[150,151]

Augenbraun et al. recently demonstrated that HSV-2 shedding was nearly four times greater in HIV-positive than in HIV-negative women and that 79% of the shedding was asymptomatic. As immunosuppression progresses (measured by declining CD4 count), shedding of HSV-2 became more common.[152]

In 12 HIV-infected men with recurrent HSV and HIV, Schacker demonstrated consistent HIV in the HSV lesions, with many containing 5000 or more copies of HIV RNA per sample.[153] There is every reason to assume that this finding occurs in women as well, and it partially explains the increased rates of HIV transmission when ulcer disease is present. Specific safer sex counseling needs to address the issue of asymptomatic viral shedding associated with HSV.

Simple mucocutaneous lesions can be treated with acyclovir or famciclovir. Severe mucocutaneous disease or any evidence of systemic disease dictates intravenous acyclovir. Nonhealing mucocutaneous lesions should prompt consideration of acyclovir resistance and necessitate use of intravenous foscarnet. Some smaller recalcitrant lesions heal well with trifluridine ophthalmic drops applied directly to the lesion, covered by an occlusive dressing.

GIANT IDIOPATHIC APTHOUS GENITAL ULCERS. Giant idiopathic apthous genital ulcers are infrequent but painful, disabling, and difficult to treat. Such ulcers should be evaluated with a full work-up for HSV, CMV, syphilis, chancroid, gonorrhea, bacterial or fungal pathogens, and malignancies. The pathogenesis may be similar to giant oral or esophageal apthous ulcers. Anecdotal reports suggest that thalidomide may be effective for esophageal ulcers, but there is negligible experience with genital ulcers in women. A rigorous application process would be required in order to give thalidomide on a compassionate-use basis.[154]

Pelvic Inflammatory Disease

HIV is prevalent in women with PID, and there have been suggestions that PID may be more severe with advanced HIV disease.[155,156] Early findings of the Multicenter HIV and PID Study Group did not confirm a substantially worse presentation. PID responded to therapy equally in HIV-infected and HIV-uninfected groups.[103,157]

HIV-positive patients may present with lower white counts. Tubo-ovarian abscess formation has been reported to occur in as many as 25% of HIV-infected women with PID versus 12% of HIV-uninfected controls with PID. Therefore, more surgical intervention is required, especially in the more advanced AIDS patients. Standard antibiotic regimens that include anaerobic coverage can be used initially. If response is poor, antibiotic coverage of anaerobes should be enhanced.[131] Most clinicians maintain a low threshold to hospitalize, especially if the HIV disease is advanced.

Menstrual Disorders

There are currently no data to suggest that diagnosis or treatment of menstrual disorders in HIV-positive women should be different from that for HIV-negative women. However, further documentation of the specific types of menstrual irregularity, the frequency, and the hormone interaction is needed. These menstrual disorders are relevant not only because of personal discomfort but because unsuspected pregnancy may masquerade as a delayed period. Menstrual irregularities make prediction of time of fertility difficult for those wishing to conceive or avoid pregnancy and may potentially increase exposure to menstrual blood for a partner.[151]

Sporadic reports suggest that HIV-infected women experience higher rates of menstrual irregularities, including amenorrhea, menorrhagia, intermenstrual bleeding, and worse premenstrual syndrome. A New York study of IV drug-using women compared 39 HIV-positive women to 39 HIV-negative women and identified more menstrual abnormalities in the HIV-positive women (41% versus 24%).[158] Amenorrhea and between-period bleeding were noted particularly. Other small studies support that approximately one third of HIV-positive women have either excessive bleeding or amenorrhea.[29,159,160]

A recent small controlled trial of HIV-negative women and HIV-positive women with midstage disease found no menstrual differences between groups.[144] The fluctuations of progesterone, estradiol, and cortisol throughout the menstrual cycle of HIV-infected women with normal cycles was identical to well-established norms in the population at large.[161]

A 1997 study[162] emanating from the WIHS looked at 2000 HIV-infected women and compared them to 500 seronegative controls. Amenorrhea (defined as no menstrual period for greater than 90 days) was noted in 7% of HIV-infected women and 5% of seronegative controls. The risk factors for amenorrhea in the study were found to be HIV infection, heroin use, low albumin, and live births. Lower CD4 lymphocyte counts, serum albumin levels of less than 3.0 gm/dl, or use of heroin or amphetamine increased the risk of amenorrhea. Many HIV-infected women (61%) reported irregular periods in the past 6 months, but this was not statistically significant when compared with controls. The majority of these women had amenorrhea on the basis of hypothalamic dysfunction, with low or normal levels of follicle-stimulating hormone and low levels of estradiol.[162]

GUIDELINES FOR THE USE OF ANTIRETROVIRAL TREATMENT EFFICACY AND TOXICITY IN WOMEN

Potential toxicity issues affecting treatment with antiretrovirals include the lower mean body weight in women, lower mean hemoglobin level (with the potentially complicating effect of zidovudine or dapsone in further inducing anemia), and absence of established controls and norms for CD4 counts in women.

Guidelines established for licensed antiretroviral therapies and prophylaxis against PCP and other opportunistic infections are derived from large national studies conducted on men and women. Although men predominate in these studies, the results led to licensure and established recommendations for persons of both sexes. Data from two large early national studies from the AIDS Clinical Trials Groups (ACTG 016 and 019)[72,98,163] comparing zidovudine versus placebo in mildly symptomatic HIV-infected patients in ACTG 016 and asymptomatic HIV-infected persons in ACTG 019 suggested no difference in benefit from zidovudine for women or nonwhite persons.[126,164]

Disappointingly, there is still a paucity of data about efficacy and toxicity of antiretroviral drugs in women. Although more recent studies have sought participation from women, their participation is still low.[72,127,165] More recently, studies have looked at both efficacy and toxicity and suggest that the current combinations appear equally effective in women. At our clinic, anecdotal experience is congruent with that finding. A recent study by Zorrilla and colleagues looked at a four-drug regimen of nelfinavir, saquinavir, stavudine, and lamivudine given in a twice- or thrice-daily regimen to antiretroviral-naive HIV-infected women with viral loads greater than 200,000 copies/ml of blood. Results are still accruing, but preliminary data suggest women are tolerating the regimen well; 84% have viral loads below the level of detection, with a median T-cell count increase of 100 cells/mm^3.[166] Currier and colleagues have reported on the toxicity of ritonavir in combination with reverse transcriptase inhibitors in 90 women versus 996 men. Both women and men experienced similar toxicity, with women having more nausea (63% vs. 56% in men), vomiting (49% vs. 31%), malaise and fatigue (47% vs. 34%), and perioral numbness and tingling (37% vs. 27%). Men were noted to experience more diarrhea (62% vs. 49%).[167] Gersten and colleagues reported on efficacy and toxicity from nelfinavir (Viracept) in 78 women and 616 men. Decreases in viral load among women and men were similar following nelfinavir treatment. Increases in CD4 lymphocytes were greater in women (116 cells/mm^3 vs. 84 cells/mm^3 in men). Diarrhea was more common in men but women had more abdominal pain (6.7% in women vs. 1.5% in men), itching (3% vs. 0.3%), and skin rash (5% vs. 2%). None of these toxicities had a predictable or obvious female-related predilection.[127,168]

Women who are using oral contraceptives containing ethinyl estradiol need to know that protease inhibitors such as ritonavir or nelfinavir or the non-nucleoside reverse transcriptase inhibitor nevirapine may substantially reduce the bioavailability of ethinyl estradiol.[166]

CLINICAL RESEARCH AND ACCESS TO CARE

Cotton and colleagues reported data from 1987 through 1990, when women accounted for only 6.7% of 11,909 ACTG clinical trial participants. Most of the women in the studies were Caucasian and only 22.6% were IDUs, which did not reflect the large amount of IDUs and women of color living with AIDS. At that time, women comprised approximately 9.8% of those with AIDS diagnoses in the United States.[169] In the early 1990s, 22.5% of ACTG trial subjects were women. However, 26% of these were in one large trial of the role of zidovudine in interrupting perinatal transmission. By 1997, 12% of the ACTG trial subjects in non-pregnancy-related trials were women.[127] Every effort should be undertaken to increase these numbers and include substantial numbers of women in upcoming clinical trials. All trials should establish guidelines for enrolling pregnant women and nonpregnant women, female-specific endpoints, and guidelines about dose, body weight, and laboratory measurements standardized for women. Because women are a smaller percentage of the overall AIDS population, a disproportionate enrollment may be needed to allow sufficient numbers to detect statistically significant differences.[72] New guidelines released by the Food and Drug Administration (FDA) in 1993 may enhance enrollment and foster evaluation of drugs in pregnant women in clinical trials.[170,171] Specifically, the FDA withdrew restrictions on participation of women of childbearing potential in early clinical trials, including clinical pharmacology studies and early therapeutic studies. The FDA also is formalizing expectations regarding inclusion of subjects of both genders in drug development, analysis of clinical data by gender, assessment of potential pharmacokinetic differences between genders, and, where appropriate, assessment of pharmacodynamics.[170,171]

SUMMARY

The increasing frequency of HIV in women has led to a considerable body of knowledge about epidemiology, transmission, and perinatal infection. Clinical management of HIV-infected pregnant and nonpregnant women requires considerable further study about pathogenesis, infections, and malignancies of the female reproductive tract. Improved methods are needed for enrolling women in epidemiologic and clinical trials to achieve statistically significant results in endpoints, mortality, and natural history. The WIHS and HIV Epidemiologic Research Study (HERS) are being conducted at eight sites in the United States and will prospectively compare several thousand HIV-infected women to HIV-uninfected women. These large controlled studies should shed additional light on some of the issues obscured by low numbers.

References

1. AIDS Control and Prevention (AIDSCAP) Project of Family Health Internal, The Francois-Xavier Bagnoud Center for Public Health and Human Rights of the Harvard School of Public Health, UNAIDS: The Status and Trends of the Global HIV/AIDS Pandemic. Final Report July 5–6. Boston, Harvard School of Public Health, 1996 (Updated report April 1998)
2. Centers for Disease Control and Prevention: HIV/AIDS Surveill Rep 9(1), 1997
3. Centers for Disease Control and Prevention: HIV/AIDS Surveill Rep 9(2), 1997
4. Centers for Disease Control: HIV/AIDS Surveill Rep 5(3), 1993
5. Centers for Disease Control and Prevention: HIV/AIDS Surveill Rep 7(1), 1995
6. Centers for Disease Control and Prevention: First 500,000 AIDS cases, United States, 1995. JAMA 274:1827, 1995
7. Saglio SD, Kurtzman JT, Radner AB: HIV infection in women: An escalating health concern. Am Fam Physician, Oct:1541–1548, 1554, 1996
8. Centers for Disease Control: Risk for cervical disease in HIV-infected women, New York City. MMWR Morbid Mortal Wkly Rep 39:826, 1990
9. Ellerbrock T, Wright TC, Chiasson MA, et al: Strong independent association between HIV infection and cervical intraepithelial neoplasia (CIN). In: Abstracts of the IXth Conference on AIDS, Berlin, 1993, Abstract WS-B07-5
10. Michaels D, Levine C: Estimates of the number of motherless youth orphaned by AIDS in the United States. JAMA 268:3456, 1992
11. Wortley PM, Fleming PL: AIDS in women in the United States. N Engl J Med 278:911, 1997
12. Conti S, Lepri AC, Farchi G, et al: AIDS: A major health problem among young Italian women. AIDS 10:407, 1996
13. Nelson KE, Vlahov D, Cohn S, et al: Sexually transmitted diseases in a population of intravenous drug users: Association with seropositivity to the human immunodeficiency virus. J Infect Dis 164:157, 1991
14. Volberding PA, Lagakos SW, Koch MA, et al: Zidovudine in asymptomatic human immunodeficiency virus infections: A controlled trial in persons with fewer than 500 CD-positive cells per cubic millimeter. N Engl J Med 322:941, 1990
15. Conway GA, Epstein MR, Hayman CR, et al: Trends in HIV prevalence among disadvantaged youth. JAMA 269:2387, 1993
16. Moss GB, Clemetson D, D'Costa L, et al: Association of cervical ectopy with heterosexual transmission of human immunodeficiency virus: Results of a study of couples in Nairobi, Kenya. J Infect Dis 64:588, 1991
17. Shevits A, Pagano M, Chiasson MA, et al: The association between youth, women, and acquired immunodeficiency syndrome. J Acquir Immune Defic Syndr 13:427, 1996
18. Fullilove RE, Fullilove MT, Bowser BP, et al: Risk of sexually transmitted disease among black adolescent crack users in Oakland and San Francisco, California. JAMA 263:851, 1990
19. Gomez MA, Fernandez D, Velazquez M, Hunter R: Psychosocial and risk features of young HIV Puerto Rican women. In: Abstracts of the 4th Conference on Retroviruses and Opportunistic Infections, Washington, DC, 1997, Abstract 327
20. Justman JE, Augenbraum M, Kalish L, et al: Hepatitis B seroprevalence among an inner-city cohort of HIV-infected and uninfected women. In: Abstracts of the XIth International Conference on AIDS, Vancouver, 1996, Abstract Mo.C.1408
21. Stock R: When older women get HIV. New York Times, Sept 31:C1, 1997
22. Padian NS, Shiboski SC, Glass OS: Heterosexual transmission of HIV in northern California: Results of a ten year study. Am J Epidemiol 146:350, 1997
23. Padian NS, Shiboski SC, Jewell NP: Female to male transmission of human immunodeficiency virus. JAMA 266:1664, 1991
24. Padian NS: Epidemiology of AIDS and heterosexually transmitted HIV in women. AIDSFile 5:1, 1991

25. Allen JR, Setlow VP: Heterosexual transmission of HIV—a view of the future [editorial]. JAMA 266: 1695, 1991

26. Plummer FA, Simones JN, Cameron DW, et al: Co-factors in male-female sexual transmission of human immunodeficiency virus type 1. J Infect Dis 163:233, 1991

27. Greenblatt RM, Barkan S, Delaphena R, et al: In: Abstracts of the XIth International Conference on AIDS, Vancouver, 1996, Abstract We.C.3402

28. Royce RA, Sena A, Cates W Jr, Cohen MS: Sexual transmission of HIV. N Engl J Med 336:1072, 1997

29. Clemetson DBA, Moss GB, Willerford DM, et al: Detection of HIV DNA in cervical and vaginal secretions: Prevalence and correlates among women in Nairobi, Kenya. JAMA 269:2860, 1993

30. Klevens RM, Fleming PL, Mays M: Patterns of reporting multiple risks for HIV infection in the United States. In: Abstracts of the 4th Conference on Retroviruses and Opportunistic Infections, Washington, DC, 1997, Abstract 306

31. Marx PA, Spira AI, Gettie A, et al: Progesterone implants enhance SIV vaginal transmission and early virus load. Nature Med 2:1084, 1996

32. Rowe PM: HIV subtypes raise vaccine anxieties. Lancet 347:603, 1996

33. Sota-Ramirez E, Renijifo B, McLane MF, et al: HIV-1 Langerhans' cell tropism associated with heterosexual transmission of HIV. Science 271:1291, 1996

34. Korvick JA, Statton P, Spino K, et al: Women's participation in AIDS Clinical Trials Group (ACTG) trials in the USA—enough or still too few? In: Abstracts of the IXth International Conference on AIDS, Berlin, Abstract PO-B44-2555

35. Kreiss J, Hopkins S: The association between circumcision and human immunodeficiency virus infection among homosexual men. J Infect Dis 168:1404, 1993

36. Anderson DJ, O'Brien TR, Politch JA, et al: Effects of disease stage and zidovudine therapy on the detection of human immunodeficiency virus 1 in semen. JAMA 267:278, 1992

37. Bergeron MG, Gagne N, Cormier H, et al: New approach in preventing sexual transmission of HIV. In: Abstracts of the 4th Conference on Retroviruses and Opportunistic Infections, Washington, DC, 1997, Abstract 343

38. Gupta P, Mellors J, Kingsley L, et al: High viral load in semen of HIV-1 infected men at all stages of disease and its reduction by antiretroviral therapy. In: Abstracts of the 4th Conference on Retroviruses and Opportunistic Infections, Washington, DC, 1997, Abstract 438

39. Hamed KA, Winters MA, Holodniy M, et al: Detection of human immunodeficiency virus type 1 in semen: Effects of disease stage and nucleoside and nucleoside therapy. J Infect Dis 167:798, 1993

40. National Institute of Allergy and Infectious Diseases: Clinical alert—important therapeutic information on the benefit of zidovudine for the prevention of the transmission of HIV from mother to infant. Bethesda, MD, National Institute of Allergy and Infectious Diseases, 1994

41. Kreiss J, Ngugi E, Holmes K, et al: Efficacy of nonoxynol-9 contraceptive sponge use in preventing heterosexual acquisition of HIV in Nairobi prostitutes. JAMA 268:477, 1992

42. Long SR, Whitfeld MJ, Eades C, et al: Bacillary angiomatosis of the cervix and vulva in a patient with AIDS. Obstet Gynecol 88:709, 1996

43. Niruthisard S, Roddy RE, Chutivongse S: The effects of frequent nonoxynol-9 use on the vaginal and cervical mucosa. Sex Transm Dis 18:176, 1991

44. Niruthisard S, Roddy RE, Chutivongse S: Use of nonoxynol-9 and reduction in rate of gonococcal and chlamydial cervical infections. Lancet 339:1371, 1992

45. Stone KM, Peterson HB: Spermicides, HIV, and the vaginal sponge [editorial]. JAMA 268:521, 1992

46. Phillips DM: Microbicide development: Progress and obstacles. In: Abstracts of the 3rd Conference on Retroviruses and Opportunistic Infections, Washington, DC, 1996, Abstract S47

47. Sonderfan AJ, Chancellor T, Buckheit RW, et al: Safety and *in vitro* efficacy of a topical microbicide gel for the prevention of HIV-1 transmission. In: Abstracts of the 4th Conference on Retroviruses and Opportunistic Infections, Washington, DC, 1997, Abstract 348

48. Mostad S, Overbaugh J, DeVange D, et al: Hormonal contraception, vitamin A deficiency, and other risk factors for shedding of HIV-1 infected cells from the cervix and vagina. Lancet 350:922, 1997

49. Marmor M, Weiss L, Lynden M, et al: Possible female-to-female transmission of human immunodeficiency virus. Ann Intern Med 105:969, 1986

50. Chu S, Buehler JW, Fleming PL, Berkelman RL: Epidemiology of reported cases of AIDS in lesbians, United States, 1980–1989. Am J Public Health 80: 1380, 1990

51. Rich JD, Buck AM, Tuomala RE, et al: Transmission of human immunodeficiency virus infection presumed to have occurred via female homosexual contact. Clin Infect Dis 17:1003, 1993

52. Kennedy MB, Scarlett MI, Duerr AC, et al: Assessing HIV risk among women who have sex with women: Scientific and communication issues. J Am Med Wom Assoc 50:103, 1995

53. Berger BJ, Kolton S, Zenilman JM, et al: Bacterial vaginosis in lesbians: A sexually transmitted disease. Clin Infect Dis 21:1402, 1995

54. Petersen LR, Doll L, White C, et al: No evidence for female-to-female HIV transmission among 960,000 female blood donors. J Acquir Immune Defic Syndr 5:853, 1992

55. Raiteri R, Fora R, Sinicco A: HIV transmission in HIV-discordant lesbian couples. In: Abstracts of the XIth International Conference on AIDS, Vancouver, 1996

56. Lemp GF, Jones M, Kellogg TA, et al: HIV Seroprevalence and risk behaviors among lesbians and bisexual women in San Francisco and Berkeley, California. Am J Public Health 85:1549, 1995

57. Barkan S, Deamant C, Young M, et al: Sexual identity and behavior among women with female sexual partners: The Women's Interagency HIV Study. In: Abstracts of the XIth International Conference on AIDS, Vancouver, 1996, Abstract Tu.C.2476

58. Norman AD, Perry MJ, Stevenson LY, et al: Lesbian and bisexual women in small cities—at risk for HIV? Public Health Rep 111:347, 1996

59. White JC: HIV risk assessment and prevention in lesbians and women who have sex with women: Practical information for clinicians. Health Care Women Int 18:127, 1997

60. Bastin L, Bennett CL, Adams J, et al: Differences between men and women with HIV-related Pneumocystis carinii pneumonia: Experience from 3,070 cases in New York City in 1987. J Acquir Immune Defic Syndr 6:617, 1993

61. Melnick SL, Sherer R, Louis TA, et al: Survival and disease progression according to gender of patients with HIV infection. JAMA 272:1915, 1994

62. Sherer R, Melnick S, Hillman D, et al: Gender, HIV-related clinical events and mortality: Preliminary observational data from the Community Programs for Clinical Research on AIDS (CPCRA). In: Abstracts of the VIIIth International Conference on AIDS, Amsterdam, 1992, Abstract 09.55

63. Anastos K, Denenberg R: Human immunodeficiency virus in women. Med Clin North Am 81:533, 1997

64. Chaisson RE, Keruly JC, Moore RD: Race, sex, drug use, and progression of human immunodeficiency virus disease. N Engl J Med 333:751, 1995

65. Turner BJ, Markson LE, McKee LJ, et al: Health care delivery, zidovudine use, and the survival of women and men with AIDS. J Acquir Immune Defic Syndr 7:1250, 1994

66. Benson C, Sha B, Urbanski P, et al: Women with HIV disease: Clinical progression and survival in a cohort followed at a university medical center. In: Abstracts of the VIIIth International Conference on AIDS, 1992, Abstract 10.15

67. Brettle RP, Leen CHS: The natural history of HIV and AIDS in women. AIDS 5:1283, 1991

68. Creagh T, Thomspon M, Morris A, et al: Gender differences in the spectrum of HIV disease. In: Abstracts of the VIIIth International Conference on AIDS, Amsterdam, 1992, Abstract 10.05

69. Msellati P, Leroy V, Lepage P, et al: Natural history of HIV-1 infection in African women: A prospective cohort study in Kigali (Rwanda) 1988–1991. In: Abstracts of the VIIIth International Conference on AIDS, Amsterdam, 1992, Abstract 10.35

70. Sacks H, Szabo S, Miller LH, et al: Gender differences in the natural history of HIV infection. In: Abstracts of the VIIIth International Conference on AIDS, Amsterdam, 1992, Abstract 09.45

71. Stein MD, Liebman BD, Wachtel TJ, et al: HIV-positive women: Reasons they are tested for HIV and their clinical characteristics on entry into the health care system. J Gen Intern Med 6:286, 1991

72. Currier JS, et al: Women and power: The impact of accrual rates of women on the ability to detect gender differences in toxicity rates and response to therapy in clinical trials. In: Abstracts of the VIIIth International Conference on AIDS, Florence, 1991

73. Farizo KM, Buehler JW, Chamberland ME, et al: Spectrum of diseases in persons with human immunodeficiency virus infection in the United States. JAMA 267:1798, 1992

74. Carpenter CJ, Mayer KH, Stein MD, et al: Human immunodeficiency virus infection in North American women: Experience with 200 cases and a review of the literature. Medicine 70:307, 1991

75. Clancy CM, Massion CT: American women's health care—a patchwork quilt with gaps [editorial]. JAMA 268:1918, 1992

76. Hankins CA, Handley MA: HIV disease and AIDS in women: Current knowledge and a research agenda. J Acquir Immune Defic Syndr 5:957, 1992

77. Laurence J: Severe manifestations of common disorders in women. AIDS Reader:147, 1991

78. Wilcox CM, Schwartz DA, Clark WS: Esophageal ulceration in human immunodeficiency virus infection. Ann Intern Med 122:143, 1995

79. Greenberg AE, Thomas PA, Landesman SH, et al: The spectrum of HIV-1-related disease among outpatients in New York City. AIDS 6:849, 1992

80. Witt DJ, Craven DE, McCable WR: Bacterial infections in adult patients with the acquired immunodeficiency syndrome (AIDS) and AIDS-related complex. Am J Med 82:900, 1987

81. Chaisson MA, Kelly KF, Williams R, et al: Invasive cervical cancer (ICC) in HIV+ women in New York City (NYC). In: Abstracts of the 3rd Conference on Retroviruses and Opportunistic Infections, Washington, DC, 1996, Abstract A412

82. Cu-Uvin S, Flanigan TP, Rich JD, et al: Human immunodeficiency virus infection and acquired immunodeficiency syndrome among North American women. Am J Med 101:316, 1996

83. Imam W, Carpenter CJ, Mayer K, et al: Hierarchical pattern of mucosal Candida infections in HIV-seropositive women. Am J Med 89:142, 1990

84. Centers for Disease Control: USPS/IDSA guidelines for the prevention of opportunistic infections in persons infected with the human immunodeficiency virus: A summary. MMWR Morbid Mortal Wkly Rep 81, 1995

85. Clarke LM, Duerr A, Feldman J, et al: Factors associated with cytomegalovirus infection among human immunodeficiency virus type-1-seronegative and seropositive women from an urban minority community. J Infect Dis 173:77, 1996

86. Lassoued K, Clauvel J, Fegueux S, et al: AIDS-associated Kaposi's sarcoma in female patients. AIDS 5:877, 1991

87. Beral V, Peterman TA, Berkelman RL, Jaffe HW: Kaposi's sarcoma among persons with AIDS: A sexually transmitted infection? Lancet 335:123, 1990

88. Weiss RA: Perspectives on HHV8 and Kaposi's sarcoma. In: Abstracts of the 3rd Conference on Retroviruses and Opportunistic Infections, Washington, DC, 1996

89. Kedes DH, Ganem D, Ameli N, Kedes D: The prevalence of serum antibody to human herpesvirus 8 (Kaposi sarcoma-associated herpesvirus) among HIV-seropositive and high risk HIV-seronegative women. JAMA 277:478, 1997

90. Whitby D, Howard MR, Tenant-Flowers M, et al: Detection of Kaposi's sarcoma-associated herpesvirus in peripheral blood of HIV-infected individuals and progression to Kaposi's sarcoma. Lancet 346:799, 1995

91. Cooley TP, Hirschhorn LR, O'Keane JC: Kaposi's sarcoma in women with AIDS. AIDS 10:1221, 1996

92. Aboulafia D, Mathisen G, Mitsuyasu R: Case report: Aggressive Kaposi's sarcoma and camphylobacteremia in a female with transfusion-associated AIDS. Am J Med Sci 301:256, 258, 1991

93. Dodd CL, Greenspan D, Greenspan JS: Oral Kaposi's sarcoma in a woman as first indication of HIV infection. J Am Dent Assoc 122:61, 1991

94. Shiboski CH, Hilton JF, Neuhaus JM, et al: Human immunodeficiency virus-related oral manifestations and gender. Arch Intern Med 156:2249, 1996

95. Macasaet MA, Duerr A, Thelmo W, et al: Kaposi sarcoma presenting as a vulvar mass. Obstet Gynecol 86:695, 1995

96. Neary B, Young SB, Reuter KL, et al: Ovarian Burkitt lymphoma: Pelvic pain in a woman with AIDS. Obstet Gynecol 88(4):706, 1996

97. Gail MH, Pluda JM, Rabkin CS, et al: Projections of the incidence of non-Hodgkin's lymphoma related to acquired immunodeficiency syndrome. J Natl Cancer Inst 3:695, 1991

98. Ioachim HL, Dorsett B, Cronin W, et al: Acquired immunodeficiency syndrome-associated lymphomas. Hum Pathol 22:659, 1991

99. Watsuba I, Behrens C, Milchgrub S, et al: Comparison of molecular changes in lung cancers in HIV-positive and HIV-indeterminate subjects. JAMA 279:1554, 1998

100. Kaplan M: The changing pattern of neoplastic disease complicating HIV infection: A new epidemic of lymphoma and unusual neoplasms in women. In: Abstracts of the 5th Conference on Retrovirus and Opportunistic Infections, Chicago, 1998, Abstract 719/session 89

101. Centers for Disease Control: AIDS in women—United States. MMWR Morbid Mortal Wkly Rep 47:845, 1990

102. Feingold PR, Vermund SH, Burk RA, et al: Cervical cytologic abnormalities and papillomavirus in women infected with human immunodeficiency virus. J Acquir Immune Defic Syndr 3:896, 1990

103. Irwin K, Rice R, O'Sullivan M, et al: The clinical presentation and course of pelvic inflammatory disease in HIV+ and HIV− women: Preliminary results of a multicenter study. In: Abstracts of the IXth International Conference on AIDS, Berlin, 1993, Abstract WS-B07-1

104. Maiman M, Fruchter RG, Segur E, et al: Human immunodeficiency virus and cervical neoplasia. Obstet Gynecol 38:377, 1991

105. Maiman M, Tarricons N, Viera J, Suarez J: Colposcopic evaluation of human immunodeficiency virus-seropositive women. Obstet Gynecol 78:84, 1991

106. Centers for Disease Control: 1993 revised classification system for HIV-infection and expanded surveillance case definition for AIDS among adolescents and adults. MMWR Morbid Mortal Wkly Rep 41(RR17):1, 1992

107. Watts D, Heather N, Spino C, et al: A comparison of gynecologic findings in HIV positive women with CD4 lymphocyte counts 200 to 500/CC and <100/CC. In: Abstracts of the XIth International Conference on AIDS, Vancouver, 1996, Abstract Th.B.4137

108. Stephens PC, Zheng ZT, Flannery HT, et al: Incident AIDS and cervical cancer in Connecticut women: An ecological examination of time trends and age period cohort effects. In: Abstracts of the IXth International Conference on AIDS, Berlin, 1993, Abstract WS-B17-1

109. Weber T, Chin K, Sidhu JS, Janssen RS, for the Sentinel Hospital Surveillance System for HIV Infection Principal Investigators: Prevalence of invasive cervical cancer among HIV-infected and uninfected hospital patients, 1994–1995. In: Abstracts of the 5th Conference on Retroviruses and Opportunistic Infections, Chicago, 1998, Abstract 717/session 89

110. Burk R, Minkoff H, Feldman J, Landesman S: The relationship of HIV serostatus and immune status to the natural history of genital tract oncogenic HPV. In: Abstracts of the 4th Conference on Retroviruses and Opportunistic Infections, Washington, DC, 1997, Abstract 695

111. Cannistra SA, Niloff JM: Cancer of the uterine cervix. N Engl J Med 334:1030, 1996

112. Kelley KF, Smith PF, Mikl J: Review of invasive cervical cancer cases for AIDS surveillance. J Acquir Immune Defic Syndr 8:102, 1995

113. Klevens RM, Fleming PL, Mays MA, Frey R: Characteristics of women with AIDS and invasive cervical cancer. Obstet Gynecol 88:269, 1996

114. Wright TC, Sun X, Ellerbrock T, et al: Human papillomavirus infection in HIV(+) and HIV(−) women: Prevalence, association with cervical intraepithelial neoplasia, and impact of CD4(+) count. In: Abstracts of the IXth International Conference on AIDS, Berlin, 1993, Abstract WS-B17-2

115. Sun XW, Ellerbrook TV, Lunglu O, et al: Human papillomavirus infection in human immunodeficiency virus-seropositive women. Obstet Gynecol 85:680, 1995

116. Sun XW, Kuhn L, Ellerbrook TV, et al: Human papillomavirus infection in women infected with the human immunodeficiency virus. N Engl J Med 337:1342, 1997

117. de Ruiter A, Carter P, Katz D, et al: A comparison between cytology and histology to detect anal intraepithelial neoplasia. In: Abstracts of the IXth International Conference on AIDS, Berlin, 1993, Abstract PO-B14-1638

118. Franco EL: Human papillomavirus and the natural history of cervical cancer. Infect Med 57, 1993

119. Heard I, Costagliola D, Kazatchkine, Orth G: High rate of persistence of HPV infection in HIV-seropositive women. In: Abstracts of the 4th Conference on Retroviruses and Opportunistic Infections, Washington, DC, 1997, Abstract 628

120. Hillemanns P, Ellerbrock TV, McPhillips S, et al: Prevalence of anal human papillomavirus infection and anal cytologic abnormalities in HIV-seropositive women. AIDS 10:1641, 1996

121. Lai KK: Incidence of cervical dysplasia and human papilloma virus infection among HIV-infected women. In: Abstracts of the XIth International Conference on AIDS, Vancouver, 1996, Abstract We.C.3405

122. Larsen C: PAP smear screening for squamous intraepithelial lesions in HIV infected women. In: Abstracts of the XIth International Conference on AIDS, Vancouver, 1996, Abstract We.B.542

123. Palefsky JM: Human papillomavirus-associated malignancies in HIV-positive men and women. Curr Opin Oncol 7:437, 1995

124. Palefsky J, Minkoff H, Kalish LA, et al: Cervicovaginal human papillomavirus infection in HIV positive and high risk HIV negative women. J Acquir Immune Defic Syndr Hum Retroviral 14:(abstr S3):A11, 1997

125. Wright TC, Ellerbrook TV, Chiasson MA, et al: Cervical intraepithelial neoplasia in women infected with human immunodeficiency virus: Prevalence, risk factors, and validity of Papanicolaou smears. Obstet Gynecol 84:591, 1994

126. Lagakos S, Fishl MA, Stein DS, et al: Effects of zidovudine therapy in minority and other subpopulations with early HIV infection. JAMA 266:2709, 1991

127. Ocamb K, Hall J, Long I: Gender matters. POZ Dec:75, 1997

128. Padian NS, Marquis L, Francis DP, et al: Male to female transmission of human immunodeficiency virus. JAMA 258:788, 1987

129. Ellerbrock TV, Bush TJ, Chamberland ME, et al: Epidemiology of women with AIDS in the United States, 1981 through 1990. JAMA 265:2971, 1991

130. Fruchter RG, Palefsky J, Riester KA, et al: Abnormal cervical cytology in HIV infected women. J Acquir Immune Defic Syndr Hum Retrovirol 14(abstr 6):A17, 1997

131. Korn AP, Landers DV: Gynecologic disease in women infected with the immunodeficiency virus type 1. J Acquir Immune Defic Syndr 9:361, 1995

132. Minkoff HL, DeHovitz JA: Care of women infected with the human immunodeficiency virus. JAMA 66:2253, 1991

133. Sedlis A, Maiman M, Fruchter RG, et al: The sensitivity of cervical cytology in HIV infected women. J Acquir Immune Defic Syndr Hum Retrovirol 14:(abstr 131):A49, 1997

134. Cote T, Schiffman M, Biggar R, et al: Invasive cervical cancer among women with AIDS: Results of a registry linkage. In: Abstracts of the IXth International Conference on AIDS, Berlin, 1993, Abstract PO-B14-1637

135. Stratton P, Guupta P, Kalish L, et al: Immune status, STD's and cervical dysplasia on Pap smear in HIV+ pregnant and nonpregnant women in the Women and Infants Transmission Study (WITS). In: Abstracts of the 3rd Conference on Retroviruses and Opportunistic Infections, Washington, DC, 1996, Abstract A426

136. Wright TC, Koulos J, Schnoll F, et al: Cervical intraepithelial neoplasia in women infected with the human immunodeficiency virus: Outcome after loop electrosurgical excision. Gynecol Oncol 55:253, 1994

137. Melbye M, Cote T, Biggar RJ, et al: High incidence of anal cancer among AIDS patients. In: Abstracts of the IXth International Conference on AIDS, Berlin, 1993, Abstract PO-B14-1636

138. Northfelt DW: Anal neoplasia in persons with HIV infection. AIDS Clin Care 8:63, 1996

139. Palefsky JM, Shiboski S, Moss A: Risk factors for anal human papillomavirus infection and cytologic abnormalities in HIV positive and HIV negative men. J Acquir Immune Defic Syndr 7:599, 1994

140. Critchlow C, Holmes K, Daling J, et al: Risk for development of anal squamous intraepithelial lesions among HIV(+) and HIV(−) gay men. In: Abstracts of the IXth International Conference on AIDS, Berlin, 1993, Abstract PO-B14-1635

141. Williams A, Darragh T, Osmond D, et al: Anal/cervical HPV infection and risk of anal/cervical dysplasia associated with HPV-1. In: Abstracts of the IXth International Conference on AIDS, Berlin, 1993, Abstract WS-B17-5

142. Boken DJ, Swindells S, Rinaldi MG: Fluconazole-resistant Candida albicans. Clin Infect Dis 17:1018, 1993

143. Duerr A, Sierra M, Clake L, et al: Vaginal candidiasis among HIV-infected women. In: Abstracts of the IXth International Conference on AIDS, Berlin, 1993, Abstract PO-B01-0880

144. Rhoads JL, Wright C, Redfield RR, et al: Chronic vaginal candidiasis in women with human immunodeficiency virus infection. JAMA 257:3105, 1987

145. Sobel JD, Schuman P, Mayer K, et al: Candida colonization and mucosal candidiasis in women with or at risk for HIV infection. In: Abstracts of the XIth International Conference on AIDS, Vancouver, 1996

146. Sobel JD: Recurrent vulvovaginal candidiasis in HIV-infected women. Clinguide to Fungal Infections 3:1, 1998

147. Spinillo A, Capuzzo E, Egbe TO, et al: *Torulopsis glabrata* vaginitis. Obstet Gynecol 85:993, 1995

148. Spinillo A, Michelone G, Cvanna C, et al: Clinical and microbiological characteristics of symptomatic vulvovaginal candidiasis in HIV-seropositive women. Genitourin Med 70:268, 1994

149. Greenblatt RM, Lukehart SA, Plummer FA, et al: Genital ulceration as a risk factor for human immunodeficiency virus infection. AIDS 2:47, 1988

150. Safrin S, Assaykeen T, Follansbee S, et al: Foscarnet therapy for acyclovir-resistant mucocutaneous herpes simplex virus infection in 26 AIDS patients: Preliminary data. J Infect Dis 161:1078, 1990

151. Centers for Disease Control: Sexually transmitted diseases treatment guidelines. MMWR Morbid Mortal Wkly Rep 42:88, 1993

152. Augenbraun M, Feldman J, Chirgwin K, et al: Increased genital shedding of herpes simplex virus type 2 in HIV-seropositive women. Ann Intern Med 123:845, 1995

153. Schacker T, Ryncarz A, Goddard J, et al: Frequent recovery of replication HIV from genital herpes simplex virus lesions in HIV-infected persons. In: Abstracts of the 4th Conference on Retroviruses and Opportunistic Infections, Washington DC, 1997, Abstract 342

154. Schuman P, Christianen C, Sobel JD: Apthous genital ulceration in three women with AIDS. In: Abstracts of the 3rd Conference on Retroviruses and Opportunistic Infections, Washington, DC, 1996, Abstract A429

155. Hoegsberg B, Abulafia O, Sedlis A, et al: Sexually transmitted disease and human immunodeficiency virus infection among women with pelvic inflammatory disease. Am J Obstet Gynecol 163:1135, 1990

156. Safrin S, Dattel BJ, Haver L, et al: Seroprevalence and epidemiologic correlates of infection in women with acute pelvic inflammatory disease. Obstet Gynecol 75:666, 1990

157. Kamenga M, Toure CK, Nghichi JM, et al: Human immunodeficiency virus infection in women with pelvic inflammatory disease (PID) in Abidjan, Ivory Coast, Africa. In: Abstracts of the VIIIth International Conference on AIDS, Amsterdam, 1992, Abstract WS-B07-2

158. Warne PA, Ehrhardt A, Schochter D, et al: Menstrual abnormalities in HIV+ and HIV− women with a history of intravenous drug use. In: Abstracts of the International Conference on AIDS, Florence, 1991, Abstract M.C.3113

159. Cohen MH, Greenblatt R, Minkoff H, et al: Menstrual abnormalities in women with HIV infection. In: Abstracts of the XIth International Conference on AIDS, Vancouver, 1996, Abstract Mo.B.540

160. Ellerbrock TV, Wright TC, Bush TJ, et al: Characteristics of menstruation in women infected with human immunodeficiency virus. Obstet Gynecol 87:1030, 1996

161. Shelton M, Adams J, Gugino L, et al: Menstrual cycle hormone patterns in HIV-infected women. In: Abstracts of the 3rd Conference on Retroviruses and Opportunistic Infections, Washington, DC, 1996, Abstract A432

162. Cohen M, Greenblatt R for the WIHS Collaborative Study Group: Menstrual adnormalities in women with HIV infection. In: Abstracts of the XIth International Conference on AIDS, Vancouver, 1996, Abstract Mo.B.540

163. Fishl MA, Richman DD, Grieco MH, et al: The efficacy of azidothymidine (AZT) in the treatment of patients with AIDS and AIDS-related complex: A double-blind, placebo controlled trial. N Engl J Med 317: 185, 1987

164. Easterbrook PJ, Keruly JC, Creah-Kirk T, et al: Racial and ethnic differences in outcome in zidovudine-treated patients with advanced HIV disease. JAMA 266:2713, 1991

165. Aboulker JP, Swart AM: Preliminary analysis of the Concorde trial. Lancet 341:889, 1993

166. Zorrilla C, Clark R, Currier J, et al: Women First: A study in HIV positive women of quadruple therapy: nelfinavir (NFV), saquinavir (SQV), stavudine (d4T) and lamivudine (3TC). In: Abstracts of the 5th Con-

ference on Retrovirus and Opportunistic Infections, Chicago, 1998, Abstract 722/session 89

167. Currier JS, Yeetzer E, Potthoff A, et al: Gender differences in adverse events on ritonavir: An analysis from the Abbott 247 study. In: Proceedings of the National Conference on Women and HIV, Pasadena, CA, 1997, Abstract 304.7

168. Gersten M, Chapman S, Farnsworth A, et al: The safety and efficacy of Viracept (nelfinavir mesylate) in female patients who participated in pivotal Phase II/III double blind randomized controlled trials. In: Proceedings of the National Conference on Women and HIV, Pasadena, CA, 1997, Abstract 304.1

169. Cotton D, Feinberg J, Finkelstein D, ACTG SDAC: Participation of women in multicenter HIV clinical trials programs in the United States. In: Abstracts of the VIIth International Conference on AIDS, Florence, 1991, Abstract Tu.D.114

170. Bennett JC: Inclusion of women in clinical trials— policies for population subgroups. N Engl J Med 329: 288, 1993

171. Merkatz RB, Temple R, Sobel S, et al: Women in clinical trials of new drugs—A change in Food and Drug Administration policy. N Engl J Med 329:292, 1993

35 | Conception, Pregnancy, and Parenthood: Maternal Health Care and the HIV Epidemic

KAREN P. BECKERMAN

The original observations of vertical transmission of HIV from mother to infant were unavoidably retrospective and readily established the association of pediatric AIDS with HIV infection in women. Because most mothers of infected children were themselves HIV infected, the inference was made that infected mothers almost always transmitted the AIDS virus to their babies—a misimpression that persists today, in both the medical and lay communities. In fact, nothing could be further from the truth. Prospective studies of HIV-1–infected pregnant women have consistently revealed that three out of four of their babies will be uninfected. Furthermore, with good prenatal care, careful attention to maternal health and nutrition, and zidovudine monotherapy for pregnant mothers and their newborns over the last 3 years, many centers now report vertical transmission rates of 8% or lower. These rates appear to approach zero at centers that offer intensive monitoring and aggressive treatment of maternal HIV disease during pregnancy.[1]

The AIDS Clinical Trials Group (ACTG) 076 trial[2] was the first to demonstrate the safety and efficacy of zidovudine prophylaxis during pregnancy, labor, and early infancy in preventing vertical transmission. Now, there is every reason to believe that, with the use of newer antiretroviral therapies both during and after pregnancy, many HIV-infected women of the developed world will be able to anticipate not only that their babies will be born uninfected, but also that they themselves will have a significant chance of living long enough to see their children grow to young adulthood.

In 1999, we are in the midst of parallel revolutions: one in the understanding of HIV disease, and one in the care and treatment of HIV infection and related illness. Ironically, much of this rapid growth in understanding and treatment of the disease has bypassed pregnant women, the population in which the efficacy of antiretroviral therapy for transmission prophylaxis was first conclusively demonstrated. This chapter is therefore intended for the primary HIV caregiver who may care for clients who are considering pregnancy, become pregnant, or present in pregnancy, and for perinatal health care providers who provide prenatal and intrapartum care for HIV-infected women. This chapter cannot provide a full course in HIV care for obstetricians and midwives, or an all-inclusive overview of high-risk obstetrics for HIV care providers; however, every attempt is made to highlight perspectives from both subspecialties that are essential to the informed decision-making process that is required of both the client and her caregivers. It also attempts to chronicle the current information, thinking, and decision-making processes that go into the reproductive counseling and care of HIV-infected women and couples. Practitioners and students of this exciting field must first understand the need to keep an ear to the ground or an eye on the Internet to stay abreast of ongoing developments.

PRECONCEPTIONAL COUNSELING

Fundamentals

Preconceptional counseling has evolved closely with the fields of perinatology and perinatal genetics. In the last 20 years, the dramatically improved outcomes of pregnancies complicated by maternal illnesses such as diabetes, chronic hypertension, systemic lupus erythematosus, and epilepsy have been due in large part to understanding the importance of highly informed, up-to-date decision making by women with these illnesses who are contemplating pregnancy. Such counseling has provided a unique opportunity to achieve preconceptional control of disease, which has invariably led to improved pregnancy outcomes. Most practitioners would agree that the essential hallmarks of any reproductive counseling are that it be supportive, nondirective, and educational. All three qualities must be the underpinnings of counseling of women and families living with chronic illness or with diseases that they could transmit to their children, including HIV infection.

Topics to address with clients requesting preconceptional counseling in the context of HIV infection are summarized in Table 35–1. When possible, two counseling sessions are preferable because there is a great deal of ground to cover if caregivers working with HIV-infected women are to enable clients to make informed decisions based on the most current information available.

Because therapeutic recommendations regarding HIV disease have been changing at a rate that far outpaces the appearance of textbooks and peer-reviewed journal articles, it is widely agreed that the best resources for learning the latest findings in both clinical and basic research is by direct consultation with experts (e.g., through clinician consultation services such as the National HIV Telephone Consultation Service [1-800-933-3413] or from constantly updated sites on the Internet, such as HIVInSite, published by the University of California, San Francisco with support from the Kaiser Family Foundation [http://www.hivinsite.ucsf.edu]).

Pregnancy does not appear to change the course of HIV disease, at least in the developed world.[3] Although case reports have identified effects of HIV infection on fetal development, only the association of transmission of the virus itself has been supported by prospective, controlled examination of HIV-infected pregnancies. The course of pregnancy does not appear to be altered by HIV infection alone, although complications of chronic immunosuppression, such as *Pneumocystis carinii* pneumonia (PCP) and other opportunistic infections (OIs), can be

---

TABLE 35–1. Guidelines for Preconceptional Counseling of HIV-Infected Women

1. Antibody testing for HIV infection available to all individuals
2. Serostatus confirmed with hard copy of two separate HIV antibody tests
3. Obstetric and gynecologic history, including sexually transmitted disease, hepatitis, and herpes history
4. Assessment of general maternal health and HIV disease: history, physical examination, and laboratory tests, including recent CD4 counts and plasma HIV RNA (viral load) assessment
5. Review of current HIV care: assessment of current and prior antiretroviral therapeutic regimens
6. Laboratory studies that are helpful to know preconceptionally:
   - Rubella and varicella antibody status
   - Toxoplasma antibody status
   - Cytomegalovirus serostatus
   - Blood type and antibody screen
   - Hepatitis serology
   - Syphilis serology, chlamydia and gonorrhea culture
   - Baseline chest radiograph
7. Assessment of need for vaccinations, and recommendation that indicated vaccinations be carried out preconceptionally
8. Recommendations for optimization of HIV and general medical care before pregnancy, including:
   - Optimization of antiretroviral therapy control of HIV replication
   - Optimization of adherence
   - Optimization of prophylaxis for opportunistic infections
   - Nutrition
9. Review of HIV-specific therapeutic options during pregnancy
10. Review of procedures for labor and delivery, neonatal care, and therapeutic recommendations for HIV-exposed infants
11. Review of HIV diagnostic testing procedures for neonates
12. Discussion of adherence issues during pregnancy and the postpartum period
13. Discussion of guardianship and other legal issues pertinent to families living with HIV
14. Discussion of fertility, conception, and safe sex issues
15. Discussion of risks of vertical transmission and pediatric HIV disease
16. Discussion of advanced maternal age, neural tube defect, and other birth defect screening programs, particularly because a positive screen may result in the question of invasive diagnostic fetal testing, such as amniocentesis
17. Discussion of access to clinical trials and other research
18. Facilitation of peer counseling and peer support

devastating in pregnant women. In time, we may see more maternal complications of pregnancy attributable to advanced HIV disease. In particular, women who present with loss of estrus and infertility as a result of wasting syndrome need to understand the importance of control of their HIV disease prior to embarking on attempts at pregnancy. Experienced workers in this area emphasize the improbability of conception when body weight falls below 100 pounds.[4]

Another consideration is advanced maternal age. Many women living with HIV who present for preconceptional counseling may have deferred childbearing because of their serostatus but are now reconsidering their reproductive options because of the promise of new therapies to both improve their own health and longevity and reduce the risk of vertical transmission. In many states, such as California, noninvasive triple-marker screening for a number of birth and genetic defects is available to all pregnant women.[5,6] However, before becoming pregnant, women should consider whether they would want triple-marker screening and, if so, need their options clarified should a triple-marker screen yield a positive result, or should their age-related risk of chromosomal anomaly be high. These options range from doing nothing to having invasive diagnostic procedures and/or detailed sonographic examinations. Invasive diagnostic procedures such as amniocentesis can rule out genetic aneuploidy and neural tube and abdominal defects with a high degree of reliability, but carry the risk of miscarriage of approximately one fetal loss for every 200 procedures. Furthermore, in the case of an HIV-infected woman, there is a theoretical risk of inoculation of the fetal compartment by the needle that must pass through infected maternal tissues. Attempts to quantitate the risk of HIV transmission resulting from invasive obstetric procedures generally focus on intrapartum procedures, and studies have demonstrated both no increased risk[7,8] and an increased risk.[9] Most practitioners agree that invasive procedures should be avoided when possible during pregnancy in HIV-infected women. However, when there would otherwise be a clear indication for genetic amniocentesis, the practice at San Francisco General Hospital (SFGH) has been not to withhold the procedure when, after thorough counseling, mothers request that it be performed. Before performing any invasive obstetric procedure, early or late in pregnancy, it has seemed prudent to check maternal plasma HIV RNA levels and to optimize antiretroviral therapy.

Evaluation of a Woman's HIV Disease

At SFGH, women are counseled that the goal of therapy is not just to protect their babies from HIV infection, but also to treat maternal HIV disease so that mothers will live to attend their child's high school graduation. This orientation has been crucial to clients' understanding the importance of adherence to their HIV therapy, both during pregnancy and during the very difficult periods of infancy and early childhood.

Evaluation and characterization of an individual woman's HIV disease activity consists of history, physical examination, and laboratory evaluation. This part of counseling not only helps in discussing the risk of having an infected baby, but helps determine whether an individual's HIV disease is under optimal control. At SFGH, "optimal control" currently implies that an individual with a measurable viral burden is taking highly active antiretroviral therapy (HAART), has a stable or increasing CD4 count, is receiving appropriate prophylaxis for OIs (based on the lowest prior CD4 count, not the current laboratory value on HAART), is consistently adhering to therapy, and has achieved maximum suppression of HIV replication.

Assessing Predictors of Vertical Transmission

The risk of vertical transmission is usually the first question most HIV-infected women wish to address when they are considering pregnancy. In fact, many women appear to be more concerned about the danger that their infection poses to the health of their baby than to their own health. Comprehensive reviews of this topic have been published.[7,10–12] In the developed world, vertical transmission rates range from 16% to 24% for women receiving no antiretroviral therapy. Zidovudine monotherapy given by mouth during pregnancy, intravenously during labor and delivery, and by mouth to the infant during the first 6 weeks of life results in transmission rates of about 8%, with cohorts in North Carolina, New York City, and France reporting rates in the 4 to 5% range.[13–15]

Although the general consensus is that perinatal transmission of HIV-1 can occur at all levels of maternal viremia, just as protection of fetuses also occurs at all levels of maternal viremia, a number of reports have appeared identifying maternal plasma HIV-1 viremia, measured by copies/mL of maternal plasma HIV-1 RNA, as strongly predictive of perinatal

HIV-1 transmission. Most recently, Shaffer et al.[15a] published results of a prospective study of 342 HIV-1 subtype E-infected, untreated Thai mothers and their perinatally exposed, formula-fed infants. Maternal plasma HIV-1 RNA levels at delivery were directly correlated with risk of vertical transmission. No transmissions were identified when maternal plasma HIV-1 RNA levels were less than 2,000 copies/ml at delivery ($n = 19$). Levels less than 10,000 copies/ml were associated with a transmission risk of 8.5%; levels greater than 10,000 copies/ml the risk was 31%. Significantly, the highest quintile of maternal plasma HIV-1 RNA (greater than 93,126 copies/ml) had an adjusted odds ratio for perinatal transmission of 24.8.

Shaffer et al. have also reported, in abstract form, maternal plasma HIV-1 RNA data from a randomized placebo-controlled trial of short course oral ZDV.[15b] The authors noted a significant two-fold reduction in perinatal transmission among mothers who were randomized to ZDV prophylaxis during the last month of pregnancy and also reported a reduction of 0.5 log plasma HIV-1 RNA during the first week of ZDV therapy. Analysis of this observed reduction in maternal viral load and its relationship to probability of transmission is ongoing.[15c]

There have been no published reports of transmission rates of mothers receiving HAART but anecdotal evidence from several health centers suggests transmission rates that are significantly less than 5% in women who receive aggressive intervention with combination antiretroviral therapy, with frequent assessment of disease activity (i.e., plasma HIV-1 RNA testing) during pregnancy.

While it may be reasonable to assume that lowering maternal plasma HIV-1 RNA using combination antiretroviral therapy will lower vertical transmission risk, data supporting this assumption[1] are retrospective and uncontrolled, and will likely remain so for the foreseeable future.

Substance Use

Substance use, especially tobacco[16] and intravenous drug use,[7] have been cited as risk factors for vertical transmission. Methadone maintenance during pregnancy is well tolerated by mothers and fetuses. Methadone withdrawal before or during pregnancy should only be considered during a period of great stability. It is fraught with risk during pregnancy because the fetus also undergoes in utero withdrawal, which

can result in fetal hypoxia, asphyxia, distress, and death. In addition, acute maternal withdrawal sharply increases the ever-present risk of return to illegal substance use behaviors.[17,18] Families need to be counseled regarding the difficulties that may surround neonatal withdrawal from methadone and the possible need for prolonged hospitalization for severely affected withdrawing babies.

In contrast, cocaine use in any form poses unique and extreme risks of morbidity and mortality to any pregnant woman and her fetus. It may be teratogenic and is associated with preterm delivery, preterm rupture of membranes, and placental abruption with risk of fatal maternal hemorrhage.[18] Issues of drug dependency are central to the prenatal care of many (but not all) HIV-infected mothers. A valuable clinical reference is published by the Maternal and Child Health Branch of the California Department of Health Services and can be obtained by telephone or by mail.[19]

Preconceptional Control of HIV Disease

The National Institutes of Health's current recommendations regarding treatment of HIV disease in women of reproductive age are quite clear:

Principle 8. Women should receive optimal antiretroviral therapy regardless of pregnancy status. Women already receiving antiretroviral therapy at the time that pregnancy is diagnosed should continue their therapy. If antiretroviral therapy is discontinued during the first trimester for any reason, all agents should be discontinued simultaneously. Once they are reinstituted, they should be introduced simultaneously.[20]

Detailed recommendations regarding antiretroviral use in pregnancy have also recently been issued by the U.S. Public Health Service[21] and stress this principle, while emphasizing the many unknowns surrounding antiretroviral drug use during pregnancy and the client-controlled decision-making process that is essential in constructing a therapeutic strategy. Clients must be advised that any interruption of therapy is very likely to be associated with rebound of plasma HIV RNA measurements to pretreatment levels or higher.

Women who are not receiving antiretroviral therapy frequently decide not to begin taking antiretroviral drugs until early in the second trimester (12 to 14 weeks' gestation) to avoid possible teratogenetic effects of these drugs on the developing fetus as well as the stresses of adherence to combination therapy at a time that they may also be experiencing the nausea and vomiting of early pregnancy. If a woman has an AIDS-defining diagnosis, however, she should be advised to avoid any interruption in or postponement of PCP prophylaxis and other indicated OI prophylaxis. Women already receiving optimal therapy usually choose to continue their current regimen through the preconceptional period and the first trimester. Adherence to therapy must be addressed and optimized before considering any changes in therapy for antiretrovirally experienced individuals before, during, or after pregnancy. In addition, collaboration with the patient's primary HIV caregiver is necessary when making any therapeutic changes.

Vaccination

Reports of readily demonstrable, transient increases in plasma HIV-1 RNA levels suggest that vaccination may lead to activation of virus replication.[22] Consequently, when possible, all indicated vaccinations (as decided upon by the caregiver and client) should be given in the preconceptional period rather than during pregnancy, and then only when viral replication is under optimal control. At SFGH, current practice is to avoid vaccination during pregnancy, the reasoning being more theoretical than based on clinical data. First, although HIV plasma viremia has not been shown to be invariably correlated with transmission rates, it has been our practice to achieve maximal suppression of HIV replication during gestation, and we are therefore reluctant to give treatments that may increase HIV viremia, even transiently. Second, because no large influenza pandemic has occurred recently, data concerning the dangers of deferring influenza vaccination during pregnancy are essentially unknown. Because treatment recommendations are in flux in this area, our practice of withholding vaccinations during pregnancy could change for any of a number of reasons.

Safe Sex and Fertility

Safe sex and fertility are now mutually exclusive terms. In general, a baby cannot be conceived without risk of acquiring sexually transmitted diseases (STDs), including HIV disease. Heterosexual transmission of HIV is highly cor-

related with transmission of other STDs and genital ulcerative disease in particular.[23] Transmission can take place even after a single sexual exposure,[24] and the correlation between the number of acts and the probability of transmission is poor.[25]

Conception appears to be a far more efficient process than heterosexual transmission of HIV. On average, the risk of HIV transmission per exposure is about 100 times lower than the probability of achieving pregnancy. HIV-infected women with uninfected partners can eliminate transmission risk by self-administering artificial insemination with their partner's sperm. Conversely, it is not clear whether conception-related male-to-female transmission risk can be reduced or eliminated with limited, ovulation-only exposure to the semen of an HIV-infected partner or by processing the semen to eliminate as much cell-associated and free HIV as possible. A French report on 104 pregnancies of 92 HIV-uninfected women with HIV-infected partners whose CD4 counts ranged from 7 to 1273 cells/mm^3 described several findings.[26] Couples received nondirective preconceptional counseling regarding the risk of heterosexual transmission. Genital infections were diagnosed and treated, a basic fertility evaluation was offered if indicated, and couples were advised to determine the exact time of ovulation with commercially available test kits in order to reduce exposure. One third of couples reported inconsistent or no condom use; 17 pregnancies occurred after only one unprotected intercourse, and 51 occurred after several timed conception attempts at ovulation. No seroconversions occurred among the women by 3 months' gestation, suggesting that seroconversion did not occur as a result of conception attempts. Four women did eventually seroconvert: two at 7 months' gestation and two postpartum. All four seroconverters reported inconsistent condom use after conception.

A technique of artificial intrauterine insemination of HIV-uninfected partners of HIV-infected men with partners' processed semen has been advocated by some investigators.[27] This technique involves centrifugating of semen and isolating of spermatozoa by a sperm migration technique. Women were evaluated for normal ovulatory activity and tubal patency, and gonadotropins were administered when indicated.[28] In a recent abstract, these investigators reported 200 pregnancies after 1000 insemination attempts using this technique in 350 couples, with no cases of female seroconversion either before or after delivery.

Several points about these studies merit careful consideration. First, both outcomes are consistent with a seroconversion rate on the order of 1:1000 episodes of unprotected intercourse reported in longitudinal studies of stable heterosexual couples.[29] Second, when unprotected intercourse is totally limited to timed-ovulation attempts, "natural conception" may be easier for couples and as safe as semen processing with intrauterine insemination. However, any endorsement of unprotected intercourse, even for conception only, could nonetheless encourage inconsistent condom use after conception, which could result in some seroconversions. Third, the semen-processing cohort is not large enough to demonstrate a protective effect of the technique, and the possibility exists that bypassing the cervical barrier during intrauterine insemination could result in a higher transmission risk. Fourth, it is unclear from published data how fertility (i.e., successful conception) rates from the two cohorts compare. Another group, the Assisted Reproduction Foundation in Massachusetts, has advocated the use of natural-cycle in vitro fertilization/embryo transfer technology for discordant couples in order to minimize or eliminate conception-associated transmission risk. Information about this program has appeared in abstract form[30] and can be found on the Internet (www.reproduction.org).[31,32]

Despite receiving a clear message from society at large that they should not get pregnant, many women living with HIV have decided not to deny themselves and their partners the fulfillment of family life, and present for care already pregnant. Others have decided to become pregnant in the safest way they could possibly devise.[33,34] Although the concept of "risk reduction" has become acceptable in many areas, such as needle exchange programs, few caregivers are comfortable discussing risk reduction behaviors for HIV-discordant couples who wish to have a child together. A summary of these considerations is provided in Table 35–2.

EARLY PREGNANCY COUNSELING AND CARE

Counseling and Testing Pregnant Women for HIV Infection

Many women go through pregnancy with little or no information about HIV and other STDs. New mothers continue to learn of their own infection after their child is diagnosed with AIDS. These situations occur despite universal agreement on the importance of making HIV counseling and testing readily available to all pregnant women, and are in large part due to lack of understanding among care providers and in society at large that HIV can infect anyone, regardless of socioeconomic status or "risk" categories. All pregnant women are at risk because they have been having unprotected sexual intercourse. Ironically, women receiving prenatal

---

TABLE 35–2. Considerations in Risk Reduction Counseling for HIV-Affected Couples Planning Pregnancy

Although there is no absolutely sure way to achieve conception and avoid heterosexual transmission of HIV, couples may use risk-reduction techniques to minimize risk of HIV transmission to a partner when they are attempting to conceive.

- Use ovulation determination kits to limit sexual exposure to HIV to the period of maximal fertility during the month.
- Sperm analysis may be helpful to rule out male-factor infertility, particularly in the setting of advanced HIV disease.
- Emphasize preconceptional optimization of HIV disease control.
- Screen for and treat STDs, including bacterial vaginosis, chlamydia, trichomoniasis, gonorrhea, syphilis, and recurrent herpes simplex virus type 2 in both partners. Vaginal candidiasis should also be treated.

Assisted reproductive technologies that could be available to HIV-discordant couples in the future include

   Uninfected mother/infected father:
- Artificial insemination with donor sperm
- Artificial insemination with processed sperm ("sperm washing"; see text)
- In vitro fertilization–embryo transfer techniques

   Uninfected father/infected mother:
- Artificial insemination with partner's sperm

NOTE: Whether one or both partners is HIV infected, all couples living with HIV should understand the importance of practicing safe sex before and after conception. The role of postexposure prophylaxis for HIV-discordant couples attempting to achieve pregnancy has not yet been established.

care through public clinics or centralized health maintenance organizations are more likely to have access to HIV counseling and testing than are women receiving care in the private sector.

Access to HIV testing should be a national priority of primary care for all individuals. Identifying HIV-infected pregnant women is urgent, not only because early administration of antiretroviral therapy can prevent transmission to the newborn, but also because maternal disease should be treated as soon as possible, thereby ensuring that the newborn will have a mother as he or she grows up. Undiagnosed advanced HIV disease in pregnancy can be devastating to maternal health, particularly when complicated by serious OIs such as PCP.

Counseling the Newly Diagnosed Pregnant Woman

Many unique issues are raised when a woman discovers she is HIV infected during pregnancy. Pregnant women have to confront the same disclosure issues that are of major importance to anyone first facing the diagnosis, but these women also may fear losing custody of their children, being abandoned, domestic violence, and loss of housing and employment. If she already has other children, they need to be tested, immediately if possible, and at the same site where the mother was tested. Chances are that other siblings are not infected, and such news can help to stabilize the situation. If siblings are infected, they need to be evaluated and cared for without delay. The partner of a newly diagnosed woman should also be counseled and given access to testing. Caregivers may face difficult ethical dilemmas about their responsibility to patient confidentiality when a woman feels she cannot disclose her HIV status to a sexual partner. Although there are no easy answers here, it is nonetheless clear that confidentiality must be maintained. Professional and peer support must be available to address the entire situation and help an individual and her family toward the goal of finding a safe environment away from abusive relationships in which disclosure is impossible.

Women attending our clinic at SFGH report receiving impressively inappropriate advice about reproduction in the past. Many have been told they must never get pregnant, whereas others have experienced difficulty finding a physician who is willing to perform an abortion. Still others have been told that they "must" terminate their pregnancy or undergo permanent ster-

ilization because of their HIV status. Reproductive counseling must always be nondirective. It should also be emphasized that, under international law, all individuals are awarded certain rights that exist in international treaties. Among these rights are the right to marry, the right to found a family, and the right to education.[35] As a society, we are generally respectful of the reproductive wishes of individuals affected by disorders or diseases that they might pass on to their children. The same respect should be accorded families and individuals affected by HIV disease.

Early Prenatal Care

Families living with HIV have complex social service needs, and all clients will eventually require social service assistance of some kind during their pregnancy. Early assessment and, where appropriate, intervention and referral are always helpful later at a time of crisis. Social workers require special skills in this setting, which include the ability to coordinate maternal and child health services and HIV services across county lines. Many women struggling with HIV disease and childbearing experience a profound sense of isolation, no matter what their social class. They can benefit enormously by participating in peer support education and other community support groups during pregnancy and when their offspring are in early childhood. Client education, of course, is the first step toward empowerment and self-determination and must be the centerpiece of any program that deals with HIV and reproduction.

Early nutritional counseling is an important part of HIV care during pregnancy because HIV disease and pregnancy both place major nutritional burdens on a woman's body. Assessment of a mother's nutritional needs and medication schedule are critical parts of this counseling, and mothers must be given all available help in coming up with realistic schemes and schedules that will enable them to cope with the difficult tasks of taking care of themselves, meeting their own nutritional needs, and adhering to complicated medication schedules.

Drug Treatment of HIV Disease in Early Pregnancy

HIV infection must be evaluated rapidly once it is diagnosed in a pregnant woman. Because many clinical decisions must be made based on gestational age, early sonographic confirmation of viability, intrauterine location, and gestational age is very helpful. Opportunistic infection, especially pulmonary disease, must be ruled out, and stage of disease must be characterized so that treatment options can be offered. Women with an AIDS-defining diagnosis should begin appropriate prophylaxis for OI immediately, as recommended in U.S. Public Health Service guidelines. In the case of PCP, prophylaxis with daily doses of trimethoprim-sulfamethoxazole (double strength) is generally safe and well tolerated in pregnancy. Theoretical concerns regarding neonatal anemia associated with this treatment late in pregnancy are far outweighed by the very real danger to the fetus of maternal PCP. There is less experience with second-line prophylactic therapies, although monthly treatment with aerosolized pentamidine appears to be well tolerated. The risk of *Toxoplasma* encephalitis and *Mycobacterium avium* complex in pregnant women with no prior history of these infections is low, and it may be prudent to delay prophylaxis for these conditions until after delivery. However, prophylaxis to prevent recurrence of these and other OIs may be urgent in women who have a history of prior OIs.

If there is no urgent medical indication for immediate antiretroviral therapy in a woman who has not yet received it, there are two important reasons why it may be reasonable to hold off until 12 to 14 weeks' gestation. First, nausea and vomiting of early pregnancy ("morning sickness") may make it difficult for women to tolerate the large number of pills required with HAART. Poor adherence during this challenging period of adjustment to new medications could undermine the success of therapy from the very beginning. Second, the effect of these drugs on the developing fetus is entirely unknown. To date, none of the Food and Drug Administration–approved antiretroviral medications in current use has been associated with birth defects or adverse pregnancy outcome. Zidovudine, the drug for which the most data are available, is associated with neonatal anemia, although this anemia is transient and generally well tolerated. However, clinical studies addressing the safety of other antiretrovirals in pregnancy are only just now underway. Because organogenesis is essentially complete by 11 weeks after the last menstrual period, many women think it is worthwhile to postpone therapy until this period of maximal risk to fetal development is past. However, therapy must not be withheld from mothers who feel it is important to start immediately.

Women in early pregnancy who are already on a regimen of antiretroviral therapy and have stable HIV disease should be counseled about the risks of stopping therapy, which include rebound of plasma viremia and emergence of viral resistance, and the risks of taking medications of unknown teratogenic potential during the first trimester. The most up-to-date information about these drugs during pregnancy is available through the Antiretroviral Pregnancy Registry (P.O. Box 13398, Research Triangle Park, NC; telephone 1-800-722-9292), which issues an interim report every 6 months. To date, numbers of babies exposed to antiretrovirals who have been reported to the registry remain very small. Overall, no patterns of birth defects have been identified among prospective and retrospective reports of antiretroviral agents under study.

PRENATAL CARE

There is currently some controversy about the best site for prenatal care of HIV-infected pregnant women. Access to a center staffed by caregivers familiar and experienced with the management of HIV-infected pregnant clients would seem optimal. Studies have shown that survival in men and women is highly correlated with increased hospital and provider experience.[36] Improved maternal and neonatal health outcomes will likely also be linked to hospital and provider experience in treating and delivering HIV-infected mothers and their exposed babies. Finally, the lack of understanding of disease pathogenesis in women and of mechanisms of transmission of HIV from mothers to their babies mandates universal access to centers where clinical trials are available for all women, especially those who are pregnant.

Initial Evaluation

The initial prenatal evaluation is similar to that described for early pregnancy. Serostatus should be confirmed, with a hard copy record of two HIV tests, baseline HIV disease stage should be determined by pretreatment CD4 count and plasma HIV RNA load, and disease activity should be assessed while on therapy. Any history of STDs, including chlamydia, herpes simplex, syphilis, and gonorrhea, must be ascertained. Physical examination should involve particular attention to manifestations of HIV disease, such as oral and vaginal candidiasis and hairy leukoplakia. A thorough pelvic examination with Pap smear and cultures must be performed, including those for any suspected genital herpes lesions. If a woman presents before 23 weeks' gestation, sonography is frequently very useful in confirming or determining gestational age and ruling out major structural anomalies, which may be of particular concern to women who have been treated with antiretroviral medications in the first trimester. All routine prenatal laboratory studies should be obtained. Hepatitis serology for hepatitis B and C should be assessed in all clients, and baseline liver function tests, including serum bilirubin values, may be very helpful. Purified protein derivative (PPD) tuberculosis skin testing should be performed. At SFGH, we have abandoned the routine use of mumps and monilia controls and order chest radiography after the first trimester for all our HIV-infected clients, regardless of their PPD status. Antituberculosis therapy is instituted as would be indicated for any nonpregnant HIV-infected individual.

Prophylaxis for Opportunistic Infections

There is general agreement that HIV disease progression is not influenced by gender alone. The risk of most OIs is similar for men and women, with the exception of bacterial pneumonia and herpes simplex virus ulceration, which reportedly occur 1.4 and 3.4 times more frequently, respectively, in women than men, and Kaposi's sarcoma, which occurs only rarely in women in Western countries.[37,38] Vigilant observation for all OIs must therefore be part of ongoing prenatal care.

Antiretroviral Therapy

We now have considerable data that suggest the safety and efficacy of zidovudine monotherapy administered per the ACTG protocol 076 during pregnancy, labor, and the neonatal period in reducing mother-to-child transmission of HIV-1.[2,39] Although reports have also appeared in the lay press suggesting that a modified, less expensive regimen of zidovudine monotherapy may be effective in preventing vertical transmission in the developing world, thus far, those studies have not appeared in a peer-reviewed journal. However, concerns persist regarding zidovudine

as a mutagen, and in vitro and animal studies have demonstrated mutagenic and carcinogenic activity of zidovudine at levels far higher than found in humans.[40] Nonetheless, the U.S. Public Health Service recommends that standard antiretroviral therapy be discussed with and offered to HIV-infected pregnant women.[21]

Early Disease

Women who present with early HIV disease (CD4 count >500 cells/mm^3 and plasma HIV RNA at undetectable levels or below 500 copies/ml) with no history of antiretroviral treatment must choose whether to take no therapy, zidovudine monotherapy, a two-drug regimen, or a three-drug regimen. The only purpose of zidovudine monotherapy in this case would be to lower the transmission risk to the fetus, because there is no plasma HIV RNA level below which there is no risk of transmission; a transmission event can occur at any level. Although the possibility of a woman developing zidovudine resistance during pregnancy monotherapy is a very real concern, it appears that, especially among women with early disease, an exposure to zidovudine alone of 6 months or less rarely results in development of resistance.[41]

Some women with early HIV disease and most women with late disease are concerned about zidovudine resistance and may opt for double or triple combination therapy. At SFGH, we stress both the theoretical and practical advantages of triple combination therapy, but find some women are reluctant to take a third agent, particularly protease inhibitors. Mothers appear to have a number of concerns about these drugs, including safety for the fetus, their own ability to adhere to dosing schedules, and lack of access to drugs postpartum. Several mothers have not wanted to start lifelong complicated drug regimens.

Until recently, many practitioners recommended adding lamivudine as a second agent during pregnancy, as well as in nonpregnant patients. Because lamivudine therapy can result in high-level resistance by selecting for variants with a valine substitution at codon 184 (M184V),[42] and such resistance can later result in zidovudine resistance (albeit only after multiple substitutions[43]), we now recommend didanosine as a second agent with zidovudine for double therapy because high-level didanosine resistance has not yet been reported. Still, we know of one mother who has decided to take the single-pill zidovudine/lamivudine preparation (Combivir) for ease of administration and increased adherence.

Moderately Advanced Disease

Women who present with moderately advanced disease (CD4 counts between 200 and 500 cells/mm^3 and plasma HIV RNA between 500 and 5000 copies/ml) comprise a group that has diverse reasonable therapeutic options. Despite the availability of triple-drug therapy at our center, a significant number of women with disease in this category have chosen double therapy, citing reasons similar to those with early disease.

Advanced Disease

When women present with plasma HIV RNA above 5000 copies/ml and/or CD4 counts less than 200 cells/mm^3, they are counseled about the importance of four issues: obtaining optimal control of their disease, forestalling development of resistant mutations with triple-drug therapy, suppressing viral replication to protect damage by HIV disease to their immune systems, and minimizing exposure of fetal tissues to HIV-infected maternal cells and infectious free HIV particles. In this situation, their attention is directed once again not only to their pregnancy, but also to their own health maintenance and preserving their ability to care for and nurture their child for many years once it is born.

At the University of California–San Francisco Bay Area Perinatal AIDS Center, first-line triple combination therapy for antiretroviral therapy–naive pregnant women currently is zidovudine 200 mg every 8 hours, lamivudine 150 mg bid, and nelfinavir 750 mg every 8 hours. This combination is a somewhat arbitrary choice, based on the following reasoning. First, clinical experience with zidovudine has shown it to be safe and well tolerated in human pregnancy. It is the only agent that has been demonstrated to prevent vertical transmission. Second, lamivudine is an effective and well-tolerated adjunct to zidovudine and, when used as part of a triple regimen, is unlikely to be associated with the emergence of resistance. Third, nelfinavir has been well tolerated by all of our patients to date and is not associated with hyperbilirubinemia, as is indinavir, for which a theoretical concern is that it may cause or exacerbate neonatal hyperbilirubinemia. Two mothers with adherence difficulties have been placed on every-12-hour regimens. This alternative (zidovudine 300 mg–lamivudine 150 mg

combination [Combivir] plus nelfinavir, 1250 mg every 12 hours) may be presented to mothers more often once we gain further experience with it outside of pregnancy and more pharmacokinetic data on protease inhibitors in pregnant women are available.

Women Already on HAART

Recommendations regarding antiretroviral therapy for pregnant women already receiving HAART are more complicated than in antiretroviral therapy–naive patients. Although women in our clinic are given the option of interrupting therapy during the first trimester, none has yet chosen to do so. Women who present with their disease optimally controlled on a triple combination regimen that includes zidovudine generally continue with that regimen. We counsel them about possible changes that they might like to make in their therapy because they are pregnant (e.g., switching from indinavir to nelfinavir to avoid the theoretical possibility of neonatal hyperbilirubinemia), but, so far, four clients who were on indinavir at the time they came to our clinic have chosen to continue its use. They and their babies have done well. In fact, all infants exposed to protease inhibitors (16 to date) have done well.

Recommendations are more difficult to make when women are on combination therapy that does not contain zidovudine. Zidovudine is the only agent that has been shown to reduce vertical transmission, and U.S. Public Health Service guidelines suggest that it be incorporated into the antiviral regimen of all pregnant women.[21] However, there are no data to suggest that other antiretrovirals are not also effective in preventing vertical transmission. In addition, in most women who are not taking it, zidovudine has usually already failed, either because of resistance, intolerance, or hypersensitivity to the drug. At SFGH, if a pregnant woman's history is suggestive of zidovudine resistance or intolerance, the drug is not added to her daily combination regimen. However, we still recommend its use intravenously during labor and by mouth for the baby in the neonatal period. If a woman has a history of hypersensitivity, we forego maternal zidovudine administration altogether, but still recommend its use in the neonate.

Problems with Protease Inhibitors

Protease inhibitors may present unique problems during pregnancy. Pregnant women may have more difficulty tolerating the gastrointestinal disturbances associated with saquinavir, ritonavir, and nelfinavir. Hyperbilirubinemia with indinavir is also of some concern. We have been monitoring maternal bilirubin levels once each trimester. Although some authorities have advocated that indinavir be discontinued during labor, we have elected to continue administering the drug with sips of water during labor, if the mother's bilirubin level is normal.

Because the ureter is markedly dilated as part of the normal physiologic changes of pregnancy, indinavir-associated nephrolithiasis would seem unlikely, but pregnant women can and do get kidney stones, and an increased incidence may someday be reported in gravidas who take this agent. Maintaining adequate hydration is important for all pregnant mothers, and is much more so for those taking indinavir.

A diabetogenic effect of protease inhibitors has been suggested in some early reports.[44] The incidence of hyperglycemia is uncommon—0.52 per 100 person-months of protease inhibitor therapy—but, when it occurs, it can be severe. Glucose intolerance is a common complication of pregnancy, and concern that the double stress of pregnancy and protease inhibitor therapy could result in an increased incidence of gestational diabetes mellitus is justifiable. Our practice is to obtain glucose challenge tests (also known as a 50-gm glucose load test) at least twice: at between 20 and 24 weeks' estimated gestational age and again at 30 to 34 weeks. It may become appropriate to check several timed postprandial glucose levels. Our limited experience thus far is that pre-existing and gestational diabetes mellitus can be challenging to manage in pregnant women who are receiving protease inhibitor therapy.

The non-nucleoside reverse transcriptase inhibitor nevirapine has been studied in late pregnancy and the neonatal period. So far it has been well tolerated, but the limited data available have not yet been published. Recent warnings have appeared that the not-yet released DMP 266 was associated with central nervous system anomalies in exposed monkeys. Practitioners considering its use in pregnant women should consult with the manufacturer regarding the latest data available.

Monitoring Plasma HIV RNA Levels

Plasma HIV viremia must be closely monitored in pregnant patients for several important reasons. First, pregnancy-specific pharmacokinetic data do not exist for most agents in use today, except for zidovudine, didanosine, and nevirapine. The intravascular blood volume is increased by 50% as early as 10 weeks' gestation. It is therefore possible that, by following adult dosing guidelines, we are inadequately treating our pregnant patients. It is important to learn as soon as possible if viral replication is inadequately suppressed so that treatment can be altered. Second, adhering to treatment during pregnancy can be challenging for clients for many reasons, such as nausea and vomiting, preoccupation with other pressing responsibilities, exhaustion, and denial. If plasma HIV RNA levels rise as a result of any of these, it is best to recognize it immediately and address issues of adherence as soon as possible. Third, because little is known about HIV viral dynamics during pregnancy and the postpartum period, we are obligated to monitor disease activity very closely. Missing a breakthrough event by several months could have a significant effect on maternal health and be disastrous in terms of the likelihood of a transmission event. At the Bay Area Perinatal AIDS Center, plasma HIV RNA is monitored monthly. However, we occasionally relax that schedule to every second month if patients have undetectable plasma HIV RNA levels and/or CD4 counts greater than 500/mm^3, or have been receiving triple combination therapy for a prolonged period and have stable CD4 counts and plasma HIV RNA levels.

Recurrent Genital Herpes

Genital herpes simplex virus type 2 (HSV2) infection, which has an incidence of 40% in the general population, is a common problem in pregnancy. Ironically, the greatest risk of fetal or neonatal infection is when a mother has no previous history of HSV2 and suffers a primary herpetic outbreak around the time of birth. Neonatal herpes is less commonly the result of a recurrent outbreak, but there is a small but definite risk (0.5 to 1 per 1000 deliveries of mothers who have had herpes in the past) of infection of the neonate during birth, even if cesarean sections are routinely performed for active maternal herpetic lesions.[45] Neonatal herpes is devastating, even when treated promptly. HIV coinfection presents additional complications. Seventy percent of HIV-infected woman are seropositive for HSV2 and are more likely to have herpes reactivation in labor.[46] Moreover, reports have appeared in abstract form that herpetic lesions shed high titers of replication competent HIV-1 in addition to HSV2,[47] so that an infant of an HIV-positive mother with a recurrent HSV2 outbreak during labor faces not only the risk of herpetic infection, but also the risk of exposure to HIV in the herpetic lesions.

Prophylactic acyclovir (400 mg PO tid) for pregnant women has been shown to be highly effective in preventing recurrent lesions in labor, is significantly more cost-effective, and causes less maternal morbidity than routine elective cesarean section.[45] For these reasons, we give acyclovir prophylaxis to pregnant women who have one episode of recurrent HSV2 in their current pregnancy. The drug is considered safe in pregnancy and has been well tolerated in our patients. The addition of acyclovir prophylaxis will mean that many women will be taking a total of four antiviral drugs, which could affect their ability to adhere to anti-HIV therapy.

MEDICAL COMPLICATIONS OF PREGNANCY IN HIV-1 INFECTED WOMEN

Few obstetricians have had extensive experience administering HAART to women to whom they deliver prenatal care. Consequently, many women will continue to have different providers for prenatal care and HIV primary care. Therefore, open lines of communication must exist between providers, and collaborative, crossdisciplinary education must be an ongoing process. HIV primary care providers can no more ignore their clients' pregnancy than obstetricians can ignore their clients' HIV status.

The following discussion covers pregnancy complications that occur with significant frequency and may greatly affect anti-HIV therapy. Ectopic pregnancy and pre-eclampsia, although common, are easy to miss, require immediate intervention, and can be life threatening to any mother. Nausea and vomiting of pregnancy may have a great impact on a woman's ability to adhere to antiretroviral therapy. Multiple gestation and/or preterm labor may affect the risk of vertical transmission. Psychiatric illness is all too often overlooked and undertreated during pregnancy, many times with disastrous outcomes.

Ectopic Pregnancy

In recent decades, ectopic pregnancy rates have markedly increased. The typical presentation of ectopic pregnancy can be misleading because the vaginal bleeding and abdominal pain are often suggestive of threatened spontaneous abortion. Without clinical suspicion of ectopic pregnancy, it cannot be diagnosed. It is therefore alarming that most women who die from an ectopic pregnancy rupture have been seen by a medical care provider within the previous several days. Early diagnosis is easier with ultrasensitive serum and urine testing for pregnancy (human chorionic gonadotropin assays) that is now the standard of care, along with pelvic sonography with use of abdominal and vaginal probes. Medical intervention is now possible before and after rupture of a tubal ectopic pregnancy, and the earlier ectopic pregnancy can be diagnosed, the less invasive and destructive surgical interventions need to be.

Nausea and Vomiting and Hyperemesis Gravidarum

Between 60% and 80% of women will experience some nausea and/or vomiting during pregnancy, but hyperemesis gravidarum, with its characteristic intractable nausea and vomiting, fluid and electrolyte imbalances, weight loss, and ketonuria, occurs in about 1:100 women. Regardless of the severity of these symptoms, the inability to tolerate food and oral medications can have serious consequences for an HIV-infected woman. Therefore, it may be prudent to delay initiating antiretroviral therapy in a medically stable patient until after the first trimester, when nausea and vomiting are likely to have resolved or at least improved. In the case of women who are already receiving therapy and elect to continue it through the first trimester, we advise them not to repeat doses of antiretroviral pills unless they can identify the pills in their emesis. We also reassure them that medications are likely to be absorbed even if vomiting is recurrent. Plasma HIV RNA can be monitored frequently to assess whether antiretroviral medication is being adequately absorbed. Nutritional counseling may be beneficial in scheduling meals and pills to enhance tolerance of both. Treating a mothers' nausea and vomiting pharmacologically should be done without hesitation. Women who show signs of dehydration or ketonuria should be admitted to the hospital because intravenous rehydration for a few hours in an emergency department is bound to fail. Several pharmacologic agents have been used successfully, and different women find different medications helpful. Common recommendations include pyridoxine (10 to 30 mg/day), promethazine rectal suppositories (25 mg every 12 hours), and trimethobenzamide (750 mg/day in divided doses). There are no reports of teratogenic effects of these antiemetics, but they must be cautiously assessed for drug–drug interactions with any antiretroviral medication that a woman might be taking.

Preterm Labor and Multiple Gestation

Preterm delivery is of particular concern with HIV-infected mothers because, for reasons not well understood, premature infants are at greater risk of being HIV infected. HIV-infected women have twins at least at the same rate as the general population, and there is some suggestion that twinning may be more common among HIV-infected mothers. Therefore, multiple gestation and other risk factors, such as previous preterm delivery, indicate the need for ongoing assessment of preterm cervical dilation and other signs of preterm labor. Many obstetricians consider bed rest to prevent preterm labor in mothers of twins extremely valuable.[48] In the case of HIV-infected women, whose lives are often chaotic and demanding, there is even greater urgency to prevent premature delivery of HIV-exposed infants. Therefore, every attempt should be made to enable women at risk of preterm delivery to reduce their activity, rest during the day, or, when indicated, adopt a modified or strict bed rest plan.

Hypertensive Disorders

Although hypertensive disorders of pregnancy are relatively common, they can be difficult to diagnose. Our greatest concern with pregnant women is pregnancy-induced hypertension and superimposed pre-eclampsia in chronic hypertensives. During the third trimester, virtually any medical abnormality must be assessed carefully to determine whether there might be a pre-eclamptic cause. For instance, abnormal liver function tests could be a sign of ritonavir hepatotoxicity, but they also could be the result of severe pre-eclampsia, as could a falling platelet count, an increased hematocrit, intravascular hemolysis, pulmonary edema, cerebral edema, right upper quadrant pain, or deteriorating renal function tests. Generally, mild pre-eclampsia at term (37 weeks or greater) or severe pre-eclampsia at any gestational age mandates delivery. Although severe pre-eclampsia is un-

likely in the absence of increased blood pressure and new-onset proteinuria, the disease can and does present atypically. All caregivers of pregnant women, whether they are directly responsible for prenatal care or are providing HIV care collaboratively, must be vigilant in looking for the signs and symptoms of pre-eclampsia.

Psychiatric Illness

Psychiatric illness must not be overlooked during pregnancy (see Chapter 15). Treatment that results in stabilizing psychiatric problems may help control other illnesses, including substance use, diabetes, and HIV disease. Control of other diseases and adherence to antiretroviral therapy are unlikely when patients' mental health needs have been neglected or deferred because of pregnancy. Psychiatric referrals should be made to practitioners who are comfortable and experienced with the use of antidepressants, antipsychotics, and antianxiety agents in pregnancy.[49] They should also be aware of possible interactions between these drugs and HIV-related drugs, especially the protease inhibitors.

Infectious Complications of Pregnancy

Caregivers must also be vigilant in looking for infectious complications of pregnancy. All pregnant women have, by definition, been having unsafe sex. STDs are reported to be associated with high risk of vertical transmission, and positive syphilis serologic results are not unusual in HIV-infected pregnant populations.

Chorioamnionitis is of particular concern. It is clear that the interval between rupture of membranes and delivery correlates directly with vertical transmission risk, and two published reports have shown an increased risk of transmission when that interval was longer than 4 hours.[7,50] Interestingly, there was no cutoff point where risk of rupture was substantially higher from one hour to the next, and one abstract report suggests that chorioamnionitis may be a more powerful predictor of transmission than length of rupture.[51] Such findings have important implications for intrapartum management (see later sections of this chapter).

INTRAPARTUM CARE

The key ingredients for smooth intrapartum management of an HIV-infected mother and her baby are meticulous attention to maternal HIV disease throughout pregnancy, close monitoring of plasma HIV RNA levels, and appropriate combination antiretroviral therapy. Our experience suggesets that other factors, such as route of delivery, method of fetal monitoring, and even duration of rupture of membranes, are secondary to whether or not the mother's HIV infection is under optimal control. Still, important intrapartum issues are addressed below.

Admission to the Hospital

HIV-infected mothers should be admitted to the hospital in labor somewhat earlier than most patients. It may be difficult to obtain intravenous zidovudine, and coordination with other drug administration schedules may be required. When all of these arrangements can be made during the calm of the early latent stage of labor, errors are less likely to occur. In no case should a mother who presents with spontaneous rupture of membranes be sent home.

Route of Delivery

Prevention of pediatric HIV infection is surrounded with controversies, but route of delivery looms as the largest, with serious implications for maternal versus fetal health issues, international health care resources, and standards of care. This one consideration highlights our profound lack of understanding of the mechanism of vertical transmission.

Recently a retrospective multicenter review has appeared[52] confirming the protective effect of zidovudine monotherapy during pregnancy against vertical transmission. A transmission rate of 6.6% was observed in mothers taking antepartum zidovudine who delivered vaginally. A select group of the zidovudine-treated mothers ($n = 133$) who received elective cesarean section, strictly defined as occurring before the onset of labor and before spontaneous rupture of membranes, showed an even lower rate of transmission (0.8%, or 1 of 133 mothers), suggesting a protective effect of elective cesarean section.

Caregivers and clients must understand important points about these interesting data. First, cesarean section offered no protective benefit when performed after the onset of labor or after rupture of membranes, or in the absence of maternal antepartum zidovudine prophylaxis. Second, confounders such as site of delivery, qual-

ity of prenatal care, and determinants of who was offered elective cesarean before the onset of labor (presumably women with excellent prenatal care and excellent dating criteria) instead of after the onset of labor (as would be offered to women with little prenatal care and unsure dating) are not discussed. Finally, maternal p24 antigenemia is reported as highly correlated with transmission, however, other more precise indicators of maternal HIV disease stage and activity, such as CD4 count and plasma HIV RNA level, are not included in the analysis. Ending as it does in 1996, the report does not include analysis of mothers receiving antiretroviral therapy for the treatment of their own disease.

Even though the idea of elective cesarean section may sound appealing, there is nothing straightforward about it in either the developed or developing world. One need only note that cesarean section for a fetal indication was unheard of until the 1950s, when cesarean-associated maternal morbidity and mortality rates became low enough to justify a possible fetal benefit of abdominal delivery. Elective cesarean delivery is fraught with hazards to both mother and baby. Among these are iatrogenic prematurity; the requirement for precise, early ultrasound-confirmed dating; increased risk of maternal hemorrhage; increased risk of placenta previa, placenta accreta, and uterine rupture in a subsequent pregnancy; the need for modern blood-banking facilities; and the frequent need for intravenous antibiotic therapies for the treatment of post–cesarean section febrile morbidity. Additionally, mothers at highest risk for transmitting HIV to their fetuses are those with the most advanced HIV disease, and their health may be most threatened by major abdominal surgery.

At SFGH, route of delivery of HIV-exposed fetuses has been determined by obstetric indications. Operative vaginal delivery and cesarean section have been performed for the same indications that they would have been in an uninfected mother.

Since the publication of the French perinatal cohort data[52] in July, 1998, we have counseled mothers regarding the potential risks and benefits of elective cesarean section prior to the onset of labor and rupture of membranes. Of the four mothers counseled to date, three have requested routine obstetric management; one of these received a repeat cesarean section for superimposed pre-eclampsia at term and prior vertical uterine incision, and one was scheduled for elective primary cesarean section at 39 weeks at her request. Our discussions with her emphasized that no benefit for prevention of vertical transmission had been demonstrated for cesarean section performed after the onset of labor or rupture of membranes, and that if she presented in labor or leaking fluid, she would receive a cesarean section for obstetrical indications only. She underwent elective primary cesarean section at 39 weeks. She required a blood transfusion postoperatively, and her infant required intravenous hydration for poor feeding and oxygen therapy for transient tachypnea of the newborn.

Anesthesia and Analgesia

HIV-infected mothers require the same access to modern obstetric anesthesia as do other pregnant women. These agents can be administered by the same routes as for uninfected mothers, with generally similar doses. There are no HIV-related contraindications to spinal anesthesia or to lumbar epidural anesthesia. Potent narcotics may have some interactions with antiretrovirals; therefore, dosages should be titrated carefully as they are in all patients. Finally, for patients with a history of narcotic dependence, availability of adequate analgesia during labor is extremely important and must not be neglected.

Antiretroviral Therapy During Labor

Antiretroviral therapy should not be interrupted during the birth process. According to the ACTG 076 protocol (Table 35–3), oral zidovudine should be replaced with intravenous zidovudine until the baby is born, at which time the oral medication is resumed. Zidovudine cannot be given in the same intravenous infusion line as oxytocin, so many mothers will require two intravenous lines during labor. At SFGH we have found it very useful to have intravenous zidovudine available in the labor and delivery suite at all times in order to avoid delays in receiving the drug from the pharmacy.

If a woman is taking zidovudine monotherapy or dual therapy only for the purpose of transmission prophylaxis, therapy should be stopped when the cord is clamped. Women receiving combination therapy for maternal health simply continue their medication through the birth process and into the postpartum period. A national trial is currently underway to examine the benefit of administering nevirapine during labor and the early neonatal period for the prevention of transmission. Because the efficacy of this intervention has not been proven, we have not recommended its use outside of a clinical trial setting.

The theoretical possibility of neonatal hyperbilirubinemia resulting from maternal indinavir use mentioned earlier underlies our current practice of obtaining a maternal bilirubin level during labor and a total bilirubin value for neonates on the second or third day of life. Although an association between protease inhibitors and glucose intolerance in pregnancy has not been established, the theoretical possibility of this complication from the double diabetogenic stress of pregnancy and protease inhibitors exists. Therefore, if mothers are taking a protease inhibitor, maternal glucose tolerance screening is performed at 20 to 24 weeks' gestation and again at 30 to 34 weeks' gestation. Chemsticks are currently being used to check for neonatal hypoglycemia at 1 and 4 hours of life in babies exposed to protease inhibitors.

Fetal Monitoring

According to contemporary standards of in-hospital obstetric care, all fetuses, regardless of exposure to HIV, are required to be monitored either electronically or by auscultation of the fetal heart rate. Occasionally, it is impossible to pick up or interpret externally generated fetal heart rate tracings. In such circumstances, an electrode is applied to the fetal scalp in order to detect and measure the fetal electrocardiographic signal.

It is difficult to make recommendations regarding the use of fetal scalp electrodes during the labor of an HIV-infected mother. Although it would seem obvious that practitioners should be reluctant to apply the electrode to the fetal scalp through the vagina of an HIV-infected mother, there may be simply no other way to ascertain fetal condition. Although the infection of a fetus by its HIV-positive mother via a fetal scalp electrode is theoretically plausible, data are lacking to prove this association. At SFGH, when a mother is HIV infected, our current practice is to apply a scalp electrode if the attending physician feels that it is necessary to monitor fetal condition and the mother agrees to its use. A common reason for difficulty with the external monitor is the presence of severe variable or late decelerations of the fetal heart rate, both of which are patterns that can be suggestive of significant fetal compromise. If the external tracing is inadequate or suspicious, and practitioners are unwilling to apply a scalp electrode

TABLE 35–3. Calculation of Zidovudine Dosing in Pregnancy to Reduce Vertical Transmission (from ACTG 076 Protocol*)

MATERNAL

Antepartum	Begin after 14 weeks' gestation
	Zidovudine 200 mg PO 3 times/d
Intrapartum	Zidovudine loading dose 2 mg/kg = _____ mg over 1 hr
	Then
	1 mg/kg/hr _____ mg/hr IV infusion
Diluent:	D_5W
Preparation:	Zidovudine 1000 mg in 250 ml D_5W
Final concentration:	4 mg/ml

INFANT

PO infant:	Zidovudine Elixir 2 mg/kg = _____ mg PO q6h × 6 wk
	Plus extra week supply
NPO infant:	Zidovudine 1.5 mg/kg = _____mg IV q6h
	Infuse over 30–60 min
Diluent:	D_5W
Final concentration:	0.5 mg/ml

*Data from Connor EM, Sperling RS, Gelber R, et al: Reduction of maternal-infant transmission of human immunodeficiency virus type 1 with zidovudine treatment. N Engl J Med 331:1173, 1994.

because of maternal HIV status, a cesarean section must be performed for presumed fetal intolerance of labor or fetal distress. There is no excuse for inadequate monitoring of a fetus simply because its mother is HIV-infected.

Rupture of Membranes

There is a clear association of length of rupture of membranes with risk of vertical transmission in cohorts of patients that have minimal exposure to zidovudine and other antiretrovirals.[50] Artificial rupture of membranes is therefore avoided during the labor of an HIV-infected mother. Amniotomy is occasionally performed if required for fetal monitoring purposes, although the majority of our patients are able to progress through labor without it.

Women who present with premature rupture of membranes at or near term should receive an oxytocin infusion for induction or augmentation of labor as soon as possible. As noted above, these mothers will require two intravenous lines, because oxytocin and zidovudine cannot be administered in the same line. It is important to note that rupture of membranes is not necessarily an indication for cesarean section. The number of vaginal examinations should be minimized after rupture of membranes (as with any patient), and all efforts should be directed at aggressive augmentation of labor strategies[53] to get the fetus delivered as soon as possible.

Occupational Exposure Issues for Labor and Delivery Staff

The use of universal precautions while caring for each and every patient is the only acceptable standard of professional conduct regarding prevention of occupational exposure to HIV during the intrapartum care of any woman, HIV infected or not. Staff need to be educated first to understand that other life-threatening illnesses such as hepatitis B and C are much more infectious than HIV and pose much greater risk to the health of caregivers, and, second, that any pregnant woman may harbor these and other infectious organisms that simply have not been diagnosed.

The knowledge that a health care facility has a strict universal precautions policy is also reassuring to expectant HIV-infected mothers. They know that they and their babies will not be singled out or treated differently because of their infection or exposure status. Staff who are uncomfortable caring for identified HIV-infected women probably should not be working with pregnant women at all.

POSTPARTUM CARE AND PLANS FOR DISCHARGE

The postpartum period is a difficult time for all mothers. HIV-infected women face even greater challenges than the usual exhaustion from child-birth, sleep deprivation, social isolation, and employment concerns and financial worries. Therefore, an essential part of discharge planning is to carefully coordinate maternal and neonatal care and support. Family and friends should be encouraged to provide support and relief, and referrals to available HIV agencies and resources for community respite care and babysitting should be coordinated. Maternal antiretroviral dosing schedules at generally 12- and 8-hour intervals should be integrated with zidovudine prophylaxis given to the newborn at 6-hour intervals. Some flexibility should be built into these schedules to make them manageable for new mothers. Liberal use of large pill boxes, beepers, timers, and other aids can be helpful. The challenges of adhering to therapy while taking care of a newborn should be dealt with in advance of delivery and on an ongoing basis. If issues of disclosure to family and friends can be resolved before delivery, they should be included in planning schedules.

A serious issue for families living with HIV is that when an HIV-infected woman must choose between attending her own medical appointment and that of her child, she will typically put the child's medical care first. For this reason, centers have been developed that offer HIV and primary care for both mothers and babies in the same clinic during the same visits, with babysitting services available.

HIV testing schedules for exposed infants are demanding, particularly in the early months of life. All HIV-exposed babies are born "HIV positive," that is, they will test positive because of the presence of maternal anti-HIV antibody in their blood. However, most of these children will not be infected. HIV DNA polymerase chain reaction (PCR) is currently the only accepted method for distinguishing between an HIV-exposed infant and an HIV-infected infant. (Chapter 33 of this book discusses this in more detail.) At SFGH, we are drawing blood for HIV DNA PCR assays within the first 48 hours of a baby's life and then at 4 to 6 weeks, 12 weeks, and 24 weeks of age. HIV antibody testing is performed in the first 48 hours of life and then, starting at 6 months, at 6-month intervals to confirm seroreversion. Consultation with local experts concerning neonatal testing recommendations is recommended. Plasma HIV RNA (viral burden) testing is not yet an accepted method of diagnosis of HIV infection in children or adults, but may be in the near future.

If infants are DNA PCR negative on all tests by 4 months of age, we counsel families that the overwhelming likelihood is that they are not infected. We still repeat the PCR test at 6 months, and continue antibody testing until infants serorevert to "HIV negative" status after loss of their maternal antibodies at 12 to 18 months of life. Parents need to be carefully educated on multiple occasions regarding the difference between an "HIV-positive" exposed but uninfected baby and an HIV-infected baby, so that they in turn will be able to educate inexperienced caregivers they may encounter in emergency situations.

CONCLUSIONS

The medical management of HIV disease has been radically changed in the last 5 years. These changes have had an enormous impact on the field of maternal and child health. Where HIV care of mothers once was confined to social and emotional support, treatment of opportunistic and other infections, and careful attention to basic prenatal care issues, we have witnessed a rapid shift of focus to the implemention of effective prophylactic strategies to prevent vertical transmission of virus, and to aggressive and complex strategies aimed at the effective treatment of maternal disease.

References

1. Beckerman KP, Shannon M, Benson M, et al: Control of maternal HIV-1 disease during pregnancy. In: Program and Abstracts of the XIIth International Conference on AIDS, 1998, Geneva, Abstract 12151
2. Connor EM, Sperling RS, Gelber R, et al: Reduction of maternal-infant transmission of human immunodeficiency virus type 1 with zidovudine treatment. N Engl J Med 331:1173, 1994
3. Burns DN, Landesman S, Minkoff H, et al: The influence of pregnancy on human immunodeficiency virus type 1 infection: Antepartum and postpartum changes in human immunodeficiency virus type 1 viral load. Am J Obstet Gynecol 178:355, 1998
4. Anderson VM: The placental barrier to maternal HIV infection. Obstet Gynecol Clin North Am 24:797, 1997
5. Phillips OP, Elias S, Shulman LP: Maternal serum screening for fetal Down syndrome in women less than 35 years of age using alpha-fetoprotein, hCG, and unconjugated estriol: A prospective 2-year study. Obstet Gynecol 80:353, 1992
6. Haddow JE, Palomaki GE, Knight GJ, et al: Reducing the need for amniocentesis in women 35 years of age or older with serum markers for screening. N Engl J Med 330:1114, 1994
7. Landesman SH, Kalish LA, Burns DN, et al: Obstetrical factors and the transmission of human immunodeficiency virus type 1 from mother to child. N Engl J Med 334:1617, 1996

8. Viscarello RR, Copperman AB, DeGennaro NJ: Is the risk of perinatal transmission of human immunodeficiency virus increased by the intrapartum use of spiral electrodes or fetal scalp pH sampling? Am J Obstet Gynecol 170:740, 1994

9. Mandelbrot L, Mayaux MJ, Bongain A, et al: Obstetric factors and mother-to-child transmission of human immunodeficiency virus type 1: The French perinatal cohorts. SEROGEST French Pediatric HIV Infection Study Group. Am J Obstet Gynecol 175:661, 1996

10. Fowler MG: Update: Transmission of HIV-1 from mother to child. Curr Opin Obstet Gynecol 9:343, 1997

11. Cao Y, Krogstad P, Korber BT, et al: Maternal HIV-1 viral load and vertical transmission of infection: The Ariel Project for the prevention of HIV transmission from mother to infant. Nat Med 3:549, 1997

12. Mofenson LM: Mother-child HIV-1 transmission: Timing and determinants. Obstet Gynecol Clin North Am 24:759, 1997

13. Thomas P, Singh T, Bornschlegel K, et al: Use of ZDV to prevent perinatal HIV in New York City. In: Program and Abstracts of the 4th Conference on Retroviruses and Opportunistic Infections, 1997, Washington, DC, Abstract 381

14. Fiscus SA, Adimora AA, Schoenbach VJ, et al: Importance of maternal ZDV therapy in the reduction of perinatal transmission of HIV. In: Program and Abstracts of the 4th Conference on Retroviruses and Opportunistic Infections, 1997, Washington, DC, Abstract 379

15. Blanche S, Mayaux MJ, Mandelbrot L: Acceptability and impact of zidovudine prevention on mother to child HIV-1 transmission in France. In: Program and Abstracts of the 4th Conference on Retroviruses and Opportunistic Infections, 1997, Washington, DC, Abstract 380

15a. Shaffer N, Roongpisuthipong A, Siriwasin W, et al: Maternal virus load and perinatal human immunodeficiency virus type 1 subtype E transmission, Thailand. J Infect Dis 179:590, 1999

15b. Shaffer N, Bhadrakom C, Siriwasin W, et al: Randomized placebo-controlled trial of short-course oral ZDV to reduce perinatal HIV transmission, Thailand. In: Program and Abstracts of the XIIth International Conference on AIDS, 1998, Geneva, Abstract 33163

15c. Shaffer N, Roongpisuthipong A, Siriwasin W, et al: Changes in plasma viral load related to short-course oral zidovudine (ZDV) during late pregnancy. In: Program and Abstracts of the XIIth International Conference on AIDS, 1998, Geneva, Abstract 33164

16. Burns DN, Landesman S, Muenz LR, et al: Cigarette smoking, premature rupture of membranes, and vertical transmission of HIV-1 among women with low CD4+ levels. J Acquir Immune Defic Syndr Hum Retrovirol 7:718, 1994

17. Ewing HH: Methadone maintenance and tapering. In Jessup M (ed): Drug Dependency in Pregnancy: Managing Withdrawal. North Highlands, CA, California Department of Health Services, Maternal and Child Health Branch, 1992, p 91

18. Kyei-Aboagye K: Treatment of cocaine dependency during pregnancy. In Jessup M (ed): Drug Dependency in Pregnancy: Managing Withdrawal. North Highlands, CA, California Department of Health Services, Maternal and Child Health Branch, 1992, p 175

19. Jessup M: Drug Dependency in Pregnancy: Managing Withdrawal. North Highlands, CA, California Depart-

ment of Health Services, Maternal and Child Health Branch, 1992. Copies may be obtained by telephone 916-973-3700 or mail. State of California Department of General Services Publications, PO Box 9015, North Highlands, CA 95660.

20. NIH Guidelines: Report of the NIH panel to define principles of therapy of HIV infection. HIVInsite Drug Advisories. Bethesda, MD, National Institutes of Health, 1997

21. Centers for Disease Control and Prevention: Public Health Service Task Force recommendations for the use of antiretroviral drugs in pregnant women infected with HIV-1 for maternal health and for reducing perinatal HIV-1 transmission in the United States. MMWR Morbid Mortal Wkly Rep 47:1, 1998

22. Staprans SI, Hamilton BL, Follansbee SE: Activation of virus replication after vaccination of HIV-1-infected individuals. J Exp Med 182:1727, 1995

23. Plummer FA. Heterosexual transmission of human immunodeficiency virus type 1: Interactions of conventional sexually transmitted diseases, hormonal contraception and HIV-1. AIDS Res Hum Retroviruses 14: S5, 1998

24. Clumeck N, Taelman H, Hermans P, et al: A cluster of HIV infection among heterosexual people without apparent risk factors. N Engl J Med 23:1460, 1989

25. Downs AM, DeVincenzi I: Probability of heterosexual transmission of HIV: Relationship to the number of unprotected sexual contacts. J Acquir Immune Defic Syndr Hum Retrovirol 11:388, 1996

26. Mandelbrot L, Heard I, Henrion-Geant E, et al: Natural conception in HIV-negative women with HIV-infected partners. Lancet 349:850, 1997

27. Semprini AE, Fiore S, Pardi G: Reproductive counselling for HIV-discordant couples. Lancet 349:1401, 1997

28. Semprini AE, Levi-Setti P, Bozzo M, et al: Insemination of HIV-negative women with processed semen of HIV-positive partners. Lancet 340:1317, 1992

29. deVincenzi I: A longitudinal study of human immunodeficiency virus transmission by heterosexual partners. N Engl J Med 331:341, 1994

30. Kiessling AA, Eyre RC, Winig P, et al: Special program of assisted reproduction (SPAR) for couples with infectious disease infertility. In: Program and Abstracts of the IFFS/American Society for Reproductive Medicine, 1998, San Francisco

31. Smith S: The fertility race, part 4: HIV and infertility. Available at: http://www.mpr.org. Accessed November 3, 1998

32. Smith S: The fertility race, part 5: Conceiving with HIV. Available at: http://www.msnbc.org under Living. Accessed November 3, 1998

33. Denison R: Where are they now? Women Organized to Respond to Life-Threatening Diseases (WORLD) Newsletter, p 6, 1996 (P.O. Box 11535, Oakland, CA 94611)

34. Denison R: The hardest decision I ever made. Women Organized to Respond to Life-Threatening Diseases (WORLD) Newsletter, p 1, 1995 (P.O. Box 11535, Oakland, CA 94611)

35. Goldman E, Miller R, Lee CA: Counseling HIV positive haemophilic men who wish to have children. BMJ 304:829, 1992

36. Laine C, Markson LE, McKee LJ, et al: The relationship of clinic experience with advanced HIV and survival of women with AIDS. AIDS 12:417, 1998

37. Melnick SL, Sherer G, Louis TA: Survival and disease progression according to gender of patients with HIV

infection. The Terri Beirn Community Programs for Clinical Research on AIDS. JAMA 272:1915, 1994

38. Philips AN, Antues F, Stergious G, et al: A sex comparison of rates of new AIDS-defining disease and death in 2554 AIDS cases: AIDS in Europe Study Group. AIDS 8:831, 1994

39. Ferrazin A, de Maria A, Gotta C, et al: Zidovudine therapy of HIV-1 infection during pregnancy: Assessment of the effect on the newborns. J Acquir Immune Defic Syndr Hum Retrovirol 6:376, 1993

40. Toltzis P, Mourton T, Magnuson T: Effect of zidovudine on preimplantation murine embryos. Antimicrob Agents Chemother 37:1610, 1993

41. Richman D, Grimes J, Lagakos S: Effect of stage of disease and drug dose on zidovudine susceptibilities of isolates of human immunodeficiency virus. J Acquir Immune Defic Syndr Hum Retrovirol 3:743, 1990

42. Schuurman R, Nijhuis M, van Leeuwen R, et al: Rapid changes in human immunodeficiency virus type 1 RNA load and appearance of drug-resistant virus populations in persons treated with lamivudine (3TC). J Infect Dis 171:1411, 1995

43. Nijhuis M, Schuurman R, de Jong D, et al: Lamivudine-resistant human immunodeficiency virus type 1 variants (184V) require multiple amino acid changes to become co-resistant to zidovudine in vivo. J Infect Dis 176:398, 1997

44. Keruly JC, Chaison RE, Moore RD, et al: Diabetes and hyperglycemia in patients receiving protease inhibitors. In: Program and Abstracts of the 5th Conference on Retroviruses and Opportunistic Infections, 1998, Chicago, Abstract 415

45. Randolph AG, Hartshorn RM, Washington AE: Acyclovir prophylaxis in late pregnancy to prevent neonatal herpes: A cost-effectiveness analysis. Obstet Gynecol 88:603, 1996

46. Hitti J, Watts DH, Burchett SK, et al: Herpes simplex virus seropositivity and reactivation at delivery among pregnant women infected with human immunodeficiency virus-1. Am J Obstet Gynecol 177:450, 1997

47. Schacker T, Ryncarz A, Goddard J, et al: Frequent recovery of replication competent HIV from genital herpes simplex virus lesions in HIV-infected persons. In: Program and Abstracts of the 4th Conference on Retroviruses and Opportunistic Infections, 1997, Washington, DC, Abstract 27

48. Komoramy B, Lampe L: Value of bed rest in twin pregnancies. Int J Gynecol Obstet 14:262, 1977

49. Hohener HC, Spielvogel AM: Teaching women's issues in psychiatric residency: Resident's attitudes. J Am Med Wom Assoc 50:14, 1995

50. Minkoff H, Burns DN, Landesman SH, et al: The relationship of the duration of ruptured membranes to vertical transmission of human immunodeficiency virus. Am J Obstet Gynecol 173:585, 1995

51. Popek EJ, Korber BT, Merritt L, et al: Acute chorioamnionitis and duration of membrane rupture correlates with vertical transmission of HIV-1. In: Program and Abstracts of the 4th Conference on Retroviruses and Opportunistic Infections, 1997, Washington, DC, Abstract 504

52. Mandelbrot L, Le Chenadec J, Berrebi A, et al: Perinatal HIV-1 transmission: Interaction between zidovudine prophylaxis and mode of delivery in the French Perinatal Cohort. JAMA 280:55, 1998

53. Peaceman AM, Socol ML: Active management of labor. Am J Obstet Gynecol 175:363, 1996

36 | HIV Disease in Substance Abusers: Treatment Issues

GERALD FRIEDLAND

EPIDEMIOLOGY

The injection of illicit drugs has played a central and expanding role in the HIV/AIDS epidemic. Several features of the epidemiology of HIV/AIDS in injection drug users have important therapeutic and public health implications. In the United States, injection drug use is the second largest risk category for reported AIDS cases. Approximately 30% of people reported with AIDS had injection drug use as their recorded risk behavior. The proportion of new AIDS cases attributable to this risk factor has increased over the course of the epidemic. Initially representing 17% of cases in 1982, injection drug users accounted for 29% of reported cases in 1996.[1] In addition, information from a number of sources suggests that HIV incidence remains highest among injection drug users.

As a result of continuing new infections and the decline in AIDS mortality, it is estimated that the number of drug users living with AIDS or HIV has increased by 10% between 1995 and 1996, a trend that is likely to continue.[1] The Centers for Disease Control and Prevention (CDC) estimates that, in 1997, 48,000 active or former injection drug users were living with AIDS and 120,000 with HIV disease.[1] Thus the numbers of drug users for whom HIV therapy will be essential will increase over the next decade.

The geographic distribution of HIV disease among injection drug users is quite varied. Whereas the seroprevalence of HIV infection among men who have sex with men is relatively evenly distributed in urban centers across the United States,[2] seroprevalence studies indicate wide geographic disparities in rates of infection and AIDS cases among drug users. Over half of new AIDS cases in Northeast urban areas, parts of the south, and Puerto Rico occur in this population, and 25% to 50% of drug users are infected with HIV in these areas. In contrast, rates of infection among drug users range from 5% to 25% in other parts of the country.[3]

Injection drug use is especially important in the HIV/AIDS epidemic among women and children. Injection drug users represent the major route for heterosexual and perinatal transmission of HIV.[2,3] Approximately half of the reported cases of AIDS in women have been the direct result of injection drug use, and currently over 60% of pediatric AIDS cases are among children whose mothers were either drug users themselves or sexual partners of drug users. Thus most cases of heterosexually acquired and perinatally acquired HIV are directly or indirectly attributable to injection drug use.[2,3]

Finally, injection drug use is a major international issue in the global HIV/AIDS pandemic. Epidemiologic trends in Europe (particularly Eastern Europe), Asia, and Latin America indicate that injection drug use is often the entry route of HIV and the initial source of its rapid spread.[3,4]

In light of the increasingly central role of injection drug use in the national and global HIV/AIDS epidemic, issues of HIV clinical care and therapeutics in this population are of great importance.[5] Of particular relevance are the special clinical features of HIV disease in drug users, the treatment of HIV disease itself, the special difficulties in providing care to drug users, and the treatment of substance abuse.

HIV DISEASE IN DRUG USERS

A wide array of studies have indicated that the natural history of HIV disease among drug users is similar to that in other transmission risk categories.[3] Before highly active antiretroviral therapy became available, progression time to AIDS and death after the acquisition of HIV infection was shown to be almost identical between drug users and men who have sex with men.[6-8] Differences in disease progression were likely related to the lack of availability or use of treatment in this population.[9] There are, however, substantial differences in the incidence of HIV-related clinical complications in injection drug users that have a great impact on clinical care and therapeutics (Table 36-1). Many of these complications are the result of prior exposure to various infectious pathogens and the mechanics and procedures associated with the unsterile injection of intravenous drugs.[2,3] As a result of these lifestyle issues, prior to the HIV/AIDS epidemic, injection drug users were known to have mortality rates 10- to 20-fold higher than age-matched non-drug-using control populations.[3] HIV disease has now rapidly outdistanced all other causes of mortality and is now the leading cause of morbidity and mortality among injection drug users.

The incidence of HIV-related complications among injection drug users differs from that in other populations. Certain AIDS diagnoses are more common, including *pneumocystis carinii* pneumonia (PCP), tuberculosis, esophageal candidiasis, HIV neuropathy, and wasting syndrome.[10] In addition, gender-specific diseases such as cervical cancer are common because of the large number of women who are injection drug users.

In contrast, certain diseases are less common among injection drug users, including cytomeg-alovirus, non-Hodgkin's lymphoma, cryptosporidiosis, and Kaposi's sarcoma[10]; the latter occurs in only 2% to 3% of injection drug users.

Although these HIV-specific complications are sources of morbidity and mortality among drug users, it is the less specific but clearly HIV-related complications outlined below that most distinguish this population clinically from others with HIV disease. Although most of these infections and other diseases were common among drug users before the HIV epidemic,[11-14] their incidence and severity have been accentuated by HIV disease. In both inpatient and outpatient settings, these are more common than specific HIV-related complications and often confound both diagnosis and treatment.

INFECTIONS ASSOCIATED WITH HIV DISEASE AMONG INJECTION DRUG USERS

Multiple features of injection drug use contribute to the increased risk of infection: (1) increased rates of skin, mucous membrane, and nasopharyngeal carriage of pathogenic organisms; (2) unsterile injection technique; (3) contamination of injection equipment or drugs with microorganisms that may be present in residual blood in shared injection equipment; (4) humoral, cell-mediated, and phagocyte defects induced by HIV infection and/or drug use; (5) poor dental hygiene that impairs gag and cough reflexes; (6) alteration of the normal microbial flora by self-administered antibiotic use; (7) increased prevalence of exposure to certain pathogens (notably *Mycobacterium tuberculosis*); (8) concomitant behaviors such as cigarette smoking, alcohol use, or exchange of sex for drugs or money; and (9) decreased access to and/or lack of appropriate use of preventive and primary health care services.

Bacterial infections are common in both inpatient and outpatient settings, and are the most common reason for hospitalization, accounting for more than one half of all hospital admissions among injection drug users with HIV disease.

Skin and Soft Tissue Infections

The high frequency of skin and soft tissue infections results from unsterile intravenous and subcutaneous injection (skin popping), combined with increased skin carriage of pathogenic organisms and adulterants that may cause tissue

---

TABLE 36-1. Expanded Spectrum of HIV-Related Disease in Injection Drug Users

Pyogenic bacterial infections
  Skin infections
  Sinusitis
  Pneumonia
    Streptococcus pneumoniae
    Haemophilus influenzae
  Bacterial endocarditis
    Staphylococcus aureus
    Streptococci
    Enteric gram-negative bacilli
Tuberculosis
Sexually transmitted diseases
  Syphilis
  Human papillomavirus infection
Hepatitis A, B, C, and D
Renal disease
Cervical cancer

Adapted from Alcabes P, Friedland GH: Injection drug use and human immunodeficiency virus infection. Clin Infect Dis 20: 1467, 1995, with permission.

necrosis. The clinical spectrum ranges from simple cellulitis and abscess to life-threatening necrotizing fasciitis and septic thrombophlebitis.[11] The clinical appearance is often atypical and subtle because of longstanding damage to the skin and to venous and lymphatic systems, resulting in underlying lymphedema, hyperpigmentation, scarring, and regional lymphadenopathy. Nevertheless, careful examination often reveals characteristic redness, warmth, and tenderness, with tender inguinal or axillary lymph nodes. Fever is variable and bacteremia is infrequent. Although the precise microbial etiology is difficult to determine, uncomplicated cellulitis is most frequently due to group A streptococci, other streptococci, or *Staphyloccus aureus*.

For injection drug users who have an established relationship with a health care provider, mild infections may be treated with oral antistaphylococcal agents on an outpatient basis; therapy should be followed by frequent visits at which time the response is assessed. In other instances, treatment should consist of hospitalization, administration of intravenous antistaphylococcal β-lactam antibiotics such as oxacillin or nafcillin, and incision and drainage in instances of abscess formation. Many experienced clinicians treat such infections with clindamycin. In areas where methicillin-resistant *S. aureus* is prevalent, vancomycin may be used empirically pending the results of susceptibility tests. The total duration of therapy is quite variable but should be at least 7 to 10 days.

More serious, indeed life-threatening skin and soft tissue infections include necrotizing fasciitis, myositis, and septic thrombophlebitis. Although infrequent, they should always be considered. Crepitus may be noted, and soft tissue radiographs or other imaging studies may reveal gas in tissues. Immediate surgical exploration is critical, and extensive drainage and debridement of infected and nonviable tissue is essential. These infections are often polymicrobial in etiology, therefore, parenteral antibiotic therapy is essential and should be aimed at gram-positive and gram-negative aerobic and anaerobic organisms. Rarely, septic thrombophlebitis may result from unsterile skin injection, requiring surgical exploration and vein ligation.

More benign indolent skin ulcers are common, particularly in women injection drug users. These result from skin popping and consist of low-grade foreign-body granulomatous inflammation and necrosis. These shallow lesions may become superinfected. They usually respond to local wound care and oral or topical antibiotics. Occasionally, the ulcers are quite extensive and require skin grafting. Hyperpigmented, depressed scars often remain at the site of healed lesions.

Other rare complications of injection drug use that result from unsterile injection include wound botulism, tetanus, malaria, and disseminated candidiasis.

Endocarditis

Bacterial endocarditis in injection drug users has received the greatest attention by clinicians and researchers,[15,16] and suspicion of its presence is among the most frequent reasons for hospitalization of drug users. Longer duration and increased frequency of intravenous drug use are associated with a cumulative increase in the risk of endocarditis. There is evidence that the incidence, rate of recurrence, and morbidity and mortality from endocarditis is greater among drug users who are HIV seropositive compared to those who are HIV seronegative.[17]

The diagnosis of endocarditis in injection drug users can be problematic in the emergency room setting, where most febrile drug users are evaluated and where this diagnosis is often suspected.[18] This is particularly so because most endocarditis is right sided and peripheral manifestations are absent.

In patients with HIV disease, the differential diagnosis is broader and even more difficult. All febrile injection drug users, with and without HIV disease, should have a detailed history and physical examination focusing on the presence of septic emboli in the skin and on mucosal surfaces, as well as the presence of regurgitant murmurs. Chest radiography to detect characteristic septic pulmonary emboli should be performed and blood cultures and cardiac imaging studies should be obtained. The latter are of variable sensitivity and specificity; false-negative results are frequent in right-sided involvement, and false-positive results also have been documented.

Staphylococcus aureus is the most commonly responsible organism; streptococci and enteric gram-negative rods are seen less frequently. After blood cultures are obtained, empirical antibiotic therapy directed toward *S. aureus* and dictated by local epidemiology should be instituted if patients are acutely ill, if left-sided endocarditis is highly suspected, and/or if septic pulmonary emboli are seen on radiographs. However, it is not necessary to institute therapy for endocarditis in all injection drug users with fever. Most will not have endocarditis.[18] It is often reasonable to withhold antibiotics and to observe the patient carefully until the results of blood cultures are known. Some patients will be found to have a minor transient illness or a pyrogenic or hypersensitivity reaction to injected drugs and will defervesce within 24 hours. In others, an alternative diagnosis will become apparent. The prognosis of right-sided staphlococcal endocarditis in this population is excellent, with only rare deaths and infrequent lack of response to medical therapy.[15] Endocarditis caused by other organisms and left-sided involvement carries a more serious prognosis with higher complication and fatality rates. These are largely determined by valve destruction with resultant congestive heart failure and the site and severity of peripheral arterial emboli. The duration of antibiotic therapy is controversial. Many experts prefer a full 4 weeks of therapy and avoidance of aminoglycoside antibiotics because of the high prevalence of underlying renal disease in this population (see below).

Pneumonia

HIV infection has dramatically increased the already high incidence of bacterial pneumonia in drug injectors. Prospective studies demonstrated that, even when they were not actively injecting drugs, HIV-infected drug users prior to an AIDS diagnosis had a four- to fivefold greater risk of bacterial pneumonia and sepsis (up to 10 cases per 100 person-years) than their HIV seronegative counterparts.[19] The increase in frequency of bacterial pneumonia begins at CD4 counts above 350 cells/mm^3 and, as with other HIV complications, increases further as the CD4 cell count falls. The organisms involved in HIV-related pneumonia among drug injectors are predominantly those reported in the earlier literature on community-acquired pneumonia in this group, that is, *Streptococcus pneumoniae* and *Haemophilus influenzae*.[20,21]

Among other infectious entities to be considered in the differential diagnosis of pulmonary disease in this population of patients are PCP, tuberculosis, and septic pulmonary emboli. A combination of historical, physical examination, radiographic, and laboratory information can usually enable the clinician to distinguish among these entities.[22] Not infrequently, however, the diagnosis is sufficiently unclear so that both PCP and bacterial pneumonia are treated empirically until bronchoscopic and/or microbiologic data provide a precise diagnosis. Intravenous trimethoprim-sulfamethoxazole will cover both entities adequately, although it is usually possible to treat specifically for bacterial

pneumonia, if strongly suspected, with a penicillin, cephalosporin, or macrolide antibiotic.

Tuberculosis

The HIV/AIDS epidemic has resulted in a secondary global epidemic of resurgent tuberculosis, predominately among injection drug users in the United States (see also Chapter 23, which deals specifically with tuberculosis infection in HIV-infected individuals). This is the result of higher levels of latent infection with *M. tuberculosis* compared to other populations infected with HIV, with consequent greater likelihood of reactivation and greater opportunity for spread to HIV-infected susceptible individuals in hospital settings and in the community.[23] In the urban northeastern United States, Puerto Rico, and the southeast, as many as 20% of drug injectors may have evidence of latent *M. tuberculosis* infection, and 40% may be infected with HIV. The overlap of these two endemic infections has resulted in an unprecedented increase in the incidence of tuberculosis since 1985, including multi-drug-resistant tuberculosis.

Pulmonary tuberculosis should always be suspected and included in the differential diagnosis in injection drug users with pneumonia. Initial airborne isolation is recommended if the etiology of pneumonia is unclear and if epidemiologic and clinical features raise the suspicion of tuberculosis. The diagnosis can be particularly difficult because chest radiographs are often atypical and extrapulmonary tuberculosis is greatly increased in frequency.[24] Initial therapy with four drugs is recommended (isoniazid, rifampin, pyrazinamide, and ethambutol) and is highly effective, but special efforts must be made to ensure long-term adherence to the regimen, including directly observed therapy (DOT).[25,26] The duration of therapy in HIV-infected patients with tuberculosis is the same as that among those who are not HIV infected.[27] A special problem in this population is the interaction between rifampin and methadone and protease inhibitor drugs. Methadone doses must be raised to avoid abrupt withdrawal.

The CDC has recommended that tuberculosis be aggressively treated first and antiretroviral therapy begun after completion of tuberculosis therapy.[28] Alternatively, rifabutin can be substituted for rifampin and antiretroviral and methadone therapy continued under careful observation for antiviral effect and methadone withdrawal.

Hepatitis

Injection drug users are at risk for hepatitis as a result of using blood-contaminated injection paraphernalia. Both hepatitis B and C are acquired early in injection drug use. Seroprevalence studies have indicated that 75% to 90% of long-term injectors have serologic evidence of past exposure to hepatitis B and C. Approximately 5% to 10% of individuals are chronic carriers of hepatitis B surface antigen. Hepatitis D virus has been documented in numerous seroprevalence studies among drug users in the United States and worldwide. Hepatitis B and C are common sources of chronic active hepatitis with persistent abnormalities of liver function and, ultimately, cirrhosis.[13] Hepatitis A has also been associated with injection drug use. Several surveillance-based investigations have indicated injection drug users may have up to 50-fold higher risk of acquiring hepatitis A than non–injection drug users. In addition, recent outbreaks of hepatitis A have been linked to groups of injection drug users in both the United States and Europe.

It is not surprising that in a variety of settings surveyed (entrants into drug treatment programs, newly incarcerated, street samples), more than 40% of injection drug users have abnormalities of liver function. As noted, hepatitis A, B, or C accounts for many of these abnormalities. In addition to infectious causes, coexisting alcohol abuse is common among injection drug users and often contributes to alterations in hepatic enzyme function. This high prevalence of hepatic disease often complicates HIV therapeutics in injection drug users. (See Chapters 13 and 26 for more discussion of hepatitis among HIV-infected individuals.)

OTHER COMMON COMPLICATIONS ASSOCIATED WITH HIV DISEASE AMONG INJECTION DRUG USERS

Neurologic Complications

The central nervous system is another important site for adverse sequelae of drug injection.[11] As a consequence, the differential diagnosis of neurologic disease is broader and often more difficult in this population than in others with HIV disease. Drug-induced altered mental status, comorbid psychiatric disease, head trauma, intracerebral hemorrhage and other stroke syndromes (especially in cocaine and amphetamine users), and septic and particulate emboli to the brain and spinal cord all enter into the differential diagnosis, in addition to HIV-related opportunistic infections and dementia. Injection drug users also commonly have neuropathic pain syndromes involving peripheral nerves and muscles. These must be added to the HIV- and therapy-related peripheral neuropathy. Diagnosis and treatment is often complicated by difficulties in pain management (see discussion later in this chapter).

Renal Disease

Severe renal disease is a frequent and characteristic complication of both injection drug use and HIV disease in injection drug users. It is rare among other populations with HIV disease. Prior to the HIV/AIDS epidemic, the entity known as "heroin nephropathy" was recognized.[11,12] The clinical features consisted of proteinuria and slowly progressive renal insufficiency, often requiring hemodialysis. Histologically, focal glomerular sclerosis was described. HIV-positive injection drug users develop a similar form of renal disease, but its course is markedly accelerated in tempo.[29] Progression from normal renal function to renal failure and need for dialysis may occur over several weeks to months. The etiology remains undetermined. Anecdotal suggestions of benefit from steroids early in the disease are currently being evaluated in controlled clinical trials. Either chronic ambulatory peritoneal dialysis or hemodialysis are required and are life sustaining. Studies indicate that, apart from a higher incidence of peritoneal infection, HIV-infected injection drug users fare as well as those receiving these therapies for other etiologies of renal failure.[30] Special therapeutic problems include the need for caution in the use of aminoglycoside antibiotics and other nephrotoxic agents in HIV-infected drug users and the absence of data on the pharmacokinetics of antiretroviral drugs in renal failure and dialysis.

TREATMENT OF HIV DISEASE IN DRUG USERS

Although declines in both mortality and morbidity from HIV disease have been seen among injection drug users, these individuals have not shared equally in the benefits and advances in

HIV therapeutics. Whereas the overall decline in AIDS mortality was 23% between 1995 and 1996, and 25% among men who have sex with men, it was only 17% and 10% in male and female injecting drug users, respectively.[1]

Despite great health needs, for drug users with HIV disease, clinical care is often difficult and inadequate. Providing care to HIV-infected injection drug users is challenging and often stressful for clinicians and other health care workers. In addition to the challenges of HIV disease, a complex array of substance abuse–related medical, psychological, and social problems often complicate the care of injection drug users. Drug users have frequent comorbid underlying psychiatric disease that may further complicate provision of care. Substance abusers may also have increased difficulties with adherence to medications.[31-37] This may be compounded by their underlying diseases, increased side effects, and drug interactions. The presence and treatment of pain and pain medication–seeking behavior present additional difficulties.[5]

Access to Care

Injection drug users as a group have had less access to and less ongoing care with HIV therapies than other populations. Recent studies indicate that, among drug users who are clinically eligible for antiretroviral therapy, only a small percentage actually receive it.[38,39] For example, in a cross-sectional survey of self-reported antiretroviral therapy during July 1996 to June 1997 among a well-characterized cohort of injection drug users in Baltimore, with CD4 cell counts below 500 cells/mm^3, 51% were on no antiretroviral therapy, 14% were on reverse transcriptor therapy alone, 23% were on combination therapy including only reverse transcriptase inhibitors, and 14% were on combination therapy that included a protease inhibitor. In this study, having a usual source of care, a consistent provider, and recent outpatient visits were associated with receiving combination therapies, including a protease inhibitor. In a similar study in Vancouver, where access to care and antiretrovirals is universal, only 40% of known injection drug users received antiretroviral therapies. Female drug users were less likely to receive antiretrovirals, and those in drug treatment were more likely.

These studies clearly point out that barriers to proper HIV care remain for injection drug users, regardless of site and system. They offer insight as well into some of the issues impeding availability and use of HIV therapies and their solution. There is real and perceived absence of access to adequate health care facilities and substance abuse treatment for drug users, and the chaotic lifestyle of drug users often makes use of existing facilities difficult and erratic.[5] Inexperience in managing HIV disease is common at sites where drug users are cared for, such as drug treatment programs and prisons; conversely, inexperience in managing substance abuse issues is likely at sites where HIV disease care is usually provided. The chronic relapsing nature of addiction as a medical disease is often not appreciated by clinicians, nor is the fact that drug users may be quite diverse and heterogeneous. Many physicians assume that drug users' antisocial behavior and drug use indicate a lifelong lack of concern for others and indifference to their own well-being, rather than a consequence of addiction. In addition, most clinicians lack information or knowledge about the treatment of substance abuse. There is often mutual suspicion between drug users and health care providers. Clinicians tend to have stereotypic views of drug users and may have negative feelings about the social worth of injection drug users. As with other "hateful" patients, physicians may come to view addicts as manipulative, unmotivated, and undeserving of care.[5,40] More than half of physicians surveyed in 1990 reported negative attitudes about treating injection drug users, and only 28% reported feeling comfortable caring for them.[5] Conversely, drug users often are distrustful of the health care system and harbor expectations that they will be treated punitively. Drug users often conceal their continuing drug use from health care professionals out of fear of rejection and in reaction to previous difficult encounters with the health care system. In turn, clinicians are sometimes reluctant to confront patients with their suspicions about substance abuse, fearing that the confrontation will compromise their relationship. However, the failure to acknowledge ongoing drug use itself will compromise the relationship because it means that one of the most important aspects of the patient's health is off limits for discussion.

There are strategies to help break the cycle of anger and frustration that too often characterizes physicians' interactions with injection drug users. As a result, many drug users have clearly benefited from current dramatic advances in HIV therapeutics,[1] principally those who have had access to or have participated in ongoing clinical care. It has been possible to engage many drug users successfully in HIV clinical care within drug treatment programs, in prisons, and in flexible outpatient settings.[41–44] Programs have been designed and executed that document successes in all of these areas. For example, in Connecticut, where 10% of the HIV-infected population is incarcerated, 70% of those initiated antiretroviral therapy in prison.[44] Tuberculosis and HIV care have been successfully provided in methadone treatment programs; drug users were shown to be compliant with clinic visits and care at the same rate as others in a clinic sensitive to their needs,[45] and homeless persons have been successfully treated in outreach programs.[46] In a recently reported study on drug users in Germany, considerable therapeutic success was obtained using a once-a-day antiretroviral regimen consisting of nevirapine, didanosine, and lamivudine, suggesting the possibility of once-a-day DOT for this population.[47]

Clinical Care Strategies to Improve the Quality of Care

An array of both structural and clinician patient strategies may improve care of injection drug users with HIV disease:

1. Establish sites where drug users may be reached and brought into ongoing HIV care. These include drug treatment programs, community sites, prisons, and flexible HIV care sites.
2. Educate clinicians about substance abuse.
3. Establish a multidisciplinary team consisting of primary care HIV specialists, substance abuse treatment experts, psychiatrists, social workers, and nurses to meet the complex treatment needs of injection drug users and to manage problematic behavior. Identify a single primary care provider to maximize consistency and continuity while minimizing the "splitting" of groups of professionals.
4. Obtain a thorough history of the patient's substance abuse history, practices, needle and syringe source, drug abuse complications, and treatment history. Nonjudgmental, clinical assessment of this information is essential as with any other medical problem. Educate the patient about his or her medical status and the effects of continued drug use. Nonjudgmental discussion of the adverse health and social consequences of drug use and the benefits of abstinence may increase the patient's understanding of his or her disease and interest in change.
5. Establish a relationship of mutual respect. Avoid moral condemnation or attribution of addiction to moral or behavioral weakness. Acknowledge that addiction is a medical disease, compounded by psychological and social circumstances. Reducing or stopping drug use is difficult, as is sustaining abstinence. Success may require several attempts and relapse is common. Complete abstinence may not be a realistic goal for many substance-abusing patients. Rather, increasing the proportion of days, weeks, and months of drug-free or controlled sobriety is an acceptable goal. Do not be discouraged or consider lack of success as the physician's failure. Relapses are common and should be anticipated and treated rather than seen as a treatment failure.
6. Work closely with a substance abuse treatment program. Clinicians should remain hopeful that patients can benefit from drug treatment and should be familiar with local resources for the treatment of HIV-infected injection drug users.
7. Define and agree on the roles and responsibilities of both the health care team and the patient. Establish a formal treatment contract that specifies the services to be provided to the patient, the caregiver's expectations about the patient's behavior, and the consequences of behavior that violates the contract. These behaviors might include "loss" of prescriptions, misuse of prescription drugs, disruptive behavior in the clinic, or use of illicit drugs during hospital stays.
8. Set appropriate limits and respond consistently to behavior that violates those limits. In the hospital setting, create a system of graduated restrictions for violation of agreed upon behavior (i.e., restrictions on unsupervised visits or visiting hours, closer supervision of visits, confinement to room, etc.). These should be imposed in a professional manner that reflects the aim of enhancing patients' well-being, and not in an atmosphere of blame or judgment.
9. Always consider acute substance administration when evaluating behavior change and neurologic disease. Use toxicologic testing to evaluate behavioral changes and to discourage illicit drug use by HIV-infected injection drug users during hospital stays.

Clinical Trials in Drug Users

Medical treatment of HIV disease in drug users is based on findings from clinical trials conducted in other populations, such as men with same-sex contact. Injection drug abusers are seriously underrepresented in most clinical trials of new therapies for HIV disease.[48,49] Studies show that drug users can participate in clinical trials if special efforts are made to recruit them.[50] It is important to appreciate that recovering drug users or those in control of their addiction can be distinguished from those who are out of control and unable to participate in trials. Treatment of drug addiction is often an essential prerequisite for participation in clinical trials.

Existing evidence indicates that the rate of HIV disease progression can be slowed among injection drug users by medical interventions.[51] Observational studies have shown benefits from of antiretroviral therapies, but retrospective subgroup analyses of large-scale HIV clinical trials have not been carried out to determine if drug users experience the same efficacy and toxicities as other populations receiving HIV therapy. In clinical practice, injection drug users who self-inject multiple daily doses of illicit drugs such as heroin and cocaine, in addition to other drugs of abuse, and who have, a high prevalence of underlying hepatic disease[13] and are often receiving pharmacotherapies for the treatment of substance abuse, may have different profiles of therapeutic efficacy, toxicity, and side effects with drugs used for the treatment of HIV.[5] Thus information derived from the study of therapies in other populations may not be fully generalizable to drug users.

Drug Interactions with HIV Therapies

Provision of drug abuse treatment is often key to successful treatment of HIV disease in this population.[5] Many drug-using patients with HIV disease must receive appropriate and adequate treatment for substance abuse in order to reverse the psychological and physiologic disruptions that perpetuate the instability of the drug-abusing lifestyle. For patients who are opioid dependent and HIV infected, the treatment of choice is substitution therapy with an opioid agonist—either methadone, L-α-acetylmethadol (LAAM), or the soon-to-be-widely-available buprenorphine.[52-56] Drug interactions between agents used for the treatment of substance-related disorders and those used for the treatment of HIV disease may influence the effectiveness of both treatment strategies. Although many studies of interactions between antiretroviral agents and other HIV therapies and other classes of drugs have been performed, interactions between HIV therapeutics and substances of abuse and their treatments have been very limited. In fact, only zidovudine (ZDV) has been carefully studied in terms of potential for interaction with opiates.[57,58]

An initial study was conducted in HIV-positive outpatients who were opioid dependent and on methadone maintainance therapy.[57] Methadone levels were obtained prior to and after starting ZDV therapy. Pharmacokinetic parameters for methadone and for ZDV, alone and in combination, were determined. Concurrent administration of ZDV did not alter methadone pharmacokinetic parameters. However, serum ZDV levels were significantly higher in methadone-maintained patients (average 43% increase in ZDV area under the time-concentration curve [AUC] relative to control patients; $p < .05$). A subsequent, more definitive within-subject study has recently been completed.[58] In this study, opioid-dependent subjects were hospitalized and detoxified with clonidine, then received ZDV and subsequently methadone. Both acute and chronic (8 weeks) effects of methadone on ZDV were studied. Acute methadone treatment increased oral ZDV AUC by 41% ($p = .03$). Chronic methadone treatment increased oral ZDV AUC by 29%. Methadone levels remained in the therapeutic range during ZDV treatment. The increase in ZDV levels appeared to have resulted primarily from inhibition of ZDV glucuronidation, but also from decreased renal clearance of ZDV. This study confirmed that methadone-maintained patients receiving standard ZDV doses experience greater ZDV exposure and may be at increased risk for ZDV side effects and toxicity. These findings have important implications for the treatment of HIV-infected patients who are also methadone-maintained. Methadone-maintained patients may complain of malaise, insomnia, and dysphoria upon initiating ZDV therapy. These symptoms are usually attributed to opiate withdrawal, which often results in the patient requesting an increase in methadone dose or not taking ZDV. The findings of this study indicate that such symptoms may be related to increased exposure to ZDV. Based on these results, increased toxicity surveillance and possibly reduction in ZDV dose are indicated when these two agents are given concomitantly.

Interactions with LAAM and buprenorphine are under investigation; preliminary data suggest that LAAM appears to elevate ZDV levels while buprenorphine has no effect on ZDV disposition (E. McCance, personal communication, July 1998). Other reverse transcriptase inhibitors (didanosine, stavudine, and lamivudine) are currently under study with regard to potential interactions with methadone. No interaction studies have been performed in a rigorous manner with any of the protease agents or non-nucleoside reverse transcriptase inhibitors. The potential for interactions is great because the metabolism of methadone, LAAM, buprenorphine, and other opiates involves *n*-demethylation by cytochrome P-450 (CYP) isoform 3A4.[59]

Protease and non-nucleoside reverse transcriptase inhibitors share metabolic pathways with opiates, and interactions may be expected to occur. Effects may vary in intensity and type among these drugs. Ritonavir may be expected to have the most profound effect because its inhibition of the function of several enzymes in the CYP oxidase system is greatest among this class of drugs.[60] Nelfinavir's inhibitory effect on this CYP system is much less than that of other protease inhibitors, including ritonavir and indinavir, and therefore may have fewer drug interactions with opioids. Nevirapine is extensively metabolized to hyroxylated metabolites by CYP3A4 and 2B6, which are in turn excreted via renal pathways. Nevirapine induces CYP activity with increased oxidative capacity noted for the 3A isoforms, which could result in decreased opioid concentrations on standard doses. This effect could be associated with a withdrawal syndrome in patients treated with this drug and maintained on an opioid. Indeed, several anecdotal reports of this phenomenon have been described (F. L. Altice and L. Cooney, personal communication, July 1998). Delavirdine also is extensively metabolized by the CYP system, primarily by the 3A4 isoform. Delavirdine also inhibits CYP3A and reduces the hepatic clearance of other drugs.[61] One study recently explored the possibility of interaction between ritonavir and methadone.[62] No effect on ritonavir was seen. However, there were several flaws in the study design that invalidate this result. Most importantly, study subjects were not opioid dependent and received only one dose of methadone, at a dose far below that given in the treatment of opiate addiction (5 mg).

Fluconazole is known to be an inhibitor of CYP metabolism. Methadone pharmacokinetics were determined in a group of patients on methadone maintenance therapy who were then begun on oral fluconazole at 200 mg/day. After 14 days, there was a 35% average increase in serum methadone AUC relative to baseline ($p = .0008$). At the same time, mean serum methadone peak and trough concentrations increased by 27% ($p = .0076$) and 48% ($p = .0023$), re-

spectively, and oral clearance of methadone was reduced by 24% ($p = .0007$).[62] This study indicated that fluconazole prophylaxis increases methadone exposure, and methadone dosage adjustment may be required.

The interaction of rifampin and methadone is well known and of great significance in the treatment of tuberculosis[63] in substance abusers. The induction of hepatic metabolism of antiretroviral agents by rifampin creates additional therapeutic dilemmas in the treatment and prophylaxis of both tuberculosis and HIV disease. Rifampin and, to a lesser extent, rifabutin induce the metabolism of methadone and result in withdrawal. Rifampin administration will therefore require emperical, rapid, and sequential increase in methadone doses to up to 50% over usual maintenance levels.[5]

There is no information about interactions among other substances of abuse, including cocaine, amphetamines, marijuana, alcohol, nicotine, and caffeine, with HIV therapies. Properly done studies to explore the presence and/or absence of interactions are crucial so that appropriate choices and doses can be established for both HIV and substance abuse therapies for opiate-dependent persons with HIV disease.

PAIN MANAGEMENT

Drug-addicted patients are concerned that they will not be given adequate pain medication. Conversely, clinicians often feel that drug users engage in manipulative pain medication–seeking behavior. This often results in contentious and confrontational interactions from which neither benefits. It is important to remember that people who are using daily opiates, including methadone, have developed a tolerance to the effects of these drugs, including the analgesic effects. However, their pain threshold may be the same as, or lower than, that of a drug-free person, and they will require as much or more analgesic medication. Nevertheless, clarity, structure, and firmness in pain medication administration is often necessary. Providing adequate pain relief will contribute substantially to the development of a trusting patient–provider relationship, while failure to do so may contribute to drug-seeking behavior.

Guidelines that may be helpful in developing an effective pain management plan for patients with addictive disease are:

1. Evaluate the pain syndrome thoroughly, paying careful attention to history and previous

treatment. It is important to remember that description may be colored by previous experiences with pain and the health care system.

2. Be clear and direct in discussions of pain and its management. Let the patient know that you take the report of pain seriously, but be honest about your concerns and firm about treatment plans.

3. For the patient on methadone maintenance, continue the usual methadone dose and treat pain with other analgesics in standard or higher-than-usual doses. Methadone's analgesic effectiveness is quite limited in the tolerant individual, and the drug should not be used for analgesia. In addition, the methadone dose is part of the therapeutic plan developed by the drug treatment team and should not be altered without their participation. Discuss pain management plans with the drug abuse treatment program staff or others involved in the care of the patient.

4. For outpatients, prescribe small quantities of medications, no more than a 2-week supply if possible. Inform the patient that prescriptions will not be refilled earlier. Record both the pain management plan and the actual medications, number prescribed, and date of prescriptions.

5. Make sure that other clinicians and providers are aware of the plan and that the patient is to receive medication from only one source, but also be sure that arrangements are in place to obtain additional medication when it is due, if that source is not available.

6. Prescribe generic formulations when possible.

7. Be clear about how long you plan to continue the medication. Periodically and regularly reevaluate the need.

8. For inpatients with acute medical problems, set up a reasonable around-the-clock dosage schedule. Discuss with the patient and be clear about amount prescribed and dosing schedule. Avoid or discourage nonscheduled requests and administrations. Reassess medication need every 24 to 48 hours.

COMMONLY USED DRUGS

The illicit drugs most closely associated with HIV infection in the United States are heroin and cocaine. More recently, the abuse of methamphetamine has raised great concerns as well. Initially encountered in the southwestern part of the United States, high levels of methamphetamine abuse are now present in many areas of the Midwest. Each of these can be administered by a variety of routes. Injection with shared contaminated needles and syringes or other injection paraphernalia carry the greatest risk for HIV disease and other complications. However, noninjection use of cocaine drives a large portion of the HIV epidemic in women through its association with the exchange of drugs for sex with multiple partners. It is important to be aware of local patterns of drug availability and use.

Heroin

There are a number of opioid drugs with abuse potential available in the United States, including heroin, methadone, and prescription analgesics. Heroin is a short-acting, semisynthetic opioid produced from opium poppies. It may be smoked, inhaled, or injected into a vein or soft tissue. Heroin has a moderately long half-life. Peak heroin euphoria begins shortly after injection and lasts approximately 1 hour, followed by 1 to 4 hours of sedation. Withdrawal symptoms commence several hours later. As a consequence, most drug users addicted to heroin inject two to four times per day. Many heroin users will mediate the sedating effects of heroin by injecting a small amount of cocaine with heroin, a mixture known as a "speedball." Heroin metabolites can be measured in the urine 24 hours after administration. Heroin itself is not a dangerous drug. Rather, the unsterile method of use, unpredictable concentrations in street samples, adulterants in the injection mixture, and lifestyle necessary to procure drugs are responsible for most heroin-associated medical complications. Table 36–2 describes the range of heroin effects.

Cocaine

Cocaine is an alkaloid extracted from the leaves of the coca plant.[64] It is available as a water-soluble hydrochloride salt that is injected or taken by nasal inhalation ("snorted"). Cocaine hydrochloride powder is destroyed by heat and therefore cannot be smoked. However, it may be chemically converted to a freebase "rock" or "crack" cocaine, which can be smoked. Pulmonary absorption of "crack" is as rapid as intravenous injection. "Crack" cocaine is marketed in small relatively inexpensive quantities, substantially escalating the cocaine epidemic in

TABLE 36–2. Heroin Effects

TYPE OF EFFECT	ACUTE	CHRONIC	WITHDRAWAL
Psychological	Euphoria Sedation Lethargy		Anxiety Restlessness Irritability Agitation
Physical	Pupillary constriction Lowered temperature Respiratory depression Peripheral vasodilation Decreased gastrointestinal motility Urinary retention Hives/pruritis	Constipation Decreased libido	Lacrimation Rhinorrhea Tachycardia Hypertension Piloerection Yawning Diaphoresis Shivering Nausea Vomiting Diarrhea Abdominal pain Myalgias Tremors (rare seizures)

Adapted from Williams AB, Friedland GH: Substance abuse issues in women with HIV. In Cotton DJ, Watts DH (eds): Medical Management of AIDS in Women. New York, John Wiley & Sons, 1996, with permission.

the United States by making it more affordable and accessible. Cocaine's half-life is short, resulting in the need for frequent administration. Active cocaine users may inject or inhale cocaine as many as 20 times a day. Cocaine can be detected in the urine for about 12 hours after administration. Cocaine induces feelings of elation, omnipotence, and invincibility and is rapidly addicting. The multiple psychological and physical effects of cocaine (Table 36–3) can

TABLE 36–3. Cocaine Effects

TYPE OF EFFECT	ACUTE	CHRONIC	WITHDRAWAL
Psychological	Euphoria Self-confidence Hyperstimulation Excitability Restlessness Delusions Hallucinations Psychosis	Paranoia Irritability Withdrawal Psychosis	Depression Anhedonia

Physical	Mild
	  Pupillary dilation
	  Elevated blood pressure
	  Nausea
	  Vomiting
	  Irregular breathing
	  Tremors
	Severe
	  Arrhythmias
	  Chest pain
	  Myocardial infarction
	  Cardiac arrest
	  Respiratory failure
	  Seizures
	  Stroke
	  Hyperthermia
	  Rhabdomyolysis, renal failure
		Loss of appetitie
		Weight loss
		Attention disturbances
		Fatigue
		Nasal septal perforation
			Muscle tremors
			Headache
			Insomnia
			Appetite changes

Adapted from Williams AB, Friedland GH: Substance abuse issues in women with HIV. In Cotton DJ, Watts DH (eds): Medical Management of AIDS in Women. New York, John Wiley & Sons, 1996, with permission.

TABLE 36–4. Methamphetamine Effects

TYPE OF EFFECT	ACUTE	CHRONIC	WITHDRAWAL
Psychological	Increased attention Decreased fatigue Increased activity Euphoria and rush Increased libido Aggression Violent behavior	Paranoia Hallucinations Mood disturbances Fatigue Repetitive motor activity Social and occupational deterioration Violent behavior	Depression Anxiety Paranoia Delusions
Physical	Decreased appetitie Increased respiration Hyperthermia Stroke	Weight loss	

completely disrupt clinical care of HIV-infected men and women and their families.

Methamphetamine

Methamphetamine is similar in chemical structure to amphetamine but has more profound effects on the central nervous system. It is easily manufactured and can be used intravenously by smoking or by snorting. It is commonly known as "speed," "meth," and, in its smoked form, "ice," "crystal," and "glass." Although its metabolic pathways differ, as with cocaine, methamphetamine use produces stimulation and feelings of euphoria. In contrast to cocaine, which is quickly removed and almost completely metabolized, methamphetamine has a longer duration of action and a larger percentage of the drug remains unchanged in the body. Thus stimulant effects can be quite prolonged, lasting from 6 to 8 hours after a single dose. However, tolerance develops rapidly and escalation of dose and frequency is required. Methamphetamine users exhibit a wide array of physical and psychological symptoms (Table 36–4).

SUBSTANCE ABUSE TREATMENT

Addiction is a chronic, relapsing, and treatable disease, characterized by compulsive drug-seeking and drug use. Although exposure to addicting substances is widespread in society, high vulnerability to addiction is more limited and is the product of biologic, psychological, and environmental influences. Thus identification of addictive disease and referral to appropriate treatment services is an essential part of the clinical care of HIV-infected patients. There

are a wide variety of treatment modalities (Table 36–5). Selection of the appropriate program is an individual decision based in part upon the drug used, the length and pattern of the patient's drug use, personal psychosocial characteristics, and local availability. Resources are limited in many communities, substantially limiting options for referral. The majority of programs have been designed for male addicts and do not take into account the special needs of women.

Opiate Withdrawal

Withdrawal from opioids involves the gradual reduction of dosage over a period of time. Although patients can be withdrawn using the drug to which they are addicted, in most instances it is easier to substitute methadone for the primary opioid of addiction. It is usually not possible to know with certainty how much drug the patient

TABLE 36–5. Drug Abuse Treatment Modalities

Pharmacologic
  Methadone
    Detoxification
    Maintenance
  LAMM
  Buprenorphine
  Narcotic antagonist: naltrexone (for acute
    intoxication)
Self-help programs
  Narcotics Anonymous
  Cocaine Anonymous
  Alcoholics Anonymous
Therapeutic communities
  Long-term, structured, residental programs
Psychological support
  Individual therapy
  Group counseling
Acupuncture

has been taking. Regardless of the amount, my-algias, diarrhea, and insomnia and irritability associated with withdrawal can be controlled with a daily oral dose of 25 to 30 mg of methadone. However, this dose will not eliminate drug craving. Decreasing the methadone dose by 20% a day after the abstinence syndrome is suppressed should maintain patient comfort. It is best to do this during acute medical admissions so as not to confuse medical problems with opiate withdrawal. Other pharmacologic agents used to mediate opiate withdrawal syndrome are clonidine, a centrally acting adrenergic agonist that suppresses symptoms of opiate withdrawal, and buprenorphine, a mixed agonist–antagonist, semisynthetic opioid that is 25 to 50 times more potent than morphine. The major challenge to remain drug free after withdrawal requires a multidisciplinary team effort over a period of time. For this reason it is important to develop close, collaborative relationships with drug treatment programs and to involve these experts in the care plan.

Treatment of Opioid Dependence

The treatment of choice for the patient who is opioid dependent and has HIV disease is maintenance with a long-acting opiate such as methadone or LAAM.[52–54] Buprenorphine is likely to become increasingly important as an opiate-dependence treatment agent in the near future.[55,56] Little is known regarding optimal pharmacotherapeutic treatment for opioid dependence in drug users with HIV disease and how this may differ from those who are not infected. There is no information about whether a specific pharmacotherapy for opioid dependence is superior to other available treatments or whether optimal opioid dependence therapy should vary based on medical status and current HIV medications. Answers to these questions would make a significant contribution to optimizing treatment for HIV-infected, opioid-dependent patients. The long-term treatment of chronic opioid dependence usually includes pharmacotherapy to assist the patient in remaining free of illicit drug use and facilitate engagement in a comprehensive drug treatment program designed to prevent the abuse of other drugs and promote rehabilitation. Agonist treatment of opioid dependence is particularly important for the patient with comorbid HIV infection because effective treatment enhances HIV treatment and may decrease the risk of virus transmission via routes of shared needle use and unprotected sexual con-

tact.[65,66] Methadone maintenance continues to be the most prevalent agonist used in the treatment of opioid dependence. However, other long-acting opioids are now being utilized with increasing frequency for maintenance therapy.

Methadone

Long-term, daily use of methadone has afforded a normal life[54] for many heroin addicts in the United States. Methadone is a semisynthetic, long-acting opioid analgesic used for opiate detoxification as described above, and for long-term treatment of opiate abuse. It is well absorbed, reaching peak plasma levels in 1 to 2 hours, and is metabolized by hepatic demethylation and cyclization. Methadone is particularly valuable for its oral bioavailability, long half-life of 24 to 36 hours, and the consistent plasma levels that are obtained with regular administration.[52] A single daily dose is given to maintain stable plasma levels. Methadone is a very safe drug. In the first 6 months of treatment some may experience side effects common to other opiates (Table 36–6), but tolerance to the majority of these effects develops rapidly. Persistent side effects include diaphoresis, constipation, and amenorrhea. Tolerance to the hypothalamic effects of methadone occurs during chronic methadone treatment, and the majority of women experience the return of menses after 12 to 18 months of therapy.[37] As a result of irregular menses, women may incorrectly believe they are infertile, fail to use contraception, and fail to identify early pregnancy. Methadone maintenance has been shown to be effective in decreasing psychosocial and medical morbidity associated with opioid dependence.[54] As a result of the stable plasma level and development of tolerance, regular methadone users do not experience euphoria and the highs and lows of the heroin cycle. Drug-seeking behavior decreases, creating the possibility for the development of more constructive behaviors and relationships. Furthermore, methadone maintenance improves overall health status and is associated with decreased criminal activity and improved social functioning, in addition to its benefit in decreasing the spread of HIV among injection drug users.[54] There is no optimal dose of methadone for treatment of opioid-dependent patients, who must be assessed individually for treatment response. Generally, doses of 30 to 60 mg daily will block opioid withdrawal symptoms, but higher doses, in the 70 to 80-mg daily range, are needed to block opioid craving and decrease

TABLE 36–6. Methadone–Drug Interactions

DRUG	EFFECT	SOLUTION
Rifampin	Increased metabolism of methadone; abrupt onset of withdrawal symptoms	Monitor for opiate withdrawal symptoms. Increase dose of methadone incrementally to 20–50% of pre-rifampin dose. Alternatively, choose another antitubercular agent if possible.
Rifabutin	Similar to rifampin, but milder and less frequently resulting in withdrawal symptoms	Monitor for opiate withdrawal symptoms and treat as above, if necessary.
Phenytoin	Increased metabolism of methadone; onset of mild withdrawal symptoms 2–4 d after initiating phenytoin	Observe and increase methadone dose if necessary.
Zidovudine	Increased ZDV exposure	Observe closely for ZDV dose-related side effects and toxicities.
Fluconazole	Increase in methadone levels	Observe for methadone-related side effects.
Other nucleoside reverse transcriptase inhibitors (RTIs)	No data	
Non-nucleoside RTIs (NNRTIs)	No data, but reduction in methadone potential; effect on NNRTI not known	Anticipate methadone withdrawal or overdose.
Protese inhibitors	No data, but reduction in methadone potential; effect on protease not known	Anticipate methadone withdrawal or overdose.

illicit drug use. These higher doses are also associated with greater retention in treatment.[67]

LAAM, a derivative of methadone, has also become available as a Food and Drug Administration–approved agent for the treatment of opioid dependence. Although similar to methadone in terms of the level of physical dependence it produces, LAAM is much longer acting than methadone and can suppress symptoms of opiate withdrawal for more than 72 hours.[68] LAAM dosing on a thrice-weekly basis has been shown by various criteria, such as reduction of opiate-positive urines, suppression of withdrawal symptoms, and retention rates, to be as effective as daily methadone maintenance in treating opioid dependence.[68] Side effects including sedation and nausea reported by patients treated with LAAM are similar to those of equivalent doses of methadone. LAAM is usually prescribed in doses of 20 to 140 mg, with an average dose being 60 mg. The major advantage to patients of LAAM treatment is the infrequent dosing relative to methadone, which allows for fewer clinic visits and more rapid integration into activities such as employment or other rehabilitative processes while obtaining equivalent benefit in terms of blocking opiate withdrawal and decreasing drug craving.[68] LAAM is rapidly being incorporated into opioid

dependence treatment programs and for many patients has become their treatment of choice.

Buprenorphine, a partial μ-opiate agonist, has demonstrated efficacy in the treatment of opioid-dependent patients.[55,56] Buprenorphine produces morphine-like subjective effects and can block the full effects of a dose of an agonist such as hydromorphone; has a long duration of action, allowing for once-a-day or an alternate-day schedule of administration; and mild withdrawal symptoms that make detoxification from buprenorphine maintenance easier than that from methadone. Its partial agonist properties provide a desirable safety profile because of its limited peak effect at maximal dose and decreased risk of respiratory depression in overdose. Side effects experienced with buprenorphine are sedation and drowsiness, but tolerance may develop to these effects. Buprenorphine has recently been shown to be equivalent to methadone in the treatment of opioid-dependent patients.[55,69] Buprenorphine is already available to practitioners as a pain reliever, and may be dosed out of physician's offices for the treatment of opioid dependence. Such a configuration of services could be of significant value to HIV-infected patients because this would enable one physician to provide all needed services, medical and substance abuse related, in addition to providing these patients an alternative to standard opioid clinic treatment. Buprenorphine appears to have no effect on ZDV disposition (E. McCance, personal communication, July 1998), and might become the preferred drug with which to treat opioid-dependent patients with HIV disease.

Cocaine Abuse Treatment

Unfortunately, treatment modalities for cocaine addiction are much less well developed than those for opiate dependence.[64] Although several pharmacologic agents, including dopaminergic agonists such as bromocriptine and amantadine as well as tricyclic antidepressants, have been proposed as supplements to counseling and other nonpharmacologic approaches, there is little evidence that these drugs are very effective in prolonging abstinence. The lack of successful, standardized treatment strategies for cocaine users is a significant problem as the cocaine epidemic grows. In the absence of effective programs to treat cocaine abuse, HIV care providers may feel helpless and frustrated when confronted with a patient who is actively using cocaine. Referral to a cocaine treatment program, if available, is essential. Although unable to help at the moment, it is important to let the patient know that you are concerned about his or her health, and will be available for the time when the addictive disease is in remission and he or she is ready to engage in care.

SPECIAL ISSUES IN PREVENTION: HARM REDUCTION

The relapsing pattern of drug use and the wide array of serious infectious and other consequences require the development of preventive harm reduction strategies. These are based on the underlying principle that injection drug use is a chronic disease that may not be cured in the individual or eliminated from society but can be conducted in a way that minimizes harm to the user and others. Reduction of drug use frequency and safer injection practices are more realistic goals for many drug users. There are several practical components to harm reduction strategies (Table 36–7). Education about and provision of equipment for more hygienic injection practices for the prevention of infectious complications of injection are essential. Needle-

TABLE 36–7. HIV Risk Reduction in Drug Users

Knowledge about risk
Self-organization
Drug addiction treatment
Harm reduction
   Availability of sterile needles and syringes
      Needle and syringe exchange
      Repeal of restrictive needle and syringe
         prescription and possession laws and regulations
     Instruction in syringe and needle cleaning and use
   Distribution and instruction in the use of condoms

and syringe-exchange programs are the most obvious example of the harm reduction approach.[70,71] This strategy has been shown to reduce HIV risk behaviors without increasing drug use. In addition to the distribution or exchange of injection equipment, these programs typically include AIDS education, condom distribution, and referral to or enrollment in a variety of drug treatment, medical, and social services. In some locations, repeal of restrictive prescription and paraphernalia laws that severely limit sterile needle and syringe availability can be of great importance and effectiveness.[72] Provision of primary medical care services linked to drug abuse treatment is a way to promote preventive regimens to enhance harm reduction.[3] In this and all other clinical settings, in addition to the treatment of HIV disease and prevention of complications, injection drug users should be routinely screened for hepatitis B and C, latent *M. tuberculosis* infection, syphilis, and other sexually transmitted diseases. They should be offered pneumococcal, influenza, tetanus, and hepatitis B immunization and (when appropriate) prophylaxis for tuberculosis.

The ultimate goal of harm reduction strategies should be the reduction or prevention of illicit drug use itself, the development of strategies that will minimize the serious medical consequences of drug abuse, and the development of strategies that will eliminate drug abuse and its root causes. Until we are successful in this arena, we stand little chance of limiting the spread and consequences of HIV disease in this and related populations.

References

1. Centers for Disease Control and Prevention: Update: Trends in AIDS incidence—United States. MMWR Morb Mortal Wkly Rep 46:861, 1996
2. Friedland GH: Parental drug users. In Kaslow RA, Francis DP (eds): The Epidemiology of Aids. New York, Oxford University Press, 1989, p 153

3. Alcabes P, Friedland GH: Injection drug use and human immunodeficiency virus infection. Clin Infect Dis 20:1467, 1995
4. Des Jarlais DC, Friedman SR, Choopanya K, et al: International epidemiology of HIV and AIDS among injecting drug users. AIDS 6:1053, 1992
5. O'Connor PG, Selwyn PA, Schottenfeld RS: Medical care for injection-drug users with human immunodeficiency virus infection. N Engl J Med 331:450, 1994
6. Rezza G, Lazzarin A, Angarano G, et al: Risk of AIDS in HIV seroconverters: A comparison between intravenous drug users and homosexual males. Eur J Epidemiol 6:99, 1990
7. Alcabes P, Munoz A, Vlahov D, Friedland GH: Maturity of human immunodeficiency virus infection and incubation period of acquired immuno-deficiency syndrome in injecting drug users. Ann Epidemiol 4:17, 1994
8. Mariotto AB, Mariotti S, Pezzotti P, et al: Estimation of the acquired immunodeficiency syndrome incubation period in intravenous drug users: A comparison with male homosexuals. Am J Epidemiol 135:428, 1992
9. Friedland GH, Saltzman B, Vileno J, et al: Survival differences in patients with AIDS. J Acquir Immune Defic Syndr Hum Retrovirol 4:144, 1991
10. Greenberg AE, Thomas PA, Landesman SH, et al: The spectrum of HIV-1-related disease among outpatients in New York City. AIDS 6:843, 1992
11. Levine DP, Sobel JD: Serious Infections in Intravenous Drug Abusers. New York, Oxford University Press, 1991
12. Friedland GH, Selwyn PS: Infections (excluding AIDS) in injecting drug users. In Isselbacher K, Braunwald E, Wilson J, et al. (eds): Harrison's Principles of Internal Medicine. New York: McGraw-Hill, 1996, p 831
13. Haverkos HS, Lange WR: Serious infections other than human immunodeficiency virus among intravenous drug users. J Infect Dis 161:894, 1990
14. Cherubin CE, Sapira JD: The medical complications of drug addiction and the medical assessment of the intravenous drug user: 25 years later. Ann Intern Med 119:1017, 1993
15. Sande MA, et al: Endocarditis in intravenous drug users. In Kaye D (ed): Infective Endocarditis. New York, Raven Press, 1992, p 345
16. Chambers HF, Horzenowski OM, Sande MA, for the National Collaborative Endocarditis Study Group: Staphylococcus aureus endocarditis: Clinical manifestations in addicts and non-addicts. Medicine 62:170, 1983
17. Hardalo C, Khoshnood K, Alcabes P, Friedland GH: High incidence and recurrence rates of bacterial endocarditis in HIV+ drug injectors. In: Abstracts of the Xth International Conference on AIDS, Yokohama, 1994, Abstract 336B
18. Marantz PR, Linzer M, Feiner CJ, et al: Inability to predict diagnosis in febrile intravenous drug abusers. Ann Intern Med 106:823, 1987
19. Selwyn PA, Feingold AR, Hartel D, et al: Increased risk of bacterial pneumonia in HIV-infected intravenous drug users without AIDS. AIDS 2:267, 1988
20. Caiaffa WT, Graham NMH, Vlahov D: Bacterial pneumonia in adult populations with human immunodeficiency virus (HIV) infection. Am J Epidemiol 138:909, 1993
21. Hirschtick RE, Glassroth J, Jordan MC, et al: Bacterial pneumonia in persons infected with the human immunodeficiency virus. N Engl J Med 333:845, 1995
22. Selwyn PA, Pumerantz AS, Durante A, et al: Clinical predictors of *Pneumocystis carinii* pneumonia, bacterial pneumonia and tuberculosis in HIV-infected patients. AIDS 12:885, 1998
23. Alland D, Kalkut GE, Moss AR, et al: Transmission of tuberculosis in New York City: An analysis by DNA fingerprinting and conventional epidemiologic methods. N Engl J Med 330:1710, 1994
24. Barnes F, Bloch AB, Davidson T, Snider DFJ: Tuberculosis in patients with human immunodeficiency virus infections. N Engl J Med 324:1644, 1991
25. Alwood K, Keruly J, Moore-Rice K, et al: Effectiveness of supervised, intermittent therapy for tuberculosis in HIV-infected patients. AIDS 8:1103, 1994
26. Weis SE, Slocum PC, Blais DX, et al: The effect of directly observed therapy on the rates of drug resistance and relapse in tuberculosis. N Engl J Med 330:1179, 1994
27. Rigsby MO, Friedland G: Tuberculosis and human immunodeficiency virus infection. In DeVita VT, Hellman S, Rosenberg SA (eds): AIDS: Eiology, Diagnosis, Treatment and Prevention. Philadelphia, Lippincott-Raven, 1997, p 245
28. Centers for Disease Control and Prevention: Treating concurrent HIV and TB. MMWR Morbid Mortal Wkly Rep 45:921, 1996
29. Rao TKS, Friedman EA, Nicastri AD: The types of renal disease in the acquired immunodeficiency syndrome. N Engl J Med 6:1062, 1987
30. Tebben JA, Rigsby MO, Selwyn PA, et al: Outcome of HIV infected patients on continuous ambulatory peritoneal dialysis. Kidney Int 44:191, 1993
31. Ferrando SJ, Wall TL, Batki SL, Sorensen JL: Psychiatric morbidity, illicit drug use and adherence to zidovudine (AZT) among injection drug users with HIV disease. Am J Drug Alcohol Abuse 22:475, 1996
32. Samet JH, Libman H, Steger KA, et al: Compliance with zidovudine therapy in patients infected with human immunodeficiency virus, type 1: A cross-sectional study in a municipal hospital clinic. Am J Med 92:495, 1992
33. Mehta S, Moore RD, Graham NMH: Potential factors affecting adherence with HIV therapy. AIDS 11:1665, 1997
34. Wall TL, Sorensen JL, Batki SL, et al: Adherence to zidovudine (AZT) among HIV-infected methadone patients: A pilot study of supervised therapy and dispensing compared to usual care. Drug Alcohol Depend 37:261, 1995
35. Muma RD, Ross MW, Parcel GS, Pollard RB: Zidovudine adherence among individuals with HIV infection. AIDS Care 7:439, 1995
36. Williams A, Friedland GH: Adherence, compliance, and HAART. AIDS Clin Care 9:51, 1997
37. Williams AB, Friedland GH: Management of addictive disease. In Cotton DJ, Watts DH (eds): Medical Management of AIDS in Women. New York, John Wiley & Sons, 1996, p 437
38. Strathdee SA, Palepu A, Cornelisse PGA, et al: Barriers to use of free antiretroviral therapy in injection drug users. JAMA 280:547, 1998
39. Celantano DD, Vlahov D, Cohn S, et al: Self-reported antiretroviral therapy in injection drug users. JAMA 280:544, 1998
40. Friedland GH: AIDS and compassion. JAMA 259:2898, 1998
41. Selwyn PA, Feingold AR, Iezza A, et al: Primary care for patients with human immunodeficiency virus (HIV) infection in a methadone maintenance treatment program. Ann Intern Med 111:761, 1989

42. O'Connor PG, Molde S, Henry S, et al: Human immunodeficiency virus infection in injection drug users: A model for primary care. Am J Med 93:382, 1992

43. Selwyn PA, Budner NS, Wasserman WC, et al: Utilization of on-site primary care services by HIV-seropositive and seronegative drug users in a methadone maintenance program. Public Health Rep 108:492, 1993

44. Altice FL, Mostashari F, Thompson AS, Friedland GH: Perceptions, acceptance and adherence to antiretrovirals among prisoners. In: Abstracts of the 4th Conference on Retroviruses and Opportunistic Infections, Washington, DC, 1997, Abstract 253

45. Gourevitch MN, Wasserman W, Panero MS, Selwyn PA: Successful adherence to observed prophylaxis and treatment of tuberculosis among drug users in a methadone program. J Addict Dis 15:93, 1996

46. Bangsberg DR, Zolopa AR, Charlebois E, et al: HIV-infected homeless and marginally housed (H/M) patients adhere to and receive early virologic benefit from protease inhibitors (PI). In: Abstracts of the 5th Conference on Retroviruses and Opportunistic Infections, Chicago, 1998, Abstract 32406

47. Harberl A, Gute P, Carlebach A, et al: Once-daily therapy (NVP/ddI/3TC) for the IVDV HIV-infected population of the Frankfurt HIV Cohort. In: Abstracts of the XIIth International Conference on AIDS, Geneva, 1998, Abstract 22398

48. El-Sadr W, Capps I: The challenge of minority recruitment in clinical trials. JAMA 267:954, 1992

49. Craven DE, Liebman HA, Fuller J, et al: AIDS in intravenous drug users: Issues related to enrollment in clinical trials. J Acquir Immune Defic Syndr S3:45, 1990

50. Morse EV, Simon PM, Besch CL, Walker J: Issues of recruitment, retention, and compliance in community-based clinical trials with traditionally underserved populations. Appl Nurs Res 8:8, 1995

51. Selwyn PA, Alcabes P, Hartel D, et al: Clinical manifestations and predictors of disease progression in drug users with human immunodeficiency virus infection. N Engl J Med 327:1697, 1992

52. Kosten TR: Current pharmacotherapies for opioid dependence. Psychopharmacol Bull 26:69, 1990

53. American Psychiatric Association: Practice guideline for the treatment of patients with substance use disorders: Alcohol, cocaine, opioids. Am J Psychiatry 152(Suppl):5, 1995

54. Hubbard RL, Marsden ME, Rachal JV: Drug Abuse Treatment: A National Study of Effectiveness. Chapel Hill, University of North Carolina Press, 1989

55. Schottenfeld RS, Pakes JR, Oliveto A, et al: Buprenorphine vs methadone maintenance treatment for concurrent opioid dependence and cocaine abuse. Arch Gen Psychiatry 54:713, 1998

56. Strain EC, Stitzer ML, Liebson IA, Bigelow GE: Buprenorphone vs methadone in the treatment of opioid dependence: Sself reports, urinalysis, and addiction severity index. J Clin Psychopharmacol 16:58, 1996

57. Schwartz EL, Brechbul A-B, Kahl P, et al: Pharmacokinetic interactions of zidovudine and methadone in intravenous drug-using patients with HIV infection. J Acquir Immune Defic Syndr 5:619, 1992

58. McCance E, Jatlow P, Rainey P, et al: Methadone effect on AZT disposition. J Acquir Immune Defic Syndr Hum Retrovirol 18:435, 1998

59. Moody DE, Alburges ME, Parker RJ, et al: The involvement of cytochrome P 450 3A4 in the n-demethylation of L-alpha-acetylmethadol (LAAM), norLAAM, and methadone. Drug Metab Dispos 25:1347, 1997

60. Kumar GN, Rodriguez AD, Buko AM, Denissen JF: Cytochrome P-450 mediated metabolism of the HIV-1 protease inhibitor ritonavir in human liver microsomes. J Pharmacol Exp Ther 277:423, 1996

61. Freimuth W: Delavirdine mesylate, a potent non-nucleoside HIV-1 reverse transcriptase inhibitor [review]. Adv Exp Med Biol 394:279, 1996

62. Cobb MN, Desai J, Brown LS, et al: The effect of fluconazole on the clinical pharmacokinetics of methadone. Clin Pharm Ther 63:655, 1998

63. Kreek MJ, Garfield JW, Gutjahr CL, Guisti LM: Rifampin induced methadone withdrawal. N Engl J Med 294:1104, 1976

64. Gawin FH, Ellinwood EH: Cocaine and other stimulants. N Engl J Med 318:1173, 1998

65. Metzger DS, Woody GE, McLellan AT, et al: Human immunodeficiency virus seroconversion among intravenous drug users in- and out-of-treatment: An 18-month prospective follow-up. J Acquir Immune Defic Syndr Hum Retrovirol 6:1049, 1993

66. Ball JC, Lange WR, Myers CP, Friedman SR: Reducing the risk of AIDS through methadone maintenance treatments. J Health Soc Behav 29:214, 1998

67. Hartel D, Schoenbaum EE, Selwyn PA, et al: Heroin use during methadone maintenance treatment: Importance of methadone dose and cocaine use. Am J Public Health 85:83, 1995

68. Prendergast ML, Grella C, Perry SM, Anglin MD: Levo-alpha-acetylmethadol (LAAM): Clinical, research, and policy issues of a new pharmacotheapy for opioid addiction. J Psychoactive Drugs 27:239, 1995

69. Fudala PH, Johnson RE, Jaffe JH: Outpatient comparison of buprenorphine and methadone maintenance. I. Effects on opiate use and self-reported adverse effects and withdrawal symptomatology. NIDA Res Monogr 105:585, 1998

70. Lurie P, Reingold AL, Bowser B, et al: The public health impact of needle exchange programs on the United States and abroad. Berkeley, University of California, 1993

71. Kaplan EH, Heimer R: HIV incidence among needle exchange participants: Estimates from syringe tracking and testing data. J Acquir Immune Defic Syndr 8:223, 1994

72. Gostin LO, Lazzarini Z, Jones TS, Flaherty K: Prevention of HIV/AIDS and other blood-borne disease among injection drug users: A national survey on the regulating of syringes and needles. JAMA 277:53, 1997

37 | AIDS in Older Persons

BRADLEY S. BENDER • DAVID W. BENTLEY

"The aging of an infected population means more cancer, neurological disorders and other infections from immune suppression among people infected with HTLV-III."

James W. Curran, M.D., 1st International Conference on AIDS, as quoted by Shilts[1]

EPIDEMIOLOGY

During the 1990s, approximately 10% to 11% of persons reported with AIDS have been 50 years of age or older.[2] Despite the fact that there are six times as many reported cases of AIDS in persons over age 50 and twice as many in persons over age 60 as compared to those under age 19, HIV in older persons has received little attention.

Early in the epidemic, most older persons who acquired HIV infection did so from transfusions.[3] The introduction of donor screening by questionnaire and serology has changed this so that in 1996, sexual transmission is now the most common HIV exposure category (Table 37–1).[2,4,5] Indeed, the demographic characteristics of older persons reported with AIDS closely resembled those of younger adults: 84% were male, 43% were black, and 36% were gay/bisexual.

Despite extensive data showing that older persons are still interested in and participate in sexual activity, they receive little HIV prevention information. Seniors do not perceive themselves to be at risk for HIV infection (or are no longer concerned about contraception). Consequently, they are one sixth as likely to use condoms during intercourse and one fifth as likely to have been tested for HIV infection as individuals in their 20s.[6] Schable et al. interviewed 556 women with heterosexually acquired AIDS and found that older women were more likely than younger women to have never used a condom before HIV diagnosis.[7] These data, coupled with the aging of the U.S. population and the longer life expectancy of HIV-positive persons, suggest that the numbers of older persons with HIV infection will continue to increase.

IMMUNOPATHOGENESIS OF HIV IN OLDER PERSONS

It is likely that the age-associated acceleration in HIV progression (Table 37–1) is immunologically based, and there are published data consistent with five possible immunologic mechanisms: (1) with aging, more virus is produced; (2) more CD4+ T cells are infected; (3) the infected cells are destroyed more rapidly; (4) these cells cannot be replaced as efficiently; or (5) there is less effective anti-HIV immune activity, resulting in higher viral burden. As in much of aging, the actual reason for the accelerated progression will likely turn out to be multifactorial.[8]

First, HIV production is under control of many cytokines; proinflammatory cytokines such as interleukin 6 and tumor necrosis factor-α up-regulate HIV production and other cytokines, such as interleukin 10, down-regulate it.[9] Long-term prognosis is inversely proportional to the amount of virus in the blood, also referred to as the "set point."[10] A recent abstract suggests that the set point could be higher in older persons.[11] If so, could this be due to the age-related increase in interleukin 6?[12]

Second, HIV preferentially infects memory T cells of both adults[13] and children[14]; these cells are characterized by the presence of CD45RO, the low-molecular-weight isoform of the leukocyte common antigen family. CD4+CD45RO+ memory T cells develop from CD4+CD45RA+ naive T cells via a post-thymic differentiation pathway. Less than 20% of the peripheral blood CD4+ T cells of neonates express CD45RO.[14] There is an age-related increase in the numbers

TABLE 37–1. Demographic Characteristics of Persons Reported with AIDS in the United States in 1996

	AGE GROUP	
CHARACTERISTIC	≥50 Years	13–49 Years
Number	7459	61,014
Men	84%	79%
Race		
White, non-Hispanic	39%	38%
Black, non-Hispanic	43%	41%
Hispanic	17%	19%
Other	1%	1%
HIV exposure category		
Men who have sex with men	36%	40%
Injection drug use	19%	26%
Heterosexual contact	15%	13%
Men who have sex with men and who are injection drug users	2%	5%
Receipt of blood or blood products	2%	1%
No risk reported	26%	16%
AIDS-defining conditions		
HIV encephalopathy	3%	1%
Wasting syndrome	7%	4%
Other opportunistic illnesses	38%	36%
Severe HIV immunosuppression	52%	58%

Data adapted from Centers for Disease Control and Prevention: AIDS among persons aged ≥50 years—United States, 1991–1996. MMWR Morb Mortal Wkly Rep 47:21, 1998.

of these cells so that about 30% to 40% of CD4+ T cells are CD45RO+ in young adults, with a further increase to 50% to 65% of CD4+ T cells in the elderly.[15] Because older persons have more susceptible targets, are more of these cells actually infected? This could be evaluated with a semiquantitative polymerase chain reaction method to detect HIV proviral DNA within purified lymphocyte populations.[14] If more cells are infected in older subjects, another contributing factor might be if there were an age-related increase in the number of viral coreceptors.[16,17]

Third, there may be more rapid destruction of infected T cells. Cellular senescence is related to loss of telomeric DNA.[18] Telomeres are highly conserved (repeats of TTAGGG) nucleoprotein structures that cap the ends of linear, eukaryotic chromosomes. Telomeres protect against exonucleases and recombination and serve as a buffer against end replication problems (i.e., the fact that during each round of replication some of the terminal DNA is not replicated). Effros et al. studied the CD28–CD8+ T-cell population of HIV-infected persons.[19] There is a progressive expansion in the number of these cells during the course of HIV disease[20] that may have significant clinical implications because CD28 is a co-stimulatory molecule that provides a second signal for cellular activation. They found that the telomeres from CD28–CD8+ T cells from HIV-infected persons were much shorter than those of uninfected control subjects and were similar in length to those observed from centenarians. This process of telomeric shortening and enhanced cellular senescence may be even more rapid in older persons.

Fourth, there may be impaired replacement of HIV-infected CD4+ T cells. Mackall et al. studied lymphocyte regeneration after chemotherapy in 15 patients age 1 to 24 years and found an inverse relation between age and the number of CD4+ T cells 6 months after therapy.[21] This was due mostly to lower numbers of regenerated CD4+CD45RA+ T cells in the older subjects. Slower regeneration probably continues throughout adult life. For example, following thermal injury, there is a marked drop in the number of circulating T lymphocytes, and it takes a 40-year-old twice as long as a 20-year-old to replenish these cells.[22] Additionally, antiretroviral treatment of children leads to a large, more sustained increase in the number of peripheral blood CD4+ T cells.[23] Data shown in Figure 37–1 later in this chapter and reported elsewhere,[24] however, suggest that older persons have a fairly robust increase in CD4+ T cells following initiation of antiretroviral therapy. It is necessary to determine whether this increase in the number of circulating T cells occurs mostly in the extrathymic-(CD4+CD45RO+)

rather than thymic-derived (CD4+CD45RA+) cells.

Fifth, older persons may have less effective anti-HIV cytotoxic T lymphocyte (CTL) activity than younger persons. This possibility is consistent with observations on other infections that are normally contained by the cellular immune system and occur more frequently in aging. For example, active tuberculosis is associated with loss of delayed-type hypersensitivity response, and increased activity of influenza correlates with lower anti-influenza CTL activity.[25] To test the hypothesis that an age-related loss of immunosurveillance leads to loss of control of the virus, genetic typing could be performed on viral isolates from individuals of varying ages. A hallmark of HIV infection is the marked genetic heterogeneity even among isolates from the same patient, a phenomenon referred to as "quasispeciation."[26] These quasispecies occur by mutation and persist through escape from immune surveillance.[27] The stronger the immune surveillance, the more quasispecies and vice versa. If, as predicted, anti-HIV CTL activity deceases with aging, then there would be less immune pressure, with more homogeneous populations of virus recovered from older persons.

CLINICAL PRESENTATION

Natural History

Aging is a powerful biologic phenomenon, and it is well recognized that there is more rapid progression of HIV infection (as measured by time to AIDS diagnosis and time to death) in older persons.[28-31] These earlier studies were limited by their relatively small numbers of older persons, fairly short follow-up periods, possible selection biases, and some uncertainty

about the exact time of diagnosis.[32] These concerns were mostly addressed by the more recent report of Darby et al.[33] They studied 1229 HIV-infected hemophiliacs from the United Kingdom; because these patients received their Factor VIII concentrates through a centralized registry, essentially all patients could be tracked and a relatively precise determination of the date of seroconversion made. (Not surprisingly, this was mostly in the fall of 1981.) Patients were grouped by their age at estimated time of seroconversion and followed for the next decade. A summary of Darby et al.'s findings is shown in Table 37–2. They found that advancing age is associated with an increased rate of progression to AIDS and decreased survival following an AIDS diagnosis. As discussed below, these findings have important implications for both the immunopathogenesis of HIV and treatment decisions.

Clinical Manifestations

The actual clinical presentation of older patients with HIV infection is similar to that of younger patients. There is a general perception, however, that HIV is frequently misdiagnosed or missed in the elderly population because many of the early symptoms of HIV, such as fatigue, anorexia, weight loss, and memory problems, are relatively nonspecific and may mimic common geriatric symptoms. For example, Gordon and Thompson found that, among 24 elderly patients who presented to a physician with signs or symptoms of HIV infection, 11 underwent extensive medical evaluations to rule out malignancies and three were initially diagnosed with organic brain syndrome.[5] In a retrospective case–control study, Skiest et al.[34] found that older HIV-positive patients had a shorter AIDS-

TABLE 37–2. Effect of Age on Progression to AIDS and Survival in HIV-Infected Hemophiliacs from the United Kingdom

AGE AT SEROCONVERSION (YEARS)	NUMBER HIV-INFECTED	NUMBER OF AIDS CASES	% AIDS-FREE AT TEN YEARS	RELATIVE RATE OF AIDS	OBSERVED DEATHS	% SURVIVAL ONE YEAR AFTER AIDS	RELATIVE MORTALITY RATE
<15	307	64	80	1.0	35	70	1.0
15–34	599	197	65	1.8	136	65	1.5
35–54	259	122	46	3.3	98	52	2.0
≥55	64	27	40	5.0	26	16	4.7
Total	1229	410	64	. . .	295	58	. . .

From Darby SC, Ewart DW, Giangrande PLF, et al, for the UK Haemophilia Centre Directors' Organisation: Importance of age at infection with HIV-1 for survival and development of AIDS in UK haemophilia population. Lancet 347:1573, 1996. Copyright 1996, The Lancet Ltd, *and* from Bender BS: HIV and aging as a model for immunosenescence. J Gerontol A Biol Sci Med Sci 52:M261, 1996. Copyright 1996 Gerontological Society of America and Copyright Clearance Center, Inc, with permission.

free interval, shorter survival time, and more HIV-related and non-HIV-related comorbidity. They also had lower CD4+ T-cell counts at time of diagnosis, which the investigators ascribed to a lack of HIV awareness but which also could be due to a more rapid loss of CD4+ cells.[34]

Another frequently stated reason for underdiagnosis of HIV in older patients is a lack of knowledge among physicians of the epidemiology of HIV in older persons. In support of this, el Sadr and Gettler performed HIV antibody testing on elderly persons with no history of HIV infection who died at Harlem Hospital (a hospital with a relatively high percentage of patients with HIV infection) and found that 13 of 257 (5%) were HIV positive.[35] No young control group was included, however, and the Hospital HIV Surveillance Group found that HIV seroprevalence was consistently highest among patients 15 to 54 years old.[36] The seroprevalence rate for persons over age 65 varied from zero to about 6%, whereas the rate for those between 15 and 44 varied from 1.3% to 39.8%.[36] Given the data presented here, however, perhaps the Centers for Disease Control and Prevention's recommendation that routine HIV screening be offered only to hospitalized patients between the ages of 15 and 54 years should be reconsidered.[36]

When the disease progresses further, there is little or no difference in the initial AIDS-defining diagnoses between younger and older adults (Table 37–1). In a study of transfusion-associated cases, the two most common opportunistic infections were *Pneumocystis carinii* pneumonia and *Candida* esophagitis in patients both younger than 65 and 65 and older, with smaller numbers of patients with other infections.[31] It does appear, however, that progression of opportunistic infections may be more rapid in older persons,[37] although these observations were made before protease inhibitors were introduced.

Two complications that deserve particular mention are Kaposi's sarcoma and primary lymphoma of the brain. Prior to the HIV epidemic, Kaposi's sarcoma was seen primarily in older men of Southern (Italian) or Eastern (Jewish) European descent. It typically involved the lower legs, lymphadenopathy was uncommonly, and it had a relatively indolent clinical course.[38–40] Central nervous system lymphoma was similarly seen in older persons.[41] Consequently, it is particularly important in persons older than age 60 with either Kaposi's sarcoma or primary lymphoma of the brain to obtain positive serol-ogy for HIV infection prior to making a diagnosis of AIDS.

Perhaps the most pernicious complication of HIV infection in older patients is progressive dementia. Although usually a late-stage manifestation, some older HIV-positive patients who have presented with altered mental status characteristic of the AIDS dementia complex have been misdiagnosed as having Alzheimer's disease.[42,43] Clinically, these two conditions may be very difficult to differentiate; patients with AIDS dementia complex tend to have more accompanying motor and sensory findings such as ataxia, reflex abnormalities, weakness, and peripheral neuropathy. Imaging of the brains of patients with AIDS dementia complex by either computer tomography or magnetic resonance imaging shows increased atrophy with age, and the cerebrospinal fluid frequently shows a mild pleocytosis and elevated protein level. Therapy of AIDS dementia usually includes high doses of zidovudine and stavudine and is discussed more fully in Chapter 14.

THERAPY

Despite their relatively large numbers, older persons are rarely included in clinical trials and there are no published recommendations on the use of the antiretrovirals in older persons. There are, however, several important considerations to bear in mind. First, the above observations on natural history showing that older persons have a more rapid progression of HIV infection suggest that older persons might require a more aggressive approach to therapy, with earlier use of combination therapies. Second, older persons appear to respond equally well to combination therapy as younger persons. In a preliminary study, in patients age 50 to 73 years combination therapy that included a protease inhibitor resulted in a mean increase in CD4+ T cells of 127 cells/μl and a drop in viral load of 2.2 $\log_{10}$ copies/ml.[24] Third, as with many other medications, drug toxicities and interactions are more common in older persons. Sundar et al reviewed the experience with zidovudine-induced lactic acidosis and hepatic failure.[44] These 14 patients were relatively older, with a mean age of 45 years (range 31 to 69). Because older persons need treatment for coexisting diseases (e.g., diabetes and hypertension), the potential for drug interactions and difficulty with compliance increase. An example from our experience was with a patient whose hypertension was well controlled with verapamil was admitted to the intensive care unit because of a junctional rhythm several days after beginning ritonavir-saquinavir combination therapy. Verapamil was withheld, but a temporary pacemaker was required until the patient's verapamil level was undetectable.

Figure 37–1 illustrates the viral and immulogic response to protease inhibitors in three older persons. Each case detailed below illustrates many of the clinical issues previously noted.

Patient 1 (age 66 years) was admitted for workup of a 25-lb weight loss and chronic diarrhea. He was found to have *Camphylobacter* in his

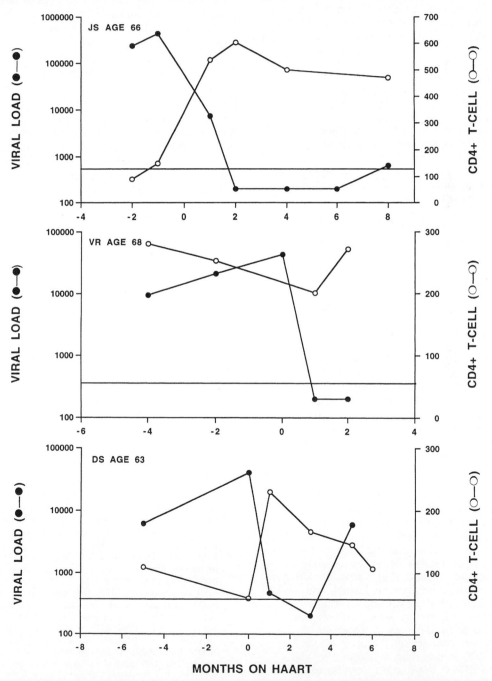

FIGURE 37–1. Response of three older persons to highly active antiretroviral therapy (HAART). Viral load is given in number of copies/per milliliter as determined by polymerase chain reaction, and CD4+ T-cell count is absolute number of cells per microliter. See text for detailed description of each patient.

stool, a normocytic, normochronic anemia, and malabsorption. Upper and lower endoscopies were unrevealing, iron studies were consistent with anemia of chronic disease, and he was treated with antibiotics and discharged to be followed in the gastrointestinal disease clinic. He was re-admitted 3 months later because of dehydration and further weight loss. Computed tomography scans of the chest and abdomen did not demonstrate a malignancy, and plasma cortisol and aldosterone levels were borderline low. He was again discharged, but was re-admitted several days later for continued dehydration; an infectious disease consultant recommended HIV testing, which returned positive. On further questioning, the patient revealed that, since his wife had died several years previously, he had frequented prostitutes about once a month. After combination therapy with lamuvidine, stavudine, and indinavir, his CD4+ T-cell count rose from 90 to 537 cells/μl and his viral load fell from 437,000 to less than 400 copies/ml. He also gained about 30 pounds and his anemia resolved.

Patient 2 (age 68 years) tested positive on routine screening prior to elective surgery and was started by another physician on zidovudine and lamuvidine. His mean corpuscular volume was 106 μm³, and his cardiologist ordered tests to determine vitamin B_{12} and folate levels. He referred himself to the infectious diseases clinic, where two viral load measurements were 9500 and 21,000 copies/ml and CD4+ T-cell counts were 253 and 201 cells/μl. His therapy was changed to stavudine, lamuvidine, and indinavir, whereupon his viral load dropped to an undetectable level and his CD4+ T-cell count rose to 272 cells/μl. He died suddenly about 3 months after starting therapy. His risk factor had been an extramarital heterosexual affair, and his wife refused testing while he was still living because she "didn't want him to feel bad [if she were positive]."

Patient 3 (age 63 years) was hospitalized for acute ischemia of his foot. He had been known to be HIV positive for about 5 years, and his former partner had died from AIDS. He had been on zidovudine and lamuvidine for over 1 year. Because of severe atherosclerosis requiring bypass surgery, it was decided after discussion with the patient to wait until after his surgery and recovery period before starting a protease inhibitor. Several months later, nelfinavir was added and zidovudine was replaced by stavudine. He had an initial drop in his viral load from 41,000 to less than 400 copies/ml and a rise in his CD4+ T-cell count from 58 to 230 cells/μl. This was relatively short lived, but the patient was moving again for personal reasons and preferred to wait prior to changing therapy.

CONCLUSIONS

In the first two decades of the evolving HIV epidemic, the virus has had a profound biologic, medical, and social impact on every segment of society, so it is not surprising that older persons are affected as well. As with other illnesses, older persons have higher numbers of comorbid conditions that make therapy more complex, and further studies are clearly needed to define their care. AIDS physicians and geriatricians should find that they have much in common. Both deal with persons with relatively limited life expectancies in which a cure is generally not expected. Rather, the main goals of therapy are to maximize functional independence and minimize hospitalization. The clinical course of both types of patients is marked by increased susceptibility to infections and tumors, and many of the investigative clinical interventions (e.g., growth hormone replacement and cytokine administration) are similar. Much of the cost of their medical care comes in the last years of life. A multidisciplinary approach utilizing the talents of physicians, pharmacists, nurses, dietitians, and social workers is required. Unfortunately, many elderly persons and HIV-infected patients are still viewed as pariahs by their families and some segments of society.[8]

REFERENCES

1. Shilts R: And the Band Played On: People, Politics, and the AIDS Epidemic. New York; St. Martin's Press, 1987
2. Centers for Disease Control and Prevention: AIDS among persons aged ≥50 years—United States, 1991–1996. MMWR Morb Mortal Wkly Rep 47:21, 1998
3. Ship JA, Wolff A, Selik RM: Epidemiology of acquired immunodeficiency syndrome in persons aged 50 years or older. J Acquir Immune Defic Syndr 4:84, 1991
4. Selik RM, Ward JW, Buehler JW: Demographic differences in cumulative incidence rates of transfusion-associated acquired immunodeficiency syndrome. Am J Epidemiol 140:105, 1994
5. Gordon SM, Thompson S: The changing epidemiology of human immunodeficiency virus infection in older persons. J Am Geriatr Soc 43:7, 1995
6. Stall R, Catania J: AIDS risk behaviors among late middle-aged and elderly Americans: The national AIDS behavioral surveys. Arch Intern Med 154:57, 1994
7. Schable B, Chu SY, Diaz T: Characteristics of women 50 years of age or older with heterosexually acquired AIDS. Am J Public Health 86:1616, 1996
8. Bender BS: HIV and aging as a model for immunosenescence. J Gerontol A Biol Sci Med Sci 52:M261, 1996
9. Fauci AS: Host factors and the pathogenesis of HIV-induced disease. Nature 384:529, 1996

10. Mellors JW, Rinaldo CR Jr, Gupta P, et al: Prognosis in HIV-1 infection predicted by the quantity of virus in plasma. Science 272:1167, 1996
11. Weissman S, Fuehrer S, Justice A: Survival differences between younger and older HIV positive patients. In Abstracts of the 5th Conference on Retroviruses and Opportunistic Infections, Chicago, 1998, Abstract 210
12. Ershler WB, Sun WH, Binkley N: The role of interleukin-6 in certain age-related diseases. Drugs Aging 5: 358, 1994
13. Schnittman SM, Lane HC, Greenhouse J, et al: Preferential infection of CD4+ memory T cells by Human immunodeficiency virus type 1: Evidence for a role in the selective T-cell functional defects observed in infected individuals. Proc Natl Acad Sci USA 87:6058, 1990
14. Sleasman JW, Aleixo LF, Morton, A, et al: CD4+ memory T cells are the predominant population of HIV-1-infected lymphocytes in neonates and children. AIDS 10:1477, 1996
15. Stulnig T, Maczek C, Bock G, et al: Reference intervals for human peripheral blood lymphocyte subpopulations from "healthy" young and aged subjects. Int Arch Allergy Immunol 108:205, 1995
16. Feng Y, Broder CC, Kennedy PE, Berger EA: HIV-1 entry cofactor: Functional cDNA cloning of a seven-transmembrane, G protein-coupled receptor. Science 272:872, 1996
17. Alkhatib G, Combadiere C, Broder CC, et al: CC CKR: A RANTES, MIP-1alpha, MIP-1beta receptor as a fusion cofactor for macrophage-tropic HIV-1. Science 272:1955, 1996
18. Harley CB, Futcher, AB, Greider CW: Telomeres shorten during aging of human fibroblasts. Nature 345: 458, 1990
19. Effros RB, Allsopp R, Chiu C-P, et al: Shortened telomeres in the expanded CD28-CD8+ cell subset in HIV disease implicate replicative senescence in HIV pathogenesis. AIDS 10:F17, 1996
20. Caruso A, Licenziati S, Canaris AD, et al: Contribution of CD4+, CD8+CD28+, and CD8+CD28− T cells to CD3+ lymphocyte homeostasis during the natural course of HIV-1 infection. J Clin Invest 101:137, 1998
21. Mackall CL, Fleisher TA, Brown MR, et al: Age, thymopoiesis, and CD4+ T-lymphocyte regeneration after intensive chemotherapy. N Engl J Med 332:143, 1995
22. Adler WH, Baskar PV, Chrest FJ, et al: HIV-1 infection and aging: Mechanism to explain the accelerated rate of progression in the older patients. Mech Aging Develop 96:137, 1997
23. Mueller BU, Butler KM, Stocker VL, et al: Clinical and pharmacokinetic evaluation of long-term therapy with didanosine in children with HIV infection. Pediatrics 94:724, 1994
24. Maruenda J, Uphold C, Bender BS: Response to protease inhibitors in older patients. In Abstracts of the 51st Annual Meeting of the Gerontological Society of America, Philadelphia, 1998
25. Powers DC: Influenza A virus-specific cytotoxic T lymphocyte activity declines with advancing age. J Am Geriatr Soc 41:1, 1993
26. Goodenow M, Huet T, Saurin W, et al: HIV-1 isolates are rapidly evolving quasispecies: Evidence for viral mixtures and preferred nucleotide substitutions. J Acquir Immune Defic Syndr 2:344, 1989
27. Phillips RE, Rowland Jones S, Nixon DF, et al: Human immunodeficiency virus genetic variation that can escape cytotoxic T cell recognition. Nature 354:453, 1991
28. Rosenberg PS, Goedert JJ, Biggar RJ: Effect of age at seroconversion on the natural AIDS incubation distribution: Multicenter Hemophilia Cohort Study and the International Registry of Seroconverters. AIDS 8:803, 1994
29. Carre N, Deveau C, Belanger F, et al: Effect of age and exposure group on the onset of AIDS in heterosexual and homosexual HIV-infected patients. SEROCO Study Group. AIDS 8:797, 1994
30. Veugelers PJ, Strathdee SA, Tindall B, et al: Increasing age is associated with faster progression to neoplasms but not opportunistic infections in HIV-infected men. AIDS 8:1471, 1994
31. Sutin DG, Rose DN, Mulvihill M, Taylor B: Survival of elderly patients with transfusion-related acquired immunodeficiency syndrome. J Am Geriatr Soc 41:214, 1993
32. Volberding PA: Age as a predictor of progression of HIV infection. Lancet 347:1569, 1996
33. Darby SC, Ewart DW, Giangrande PLF, et al, for the UK Haemophilia Centre Directors' Organisation: Importance of age at infection with HIV-1 for survival and development of AIDS in UK haemophilia population. Lancet 347:1573, 1996
34. Skiest DJ, Rubinstein E, Carley N, et al: The importance of cormorbidity in HIV-infected patients over 55: A retrospective case-control study. Am J Med 101:605, 1996
35. el Sadr W, Gettler J: Unrecognized human immunodeficiency virus infection in the elderly. Arch Intern Med 155:184, 1995
36. Janssen RS, St Louis ME, Satten GA, et al: HIV infection among patients in U.S. acute care hospitals: Strategies for the counseling and testing of the hospital patients. The Hospital HIV Surveillance Group. N Engl J Med 327:445, 1992
37. McCormick W, Wood R: Clinical decisions in the care of elderly persons with AIDS. J Am Geriatr Soc 40: 917, 1992
38. Rothman S: Some clinical aspects of Kaposi's sarcoma in European and North American population. Acta Un Int Contra Cancrum 18:364, 1962
39. Rothman S: Remarks on sex, age and racial distribution of Kaposi's sarcoma and on possible pathogenetic factors. Acta Un Int Conta Cancrum 18:326, 1962
40. DiGiovanni JJ, Safai B: Kaposi's sarcoma: Retrospective study of 90 cases with particular emphasis on the familial occurrence, ethnic background and prevalence of other diseases. Am J Med 71:779, 1981
41. Hochberg FH, Miller DC: Primary central nervous system lymphoma. J Neurosurg 68:835, 1988
42. Weiler PG, Mungas D, Pomerantz S: AIDS as a cause of dementia in the elderly. J Am Geriatr Soc 36:139, 1988
43. Rosenzweig R, Fillit H: Probable heterosexual transmission of AIDS in an aged woman. J Am Geriatr Soc 40:1261, 1992
44. Sundar K, Suarez M, Banogon PE, Shapiro JM: Zidovudine-induced fatal lactic acidosis and hepatic failure in patients with acquired immunodeficiency syndrome: Report of two patients and review of the literature. Crit Care Med 25:1425, 1997

38 | Alternative Therapies

DONALD I. ABRAMS

The history of the alternative therapy movement in HIV/AIDS has been intricately associated with the availability and perceived effectiveness of orthodox antiretroviral interventions.[1–5] While the current fascination with alternative therapies continues to sweep the nation, interest in such interventions among people living with HIV infection may be on the decline. Sales of melatonin and dehydroepiandosterone (DHEA) may be skyrocketing in the nation's pharmacies, supermarkets, and health food stores, but the situation at the HIV therapies buyer's clubs—the sites where alternative therapies were usually purchased—appears less sanguine.

We are currently in a new era of HIV therapeutics, with 13 or 14 available antiretroviral agents and several other new drugs in late stages of clinical trials. The hope of benefit from triple combination therapies—especially regimens that contain protease inhibitors—has all but negated the need to seek alternative interventions from buyer's clubs. As a testament to this paradigm shift, the two former directors of the San Francisco Healing Alternative Buyer's Club have both taken positions in the AIDS Program at San Francisco General Hospital within the past 6 months as outreach workers, encouraging enrollment of patients into antiretroviral clinical trials.

SURVEYS OF ALTERNATIVE THERAPY USE

Numerous studies have investigated the use of alternative therapies by patients with HIV infection.[6–8] Most of this research was conducted prior to the wide availability of highly active antiretroviral regimens including combinations of protease inhibitors. Studies have estimated that anywhere from 40% to 70% of patients with HIV infection in the United States utilize alternative or complementary therapies,

with similar percentages emanating from studies in Europe.[9–11] A recent evaluation of patterns of alternative therapy use in British Columbia benefited from the fact that patients with HIV infection received their drug treatments from a central provincial program.[12] In a survey of 1019 participants receiving antiviral drugs, 34% noted that they had ever used complementary treatments. Of these, 53% reported using dietary supplements and vitamins and 43% had ingested other agents. In comparing those who used alternative therapies to those who had not, the users were more likely to have an AIDS diagnosis, moderate or severe pain, and more educational degrees and were not currently on antiretroviral therapies. A Stanford University study of "nontraditional" treatment used by those receiving traditional care followed 1467 HIV-positive participants over 5 years.[13] Data on the frequency and type of nontraditional therapy were updated every 3 months, with a mean follow-up of 21 months at the time the study was reported in 1996. Herbs (44%), acupuncture (41%) chiropractic (40%), and other nonsanctioned drugs (19%) were the most frequently utilized agents reported. Of the respondents, 42% used multiple types of alternative therapies. A survey of 1049 HIV-positive women enrolled in the Women's Interagency HIV Study found that use of complementary and alternative medicine was similar in the HIV-positive women compared to a group of 236 HIV-negative controls.[14] Those using alternatives tended to be older, with higher education and income, and less frequently, to be women of color. Spiritual practices, regular exercise, and Chinese herbs were the most frequent alternatives reported. Seventy percent of the women using the complementary and alternative medicines did not disclose it to their health provider.

Researchers at the University of California, San Diego Neuro-Behavioral Research Center queried 145 HIV-positive participants in an HIV

Cost and Services Utilization Study survey.[15] They documented that 76% of the respondents had reported recently using some type of complementary and alternative medicine. Of those who had used such an intervention, 44% did not disclose it to their medical provider and 14% stated that they used the alternative therapy in lieu of traditional treatment. The investigators sought to determine whether there were any differences between the cohort of patients who used these interventions in lieu of traditional treatment (i.e., strictly alternative) and those who used them to complement their prescribed medications. They found that those substituting alternatives for conventional therapy were more optimistic ($p < .05$), expected to live longer ($p < .001$), were less likely to have any advance directive ($p < .05$), and were less interested in making end-of-life preparations ($p < .001$). Substitution was related to negative attitudes toward taking zidovudine in particular and antiretroviral therapy in general. Again it must be noted that the study was conducted and the results reported prior to the widespread utilization of protease inhibitor–containing antiretroviral therapies. It would be most interesting to see this study duplicated to compare current results to the previous findings.

In 1990 Eisenberg et al. conducted a telephone survey of 1539 adults in the United States and found that 34% reported using at least one unconventional therapy.[16] Nearly three quarters of those using unconventional therapies did not inform their primary care provider. The highest use of alternatives was found in non-blacks age 25 to 49 years with higher education and income levels. The out-of-pocket expenditures for visits to providers of alternative interventions surpassed the cost of visits to traditional primary care providers in this 1990 survey.

THE CYCLE OF ORTHODOX AND ALTERNATIVE TREATMENT USE

At the beginning of the AIDS epidemic, before the etiologic agent was identified, early alternative therapies, largely being used by gay men, who comprised the main group of infected individuals, included high-dose intravenous or oral vitamin C and topical application of the sensitizer dinitrochlorobenzene.[17-21] At the same time that clinical trials of immunomodulators and antivirals such as isoprinosine and ribavirin were getting underway at the research centers,

they were also being obtained over the counter in easily accessed foreign markets. With no standard treatment available for HIV/AIDS during the first 5 years of the epidemic, the search was on for alternative therapies that offered any hope.

Late in 1986, zidovudine was approved, and an orthodox treatment was now available by prescription for the first time.[22] Interest in alternatives slowed down for awhile, and hopes ran high that additional antiretrovirals would soon be released. However, when none emerged, interest in alternative therapies surged from 1987 through 1989. In 1989, results of large clinical trials demonstrated that zidovudine was useful in patients with earlier stages of HIV infection.[23,24] Expanded access programs for additional nucleoside analogs were also established at this time, which gave patients for whom zidovudine failed or whose disease progressed access to other potentially beneficial therapeutic agents.[25,26] Once again, the availability of orthodox treatments ushered in a period of decreased interest in alternative interventions, although some individuals continued to use alternative treatments, which they often described as "complementary" to their prescribed antiretroviral medication.

Interest in alternative therapies picked up again in 1993, following preliminary reports of disappointing results from the large collaborative Concorde trial, which evaluated early versus deferred zidovudine therapy in patients with asymptomatic HIV infection.[27,28] The results of other clinical trials reported at the 1993 International Conference on AIDS were also disappointing. Disenchantment over available "orthodox" treatments led increasing numbers of patients to once again seek alternative therapy for their HIV infection.

Only 2 years later, caregivers and patients found themselves in the current era of hope, which began in 1995 with promising surrogate marker information from trials combining zidovudine and lamivudine, followed by even more impressive responses when a protease inhibitor was added.[29-33] The anti-HIV arsenal has dramatically increased with the rapid licensure and approval of four protease inhibitors and three non-nucleoside reverse transcriptase inhibitors. As might be expected then, the consequent hope that the virus might be suppressed by prescribed medication has virtually supplanted the need to obtain potential antiretroviral interventions from the buyer's clubs. However, therapies are still sought for some of the manifestations of HIV disease for which orthodox medicine has little to offer. Immune reconstitution and wasting are two current areas where the highest interest in alternative intervention remains.

WHY PATIENTS SEEK ALTERNATIVE THERAPIES

According to Eisenberg, of the Center for Alternative Medicine and Research at the Beth Israel Deaconess Medical Center in Boston, there are five possible reasons why patients seek alternative therapies[34]: (1) for the purpose of health promotion and disease prevention, (2) when conventional therapies have been exhausted, (3) when conventional therapies have questionable efficacy or are associated with significant adverse effects, (4) when no conventional therapy exists to relieve the patient's condition, (5) and where the conventional approach is held to be "emotionally or spiritually without benefit." Regardless of the reason, Eisenberg suggests that primary care providers be aware of the possibility and question the patient directly to establish a sense of shared decision making about the use of alternative therapies.

The need for this kind of openness is particularly apparent with the current protease inhibitors, which are so intricately linked to hepatic metabolism via the cytochrome P-450 system. In this era of antiviral regimens that contain protease inhibitors, drug–drug interactions, especially those mediated through the hepatic cytochrome P-450 system, have become increasingly important. Unfortunately, there have been no pharmacokinetic interaction trials looking at the effects of various alternative treatment regimens. Therefore, whether the alternative therapies a patient is taking share hepatic metabolic pathways will largely be unknown because of lack of study. This makes it all the more imperative that providers question patients carefully about their use of complementary and alternative medicine. Unsuspected interactions between orthodox regimens containing protease inhibitors and other treatments may lead to decreased efficacy or increased toxicity of the combination antiretroviral therapy regimen. Providers with patients on these complex regimens should be aware of all the additional substances that patients are ingesting.

The best way to integrate questions regarding the use of alternative therapies into the standard medical interview is to maintain neutrality, thereby encouraging the most honest responses. Eisenberg advises that it is not necessary to use a label that may be perceived as judgmental, such as "alternative," "complementary," or "unorthodox," in discussing the "other therapies" that patients may be using. He also recommends that providers document use of alternative regimens in the patient's medical record.

ALTERNATIVE THERAPY IN A GLOBAL CONTEXT

Alternative therapy use by patients with HIV infection must be viewed in light of the fact that AIDS is a global pandemic. Therefore, what might be considered to be "alternative" therapy in one culture is actually "traditional" in another. This was first highlighted for HIV/AIDS by a small study in Rwanda of traditional versus modern medicine for the treatment of AIDS.[35] Factors and perceptions determining choice between a traditional healer and western medicine were assessed among 45 urban African women with AIDS. The majority reported concurrent use of both traditional healers and western medicine. Although all of the women reported that traditional healers treat certain illnesses better than western medicine, they consulted western providers for their perceived appropriateness in treating specific illnesses and access to diagnostic medical technology. For these women, western medicine may in fact be considered the "alternative" to "conventional" therapy. A subsequent randomized trial directly compared the effectiveness of traditional herbal medicines with the best available medical therapy, including acyclovir, for treatment of chronic diarrhea and herpes zoster.[36] Among the 272 patients with herpes zoster, the lesions healed at the same rate whether the patients were receiving herbal therapy or medical therapy with acyclovir. Fewer patients treated with the herbal preparation by the traditional healers suffered postherpetic neuralgia than did those receiving acyclovir (11% vs. 44%; $p < .005$). Patients with chronic diarrhea ($n = 387$) also responded significantly more often to the herbal preparation than to the conventional therapy (73% vs. 29%; $p < .005$), with faster responses also being reported. CD4 cell declines were noted equally in all groups.

As the population affected by HIV infection expands worldwide into diverse ethnic groups and global information exchange becomes more easily accomplished, the lines separating alternative and orthodox therapies will likely continue to blur.

Many of the drugs in common use, as well as a number of potent cytotoxic chemotherapy agents, are derived from the world's flora. Therefore, the medicinal potential of plants, including herbs, cannot be ignored by even those most skeptical of alternative therapies. A recent meta-survey of plant and herb material as treatment for HIV infection found that, of tens of thousands of substances screened, 70 compounds and 76 crude extracts from 123 species reportedly exhibited HIV-inhibitory activity in vitro, and 63 of the bioactive ingredients were listed in the Chinese Materia Medica.[37] The classes of compounds reported were terpenes, flavonoids, polysaccharides, coumarins, tannins, lectins, quinolones, peptides, and other alkaloids. The natural substances were reported to have activity inhibiting reverse transcriptase and protease enzymes as well as interfering with infection at the level of viral entry into the cell. Of note, a fungal extract and the dicaffeoylquinic acids derived from Bolivian medicinal plant extracts are currently being evaluated as possible inhibitors of HIV intergrase.[38]

COMMONLY USED ALTERNATIVE THERAPIES

The popularity of a number of alternative therapies has waxed and waned over the past 15 years. With the current abundance of available antiretroviral agents, alternative therapies are now more frequently sought for conditions without truly effective interventions, such as some of the symptomatic manifestations of HIV disease, as well as to augment the immune system and to counteract the wasting syndrome. Providers should become familiar with some of the common complementary and alternative agents in current use (Table 38–1).

Chinese Herbs and Acupuncture

Especially in the San Francisco Bay Area, where much traditional Chinese medicine is practiced by the large local Asian community, patients with HIV infection often seek herbal therapies and/or acupuncture as adjuncts to their orthodox treatments. These therapies are generally sought not as specific antiretroviral or immunomodulating interventions, but to treat certain symptomatic manifestations of HIV disease, including wasting, nausea, sleep disturbances, and pain syndromes. Anecdotal reports of the effectiveness of these interventions in patients for whom previous western treatments have failed are abundant.

To obtain pilot information on the efficacy of Chinese herbal therapies in patients with symptomatic HIV infection, a placebo-controlled, randomized, double-blind trial in 30 HIV-positive patients with CD4 cell counts between 200 and 500/mm^3 without a prior AIDS-defining diagnosis was conducted in the AIDS Clinic at San Francisco General Hospital.[39] The trial tested a 31-herb combination based on two preparations, Enhance and Clear Heat, which have been used widely in the treatment of patients with HIV infection. The herbs included in the mixture were selected for their purported antiviral and immunomodulatory properties. Patients were required to have at least two HIV-related symptoms to be eligible for the trial, and were randomized to receive either 28 pills of the Chinese herbal preparation or placebo daily for 12 weeks. Outcome variables included changes from baseline in overall well-being, physical and social functioning, and symptoms. Compliance over the course of the trial was excellent, and the only adverse reaction noted was the development of diarrhea, which required that treatment be discontinued in one placebo recipient. Only a single case of transaminase elevations

TABLE 38–1. Currently Used Alternative Therapies

AGENT	NATURE OF AGENT	PROPOSED ACTIVITY	SIDE EFFECTS
Chinese herbs	Traditional herbal mixture	Symptom palliation	Generally none seen, but many possible
Vitamin C	Antioxidant	Free radical scavenger, antiviral	Gastrointestinal distress at high doses
N-acetylcysteine	Cysteine precursor, mucolytic, acetaminophen antidote	Tumor necrosis factor inhibitor, antiviral	None reported
Allicin	Chinese garlic concentrate	Antibiotic vs. parasites, antifungal	Garlic taste, smell
Malaleuca	Tea tree extract	Antifungal	Oral blisters, nausea if swallowed

requiring cessation of therapy was reported, also in a placebo recipient. No significant changes were seen in any of the major outcome variables studied. The mean number of symptoms was reduced from the baseline 14 by two in the subjects on herbs but was unchanged in placebo recipients. There was a greater change in median score on a "life satisfaction" scale in the herbal group as well. At the end of 12 weeks, CD4 cells counts had declined somewhat more in the herbal recipients and the placebo recipients appeared to gain slightly more weight. One criticism of these findings, from a practitioner from China, was that it is not possible to evaluate Chinese herbal interventions in a placebo-controlled manner and that one should not expect isolated herbal preparations to work in the absence of the entire herb and removed from the context of a regimen that includes acupuncture. In any event, we have now embarked on a trial of Chinese preparations for treatments of *Cryptosporidium*-negative diarrhea and for mild anemia, the latter funded by the Office of Alternative Medicine (OAM) of the National Institutes of Health (NIH). These were originally placebo controlled, but we had to jettison the placebo in both because patients with diarrhea and anemia were not interested in participating in a placebo-controlled trial.

Aware that acupuncture was being widely used to treat peripheral neuropathy in patients for whom analgesics gave unsatisfactory relief, the Community Program for Clinical Research on AIDS (CPCRA) conducted a nationwide trial of a standard acupuncture regimen and amitriptylene, in which 250 patients were initially randomized to receive one of the four treatment arms for 14 weeks, as follows: amitriptylene 75 mg/day or placebo, in combination with standardized acupuncture with spleen 9, 7, and 6 (Lower Three Kings) or alternate-points acupuncture (Lower Three Jesters); standardized additional points could be used with the Lower Three Kings, depending on patient symptoms.[39a] The primary endpoint was the change in pain from baseline to 6 and 14 weeks. Patients graded their pain using a standardized pain scale consisting of 13 words that were each associated with a numerical value. The results indicated that nearly 50% of both the standardized acupuncture and the sham acupuncture groups reported at least moderate pain relief at both the 6-week and 14-week evaluation points. There was no statistically significant difference between the two groups with regard to the reduction of neuropathic pain. Amitriptylene fared no better than placebo in the final analysis. The in-vestigators note that, although there are numerous acupuncture regimens that could be used to treat HIV-related peripheral neuropathy, the one used in this study was not clearly effective in providing pain relief. Conclusions regarding the efficacy of any other acupuncture regimens could not be extrapolated from this trial. Acupuncture proponents will note that the intervention was given in a standardized fashion to all patients rather than being individualized on the basis of an antecedent traditional Chinese medicine diagnosis. The absence of concurrent herbal adjunctive therapy may also be cited as a flaw in the trial design. Nonetheless, the fact that the study was conducted by a federally funded HIV clinical trials group speaks for the viability of evaluating alternative therapies in the mainstream clinical research infrastructure.

Vitamin C and Antioxidants

Vitamin C, one of the first interventions proposed as a potential alternative therapy, is still consumed by a significant segment of the HIV-infected population for its potential antiviral and antioxidant activities.[3,40] Early in the epidemic, before any conventional antiviral therapies were available, high doses of vitamin C (up to 50 gm/day) were taken orally or intravenously. The rationale was based on anecdotal observations of broad antiviral activity as well as in vitro activity demonstrated against a human retrovirus.[17,18] Patients were advised by proponents of the therapy to ingest as much vitamin C as possible, titrating the dose to the intolerability of the resultant diarrhea. However, when many early proponents of high-dose vitamin C therapy died as a result of AIDS-related illnesses, enthusiasm for this intervention in the community waned.

Interest in the potential therapeutic utility of antioxidants in general and vitamin C in particular resurged in 1990, after the NIH sponsored a conference to review the biologic and clinical actions of vitamin C.[40] The NIH summarized the existing evidence as follows: Oxidative stress is postulated to be toxic to lymphocytes, thus potentiating the destructive effect of HIV in infected patients. Vitamin C is believed to be one of the first-line defenses against free radical damage, as well as having a potential role in preserving immune function. In vitro studies support the anecdotal observations of antiretroviral activity. Viral replication in both chronically and acutely infected cell lines has been shown to be inhibited by continuous exposure of HIV-infected cells to noncytotoxic ascorbate concentrations.[17] Another potential pathway of benefit for vitamin C's activity is its ability to raise intracellular glutathione levels,[18] which may foster synergistic activity when ascorbate is combined with *N*-acetylcysteine (NAC).

The new wave of enthusiasm has convinced vitamin C treatment activists moreso than before that, because vitamins are not patentable, they will never be seriously studied in clinical trials because they pose a threat to the pharmaceutical industry and the mainstream medical profession. Nonetheless, the CPCRA did develop a protocol to investigate the utility of vitamin C in patients with HIV infection, but further investigation of the antiretroviral potency of vitamin C waned with the advent of the new and more effective conventional antiviral treatments that featured protease inhibitors.

Tumor Necrosis Factor Inhibitors

Cysteine is an essential amino acid that is utilized in the biosynthesis of the peptide glutathione. NAC is the *N*-acetyl derivative of cysteine that, in aerosolized form, is used as a mucolytic treatment for bronchitis in Europe. In the United States it is given orally or intravenously (Mucomyst) to treat acetaminophen overdosage. Patients with HIV infection have decreased stores of intracellular glutathione,[41–43] and cysteine precursors may indirectly inhibit HIV replication by raising intracellular glutathione levels.[44] Evidence for this comes from in vitro studies in persistently infected cell lines, which have demonstrated that cysteine and NAC raise intracellular glutathione and inhibit HIV replication. These actions may be secondary to blocking the effects of tumor necrosis factor (TNF) in the HIV-infected cells.[45–47] TNF levels are elevated in people with advanced HIV infection and may be associated with increased HIV replication.[47,48] TNF-α has also been implicated as a cytokine that may contribute to the pathogenesis of a number of the manifestations of HIV infection, including HIV-related wasting.[49] Consequently, agents that may block TNF-α are good candidates for clinical trials. Several other agents that have been popular alternative therapies over the years have had TNF blockade as their presumed mechanism of action. However, because of NAC's wide availability in foreign markets, its biochemical rationale, and the lack of significant toxicity associated with therapy (occasional dyspepsia, diarrhea), it continues to rank as one of the largest selling items in the buyer's clubs nationwide. Therefore, the National Institute of Al-

lergy and Infectious Diseases (NIAID) conducted a small study of intravenous and oral preparations in an effort to ascertain the safety, pharmacokinetics, and antiviral activity of NAC in HIV-infected patients with CD4 counts less than 500 cells/mm^3.[50] Patients received 6 weeks of escalating doses of intravenous NAC three times a week, followed by 6 weeks of escalating oral doses from 600 to 4800 mg daily. Although the results suggested there was little or no oral bioavailability, NAC supporters explain that, once ingested, the substance is rapidly converted into cysteine and subsequently glutathione, and therefore it is not surprising that blood levels should be difficult to measure. In addition, if NAC were not being absorbed by mouth, how can its efficacy as a mucolytic agent or an antidote to acetaminophen be explained? The NIAID study found no significant benefits from NAC with regard to changes in CD4 cell counts, p24 antigen levels, HIV plasma viremia, or plasma cysteine levels. A subsequent in vitro evaluation demonstrated that both NAC and glutathione actually enhanced replication of HIV-1 in macrophages by up to 160%, leading the investigators to conclude that oxygen radical scavengers "other than NAC should be considered as therapeutic agents in AIDS."[51]

In a recent study, the vasodilating agent pentoxifylline, another TNF inhibitor formerly in wide use as an alternative therapy, was found to synergistically promote cytomegalovirus replication.[52] The study investigators specifically advise against the use of pentoxifylline in patients with a defective T-cell response, such as those with advanced HIV infection.

Nonetheless, proponents of NAC continue to believe that it has the potential to prolong the life of patients with HIV infection. Glutathione deficiency in CD4 lymphocytes from patients with HIV infection was recently associated with markedly decreased survival 2 to 3 years after baseline data collection.[53] Despite the fact that the NIAID trial showed no apparent benefit in any of the endpoints measured, the NAC proponents conducted a clinical trial designed to determine whether orally administered NAC could replenish glutathione in subjects with low intracellular levels. They used a fluorescence-activated cell sorter technique to assay intracellular glutathione levels. Patients with HIV infection and CD4 cell counts greater than 200/mm^3 had higher levels of intracellular glutathione than those with CD4 counts less than 200/mm^3. A logistic regression analysis demonstrated a close relationship between baseline intracellular glutathione level and survival 2 to

3 years later. Subjects with CD4 counts less than 200/mm^3 who took NAC for 8 to 32 weeks survived significantly longer than a comparable group who were not offered or did not choose to take NAC. The authors concluded that "the association of oral NAC administration (consequently GSH replenishment) with greater survival is consistent with the dramatically better survival of individuals with higher GSB levels."[53] The authors also warned that the study was not a formal placebo-controlled evaluation and suggested that such a trial be conducted before reaching any definitive conclusions about the effect of NAC on survival. However, interpretation of data even from that study is hampered by the inability to ascertain exactly how many patients were receiving NAC. Also unclear is whether the intracellular glutathione level is simply an epiphenomenon marking patients with advanced HIV disease and low CD4 counts or is pathogenic and warrants therapeutic intervention.

Thalidomide

Thalidomide, the sedative previously associated with birth defects when taken by pregnant women, is another TNF-α inhibitor that achieved significant popularity as an alternative for HIV. Thalidomide continues to be used as a treatment for erythema nodosum leprosum.[54] Its mechanism of action is thought to be enhancement of the degradation of TNF-α messenger RNA.[55]

Thalidomide was initially used in HIV-infected patients to treat individuals with HIV, tuberculosis, and wasting in Thailand.[56] Patients treated with thalidomide in addition to their antituberculosis therapy gained significantly more weight than those receiving antibiotics alone. By down-regulating TNF-α, thalidomide has also been shown to reduce HIV-1 production in acutely infected human monocytes in vitro.[57,58]

When news of these potential beneficial properties of thalidomide spread, alternative therapy activists began to obtain thalidomide from foreign markets for distribution through the buyer's club network.[59] At the same time, a double-blind, placebo-controlled clinical trial of thalidomide as therapy for idiopathic aphthous stomatitis and esophagitis was being conducted by the AIDS Clinical Trials Group. After a 4-week course of thalidomide 200 mg daily or placebo,[60] 55% of the thalidomide group had complete healing of their aphthous ulcers, as com-

pared with 7% of the placebo group ($p <. 001$). Thalidomide recipients also reported diminished pain and improved ability to eat. The main adverse effects seen in patients treated with thalidomide included somnolence and rash. Unexpectedly, thalidomide treatment was also associated with an increase in the plasma concentration of TNF-α as well as a median 0.42 log increase in HIV-RNA levels when compared with placebo ($p = .04$). The early termination of the oral ulcer trial increased community interest in obtaining wider access to the agent, but the U.S. Food and Drug Administration (FDA) was becoming increasingly concerned about the widespread uncontrolled distribution through buyer's clubs of this emotionally charged drug. They demanded that the groups cease sales of thalidomide. The pharmaceutical manufacturer subsequently developed a placebo-controlled trial for patients with HIV-related wasting syndrome that has now been fully accrued and will soon undergo analysis. In response to increased pressure from the AIDS treatment activist community, the company and the FDA established a compassionate use program for individuals with severe HIV-related weight loss. The potential teratogenic effect continues to be of concern in women with childbearing potential who are infected with HIV. Because of the recently re-established efficacy of thalidomide as a pharmaceutical agent, an FDA Advisory Committee recommended that thalidomide should be introduced again into the United States formulary, with limited distribution and increased efforts to "assist in preventing birth defects and other side effects of thalidomide exposure."[61]

Other Alternative Treatments for Wasting

The lack of truly effective available therapies for HIV-associated wasting and weight loss has led the alternative treatment community to seek treatments in addition to TNF inhibitors (Table 38–2). The unsatisfactory effects of the two licensed appetite stimulants available and the cost of recombinant human growth hormone, which must be injected subcutaneously, have led to efforts to find more effective and economical treatments.[62–66] Testosterone and its derivatives have been used increasingly in an attempt to increase lean body mass.[67] Testosterone supplementation has been used by HIV-infected men who are also hypogonadal, as well as in eugonadal men to counteract wasting.[68] Intramuscular or transdermal testosterone preparations require

TABLE 38–2. Alternative Therapies for HIV Wasting

AGENT	NATURE OF AGENT	PROPOSED ACTIVITY	SIDE EFFECTS
Thalidomide	Sedative	TNF inhibitor, antiviral	Sedation, teratogenecity
Anabolic steroids	Androgens	Increased lean body mass	Androgenizing effects
DHEA	Adrenal hormone	Androgen precursor	Mild androgenizing effects
Marijuana	Cannabis	Appetite stimulant	Mental status, pulmonary (?) drug–drug interactions (?)

prescription and cooperation of a primary care provider.[69] To get around this, individuals who seek a testosterone-like benefit have been turning to DHEA, a naturally occurring adrenal steroid that had been studied for its possible immunomodulatory and/or antiretroviral activity when early reports found AIDS patients to have depleted stores.[70] A 16-week Phase I dose-escalating trial of patients treated with oral DHEA 250 to 750 mg three times daily with surrogate marker endpoint monitoring found no changes in lymphocyte subsets or p24 antigen levels and a transient decrease in serum neopterin levels.[71] Although these disappointing results may have thwarted future clinical trials of DHEA, it has nonetheless has become an increasingly popular buyer's club item. Although the side effects (insomnia, fatigue, and nasal congestion) observed with DHEA in the clinical trial were rare, there is anecdotal evidence that women may develop hirsuitism and deepening of the voice. Whether or not commercially available oral DHEA may be associated with the progression of Kaposi's sarcoma lesions has not been carefully studied to date.

Injectable anabolic steroids, particularly nandralone, usually in conjunction with testosterone, are also gaining popularity as an alternative therapy for HIV-related weight loss and wasting.[72] Controlled clinical trials of the intervention are being conducted in both men and women with HIV-associated wasting.

Δ^9-Tetrahydrocannabinol (dronabinol), the active component of marijuana, is a licensed therapy for the anorexia associated with HIV-related wasting.[62,65] However, some individuals prefer to inhale their cannabinoids rather than ingest them.[73] In the San Francisco Bay Area, the number of cannabis buyers' clubs increased when legislation was passed that allows for the use of marijuana as medicine.[74] At these clubs, a physician's letter confirming the diagnosis of one of the indicated conditions, which include AIDS and wasting, enables an individual to purchase, for medical use, from a variety of different vintages of marijuana. The Community Consortium, the Bay Area community-based clinical trials organization, recently conducted a survey of the utilization of marijuana by clients of the cannibis buyers' clubs.[74a] Preliminary analysis of 150 patients with and without HIV infection demonstrates clearly that patients with HIV report appetite stimulation (75%) as the most frequent reason for their use of inhaled marijuana. Only 18% of HIV-negative clients answered that they were purchasing marijuana for appetite stimulation. Individuals reported smoking three times daily, consuming one marijuana cigarette at each interval for a daily consumption of approximately 1 gm. The survey sought this information in order to determine the best dose for investigation in a controlled clinical trial evaluating the safety and effectiveness of inhaled marijuana in patients with AIDS-related wasting syndrome.[75–77] The mechanism of action of cannabinoids and appetite stimulation remains unclear, but the effect may be related to increasing the sensory appeal of food or decreasing satiety.[78] Clinical trials have demonstrated that, in a controlled residential setting, individuals inhaling marijuana increased their caloric intake and weight over time.[79] The major obstacle to the Community Consortium's attempts to investigate inhaled marijuana has been finding a legal source of the drug.[75–77] With the widespread availability of protease inhibitors, it is all the more imperative that the safety of inhaled marijuana as well as oral tetrahydrocannabinol be evaluated, because the cannabinoids are also metabolized by the hepatic cytochrome P-450 system. The Community Consortium has recently been awarded an NIH grant to investigate the pharmacokinetic interaction between oral and smoked THC and protease inhibitors. Either or both may increase or inhibit protease inhibitor metabolism, leading to either loss of antiviral activity or increased toxicities. In the era of combination therapy with protease inhibitor–containing regimens, it becomes all the more critical for providers to query patients in full detail regarding their use of other substances that have an impact on hepatic metabolic pathways.

Allicin and Malaleuca

Whereas many of the reported trials of alternative interventions over the years have produced either negative results or data that are inherently biased by the interpretation of the investigator, two agents presented in results of small pilot studies at the 1996 International AIDS Conference in Vancouver warrant mention. Allicin is a high-dose garlic concentrate from China, used there mainly to treat refractory diarrhea.[80] It is generally well tolerated but does produce a strong garlic taste and smell in those who use it. A 6-week pilot study of allicin 30 mg twice daily was conducted in 20 patients with intractable *Cryptosporidium parvum* diarrhea by the Los Angeles community-based clinical trials group Search Alliance. The median CD4 cell count was $18/mm^3$ and all patients were on antiretroviral therapy and prophylaxis for opportunistic infections. Cryptosporidium was newly diagnosed in five patients; an additional five were within a month of being diagnosed. Of 16 evaluable patients, 10 reported a decrease in stool frequency with stable or increased body weight. Patients who showed clinical improvement were allowed to extend their participation beyond the initial 6-week pilot period. Stools became negative for *Cryptosporidium* organisms in four of the eight patients who received treatment for more than 8 weeks. Spontaneous resolution of cryptosporidiosis would not expected in patients with such marked immune suppression and low CD4 lymphocyte counts.

Tea tree oil, an extract from an Australian bush (*Malaleuca*), is but one malaleuca extract used as a natural remedy and appreciated for its broad antibiotic activities. It has shown excellent in vitro activity against isolates of *Candida* species. Malaleuca products, including soaps, impregnated dental floss and toothpicks, and mouthwashes, are available over the counter in natural food stores. A trial of 15 ml of malaleuca oral solution (Breathaway) used in a "swish and spit" fashion four times a day for 2 to 4 weeks in 14 patients with clinical and mycologic resistant thrush found that 5 of the 12 evaluable patients were cured, 5 improved, and 2 had no response.[81] A mycologic response with clearing of *Candida* was documented in eight patients, all of whom had responded clinically. There were no relapses perceived 4 weeks off treatment. The treatment was well tolerated, although nausea may result if the solution is inadvertently swallowed. Oral blistering was rare. The CPCRA has been attempting to conduct a controlled clinical trial comparing malaleuca mouthwash to other interventions in patients with refractory oral *Candida*, but the trial has been postponed because of regulatory obstacles.

Massage Therapy

Another study reported at the 1996 International AIDS Conference had less positive results than the allicin and malaleuca trials. Although massage has frequently been used to provide general relaxation of the body, its effect on immune function has received little study. Therefore, 42 HIV-infected individuals with no active medical symptoms (median CD4 lymphocyte count at entry was $355/mm^3$) were evaluated in a study to assess the effects of massage therapy alone or in combination with either exercise training or stress management counseling on immune function and quality of life.[82] The investigators hypothesized that immune function may be further suppressed by chronic anxiety and depression. Patients were randomized to receive, for 12 weeks, either massage only, massage and exercise, massage and stress management, or nothing at all (control). Only the control group demonstrated an increase in CD4+ lymphocytes; the massage and exercise and massage and stress management cohorts sustaining a drop in CD4 counts, and the massage-only group showed no significant change. Neither CD8+ lymphocyte nor natural killer cell counts changed significantly in any group. No significant differences were found among the groups on any of the quality-of-life measures comparing pre- and poststudy values. The authors concluded that short-term massage therapy alone or combined with either exercise training or stress management counseling did not have any significant impact on immune function or quality-of-life measures and that "these alternative therapies, while not harmful, should not be used as substitutes for more conventional therapies for HIV infected persons."[82] As is the case with any attempt to investigate alternative interventions scientifically, proponents of massage therapy may question the power of the study based on the sample size enrolled, whether the appropriate massage techniques were used, whether the appropriate patient population was investigated, and whether the correct immune variables were monitored. However, massage therapy is not likely to be a detrimental intervention in patients with HIV infection. Therefore, as with most of the other alternatives in current widespread use, clinical investigations are not likely to influence those who strongly adhere to their favorite alternative intervention.

THE OFFICE OF ALTERNATIVE MEDICINE

In 1993 the NIH established the Office of Alternative Medicine.[83] In 1995, Bastyr University in Seattle, a naturopathic institution, received funding from the OAM to become a center for HIV alternative studies, and has established a national data base cohort of HIV-infected individuals who are using alternative therapies.[84] Follow-up information on outcome measures is being collected on patients who use a wide variety of alternative interventions. In addition, the OAM has provided seed funding to investigators conducting small pilot interventional trials in patients with HIV. An ad hoc subcommittee reviewing the NIH response to AIDS recommended that the OAM work closely with the FDA to set up guidelines for investigation of alternative treatment interventions. They suggested that the FDA review their regulatory requirements and evaluate whether or not they are appropriate in the investigation of alternative therapies, and recommended that individuals with expertise in the fields of complementary and alternative medicine be integrated into NIH review panels and advisory committees.

CONCLUSIONS

The history of the alternative therapies movement over the past 15 years suggests that the current lull in the popularity of alternative therapies among patients with HIV infection may in fact be transient. Even though potent combination antiretroviral drug regimens are available, individuals with HIV infection are still interested in treatments complementary to their orthodox therapies, especially for manifestations of HIV infection for which satisfactory agents are not being prescribed by their physicians. Obviously, pharmacokinetic interaction studies cannot be undertaken on every alternative treatment a patient with HIV infection might ingest. However, the possibility of hepatic damage or drug–alternative therapy interactions that may alter the concentration of antiretroviral agents, particularly protease inhibitors, increases the stakes in the current era of HIV therapeutics. Providers should therefore question their patients regarding the use of alternative therapies,

counsel them as completely as possible regarding possible concerns, and document use of these interventions in the patient's medical record. To do so effectively, caregivers must stay informed about agents in widespread use, consulting available references and resources to ensure, as much as possible, the continued well-being of patients who use alternative therapies for their HIV infection.

References

1. Abrams DI: Dealing with alternative therapies for HIV. In Sande MA, Volberding P (eds): The Medical Management of AIDS, 5th ed. Philadelphia, WB Saunders Company, 1997, p 143
2. Abrams DI: Alternative therapies. In Repoza NP (ed): HIV Infection and Disease: Monographs for Physicians and Other Health Care Workers. Chicago, AMA Press, 1989, p 163
3. Abrams DI: Alternative therapies in HIV infection. AIDS 4:1179, 1990
4. Abrams DI: Dealing with alternative therapies for HIV. In Sande MA, Volberding P (eds): The Medical Management of AIDS, 4th ed. Philadelphia, WB Saunders Company, 1995, p 183
5. Abrams DI: Alternative therapies. In Wormser G (ed): A Clinical Guide to AIDS and HIV. Philadelphia, Lippincott-Raven, 1996, p 379
6. Greenblatt RM, Hollander H, McMaster JR, et al: Polylypharmacy among patients attending an AIDS clinic: Utilization of prescribed, unorthodox, and investigational treatments. J Acquir Immune Defic Syndr 4:136, 1991
7. Mayer K, Seage G, Gross M, et al: Predictors of therapeutic choices among HIV-infected homosexual males. In Abstracts of the IXth International Conference on AIDS, Berlin, 1993, Abstract PO-B32-2236
8. Anderson WH: Patient use and assessment of conventional and alternative therapies for HIV infection and AIDS. AIDS 74:561, 1993
9. Laifer G, Ruettimann S, Langewitz W, et al: Frequent use of alternative therapies and higher subjective benefit compared to traditional medicine in HIV-infected patients. In Abstracts of the VIIIth International Conference on AIDS, Amsterdam, 1992, Abstract PO-B-3395
10. Valentine C, Weston R, Kitchen V, et al: Anonymous questionnaire to assess consumption of prescribed and alternative medication and patterns of recreational drug use in an HIV positive population. In Abstracts of the VIIIth International Conference on AIDS, Amsterdam, 1992, Abstract TH-B-1508
11. Van Dam F, De Boer J, Cleijne W, et al: The use of remedies and alternative therapies by patients with symptomatic HIV infection. In Abstracts of the VIIIth International Conference on AIDS, Amsterdam, 1992, Abstract PO-B-3402
12. Ostrow M, Cornelisse PGA, Hogg RS, et al: Patterns of complementary therapy use in a province wide HIV/AIDS drug distribution program. In Abstracts of the XIth International Conference on AIDS, Vancouver, 1996, Abstract Th.B.4095
13. Lubeck D, O'Driscoll PT, Morfeld DH, Williams CA: Use of "non-traditional" treatments by persons with

HIV infection who are receiving "traditional" care from primary care physicians. In Abstracts of the XIth International Conference on AIDS, Vancouver, 1996, Abstract Th.D.5119

14. Berrier J, Young M, Barkan S, et al: Use of complementary/alternative therapies by HIV+ women: The Women's Interagency HIV Study (WIHS). In Abstracts of the XIth International Conference on AIDS, Vancouver, 1996, Abstract Th.D.5120

15. Collins RL, Kanouse DE, Senterfitt JW, et al: Use of alternative treatment for HIV: Patterns and correlates. In Abstracts of the XIth International Conference on AIDS, Vancouver, 1996, Abstract Mo.B.183

16. Eisenberg DM, Kessler RC, Foster C, et al: Unconventional medicine in the United States: Prevalence, costs and patterns of use. N Engl J Med 328:246, 1993

17. Harakeh S, Jariwalla RJ, Pauling L: Suppression of human immunodeficiency virus replication by ascorbate in chronically and acutely infected cells. Proc Natl Acad Sci U S A 87:7245, 1990

18. Jariwalla RJ, Harakeh S: HIV suppression by ascorbate and its enhancement by glutathione precursor. In Abstracts of the VIIIth International Conference on AIDS, Amsterdam, 1992, Abstract PO-B-3697

19. Mills BL: Stimulation of T-cellular immunity by cutaneous application of dinitrochlorobenzene. J Am Acad Dermatol 6:1089, 1986

20. Stricker RB, Elswood BF, Abrams DI: Dendritic cells and dinitrochlorobenzene (DNCB): A new treatment approach to AIDS. Immunol Lett 29:191, 1991

21. Stricker RB, Elswood BF: Topical dinitrochlorobenzene in HIV disease. J Am Acad Dermatol 28:796, 1993

22. Fischl MA, Richman DD, Hansen N, et al: Azidothymidine (AZT) in the treatment of patients with AIDS and AIDS-related complex: A double-blind, placebo-controlled trial. N Engl J Med 317:185, 1987

23. Fischl MA, Richman DD, Hansen N, et al: The safety and efficacy of zidovudine (AZT) in the treatment of subjects with mildly symptomatic human immunodeficiency virus type 1 (HIV) infection: A double-blind, placebo trial. Ann Intern Med 112:727, 1990

24. Volberding PA, Lagakos SW, Koch MA, et al: Zidovudine in asymptomatic human immunodeficiency virus infection: A controlled trial in persons with fewer than 500 CD4-positive cells per cubic millimeter. N Engl J Med 322:941, 1990

25. Cooley TP, Kunches LM, Saunders CA, et al: Once-daily administration of 2,3-dideoxyinosine (ddI) in patients with acquired immunodeficiency syndrome or AIDS-related complex. Results of a Phase I trial. N Engl J Med 322:1340, 1990

26. Lambert JS, Seidlin N, Reichman RC, et al: 2',3'-dideoxyinosine (ddI) in patients with the acquired immunodeficiency syndrome or AIDS-related complex: A phase I trial. N Engl J Med 322:1333, 1990

27. Aboulker JR, Swart AM: Preliminary analysis of the Concorde trial. Lancet 341:889, 1993

28. Concorde Coordinating Committee. Concorde: MRC/ANRS randomised double-blind controlled trial of immediate and deferred zidovudine in symptom-free HIV infection. Lancet 343:871, 1994

29. Eron JJ, Benoit SL, Jemsek J, et al: Treatment with lamivudine, zidovudine, or both in HIV-infected patients with 200 to 500 CD4+ cells per cubic millimeter. N Engl J Med 333:1662, 1995

30. Kitchen VS, Skinner C, Ariyoshi K, et al: Safety and efficacy of saquinavir in HIV infection. Lancet 345: 952, 1995

31. Markowitz M, Saag M, Powderly WG, et al: A preliminary study of ritonavir, an inhibitor of HIV-1 protease, to treat HIV-1 infection. N Engl J Med 333: 1534, 1995

32. Danner SA, Carr A, Leonard JM, et al: A short term study of the safety, pharmacokinetics, and efficacy of ritonavir, an inhibitor of HIV-1 protease. N Engl J Med 333: 1528, 1995

33. Gulick R, Mellors J, Havir D, et al: Potent and sustained antiretroviral activity of indinavir in combination with zidovudine and lamivudine. In Abstracts of the 3rd Conference on Retroviruses and Opportunistic Infections, Washington, DC, p 162

34. Eisenberg DM: Advising patients who seek alternative medical therapies. Ann Intern Med 127:61, 1997

35. King R, Homsy J, Serufilira A, et al: Traditional medicine vs. modern medicine for AIDS. In Abstracts of the VIIIth International Conference on AIDS, Amsterdam, 1992, Abstract PO-B-3394

36. Homsy J, Kabatesi D, Kwamya L, et al: Traditional medicine is a valid local alternative for the treatment of chronic diarrhea and herpes zoster in AIDS patients in Kampala, Uganda. In Abstracts of the XIth International Conference on AIDS, Vancouver, 1996, Abstract Mo.B.300

37. Chang RY, Kong XB: Meta-survey of plant and herb material as treatment for HIV. In Abstracts of the XIth International Conference on AIDS, Vancouver, 1996, Abstract Mo.B.303

38. Hazadu D, Blau C, Felock P, et al: Isolation and characterization of a novel class of human immunodeficiency virus integrase inhibitors from natural product screening. In Abstracts of the XIth International Conference on AIDS, Vancouver, 1996, Abstract Mo.A.1020

39. Burack JH, Cohen MR, Hahn JA, Abrams DI: A pilot randomized controlled trial of Chinese herbal treatment for HIV-associated symptoms. J Acquir Immune Defic Syndr 12:386, 1996

39a. Shlay JC, Chaloner K, Max MB, et al: Acupuncture and amitriptyline for pain due to HIV-related peripheral neuropathy. JAMA 280:1590, 1998

40. Block G, Henson DE, Levine M: Vitamin C: A new look. Ann Intern Med 114:909, 1991

41. Buhl R, Ari Jaffe H, Holroyd KS, et al: Systemic glutathione deficiency in symptom-free HIV-seropositive individuals. Lancet 2:1294, 1989

42. Staal FJT, Ela SW, Roederer M, et al: Glutathione deficiency and human immunodeficiency virus infection. Lancet 339:909, 1992

43. Staal JFT, Roederer M, Anderson MT, et al: Intracellular glutathione deficiency in AIDS: Implication for therapy. In Abstracts of the VIIIth International Conference on AIDS, Amsterdam, 1992, Abstract PO-A-2400

44. Roderer M, Stahl FJI, Raju PA, et al: Cytokine-stimulated human immunodeficiency viruses replication is inhibited by N-acetyl-L-cysteine. Proc Natl Acad Sci USA 87:4884, 1990

45. Kalebic T, Kinter A, Poli G, et al: Suppression of human immunodeficiency virus expression in chronically infected monocytic cells by glutathione, glutathione ester and N-acetylcysteine. Proc Natl Acad Sci USA 88:986, 1991

46. Mihm S, Ennen J, Pessara U, et al: Inhibition of HIV-1 replication and NF-nB activity by cysteine and cysteine derivatives. AIDS 5:497, 1991

47. Lahdevirta J, Maury CP, Teppo AM, et al: Elevated levels of circulating cachectin/tumor necrosis factor in

patients with acquired immunodeficiency syndrome. Am J Med 85:289, 1988

48. Folks TM, Clouse KA, Justement J, et al: Tumor necrosis factor alpha induces expression of human immunodeficiency virus in a chronically infected T cell clone. Proc Natl Acad Sci USA 86:2365, 1989

49. Fauci AS: Multifactorial nature of human immunodeficiency virus disease: Implication for therapy. Science 262:1011, 1993

50. Walker RE, Lane H, Boenning C, et al: The safety, pharmacokinetics, and antiviral activity of N-aceylcysteine in HIV-infected individuals. In Abstracts of the VIIIth International Conference on AIDS, Amsterdam, 1992, Abstract MO-B-0022

51. Nottet HSLM, van Asbeck BS, de Graaf L, et al: Role for oxygen radicals in the self-sustained HIV-1 replication in monocyte-derived macrophages: Enhanced HIV-1 replication by N-acetyl-L-cysteine. In Abstracts of the IXth International Conference on AIDS, Berlin, 1993, Abstract PO-A12-0199

52. Staak K, Prosch S, Stein J, et al: Pentoxifylline promotes replication of human cytomegalovirus in vivo and in vitro. Blood 89:3682, 1997

53. Herzenberg LA, DeRosa SC, Dubs JG, et al: Glutathione deficiency is associated with impaired survival in HIV disease. Proc Natl Acad Sci USA 94:1967, 1997

54. Sampaio EP, Moreira AL, Sarno EN, et al: Prolonged treatment with recombinant interferon-γ induces erythema nodosum leprosum in lepromatous leprosy patients. J Exp Med 175:1729, 1992

55. Moreira AL, Sampaio EP, Zmuidzinas A, et al: Thalidomide exerts its inhibitory action on TNF-alpha by enhancing mRNA degradation. J Exp Med 177:1675, 1993

56. Tramontana JM, Utzipatu M, Molloy A, et al: Thalidomide treatment reduces tumor necrosis factor production and enhances weight gain in patients with pulmonary tuberculosis. Mol Med 1:384, 1995

57. Makonkawkeyoon S, Limson-Probre RNR, Moreira AL, et al: Thalidomide inhibits replication of human immunodeficiency virus type 1. Proc Natl Acad Sci USA 90:5974 1993

58. Moreira AL, Ye W, Shen Z, et al: Thalidomide reduces HIV-1 production in acutely infected human monocytes in vitro. In Abstracts of the 3rd Conference on Retroviruses and Opportunistic Infections, Washington, DC, 1996, Abstract 313

59. Cooper S: Thalidomide, gentrified: Notes from the Underground: The PWA Health Group Newsletter 31: 1, 1996

60. Jacobson JM, Greenspan JS, Spritzler J, et al: Thalidomide for the treatment of oral aphthous ulcers in patients with human immunodeficiency virus infection. N Engl J Med 336:1487, 1997

61. FDA Talking Paper: Advisory Committee recommends thalidomide approval. Washington, DC, Food and Drug Administration, 1997

62. Gorter R, Seefried M, Volberding P: Dronabinol effects on weight in patients with HIV infection. AIDS 6:127, 1992

63. Mulligan K, Grunfeld C, Hellerstein MK, et al: Anabolic effects of recombinant human growth hormone in patients with weight loss associated with HIV infection. J Clin Endocrinol Metab 77:956, 1993

64. Oster MH, Enders SH, Samuels ST, et al: Megestrol acetate in patients with AIDS and cachexia. Ann Intern Med 121:400, 1994

65. Struwe M, Kaemfper SH, Geiger CF, et al: Effect of dronabinol on nutritional status in HIV infection. Ann Pharmacol 27:827, 1993

66. von Roenn JH, Armstrong D, Kotler DP, et al: Megestrol acetate in patients with AIDS related cachexia. Ann Intern Med 121:393, 1994

67. Bhasin S, Storer T, Berman N, et al: The effects of supraphysiologic doses of testosterone on muscle size and strength in normal men. N Engl J Med 335:1, 1996

68. Dobs AS, Dempsy MA, Landenson PW, et al: Endocrine disorders in men infected with HIV. Am J Med 84:611, 1988

69. Place VA, Atkinson L, Prather DA, et al: Transdermal testosterone replacement through genital skin. In Nieschlag E, Behre HM (eds): Testosterone — Action, Deficiency, Substitution. Berlin, Springer-Verlag, 1990, p 165

70. Merril CR, Harrington MG: Plasma dehydroepiandrosterone levels in HIV infection. JAMA 261:1149, 1989

71. Dyner TS, Lang W, Geaga J, et al: An open-label dose-escalation trial of oral dehydroepiandrosterone tolerance and pharmacokinetics in patients with HIV disease. J Acquir Immune Defic Syndr 6:459, 1993

72. Gold J, High H, Li Y, et al: Safety and efficacy of nandralone decanoate for treatment of wasting in patients with HIV infection. AIDS 10:745, 1996

73. Grinspoon L, Bakalar JB, Doblin R: Marijuana as medicine: A plea for reconsideration. JAMA 273: 1875, 1995

74. Kassirer JP: Federal foolishness and marijuana. N Engl J Med 336:366, 1997

74a. Child CC, Mitchell TF, Abrams DI: Patterns of therapeutic marijuana use in two community-based cannabis buyers' cooperatives. In Abstracts of the 12th World AIDS Conference, Geneva, 1998, Abstract 60569, p 1105

75. Abrams DI, Child CC, Mitchell TF: Marijuana, the AIDS wasting syndrome, and the U.S. government [response]. N Engl J Med 333:671, 1995

76. Grinspoon L, Bakalar JB, Doblin R: Marijuana, the AIDS wasting syndrome, and the U.S. Government. N Engl J Med 333:670, 1995

77. Steele FR: Keeping a lid on marijuana research. Nat Med 1:853, 1995

78. Hollister LE: Hunger and appetite and single doses of marijuana, alcohol, and dextroamphetamine. Clin Pharmacol Ther 12:44, 1971

79. Greenberg I, Kuenhle J, Mendelson JH, Bernstein JG: Effects of marijuana use on body weight and caloric intake in humans. Psychopharmacology 49:79, 1976

80. Search Alliance: Allicin in cryptosporidium diarrhea. Searchlight, Spring 1994

81. Vasquez JA, Vaishampayan J, Arganoza MT, et al: Use of an over-the-counter product, Breathaway® (Malaleuca oral solution) as an alternative agent for refractory oropharyngeal candidiasis in AIDS patients. In Abstracts of the XIth International Conference on AIDS, Vancouver, 1996, Abstract We.B.3305

82. Birk TJ, MacArthur RD, McGrady A, Khuder S: Lack of effect of 12 weeks of massage therapy on immune function and quality of life in HIV-infected persons. In Abstracts of the XIth International Conference on AIDS, Vancouver, 1996, Abstract Th.B.4105

83. Marwick C: Alternative medicine office urged to act rapidly. JAMA 270:1409, 1993

84. Standish LJ, Calabrese C, Reeves C: Nationwide longitudinal outcomes study of HIV/AIDS alternative therapies. In Abstracts of the XIth International Conference on AIDS, Vancouver, 1996, Abstract Mo.B.181

Index

Note: Page numbers in *italics* refer to illustrations; page numbers followed by t refer to tables.

Abacavir (ABC), 99t, 103
  combination therapy with, 101t, 103
  dosage of, 98t
  for AIDS dementia, 227
  HIV mutations and, *55,* 99t
Abdominal girth, enlargement of, from antiretroviral therapy, 292
ABVD therapy, for Hodgkin's disease, 485, 486
Acanthamoebiasis, 189
ACE (angiotensin-converting enzyme) inhibitors, 300
Acquired immunodeficiency syndrome (AIDS). See *Human immunodeficiency virus (HIV) disease.*
  in children. See *Pediatric AIDS.*
Acupuncture, in HIV disease management, 604–605
Acute necrotizing ulcerative gingivitis (ANUG), 161
Acyclovir, adverse effects of, depression from, 244
  for HSV, 162, 186t, 197t, 198, 200, 441–442, 442t, 444, 444t, 445, 446, 547, 603
    dosage adjustment for, in renal dysfunction, 442, 442t
    in pregnancy, 565–566
    ocular, 174
    prophylactic, 132, 446, 565–566
    resistance to, 441, 445–446
  for VZV, 186t
    ophthalmic, 171, 447, 448t
Addison's disease, 287
Adenoviruses, gastrointestinal infections with, 200
Adolescents, HIV infection in, 532. See also *Children, HIV infection in.*
Adrenal disease, 286–288, 297
Adrenal insufficiency, fatigue from, 256t
Adrenocorticotropin (ACTH), 286, 287
Adriamycin, cardiomyopathy from, 280
Africa, sub-Saharan, HIV 2 in, 3–4
  HIV infection in, 3, *4,* 499
  HIV prevention programs in, 506
African Americans, female, HIV infection in, 537
  HIV infection in, 6, 7, 13–14
    by age, 594t
AIDS (acquired immunodeficiency syndrome). See *Human immunodeficiency virus (HIV) disease.*
  pediatric. See *Pediatric AIDS.*
AIDS cholangiopathy, 207–208, 208t
AIDS dementia complex (ADC), 221, 222–227, 223t, 431
  classification of, 222, 223t
  clinical presentation of, 223–224, 223t
  CSF examination in, 224, 226
  depression and, 250

AIDS dementia complex (*Continued*)
  differential diagnosis of, 222
  etiology and pathogenesis of, 226–227
  in older patients, 596
  neuroimaging in, 224, 225t
  neuropathology of, 226
  neuropsychological profile in, 224
  treatment of, 227, 250
AIN. See *Anal intraepithelial neoplasia (AIN).*
Alcohol use, nonadherence to antiretroviral therapy and, 117
Aldosterone deficiency, 287
Allicin, 609
Alprazolam, 252, 252t
  drug interactions with, 88t
Alternative Medicine, Office of, 610
Alternative therapies, for HIV disease, 601–610. See also individual therapies, e.g., *Acupuncture.*
Amenorrhea, HIV infection and, 547–548
Amikacin, for *Mycobacterium avium*-complex, 345, 346
  in gastrointestinal disease, 201
  for *Mycobacterium tuberculosis,* 356t
Amitriptyline, 246, 248
  acupuncture therapy vs., 605
  dosage of, 247t
Amniocentesis, 557
Amoxicillin, for gingivitis and periodontitis, 161
  for *Streptococcus pneumoniae,* 333, 333t
Amoxicillin-clavulanate, for gingivitis and periodontitis, 161
Amphetamines, 584, 586
  drug interactions with, 88t
  effects of, 586t
Amphotericin B, adverse effects of, 365, 368
  for aspergillosis, 336
  for candidiasis, 158
  for coccidioidomycosis, 338, 374
  for cryptococcosis, 336, 338, 365, 366t, *367,* 367–368, 368t
    maintenance regimen of, 369–370
  for histoplasmosis, 338, 372, 372t
  for *Penicillium marneffei,* 425
  for pneumonia, 341
Amplicor HIV-1 RNA Monitor assay, 52
Amprenavir, 105
  adverse effects of, 98t
  dosage of, 98t
  HIV mutations and, *55,* 99t
  resistance to, 105
Anabolic steroids, for wasting syndrome, 608, 608t
Anal intercourse, HIV transmission via, 505, 538, 539t
  neoplasia and, 545–546

Anal intraepithelial neoplasia (AIN), 129. See also *Anogenital neoplasms.*
  in homosexuals, 129, 488
  in women, 545–546
Anemia, 266–268, 267t
  drug-induced, 267t, 268
    by ganciclovir, 435, 436t
    by zidovudine, 79
    in pregnancy, 561
  etiology and diagnosis of, 267–268, 267t
  fatigue from, 256t
  macrocytic, 267t
  microcytic, 267t
  normocytic, 267t
  of chronic disease, 265–266
Angiosarcoma, differential diagnosis of, 416
Angiotensin-converting enzyme (ACE) inhibitors, 300
Angle-closure glaucoma, 175
Anisopoikilocytosis, 266
Anogenital neoplasms, 128–129, 468, 486, 488–489
  HPV and, 486, 488–489
  screening for, 128–129, 489t
Anorectal infections, from HSV, 439–440, *440,* Color Plate IIF
Anorexia, AIDS-related, 291
Antibody tests, for HIV, *46,* 46–49, *47*
Anticonvulsant drugs, adverse effect(s) of, depression as, 244
  mania as, 254
  psychosis as, 255
Antidiuretic hormone, syndrome of inappropriate secretion of, 286, 297
Antiemetic agents, for pregnant women, 566
Antigen test with p24 protein, 44, *45,* 49–50, *50, 53,* 53t, 70–71, 517
  acidified procedure for, 50
  for primary HIV infection, 70–71, 72, 74
  in children, *527*
Antihistamines, drug interactions with, 90t
Antimania drugs, 254, 254t
Antimotility agents, 201
Antineoplastic agents. See also specific agents and combination therapies.
  for Hodgkin's disease, 485
  for Kaposi's sarcoma, 473–474, 473t, 477t
  for non-Hodgkin's lymphoma, 480, 481t, 482
Antioxidants, in HIV disease management, 604t, 605–606
Antipsychotic medications, 251, 252t
  drug interactions with, 90t
Antiretroviral Pregnancy Registry, 562
Antiretroviral therapy, 97–113, 129. See also individual drugs.
  adherence to, 117–121
  failure of, HIV resistance from, 117
    risk factors in, 117–118
    for suppression of HIV replication, 118–119
    importance of, 117, *118*
    improving, 119–120
    problems with, 109
    success rates in, 119
  adverse effects of, 79–83, 80t
    abnormal fat distribution from, 292
    cutaneous, 190
    depression from, 244
    gastrointestinal, 195, 201–203, 202t
    hematologic, 270–271
    hepatic, 205–207, 206t
    in pregnancy, 562, 564–565

Antiretroviral therapy (*Continued*)
    toxic axonal neuropathy from, 231–232
  choice of agents for, 109–110, 110t
  combination. See also individual drugs.
    for AIDS dementia, 227, 250
    for children, 528–531, 530t
    for HIV-related thrombocytopenia, 269
    for primary HIV disease, 67, 75, 110
    for women, 112, 548
      pregnant, 112, 563–565
    Mycobacterium avium-complex and, 344, 347–348
    recommendations for, 109–110, 110t
    trials of, 100t–101t
  dermatologic conditions and, 185, 193
  drug interactions with, 83–93
    and illicit drugs, 582–583
  failure of, risk factors for, 111t
  for AIDS dementia, 227, 250
  for children, 528–531
    changing, 531
    initial, 529–531, 530t
    principles for, 528–529
    starting, 529
  for Kaposi's sarcoma, 468, 475–476, 477t
  for older patients, 596–598
  for primary HIV disease, 67, 75, 112
  for women, 548
  gastrointestinal infections and, 210
  HIV pathogenesis and, 97
  HIV quantitation and, 99
  in pregnancy, 112, 499, 504–505, 519, 561–565
    adverse effects of, 562, 564–565
    for advanced disease, 564
    for early disease, 563
    for moderately advanced disease, 563
    intrapartum, 569, 570t
  in prison, 581
  individualization of, 120
  initiation of, 109
  key clinical questions regarding, 109–112
  modification of, 110–111, 111t
  patient education regarding, 120
  prophylactic use of, 503
    perinatal, 112, 499
    postexposure, 111–112, 518–521, 520t, 521t
  stopping, 111
Antituberculous agents, 355–358, 356t, 578. See also individual drugs.
  adverse effects of, 356t
  combination regimens with, 355, 356t, 357t
  dosages for, 356t, 357t
  drug interactions with, 356–357
  empiric use of, 341
  for drug users, 578
  nonadherence to, 118
  resistance to, 357–358
ANUG (acute necrotizing ulcerative gingivitis), 161
Anxiety, in HIV-infected patients, 241, 252–253
  treatment of, 252–253, 252t
Anxiolytics, 252–253, 252t
Aphthous ulcers, diagnosis and treatment of, 197t
  esophageal, 198
  genital, in women, 547
  recurrent, 159t, 164
Arrhythmias, 281
Arthralgia, in primary HIV infection, 67, 68t
Arthropod-borne disease, *Bartonella* from, 421
Artificial insemination, 559
Asia, HIV infection in, 3, *4*

Aspergillosis, chest films of, 145
  choroiditis from, 177
  esophageal, 197t
  oral, 159t
  orbital manifestations of, 178
  pulmonary, 336, 337t
    differential diagnosis of, 422
    treatment of, 336
  thyroid disease from, 288
Aspirin, drug interactions with, 85
Astemizole, drug interactions with, 88t
  for eosinophilic folliculitis, 186t
Atovaquone, adverse effects of, 318t, 322
  drug interactions with, 85
  for *Pneumocystis carinii,* 317, 318t, 321–322
    prophylactic, 131, 131t, 324t, 325
  for toxoplasmosis, 386t, 388
    in maintenance therapy, 389, 389t
Augmentin, for *Mycobacterium tuberculosis,* 356t
Azithromycin, for *Haemophilus influenzae,* 334
  for *Mycobacterium avium*-complex, 345, 346, 347t
    in gastrointestinal disease, 201
    prophylactic, 131t, 132, 348
  for toxoplasmosis, 386t, 388, 389
    in maintenance therapy, 389, 389t
AZT. See *Zidovudine (AZT).*

Bacillary angiomatosis, 411–422
  clinical presentation of, 411–416
  cutaneous, 412, *413–414*
    treatment of, 420
  diagnosis of, 186t
  gastrointestinal, 412–413
  hepatic, 412
    treatment of, 420
  history of, 411
  lymphatic, 412, 413
  ocular, 177
    differential diagnosis of, 172
  oral, 162
  osseous, 412, *413*
    treatment of, 420
  respiratory, 412–413
  splenic, 412
    treatment of, 420
  treatment of, 186t, 418–420, *419,* 420t
Bacillus, keratitis from, 174
BACTEC system, for *Bartonella,* 417
  for *Mycobacterium avium*-complex, 345
Bacteremia, from *Bartonella,* 411, 415–416, 417
  from *Rhodococcus equi,* 422–423
Bacterial infections. See also individual infections.
  cutaneous, 185, 186t, 187–188
  gastrointestinal, 200–201
  keratitis from, 174
  oral, 159t
  pneumonia from, 132, 331–335, 332t
    in drug users, 578
  prophylaxis for, 132
  retinitis from, 177
Bartonella, bacteremia from, 411, 415–416, 417
    treatment of, 420–421
  diagnosis of, 416–418
    cultures for, 417–418
    histopathologic, 416, *417*
    serologic, 416
  infections with, 411–422. See also *Bacillary angiomatosis.*

Bartonella (Continued)
  clinical presentation of, 411–416
  epidemiology of, 421
  neuropsychiatric manifestations of, 413
  prevention of, 421–422
  treatment of, 418–421
    antibiotics for, 418, *419,* 420t
    for relapses, 420
Bartonella bacilliformis, 411, 416
Bartonella clarridgeiae, 411
Bartonella dashiae, 411
Bartonella elizabethae, 411
  bacteremia from, 416
Bartonella grahamii, 411
Bartonella henselae, 411, 412, 417
  epidemiology and prevention of, 421
  peliosis hepatis from, 205, 411, 412
  treatment of, 418, 420
Bartonella quintana, 411, 412
  bacteremia from, 415, 416, 417
  epidemiology and prevention of, 421
  treatment of, 418, 420
Bartonella taylorii, 411
Bartonella vinsonii, 411
Behavior change interventions, for prevention of HIV transmission, 500–502
Bereavement, 257
  Beta$_2$-microglobulin, HIV and, 57
Biliary manifestations, in HIV disease, 207–208, 208t
Bisexuals, HIV infection in, 14. See also *Lesbians; Men who have sex with men.*
  transmission of, 540–541, 541t
  syphilis in, 453
Bladder incontinence, in AIDS dementia, 224
Blastomycosis, 336
Bleomycin, for Hodgkin's disease, 485
  for Kaposi's sarcoma, 473t, 474
  for non-Hodgkin's lymphoma, 481t, 482
Blood-brain barrier, antiretroviral therapy and, 227
Blood count, for HIV-infected patient, 128
Blood cultures, for *Bartonella,* 417–418
  for *Haemophilus influenzae,* 334
  for *Pseudomonas aeruginosa,* 335
  for *Streptococcus pneumoniae,* 332
Blood products, radiolabeled, accidental infusion of HIV-infected, 515–516
Blood transfusions, for drug-induced anemia, 79
Body lice, and *Bartonella,* 421
Body substance isolation (BSI), 516
Bone disease, in bacillary angiomatosis, 412, *413,* 420
  in syphilis, 455
Bone marrow, antiretroviral therapy toxicity to, 270–271
  biopsies of, 265, 266
  disorders of, 265–266
    diagnosis of, 266
    morphology of, 265
    nutrition and, 265–266
  in bacillary angiomatosis, 413–414
Bowel incontinence. See also *Diarrhea.*
  in AIDS dementia, 224
Brachial plexopathy, 218
Brain abscess, from *Rhodococcus equi,* 423
Brain biopsy, for toxoplasmosis, 381, 383, *385, 480*
Brain disease, diffuse, 221–227
  focal, 225t, 227–230, 227t
Branched-chain DNA assay, for HIV, 50, 52, *53, 60,* 125
Breast enlargement, from protease inhibitors, 106
Breast milk, HIV transmission by, 67, 505
Bronchiectasis, 147

Bronchitis, chest films of, 147, *147*
   incidence of, 332t
   prevention of, 132
Bronchoalveolar lavage, for *Cryptococcus,* 336
   for *Pneumocystis carinii,* 139, 305–306, *314,* 315
   for *Rhodococcus equi,* 423
   for *Toxoplasma gondii,* 382
Bronchogenic carcinoma, chest films of, 148–149
Bronchopleural fistula, from *Pneumocystis carinii* pneumonia, 312, 313
Bronchoscopy, in pneumonia, 339
"Buffalo hump," from protease inhibitors, 106, 292
Bullous impetigo, 187
Buprenorphine, 587, 588–589
   adverse effects of, 588
   antiretroviral therapy interaction with, 582
Bupropion, 246, 248
   dosage of, 247t
   mania from, 254
Burkitt's lymphoma, 478
Buspirone, for anxiety, 252–253, 252t
   mania from, 254
   psychosis from, 255

Calcium channel blockers, drug interactions with, 88t
Calmette-Guérin vaccine, 130
Campylobacter jejuni, clinical manifestations of, 201
   differential diagnosis of, 432
Cancer. See *Neoplasms*; specific neoplasm, e.g., *Lymphoma.*
Candida albicans, 158
Candida glabrata, 158
Candida krusei, 158
Candida tropicalis, 158
Candidiasis, choroiditis from, 177
   erythematous, *157, 159t,* 160
   esophageal, 196, 197t, 198
     and progression of HIV disease, 126
     differential diagnosis of, 432, 440
     epidemiology of, 11
     in drug users, 576
     in older patients, 596
     in women, 542
   gastrointestinal, 200
   in primary HIV infection, 68t, 69, 126
   keratitis from, 174
   oral, 157–158, 159t, *160*
   pneumonia from, 336, 337t
   pseudomembranous, *157, 159t,* 160
   treatment of, 197t
     Malaleuca for, 609
   vaginal, 546
Capnocytophaga, keratitis from, 174
Capreomycin, for *Mycobacterium tuberculosis,* 358
   dosage of, 356t
Caprine arthritis–encephalitis virus, 24
Carbamazepine, 254, 254t
   drug interactions with, 88t
Cardiac tamponade, 277
Cardiomyopathy, treatment of, 280–281
Cardiovalvular disorders, 276, 281
Cardiovascular complications, of HIV disease, 275–283. See also specific disorders.
Cardiovascular examination, 276–277
Cardiovascular procedures, in HIV-infected patients, 282
Caregiver issues, 257–258
Case management, for HIV-infected patients, 133–134
Cat-scratch disease, 411, 421

Cats, *Bartonella* and, 421
CCR5 chemokine receptor, 25–26, *26, 27*
   AIDS dementia and, 226
CD3 T cells, 57
CD4+ T cells, as targets of HIV, 25–27, 29, 33, 400
     testing for, 44–45
   declining count of, 23, 27, 29, *53,* 57, 58
     and CMV infections, 430
     and gastrointestinal disease, 210
     and HPV-related neoplasms, 488
     and initiation of antiretroviral therapy, 58, 97, 109
       in children, 529, 531, 532
     and Kaposi's sarcoma, 471, *471,* 472t
     and non-Hodgkin's lymphoma, 479
     and pneumonia, 339, 340t
       from *Pneumocystis carinii,* 307–309, 323–324
     and toxoplasmosis, 380
     and tuberculosis, 354
   evaluation of, 57, 127, 127t, 128
     in HIV-infected children, 526, 526t, 531
       and initiation of antiretroviral therapy, 529, 531, 532
     in older HIV-infected individuals, 593–594
     in pregnancy, 563–564
     in primary HIV disease, 69, 73, 74
       in children, 531
   fluorescent antibody cell sorting of, 57
   gastrointestinal, 195–196
   interferon α and, 406, 408
   measurement of, periodic, 61, 61t
CD8+ T cells, and primary HIV disease, 73, 74
   HIV and, 44–45, 57
CD45RO, 593–594
CD4/CD8 ratio, 57
   and gastrointestinal disease, 196
   in primary HIV infection, 69
Cefotaxime, for pneumonia, 341
   for *Streptococcus pneumoniae,* 333, 333t
Ceftizoxime, for *Bartonella,* 418, 420t
Ceftriaxone, for pneumonia, 341
   for syphilis, 460, 461
Cefuroxime, for pneumonia, 341
Cell-mediated immunity. See specific cells, e.g., *CD4+ T cells.*
Cellulitis, in drug users, 577
   preseptal, 173
   staphylococcal, 187
Central nervous system lymphoma. See *CNS lymphoma, primary.*
Cephalosporins, for staphylococcal dermatitis, 187
Cerebrospinal fluid (CSF), examination of, for *Bartonella,* 413
   for CMV, 430–431
   for *Cryptococcus,* 362–363, 363t, *364*
   for *Toxoplasma gondii,* 382
   for *Treponema pallidum,* 453, 457, 458, 461
   in AIDS dementia complex, 224, 226
   in early HIV infection, 218
Cervical neoplasia, 128, 467, 468t, 486–488, 544–545
   HPV and, 486–488, 544
   screening for, 128, 489, 489t, 544–545, 545t
   treatment of, 545
Cesarean section, 568
   for HIV transmission prevention, 526
C31G, 539
Chancroid, and HIV transmission, 500
Cheilitis, angular, 158
Chest x-rays, in HIV disease, 139–151. See also individual diseases.
   lymphocytic and nonspecific interstitial pneumonitis and, 149–150, *151*

Chest x-rays (*Continued*)
  neoplasms and, 147–149, *148–150*
  opportunistic infections and, 139–147, *140–147*
  pneumonia and, 339, 340t
Children, HIV infection in, 525–533
  antiretroviral therapy for, 528–531, 569, 569t
    changing, 531
    initial, 529–531, 530t
    principles for, 528–529
    starting, 529
    CD4+ T cell count in, 526, 526t, 531
      and initiation of antiretroviral therapy, 529, 531, 532
    diagnosis of, 527
    epidemiology of, 3, 7, 525
      in United States, 7
    management of, 527–528, 532
    monitoring of, 527–528, 528t
    mortality from, 525
    natural history of, 526–527, 526t
    plasma viral load and, 526–527
    prophylaxis in, for opportunistic infections, 532
      for PCP, 527–528
    risk factors for, 525–526
    timing of contraction of, 526, 526t
    vaccinations and, 528
Chinese herbs, 603, 604–605, 604t
Chlamydia pneumoniae, pneumonia from, 332t, 335
Chlamydia trachomatis, prevention of, 506
Cholangiopancreatography, endoscopic retrograde, 207, 208
Cholangiopathy, AIDS-related, 207–208, 208t
Cholangitis, infectious, 207–208
  primary sclerosing, 208t
Cholecystitis, acalculous, 207
CHOP therapy, for non-Hodgkin's lymphoma, 481t, 482
Chorioamnionitis, 567
Chorioretinitis. See also *Retinochoroiditis.*
  from CMV, 176, 429–430, *430,* Color Plate 3B, Color Plate IF
  from syphilis, 175, 177, 455
Choroidal effusion syndrome, 175
Choroiditis, infectious, 177
Cidofovir, adverse effects of, 437
  for CMV, 176, 197t, 437
  for HSV, 444
  for molluscum contagiosum, 189
Cimetidine, drug interactions with, 87
Ciprofloxacin, for *Mycobacterium avium*-complex, 345, 346
  in gastrointestinal disease, 201
  for *Mycobacterium tuberculosis,* 356t
  for *Rhodococcus equi,* 423
  psychosis from, 255
Circumcision, lack of, and HIV transmission, 499, 539
Cisapride, drug interactions with, 88t
Clarithromycin, adverse effects of, 346
  for *Mycobacterium avium*-complex, 345, 346, 347t
    in gastrointestinal disease, 201
    prophylactic, 131t, 132, 348
  for *Streptococcus pneumoniae,* 333t, 334
  for toxoplasmosis, 386t, 388
    in maintenance therapy, 389, 389t
Clindamycin, for gingivitis and periodontitis, 161
  for staphylococcal dermatitis, 187
  for toxoplasmosis, 386, 386t, 389
    in maintenance therapy, 389, 389t
Clindamycin-primaquine, adverse effects of, 317t, 318t, 319
  for *Pneumocystis carinii,* 317, 317t, 318t, 319–320

Clobetasol, for aphthous ulcers, 164
Clofazimine, for *Mycobacterium avium*-complex, 345, 347
  for *Mycobacterium tuberculosis,* dosage of, 356t
Clonazepam, 252, 252t
Clonidine, 587
Clostridium difficile, clinical manifestations of, 201
Clotrimazole, for antifungal prophylaxis, 375
  for candidiasis, 158
  for seborrheic psoriasis, 158
CMV. See *Cytomegalovirus (CMV).*
CNS lymphoma, primary, 219, 225t, 227, 227t, 228, 229. See also *Non-Hodgkin's lymphoma.*
  differential diagnosis of, 384
  etiology and diagnosis of, 228, 479–480
  treatment of, 484, 484t
Coagulopathies, HIV-associated, 269–270
Cocaine use, 584–586. See also *Drug users.*
  effects of, 585t
  in pregnancy, 558
  treatment of, 589
Coccidioidomycosis, 373–374, Color Plate IIE
  chest films of, 144
  clinical manifestations of, 373–374
  diagnosis of, 374
  epidemiology and pathogenesis of, 373
  pulmonary, 336, 337t, 338, 373–374
  treatment of, 338, 374
Colitis, from CMV, 199–200, 432, *432*
  from HSV, 200
Colonoscopy, 203
Colony-stimulating factors, therapeutic use of, 271, 271t
COMLA therapy, for non-Hodgkin's lymphoma, 481t, 482
COMP therapy, for non-Hodgkin's lymphoma, 481t, 482
Computed tomography (CT), for AIDS dementia, 224
  for cryptococcosis, 362, 363t, *364*
  for neurologic diseases, 218
  for non-Hodgkin's lymphoma, 479
  for *Pneumocystis carinii,* 139, 313–314, *315*
  for primary CNS lymphoma, 228
  for toxoplasmosis, 382–383, 384, *385*
Condoms, female, 502, 539
  for HIV transmission prevention, *501,* 501–502, 505, 507, 538
Congenital infections, with toxoplasmosis, 381
Congestive heart failure, treatment of, 280–281
Conjunctival diseases, 171–173
Conjunctival intraepithelial neoplasia, 172
Conjunctival lymphoma, 172
Conjunctival microvasculopathy, 173
Conjunctivitis, 173
Contraceptives. See also *Condoms.*
  and HIV transmission, 538, 539–540, 539t
Conus medullaris syndrome, toxoplasmosis and, 380
Corneal phospholipidoses, 175
Corticosteroids, adverse effects of, depression from, 244
  for *Pneumocystis carinii,* 322–323
  for toxoplasmosis, 384, 386
  mania from, 254
  psychosis from, 255
Cortisol deficiency, 286
Cotton-wool spots, 430
"Crack" cocaine, 584–586
Cranial neuropathy, 218
"Crix belly," from antiretroviral therapy, 82, 292
Crotamiton, for scabies, 190
Cryotherapy, for Kaposi's sarcoma, 473
Cryptococcal antigen (CRAG) test, 363–364, 363t
Cryptococcoma, 228

Cryptococcosis, 361–370
  adrenal, 286
  and progression of HIV disease, 126
  chest films of, 144, 145, *146*
  choroiditis from, 177
  clinical manifestations of, 362, 363t
  conjunctivitis from, 173
  CSF examination for, 362–363, 363t, *364*
  diagnosis of, 362–364, *364*
  differential diagnosis of, 362, 364, 440
  epidemiology of, 11, 361–362
  meningeal, 220, 225t, 362–363, 363t, *364,* 365
    clinical manifestations of, 363t
    computed tomography of, 362, 363t, *364*
    laboratory findings in, 363t
    prognosis for, 365
  microbiology of, 361
  neuro-ophthalmic manifestations of, 178
  oral, 159t
  pancreatic abscesses from, 209
  prophylaxis against, 132–133
    in children, 532
  pulmonary, 336, 337t, 338, 362
    diagnosis of, 336, 337t
    treatment of, 336, 338
  thyroid disease from, 288
  treatment of, 365–370
    acute, 366–368, 366t, *367,* 368t
    antifungal agents in, 365–368
    chronic, 369–370
    management of intracranial hypertension in, 368–369
Cryptococcus neoformans var. *gattii,* 361
Cryptococcus neoformans var. *neoformans,* 361
Cryptosporidiosis, biliary disease from, 207–208
  gastrointestinal, 200
    differential diagnosis of, 432
  in drug users, 576
  pancreatic abscesses from, 209
  treatment of, allicin for, 609
CSF. See *Cerebrospinal fluid.*
CT. See *Computed tomography (CT).*
Cuba, HIV prevention program in, 505
Cultures, for HIV, 43–45, *45*
Cushing's syndrome, 292
Cutaneous exposure, to HIV, 514
CXCR4 chemokine receptor, 26, *26,* 73
Cyclophosphamide, for non-Hodgkin's lymphoma, 481t, 482
Cycloserine, for *Mycobacterium tuberculosis,* 358
  dosage of, 356t
CYP3A enzymes, drug interactions and, 85, 88, 89, 89t, 90t, 92t, 93, 105–106
Cytochrome P-450, drug interactions and, 104, 105–106, 107, 603
Cytokines, AIDS dementia and, 226
  and HIV disease, 593
    primary, 74
  glucocorticoid deficiency and, 286, 287
  myocarditis and, 280
  neurotoxicity mediated by, 231
Cytomegalovirus (CMV), 429–438
  adrenal disease from, 286
  biliary disease from, 207–208
  chest films of, 145–146, 433
  chorioretinitis from, 176, 429–430, *430,* Color Plate 3B, Color Plate IF
  dementia from, 431
  differential diagnosis of, 199, 384
  distal neuropathy from, 432

Cytomegalovirus (*Continued*)
  encephalitis from, 221–222, 225t, 431
  epidemiology of, 11
  esophageal, 196, 197t, 198
    differential diagnosis of, 440
  gastrointestinal infections with, 198, 199–200, 432, *432*
    antiretroviral therapy and, 210
  hepatic disease from, 204
  in drug users, 576
  in women, 543
  iridocyclitis from, 175
  keratitis from, 174
  mononeuritis multiplex from, 431–432
  myelitis from, 430–431
  myocarditis from, 279–280
  neuropathies from, 231, 231t, 430
  oral ulcers from, 162
  pancreatic abscesses from, 209
  PCR of, 231
  polyradiculopathy from, 230, 230t, 430–431
  prophylaxis for, 133, 437–438
    ganciclovir for, 437–438
  pulmonary manifestations of, 432–433
  treatment of, 197t, 199–200, 433–437
    cidofovir in, 437
    combination therapies in, 437
    foscarnet in, 436–437
    ganciclovir in, 433–436, 434t, *435,* 436t
  ventriculoencephalitis from, 431
Cytopenias, colony-stimulating factors for, 271, 271t
  peripheral, 266–269
Cytosine arabinoside, for non-Hodgkin's lymphoma, 481t, 482

Dacarbazine, for Hodgkin's disease, 485
Danazol, 269
Dapsone, adverse effects of, depression from, 244
    psychosis from, 255
  for *Pneumocystis carinii,* prophylactic, 131, 131t, 324–325, 324t
  for toxoplasmosis, 386t, 388
    in maintenance therapy, 389, 389t
Dapsone + pyrimethamine, for *Pneumocystis carinii,* prophylactic, 324, 324t
  for toxoplasmosis, prophylactic, 131–132, 131t
Darkfield microscopy, for syphilis, 456
Daunorubicin, for Kaposi's sarcoma, 473–474, 473t
ddc. See *Zalcitabine.*
ddI. See *Didanosine.*
DEET (diethyltoluamide), 190
Dehydroepiandrosterone (DHEA), 601
Dehydroepiandrosterone (DHEA), for wasting syndrome, 608, 608t
Delavirdine, 107–108
  adverse effects of, 80t, 82, 98t, 107
  combination therapy with, 101t, 106t, 108, 110, 110t
  dosage of, 98t, 106t
  drug interactions with, 88–89, 88t, 107, 108, 356
  HIV mutations and, *55,* 99t, 108
Delirium, in HIV-infected patients, 241, 253–254
  organic brain disease and, 250
Dementia, 221–227, 249–252. See also *AIDS dementia complex.*
  from CMV, 431
  in drug users, 578
  milieu management for, 250–251
  treatment of, 251–252, 252t
17-Deoxysteroid, 287

Depression, fatigue from, 256t
  in AIDS dementia, 224
  in HIV-infected patients, 241, 242, 243–249
    diagnosis of, 244–245
    etiology of, 244
    treatment of, 245–249, 247t
      failure of, 249
  organic brain disease and, 250
Dermatologic disorders, in HIV disease, 185–194, 186t.
      See also specific diseases.
    drug-induced, 190, *190*
    hypersensitive, 190–191
    infectious, 185–189
    papulosquamous, 192–193, *193, 194*
    photosensitive, 191
    pruritic, 191–192, *192*
Dermatomyositis, 232
Desipramine, dosage of, 247t
Dexamethasone, for aphthous ulcers, 164
  for non-Hodgkin's lymphoma, 481t, 482
Dextroamphetamine, 248
  dosage of, 247t
DFA (direct fluorescent antibody) test, for syphilis, 456
d4T. See *Stavudine.*
DHEA (dehydroepiandosterone), 601
  for wasting syndrome, 608, 608t
Diabetes mellitus, from megestrol acetate, 290
  from protease inhibitors, 282
    in pregnancy, 565
  gestational, 565
Diarrhea, 199–203
  and progression of HIV disease, 126
  drug-induced, 201–203, 202t
    by ganciclovir, 435
    by nelfinavir, 83
    by protease inhibitors, 201–203, 202t
    in women, 548
  evaluation of, in HIV-infected patients, 203, 203t
  from adenovirus, 200
  from bacteria, 200–201
  from CMV, 199–200
  from fungi, 200
  from HIV enteropathy, 201
  from HSV, 200
  from protozoa, 200
Dicloxacillin, for staphylococcal folliculitis, 186t
Didanosine (ddI), 27, 102
  adverse effects of, 80, 80t, 98t, 102
    gastrointestinal, 202t
    hepatic, 206t, 207
    pancreatic, 209
    toxic axonal neuropathy from, 231–232
  combination therapy with, 100t, 101t, 102, 110, 110t
    in pregnancy, 563–564
  dosage of, 98t, 106t
  drug interactions with, 86–87, 86t
    ganciclovir and, 436
  food and, 93, 93t
  for primary HIV disease, 75
  HIV mutations and, *55,* 99t
2',3'-Dideoxyinosine. See *Didanosine.*
Diethyltoluamide (DEET), 190
Diphtheria-tetanus-pertussis (DTP) vaccine, 528
Diphtheria/tetanus (dT) vaccine, 131
Direct antiglobulin test, 268
Direct fluorescent antibody (DFA) test, for syphilis, 456
Disability issues, 258–259
DNA probe, for HIV, 50–54
  for *Mycobacterium avium*-complex, 345

Doppler echocardiography, 276
Doxepin, 246
  dosage of, 247t
Doxorubicin, for Hodgkin's disease, 485
  for Kaposi's sarcoma, 473–474, 473t
  for non-Hodgkin's lymphoma, 481t, 482
Doxycycline, for bacillary angiomatosis, 186t
  for *Bartonella,* 418, *419,* 420, 420t, 421
  for syphilis, 459, 459t, 460
  for toxoplasmosis, 388
Dronabinol, 291
Drug resistance, by HIV. See also *Human immunodefi-
      ciency virus (HIV) 1, mutations of;* and individual
      drugs.
    nonadherence to therapy and, *117*
    testing for, 54–57, *55*
Drug users, health care access for, 580–581
  intravenous, access to health care care for, 580–581
    behavior change for, 504, 589
    female, HIV infection in, 537, 540, 541
      pregnant, 558
    HIV infection in, 3, *14,* 14–15, 16, 575–589
      by age, 594t
      clinical trial for, 581–582
      drug interactions with antiretroviral therapy for,
          582–583
      endocarditis and, 577–578
      epidemiology of, 575
      hepatitis and, 579
      natural history of, 575–576
      neurologic disease and, 579
      opportunistic infections and, 576–579, 576t
      pneumonia and, 578
      renal disease and, 579
      skin and soft tissue infections and, 576–577
      transmission of, 499, 504
      treatment of, 579–583
      tuberculosis and, 578
    HIV postexposure prophylaxis for, 519–521, 521t
    Hodgkin's disease in, 485
    nonadherence to therapy among, 117
    pain management for, 583–584
    risk reduction for, 589, 589t
    treatment of dependence in, 587–589
    withdrawal syndrome in, 588–589
Drug-drug interactions, in HIV treatment, 83–93. See also
      individual drugs.
    absorption and, 84
    distribution and, 84
    excretion and, 84
    hepatic biotransformation and, 84–85
    nutrients and, 91–93
    pharmacodynamic, 83
    pharmacokinetic, 83–85, 84t
    with NNRTIs, 87–89, 88t
    with NRTIs, 85–87, 86t
    with PIs, 89–91, 89t, 90t, 92t
Drug-induced disorders. See also individual drugs.
    anemia from, 267t, 268
    depression from, 244
    dermatologic, 190, *190*
    diarrhea from, 201–203, 202t
    hepatotoxic, 205–207, 206t
    mania from, 254
    myelosuppression from, 268, 268t
    psychosis from, 255
    renal failure from, 299t
d4T. See *Stavudine.*
dT (diphtheria/tetanus) vaccine, 131

DTP (diphtheria-tetanus-pertussis) vaccine, 528
Dysphagia, 196

EBV. See *Epstein-Barr virus (EBV).*
Echocardiography, 276, 279, 280
Ecthyma, 187
Ectopic pregnancy, 566
Efavirenz, 108
  adverse effects of, 98t, 108
  combination therapy with, 101t, 106t, 108, 110, 110t
  dosage of, 98t, 106t
  HIV mutations and, *55,* 99t, 108
  resistance to, 108
Electrolyte disorders, in HIV-infected patient, 128
  delirium from, 253
ELISA. See *Enzyme-linked immunosorbent assay (ELISA).*
Emotional well-being, of HIV-infected individuals, 242.
  See also *Psychiatric syndromes.*
Encephalitis, differential diagnosis of, 440
  from CMV, 221–222, 225t, 431
  from cryptococcosis, 440
  from HSV, 222, 440–441
  from toxoplasmosis, 221, 379, 380, 383, 384, 440
  from VZV, 447
  multinucleated-cell, in AIDS dementia, 226
Encephalitozoon intestinalis, manifestations of, 200
  treatment of, 208
Encephalopathies, differential diagnosis of, 245
  diffuse, 221–222
  HIV, 178
    by age, 594t
    in primary infection, 217–218
Endocarditis, chest radiograph in, 577
  from *Staphylococcus aureus,* 334, 577–578
  in drug users, 577–578
  infective, 281
  marantic, 281
Endocrinologic manifestations, of HIV disease, 285–292
  adrenal, 286–288
  gonadal, 289
  hypothalamic-pituitary, 285–286
  of lipid metabolism, 290–291
  of mineral homeostasis, 290
  pancreatic, 289–290
  thyroid, 288–289
  wasting syndrome and, 291
Endoscopic retrograde cholangiopancreatography (ERCP), 207, 208
Endoscopy, for esophageal disease, 198t
Entamoeba histolytica infection, differential diagnosis of, 432
Enterobacter, oral disease from, 162
Enterocolitis, from CMV, 432, *432*
Enterocytozoon bieneusi, cholangitis from, 207–208
  gastrointestinal manifestations of, 200
env gene, 24, *24,* 31
Env protein, 27
Enzyme-linked immunosorbent assay (ELISA), for HIV, 43, 46, *46,* 49, 70–71, 72, 504, 517
  false-positive, 59–60, *61*
Eosinophilic folliculitis, diagnosis and treatment of, 186t, 191–192, *192*
Epstein-Barr virus (EBV), differential diagnosis of, from primary HIV infection, 69–70, 71t
  myocarditis from, 279–280
  non-Hodgkin's lymphoma and, 478, 479
  oral hairy leukoplakia and, 162, 163
  primary CNS lymphoma and, 229, 479

Equine infectious anemia virus, 24
ERCP (endoscopic retrograde cholangiopancreatography), 207, 208
Ergot derivatives, drug interactions with, 90t
Erythema multiforme, drug-induced, 190, *190*
Erythrocytes, disorders of, 266–268, 267t
Erythromycin, for bacillary angiomatosis, 186t
  for *Bartonella,* 418, *419,* 420, 420t, 421
  for pneumonia, 341
  for *Rhodococcus equi,* 423
Erythropoietin, human recombinant, 271, 271t
  for drug-induced anemia, 79
Escherichia coli infection, clinical manifestations of, 201
Esophageal disorders, 196–198
  pathogenesis of, 196–198, 197t
  treatment of, 197t, 198
Esophageal ulcers, 196, 197t, 198
Esophagitis, 196, 197t, 198
  differential diagnosis of, 432, 440
  pill-induced, 198
  with HSV, 196, 197t, 198, 440, *441*
Esophagogastric varices, 199
Estradiol, 289
Ethambutol, for *Mycobacterium avium*-complex, 345, 346, 347
  in gastrointestinal disease, 201
  for *Mycobacterium tuberculosis,* 356–357, 356t, 578
  dosage of, 356t
Ethical issues, 255–256
Ethionamide, for *Mycobacterium avium*-complex, 345, 346
  for *Mycobacterium tuberculosis,* dosage of, 356t
Etoposide, for Kaposi's sarcoma, 473t, 474
  for non-Hodgkin's lymphoma, 481t, 482
Europe, HIV infection in, 3, *4*
Exportin 1/Crm 1 protein, 31
Extrapyramidal symptoms, 253
Eye disease, 171–178. See also specific diseases, e.g., *Retinitis.*
Eyelid diseases, 171–173

Famciclovir, for HSV, 443, 443t, 444, 445, 446, 547
  dosage adjustment for, in renal dysfunction, 443, 443t
  ocular, 174
  for VZV, 447
  ophthalmic, 171, 447
Fat distribution, abnormal, 292
  from indinavir, 82, 292
  from protease inhibitors, 106, 292
Fatigue, 256–257
  causes of, 256t
Fatty liver, 205
Feline immunodeficiency virus, 24
Fellatio, HIV transmission via, 505
Fetal monitoring, for HIV infection, 569–570
Fever, and progression of HIV disease, 126
  in primary HIV infection, 67, 68t
Fibroblast growth factor, basic, and Kaposi's sarcoma, 473
Filgastrim, drug interactions with, ganciclovir and, 436
Fluconazole, drug interactions with, 85
  opioid substitutes and, 583, 588t
  for antifungal prophylaxis, 374–375
  for candidiasis, 158, 197t, 198
  for coccidioidomycosis, 374
  for cryptococcosis, 366, 366t, 367, *367,* 368, 368t
  maintenance regimen of, 369–370
  prophylactic, 132–133
  for histoplasmosis, 373

Flucytosine, adverse effects of, 365
  for cryptococcosis, 365, 366t, 368, 368t
Fluocinonide, for aphthous ulcers, 164
Fluoroquinolones, for *Streptococcus pneumoniae,* 333, 333t
Fluoxetine, 247
  dosage of, 247t
Fluvoxamine, 247
  dosage of, 247t
Folate deficiency, 265
Folinic acid, for toxoplasmosis, 386t, 387
Follicle-stimulating hormone, 289
Follicular-associated epithelium, HIV transmission and, 196
Folliculitis, eosinophilic, 186t, 191–192, *192*
  diagnosis and treatment of, 186t
  pruritic, 191–192, *192*
  staphylococcal, 186t, 187, *187*
Food, antiretroviral drugs to be taken with or without, 93t
Food-borne disease, toxoplasmosis from, 379
Foreign-body granulomas, in drug users, 577
Foscarnet, adverse effects of, 200, 436, 444
    hypocalcemia and other mineral disorders from, 290, 436, 444
  for CMV, 176, 197t, 198, 199–200, 436–437
  for HSV, 162, 186t, 200, 443–444, 444t, 445–446
    drug resistance and, 445–446
    prophylactic, 446
  for VZV, 447, 448, 448t
Fungal infections. See also individual infections, e.g., *Candidiasis.*
  bone marrow biopsy in, 266
  gastrointestinal, 200
  keratitis from, 174
  oral, 159t
  pneumonia from, 336–338, 337t
  prophylaxis for, 132–133
  retinitis from, 177

gag gene, 24, *24,* 32
Gag protein, 31, 48
Gait disorder, in AIDS dementia, 224
Gallium scanning, for *Pneumocystis carinii* pneumonia, 314
Ganciclovir, adverse effects of, 200, 435–436, 436t
  clinical use of, 434
  drug interactions with, 435–436
  for CMV, 176, 197t, 199–200, 433–436, 434t, *435,* 436t
    intravitreal implants with, 434
    prophylactic, 437–438
    resistance to, 434–435
  pharmacology and dosage of, 433–434, 434t
    renal dysfunction and, 434t
  psychosis from, 255
  structure and mechanism of action of, 433
  virologic response to, 434, *435*
Gastric disease, 198–199
Gastroenteritis. See also *Diarrhea.*
  bacterial, prevention of, 132
Gastroesophageal reflux, 198
Gastrointestinal bleeding, 199
Gastrointestinal manifestations, of CMV infection, 198, 199–200, 432, *432*
  of HIV infection, 196–203. See also individual disorders.
    prevention of, 210
Gastrointestinal mucosa, HIV infection and, 195–196
  immunology of, 195–196
General paresis, 455
Genital ulcers, and HIV transmission, 539t
  from HSV, 439

Genital ulcers (*Continued*)
  from syphilis, 455–456
  in women, 546–547
Genital warts, 189
  in women, 545
Gentamicin, for *Rhodococcus equi,* 423
Geotrichosis, oral, 159t
Giardiasis, differential diagnosis of, 432
Gingival erythema, linear, 159t
Gingivitis, 158, 161, *161*
  acute necrotizing ulcerative, 161
Gingivostomatitis, from HSV, 439
Glaucoma, angle-closure, 175
Glomerulonephritis, cryoglobulinemic, from hepatitis C virus, 298–299
Glomerulosclerosis, focal and segmental, 299–300
Glucocorticoid deficiency, 286–287
Gonadal disease, 289
  from ganciclovir, 436
Gonorrhea, prevention of, 506
gp41 protein, 24, 25, *25, 26,* 27, 32, 48, 71
  and AIDS dementia, 226
gp120 protein, 25, *25,* 26, *26,* 27, 32, 48, 400
  and AIDS dementia, 226
gp160 protein, 32, 33, 48, *59*
Granulocyte colony-stimulating factor, chemotherapy and, 474
  therapeutic use of, 271, 271t
Granulocyte-macrophage colony–stimulating factor, chemotherapy and, 474, 476
Granulocytopenia, from zidovudine, 79
Grapefruit juice, antiretroviral drugs and, 93
Growth failure, 285
  in HIV-infected children, 531
Growth hormone, 285, 291
Guillain-Barré syndrome, 218
Gut-associated lymphoid tissue (GALT), 195–196
Gynecologic care, for HIV-infected women, 545, 545t

HAART (highly active antiretroviral therapy). See *Antiretroviral therapy.*
Haemophilus influenzae, in drug users, 578
  pneumonia from, 332t, 334
    chest films of, 146–147, 334
    treatment of, 334
Haemophilus influenzae type B vaccine, 334
  for children, 528
Haloperidol, for delirium, 254
HBV. See *Hepatitis B virus.*
HCV. See *Hepatitis C virus.*
HDAraC/HD MTX therapy, for non-Hodgkin's lymphoma, 481t, 482
Headache, from HIV-1, 219–221
  in primary HIV infection, 68, 68t
Health care worker exposures, to HIV, 75, 499, 504, 513–521. See also *Needlestick injuries; Occupational exposures to HIV.*
  antiretroviral therapy for, 111, 519
  prevention of, 513–521
  testing for, 516–517
Helicobacter cinaedi, 188
Helicobacter pylori, clinical manifestations of, 199
Hematologic complications, of HIV disease, 265–271. See also specific disorders.
Hemophiliacs, HIV infection in, 595, 595t
Hepatic disease, in bacillary angiomatosis, 412, 420
  in HIV disease, 203–207
    granulomatous, 204

Hepatic disease (*Continued*)
  inflammatory. See *Hepatitis.*
  neoplastic, 205
  vascular, 205
Hepatic transaminase levels, in bacillary angiomatosis, 412
  in primary HIV infection, 73
Hepatitis, 203–204. See also individual viruses.
  from didanosine, 80
  in drug users, 579, 589
Hepatitis A vaccine, for HIV-infected patients, 130
Hepatitis A virus (HAV), in drug users, 579
Hepatitis B vaccine, 128, 130
  for children, 528
Hepatitis B virus (HBV), 203–204
  antiretroviral therapy and, 210
  in drug users, 579
  occupational exposures to, 570
  testing for, 128
    in pregnancy, 562
  transmission of, 515
Hepatitis C virus, 203–204, 270, 399–408
  coinfection with HIV, 399, 401–405, 517
    and influence on chronicity of HCV, 403
    and influence on HCV diversity, 402
    and influence on HCV-related liver disease, 402–403
    and influence on HIV replication, 401–402
    and influence on natural history of HIV immunodeficiency, 403–405, 404t
    vertical and sexual transmission in, 405
  diagnosis of, 204, 400–401
  epidemiology of, 399–400
  glomerulonephritis from, 298–299
  in drug users, 579
  occupational exposures to, 570
  pathogenesis of, 400, 400t
  testing for, 128
    in pregnancy, 562
  transmission of, 204, 517
  treatment of, 406–408, 407t
Hepatosplenomegaly, in bacillary angiomatosis, 413
Hepatotoxicity, drug-induced, 205–207, 206t
  from nevirapine, 81–82
Herbal medicines, 603, 604–605, 604t
Heroin use, 584, 585t. See also *Drug users.*
  effects of, 585t
Herpes simplex virus (HSV), 438–446
  and progression of HIV disease, 126
  anorectal infections with, 439–440, *440,* Color Plate IIF
  brain disease from, 230
  clinical presentation of, 438–441
  cutaneous, 186t, 188
  differential diagnosis of, 432, 440
  drug-resistant, 441, 445–446
    management of, 445–446
  encephalitis from, 222, 440–441
  epidemiology of, 11
  esophageal, 196, 197t, 198, 440, *441*
    differential diagnosis of, 432, 440
  gastrointestinal infections with, 198–199, 200
  genital infections with, 439
    in women, 546–547
      pregnant, 563, 565–566
  in women, 546–547
  iridocyclitis from, 175
  keratitis from, 174
  neonatal, 565–566
  orolabial, 159t, 162, 438–439
  pancreatic abscesses from, 209

Herpes simplex virus (*Continued*)
  prophylaxis for, 132, 445–446
    in pregnancy, 565–566
  retinitis from, 177, 430
  treatment of, 197t, 200, 441–446, 444t, 547
    acyclovir in, 441–442, 442t, 444, 444t, 445, 446, 547, 565–566
      resistance to, 441, 445–446
    cidofovir in, 444
    famciclovir in, 443, 443t, 444, 445, 547
    foscarnet in, 443–444, 444t, 445–446
    in pregnancy, 565–566
    penciclovir in, 445
    valacyclovir in, 442–443, 443t, 444, 445
Herpes zoster, 446. See also *Varicella-zoster virus.*
  and progression of HIV disease, 126
  diagnosis of, 186t, 188
  management of, 186t, 188, 447–448, 448t
  neuropathy from, 231
  ophthalmicus, 171, 446
  oral, 159t, 162
  sine herpete, 174
Herpesviruses. See also individual species.
  infections with, 429–448
Heterosexual transmission. See also *Sex workers; Sexual practices.*
  of hepatitis C virus, and coinfection with HIV, 399, 405
  of HIV, 499–500, 505–507, *506, 507*
    to women, 537–541, 539t
      risk factors for, 538–539, 539t
Hidradenitis suppurativa, 187
Highly active antiretroviral therapy (HAART). See *Antiretroviral therapy.*
Hispanic Americans, female, HIV infection in, 537
  HIV infection in, 6, 7, 13–14, 16
    by age, 594t
Histamine-2 receptor antagonists, adverse effects of, depression from, 244
Histoplasma antigen test, 371–372, 371t
Histoplasmosis, 370–373
  chest films of, 144, *145,* 371
  choroiditis from, 177
  clinical manifestations of, 370–371
  diagnosis of, 337t, 338, 371–372, 371t
  epidemiology of, 11, 370
  gastrointestinal, 200
  neurologic, 370–371
  oral, 159t
  pathogenesis of, 370
  pneumonia from, 336, 337t, 338, 370
  progressive disseminated, 370
  treatment of, 272t, 338, 372–373
HIV, infection with, See *Human immunodeficiency virus (HIV) disease.*
  type 1, See *Human immunodeficiency virus (HIV) 1.*
  type 2, See *Human immunodeficiency virus (HIV) 2.*
HIV encephalopathy, 178
  by age, 594t
HIV enteropathy, clinical manifestations of, 201
HIV headache, 220
HIV-associated coagulopathies, 269–270
HIV-1–associated cognitive/motor complex, 222–223, 223t. See also *AIDS dementia complex.*
HIV-associated dementia. See *AIDS dementia complex.*
HIV-associated immune-mediated renal disease, 298–300
HIV-associated lymphoma, oral, 164
HIV-associated nephropathy (HIVAN), 298–300
HIV-related thrombocytopenia, 268–269
HIV retinopathy, 176, Color Plate 3A

Hodgkin's disease, 468t, 485–486
Home care services, for HIV-infected patients, 134
Homeless individuals, access to care for, 581
　Bartonella in, 421
　nonadherence to antiretroviral therapy among, 118
Homosexuals, anal neoplasia in, 129, 488
　CMV encephalitis in, 431
　Helicobacter cinaedi in, 188
　hepatitis C virus in, 399–400
　herpes simplex in, 438, 439
　HIV infection in, 3, 6–7, 13, 14, 15–16, 23, 539
　　by age, 594t
　Hodgkin's disease in, 485
　syphilis in, 453
　uncircumcised, 539
　warts in, 189
HPV. See *Human papillomavirus (HPV)*.
HSV. See *Herpes simplex virus (HSV)*.
HTLV (human T-cell leukemia virus), myelopathy from, 230, 230t
Human herpesvirus 8, 468–469, *469*, 543. See also *Kaposi's sarcoma*.
　in women, 543
　sexual transmission of, 543
Human immunodeficiency virus (HIV), type 1. See *Human immunodeficiency virus (HIV) 1*.
　type 2. See *Human immunodeficiency virus (HIV) 2*.
Human immunodeficiency virus (HIV) 1, adaptor proteins and, 33, *33*
　AIDS dementia from, 226–227. See also *AIDS dementia*.
　antibody tests for, *46*, 46–49, *47*
　cultures of, 43–45
　　quantitative cell, 44, *45*
　　quantitative plasma, 44, *45*
　　ultrasensitive cell, 44–45
　demyelinating neuropathy from, 218–219
　drug resistance of, assessment of, 54–57
　　clinical use of, 56–57
　　genotypic, 54–56, *55*
　　phenotypic, 56
　　nonadherence to therapy and, 117
　early expression of regulatory genes of, 29–31, *30*, 31
　env gene and, 24, *24*
　env protein and, 27
　esophageal ulcers from, 198
　gag gene and, 24, *24*, 32
　gag protein and, 31, 48
　genetic subtypes of, 3–5, *5*
　genomic structure of, 24, *24*
　gp41 protein of, 24, 25, *25*, *26*, 27, 32, 48, 71
　　and AIDS dementia, 226
　gp120 protein of, 25, *25*, 26, *26*, 27, 32, 48, 400
　　and AIDS dementia, 226
　gp160 protein of, 32, 33, 48, *59*
　group M, 4–5, *5*
　group O, 4, 5, *5*
　hepatitis C virus coinfection with, effects of, 399, 401–405
　infectiousness of, duration of, 500
　intravenous drug user exposure to, prophylaxis for, 519–521, 521t
　karyophilic properties, 27–28
　laboratory testing for, 43–62. See also individual tests, e.g., *Western blot assay*.
　　false-positive and false-negative, 58–60, 60t
　　interpretation of, *53*, 58, *61*
　　methodologies for, 43–58
　　misleading results from, 58–60, 60t
　　sensitivity and specificity of, 58–62, 60t
　　use of markers in, 53t, 60–62, 61t

Human immunodeficiency virus 1 (*Continued*)
　latency of, 29
　life cycle of, 25–33
　molecular aspects of, 23–33
　mutations of, 27
　　drug resistance and, 54, *55*, 99, 99t, 117. See also individual drugs.
　nef gene and, 24, *24*
　nef protein and, 27–28, 29–33, *33*
　neurologically asymptomatic infection with, 219
　occupational exposures to, 513–515, 514t
　　management of, 516–518
　　prophylaxis for, 518–519, 520t
　　risk reduction for, 516
　　universal precautions for, 516
　p7 protein of, 25, *25*
　p17 protein of, 25, *25*
　p24 protein of, 25, *25*, 44, *45*, 58, *59*, 60
　　antigen test with, 44, *45*, 49–50, *50*, 70–71, 517
　　in children, *527*
　pol gene and, 24, *24*
　pol protein and, 31, 32
　polymerase chain reaction for, 50, *51*, 51–52, 60, 125, 517
　　genotypic drug resistance and, 54–56
　　in children, 527, 528t
　　in neonates, 572
　　in pregnancy, 525
　　phenotypic drug resistance and, 56
　　quantitative, 52, 53t
　postexposure prophylaxis for, 518–521, 520t, 521t
　preintegration complex of, 27, 28–29
　quantitative viral RNA and DNA assays for, 50–54, 72–73
　replication of, 27
　rev gene and, 24, *24*
　rev protein and, 28, 29–31, *30*
　　as viral RNA export factor, 31, *32*
　　mutation of, 31, *32*
　　response element of, 31
　reverse transcription and integration of, 27
　screening for, in pregnancy, 560
　sexual exposure to, prophylaxis for, 519–521, 521t
　subtypes of, and heterosexual transmission, 538–539
　tat gene and, 24, *24*
　tat protein and, 29–31, *30*
　transactivation response element of, 30, *31*
　transmission of, 67, 499–500
　　behavior change to reduce, 500–502, *501*
　　blood-borne, 503–504
　　by IV drug users, 499
　　determinants of, 499–500
　　eliminating cofactors of, 503
　　gastrointestinal mucosa and, 195–196
　　heterosexual, 538–541, 539t
　　in utero, 526
　　patient-to-patient, 515
　　patient-to-provider, 513–515, 514t
　　perinatal, 10–11, *12*, 504–505, 525–526
　　prevention of, 127t, 499–508, 518–521
　　　antiretroviral prophylaxis for, 503, 518–521, 520t, 521t
　　　behavior change in, 500–502, *501*
　　　biomedical strategies for, 502–503
　　　blood-borne, 503–504, 519–521, 521t
　　　infection control for, 516
　　　occupational, 518–519, 520t
　　　perinatal and breast feeding, 504–505
　　　postexposure prophylaxis for, 518–519, 520t, 521t

Human immunodeficiency virus 1 (*Continued*)
    sexual, 505–507, *506, 507,* 519–521, 521t
      vaccine research and, 502–503
    provider-to-patient, 515
    sexual, 499–500, 505–507, *506, 507.* See also *Heterosexual transmission; Homosexuals.*
    strain selection in, 73
    vaccine research on, 502–503
    vif gene and, 24, *24*
    vif protein and, 27–28, 39–31
    viral load of, 29, 125
      and initiation of therapy, 99
        in children, 529–530
      and transmission, 503
        perinatal, 525–526
      in pregnancy, monitoring of, 503
    virion of, 24–25, *25*
      attachment of, 25–27, *26*
      internalization of, 27
      morphogenesis of, *25, 26,* 32
    vpr gene and, 24, *24*
    vpr protein and, 28, 31
    vpu gene of, 24, *24*
    vpu protein and, 31, 32–33, *33*
    Western blot for, 46–48, *47*
      false-positive, 59–60, *61*
Human immunodeficiency virus (HIV) 2, genetics of, 3–4
  testing for, 49
Human immunodeficiency virus (HIV) disease, alternative therapies for, 601–610. See also individual therapies.
    cycles of, 602–603
    global context of, 603–604
    reasons for seeking, 603
    surveys of, 601–602
  antiretroviral therapy for, 97–113, 129. See also *Antiretroviral therapy.*
    opportunistic infections and, 210
  biliary manifestations in, 207–208
  cancer screening in, 128–129
  cardiovascular complications of, 275–283
  chest films in, 139–151
  counseling on, 127t
  dermatologic care in, 185–194. See also specific diseases.
  endocrinologic manifestations of, 285–292
  epidemiology of, 3–17
    in children, 3, 7, 525
    in older individuals, 593, 594t
    opportunistic infections and, 11–17
  evaluation of immunologic status in, 57–58. See also *CD4+ T cells.*
  gastrointestinal manifestations in, 195–203. See also specific diseases.
  global impact of, 3, *4*
  hematologic complications of, 265–271
  hepatic manifestations in, 203–207
  hepatitis viruses and, 399–400, 402–403
  in children, 525–533
    antiretroviral therapy for, 528–531
      CD4+ count and, 526, 526t, 531
        changing, 531
      initial, 529–531, 530t
      principles for, 528–529
      starting, 529
    diagnosis of, 527
    epidemiology of, 3, 7, 525
      in United States, 7
    management of, 527–528, 532

Human immunodeficiency virus (*Continued*)
    monitoring of, 527–528, 528t
    mortality from, 525
    natural history of, 526–527, 526t
    plasma viral load and, 526–527
    prophylaxis for, against opportunistic infections, 532
      against PCP, 527–528
    risk factors for, 525–526
    timing of contraction of HIV infection, 526, 526t
    transmission to, 10–11, 12, 503–504, 525–526
    vaccinations and, 528
  in older individuals, 593–598
    antiretroviral therapy for, 596–598
    clinical manifestations of, 595–596
    epidemiology of, 593, 594t
    immunopathogenesis, 593–595
    natural history of, 595
  initial evaluation of, 126–129, 127t
  laboratory evaluation in, 127t, 128. See also specific tests and measures.
  latent, 29
  management of, 41–121. See also specific drugs and opportunistic infections.
    antiretroviral therapy for, 97–113, 129. See also *Antiretroviral therapy.*
      adverse effects of, 79–83, 80t
    chest films in, 139–151
    for occupational exposures, 516–518
    model for, 133–134
  morbidity and mortality trends from, 7–10, *8–10*
  natural history of, 52, *53,* 125–126
    in children, 526–527, 526t
    in drug users, 575–576
    in older patients, 595
  neurologic complications of, 217–232. See also specific disorders.
  ocular complications of, 171–178. See also specific diseases.
  opportunistic infections and. See also individual infections.
    antiretroviral therapy and, 210
    screening and prevention of, 129–133
  oral complications of, 157–165. See also specific diseases.
  pancreatic manifestations in, 208–209
  partner notification on, 501
  pathogenesis of, 23–33
    and initiation of therapy, 97
  pediatric, 525–533. See also *Pediatric AIDS.*
  prevalence and incidence of, 12–17
  prevention of transmission of, 127t, 499–508, 518–521
    antiretroviral prophylaxis for, 503, 518–521, 520t, 521t
    behavior change in, 500–502, *501*
    biomedical strategies for, 502–503
    blood-borne, 503–504, 519–521, 521t
    infection control for, 516
    occupational, 518–519, 520t
    perinatal and breast feeding, 504–505
    postexposure, 518–519, 520t, 521t
    sexual, 505–507, *506, 507,* 519–521, 521t
    vaccine research and, 502–503
  primary, 67–75
    antibody testing in, 70–71, 71t, 517
    B$_2$-microglobulin in, 73
    CD4+ T cells and, 73, 74
    CD8+ T cells and, 73, 74
    clinical manifestations of, 67–69, 68t, *69,* 70t, 517
    cytokines and, 74

Human immunodeficiency virus (*Continued*)
  definition of, 67
  diagnosis of, 69–70, 70t
  differential diagnosis of, 70t, 71t
  HIV RNA and DNA detection in, 72–73
  HIV strain selection in, 73
  immunoblotting of, 71–72, 72
  immunology in, 73, 74
  laboratory features of, 70–73
  lymph node biopsies in, 73
  neutralizing antibodies and, 74
  p24 antigen testing in, 70–71, 72, 74, 517
  predisposing factors for, 69
  prognosis for, 75
  serology for, 70–72
  treatment of, 75. See also specific drugs.
  virology of, 72–73
  progression of, 125–126
    hepatitis C virus infection and, 404–405, 404t
    in children, 526–527, 526t
    in older patients, 593–595
    in women, 541–542
    predictors of, 125–126
    viral load and, 29, 125
  psychiatric syndromes in, 241–255. See also *AIDS dementia complex.*
  psychosocial issues in, 255–259
  referrals in, 127t, 128
  renal complications of, 297–300
  staging of, and perinatal transmission, 525
    determination of, 126
  transmission of. See *Human immunodeficiency virus (HIV) 1, transmission of.*
  viral load in, and disease progression, 29, 125
    and initiation of therapy, 99
    and transmission, 500
      perinatal, 525–526
    in children, 526–527
Human papillomavirus (HPV), 185, 486–489
  anal cancer from, 128–129, 468, 486, 488–489, 545–546
  cervical cancer from, 128, 467, 468t, 486–488, 544–545
  diagnosis and treatment of, 189
  genital warts from, 189
    in women, 545
  oral warts from, 159t, *163,* 163–164
Human T-cell leukemia virus (HTLV), myelopathy from, 230, 230t
Hydrocortisone, for seborrheic dermatitis, 186t
Hydroxyurea, 108–109
  combination therapy with, 100t, 108
  dosage of, 109
Hyperbilirubinemia, from indinavir, 207, 564
Hypercalcemia, drug-induced, 290
Hypercholesterolemia, 275, 281–282, 290–291
  from protease inhibitors, 106
Hyperemesis gravidarum, 566
Hypergammaglobulinemia, 268
Hyperglycemia, 290
  from protease inhibitors, 83, 290
Hyperinsulinemia, 289–290
Hyperkalemia, 287, 297
  delirium from, 253
  drug-induced, 287
  treatment of, 297
Hyperlipidemia, 275, 281–282, 290–291
  from protease inhibitors, 83
Hypersensitive dermatologic disorders, 190–191
Hypertension, in pregnancy, HIV infection and, 567
Hypertrichosis, of eyelashes, 172–173

Hypertriglyceridemia, 275, 281–282, 290–291
  from protease inhibitors, 106, 282, 292
Hypocalcemia, drug-induced, 290
Hypoglycemia, delirium from, 253
  drug-induced, 290
Hypogonadism, 289
  depression from, 245
  fatigue from, 256t
Hypokalemia, 297
Hypomagnesemia, drug-induced, 290
Hyponatremia, 286, 287, 297
  delirium from, 253
Hypotension, delirium from, 253
Hypothalamic-pituitary axes, 285–286
Hypothyroidism, 288
Hypoxemia, delirium from, 253
  from *Pneumocystis carinii* pneumonia, 312

Idoxuridine, for ocular HSV, 174
Imipenem, for *Rhodococcus equi,* 424
Imiquimod, for molluscum contagiosum, 189
Immune thrombocytopenia, HIV-related, 268–269
Immunoglobulin, intravenous, 269
Impotence, 289
Indinavir, 104–105
  adverse effect(s) of, 80t, 82, 98t, 104
    diarrhea as, 201, 202t
    gastrointestinal, 202t
    hepatic, 206t, 207
    hyperbilirubinemia as, 207, 564
    hyperglycemia as, 290
    lipodystrophy as, 281–282
    nephrolithiasis as, 82, 104, 564
  combination therapy with, 101t, 104, 106t
    for children, 530, 530t
  dosage of, 98t, 106t
  drug interactions with, 89t, 90–91, 334, 355
  food and, 93, 93t
  for primary HIV disease, 75
  HIV mutations and, *55,* 99t
  resistance to, 105
Indirect fluorescent antibody (IFA) test, for *Bartonella,* 416
  for HIV, 48
Indomethacin, drug interactions with, 85
Infectious mononucleosis, differential diagnosis of, 69–70, 71t
Influenza vaccine, for HIV-infected patients, 130
  children, 528
  pregnant, 559
Insect bite reactions, diagnosis and treatment of, 186t
Insulin-like growth factor I, 285–286
Insulin resistance, from protease inhibitors, 282
Interferon α, adverse effect(s) of, depression as, 244
  cardiomyopathy from, 280
  CD4+ cell count and, 406
  for hepatitis C virus, 406, 407t
  for Kaposi's sarcoma, 474–476, 475t, 477
    with zidovudine, 475–476, 475t
  in primary HIV infection, 74
Interferon β, drug interactions with, 85
Interferon γ, for toxoplasmosis, 388
  Mycobacterium avium-complex and, 344
Interleukin 1, glucocorticoid deficiency and, 286, 287
Interleukin 2, cardiomyopathy from, 280
  Mycobacterium avium-complex and, 344
Interleukin 6, and HIV, 593
  and Kaposi's sarcoma, 473
  and non-Hodgkin's lymphoma, 478

Interleukin 10, and HIV, 593
  and non-Hodgkin's lymphoma, 478
Interleukin 12, *Mycobacterium avium*-complex and, 344
Interstitial pneumonitis, lymphocytic, chest films of, 149–150, *151*
  nonspecific, chest films of, 149–150
Intracranial hypertension, from cryptococcosis, management of, 368–369
Intrauterine devices, and HIV transmission, 538
Intravenous drug users. See *Drug users, intravenous.*
Iridocyclitis, 174, 175
Iron deficiency, 265, 267
Isoniazid, adverse effects of, 356t
  for *Mycobacterium tuberculosis,* 355, 356–357, 356t, 357t, 578
    dosage of, 356t
    prophylactic, 130, 358
  psychosis from, 255
Isospora belli, cholecystitis from, 207
Itraconazole, drug interactions with, 87, 366, 373
  for candidiasis, 158
  for coccidioidomycosis, 374
  for cryptococcosis, 366, 368t
  for eosinophilic folliculitis, 192
  for histoplasmosis, 372–373t
  for *Penicillium marneffei,* 425
IV drug users. See *Drug users, intravenous.*

Jarisch-Herxheimer reaction, in treatment of *Bartonella,* 418
  in treatment of *Treponema pallidum,* 459, 460
JC virus, and progressive multifocal encephalopathy, 229
  PCR of, 229

Kanamycin, for *Mycobacterium tuberculosis,* 356t
Kaposi's sarcoma, 467, 468–477, 468t
  adrenal, 286
  and progression of HIV disease, 126
  bone marrow biopsy in, 266
  chest films of, 147–148, *148, 149,* 470
  cholangitis from, 207
  clinical presentation of, 469–471, Color Plates IE and IG
  cutaneous manifestations of, 185
  differential diagnosis of, 172, 384, 412, 416, 470
  epidemiology of, 11–12, 468
  esophageal, 198
  gastric, 198–199
    differential diagnosis of, 432
  hepatic, 205
  in drug users, 576
  in women, 543
  myocardial, 281
  ocular, 172
  oral, 159t, 164
  pathogenesis of, 468–469, *469*
  pericardial effusion from, 277
  pulmonary, 323, 470
    in older patients, 596
  staging of, 471, *471,* 471t, 472t
  thyroid disease from, 288
  treatment of, 471–477
    antineoplastic agents for, 473–474, 473t, 477t
    antiretroviral drugs and, 468, 476, 477t
    cryotherapy for, 473
    interferon for, 474–476, 475t, 477, 477t
    intralesional chemotherapy for, 473
    local therapy in, 472–473

Kaposi's sarcoma (*Continued*)
    photodynamic therapy for, 473
    radiation therapy for, 472–473, 477t
    recommendations on, 476–477, 477t
    systemic therapy for, 473–476, 477t
Kaposi's sarcoma herpesvirus, 468–469, *469.* See also *Human herpesvirus 8.*
Keratitis, infectious, 173–174
Keratoconjunctivitis sicca, 173
Ketoconazole, adverse effects of, 372
    adrenal, 287
    hypogonadism from, 289
  drug interactions with, 87, 365
  for candidiasis, 158, 197t
  for cryptococcosis, 365
  for histoplasmosis, 372
  for seborrheic dermatitis, 186t, 193
  psychosis from, 255
Kidney(s). See *Renal* entries.
Klebsiella pneumoniae, keratitis from, 174
  pneumonia from, 332t
  stomatitis from, 159t, 162

L-α-actylmethadol (LAAM), 587, 588
  antiretroviral therapy interaction with, 582
L-asparaginase, for non-Hodgkin's lymphoma, 481t, 482
Lactate dehydrogenase (LDH), *Pneumocystis carinii* pneumonia and, 310
Lamivudine (3TC), 27, 103
  adverse effects of, 80t, 81, 98t
  combination therapy with, 100t, 101t, 103, 110, 110t
    for children, 530, 530t
    for women, 548
      pregnant, 563–564
  dosage of, 98t
  drug interactions with, 86t, 87
  for AIDS dementia, 227
  for primary HIV disease, 75
  HIV mutations and, *55,* 99t
  resistance to, 563
Langerhans cells, HIV transmission and, 538, 540
Large intestine, opportunistic infections of, 199–203
Laryngeal disease, in bacillary angiomatosis, 413
Latin America, HIV infection in, 3, *4*
Legal issues, 255–256
Legionella, 335
Leiomyosarcoma, 468t
Lentiviruses, characteristics of, 24
Lesbians, HIV transmission among, 538, 540–541, 541t
Leucovorin, adverse effects of, 317t, 318t
  for non-Hodgkin's lymphoma, 481t, 482
  trimetrexate with, for *Pneumocystis carinii,* 317t, 318t
Leukocytes, disorders of, 268, 268t
Leukoencephalopathy, progressive multifocal, 178, 227, 227t, 228, 229–230
  differential diagnosis of, 225t, 228, 229
Leukopenia, from ganciclovir, 435, 436t
Levofloxacin, for *Mycobacterium tuberculosis,* 356t
Lindane, for scabies, 190
Lipid metabolism, 290–291
Lipodystrophy, from protease inhibitors, 83, 281–282, 292
Lipomatosis, benign symmetrical, from antiretroviral therapy, 292
Listeriosis, meningeal, 221
Lithium, 254, 254t
Liver biopsy, 208
  in bacillary angiomatosis, 416

Lorazepam, 252, 252t
Lumbosacral polyradiculopathy, idiopathic, 431
Lung(s). See also *Pulmonary* entries.
   cancer of, 467
Lupus anticoagulant, 270
Luteinizing hormone (LH), 289
Lymph node biopsy, in bacillary angiomatosis, 416
   in primary HIV disease, 73
Lymphadenopathy, generalized, and progression of HIV
     disease, 126
   in primary HIV infection, 68, 68t
   inguinal, from HSV, 439
Lymphatic disease, in bacillary angiomatosis, 412, 413
Lymphedema, from Kaposi's sarcoma, 472
Lymphocytes, of intestinal lamina propria, 195–196
   T. See specific T cells, e.g., *CD4+ T cells.*
Lymphocytic interstitial pneumonitis, chest films of, 149–
     150, *151*
Lymphocytopenia, in primary HIV infection, 73
Lymphocytosis, in primary HIV infection, 73
   and polyneuropathy, 218–219
Lymphoma, adrenal, 286
  and progression of HIV disease, 126
  cholangitis from, 207
  esophageal, 198
  intraocular, 177
  meningeal, 221
  non-Hodgkin's. See *Non-Hodgkin's lymphoma.*
  oral, 164
  primary CNS, 219, 225t, 227, 227t, 228, 229. See also
     Non-Hodgkin's lymphoma.
    differential diagnosis of, 384
    etiology and diagnosis of, 228, 479–480
    treatment of, 484, 484t

M cells, HIV transmission and, 196
Macrophages, HIV infection of, 25
Maedi virus, 24
Magnetic resonance imaging (MRI), for CMV, 431
  for neurologic diseases, 218
  for non-Hodgkin's lymphoma, 479
  for primary CNS lymphoma, 228
  for toxoplasmosis, 382–383, 384
  in AIDS dementia, 224
  in bacillary angiomatosis, 413, *415*
Malaleuca, 609
Malnutrition, fatigue from, 256t
Managed care programs, and care for HIV-infected patients,
    133–134
Mania, in HIV-infected patients, 241, 254–255
  treatment of, 254, 254t
  organic brain disease and, 250
Manic-depressive disorders, 249
Mantoux test, 129–130
MAO (monoamine oxidase) inhibitors, 248
Marantic, endocarditis, 281
Marijuana, for wasting syndrome, 608, 608t
Massage therapy, 609–610
m-BACOD therapy, for non-Hodgkin's lymphoma, 481t,
    482–483
Measles vaccine, for children, 528
Mechanical ventilation, for *Pneumocystis carinii* pneumo-
    nia, 312
Medical caregivers, burnout of, 258
Megestrol acetate, 291
  adverse effects of, 290
Melatonin therapy, 601

Men who have sex with men (MSM). See also *Homo-*
    sexuals.
  HIV infection in, 6–7, *13,* 13–14, 16, 517
   by age, 594t
  opportunistic infections in, 11
Meningitis, from bacillary angiomatosis, 413
  from cryptococcosis, 220, 225t, 362–363, 363t, *364,*
    365
  from histoplasmosis, 371
  from HIV-1, 219–220
  from syphilis, 455
  in late HIV disease, 220–221
  pyogenic, 221
Meningovascular syphilis, 220–221, 454, 455
Menstrual disorders, in HIV-infected patients, 289, 547–
    548
Metabolic acidosis, 298
Methadone therapy, 587–589, 588t
  drug interactions with, 588t
   antiretroviral therapy and, 582–584, 588t
  for cocaine withdrawal, 587
  in pregnancy, 558
Methamphetamine use, 584, 586
  effects of, 586t
Methemoglobinemia, fatigue from, 256t
Methylphenidate, 248
  dosage of, 247t
Methyltestosterone, for hypogonadism, 256t
Metoclopramide, mania from, 254
Metronidazole, for *Clostridium difficile,* 201
  for gingivitis and periodontitis, 161
  psychosis from, 255
Micrococcus, keratitis from, 174
Microhemagglutination–*T. pallidum* (MHA-TP) test, 457
Microsporidiosis, keratitis from, 174
Midazolam, drug interactions with, 88t
Mineralocorticoid hormone deficiency, 287–288
Mitogen-activated protein kinase (MAPK), 28
Mitral valve prolapse, 281
Molluscum contagiosum, 185, *188,* 188–189
  diagnosis and treatment of, 186t, 189
  ocular, 172
Monoamine oxidase (MAO) inhibitors, 248
Mononeuritis multiplex, 231
  of CMV, 431–432
MOPP therapy, for Hodgkin's disease, 485
Motor abnormalities, in AIDS dementia, 224
MRI. See *Magnetic resonance imaging (MRI).*
MSM. See *Men who have sex with men (MSM).*
Mucocutaneous infections, from HSV, 438
  from syphilis, 455–456
Mumps vaccine, for children, 528
Myalgia, in primary HIV infection, 67, 68t
Mycobacterial infections. See also individual species.
  atypical, 343–349
  bone marrow biopsy in, 266
Mycobacterium avium-complex, 343–348
  adrenal infections with, 286
  and progression of HIV disease, 126
  anemia from, 267
  antiretroviral therapy and, 344
  chest films of, 142, 143
  cholangitis from, 207
  choroiditis from, 177
  clinical manifestations of, 344–345, 345t
  diagnosis of, 345
  dissemination of, 343, 344, 345t
  epidemiology of, 11, 343–344
  esophageal disease from, 196, 197t, 198

Mycobacterium avium-complex (*Continued*)
  gastrointestinal manifestations of, 198–199, 200–201, 345t
  hepatic disease from, 204
  in women, 542
  oral manifestations of, 159t, 162
  pancreatic abscesses from, 209
  pathogenesis of, 344, Color Plate ID
  pericardial effusion from, 277
  prophylaxis for, 131t, 132, 343, 348
    in children, 532
  treatment of, 197t, 201, 341, 345–348, 346t, 347t
Mycobacterium celatum, 348–349
Mycobacterium chelonei, 349
Mycobacterium fortuitum, 349
Mycobacterium genavense, 204, 341, 349
Mycobacterium gordonae, 341, 349
Mycobacterium haemophilum, 341, 348, 349
Mycobacterium kansasii, 204, 348–349
  chest films of, 143–144
  pneumonia from, differential diagnosis of, 422
  treatment of, 341, 349
Mycobacterium malmoense, 341, 349
Mycobacterium marinum, 348–349
Mycobacterium scrofulaceum, 348–349
Mycobacterium simiae, 341, 348–349
Mycobacterium szulgai, 341
Mycobacterium tuberculosis, 353–359. See also *Tuberculosis.*
  multidrug-resistant, 130, 353–354, 357–358
Mycobacterium xenopi, 204, 341, 348–349
Mycoplasma pneumoniae, pneumonia from, 332t, 335
Myelitis, from CMV, 430–431
Myelopathy(ies), 230, 230t
  in AIDS dementia, 226
  progressive vacuolar, 230, 230t
Myelosuppression, drug-induced, 268, 268t
  from zidovudine, 270–271
Myocardial biopsy, 280–281
Myocardial disease, 275, 278–281
  autoimmune, 280
  diagnosis of, 279
  opportunistic infections and, 279–280
  treatment of, 280–281
Myopathies, 232, 232t
Myositis, in drug users, 577

N-acetylcysteine (NAC), 606–607
NASBA (nucleic acid–based amplification), for HIV, 50, 52
Nausea and vomiting, from didanosine, 80
  from ganciclovir, 435
  from indinavir, 82
  from ritonavir, 83
  from saquinavir, 82
  in pregnancy, 566
Necrotizing fasciitis, in drug users, 577
Necrotizing stomatitis, 159t
Necrotizing ulcerative gingivitis, acute, 161
Necrotizing ulcerative periodontitis, 159t, 161
Needlestick injuries, antiretroviral therapy for, 111, 519
  HIV from, 75, 499, 504, 516, 519
    testing for, 516–517
  prevention of, 513–515, 514t, 516
nef gene, 24, *24*
Nef protein, 27–28, 29–33, *33*
Nefazodone, 248
  dosage of, 247t

Nelfinavir, 105
  adverse effect(s) of, 80t, 83, 98t, 548
    diarrhea as, 201, 202t
    gastrointestinal, 202t
    hepatic, 206t
    hyperglycemia as, 290
  combination therapy with, 101t, 105, 106t
    for children, 530, 530t
    for women, 548
      pregnant, 564
  dosage of, 98t, 106t
  drug interactions with, 89t, 91, 355, 548
    opioid substitutes and, 583
  food and, 93, 93t
  for primary HIV disease, 75
  HIV mutations and, *55,* 99t
Neoplasms. See also specific neoplasm, e.g., *Lymphoma.*
  in HIV disease, 467–490, 468t
    chest films of, 147–149, *148–150*
    epidemiology of, 11–12
    hepatic, 205
    neurologic, 218t
    oral, 159t
    screening for, 128–129
Neopterin, HIV infection and, 58
  primary, 74
Nephrolithiasis, from indinavir, 82, 104, 564
Nephropathy, HIV-associated, 298–300
Nephrotoxicity, from cidofovir, 437, 444
  from foscarnet, 436
Neuroimaging, 218
  in AIDS dementia complex, 224, 225t
Neuroleptic drugs, for HIV-infected patients, 221, 252t
Neuroleptic malignant syndrome, 253
Neurologic disease(s), 217–232. See also specific manifestations.
  classification of, 218t
  focal brain disease as, 225t, 227–230, 227t
  in asymptomatic phase of HIV infection, 218–219
  in late HIV disease, 219–227
  in primary HIV infection, 217–218
  myelopathies as, 230, 230t
  myopathies as, 232, 232t
  peripheral neuropathies as, 230–232, 231t
Neuro-ophthalmic manifestations, of HIV disease, 178
Neuropathy(ies), distal, predominantly sensory, 231
  demyelinating, HIV-related, 218
  from cytomegalovirus, 231, 231t, 430, 432
    distal, 432
  from didanosine, 80
  from stavudine, 81
  from zalcitabine, 80
  in primary HIV infection, 217–218
  pain control for, 257
  peripheral, 230–232, 231t. See also *Peripheral neuropathy.*
Neurosyphilis, 454–455, 462
  diagnosis of, 457–458
  treatment of, 459–460
    failure of, 461–462
Neutropenia, colony-stimulating factors for, 271, 271t
  drug-induced, 268, 268t
    from ganciclovir, 435, 436t
    from zidovudine, 79
Nevirapine, 107
  adverse effects of, 80t, 81–82, 107
  combination therapy with, 101t, 106t, 110, 110t
    in pregnancy, 565

Nevirapine (*Continued*)
dosage of, 106t
drug interactions with, 87–88, 88t, 107, 548
opioid substitutes and, 583
for AIDS dementia, 227
HIV mutations and, *55,* 73, 99t, 107
resistance to, 107
NF-κB/Rel factors, 29
NNRTIs. See *Non-nucleoside reverse transcriptase inhibitors.*
Nocardia, pneumonia from, 332t
differential diagnosis of, 422
Non-Hodgkin's lymphoma, 467, 468t, 477–485
bone marrow biopsy in, 266
chest films of, 148, *150*
clinical features of, 478–480, Color Plate IIB
differential diagnosis of, 479, 480
epidemiology of, 477–478
hepatic, 205
in drug users, 576
in women, 543
ocular, 172, 177
oral, 159t, 164
pathogenesis and etiology of, 478
primary CNS, 219, 225t, 227, 227t, 228, 229
differential diagnosis of, 384
etiology and diagnosis of, 228, 479–480
treatment of, 484, 484t
treatment of, 480–484, *481,* 481t, 483t
recommendations for, 484–485
Non-nucleoside reverse transcriptase inhibitors, 106–108.
See also individual drugs.
adverse effects of, 80t, 81–82, 98t
combination therapy with, 100t–101t, 110, 110t
for children, 531
dosages for, 98t
drug interactions with, 87–89, 88t, 355–356
Nonoxynol-9, 506, *506,* 539
Nonspecific interstitial pneumonitis, chest films of, 149–150
Nonsteroidal anti-inflammatory drugs (NSAIDs), depression from, 244
psychosis from, 255
North America, HIV infection in, 3, *4*
Nortriptyline, 248
dosage of, 247t
Norwegian scabies, 190
Nosocomial transmission, of HIV. See *Occupational exposures, to HIV.*
NRTIs. See *Nucleoside reverse transcriptase inhibitors.*
Nucleic acid–based amplification (NASBA), for HIV, 50, 52
Nucleoside reverse transcriptase inhibitors, 98–103. See also individual drugs.
adverse effects of, 79–81, 80t, 98t
gastrointestinal, 202t
hematologic, 270–271
hepatic, 205, 206t, 207
pancreatic, 209
combination regimens with, 100t–101t, 110, 110t
for children, 530–531, 530t
dosages for, 98t
drug interactions with, 85–87, 86t
methadone and, 588t
Nutrients, drug interactions with, 91–93
Nutrition, for prevention of wasting syndrome, 128
Nutritional assessment, for HIV-infected patient, 128
in pregnancy, 561
Nystatin, for candidiasis, 158

Obsessive-compulsive disorder, 253
Occupational exposures, to HIV, 75, 499, 504, 513–521.
See also *Needlestick injuries.*
antiretroviral therapy for, 111, 519
in labor and delivery, 570
management of, 517–518
patient-to-patient, 515
patient-to-provider, 513–515, 514t
prevention of, 513–521
provider-to-patient, 515
testing for, 516–517
Ocular complications, of HIV disease, 171–178. See also
individual disorders.
adnexal, 171–173
in anterior section, 173–175
in orbit, 178
in posterior section, 176–178
neural, 178
Odynophagia, 196
Office visit, by HIV-infected patient, 126–128, 127t
Opiate withdrawal syndrome, 585t, 586–587
management of, 586–587, 586t
Opiates, abuse of. See *Drug users, intravenous; Heroin.*
antiretroviral therapy interaction with, 582
Opportunistic infections, in HIV disease. See also individual infections.
chest films of, 139–147, *140–147*
epidemiologic trends in, 11–17
in IV drug users, 576–579, 576t
in women, 542–543
pregnant, 562–563
neurologic, 218t
prophylaxis for, 131–133
in children, 532
in pregnancy, 562–563
screening for, 129–130
Optic neuritis, from didanosine, 80
Oral complications, of HIV disease, 157–165, 158t. See also individual diseases.
Oral hairy leukoplakia, 159t, 162–163, *163,* Color Plate 1B
and progression of HIV disease, 126
Oral sex, HIV transmission via, 505
Orbital manifestations, of HIV disease, 178
Organic brain disease, differential diagnosis of, 245
in HIV-infected patients, 241, 249–252
Orolabial infections, with HSV, 159t, 162, 438–439
Oxacillin, for *Staphylococcus aureus,* 334

p7 protein, 25, *25*
p17 protein, 25, *25*
p24 protein, 25, *25,* 44, *45,* 58, *59,* 60
antigen test with, 44, *45,* 49–50, *50, 53,* 53t, 70–71, 517
acidified procedure for, 50
for primary HIV infection, 70–71, 72, 74, 517
in children, *527*
Paclitaxel, for Kaposi's sarcoma, 473t, 474, 477t
Pain control, 257
Pancreatic manifestations, of HIV disease, 208–209, 289–290
drug-induced, 80, 81, 201, 209. See also *Pancreatitis, drug-induced.*
infectious and neoplastic, 209
pathogenesis of, 208–209, 209t
Pancreatitis, drug-induced, 80, 81, 201, 209
from didanosine, 80, 209
from lamivudine, 81
from stavudine, 81

Pancreatic manifestations (*Continued*)
    from zalcitabine, 81, 209
    triglycerides and, 290
Panic disorder, in HIV-infected patients, 241, 252–253
    treatment of, 252–253, 252t
Pap smears, for anogenital neoplasia, 129, 489, 489t
    in HIV-infected women, 544, 545
Papulosquamous disorders, 192–193, *193, 194*
Para-aminosalicylic acid, for *Mycobacterium tuberculosis,*
    356t
Parasitic infections. See also specific parasites.
    cutaneous, 189
Parotid enlargement, 159t, 164–165, *165*
Paroxetine, 247
    dosage of, 247t
Partner notification policies, on HIV infection, 501
Parvovirus B19, anemia from, 267
PCP. See *Pneumocystis carinii, pneumonia from.*
PCR. See *Polymerase chain reaction (PCR).*
Pediatric AIDS, 525–533
    antiretroviral therapy for, 528–531
        CD4+ cell count and, 526, 526t, 531
        changing, 531
        initial, 529–531, 530t
        principles for, 528–529
        starting, 529
    diagnosis of, 527
    epidemiology of, 3, 7, 525
        in United States, 7
    management of, 527–528, 532
    monitoring of, 527–528, 528t
    mortality from, 525
    natural history of, 526–527, 526t
    plasma viral load and, 526–527
    prophylaxis for, against opportunistic infections, 532
        against PCP, 527–528
    risk factors for, 525–526
    timing of contraction of HIV infection in, 526, 526t
    vaccinations and, 528
Peliosis hepatis, 205, 411, 412
Pelvic inflammatory disease, 547
Penciclovir, for HSV, 443, 445
Penicillin(s), for *Streptococcus pneumoniae,* 333, 333t
    for syphilis, 458–459, 459t, 461, 462
Penicillium marneffei, 424–425
    clinical presentation of, 424
    diagnosis of, 424–425
    treatment and prevention of, 425
Pentamidine, adverse effect(s) of, 317t, 318t, 319
        hypoglycemia as, 290
        pancreatitis as, 209
    for *Pneumocystis carinii,* 141–142, 317, 317t, 318–319,
        318t, 322
        aerosolized, 322
            for prophylaxis, 324–325, 324t
            tuberculosis transmission from, 353, 359
        dosage of, 317t, 318t
Pentoxifylline, 606
Pericardial effusion, 277–278
Pericarditis, 275, 277–278
    treatment of, 277–278
Perinatal transmission, of HCV, 405
    of HIV, 10–11, *12,* 504–505, 525–526. See also *Pediatric AIDS; Pregnancy.*
        antiretroviral therapy and, 11, 499, 504, 519, 548,
            557–558
        predictors of, 557–558
        prevention of, 504–505
        risk factors for, 525–526

Periodontitis, 158, 161, *161*
    necrotizing ulcerative, 159t, 161
Peripheral blood mononuclear cells (PBMCs), HIV and,
    43–44, *45*
Peripheral neuropathy(ies), 230–232, 231t
    from didanosine, 80
    from stavudine, 81
    from zalcitabine, 80
    in drug users, 578
    pain control for, 257
Permethrin, for scabies, 190
Pharyngitis, from Kaposi's sarcoma, 472
    in primary HIV infection, 67, 68t
Phenobarbital, drug interactions with, 88t
Phenytoin, drug interactions with, 88t
    methadone and, 588t
Phosphonoformate. See *Foscarnet.*
Photodynamic therapy, for Kaposi's sarcoma, 473
Photosensitivity reactions, 191
    diagnosis and treatment of, 186t
Phototherapy, for eosinophilic folliculitis, 192
Phytohemagglutinin responses, in primary HIV infection,
    74
PIs. See *Protease inhibitors.*
Plasmacytoma, 468t
Platelets, disorders of, 268–269
PML (progressive multifocal leukoencephalopathy), 178,
    227, 227t, 228, 229–230
Pneumococcal pneumonia, 331–334, 332t
    diagnosis of, 332–333
        chest films in, *146,* 146–147, 332
    treatment of, 333–334, 333t
Pneumococcal vaccine, 334
    for children, 528
    for HIV-infected patients, 130
Pneumocystis carinii, biology of, 305–306
    choroiditis from, 177
    epidemiology of, 306–307
    extrapulmonary manifestations of, 313
    history of, 305
    host defenses against, 307–308
    orbital manifestations of, 178
    pancreatic abscesses from, 209
    pathophysiology of, 308
    pneumonia from, 305–325
        and progression of HIV disease, 126
        chest films of, 139–142, *140–144, 310,* 310–311, *311,*
            313, *314*
            trimethoprim-sulfamethoxazole and, 139
        chronic airway disease in, 313
        clinical presentation of, 309–312, *310, 311*
        complications of, 312–313
        diagnosis of, 313–316, *314, 315*
        differential diagnosis of, 139, 311, 380, 432
        epidemiology of, 11, 332t
        headache in, 219–220
        hypoxemia and respiratory failure in, 312
        in drug users, 576, 578
        in older patients, 596
        in pregnancy, 556–557
        in women, 541, 542–543
        incidence of, 308
        pneumothorax in, 312–313
        prophylaxis of, 58, 131, 131t, 323–325, 324t, 375
            in children, 527, 528, 528t, 532
            in pregnancy, 561
        risk factors for, 308–309
        treatment of, 316–323, 317t, 318t
            atovaquone in, 317, 318t, 321–322

Pneumocystis carinii (*Continued*)
      clindamycin-primaquine in, 317, 317t, 318t, 319–320
      corticosteroids in, 322–323
      empiric, 316, 316t
      failure of, 323, 323t
      pentamidine in, 317, 317t, 318–319, 318t, 322
      trimethoprim-dapsone in, 317t, 318t, 321
      trimethoprim-sulfamethoxazole in, 316–318, 317t, 318t
      trimetrexate in, 317t, 318t, 320–321
  transmission of, 306–307
  trophozoites of, 305–306
Pneumonia. See also individual causative agents.
  approach to patient with, 338–341
  chest films in, 340t
  community-acquired, in HIV-infected patients, 338–339
  diagnostic evaluation in, 339, 340t
  empiric treatment of, 341
  etiologic diagnosis of, 339–341
  from bacteria, 331–335, 332t
    prevention of, 132
  from CMV, 432–433
  from fungi, 336–338, 337t
  from *Pneumocystis carinii*, 305–325. See also *Pneumocystis carinii*, *pneumonia from*.
  from *Rhodococcus equi*, 147, 422, *422*
  from *Streptococcus pneumoniae*, 331–334, 332t, 333t. See also *Pneumococcal pneumonia*.
  from VZV, 446
  hospitalization for, 339
  in drug users, 578
Pneumothorax, from *Pneumocystis carinii* pneumonia, 140, *142, 143,* 312–313
Pokeweed mitogen responses, in primary HIV infection, 74
pol gene, 24, *24*
Pol protein, 31, 32
Polymerase chain reaction (PCR), for CMV, 231
  for Epstein-Barr virus, 479–480
  for herpes simplex virus, 441
  for HIV, 50, *51,* 51–52, 60, 125, 517
    genotypic drug resistance and, 54–56
    in children, 527, 528t
    in neonates, 572
    in pregnancy, 525
    phenotypic drug resistance and, 56
    quantitative, 52, 53t
  for JC virus, 229
  for toxoplasmosis, 382
Polymyositis, 232
Polyneuropathy, predominantly sensory, 231
Polyradiculopathy, from CMV, 230, 230t, 430–431
  from VZV, 447
  severe ascending, 231, 231t
PORN (progressive outer retinal necrosis), 176–177, Color Plate 3C
Postherpetic neuralgia, 171, 447. See also *Herpes zoster*.
  management of, 257, 448
Power of attorney, 255, 256
PPD skin test, 129–130, 358
  in pregnancy, 562
Pre-eclampsia, HIV infection and, 567, 568
Prednisone, for esophageal ulcers, 197t, 198
  for Hodgkin's disease, 485
  for non-Hodgkin's lymphoma, 481t, 482
Pregnancy, bacillary angiomatosis in, 415
  ectopic, HIV infection and, 566
  HCV infection in, 405

Pregnancy (*Continued*)
  HIV infection in, 10–11, *12,* 504–505, 519, 525–526. See also *Children, HIV infection in; Perinatal transmission of HIV.*
    antiretroviral therapy for, 112, 504–505, 519, 561–562, 563–565, 568
      adverse effects of, 564–565
      for advanced disease, 564
      for early disease, 563
      for moderately advanced disease, 564
      intrapartum, 569, 570t
    assessing predictors of vertical transmission of, 557–558
    counseling on, 560–562
      preconceptional, 555–560, 556t, 560t
    delivery alternatives for, 568
    diagnosis of, 556–557, 560
    evaluation of, 557
    fetal monitoring and, 569–570
    genital herpes and, 565–566
    hypertension and, 567
    infections and, 567
    intrapartum care for, 567–570
      anesthesia and analgesia in, 569
      antiretroviral therapy in, 569, 570t
      delivery routes in, 568
    medical complications of, 566–567
    multiple gestation and, 567
    nausea and vomiting of, 566
    obstetric decisions for, 526
    occupational exposures and, 570
    postpartum care and discharge plans for, 570–571
    prenatal care in, 562–566
      counseling for, 561
      initial evaluation for, 562
    preterm labor and, 567
    prophylaxis for opportunistic infections in, 561, 562–563
    psychiatric illness and, 567
    rupture of membranes and, 570
    substance abuse and, 558
    testing for, 560
    vaccinations and, 559
    viral load monitoring in, 565
  preconceptional counseling for, 555–560, 556t
  toxoplasmosis in, 381
Prenatal care, for HIV-infected women, 561, 562–566
Preterm labor, 567
Primaquine, adverse effects of, 317t, 318t, 319–320
  clindamycin with, for *Pneumocystis carinii*, 317, 317t, 318t, 319–320
Primary CNS lymphoma, 219, 225t, 227, 227t, 228, 229. See also *Non-Hodgkin's lymphoma*.
  differential diagnosis of, 384
  etiology and diagnosis of, 228, 479–480
  treatment of, 484, 484t
Primary HIV disease, 67–75. See also *Human immunodeficiency virus (HIV) disease, primary*.
Prison, antiretroviral therapy in, 581
Probenecid, drug interactions with, 85, 87
  for syphilis, 460
Procarbazine, for Hodgkin's disease, 485
Proctitis, from HSV, 200
Progressive multifocal leukoencephalopathy (PML), 178, 227, 227t, 228, 229–230
  differential diagnosis of, 225t, 228, 229
Progressive outer retinal necrosis (PORN), 176–177, Color Plate 3C
Prolactin, 286

ProMace-MOPP therapy, for non-Hodgkin's lymphoma, 481t, 482
Promethazine, for pregnant women, 566
Propionibacterium, orbital manifestations of, 178
Protease inhibitors, 103–106, 106t. See also individual drugs.
  adverse effect(s) of, 80t, 82–83, 98t, 564–565
    abnormal fat distribution as, 292
    diabetes and insulin resistance as, 282
    diarrhea as, 201–203, 202t
    gastrointestinal, 202t
    hepatic, 206t, 207
    hyperglycemia as, 83, 290
    in pregnancy, 564–565, 569
    lipodystrophy as, 83, 281–282, 292
    long-term, 106
  combination regimens with, 100t–101t, 105, 106t, 110, 110t
    for children, 530, 530t
  dosages for, 98t, 106t
  drug interactions with, 89–91, 89t, 90t, 92t, 105–106, 355–356, 548
    methadone and, 588t
    opioid substitutes and, 583
  for primary HIV disease, 75
  gastrointestinal infections and, 210
Protease paunch, 82, 292
Protozoal infections, gastrointestinal, 200
Pruritic folliculitis, 191–192, *192*
Pseudomonas aeruginosa, keratitis from, 174
  orbital manifestations of, 178
  pneumonia from, 332t, 335
    chest films of, 147
    differential diagnosis of, 422
Psoriasis, 185
  diagnosis and treatment of, 186t, 192–193, *194*
Psychiatric syndromes, 241–255. See also individual syndromes.
  in drug users, 579
  pregnancy and, 567
  principles of assessment for, 243
Psychosis, drug-induced, 255
  in AIDS dementia, 224
  in HIV-infected patients, 241, 255
Psychosocial issues, 126, 255–259
Psychotherapy, for HIV-infected individuals, 249
Pulmonary disease. See specific disease, e.g., *Pneumonia.*
Pulmonary embolism, 281
Pulmonary hypertension, 275, 278
  treatment of, 275, 278
Pulmonary Kaposi's sarcoma, 147–148, *148, 149,* 323, 470
  treatment of, 472
Pulmonary nodules, in bacillary angiomatosis, 413
Purified protein derivative (PPD) test, 129–130, 358
  in pregnancy, 562
Purpura, thrombotic thrombocytopenic, 270
PUVA phototherapy, for eosinophilic folliculitis, 192
Pyogenic granuloma, differential diagnosis of, 416
Pyrazinamide, for *Mycobacterium tuberculosis,* 356–357, 356t, 357t, 578
  dosage of, 356t
Pyrimethamine, adverse effects of, 387
  for toxoplasmosis, 386, 386t, 387, 389
    in maintenance therapy, 389, 389t
Pyrimethamine-dapsone, for toxoplasmosis, prophylactic, 390, 391t
Pyrimethamine-sulfadoxine, for toxoplasmosis, as maintenance therapy, 389, 389t, 390
  prophylactic, 390, 391t

Quellung test, 332, 340

Radiation therapy, for Kaposi's sarcoma, 172
Radioimmunoprecipitation assay (RIPA), for HIV, 48
Rapid plasma reagin (RPR) test, 128, 454, 456, 457, 460, 462
Rash, from delavirdine, 82, 107, 108
  from nevirapine, 81, 107
  from syphilis, 456
  from VZV, 446
  in primary HIV infection, 67, 68, 68t, *69*
Recombinant immunoblotting assay (RIBA), for hepatitis C virus, 401
Reflexes, abnormal, in AIDS dementia, 224
Reiter's syndrome, diagnosis and treatment of, 186t, 192–193, *194*
Renal disease, end-stage, 297
  in drug users, 579
  in HIV-infected patients, 297–300
Renal failure, acute, 298, 299t
    drug-induced, 299t
  chronic, 298–300
Renin deficiency, 287
Respiratory failure, from *Pneumocystis carinii* pneumonia, 312
Resting-energy expenditure (REE), 291
Retinal artery occlusion, 178
Retinal microvasculopathy, 176
Retinal necrosis, progressive outer, 176–177, Color Plate 3C
Retinal vein occlusion, 178
Retinitis, differential diagnosis of, 430
  from CMV, 176, 429–430, *430,* Color Plate 3B, Color Plate IF
    treatment of, 433–434, 436–437
  from HSV, 177, 430
  from syphilis, 455
  infectious, 176–177
Retinochoroiditis. See also *Chorioretinitis.*
  differential diagnosis of, 430
  from toxoplasmosis, 175, 177, 380, Color Plate 3D
Retinoic acid, for molluscum contagiosum, 189
Return-to-work issues, 258–259
rev gene, 24, *24*
Rev protein, 28, 29–31, *30*
  as viral RNA export factor, 31, *32*
  mutation of, 31, *32*
  response element of, 31
Rhizopus, orbital manifestations of, 178
Rhodococcus equi, clinical presentation of, *422,* 422–423
  diagnosis of, 423
  epidemiology and prevention of, 424
  pneumonia from, chest films of, 147, 422, *422*
  treatment of, 423–424
Ribavirin, drug interactions with, 86, 86t
Rifabutin, drug interactions with, 88t, 90, 105, 355, 356
    methadone and, 588t
  for *Mycobacterium avium*-complex, 345, 347, 347t
    in gastrointestinal disease, 201
    prophylactic, 131t, 132, 348
  for *Mycobacterium tuberculosis,* 356–357, 356t, 357t
  iridocyclitis from, 175
Rifampin, adverse effects of, 356t, 357
  adrenal, 287
  drug interactions with, 85, 86t, 90, 355–356, 365
    opioid substitutes and, 583, 588t
  for *Bartonella,* 418, 420t
  for *Mycobacterium avium*-complex, 345, 346
    in gastrointestinal disease, 201

Rifampin (*Continued*)
 for *Mycobacterium tuberculosis,* 355, 356t, 357t, 578
  dosage of, 356t
 for *Rhodococcus equi,* 423
 for staphylococcal folliculitis, 186t
 thyroid clearance and, 289
RIPA (radioimmunoprecipitation assay), for HIV, 48
Risk reduction counseling, for prevention of HIV transmission, 501–502
Risperidone, for delirium, 254
Ritonavir, 104
 adverse effect(s) of, 80t, 83, 98t, 104, 548
  diarrhea as, 201, 202t
  gastrointestinal, 202t
  hepatic, 206t
  hyperglycemia as, 290
  lipodystrophy as, 281–282
 combination regimen with, 104, 106t, 110, 110t
  for children, 530, 530t
  for older patients, 597
  for women, 548
 dosage of, 98t, 106t
 drug interactions with, 89t, 91, 92t, 104, 334, 355, 356, 548
  opioid substitutes and, 583
 food and, 93, 93t
 for primary HIV disease, 75
 HIV mutations and, *55,* 99t, 104
 resistance to, 104
RNA assays, for HIV, 50–54
 sensitivity and specificity of, 53–54
Roxithromycin, for toxoplasmosis, 388, 389
RPR test, 128, 454, 456, 457, 460, 462
Rubella vaccine, for children, 528

Safer sex practices, 505, 513, 559
Salivary gland disease, 159t, 164–165, *165*
Salmonellosis, gastrointestinal manifestations of, 201
Saquinavir, 103–104
 adverse effect(s) of, 80t, 82, 98t
  diarrhea as, 201, 202t
  gastrointestinal, 202t
  hepatic, 206t
  hyperglycemia as, 290
  lipodystrophy as, 281–282
 combination regimen with, 104, 106t, 110, 110t
  for children, 530, 530t
  for older patients, 597
  for women, 548
 dosage of, 98t, 106t
 drug interactions with, 89t, 90, 355, 356
 food and, 93, 93t, 104
 HIV mutations and, *55,* 99t
Scabies, diagnosis and treatment of, 186t, 190
Seborrheic dermatitis, diagnosis and treatment of, 186t, *192,* 192–193, *193*
Sedatives, drug interactions with, 90t
Seizures, from toxoplasmosis, 379–380
Selective serotonin reuptake inhibitors (SSRIs), 246–248, 253
 dosage of, 247t
 for pain, 257
Seminoma, 468t
Septic thrombophlebitis, in drug users, 577
Sertraline, 247
 dosage of, 247t
Sex workers, HIV infection in, 3, 505, 540
 HIV prevention programs for, 506
 Kaposi's sarcoma in, 543

Sexual exposure to HIV, prevention of, 505–507, *506, 507*
 prophylaxis for, 519–521, 521t
 single, antiretroviral therapy for, 111
Sexual practices, and HIV transmission, 538, 539t. See also specific practices.
 safer, 505, 513, 559
Sexual transmission, of hepatitis C virus, and coinfection with HIV, 399, 405
 of HIV, 499–500, 505–507, *506, 507*
  in homosexuals. See *Homosexuals.*
  to women, 537–541, 539t
   risk factors for, 538–539, 539t
Sexually transmitted diseases (STDs), 70. See also specific diseases, e.g., *Syphilis.*
 and HIV transmission, 70, 499
 clinics for, HIV surveys in, 12–13, *13*
  risk reduction counseling in, 501
Shigellosis, differential diagnosis of, 432
 gastrointestinal manifestations of, 201
Sigmoidoscopy, 203
Simian immunodeficiency virus (SIV), 24, 27–28, 499, 539
Sinusitis, prevention of, 132
Skin popping, 576
Small intestine, opportunistic infections of, 199–203
Soft tissue infections, in drug users, 576–577
Spiramycin, for toxoplasmosis, 387–388
Splenic disease, in bacillary angiomatosis, 412, 420
Sputum examination, in pneumonia, 339–340
 for fungi, 337t
 for *Haemophilus influenzae,* 334
 for *Pneumocystis carinii, 314–315,* 314–315
 for *Pseudomonas aeruginosa,* 335
 for *Rhodococcus equi,* 423
 for *Streptococcus pneumoniae,* 332–333
 in tuberculosis, 354, 357
Squamous cell carcinoma, conjunctival, 468t
 ocular, 172
 oral, 159t, 164
SSRIs. See *Selective serotonin reuptake inhibitors (SSRIs).*
Staphylococcal folliculitis, 186t, 187, *187*
Staphylococcus aureus, in drug users, 577
 pneumonia from, 332t, 334
  chest films of, 147, 334
 preseptal cellulitis from, 173
Staphylococcus epidermidis, keratitis from, 174
Stavudine (d4T), 27, 102–103
 adverse effect(s) of, 80t, 81, 98t
  toxic axonal neuropathy as, 231–232
 combination therapy with, 100t, 102–103, 110, 110t
  for children, 530, 530t
  for women, 548
 dosage of, 98t
 drug interactions with, 86t, 87
 for AIDS dementia, 227
 HIV mutations and, *55,* 99t
 resistance to, 103
STDs. See *Sexually transmitted diseases (STDs).*
Steatohepatitis, 205
Stevens-Johnson syndrome, 81
Stimulants, as antidepressants, 247t, 248
Streptococcus, keratitis from, 174
Streptococcus pneumoniae, 331–334, 332t
 diagnosis of, 332–333
  chest films for, *146,* 146–147
 in drug users, 578
 treatment of, 333–334, 333t
Streptomycin, for *Mycobacterium tuberculosis,* 356t
Strongyloidiasis, differential diagnosis of, 432

Subcutaneous nodules, in bacillary angiomatosis, 412, *414*
Substance abusers. See *Drug users.*
Suicide, by HIV-infected individuals, 241–242
   rational, 255–256
Sulfadiazine, adverse effect(s) of, 387
   for toxoplasmosis, 386, 386t, 387
Sulfonamides, adverse effect(s) of, 387
      depression as, 244
      hyperkalemia as, 287
Surgery, prevention of HIV transmission in, 513–514
Syphilis, 453–462
   chorioretinitis from, 175, 177, 455
   clinical manifestations of, 454–456
   CSF examination for, 453, 457, 458
   diagnosis of, 456–458
   education on, 463
   epidemiology of, 453–454
   gummatous, 456
   meningeal, 220–221, 454, 455
   mucocutaneous, 455–456
   neuro-, 178, 454–455, 462
      diagnosis of, 457–458
      treatment of, 459–460
         failure of, 461–462
   ocular, 178, 455
   orbital manifestations of, 178, 455
   pathogenesis of, 454
   persistence of treponemes and, 462
   prevention of, 506
   testing for, 128
      in HIV-infected patients, 458
   treatment of, 458–460, 459t
      alternatives for, 460
      failure of, 461–462
      follow-up in, 460–461
      for sexual contacts, 462–463

T cells. See specific T cells, e.g., *CD4+ T cells.*
Tabes dorsalis, 455
tat gene, 24, *24*
Tat protein, 29–31, *32*
Tea tree oil, 609
Teratogenicity, of ganciclovir, 436
Terfenadine, drug interactions with, 88t
Testicular atrophy, 289
Testosterone, for hypogonadism, 256t
   for wasting syndrome, 607–608, 608t
Tetracycline(s), for *Bartonella,* 418, *419,* 420t
Tetrahydrocannabinol, for wasting syndrome, 608, 608t
Thalidomide, 607
   for esophageal ulcers, 197t, 198
3TC. See *Lamivudine (3TC).*
Thrombocytopenia, HIV-related, 268–269
      management of, 269
Thrombocytopenic purpura, immune, 159t, 164
Thrombophlebitis, septic, in drug users, 577
Thrombotic thrombocytopenic purpura (TTP), 270
Thyroid-binding globulin, 289
Thyroid disease, 288–289
Thyroid-stimulating hormone, 288
Thyroiditis, 288
Thyroxine, 288
Torsade de pointes, 281
Total energy expenditure (TEE), 291
Toxic axonal neuropathy, 231–232
Toxoplasma gondii, oocysts of, 379, 383
   tachyzoites of, 383

Toxoplasmosis, 379–391
   adrenal, 286
   and progression of HIV disease, 126
   cerebral, 219, 221, 225t, 227, 228–229
      diagnosis of, 228–229, 229
      differential diagnosis of, 225t, 479, 480
      treatment of, 229
   clinical presentation of, 379–380
   congenital, 381
   diagnosis of, 381–384, 381t
      DNA detection for, 382
      histopathology for, 383–384
      isolation studies for, 382
      neuroradiologic studies for, 382–383
      serology for, 381–382
   differential diagnosis of, 380, 384
   encephalitis from, 221, 379, 380, 383, 384
      differential diagnosis of, 440
      management of, 384
   endocrinopathies from, 380
   epidemiology of, 11
   gastric disease from, 198–199
   in pregnancy, 381
   management of, 229, 384–390, *385*
      investigational drugs for, 387–389, 388t
      maintenance therapy for, 389–390, 389t
      primary therapy for, 386–387, 386t
   myelopathy from, 230, 230t
   myocarditis from, 279–280
   neuro-ophthalmic manifestations of, 178, 380
   orbital manifestations of, 178
   pancreatic abscesses from, 209
   prophylaxis for, 131–132, 131t, 229, 390–391, 390t, 391t
      in children, 532
      in pregnancy, 561
   pulmonary, 209
   reactivation of, 379
   retinochoroiditis from, 175, 177, 380, Color Plate 3D
   seizures from, 379–380
   testing for, 128
   transmission of, 379
Transverse myelitis, 230, 230t
   toxoplasmosis and, 380
Travel history, of HIV-infected patient, 126
   diarrhea and, 203
Treponema pallidum infection. See *Syphilis.*
Triamcinolone, for psoriasis, 186t, 193
Triazolam, drug interactions with, 88t
Trichomegaly, 172–173
Trichomoniasis, 506
Tricyclic antidepressants, 245, 246, 247t
   dosage of, 245, 246, 247t
   drug interactions with, 246
   for pain, 257
Trifluridine, for ocular HSV, 174
Trimethobenzamide, for pregnant women, 566
Trimethoprim-dapsone, adverse effects of, 318t, 321
   for *Pneumocystis carinii,* 318t, 321
Trimethoprim-sulfamethoxazole, adverse effect(s) of, 317t, 318, 318t, 387
      cutaneous, 190
      hyperkalemia as, 287
      in pregnancy, 561
   drug interactions with, 85
   for bacterial pneumonia, prophylactic, 132
   for *Bartonella,* 418, 420t
   for *Haemophilus influenzae,* 334
   for *Pneumocystis carinii,* 316–318, 317t, 318t

Trimethoprim-sulfamethoxazole (*Continued*)
   and chest film, 139
     dosage of, 317t, 318t
     prophylactic, 131, 131t, 324–325, 324t
       in children, 528
   for *Staphylococcus aureus,* 334
   for toxoplasmosis, 386t, 387
     prophylactic, 131–132, 131t, 229, 390, 391, 391t
Trimetrexate, adverse effects of, 317t, 318t
   for *Pneumocystis carinii,* 317t, 318t, 320–321
   for toxoplasmosis, 388
TTP. See *Thrombotic thrombocytopenic purpura (TTP).*
Tuberculosis, 353–359
   adrenal, 286
   chemoprophylaxis for, 129–130, 358–359
   chest films of, 142–143, *144, 145,* 354–355
   clinical presentation of, 354–355
   diagnosis of, 354–355
   differential diagnosis of, 310
   epidemiology of, 353–354
   esophageal, 196, 197t, 198
   extrapulmonary, 354–355
   hepatic granulomas from, 204
   in drug users, 576, 578, 589
   incidence of, in HIV-infected patients, 332t
   meningeal, 220
   multidrug-resistant, 130, 353–354, 357–358
   pancreatic abscesses from, 209
   pathogenesis of, 354
   pericardial effusion from, 277
   prevention of, 358–359
   screening for, 129–130, 358–359
   treatment of, 355–358, 356t, 578
     adverse effects of, 356t
     combination regimens for, 355, 356t, 357t
     dosages for, 356t, 357t
     drug interactions with, 356–357
     drug resistance in, 357–358
     empiric, 341
     in drug users, 578
     nonadherence to, 118
Tubo-ovarian abscess, 547
Tumor necrosis factor, glucocorticoid deficiency and, 286, 287
   HIV infection and, 593
     inhibitors of, 606–607
     primary, 74
   Mycobacterium avium-complex and, 344

United States, epidemiology of HIV in, *6,* 6–11
Universal precautions, in infection control, 516
Uveal effusion syndrome, 175

Vaccinations. See also specific vaccines, e.g., *Varicella-zoster vaccine.*
   for HIV-infected patients, 130
     children, 528
     in pregnancy, 558–559
Vaginal candidiasis, 546
Vaginal microbicides, against HIV, 539
Valacyclovir, adverse effects of, 444, 447
   for HSV, 442–443, 443t, 444, 445, 446
     dosage adjustment for, in renal dysfunction, 443–444, 444t
   for VZV, 447
     ophthalmic, 171, 447

Valproic acid, 254, 254t
   drug interactions with, 85
Vancomycin, for *Clostridium difficile,* 201
   for *Rhodococcus equi,* 423, 424
   for *Staphylococcus aureus,* 334
   for *Streptococcus pneumoniae,* 333, 333t
Varicella, 446. See also *Varicella-zoster virus.*
Varicella-zoster immune globulin (VZIG), 448
Varicella-zoster vaccine, 448
Varicella-zoster virus (VZV), 446–448
   brain disease from, 230, 447
   complications of, 446–447
   drug-resistant, treatment of, 448
   iridocyclitis from, 175
   management of, 447–448, 448t
   myelopathy from, 230, 230t
   neuropathy from, 231, 447
   ocular disease from, 171, 430, 446
     keratitis in, 174
     retinitis in, 176–177
   pneumonia from, 446
   prevention of, 448
   primary infection with, 446
   recurrence of, 446. See also *Herpes zoster.*
Venereal Disease Research Laboratories (VDRL) test, 128, 454, 456, 457, 460, 461, 462
Venlafaxine, 248
   dosage of, 247t
   for panic attacks, 253
Venous thrombosis, 281
Ventriculoencephalitis, from CMV, 431
Vertical transmission, of hepatitis C virus, and coinfection with HIV, 399, 405
   of HIV, 10–11, *12,* 504–505, 525–526. See also *Pediatric AIDS.*
     antiretroviral therapy and, 11, 499, 504, 519, 557–558, 564, 568
     assessing predictors of, 557–558
     predictors of, 557–558
     risk factors for, 525–526
   of toxoplasmosis, 381
Vidarabine, for ocular HSV, 174
vif gene, 24, *24*
Vif protein, 27–28, 29–31
Vinblastine, for Hodgkin's disease, 485
   for Kaposi's sarcoma, 473, 473t
Vincristine, for Hodgkin's disease, 485
   for Kaposi's sarcoma, 473t, 474
   for non-Hodgkin's lymphoma, 481t, 482
Vinorelbine, for Kaposi's sarcoma, 473t, 474
Vomiting. See *Nausea and vomiting.*
Viral infections. See also specific viruses.
   cutaneous, 188–189
   oral, 159t
Visna virus, 24
Vitamin B_{12} deficiency, 265, 266
Vitamin C, in HIV disease management, 604t, 605–606
vpr gene, 24, *24*
Vpr protein, 28, 31
vpu gene, 24, *24*
Vpu protein, 31, 32–33, *33*
Vulvovaginitis, candidal, 546
VZV. See *Varicella-zoster virus (VZV).*

Warts. See also *Human papillomavirus (HPV).*
   diagnosis and treatment of, 189
   genital, 189
     in women, 545
   oral, 159t, *163,* 163–164

Wasting syndrome, 291
  alternative therapy for, 607–608, 608t
  by age, 594t
  prevention of, 133
Weight loss, and progression of HIV disease, 126
Western blot assay, for HIV, 46–48, *47*
  false-positive, 59–60, *61*
Wills, 255
Women, HIV infection in, age and, 538
    anal squamous intraepithelial lesions and, 545–546
    antiretroviral therapy for, 548
    aphthous genital ulcers and, 547
    cervical neoplasia and, 544–545
      treatment of, 545
    clinical manifestations of, 542–548
    clinical research on, 548–549
    cytomegalovirus and, 543
    epidemiology of, 3, 8, *9,* 15, *16,* 537–538
    genital ulcers and, 546–547
    genital warts and, 545
    gynecologic care for, 545, 545t
    herpes simplex virus and, 546–547
    increases in, 537–538
    IV drug use and, 537, 540, 541
    Kaposi's sarcoma and, 543
    menstrual disorders and, 547–548
    opportunistic infections and, 542–543
    Pap smears and, 544, 545
    pelvic inflammatory disease and, 547
    progression of, 541–542
    resources for, 542
    transmission of, 538–541
      risk factors for, 538–539, 539t
    vaginal candidiasis and, 546
  lesbian, HIV transmission among, 538, 540–541, 541t
  older, HIV transmission in, 538
  pregnant, HIV infection in, 10–11, *12,* 504–505, 519,
      525–526. See also *Pregnancy, HIV infection in.*
  young, HIV transmission in, 538

Zalcitabine (ddC), 27, 102
  adverse effects of, 80–81, 80t, 98t
    gastrointestinal, 202t
    hepatic, 206t, 207
    pancreatic, 209

Zalcitabine (*Continued*)
    toxic axonal neuropathy from, 231–232
  combination therapy with, 100t, 101t, 102, 110, 110t
  dosage of, 98t
  drug interactions with, 86t, 87
  HIV mutations and, *55,* 99t
ZDV. See *Zidovudine.*
Zidovudine (AZT), 27, 99, 99t, 102
  adverse effects of, 79, 80t, 86, 98t
    depression from, 244
    gastrointestinal, 202t
    hematologic, 270–271
    hepatic, 206t
    in older patients, 596
    mania from, 254
    myelosuppression from, 268, 268t
    myopathy from, 232
    ventricular dysfunction from, 280
  combination therapy with, 100t, 101t, 102, 110, 110t
    for children, 530, 530t
    in older patients, 596
    in pregnancy, 563–564, 569
  dosage of, 98t
  drug interactions with, 85–86, 86t
    ganciclovir and, 435–436
    methadone and, 588t
    opioid substitutes and, 582–583
  for AIDS dementia, 227, 250
  for children, 527, 528t, 530, 530t
  for HIV-associated nephropathy, 300
  for prevention of HIV transmission, in children, 527
    intrapartum use of, 569, 569t
    perinatal, 11, 504, 519, 526, 548, 557–558, 563–564,
      568, 569, 569t
    postexposure, 503, 518–519
  for primary HIV disease, 75
  history of, 602
  HIV mutations and, *55,* 73, 99t
  hostility to use of, 602
  monotherapy with, 100t, 102
    in pregnancy, 504–505, 526, 557–558, 563, 564, 569,
      569t
  PCR testing and, 52, 53t
  resistance to, 102, 519
    in pregnancy, 563
  with interferon α, for Kaposi's sarcoma, 475–476, 475t
Zoster ophthalmicus, 171, 446